TOTAL JOINT REPLACEMENT

Dedication

To my family—Betty, David, Mark, and Julie—
whose love and support make all things possible.

Contributors

Harlan C. Amstutz, M.D. Professor of Orthopaedic Surgery, University of California, Los Angeles, School of Medicine, Los Angeles, California.

Donald L. Bartel, PH.D. Professor, Cornell University in Ithaca; Senior Scientist, Hospital for Special Surgery, New York, New York.

Stanley A. Brown, D.ENG. Associate Professor, Biomedical Engineering, Case Western Reserve University, Cleveland, Ohio.

Larry K. Chidgey, M.D. Assistant Professor, Department of Orthopaedics, University of Florida College of Medicine, Gainesville, Florida.

Paul C. Dell, M.D. Professor and Chief, Division of Hand and Microsurgery, Department of Orthopaedics, University of Florida College of Medicine, Gainesville, Florida.

C. McCollister Evarts, M.D. Professor of Orthopaedics, Pennsylvania State University College of Medicine, Hershey, Pennsylvania.

Harry E. Figgie, III, M.D. Assistant Professor of Biomechanics, Department of Orthopaedics, Case Western Reserve University School of Medicine, Cleveland, Ohio.

Mark P. Figgie, M.D. Instructor in Orthopaedic Surgery, Cornell University Medical College; Assistant Attending Orthopaedic Surgeon, Hospital for Special Surgery, New York, New York.

Peter F. Gearen, M.D. Associate Professor, Department of Orthopaedics, University of Florida College of Medicine, Gainesville, Florida.

Nikolaus Gravenstein, M.D. Associate Professor of Anesthesiology and Neurosurgery, University of Florida College of Medicine, Gainesville, Florida.

Marj M. Heare, M.D. Assistant Professor of Radiology, University of Florida College of Medicine, Gainesville, Florida.

Timothy Hupfer, M.D. Indiana Orthopaedic and Sports Medicine, Indianapolis, Indiana.

Allan E. Inglis, M.D. Professor of Clinical Surgery, Cornell University Medical College, Ithaca, New York.

Matthew J. Kraay, M.D. Hospital for Special Surgery, New York, New York.

Kenneth A. Krackow, M.D. Professor of Orthopaedic Surgery, Johns Hopkins University, Baltimore, Maryland.

Jack E. Lemons, PH.D. Professor and Chairman, Department of Biomaterials and Surgery; Director of Orthopaedic Research, University of Alabama at Birmingham, Birmingham, Alabama.

Edward McElfresh, M.D. Clinical Professor of Orthopaedic Surgery, University of Minnesota; Chief, Hand Surgery, Veterans Administration Medical Center (Minneapolis); Orthopaedic Surgeon, St. Anthony Orthopaedic Clinic, St. Paul, Minnesota.

Katharine Merritt, PH.D. Associate Professor, Biomedical Engineering, Case Western Reserve University, Cleveland, Ohio.

Gary J. Miller, PH.D. Associate Professor of Orthopaedics and Mechanical Engineering, University of Florida College of Medicine and College of Engineering, Gainesville, Florida.

William J. Montgomery, M.D. Associate Professor and Chief, Musculoskeletal Radiology, University of Florida College of Medicine, Gainesville, Florida.

J. Phillip Nelson, M.D. Associate Professor of Orthopaedic Surgery, Mayo Medical School, Rochester, Minnesota. Consultant in Orthopaedic Surgery, Mayo Clinic Scottsdale, Scottsdale, Arizona.

William Petty, M.D. Professor and Chairman, Department of Orthopaedics, University of Florida College of Medicine, Gainesville, Florida.

Nelson Scarborough, PH.D. Assistant Professor and Director, Tissue Bank, Department of Orthopaedics, University of Florida College of Medicine, Gainesville, Florida.

Thomas P. Sculco, M.D. Associate Clinical Professor Orthopaedic Surgery, Cornell University Medical College; Associate Director, Department of Orthopaedic Surgery, Hospital for Special Surgery, New York, New York.

Suzanne Spanier, M.D. Associate Professor, Department of Orthopaedics, University of Florida College of Medicine, Gainesville, Florida.

Dempsey S. Springfield, M.D. Associate Professor in Orthopaedics, Harvard Medical School, Boston, Massachusetts.

Bernard Stulberg, M.D. Associate Professor of Orthopaedic Surgery, Case Western Reserve University, Cleveland, Ohio.

David Stulberg, M.D. Department of Orthopaedic Surgery, Northwestern University, Chicago, Illinois.

James A. Turner, M.D. Attending Surgeon, Department of Hand and Upper Extremity Surgery, Pacific Presbyterian Medical Center, San Francisco, California.

Anthony S. Unger, M.D. Associate Clinical Professor of Orthopaedic Surgery, George Washington University, Washington, D.C.

Robert A. Vander Griend, M.D. Associate Professor, Department of Orthopaedics, University of Florida College of Medicine, Gainesville, Florida.

Timothy M. Wright, PH.D. Associate Professor, Cornell University Medical College; Associate Scientist, Hospital for Special Surgery, New York, New York.

Preface

Over the past three decades, tremendous strides have been made in the treatment of severely damaged joints. The first successful hip joint replacement was pioneered by Sir John Charnley, an innovative clinician and researcher from England. In the years that followed, the principles behind his remarkable achievement were applied to replacement of other joints, as well.

Although total joint arthroplasty has improved the quality of life for legions of patients, many procedures were, and continue to be, followed by complications or failures—as orthopaedic surgeons know too well. Since Charnley's first prosthesis was implanted in 1958, orthopaedic surgeons and their colleagues in related disciplines have done extensive research in their efforts to make the implantation of prostheses safer and to prolong their durability. This challenge has resulted in published articles that now number in the thousands.

Because the abundance of data is difficult for even experienced orthopaedic surgeons to assimilate, the medical publisher, W. B. Saunders Company, asked me to serve as editor of a comprehensive volume, *Total Joint Replacement*. I agreed that the time was ripe for such a text. Not only did the plethora of information on joint replacement need to be summarized and condensed, but it required critical evaluation. Consequently, I contacted outstanding authorities in various types of joint replacement, inviting them to contribute chapters to this textbook.

Total Joint Replacement is intended to provide orthopaedic surgeons, residents, and others interested in joint arthroplasty with comprehensive, up-to-date information about all aspects of the subject. The contributors from the various areas of specialization discuss prosthetic options and surgical techniques; they describe the scientific principles behind prosthesis design and insertion; and they provide the basic information necessary for the successful management of patients with severely damaged joints.

It is my hope that this volume will not only provide current information to help orthopaedic surgeons in the management of patients with damaged joints but that it will also help point the way toward future research.

WILLIAM PETTY, M.D.

Acknowledgments

As editor of *Total Joint Replacement,* I thank the many contributors whose commitment made this comprehensive text possible. Not only did these men and women offer their knowledge and expertise as leaders in the rapidly changing field of orthopaedics, but they met our tight deadlines for manuscript submission.

My task as editor was lightened by the assistance of Barbara Cox, Biomedical Editor, and her colleagues at MedEdit Associates, who improved the organization and readability of the various chapters. Trish Moran, a talented medical illustrator, was responsible for the excellent original artwork. The encouragement and support of W. B. Saunders Company's staff members were invaluable at all stages of the publication process. I am especially grateful to Edward H. Wickland, Jr., Senior Medical Editor, and Kathleen McCarthy, Assistant Developmental Editor.

Finally, I am indebted to Marita Wilkinson and Ginny Payne, members of my staff in the Department of Orthopaedics, University of Florida. Both were gracious under pressure at all times and went far beyond the call of duty to make this book a reality. In addition to their regular responsibilities, Marita and Ginny checked and organized references, helped with editing, designed tables, and tracked manuscripts—often working nights and weekends to keep the book on schedule.

Contents

SECTION VII LOWER EXTREMITY REPLACEMENT: THE KNEE 465

SECTION I

ORIGINS

CHAPTER 1

History of Arthroplasty

EDWARD McELFRESH

Medicine, like all knowledge, has a past as well as a present and a future, and . . . in that past is the indispensable soil out of which improvement must grow.

Alfred Stillé (1813–1900)[185]

RESECTION ARTHROPLASTY

Ambroise Paré (Fig. 1–1), the famous French barber-surgeon of the Renaissance, performed the first recorded joint excision in 1536. Accounts tell us that he excised the elbow joint of a patient with a destructive infection.[14, 155] Two centuries passed before another joint resection was reported. In 1762, Filkin,[62] a surgeon living in Northwick, England, successfully resected a knee joint that had been partially destroyed by tuberculosis. That same year, a German military surgeon, Beyer, resected the wrist joint of a young man injured in battle.[133]

Six years later, Charles White,[219] a physician in Manchester, England, treated a patient whose humerus had been partially destroyed by chronic osteomyelitis. After excising the head of the humerus and 10 cm of the proximal humerus, White placed the patient's arm in a sling. Within 4 months, enough bone had regenerated to permit good function. Encouraged by his success, White performed experimental resection arthroplasties on the hips of human cadavers in the year that followed. However, he apparently never excised a hip joint in a living patient.[14]

Joint excision rapidly found a place in the treatment of severely diseased joints. In 1783, Henry Park[14] of the Liverpool Infirmary is reported to have excised larger joints, including the hip, knee, and shoulder, in patients crippled with septic and other forms of arthritis. He gained considerable recognition from his medical colleagues for his method of treatment. In France, P. F. Moreau and his son performed similar procedures. In fact, the senior Moreau[139] published a volume entitled *The Resection of Articulations Affected by Caries* in 1805. In it, he described excision of all the major joints. In the early phases of arthritis, Moreau advised, joint surfaces should simply be removed along with any adjacent pathologic bone that could be reached easily. In Moreau's technique, no effort was made to reform articular surfaces. The ankylosis that usually resulted was often desired or anticipated. In 1812, another Frenchman, Philibert-Joseph Roux,[174] recommended resection for chronic

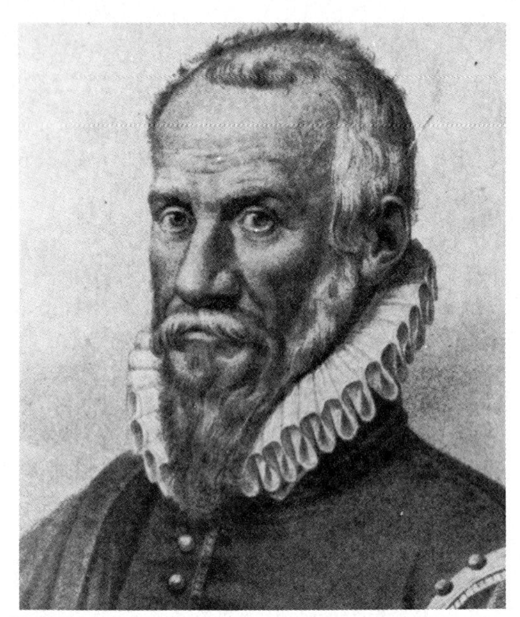

FIGURE 1–1. Ambroise Paré (1510–1590). (Garrison, F. H.: An introduction to the History of Medicine, 4th ed. Philadelphia, W. B. Saunders Company, 1929. By permission.)

arthropathies. In 1830, he published the results of his treatment.

Across the English Channel, Anthony White[199] of London excised the diseased femoral head of a young boy with tuberculosis in 1822. The boy survived for 12 years after the operation, then died of tuberculosis. The year before Anthony White performed this operation, Charles White[199]— still alive 53 years after his historic operation on a patient with chronic osteomyelitis—suggested excision of the femoral head for a condition he called "caries coxae."

The credit for introducing resection of the joints into universal general practice goes to James Syme (Fig. 1–2),[193] professor of clinical surgery at the University of Edinburgh. In 1831, he published his famous book, *The Excision of Diseased Joints*. By that time he had performed 14 resections of the elbow joint.[14, 193]

Reports of other joint resections followed, some of them from the New World. In 1834, John Collins Warren[216] of Boston resected an elbow. Henry Jacob Bigelow,[15] also of Boston, excised a hip joint in 1852. Foch attempted resection of the femoral neck for degenerative arthritis 7 years later, placing the diaphyseal stump into the acetabulum. The patient's infected wound healed 7 weeks later, and by 10 weeks he was walking with crutches. Because of the flail joint, however, he needed crutches for the rest of his life. By 1861, Foch[65] reported his results in 78 cases of femoral head excision, noting that 26 patients failed to survive the postoperative course. The year before Foch's report appeared, Textor[196] performed the first successful knee arthroplasty. Ferguson[60] followed with a similar success within a year.

In 1826, a sailor came to John Rhea Barton,[11] a Pennsylvania physician, with an ankylosed hip. An old fracture that had become infected produced ankylosis in adduction, internal rotation, and flexion. Barton performed a trochanteric osteotomy—a procedure that lasted 7 minutes and resulted in pseudoarthrosis (Fig. 1–3). On the 20th day after surgery, the hip was manipulated and by 6 weeks showed active motion. Three months after the operation, the patient could walk with a cane, using the motion obtained at the osteotomy site. However, 6 years later, all motion had been lost; 10 years after the operation, the patient died of tuberculosis. John Kearney Rodgers,[173] a New York surgeon, adopted Barton's surgical technique but resected wider areas of bone. He also instituted

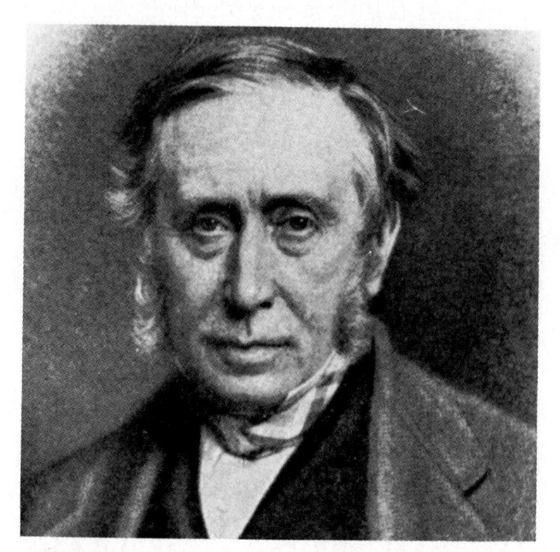

FIGURE 1–2. James Syme (1799–1870). (Garrison, F. H.: An Introduction to the History of Medicine, 4th ed. Philadelphia, W. B. Saunders Company, 1929. By permission.)

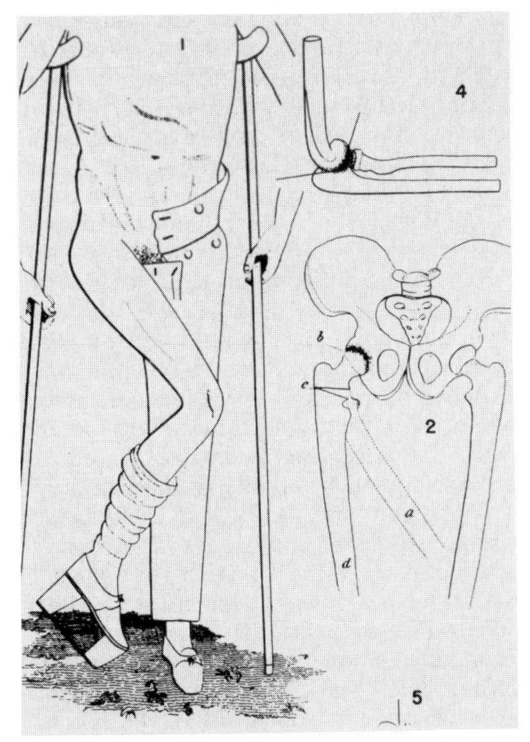

FIGURE 1–3. John Rhea Barton's drawing of his first hip osteotomy. (Barton, J. R.: Clin. Orthop. 6:4, 1955. By permission.)

early passive motion to obtain arthroplasties.

With the turn of the century came more reports of excisional arthroplasty. G. R. Girdlestone[76] reported resection of the femoral head and neck. Henry Milch[135] combined an osteotomy of the upper part of the diaphysis of the femur with a resection. After World War I, Willis Campbell[109] devised an elbow excisional arthroplasty, in which he used the triceps and anterior capsule for interposition.

Reports of excision of the distal ulna began to appear as early as the late 1700s, the first report coming from a French physician, Pierre-Joseph Desault[49] in 1791. Other reports were made by E. M. Moore[138] (1880), G. A. van Lannep[205] (1897), H. B. Angus[5] (1908), and William Darrach[44–45] (1912). Resection arthroplasties in the hand were described by Isodore Kestler,[85] Sterling Bunnell,[23] Benjamin Fowler and Daniel Riordan,[67, 171] Kauko Vainio,[203] Stewart Harrison,[90] and Jack Tupper.[12, 18, 201]

INTERPOSITIONAL ARTHROPLASTY

John Murray Carnochan,[30] a New York surgeon, is credited with the idea of interposing material between surfaces of a joint. In 1840, he reported an attempt to mobilize a patient's ankylosed jaw by placing a small block of wood between the raw bony surfaces of the mandibular joint after resecting the neck of the joint. Two decades later, Aristide A. S. Verneuil,[208] a French surgeon, described the use of soft parts for interpositional arthroplasty. Between 1878 and 1890, Louis X. E. L. Ollier (Fig. 1–4)[150–154] wrote several papers describing the use of adipose tissue as a soft cushion for interposition in noninfected joints. His classic work, *On Resections and Conservative Operations on the Osseous System,* was published in 1885.[154]

A German physician, Herman Helferich,[91] was the first to describe a pedicle flap of muscle or connective tissue as an interposing material. In 1893, he performed the procedure in an attempt to restore motion to a patient's fused temporomandibular joint. The operation was repeated the following year by Johann Mikulicz-Radecki.[134] In 1894, the use of thin platinum plates was attempted by Jules Emile

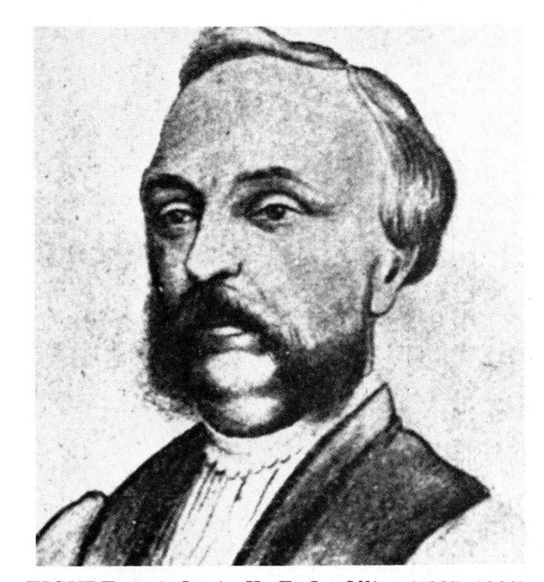

FIGURE 1–4. Louis X. E. L. Ollier (1825–1900). (Osgood, R. B.: The Evolution of Orthopaedic Surgery. St. Louis, C. V. Mosby, 1925. By permission.)

Pean[157] of Paris. He succeeded in restoring early motion of joint surfaces. In 1896, another French surgeon, Foedre,[66] applied pig's bladder as an interposing membrane.

Some of the early animal studies were published in 1900, when V. Chlumsky[38] reported his classic experiments on the placement of foreign materials in animal joints. He tested the reaction of animal tissues to magnesium, tin, zinc, silver, celluloid, rubber, collodion, and even decalcified bone. Robert Jones[100] of Liverpool, attempting the use of gold foil in a human patient, covered the femoral head for arthroplasty of an ankylosed hip joint. His patient did well for over 20 years. That same year, Pupovac[163] reported employing a magnesium plate in an arthroplasty—even though Chlumsky's report showed that magnesium appeared to stimulate excessive osteogenesis.

A Chicago surgeon, John Benjamin Murphy (Fig. 1–5),[143] first tried fascia lata as the interposing material in arthroplasty in 1902. Murphy emphasized the importance of covering the entire articular surface of

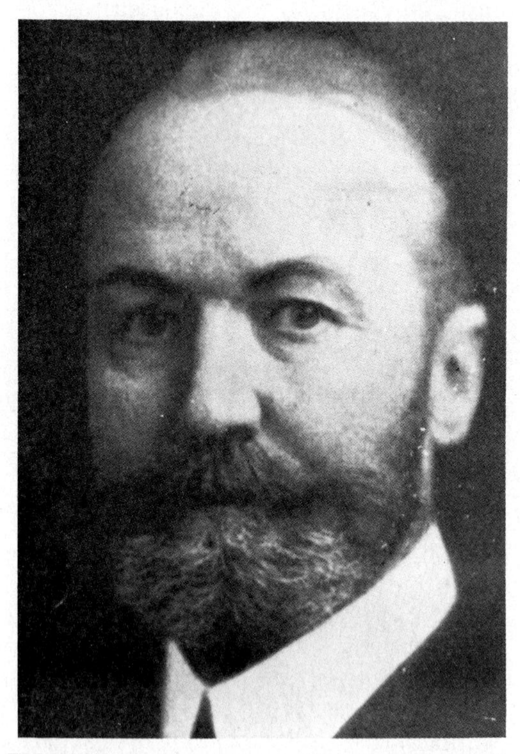

FIGURE 1–5. John Benjamin Murphy (1857–1916). (Major, R. H.: A History of Medicine, 1954. Springfield, IL, Charles C Thomas. By permission.)

the bone, but he warned that the fascia lata must be attached to only one bone. He is considered the leader of his era in interposition arthroplasty. In 1906, periosteum was transplanted as the interposing material by Hofman.[92] That same year, Erich M. Lexer,[85] a German surgeon, advocated the application of free fat and fascia. His most important contribution was his report of the transplantation of articular ends of homoplastic bones in 1908 and 1909. In Lexer's first patient, he resected the proximal humerus for a bone cyst, replacing it with the humerus of a cadaver. Although the outcome was somewhat unsatisfactory, Lexer laid the groundwork for procedures that have been tried only in later decades.

N. Allison and B. Brooks,[2] physicians with considerable experience in animal experiments, reported in 1913 that most of the materials selected for interpositional purposes deteriorated, but that this was of secondary importance. They believed that connective tissue grew from the raw surfaces of resected bone. Five years later, their theory was confirmed by Dallas B. Phemister and E. M. Miller.[159] These researchers also stated that pedunculated interposition flaps were of no value.

As medicine moved into the 20th century, more animal research was reported. In 1918, William S. Baer[9] of Johns Hopkins took Foedre's concept and described the utilization of chromatized submucosa of a pig's bladder. In 1920, an Italian physician, Vittorio Putti,[164–165] reported the use of fascia lata for interpositioning. Willis T. Campbell[26] of Memphis tried prepatellar bursa for knee interposition arthroplasty. Between the pre-World War I era and 1950, the following had been tried: injections of wax and lanolin,[195] epidermis of skin,[115] glass and Pyrex,[115] celluloid,[180] sheets of rubber,[75] amniotic membrane (Amnioplastin),[39] plastics such as Lucite and Plexiglas,[88] cellophane,[176] and sheets of nylon.[108]

In 1923, a Boston surgeon, Marius Nygaard Smith-Petersen (Fig. 1–6),[180] experimented with a unique approach to interposition. He began with glass cups in hip reconstructive surgery. Discouraged by how easily the glass cups broke, he tried Bakelite, a form of celluloid. This produced too much foreign body reaction. In 1933, he decided to try glass again—but a new,

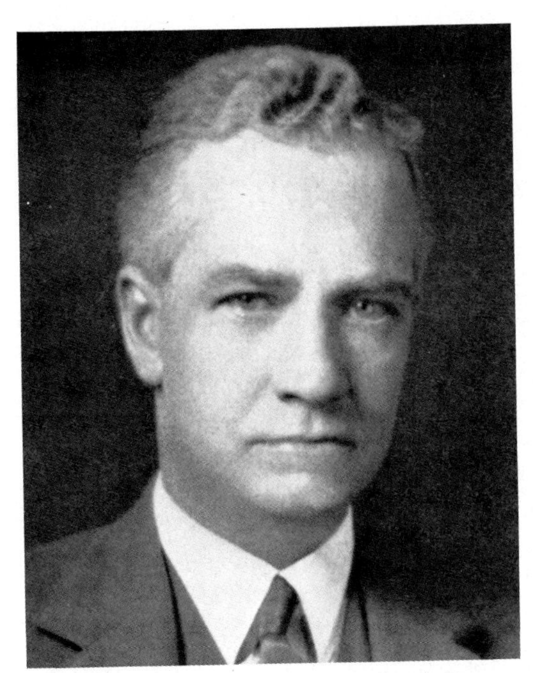

FIGURE 1–6. Marius Nygaard Smith-Petersen (1886–1953). (J. Bone Joint Surg. 35A:1043, 1953. By permission.)

extra hard type of glass called Pyrex. Still he had occasional breakage. This experience led him to experiment with a chromium-cobalt alloy in 1937 (Fig. 1–7). The next year he inserted his first mold arthroplasty cup. Before the year was over, he reported on his first 29 arthroplasties.[4, 180] The results in 1000 patients on whom the Smith-Peterson team performed this procedure were reported by Otto Aufranc[8] in 1957.

Earlier (1940), Willis T. Campbell[27] had tried Vitallium plates. He reported results in two patients in whom the plates conformed to the femoral condyles in knee arthroplasties. Campbell was disappointed in the amount of motion obtained, however, and gave up the procedure. Michael S. Burman[24] of the Hospital for Joint Disease in New York described a cup arthroplasty for the metacarpal head in 1940.

PROSTHETIC ARTHROPLASTY

In 1890, Themistocles Glück[77, 78] gave a series of lectures to Berlin physicians in which he described a remarkable system of total joint arthroplasties that involved ivory prosthetic units (Fig. 1–8). Stabilization, he said, could be achieved with a cement made of colophony, pumice, and gypsum.[77, 78, 169] Never before had a filler been considered for securing a prosthesis for the temporomandibular joint. Glück is also said to have performed the first total hip replacement consisting of an ivory ball-and-socket joint with a cement filler. According to Jules Emile Pean (Fig. 1–9),[13, 157] these prostheses were readily absorbed. The next report of a prosthetic arthroplasty came from Paris 4 years later. Pean replaced the shoulder joint and proximal humerus of a patient with an articulated prosthesis made of platinum (Fig. 1–10).

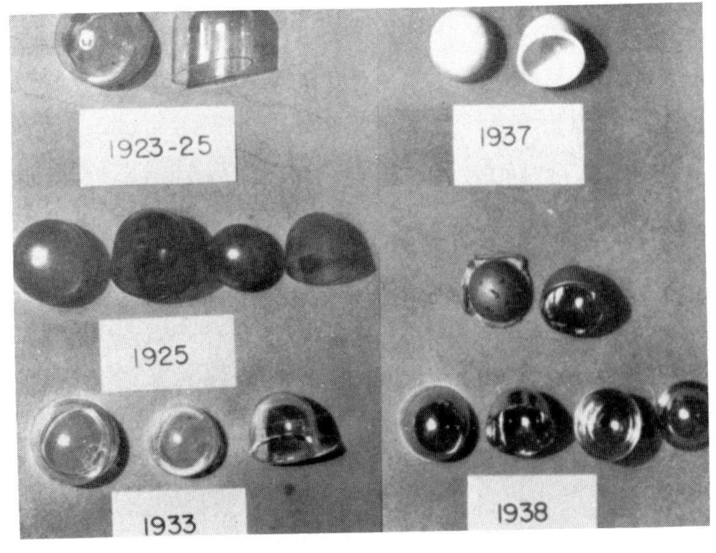

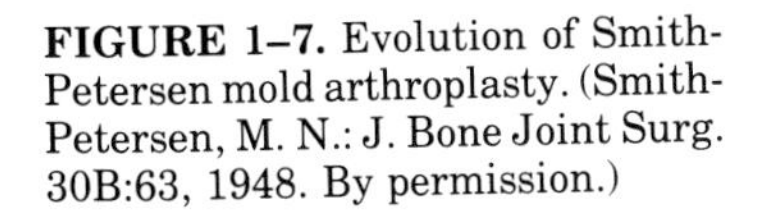

FIGURE 1–7. Evolution of Smith-Petersen mold arthroplasty. (Smith-Petersen, M. N.: J. Bone Joint Surg. 30B:63, 1948. By permission.)

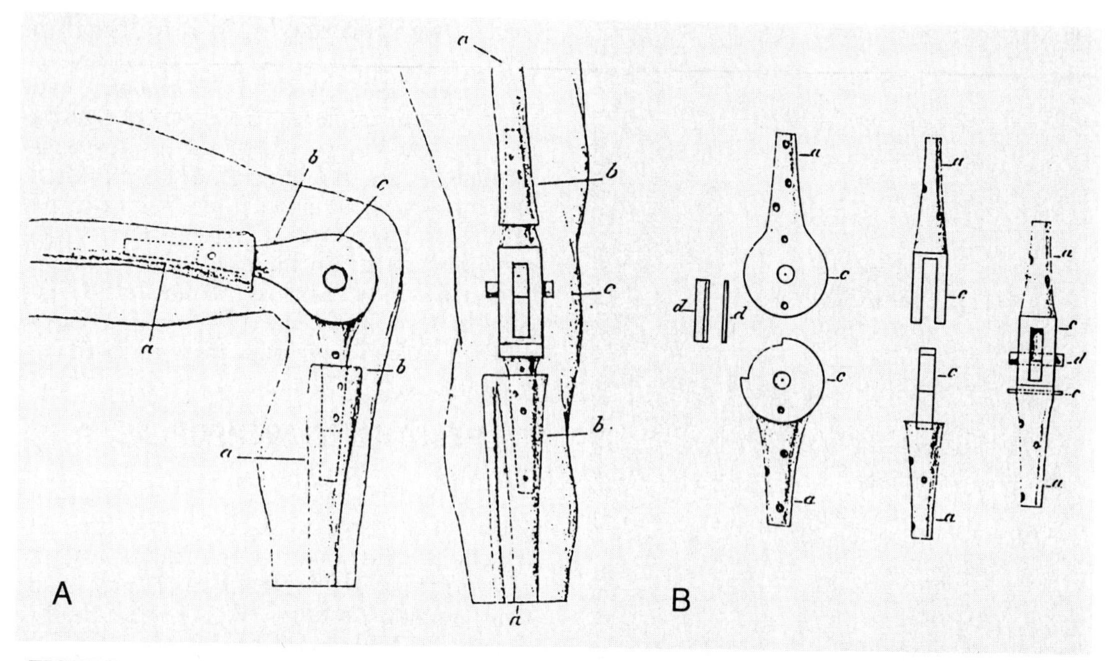

FIGURE 1–8. *A*, Glück's ivory total knee arthroplasty held in place with cement of colophony, pumice, and gypsum. *B*, Component parts of Glück's knee prosthesis. (Glück, T.: Arch. Klin. Chir. 41:186, 1891.)

He chose platinum because he had previously tried iron and steel to replace bone and cartilage structures of the nose, as had Ollier, and found them to be corrosive.

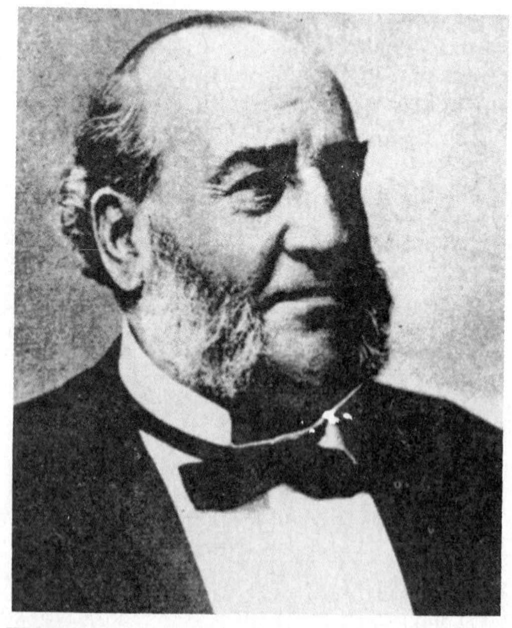

FIGURE 1–9. Jules Emile Pean (1830–1898). (Bick, E. M.: Classics of Orthopaedics. Philadelphia, J. B. Lippincott Company, 1976. By permission.)

Stainless steel was tried by Phillip W. Wiles (Fig. 1–11)[178, 188] in 1938. Ground precisely to fit, stainless steel parts replaced both the acetabular and femoral elements of the hip joint, with fixation accomplished by screws and a buttress plate. The femoral component was bolted to the femoral neck. Unfortunately, the fastening devices became loose and broke, and Wiles abandoned the procedure.

To investigate new materials for prostheses, Charles Venable and Walter Stuck[206] conducted animal experiments in Texas. The aforementioned chromium-cobalt alloy they developed was named Vitallium, consisting of 30 percent chromium, 5 percent molybdenum, and 65 percent cobalt. It proved to be nonreactive and strong enough to meet prosthesis requirements, and it could still be shaped as desired. The value of the alloy developed by Venable and Stuck was confirmed by Harold Ray Bohlman (Fig. 1–12),[17] who wished to apply it in hip replacements. First, however, he buried a Vitallium femoral head prosthesis he had designed in soil to test its noncorrosive properties. Along with it he buried control metal alloys. Satisfied with the nonreactivity of Vitallium, he employed his femoral head

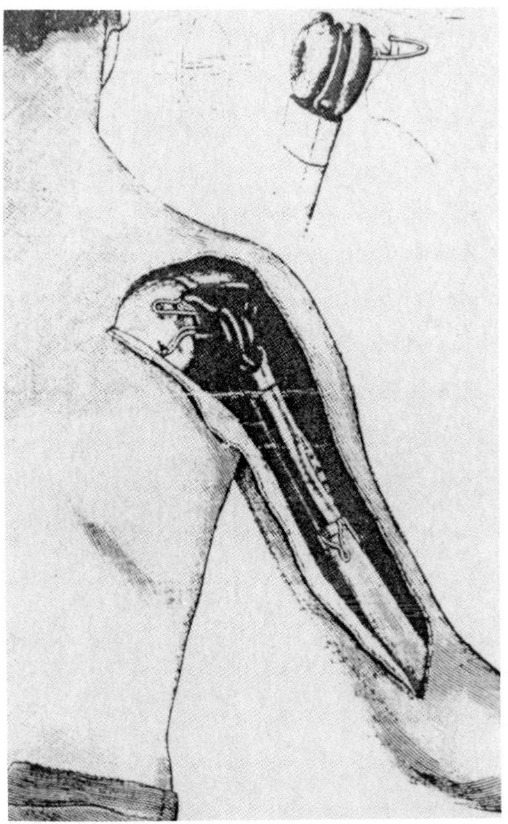

FIGURE 1–10. Pean's total shoulder arthroplasty made of platinum. (Bick, E. M.: Classics of Orthopaedics, Philadelphia, J. B. Lippincott Company, 1976. By permission.)

prosthesis in the hip joints of seven patients with nonhealing femoral neck fractures. In 1940, a fellow surgeon, J. Austin Talley Moore (Fig. 1–13),[137] asked him to help replace 30 cm of the upper end of the femur in a patient with recurrent giant cell tumor. Together they implanted a specially made Vitallium prosthesis. After surgery, the patient was able to walk without a cane except for long walks. When the patient died of a heart attack 2 years later, autopsy examination revealed no tumor recurrence in the femur and no evidence of corrosion of the prosthesis (Fig. 1–14).

Prosthetic design continued to advance. In 1950, the Judet brothers of Paris reported 300 hip arthroplasties employing a new endoprosthesis made of acrylic bound to a chromium steel rod (Fig. 1–15).[102, 103] The rod passed through the neck of the femur to the outer cortex of the greater trochanter. However, their prosthesis, like

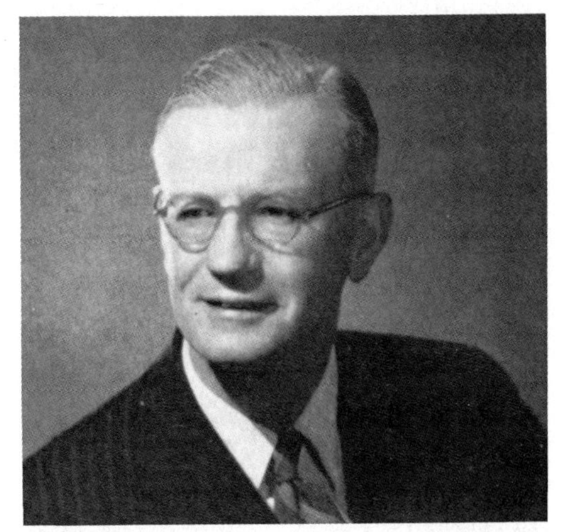

FIGURE 1–11. Phillip W. Wiles (1899–1967). (J. Bone Joint Surg. 49B:580, 1967. By permission.)

that designed by Austin Moore, had problems with mechanical loosening. In many patients, the chromium-cobalt prosthesis protruded into the acetabulum, whereas the acrylic prosthesis was subject to rapid wear and breakage.

A slightly different type of chromium-

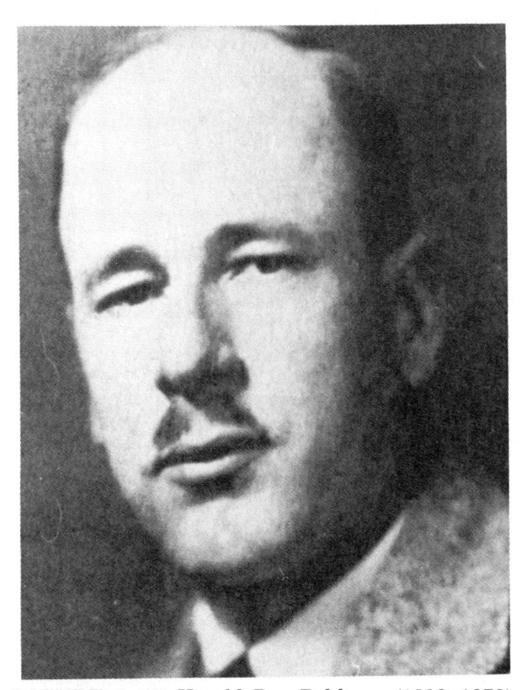

FIGURE 1–12. Harold Ray Bohlman (1893–1979). (Moore, A. T. and Bohlman, H. R.: Clin. Orthop. 176:4, 1983. By permission.)

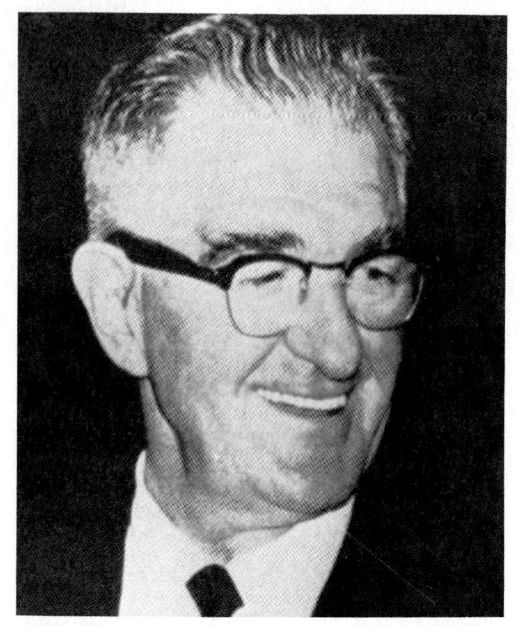

FIGURE 1–13. J. Austin Talley Moore (1899–1963). (Moore, A. T. and Bohlman, H. R.: Clin. Orthop. 176:4, 1983. By permission.)

cobalt femoral prosthesis was designed by Frederick R. Thompson[197–199] in 1951. The head and neck were fashioned with an intramedullary stem that curved to fit the

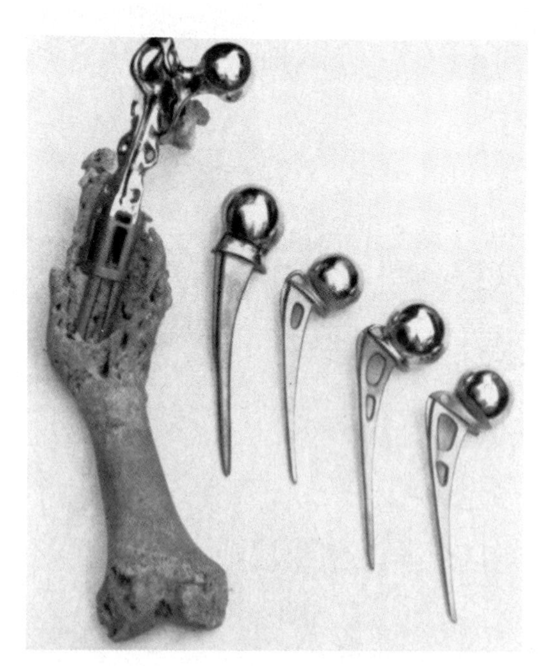

FIGURE 1–14. Evolution of the Moore prosthesis from 1939 to 1951 including the first prosthesis removed at autopsy. (Moore, A. T.: J. Bone Joint Surg. 39A:815, 1957. By permission.)

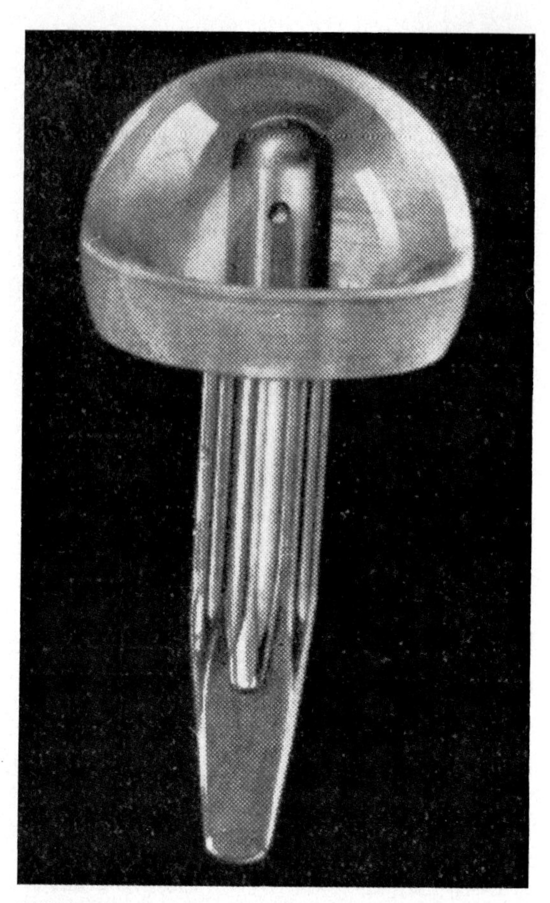

FIGURE 1–15. The Judet acrylic hip prosthesis. (Judet, J. and Judet, R.: J. Bone Joint Surg. 32B:167, 1950. By permission.)

upper shaft of the femur. Other early prostheses of similar design were reported by Peterson,[158] Evans and Reilly,[199] Eicher,[199] McBride,[125] Lippmann,[114] Thomson,[200] and d'Aubigne and Postel.[43] Several surgeons attempted to place the Thomson or Austin Moore prosthesis inside a large Smith-Petersen cup[199] but found that the constant friction of metal on metal caused debris accumulation. Others made independent attempts to produce a separate acetabular prosthesis to fit a Thompson or Austin Moore prosthesis.[126, 199, 202]

In the early 1950s, the idea of utilizing dental acrylic occurred to Edward J. Haboush[87] from the Hospital for Joint Disease in New York. The fast-setting acrylic was a monomer-polymer dough used for molding and fabrication of dentures since 1928. Haboush employed it for fixation of a Vitallium proximal femoral prosthesis. In the 1960s, G. K. McKee and J. Watson-

Farrar[127, 128] added acrylic cement to hold a prosthesis in place that they had developed several years earlier—an acetabular cap fitted over a Thomson prosthesis. In 1966, P. A. Ring[170] described a prosthesis in which the metal acetabular cup was screwed into the pelvis.

In the 1950s, Sir John Charnley (Fig. 1–16),[32–36] a surgeon practicing in a small community near Manchester, England, became interested in total hip replacement. In the first prosthesis he designed, he retained the femoral head and refashioned it as a "spigot." However, his patient developed ischemic necrosis of the inner sphere, with consequent loosening of the prosthesis. Charnley's next step was to develop a femoral prosthesis that could be cemented with polymethyl methacrylate. The purpose was to more uniformly transfer the body weight to the cancellous bone of the neck and upper end of the femur.[32, 34] By reducing the femoral head radius Charnley was able to reduce the "moment" of frictional force. He made the radius of the exterior of the acetabular component as large as possible to lessen the tendency for the socket to rotate.[35]

When Charnley first performed total hip replacements in 1958, he used Teflon (polytetrafluorethylene) for the acetabular cup. He changed to high-density polyethylene in 1960, because it possessed a low coefficient of friction with stainless steel. Charnley performed an osteotomy of the trochanter that he reattached with a double wire loop. Shortly thereafter, M. E. Müller[142] modified the Charnley prosthesis. He used screw fixation to secure the trochanteric osteotomy. Since the early 1970s, numerous modifications of total hip replacements have been described. Early contributors in the United States include Mark B. Coventry and coworkers,[42] Philip Wilson, Jr. and coworkers,[220] Frank E. Stinchfield,[186, 187] William R. Murray,[144] William H. Harris and S. D. Stulberg,[89] Charles M. Evarts,[55] Harlan C. Amstutz,[3] and Jorge Galante and coworkers.[72]

In 1966, Heinz Wagner[212] performed the first surface replacement arthroplasty of the hip. In 1971, M. Paltrienieri and C. Trentani[4, 70] introduced fixed acrylic surface replacement to Italy. Other early investigations were conducted by Kohtaro Furuya and associates,[71] William N. Capello and P. O. Eicher and associates,[29] Seisuke Tanaka,[194] M. A. Freeman and associates,[69, 70] and Harlan Amstutz and I. C. Clarke and associates.[4]

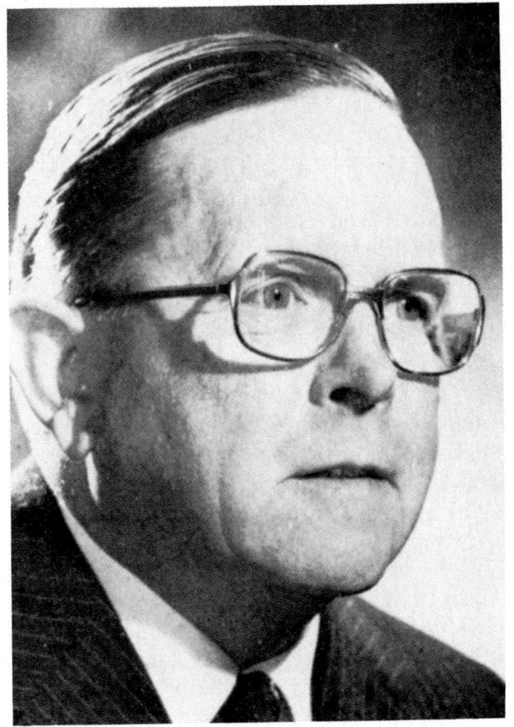

FIGURE 1–16. Sir John Charnley (1911–1982). (J. Bone Joint Surg. 65B:84, 1983. By permission.)

In 1958, D. L. MacIntosh[119] started placing an acrylic tibial plateau prosthesis similar to that of Jansen[169] in Denmark. Duncan C. McKeever[131] designed a chromium-cobalt plate for the tibial plateau in 1960. This plate was anchored with two metal blades placed at right angles to each other. Replacement of the distal femur was described by Otto Aufranc, W. Jones, and W. L. Kermond,[101] in 1964. They used a bicondylar cap anchored to the shaft by a long metal intramedullary stem. In 1967, G. Platt and C. Peppler[160] constructed a cap that was simply placed on the end of the femur without stem fixation. A similar cap, secured with a screw, was described by R. Gariepy[73] in 1968.

McKeever[130] described a metal prosthesis that was screwed in place. Bechtol[85] made a prosthesis for the patellofemoral joint. The Judet[102] brothers designed an acrylic hinged knee joint in 1947, but never applied it in clinical practice. In 1949, J.

M. Majnoni d'Intignano,[121] an Italian surgeon, employed a hinged total joint. Börje Walldius[214, 215] started using acrylic hinged knee joints in 1951 but changed to metal joints before 1958. Others who contributed to prosthetic design in the 1950s and 1960s included Merle d'Aubigne,[85] E. J. Moeys,[136] F. Anstett and colleagues,[6] Herbert Seddon,[85] William B. MacAusland,[118] L. G. P. Shiers,[179] A. von Hellens,[211] and Herman H. Young.[222] A major problem with fixed hinge joints was heavy mechanical strain in joints with multicentric axes of motion. As a result, they frequently loosened or broke. Eventually, Young[223] stated that prosthetic knee joints should no longer be used.

The first nonhinged total knee unit was designed by Frank H. Gunston (Fig. 1–17)[86, 169] in 1968, when he was working in England with John Charnley. Gunston tried to design a prosthesis that would retain the collateral and cruciate ligaments with a minimal resection of bone. In this way, an arthrodesis could be performed should the arthroplasty fail. He performed his first operation on February 19, 1968. Two Mayo Clinic surgeons, Richard S. Bryan and Lowell F. A. Peterson,[20] modified the Gunston prosthesis by changing the femoral component slightly and placing a slight posterior slope on the tibial component rather than a slight medial and lateral slope. They performed their first operation in 1970. H. W. Buccholz and E. Engelbrecht[22, 52, 53] of Hamburg helped design the "St. Georg" unit in 1969. It consisted of four pieces that contoured the femoral condyles and acted as a sledge for the tibial components. In 1970, Michael Freeman and S. A. V. Swanson and associates[68] tried their new prosthetic design. It required sacrifice of the cruciate ligaments and provided some stability with a roller into trough articulation. Five American orthopaedists—Mark B. Coventry, Lee H. Riley, Gerald A. Finerman, Roderick H. Turner, and Jackson E. Upshaw[41]—designed the geometric total knee arthroplasty, which was first utilized in 1971. Other designs of nonhinged units that followed included the modular knee,[122] the UCI,[217] the duocondylar,[94, 166, 213] the unicondylar,[20, 95] and total condylar.[96]

Hinged knee units did continue to be used. In 1970, the GUEPAR unit, held with polymethyl methacrylate, was first placed in a patient. It had been developed by a group of orthopaedists in Paris.[221] A spherocentric knee was reported by Herbert Kaufer, D. A. Sonstegard, and Larry S. Matthews.[124] Their prosthesis had a contained ball-and-socket joint that represented an attempt to achieve the stability of a hinge joint without the disadvantage inherent in a fixed hinge. For replacement of the articular surface of the patella, H. B. Groeneveld[80] developed a plastic endoprosthesis that was combined with the GUEPAR or Walldius hinged prosthesis.

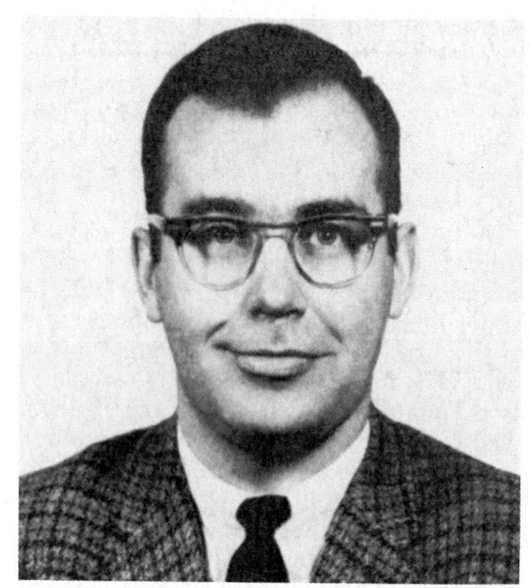

FIGURE 1–17. Frank H. Gunston. (Gunston, F. H.: Clin. Orthop. 205:4, 1986. By permission.)

In 1890, T. Glück[77] designed an ankle implant. His procedure involved resection of part of the talus and insertion of prongs into bone for fixation. Unfortunately, his patient's prosthesis rapidly loosened. Over the years, ankle prostheses have been designed by E. Engelbrecht and associates,[21] Michael Freeman and associates,[104] R. C. Smith and associates,[1] and others,[81, 147, 156, 182, 218] but none has proved very satisfactory. Therefore, arthrodesis remains the most widely employed procedure in destructive arthritic conditions of the ankle.

Pean first attempted replacement of the shoulder joint in 1894.[157] Not until the early 1950s, however, were numerous humeral prostheses described.[51, 97, 106, 168, 202] Charles Neer,[145, 146] a New York surgeon, designed a proximal humeral prosthesis in

1952. Other prostheses were developed by A. F. DePalma, James Bateman, and H. F. Moseley.[146] Stillbrink[146] utilized a high-density polyethylene glenoid component with the Neer proximal humeral prosthesis in four patients. Kenmore[146] employed it in three patients. Eventually, Neer designed his own glenoid component. Other total shoulder arthroplasties were developed in the 1970s and early 1980s by B. Reeves and coworkers,[167] J. Zippel,[224] A. W. F. Lettin and J. T. Scales,[110] Y. Gérard,[74] R. Kölbel and G. Friedebold,[105] M. Salzer and coworkers,[175] J. M. Fenlin, Jr.,[59] E. Engelbrecht and G. Stillbrink,[54] Roger Dee,[48] Ian Macnab,[120] Ronald Linscheid and Robert Cofield,[113] Melvin Post and coworkers,[161] and Anthony Gristina and L. X. Webb.[79]

In 1925, R. Robineau[172] placed the first elbow prosthesis. It was fabricated of metal and covered by dental vulcanized rubber. The first prosthesis to replace both sides of the elbow joint was utilized by I. Boerma and D. J. de Waard[16] in 1942. Acrylic prostheses were used by R. H. Mellen and George S. Phalen[132] in 1947, and nylon prostheses were used by William R. MacAusland[117] in 1954. Custom prostheses have also been designed for specific deficits.[10, 50, 98, 189, 207] Hinged prostheses of the elbow include those designed by Roger Dee[46, 181] in 1969, C. Chatzidakis[37] in 1970, N. Gschwend and H. Scheier[84] in 1974, and F. Mazas[85] in 1975.

In the early 1970s, Ralph Coonrad,[40] a Duke University surgeon, started working on a constrained total elbow arthroplasty that was eventually modified by Bernard Morrey and Richard S. Bryan and colleagues[140, 141] (1979) at the Mayo Clinic. Constrained elbow prostheses were developed by Roger Dee[47] (1972) and G. K. McKee[129] (1973). Another constrained design was the "Stanmore"[99] prosthesis (1984). Semiconstrained elbow prostheses that were introduced included the triaxial,[61, 93] Pritchard-Walker,[93, 162] Arizona Radio-Capitellar,[210] and the Schlein.[177] Nonconstrained total elbow prostheses developers, all in 1980, include Fred Ewald,[56, 57, 58] James London,[116] and Kudo and associates.[107] In 1951, C. R. Carr and J. W. Howard[31] reported a metallic cap replacement for a fractured radial head. Alfred Swanson and associates[192] also introduced a Silastic replacement for the radial head.

The first total wrist arthroplasty was attempted by N. Gschwend and P. Lalive[82] in 1969. H. C. Meuli,[133] in 1973, introduced his articulated nonhinged prosthesis of the ball-and-socket trunnion design. In 1976, Robert G. Volz[209] developed an articulated nonhinged prosthesis that worked as a dorsovolar tracking design. Alfred Swanson[191] utilized a larger Silastic prosthesis hinge, similar to his metacarpophalangeal prostheses in design, to act as a spacer for a resection arthroplasty of the wrist.

Some of the first joints for the hand began to appear in the late 1950s. In 1959, Earl W. Brannon and G. Klein[19] developed a metal hinge joint for the metacarpophalangeal joint. The following year, Adrian Flatt[63] introduced his hinged prosthesis. In 1968, Alfred B. Swanson[190] introduced Silastic hinged prostheses for the metacarpophalangeal joints and interphalangeal joints. They acted as spacers for resection arthroplasties. In 1971, John J. Niebauer and associates[149] described a Silastic prosthesis with a Dacron core that was sutured into place. Propylene prostheses were designed by Calnan and Reis[25] in 1968, and later, in 1972, in collaboration with Nicolle.[148] With the success of total joint arthroplasties of other joints held with methyl methacrylate, Arthur Steffee and coworkers[183] designed a prosthesis that was fixated into bone with bone cement. By the mid-1970s, cemented hand prostheses began to fall into disfavor because of loosening and other complications.

SUMMARY

Some prostheses that were developed early in the history of arthroplasty for a specific joint are still being used, but most have been supplanted by prostheses of more modern design. Those that are still in use today and those that are no longer used have been critical to the development of total joint replacement surgery. The success of total joint replacement today is in large measure due to the pioneering efforts of the innovative surgeons and other scientists who have contributed to the early development of prostheses and arthroplasty procedures.

References

1. Alexakis, P., Smith, R. C., and Wellisch, M.: Indications for ankle fusion versus total ankle replacement versus pantalar fusion. Orthop. Trans. 1:87, 1977.
2. Allison, N. and Brooks, B.: Ankylosis: An experimental study. J.A.M.A. 64:391, 1915.
3. Amstutz, H. C.: Complications of total hip replacement. Clin. Orthop. 72:123–137, 1970.
4. Amstutz, H. C., Clarke, I. C., Christie, J., and Graff-Radford, A.: Total hip articular replacement by internal eccentric shells. Clin. Orthop. 128:261–284, 1977.
5. Angus, H. B.: Dislocation of head of ulna caused by a "backfire" in starting a motor car. North Humberland and Durham Med J. 18:23, 1908–1909.
6. Anstett, F., Borner, R., Heinze, R., et al. (eds.): Klinische Anwendung Von Kunststoffen in der Medizin. Leipzig, J. A. Barth, 1955.
7. Aufranc, O. E.: Arthroplasty: Constructive hip surgery with mold arthroplasty. Am. Acad. Orthop. Surg. Inst. Course Lect. 11:163–187, 1954.
8. Aufranc, O. E.: Constructive hip surgery with the Vitallium mold. A report of 1000 cases of arthroplasty of the hip over a fifteen-year period. J. Bone Joint Surg. 39A:237–248, 1957.
9. Baer, W. S.: Arthroplasty with the aid of animal membrane. Am. J. Orthop. Surg. 16:1, 94, 171, 1918.
10. Barr, J. S. and Eaton, R. G.: Elbow reconstruction with a new prosthesis to replace the distal end of the humerus: A case report. J. Bone Joint Surg. 47-A:1408–1413, 1965.
11. Barton, J. R.: On the treatment of ankylosis by the formation of artificial joints. N. Am. Med. Surg. J. 3:279–292, 1827.
12. Beckenbaugh, R. D. and Linscheid, R. L.: Arthroplasty in the Hand and Wrist. Operative Hand Surgery, 2nd ed. Edited by D. P. Green. New York, Churchill Livingstone, 1988.
13. Bick, E. M. (ed.): Classics of Orthopaedics. Philadelphia, J. B. Lippincott Company, 1976.
14. Bick, E. M.: Source Book of Orthopaedics, 2nd ed. New York, Haftner Publishing Company, 1968.
15. Bigelow, H. J.: Resection of the head of the femur. Am. J. Med. Sci. 24:90, 1852.
16. Boerma, I. and deWaard, D. J.: Osteoplastiche Verankerung von Metallprothesen bei Pseudarthrose und be: Arthroplastik. Acta Chir. Scand. 86:511, 1942.
17. Bohlman, H. R. and Moore, A. T.: Metal hip joint: A case report. J. Bone Joint Surg. 25:688, 1943.
18. Boyes, J. H.: Bunnell's Surgery of the Hand, 5th ed. Philadelphia, J. B. Lippincott Company, 1970.
19. Brannon, E. W. and Klein G.: Experiences with a finger-joint prosthesis. J. Bone Joint Surg. 41-A:87–102, 1959.
20. Bryan, R. S. and Peterson, L. F. A.: Polycentric total knee arthroplasty. Orthop. Clin. North Am. 4:575–584, 1973.
21. Buchholz, H. W., Engelbrecht, E., and Siegl, A.: Totale Sprunggelenksendoprothese Modell "St. Georg." Chirurg 44:241, 1973.
22. Buccholz, H. W. and Engelbrecht, E.: Die Intracondyläre Totale Kniegelenk-endoprothese "Modell St. Georg," Chirurg 44:373, 1973.
23. Bunnell, S.: Surgery of the Hand. Philadelphia, J. B. Lippincott Company, 1944.
24. Burman, M. S.: Vitallium cup arthroplasty of metacarpophalangeal and interphalangeal joints of the fingers. Bull. Hosp. Joint Dis. 1:79–89, 1940.
25. Calnan, J. S. and Reis, N. D.: Artificial finger joints in rheumatoid arthritis. Ann. Rheum. Dis. 27:207, 1968.
26. Campbell, W.: Arthroplasty of the knee—Report of cases. J. Orthop. Surg. 3:430, 1921.
27. Campbell, W.: Interposition of Vitallium plates in arthroplasties of the knee. Am. J. Surg. 47:639, 1940.
28. Cannon, S. L.: The role of bone cements in total joint replacement. Preliminary report of effort to toughen acrylic. Orthop. Rev. 7:63, 1978.
29. Capello, W. N., Ireland, P. H., Trammell, T. R., and Eicher, P.: Conservative total hip arthroplasty—A procedure to conserve bone stock. Clin. Orthop. 134:59–74, 1978.
30. Carnochan, J. M.: Arch de Med. 284, 1860.
31. Carr, C. R. and Howard, J. W.: Metallic cup replacement of the radial head following fracture. West J. Surg. Ob. Gyn. 59:539–546, 1951.
32. Charnley, J.: Anchorage of the femoral head prosthesis to the shaft of the femur. J. Bone Joint Surg. 42B:28–30, 1960.
33. Charnley, J.: Arthroplasty of the hip: A new operation. Lancet 1:1129–1132, 1961.
34. Charnley, J.: The bonding of prostheses to bone by cement. J. Bone Joint Surg. 46B:518–529, 1964.
35. Charnley, J., Kamangar, A., and Longfield, M. D.: The optimum size of prosthetic heads in relation to the wear of plastic sockets in total hip replacement. Med. Biol. Engin. 7:31, 1969.
36. Charnley, J.: Low-friction arthroplasty. Clin. Orthop. 72:7–21, 1970.
37. Chatzidakis, C.: Arthroplasty of the elbow joint using a Vitallium prosthesis. Int. Surg. 53:119, 1970.
38. Chlumsky, V.: Über die Wiederherstellung der Beweglichkeit des Gelenkes bei Ankylose. Zentralbl f. Chir. 27:921, 1900.
39. Chow, Y-C., Humphreys, S., and Penfield, W.: Br. Med. J. 517, 1940.
40. Coonrad, R. W.: Seven-year Following of Coonrad Total Elbow Replacement. Upper Extremity Joint Replacement (Symposium on Total Joint Replacement of the Upper Extremity, 1979). Edited by A. E. Inglis. St. Louis, C. V. Mosby Company, 1982.
41. Coventry, M. B., Finerman, G. H., Riley, L. H., et al.: A new geometric knee for total knee arthroplasty. Clin. Orthop. 83:157–162, 1972.
42. Daniel, W. W., Coventry, M. B., and Miller, W. E.: Pulmonary complications after total hip arthroplasty with Charnley prosthesis as revealed by chest roentgenograms. J. Bone Joint Surg. 54A:282–283, 1972.
43. D'Aubigne, R. M. and Postel, M.: Functional results of hip arthroplasty with acrylic prosthesis. J. Bone Joint Surg. 34A:451–475, 1954.
44. Darrach, W.: Forward dislocation at the inferior radio-ulnar joint, with fracture of the lower

third of the shaft of the radius. Ann Surg. 56:801, 1912.
45. Darrach, W.: Anterior dislocation of the head of the ulna. Ann Surg. 56:802–803, 1912.
46. Dee, R.: Elbow arthroplasty. Proc. R. Soc. Med. 61:1031–1035, 1969.
47. Dee, R.: Total replacement arthroplasty of the elbow for rheumatoid arthritis. J. Bone Joint Surg. 54B:88–95, 1972.
48. Dee, R.: What's New In Joint Replacement in England? Symposium on Osteoarthritis. St. Louis, C. V. Mosby Company, 1976.
49. Desault, P.: Extrait d'un Memoire de M. Desaultsur la Luxation de l'Extremite Inferieure dn Radius. J. Chir I:78, 1791.
50. Driessen, A. P. P. M.: Thirty years with a complete elbow prosthesis. Arch. Chir. Neerl. 24–II:87, 1972.
51. Edelman, G.: Traitement Immèdiat des Fractures Complexes de l'Extrémité Supérieurede l'Humérus Par Prothèse Acrylique. Presse Med. 59:1777–1778, 1951.
52. Engelbrecht, E.: The intra-articular total endoprosthesis of the knee joint (Design “St. Georg”). Excerptea Med. 293:33, 1973.
53. Engelbrecht, E. and Zippel, J.: The sledge prosthesis “Model St. Georg.” Acta Orthop. Belg. 39:203, 1973.
54. Engelbrecht, E. and Stillbrink, G.: Totale Schulterendeoprothese Modell “St. Georg.” Chirurg. 47:525, 1976.
55. Evarts, C. M., Gramer, L. J., and Bergfield, J. A.: The ring total hip prosthesis—Comparison of results at one and three years. J. Bone Joint Surg. 54A:1677–1682, 1972.
56. Ewald, F. C.: Total elbow replacement. Orthop. Clin. North Am. 6:685–696, 1975.
57. Ewald, F. C.: Capitellocondylar total elbow arthroplasty. J. Bone Joint Surg. 62A:1259, 1980.
58. Ewald, F. C.: Total elbow arthroplasty. Clin. Orthop. 182:137–142, 1982.
59. Fenlin, J. M., Jr.: Total glenohumeral joint replacement. Orthop. Clin. North Am. 6:565–584, 1975.
60. Ferguson, M.: Excision of the knee joint: Recovery with a false joint and a useful limb. Med. Times Gazette 1:601, 1861.
61. Figgie, H. E., Inglis, A. E., and Mow, C.: Total elbow arthroplasty in the face of significant bone stock or soft tissue losses. J. Orthop. 1(2):71, 1986.
62. Filkin.: J. de Méd. 84:400, 1762.
63. Flatt, A. E.: Restoration of rheumatoid finger-joint function. Interim report on trial of prosthetic replacement. J. Bone Joint Surg. 43-A:753–774, 1961.
64. Flatt, A. E.: Care of the Arthritic Hand, 4th ed. St. Louis, C. V. Mosby Company, 1983.
65. Foch, C.: Bemerkungen und Erfahrungen Hüftgelenk Langenbecks. Arch Chir. 1:172, 1861.
66. Föderl, O.: Über Kunstliche Gelenkbildung. Zentralbl f. Chir. 23:104, 1896.
67. Fowler, S. B. and Riordan, D. C.: Surgical treatment of rheumatoid deformities of the hand. J. Bone Joint Surg. 40A:1431–1432, 1958.
68. Freeman, M. A., Swanson, S. A., and Tood, R. C.: Total replacement of the knee designs: Consideration and early clinical results. Acta Orthop. Belg. 28:181, 1973.
69. Freeman, M. A. R., Swanson, S. A. V., Day, W. H., and Thomas, R. J.: Conservative total replacement of the hip. J. Bone Joint Surg. 57B:114, 1975.
70. Freeman, M. A. R.: Editorial comment—Total surface replacement hip arthroplasty. Clin. Orthop. 134:2–4, 1978.
71. Furuya, K., Kawachi, S., Higuchi, F., et al.: Newly designed artificial socket and cup arthroplasty. J. Jpn. Orthop. Assoc. 47:1228, 1973.
72. Galante, J. O., Rostoker, W., and Doyle, F. M.: Failed femoral stems in total hip prostheses. J. Bone Joint Surg. 57A:230–236, 1975.
73. Gariépy, R.: Arthroplasty of the Knee in Rheumatoid Arthritis with Femoral Mould. Synovectomy and Arthroplasty in Rheumatoid Arthritis. Edited by G. Chapchal. Stuttgart, Thieme, 1968.
74. Gérard, Y.: Une Prothèse Totale d'Epaule. Chirurgie 99:655, 1973.
75. Giangrasso, G.: Plastiche Con Laminae di Gomma in Lesioni Articolari Sperimentale. Ann Ital. d', Chir. 19:289, 1940.
76. Girdlestone, G. R.: Pseudarthrosis. Proc. R. Soc. Med. 38:363, 1945.
77. Glück, T.: Die Invaginationsmethode der Osteo- und Athroplastik, Berl. Klin. Wochenschr. Circulation 33:752, 1890.
78. Glück, T.: Referat Über die Durch das Moderne Chirurgische Experiment Gewonnenen Positiven Resultate, Betreffenddie Naht und den Ersatz von Defecten Höherer Gewebe, Sowie Über die Verwerthung Resorbirbarer und Lebendiger Tampons in der Chirurgie. Arch. Klin. Chir. 41:186, 1891.
79. Gristina, A. C. and Webb, L. X.: Proximal humeral and monospherical glenoid replacement: Surgical technique. Rutherford, N. J., Howmedica, Inc., 1982.
80. Groeneveld, H. B.: Combined femoro-tibial-patellar endoprosthesis of the knee joint preserving the ligaments. Acta Orthop. Belg. 39:210, 1974.
81. Groth, H. E., Shen, G. S., and Fagan, P. J.: The Oregon ankle: A total ankle designed to replace all three articular surfaces. Orthop. Trans. 1:86, 1977.
82. Gschwend, N. and Lalive, P.: Das Handgelenk des Polyarthritikers: Probleme der Operativen Behandlung. Handchirurgie 1:209, 1969.
83. Gschwend, N. and Scheier, H.: Die GSB-Handgelenkprothese. Orthopäde 2:46, 1973.
84. Gschwend, N. and Scheier, H.: Elbow-arthroplasty with the new GSB-prosthesis. Scand. J. Rheum. 3:177, 1974.
85. Gschwend, N.: Surgical Treatment of Rheumatoid Arthritis. Philadelphia, W. B. Saunders Company, 1980.
86. Gunston, F. H.: Polycentric knee arthroplasty. Clin. Orthop. 94:128–135, 1973.
87. Haboush, E. J.: A new operation for arthroplasty of the hip based on biomechanics, photoelasticity, fast-setting dental acrylic, and other considerations. Bull. Hosp. Joint Dis. 14:242, 1953.
88. Harmon, P. H.: Arthroplasty of the hip for osteoarthritis utilizing foreign body cups of plastic. Surg. Gynecol. Obstet. 76:347, 1943.
89. Harris, W. A. and Stulberg, S. D.: Total hip replacement for arthritis secondary to congeni-

tal hip disease. J. Bone Joint Surg. 55A:1765, 1973.
90. Harrison, S. H.: Excision arthroplasty of the metacarpophalangeal joints. Hand 1:14–16, 1969.
91. Helferich, H.: Arch f. Klin. Chir. 48:864, 1894.
92. Hofman: Zeitschr. f. Ortho. Chir. 17:1, 1906.
93. Inglis, A. E. and Pellicci, P. M.: Total elbow replacement. J. Bone Joint Surg. 62A:1252–1258, 1980.
94. Insall, J., Ranawat, C., Aglietti, P., and Shine, J.: A comparison of four different total knee replacements. J. Bone Joint Surg. 56A:1541, 1974.
95. Insall, J. and Walker, P.: Unicondylar knee replacement. Clin. Orthop. 120:83–85, 1976.
96. Insall, J., Ranawat, C. J., Scott, W. N., and Walker, P.: Total condylar knee replacement—Preliminary report. Clin. Orthop. 120:149–154, 1976.
97. Jacobssom, A.: Fracture of the capitellum of the humerus in adults. Treatment with intra-articular chrome-cobalt-molybdenum prosthesis. Acta Orthop. Scand. 26:184, 1957.
98. Johnson, E. W., Jr. and Schlein, A. P.: Vitallium prosthesis for the olecranon and proximal port of the ulna. Case report with thirteen-year follow-up. J. Bone Joint Surg. 52A:721–724, 1970.
99. Johnson, J. R., Goetty, C. J. M., Lettin, A. W. F., and Glasgow, M. M. S.: The Stanmore total elbow replacement for rheumatoid arthritis. J. Bone Joint Surg. 66B:732–736, 1984.
100. Jones, R. and Lovett, R. W.: Orthopaedic Surgery. Baltimore, Wm. Wood, 1929.
101. Jones, W. N., Aufranc, O. E., and Kermond, W. L.: Mould arthroplasty of the knee. J. Bone Joint Surg. 49A:1022, 1967.
102. Judet, J., Judet, R., and Crepin, G. T.: Essais de Prosthese Ostéo-articulaire. Pressé Med. 52:302, 1937.
103. Judet, J. and Judet R.: The use of an artificial femoral head for arthroplasty of the hip joint. J. Bone Joint Surg. 32B:166–173, 1950.
104. Kempson, G. E., Freeman, M. A. R., and Tuke, M. A.: Engineering considerations in the design of an ankle joint. Biomed. Eng. 10:166, 1975.
105. Kölbel, R. and Friedebold, G.: Schultergelenkersatz. Z. Orthop. 113:452, 1975.
106. Krueger, F. J.: A Vitallium replica arthroplasty of the shoulder: A case report of aseptic necrosis of the proximal end of the humerus. Surgery 30:1005–1011, 1951.
107. Kudo, H., Iwano, K., Watanabe, S., and Prefecture, K.: Total replacement of the rheumatoid elbow with a hingeless prosthesis. J. Bone Joint Surg. 62A:277–285, 1980.
108. Kuhns, J. G. and Potter, T. A.: Nylon arthroplasty of the knee joints in chronic arthritis. Surg. Gynecol. Obstet. 91:351, 1950.
109. Leber, C. and Melone, C. P., Jr.: Total Elbow Replacement. Orthop. Rev. 27:857–863, 1988.
110. Lettin, A. W. F. and Scales, J. T.: Total replacement of the shoulder joint (two cases). Proc. R. Soc. Med. 65:373, 1972.
111. Lexer, E.: Über Gelenktransportation. Med. Klin. 4:817, 1908.
112. Lexer, E.: Über Gelenktransplantationen. Arch. Klink. Chir. 90:263, 1909.
113. Linscheid, R. L. and Cofield, R. H.: Total shoulder arthroplasty: Experimental but promising. Geriatrics 31:64–69, 1976.
114. Lippmann, R. K.: The transfixion hip prosthesis. Observations based upon five years of use. J Bone Joint Surg. 39A:759–785, 1957.
115. Loewe, O.: Über Haut-Tiefenplastik. München Med. Wschr. 76:2125, 1929.
116. London, J. T.: Resurfacing total elbow arthroplasty. Orthop. Trans. 2:217, 1978.
117. MacAusland, W. R.: Replacement of the lower end of the humerus with a prosthesis. A report of four cases. West J. Surg. Gynecol. Obstet. 62:557, 1954.
118. MacAusland, W. R.: Total replacement of the knee joint by a prosthesis. Surg. Gynecol. Obstet. 104:579, 1957.
119. MacIntosh, D. L.: Hemiarthroplasty of knee using space occupying prosthesis for painful varus and valgus deformities. J. Bone Joint Surg. 40A:1431, 1958.
120. Macnab, I.: Development of a glenohumeral arthroplasty for severely destroyed shoulder joint. J. Bone Joint Surg. 58B:137, 1976.
121. Majnoni d'Intignano, J. M.: Articulations Totalesen Résine Acrylique. Rev. Orthop. 36:535, 1950.
122. Marmor, L.: The modular knee. Clin. Orthop. 94:242–248, 1973.
123. Mathys, R.: Standder Verwendung von Kunststoffen für Künstliche Gelenke. Akt. Traumatol. 3:253, 1974.
124. Matthews, L. S., Sonstegard, D. A., and Kaufer, H.: The spherocentric knee. Clin. Orthop. 94:234–241, 1973.
125. McBride, E. D.: A femoral-head prosthesis for the hip joint. Four years experience and the results. J. Bone Joint Surg. 34A:989–996, 1952.
126. McBride, E. D.: The flanged acetabular replacement prosthesis. Arch. Surg. 83:721, 1961.
127. McKee, G. K. and Watson-Farrar, J.: Replacement of arthritic hips by the McKee-Farrar prosthesis. J. Bone Joint Surg. 48B:245–249, 1966.
128. McKee, G. K.: Development of total prosthetic replacement of the hip. Clin. Orthop. 72:8–103, 1970.
129. McKee, G. K.: Total replacement of the elbow. Proceedings of the 12th Congress of the International Society of Orthopaedic Surgery and Traumatology, Amsterdam, 1973.
130. McKeever, D. C.: Patellar prosthesis. J. Bone Joint Surg. 37A:1074–1084, 1955.
131. McKeever, D. C.: Tibial plateau prosthesis. Clin. Orthop. 18:86–95, 1960.
132. Mellen, R. H. and Phalen, G. S.: Arthroplasty of the elbow by replacement of the distal portion of the humerus with an acrylic prosthesis. J. Bone Joint Surg. 29:348, 1947.
133. Meuli, H. C.: Arthroplastic due Poignet. Ann Chir. 27:527–530, 1973.
134. Mikulicz, J.: Verhandl d. Deutsch Gesellsch, f. Orth. Clin. 24:350, 1895.
135. Milch, H.: The "pelvic support" osteotomy. J. Bone Joint Surg. 23:581, 1941.
136. Moeys, E. J.: Metal arthroplasty of the knee joint. An experimental study. J. Bone Joint Surg. 36A:363–367, 1954.

137. Moore, A. T.: Hip joint surgery: An outline of progress made in the past forty years. Columbia, S. C., 1963.
138. Moore, E. M.: Three cases illustrating luxation of the ulna in connection with Colles' fracture. Med. Rec. N.Y. 17:305–308, 1880.
139. Moreau, P. F.: Observations Pratiques Relative á la Résection des Articulations Affectées de Carie. Paris, 1805.
140. Morrey, B. F. and Bryan, R. S.: Total joint arthroplasty: The elbow. Mayo Clin. Proc. 54:507–512, 1979.
141. Morrey, B. F., Bryan, R. S., Dobyns, J. H., and Linscheid, R. L.: Total elbow arthroplasty: A five-year experience at the Mayo Clinic. J. Bone Joint Surg. 63A:1050–1063, 1981.
142. Müller, M. E.: Total hip prostheses. Clin. Orthop. 72:46–68, 1970.
143. Murphy, J. B.: Ankylosis, arthroplasty, clinical and experimental. J.A.M.A. 44:1573, 1905.
144. Murray, W. R.: Results in patients with total hip replacement arthroplasty. Clin. Orthop. 95:80–90, 1973.
145. Neer, C. S.: Articular replacement of the humeral head. J. Bone Joint Surg. 37A:215–228, 1955.
146. Neer, C. S.: Replacement Arthroplasty for Glenohumeral Osteoarthritis. J. Bone Joint Surg. 56A:1–13, 1974.
147. Newton, S. E., III: Total ankle arthroplasty, a four-year study. Orthop. Trans. 1:86, 1977.
148. Nicolle, F. V. and Calnan, J. S.: A new design of finger joint prosthesis for the rheumatoid hand. Hand 4:137–146, 1972.
149. Niebauer, J. J., Shaw, J. L., and Doren, W. W.: Silicone-Dacron hinge prosthesis. Design, evaluation, and application. Ann. Rheum. Dis. Suppl. 28:56–58, 1968.
150. Ollier, L.: De la Résectiondu Conde Dans les Cas d'Ankylose. Rev. Mens. de Méd et de Chir. 6:12, 1878.
151. Ollier, L.: De la Résection de la Hanche. Rev. de Chir. 3, 5, 7, 1881.
152. Ollier, L.: Démonstration Anatomique de la Réconstituion du Coude Après la Résection Sons-Periosteé. Bull. de l'Acad. 16, 1882.
153. Ollier, L.: Des Opérations Conservatives Dans la Tuberculose Articulaire, Arthrotomie Evidement Résection Typique. Rev de Chir. 3, 1885.
154. Ollier, L.: Traite des Resections et des Operations Conservatrices qu'on peut Practiquer sur le Systeme Osseux. Paris, G. Masson, 1885–1889.
155. Osgood, R. B.: The Evolution of Orthopaedic Surgery. St. Louis, C. V. Mosby Company, 1925.
156. Pappas, M., Buechel, F. F., and DePalma, A. F.: Cylindrical total ankle joint replacement: Surgical and biomechanical rationale. Clin. Orthop. 118:82–92, 1976.
157. Pean, J. E.: Des moyens Prosthetiques Destinés a Obtenir la Reparation de Parties Osseuses. Gaz. de Hop., Paris, 67:291, 1894.
158. Peterson, L. T.: The use of a metallic head. J. Bone Joint Surg. 33A:65–75, 1951.
159. Phemister, D. B. and Miller, E. M.: The method of new joint formation in arthroplasty. Surg. Gynecol. Obstet. 26:406, 1918.
160. Platt, G. and Peppler, C.: Mould arthroplasty of the knee. J. Bone Joint Surg. 51B:76–87, 1969.
161. Post, M., Jablon, M., Miller, H., and Singh, M.: Constrained total shoulder joint replacement: A critical review. Clin. Orthop. 144:135–150, 1979.
162. Pritchard, R. W.: Semi-constrained elbow prosthesis: A clinical review of five years experience. Orthop. Rev. 8:33, 1979.
163. Pupovac, D.: Zur Technik der Nearthrosenbildung Bei Ankylosierten Gelenken. Wien. Klin. Wchnschr. 34, 1902.
164. Putti, V.: Arthoplasty of the knee joint. J. Bone Joint Surg. 2:530, 1920.
165. Putti, V.: Arthroplasty. Am. J. Orthop. Surg. 3:421, 1921.
166. Ranawat, C. S. and Shine, J. J.: Duocondylar total knee arthroplasty. Clin. Orthop. 94:185–195, 1973.
167. Reeves, B., Jobbins, B., Dowson, D., et al.: The Development of a Total Shoulder Joint Endoprosthesis. Cited by Gschwend, N.: Surgical Treatment of Rheumatoid Arthritis. Philadelphia, W. B. Saunders Company, 1980.
168. Richard, A., Judet, R., and René, L.: Reconstruction Prothétique Acrylique de l'Extrémité Supérieure de l'Humérus Spécialement au Cours des Fractures—Luxations. J. Chir. (Paris) 68:537–547, 1952.
169. Riley, L. H., Jr.: The evolution of total knee arthroplasty. Clin. Orthop. 120:7–10, 1976.
170. Ring, P. A.: Complete replacement arthroplasty of the hip by the ring prosthesis. J. Bone Joint Surg. 50B:720–731, 1968.
171. Riordan, D. C. and Fowler, S. B.: Surgical treatment of rheumatoid deformities of the hand (Abstract). J. Bone Joint Surg. 40A:1431–1432, 1958.
172. Robineau, R.: Contribution of al'Etude des Prosthesis Osseuses. Bull. Soc. Nat. Chir. 53:886, 1927.
173. Rodgers, J. K.: Treatment of ankylosis. N.Y. J. Med. Surg. 1840.
174. Roux, P. J.: Rev de Méd. 1830.
175. Salzer, M., Locke, H., Engelhardt, H., et al.: Keramische Endoprosthesen der Oberen Extremität. Z. Orthop. 113:458, 1975.
176. Samson, J. E.: Arthroplasty of the knee joint. J. Bone Joint Surg. 31B:50–52, 1949.
177. Schlein, A. P.: Semi-constrained total elbow arthroplasty. Clin. Orthop. 121:222–229, 1976.
178. Shands, A. R., Jr.: Historical milestones in the development of modern surgery of the hip joint. The Hip, St. Louis, C. V. Mosby Company, 1976.
179. Shiers, L. G. P.: Hinge arthroplasty of the knee. J. Bone Joint Surg. 36B:553–560, 1954.
180. Smith-Petersen, M. N.: Evolution of mould arthroplasty of hip joint. J. Bone Joint Surg. 30B:59–75, 1948.
181. Souter, W. A.: Arthroplasty of the elbow, with particular reference to metallic hinge arthroplasty in rheumatoid patients. Orthop. Clin. North Am. 4:395–413, 1973.
182. Stauffer, R. N.: Total ankle joint replacement. Arch. Surg. 112:1105, 1977.
183. Steffee, A. D., Beckenbaugh, R. D., Linscheid, R. L., and Dobyns, J. H.: The development, technique, and early clinical results of total joint replacement for the metacarpophalangeal joint of the fingers. Orthopedics 4(2):175–180, 1981.
184. Stillbrink, G., Zippel, J., and Englert, M.: Fin-

gergelenkprothesen Modell "St. Georg." Hand Chirurgie 3:83, 1971.
185. Stillé, A.: Medical News 44:433, 1884.
186. Stinchfield, F. E.: Low-friction total hip replacement. Clin. Orthop. 72:36–39, 1970.
187. Stinchfield, F. E.: Editorial comment—total hip replacement. Clin. Orthop. 95:2–3, 1973.
188. Stinchfield, F. E.: Introduction. The Hip. St. Louis, C. V. Mosby Company, 1973.
189. Street, D. M. and Stevens, P. S.: A humeral replacement prosthesis for the elbow. Results in ten elbows. J. Bone Joint Surg. 56A:1147–1158, 1974.
190. Swanson, A. B.: Silicone rubber implants for replacement of arthritic or destroyed joints in the hand. Surg. Clin. North Am. 48:1113–1127, 1968.
191. Swanson, A. B.: Flexible implant arthroplasty for arthritic disabilities of the radiocarpal joint: A silicone rubber intramedullary stemmed flexible hinge implant for the wrist joint. Orthop. Clin. North Am. 4:383–394, 1973.
192. Swanson, A. B., Jaeger, S. H., and LaRochelle, D.: Comminuted fractures of the radial head: The role of silicone—implant replacement arthroplasty. J. Bone Joint Surg. 63A:1039–1049, 1981.
193. Syme, J.: The Excision of Diseased Joints. Edinburgh, 1831.
194. Tanaka, S.: Surface replacement of the hip joint. Clin. Orthop. 134:75–79, 1978.
195. Taylor, R. T.: Restoring mobility after bony ankylosis of the joints. N.Y. Med. J. May 31, 1912.
196. Textor, K.: Resection des Kniegelenks, Verhandl. d. Gesellsch. Deutsch. Naturf. u. Ärzte 31:177, 1860.
197. Thompson, F. R.: Vitallium intramedullary hip prosthesis. Preliminary report. N.J. State J. Med. 52:3011, 1952.
198. Thompson, F. R.: Two and half years experience with a Vitallium intramedullary hip prosthesis. J. Bone Joint Surg. 36A:489–502, 1954.
199. Thompson, F. R.: An essay on the development of arthroplasty of the hip. Clin. Orthop. 44:73–82, 1966.
200. Thomson, J. E. M.: Prosthesis for femoral head. J. Bone Joint Surg. 34A:175–182, 1952.
201. Tupper, J.: Volar plate-plasty. Am. Soc. Surg. Hand Letters, April, 1969.
202. Urist, M. R.: The principles of hip socket arthroplasty. J. Bone Joint Surg. 39A:786–810, 1957.
203. Vainio, K.: Surgery of rheumatoid arthritis. Surg. Ann. 6:309–335, 1974.
204. Van der Ginst, M. and Houssa, P.: Prothèses Acryliques et Fractures de l'Extrémité Supérieure des Membres. Acta Chir. Belg. 42:31–40, 1951.
205. Van Lannep, G. A.: Dislocation forward of the head of the ulna at the wrist joint. Fracture of the styloid process of the ulna. Hahnemannian Monthly 32:350–354, 1897.
206. Venable, C. S. and Stuck, W. G.: Electrolysis controlling factor in the use of metals in treating fractures. J.A.M.A. 111:1349, 1938.
207. Venable, C. S.: An elbow and an elbow prosthesis: Case of complete loss of the lower third of the humerus. Am. J. Surg. 83:371, 1952.
208. Verneuil, A.: De la Creationd'une Fausse Articulation par Section ou Resection Partielle de l'os Maxillaire Inferieur, Comme Moyen de Remedier L'Ankylose Orale de Faussede la Machiore Inferieur. Arch. Gen. Med. 15:284, 1860.
209. Volz, R. G.: Total wrist arthroplasty. A new approach to wrist disability. Clin. Orthop. 128:180–189, 1977.
210. Volz, R. G.: Clinical experience with a new semiconstrained elbow prosthesis. Orthop. Trans. 3:394, 1980.
211. Von Hellens, A.: Arthroplasty of the knee using an endoprosthesis. Ann. Chir. et Gynec. Fennaie 50:132–139, 1961.
212. Wagner, H.: Der Alloplastische Gelenkflächenersatz am Hüftgelenk. Arch Orthop. Unfallchir. 82:101, 1975.
213. Walker, P., Ranawat, C., and Insall, J.: Fixation of the tibial component of condylar replacement knee prostheses. J. Biomechan. 9:269, 1976.
214. Walldius, B.: Arthroplasty of the knee joint using an acrylic prosthesis. Acta Orthop. Scand. 23:121, 1953.
215. Walldius, B.: Arthroplasty of the knee using an endoprosthesis. Acta Orthop. Scand. [Suppl.] 24, 1957.
216. Warren, J. C.: Boston Med. Surg. J. 20:210, 1839.
217. Waugh, T. R., Smith, R. C., Orofino, C. F., et al.: Indications, techniques, and results of knee arthroplasty using the UCI prosthesis. J. Bone Joint Surg. 56A:1302, 1974.
218. Waugh, T. R., Evanski, P. M., and McMaster, W. C.: Irvine ankle arthroplasty, prosthetic design, and surgical technique. Clin. Orthop. 114:180, 1976.
219. White, C.: Phil. Trans. London, 59:39, 1769.
220. Wilson, P. D., Jr., Amstutz, H. C., Czerniecki, A., et al.: Total hip replacement with fixation by acrylic cement—A preliminary study of 100 consecutive McKee-Farrar prosthetic replacements. J. Bone Joint Surg. 54A:207–236, 1972.
221. Witvoet, J.: GUEPAR total knee prosthesis. Excerpta Med. 298:28, 1973.
222. Young, H. H.: Use of a hinged Vitallium prosthesis for arthroplasty of the knee. J. Bone Joint Surg. 45A:1627–1642, 1963.
223. Young, H. H.: Use of a hinged vitallium prosthesis (young type) for arthroplasty of the knee. J. Bone Joint Surg. 53A:1658–1659, 1971.
224. Zippel, J.: Vollständiger Schultergelenkersatz aus Kunststoff und Metall. Biomed. Tech. 17:87, 1972.

SECTION II

MATERIALS FOR TOTAL JOINT REPLACEMENT

GARY J. MILLER

CHAPTER 2

Metals and Alloys

JACK E. LEMONS

Materials used for total joint replacement prostheses include naturally occurring metals and their alloys. These may be constructed in cast or wrought forms. The biomechanical and chemical properties of these materials are important considerations in the design of devices for total joint replacements.

HISTORICAL OVERVIEW

Noble Metals

The early use of metals as surgical implants was dependent on the availability of naturally occurring substances.[27] Gold, which was mined as a pure element, could be fabricated into wire, rod, sheet, or plate forms because of its inherent ductility and clean, or nonoxidized, surface. The clean surface condition made possible adhesion cold welding through interference contact of components, a process that is still applied to taper-lock interference fit systems for industrial and orthopaedic devices. The chemical inertness of gold, especially in saline environments, allowed its *in vivo* utilization for musculoskeletal reconstructions.[41] This characteristic also led to the evaluation of platinum, iridium, and palladium. In each case, however, limitations were soon recognized because of the relatively low mechanical strengths of these metals.

Another key factor was cost. The noble, or inert, metals have high densities and are relatively expensive because cost is determined by weight.[30] Most currently available implant materials, including ceramics and polymers, have much lower densities.

With the introduction of the lost-wax casting method, more complex geometric forms could be fabricated at lower cost.[35] The noble metals were ideal for these type castings because their relative inertness simplified the melting, casting, and finishing procedures. The major limitations remained the cost of the metals and their low mechanical strengths. Dental applications of this process continued into the 19th and 20th centuries, but medical applications did not.[10, 24]

In industrial applications, alloys demonstrated advantageous mechanical properties. Much of the chemical inertness of the primary noble metals was retained. Adding silver and copper to gold decreased the cost and significantly increased the strength. However, the dilute corrosion products, which included copper, resulted in unacceptable biologic reactions in laboratory animals. Interestingly, because of host and environmental factors, these same biodegradation products, in limited quantities, did not result in adverse reactions within the oral cavity.

Alloy Systems

A variety of alloys used for marine hardware based on copper, nickel, iron, and cobalt were evaluated for biomedical applications.[41] Unlike alloys of noble metals, these alloys were not inert electrochemically and depended on surface films, mainly oxides, for passivity to corrosion in saline environments.[17] Experiments in laboratory animals showed that the standard industrial-grade alloys—brasses and bronzes, nickel-chromium, and carbon steels—were not sufficiently inert to biodegradation. Both biochemical and biomechanical limitations were identified.[25]

The Stellite (cobalt-chromium-molybdenum) cast form and the stainless steel (iron-chromium-nickel) wrought form alloys were found to be acceptable for musculoskeletal applications.[38] These alloys depended on surface films for relative inertness and therefore were quite different from the noble metal systems used previously.

Technologic developments in the materials field resulted in the introduction of controlled-property reactive group metals and alloys (e.g., titanium and zirconium) in the 1950s. During the 1960s, biocompatibility research emphasized chemical and biochemical inertness, which resulted in major investigations of inert ceramics and carbons for surgical implants. High-purity fired ceramics were developed in the 1960s. Biomedical-grade carbons and graphites and high molecular weight polymers then debuted.[24, 39, 41] In the 1970s bioactive substances were introduced for *in vivo* bonding to bone, and emphasis shifted to the interactions between synthetic biomaterials and tissues.

A major change in direction occurred in the 1980s, as synthetic biomaterials were constituted and fabricated for specific implant applications. Previously, materials available from industrial applications had been redirected to biomedical devices. Specially constituted and designed substances for implants will play a major role in the future.

TYPES OF METALS AND ALLOYS FOR TOTAL JOINT REPLACEMENTS

Properties of various metals and alloys employed in orthopaedic implants are summarized in Table 2–1.

Cobalt-Based Casting Alloys

The first cast alloy system to have extensive applications was derived from the Stellite alloy group and was cast in air using lost-wax methods. Cobalt (Co), chromium (Cr), and molybdenum (Mo) were the primary elements of this system. Refining of cobalt utilizing standard industrial practices results in about 1 percent nickel within the cobalt composition.[30] Most of this nickel is retained in the final alloy composition. The cobalt within the Co-Cr-Mo alloy provides the primary element of the matrix phase. The chromium adds strength and, most importantly, chemical inertness through a chromium oxide sur-

Table 2–1. PROPERTIES OF METALS AND ALLOYS FOR ORTHOPAEDIC SURGICAL IMPLANTS

Material	Nominal Analysis (w/o)	Modulus of Elasticity GN/m^2 (*psi* × 10^6)	Ultimate Tensile Strength MN/m^2 (*psi* × 10^3)	Elongation to Fracture (%)	Surface
Ti	99 + Ti	97 (14)	240–550 (25–70)	>15	Ti Oxide
Ti-Al-V (Wrought)	90Ti-6Al-4V	117 (17)	860–896 (125–130)	>12	Ti Oxide
Ti-Al-V (Cast)	90Ti-6Al-4V	117 (17)	860 (125)	>8	Ti Oxide
Stainless Steel (316L)	70Fe-18Cr-12Ni	193 (28)	480–1000 (70–145)	>30	Cr Oxide
Co-Cr-Mo (Cast)	66Co-27Cr-7Mo	235 (34)	655 (95)	>8	Cr Oxide
Co-Cr-W-Ni	55Co-20Cr-15W-10Ni	235 (34)	860 (125)	>30	Cr Oxide
Co-Ni-Cr-Mo	45Co-35Ni-20Cr-10Mo	235 (34)	793–1793 (115–260)	50–8	Cr Oxide
Co-Ni-Cr-Mo-W	52Co-20Ni-20Cr-4Ni-4W	235 (34)	600–1310 (87–190)	50–12	Cr Oxide
Zr	99^+Zr	97 (14)	552 (80)	20	Zr Oxide
Au	99^+Au	97 (14)	207–310 (30–45)	>30	Au

Minimum values are from the American Society for Testing and Materials. Selected products provide a range of properties. (w/o = weight percent of elements; GN/m^2 = Newtons per meter squared × 10^9; MN/m^2 = Newtons per meter squared × 10^6.)

face film (passive oxide layer). The molybdenum provides resistance to bulk corrosion, especially to pitting and crevice corrosion, plus solid-state strengthening.

Carbon and other minor additives interact with the primary elements to form secondary phases such as carbides. These secondary phases usually are isolated regions within the primary matrix, and they contribute resistance to abrasive wear. Carbon must be present only in a low concentration to avoid a continuous carbide phase within the alloy, which would reduce mechanical strength and ductility. Heat treatment, or annealing, is often used to make the carbide phases spheroid and to improve alloy ductility.

Advantages of cobalt cast alloys include hardness and wear resistance, and their metallurgic properties permit polishing to a smooth surface. Such alloys continue to be utilized for articulating surfaces of total joint prostheses.

Wrought Alloys of Cobalt, Iron, and Titanium

Although the mechanical properties of the cast cobalt-based alloys are adequate for some total joint components, their relative strengths and ductilities are lower than those of the wrought alloy groups.[29] Wrought describes mechanically fabricated conditions produced by techniques such as rolling, forging, swaging, and drawing. The wrought cobalt-based alloys, which contain altered quantities of nickel, molybdenum, and tungsten, demonstrate enhanced mechanical properties. Similarly, castings of alloys based on iron have lower strengths and ductilities than the wrought alloys based on iron.[29]

The wrought surgical stainless steel of the Austenitic 316L material is both strong and ductile. However, this wrought alloy, when annealed, does not demonstrate the high magnitude of strength of the wrought cobalt or titanium alloy system. Both the cast and wrought stainless steels are subject to crevice and pitting if the chromium oxide surface film is disrupted or dissolved or if the alloy is subjected to fatigue (cyclic loading) or fretting (motion along the contacting surfaces, producing localized wear debris).[21] Because of the susceptibility to crevice and pitting corrosion, neither the cast nor the wrought type of stainless steel can be utilized *in vivo* with a very rough or porous surface.

The alloy of titanium (Ti), aluminum (Al), and vanadium (V) (Ti-6Al-4V) combines relatively high mechanical strength and ductility and resistance to pitting and crevice corrosion.[29] Because titanium is a reactive group metal, this alloy spontaneously forms a surface oxide in air or tissue fluids.[8] In some applications, this characteristic has proved to be advantageous.[36] The titanium alloy, in contrast to the cobalt- and iron-based alloys, is very sensitive to fretting corrosion. In industrial applications, the alloy is known to exhibit galling, or surface abrasion associated with wear. This phenomenon explains reports of discolored tissues adjacent to titanium or titanium alloy prostheses.[16, 28, 40] The zones of discoloration were associated with relative motion along the tissue-biomaterial interface.[37]

Concerns have been expressed about titanium alloys for the articulating surface in total joint replacement. Laboratory data from joint simulators show titanium alloys to be more subject to contact surface wear when articulating with polyethylene.[1, 7, 11, 12] To produce a more wear-resistant surface, most titanium alloy surfaces are either nitrided or ion implanted, most often with nitrogen.

Physical, Mechanical, and Chemical Properties

The cobalt-, iron-, and titanium-based alloys are similar in color when polished. The iron and cobalt alloys are similar in density (8 to 10 gm/cc), whereas titanium is less dense (3 to 4 gm/cc). All of the alloys can be obtained in wrought or cast metallurgic conditions. As with other metals, all are conductors of heat and electricity. Mechanical properties are highly dependent on metallurgic conditions, with the wrought forms being stronger and more ductile than the cast forms. The iron and cobalt alloys have similar elastic moduli, which are about twice those of the titanium alloys. The cobalt alloys are hardest and most resistant to wear. The titanium alloys are most notch sensitive and may fracture under notch- or crack-induced fatigue loading. Of course, sharp angles, notches, and surface features such as cracks must be avoided for all prostheses.

Titanium alloys are the most chemically inert, but both cobalt and titanium alloys are sufficiently inert to be used as porous surfaces for tissue ingrowth. In contrast, the iron alloys are subject to *in vivo* pitting and crevice corrosion. Corrosion potentials for porous and nonporous titanium and cobalt alloys are not significantly different, corrosion rates being somewhat proportional to the relative increase in surface area for porous materials. The titanium alloys are most subject to wear, whereas the cobalt alloys are the least. Both titanium and iron alloys can be subject to fretting corrosion with metal-metal wear couples.[18]

Biologic tissue responses to these alloys and their corrosion and wear products show that titanium is less reactive than the cobalt and iron alloys.[3, 26] At higher concentrations, all of the metallic debris induces tissue reactions. Because corrosion products of cobalt and iron alloys contain nickel, these alloys should be avoided for patients who exhibit hypersensitivity reactions to nickel. Concerns have been raised about the toxicities of aluminum and vanadium from the titanium alloy.[22] In the considerable literature on this topic,[32] minimal tissue response has been demonstrated to dilute concentrations of these elements in quantities similar to those in corrosion products. Metal ion tumor production, of course, is always a concern, and questions have been raised about the various alloys.[15] At this time, the available literature does not demonstrate a direct correlation between sarcoma and total joint prostheses (see Chapter 12, *Histology and Pathology of Total Joint Replacement*).[19]

CONSIDERATIONS FOR TOTAL JOINT REPLACEMENT

Biomaterial and biomechanical properties must be considered when designing any joint replacement system.

Articulating Surfaces, Corrosion, and Wear

The detailed macroscopic and microscopic surface topographies of total joint prostheses and the materials of the articulating counterfaces are important. Polished surfaces with roughness values within the microinch range (0.025 μm) are normally selected for metallic surfaces within areas of counterface contact. All sharp corners, ridges, and other abrupt contours are avoided. The alloy-alloy combinations are the most subject to wear, and ceramics and polymers demonstrate some advantages compared with other materials.[7] When third-body abrasion is not present, the ceramics demonstrate low wear rates. However, with some devices, ceramic-ceramic combinations have shown third-body abrasive wear, that is, loss of particulate from some regions because of inadequate grain size control.[14] Reduced coefficients of friction and wear rates have been reported with ceramic-polymer combinations (see Chapter 4, *Ceramics*).[14] In general, alloy-polymer combinations with ultrahigh molecular weight polyethylene have been most popular.[29, 39] The polymer is utilized as the concave part of the geometric combination for most standard prostheses.

The iron alloys demonstrate minimal localized wear along the alloy-polymer articulation regions[6] but are not as wear resistant as the cobalt alloys. This finding is most readily explained by the presence and distribution of carbide phases within the cobalt alloy, by the differences in indentation hardness, and by the mechanical and chemical stabilities of the surface oxide.

The titanium alloys are most subject to abrasive wear along the alloy-polymer contact zone. Several surface treatments, for example, metallic ion implantation, have been attempted to minimize metallic wear.[23] However, the various metallic surface treatments for titanium alloy may improve wear resistance of an articulating surface only for a few years.[11, 12] This factor would most probably be evident in the presence of third-body abrasive particulates. The presence of polymeric, metallic, or osseous debris between the alloy and polyethylene articulating surfaces would significantly increase wear rates and particulate generation. Obviously, such debris should be kept to a minimum.

Charnley[6] selected metal-polymer articulation on the basis of laboratory measurements of coefficients of friction. Although these measurements are useful, they provide only part of the information required for material and design selections. Data from continued laboratory studies have shown relatively low coefficients of friction for the ceramic-ceramic and ceramic-polymer couples.[7, 12] Because of material and design considerations some manufacturers and surgeons choose these materials for selected total joint replacement devices.

Component and Stem Strength, Modulus, and Fixation

Cast structures have limitations in some device stems. Therefore, total hip device stems are usually fabricated from wrought high-strength alloys, typically cobalt or titanium alloys.[29] Metallic backings for acetabular components and total knee femoral and tibial parts have been fabricated from castings of iron, cobalt, or titanium alloys. The cast cobalt alloy has been employed extensively for total knee femoral components.[20]

Macroscopic stress and strain distributions are best controlled through design.[13] Shape changes can yield a stiffer or a more flexible device for any material. Whereas size and shape (section modulus) are more important for control of macroscopic strain distribution, the material and its surface have the most influence on the microscopic strain distribution along the tissue interface. For example, titanium alloys have an elastic modulus 5.7 times greater than that of compact bone, or about half the elastic moduli of iron and cobalt alloys (approximately 9.3 to 11 times that of compact bone).

Under some conditions, smooth surfaces of titanium oxide can integrate with bone. Chromium oxide on cobalt alloys may not have this capability. Integration could directly influence interfacial force transfer and thereby strain distributions within the prosthesis and associated tissues.

The fixation of one component to another utilizing grooved, undercut, snap-in, or taper-lock features has become routine in the era of modular device systems. Notch sensitivity (susceptibility to regional fracture) of the alloys is important for these complex configurations. The stress magnitudes and design features must be controlled to avoid localized fretting and fracture. Mechanical decoupling (separation of parts *in vivo*) and cyclic fatigue-induced fractures have been reported infrequently.[31, 34]

Because specifications and component tolerances are not the same for all manufacturers, parts cannot be routinely interchanged among devices, even though they look similar.

Attachment to Bone and Porous Surfaces

Most total joint replacements in the 1960s and 1970s were fixed within the bone using autocuring polymethyl methacrylate (PMMA) bone cement.[9] Manufacturers often stated that metallic surfaces, roughness, or porosities improved the strength of the device's attachment to bone cement. Later methods to decrease internal porosities within the PMMA, such as centrifuging and vacuum degassing, have also resulted in increased mechanical strength. (See Chapter 3, *Polymers,* and Chapter 7, *Fixation Methods.*)[33]

The concepts of ingrowth and mechanical strain transfer to stabilize bone interfaces emphasize the importance of design and material properties. Porous surfaces, including metals and alloys, ceramics, and polymer-based composites, enhance mechanical attachment to PMMA and furnish regions for tissue ingrowth.[26] Available surface configurations include sintered or pressure-sintered spheric beads, irregularly shaped particles and wires, and plasma- or flame-sprayed coatings. These coatings have been evaluated extensively for porosity dimensions, topology, corrosion resistance, and mechanical strength.[26, 39] Although questions remain about long-term clinical results, laboratory, animal, and human studies have already produced some significant correlations.[26] A variety of tissue types have been shown to invest the porous surfaces, with most including a mixture of fibrous tissue and bone.[31, 34]

Porous surfaces on cobalt and titanium

alloys reduce the mechanical strengths of the components to which the coating is applied.[26] Fatigue tests have revealed up to a 75-percent reduction in material strength with the introduction of porous surface coatings. These reductions are caused by both the metallurgic processing conditions required to bond the coating through sintering (high temperature exposure) and the alterations in surface topography (notches due to the pore geometries). Because of the altered mechanical strength, surface tensile and shear stresses must be kept to a minimum. Cyclic fatigue properties of the final construct and the *in vivo* stress and strain patterns are, of course, also important.

Concern about long-term tissue responses, mechanical properties of the device, and tissue conditions if revision should be required has led to recommendations for press-fit designs.[4] An interesting extension of this basic design concept, which in theory should be possible for total joint replacement devices, is osteointegration along interfaces with titanium oxide[2] or calcium phosphate[14] coating. For this process to occur, surfaces must be mechanically and chemically clean at the time of tissue contact. Mechanical fixation is required during healing to minimize localized motion along the biomaterial-tissue interface. Design and material concepts from dental implant devices have encouraged clinical investigations for such devices in musculoskeletal reconstruction (see Chapter 7, *Fixation Methods*).[5]

TRENDS IN ALLOY SYSTEMS

Metallic materials have a long history of *in vivo* application in orthopaedic reconstructive surgery. In general, they provide longevity under somewhat severe and complex mechanical and chemical environmental conditions.

A general trend in total joint replacements has been the development of alloys with increased mechanical strengths and ductilities. This development has been accomplished through alloy compositions, microstructure, residual strain, and heat treatment control. A variety of surface treatments have also been introduced. Computer-assisted design and machining systems are changing the general methodology for designing custom devices. Modular designs based on metallic parts, including systems with stacked interlocking parts, are being used for complex revision surgeries. Metallic materials, because of machinability and toughness, continue to dominate this evolving area. Utilization of alloys based on reactive group metals should continue to expand.

Research supports a move to surface-modified alloys or ceramics for articulating and bone-bonding interfaces. Risks increase as these technologies transfer from the laboratory to the clinical setting. The trend to eliminate laboratory animal testing, in which devices have been exposed to *in vivo* function for relatively long periods of time, further increases the risk. Advanced biocompatibility testing for toxicity, hypersensitivity, and carcinogenicity will be required to answer the complex questions about biomaterial and biomechanical interactions (see Chapter 6, *Biocompatibility*). Obviously, more comprehensive, prospective human clinical research protocols will be needed.

References

1. Bacon, R. K.: The Effect of Ion Implantation on the Corrosive-Wear Resistances of Ti-6A1-4V. Thesis, Dept. of Materials Engineering, University of Alabama at Birmingham, 1983.
2. Branemark, P. I., Zarb, G., and Albrektsson, T.: Tissue Integrated Prostheses. Chicago, Quintessence Publishing Company, 1985.
3. Brown, S. A. (ed.): Am. Soc. Testing Mat. STP, Vol. 810. Philadelphia, ASTM Press, 1983.
4. Burnstein, A. H.: Shands Award Paper. ORS-AAOS Annual Meeting, Las Vegas, 1989.
5. Carlsson, L. V.: On the Development of a New Concept for Orthopaedic Implant Fixation. Ph. D. Dissertation, Göteborg, Sweden, 1989.
6. Charnley, J.: Factors in the Design of An Artificial Hip Joint. Lubrication and Wear in Living and Artificial Joints. London, Institute of Mechanical Engineering, 1967.
7. Clark, I. C. and McKellop, H. A.: Wear Testing. Handbook of Biomaterials Evaluation. Edited by A. von Recum. New York, MacMillan, 1986.
8. Collings, E. W.: The Physical Metallurgy of Titanium Alloys. Metals Park, OH, American Society for Metals, 1984.
9. Consensus Conference and Proceedings on Total Hip Replacements, March 1982. Washington, D.C., NIH and AAOS, 1982.
10. Craig, R. G.: Restorative Dental Materials. St. Louis, C. V. Mosby Company, 1985.
11. Crowinshield, R., Lower, J., Gilbertson, L., et al.:

Simulating total knee replacement wear in vitro: comparison of Ti-6A1-4V and ion implanted Ti-6A1-4V. Trans. Orthop. Res. Soc. 15:470, 1990.
12. Davidson, J. A., Kovacs, P., and Lanzer, W. L.: Metal ion release during articulation of ion implanted Ti-6A1-4V alloy against UHMW-Polyethylene. Trans. Orthop. Res. Soc. 15:460, 1990.
13. Dieter, Jr., G. E.: Mechanical Metallurgy. New York, McGraw Hill, 1961.
14. Ducheyne, P. and Lemons, J. E. (eds.): Bioceramics: Material Characteristics Versus In Vivo Behavior. New York, New York Academy of Sciences, 1988.
15. Editorial: Does corrosion matter? J. Bone Joint Surg. 70B:517–520, 1988.
16. Ferguson, A. B., Akahoshi, Y., Laing, P. G., et al.: Characterization of trace ions released from embedded implants in rabbit. J. Bone Joint Surg. 44A:323, 1962.
17. Fontana, M. G. and Greene, N. D.: Corrosion Engineering. New York, McGraw Hill, 1967.
18. Fraker, A. and Griffin, C.: Corrosion and Degradation of Implant Materials, Am. Soc. Testing Mat. STP, Vol. 859. Philadelphia, ASTM Press, 1985.
19. Gillespie, W. J., Frampton, C. M. A., Henderson, R. J., et al.: The incidence of cancer following total hip replacement. J. Bone Joint Surg. 70B:539–542, 1988.
20. Goldberg, V. (ed.): Controversies of Total Knee Arthroplasty: Issues for the Nineties. Phoenix, Symposium Proceedings, November 1989. (In press.)
21. Griffin, C. D., Buchanan, R. A., and Lemons, J. E.: *In vitro* electrochemical corrosion study of coupled surgical implant materials. J. Biomed. Mater. Res. 17:489–500, 1983.
22. Hensten-Petterson, A.: General Toxicology. International Workshop on Biocompatibility, Toxicity and Hypersensitivity to Alloy Systems Used in Dentistry. Edited by B. R. Lang, H. F. Morris, and M. E. Razzoog. Ann Arbor, University of Michigan Press, 1985.
23. Hockman, R. F., Solnick-Legg, H., and Legg, K.: Ion Implantation and Plasma Assisted Processes. Metals Park, OH, American Society For Metals, 1988.
24. Leinfelder, K. F. and Lemons, J. E.: Clinical Restorative Materials and Techniques. Philadelphia, Lea & Febiger, 1988.
25. Lemons, J. E.: General Characteristics and Classifications of Implant Materials. Perspectives in Biomaterials. Edited by O. Lin and E. Chao. Amsterdam, Elsevier, 1986.
26. Lemons, J. E. (ed.): Quantitative Characterization and Performance of Porous Implants for Hard Tissue Applications. Am. Soc. Testing Mat. STP, Vol. 953. Philadelphia, ASTM Press, 1987.
27. Levert, H. S.: Experiments on the use of metallic ligatures as applied to arteries. Am. J. Med. Sci. 4:17, 1829.
28. Mears, D. C.: Materials and Orthopaedic Surgery. Baltimore, Williams & Wilkins, 1979.
29. Medical Devices, Vol. 13.01. Philadelphia, American Society for Testing and Materials, 1989.
30. Metals Handbook, Vol. 1. Metals Park, OH, American Society for Metals, 1961.
31. Morrey, B. F. (moderator): What Should be Done with the Implants I Take Out? Symposium Proceedings, AAOS Annual Meeting, Atlanta, February 1988.
32. Natiella, J. R.: Local Tissue Reaction and Carcinogenicity. International Workshop on Biocompatibility, Toxicity and Hypersensitivity to Alloy Systems Used in Dentistry. Edited by B. R. Lang, H. F. Morris, and M. E. Razzoog. Ann Arbor, University of Michigan Press, 1985.
33. O'Connor, D. O., Burke, D. W., Zelenski, E. E., et al.: Study of fatigue behavior of cemented total hip replacements under conditions simulating gait. Trans. Soc. Biomat. 12:50, 1988.
34. Retrieval and analysis of surgical implants and biomaterials. Trans. Soc. Biomat. Special Symp. 11, 1988.
35. Skinner, E. W. and Phillips, R. W.: The Science of Dental Materials. Philadelphia, W. B. Saunders Company, 1967.
36. Smith, D. C. and Williams, D. F.: Biocompatibility of Dental Materials, Vol. 4. Boca Raton, FL, CRC Press, 1982.
37. Solar, R. J., Pollack, S. R., and Korostoff, E.: *In vitro* corrosion testing of titanium surgical implant alloys: an approach to understanding titanium release from implants. J. Biomed. Mater. Res. 13:217, 1979.
38. Venable, C. S. and Stuck, W. G.: The Internal Fixation of Fractures. Springfield, Charles C Thomas, 1947.
39. Von Recum, A.: Handbook of Biomaterials Evaluation. New York, MacMillan, 1986.
40. Williams, D. F.: Biocompatibility of Clinical Implant Materials, Vol. 1. Boca Raton, FL, CRC Press, 1981.
41. Williams, D. F. and Roaf, R. (eds.): Implants in Surgery. Philadelphia, W. B. Saunders Company, 1973.

CHAPTER 3

Polymers

STANLEY A. BROWN

Currently, three types of polymers are used in total joint replacements: ultrahigh molecular weight polyethylene, polymethyl methacrylate (PMMA), and silicone elastomer. Polyethylene is unsurpassed by any material for wear resistance, toughness, low coefficient of friction, and self-lubrication. However, fatigue cracking has been observed. Polymethyl methacrylate is the polymer utilized in bone cement. It was first employed by Charnley in the 1960s; Smith, a Toronto dental materials scientist, conceived the idea of using self-curing PMMA.[17] Silicone elastomer is a polymer from which bone plugs and many one-piece flexible hinge joints (fingers and toes) are fabricated.

ULTRAHIGH MOLECULAR WEIGHT POLYETHYLENE

Polyethylenes are formed by addition polymerization of the monomer ethylene. During the polymerization reaction, chains may grow in length and may form side chains. Low-density polyethylenes typically have extensive side branching that prevents the formation of a compact structure. High-density polyethylenes are long-chain polymers with little or no side branching. Their density is usually in the range of 0.958 gm/ml, and their molecular weight ranges from 200,000 to 400,000.

Ultrahigh molecular weight polyethylene is manufactured by modified Ziegler catalyst systems and is supplied to fabricators as a fine powder. The nominal molecular weight is 3 million or higher. Owing to its high molecular weight, the American Society for Testing and Materials specification F648 provides a solution viscosity correlating with a molecular weight of greater than 3 million.[1] According to the specification, density is 0.930 to 0.944, yield strength is 19 Mega Pascals (MPa), and ultimate tensile strength is 27 MPa, with an elongation of 200 percent.

Devices are fabricated from these polyethylenes at high temperatures under a pressure molding process. The molding temperature has a significant effect on the final molecular weight and wear resistance of the fabricated device.[25] The highest molecular weights and lowest wear rates appear to be produced at 204°C, the lowest temperature utilized in experiments. Joint simulator studies have confirmed that low wear rates and the release of small wear particles are associated with high molecular weight materials.[24] Clinical studies of retrieved joint prostheses have shown wear problems due to incomplete fusion between the particles.[11, 22] Tearing of microfibrils between particles has been observed.[22] Carbon fiber reinforcing seems to exacerbate the particle fusion problem.[33]

Having a low heat distortion temperature, the polyethylene in joint replacements is normally sterilized by gamma radiation at 2.5 Mrad. Although radiation can potentially break the polymer chain (scission), this effect is probably inconsequential in the crystalline regions of ultrahigh molecular weight polyethylene, as the chains will reform. However, chain scission can lead to cross-linking in amorphous regions.[19] Radiation-induced formation of hydrophilic carbonyl groups can increase the water absorption of the polymer.[19] If radiation exceeds 5 Mrad (e.g., in repeated sterilization), wear resistance decreases.[24] Wear rate studies of samples sterilized at 20 Mrad show an initial high wear rate followed by a plateau,[24] suggesting a degraded outer surface with poor wear resistance. Similar surface damage effects due to oxidative chain scission have been observed in cups tested in joint simulators.[9] These radiation effects are much less pronounced when sterilization is conducted in a nitrogen environment rather than in air.[24]

Wear of ultrahigh molecular weight polyethylene may be due to a number of mechanisms. Much of what is observed as wear radiographically may actually be a result of creep.[23] Scratching and pitting often seen on retrieved specimens can result from processing (discussed previously). As depicted in Figure 4–1, hard particles can get between the bearing surfaces. Wear due to three-body wear can result from trapped PMMA or bone particles.[14, 26, 32] When polyethylenes are utilized, particles may become embedded in the material and cause a plowing type of wear. The problem can be minimized by careful removal of all loose PMMA or any cement that may fracture later and become interposed between the articular surfaces.

The size of the contact area between components also affects wear, as demonstrated by Charnley and colleagues[7] in their analysis of the severe wear of total hip sockets fabricated with polytetrafluoroethylene. Small-diameter femoral heads were associated with high linear wear rates and large-diameter femoral heads with high volumes of wear particle release. Linear wear rates determine the length of time before the polymeric component wears out. The total volume of particles released determines the degree of inflammatory response and the possibility of implant loosening (see Chapter 6, *Biocompatibility*, and Chapter 12, *Histology and Pathology of Total Joint Replacement*).

Wear due to subsurface shear stress and subsequent delamination has also been observed, as depicted in Figure 3–1.[26, 32] The importance of stress levels has been demonstrated with computer modeling studies of hips and tibial plateaus. Stress levels are especially critical in the tibia, where stress reverses during gait and is tensile near the edge.[2] Shear stresses are greatest on the surface of the acetabular cup. On the tibia they occur 1 to 2 mm below the surface (Fig. 3–1A). The stresses on the tibial components have been shown to increase rapidly for polyethylene components less than 10 mm thick,[2] an analysis supported by clinical retrieval.[14] Wear rates are reported to correlate with the time of implantation and patient activity.[14, 32]

Although ultrahigh molecular weight polyethylene is a very tough, ductile material, fatigue cracking has been demonstrated in laboratory tests.[6, 20] Reinforcement with carbon fibers does not improve its resistance to crack propagation.[6] Once

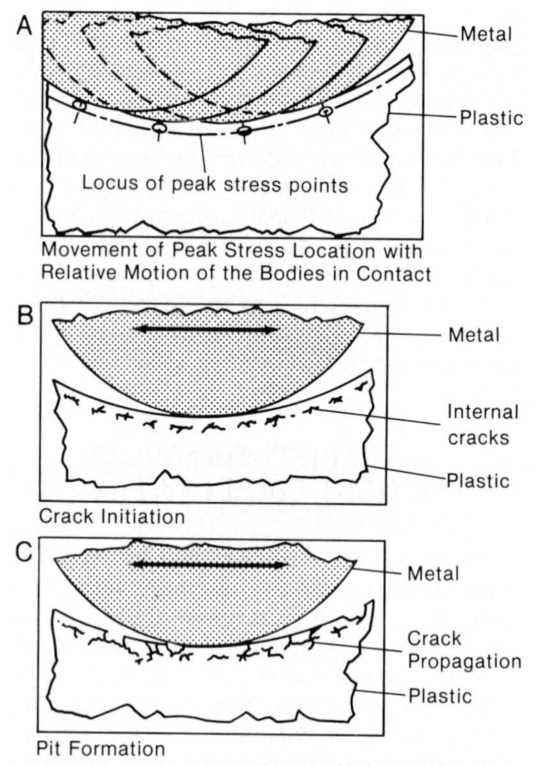

FIGURE 3–1. Wear initiation due to subsurface stress. *A*, The sequence of events involves the generation of subsurface shear stresses due to relative motion. *B*, These stresses lead to initiation of cracks. *C*, These coalesce to delamination and pit formation. (Pappas, M. J., Makris, G., and Buechel, F. F.: Biomedical Engineering Trust, Technical Report #003, January, 1986.)

a crack has formed, it spreads almost ten times faster in the composite than in the unreinforced material. Cracking of acetabular cups has been attributed to stress riser effects, due either to grooves in the back for cement retention[5, 14, 27] or to cement key holes drilled in the ilium.[13] Numerous cases of cracking of metal-backed patellar components have been reported.[3, 18] The problem has been attributed to wear and design problems of the metal back cutting the polyethylene.[28] As with most material problems, failure is related to patient weight and activity and device design.

POLYMETHYL METHACRYLATE

The idea for a prosthetic luting or grouting agent in total joint replacement was conceived by Charnley, who used pink dental acrylic in his first procedures. Since then, the pink color additive has been removed and radiopaque materials such as barium sulfate have been added, but the chemical composition has remained essentially unchanged.

Orthopaedic bone cement is provided as a combination of powder and liquid, generally 40 gm of powder and 20 gm of liquid.[17] The powder particles range from 30 to 150 μ in diameter. Radiopaque powders consist of approximately 90 percent polymer, either PMMA or a random copolymer with small amounts of styrene. The remaining 10 percent consists of a radiopacifier and a small amount of a polymerization initiator, benzoyl peroxide. The liquid contains approximately 97 percent methyl methacrylate monomer plus an inhibitor, hydroquinone, and an activator, dimethyl-*p*-toluidine. The inhibitor prevents polymerization of the monomer during storage, whereas the activator causes benzoyl peroxide to initiate polymerization after mixing.

Polymerization of PMMA occurs by free radical addition polymerization. The methyl methacrylate monomer has a double bond, which is broken by a free radical, leading to chain growth. The hydroquinone in the monomer acts as a scavenger for free radicals, thus minimizing polymerization of the monomer during storage. However, the monomer does polymerize slowly over time; therefore, the manufacturer's recommended shelf life must be observed carefully.

When the liquid and powder are mixed, the monomer softens the polymeric beads to form a gel. The dimethyl-*p*-toluidine in the liquid reacts with the benzoyl peroxide in the powder to produce reactive benzoyl free radicals. As these radicals react with the monomer, breaking the double bonds, polymerization is started. The molecular weight distribution of cured PMMA is slightly higher than that of the original powder, indicating that the matrix that forms when the liquid polymerizes has a higher molecular weight than the powder that it cements together.[12] Some monomer is lost by evaporation during mixing; a ratio of powder to liquid of 2 to 1 produces the lowest evaporation.[17] Upwards of 2.5 percent residual unreacted monomer may be present for as long as 200 days after mixing.[12]

Polymerization of PMMA releases 130 cal/gm of monomer, with most of the exothermic heat generated given off during the setting phase of polymerization. Higher ambient temperatures hasten polymerization,[4, 17] and both dough and set times decrease significantly. Higher ambient temperature and larger cement masses also raise the maximum temperature reached during setting; temperatures as high as 107°C have been recorded in a block 10 mm thick.[17] As the reaction temperature rises, the rate of chain nucleation increases; thus, the average molecular weight of the final cement declines.[4] This effect, in turn, lowers the mechanical strength of the cement.[4] In practical terms, a thin cement mantle will not get as hot and will be stronger than a thick cement mantle. However, bone cement undergoes a volume shrinkage of approximately 8 percent,[12] causing a hoop stress around a prosthesis; therefore, the cement must be thick enough to avoid cracking during shrinkage.

The final cement mass is essentially a composite of powder cemented together by the polymerized monomer and entrapped air bubbles.[11] Differences between cements due to their composition and porosity have been shown.[8] When PMMA is centrifuged to reduce porosity, fatigue strength is improved significantly.[8] Owing to differences in the composition of various cements and their viscosities, the techniques for optimum strength gained by centrifugation vary. A limit exists to how much the cement can be centrifuged, however, because it continues to polymerize while being spun. By the time very low porosity is achieved, the cement may be too doughy to be workable.

Various cements differ markedly in viscosity.[15] The rate at which a cement polymerizes and thus increases in viscosity depends on the type. It is important that orthopaedic surgeons understand the cements they employ as well as the effects of ambient temperature. Polymethyl methacrylate is a non-Newtonian fluid, that is, its viscosity changes with a change in shear rate.[15] This material behaves as a pseudoplastic fluid and becomes more fluid when injected at a faster rate or higher pressure. When injected quickly with a cement gun, such as a caulking gun, the cement flows more readily and penetrates better. Although the tensile strength of a finger-packed bone-cement interface after high-pressure pulsatile lavage does not differ significantly from that produced by pressure injection, the shear strength is significantly less[16] (see Chapter 7, *Fixation Methods*).

SILICONE ELASTOMER

Silicone elastomer is synthesized from silicon dioxide (sand). Through a series of steps, the silicon dioxide is converted to a polymer with silicon and oxygen as repeating elements on the backbone chain. Two methyl (CH_3) groups are attached to each silicon, which has a valence of 4; hence, the name polydimethylsiloxane. In its low molecular weight form, polydimethylsiloxane is an oil (silicone oil). As the molecular weight increases, the compound becomes gum like. Medical-grade silicone elastomers are prepared from polysiloxane (MW 750,000) with reactive organic silicone ligands, typically vinyl, for cross-linking. The gum is compounded with fumed silica that has a large surface area (400 m^2/gm); it is then cross-linked by heat vulcanizing with trace quantities of rare metals or peroxides as catalysts.[10] Typical cross-linking density is 1 per 325 silicon atoms. The result is a three-dimensional giant molecule. Post-curing assures that vulcanizing is complete and volatile substances are removed.[10]

Typical mechanical properties of Dow 372 Silastic are tensile strength of 9.57 MPa, modulus of 350 MPa, and elongation of more than 400 percent. Studies in dogs employing 6- to 7-month subcutaneous implantations have shown a 7 percent decrease in strength, a 10 percent decrease in elongation, and an 8 percent increase in modulus. Similar changes were seen after an additional 1.5 years *in vivo*.[30]

Failure of early finger joint replacements employing silicone elastomer was associated with discoloration and lipid absorption.[21, 29] Thermodynamic studies demonstrated a pumping action of silicone flexing as a cause of lipid absorption.[21] Laboratory simulator studies of lipid absorption failed to produce fractures or lipid absorption after 7×10^6 cycles in serum for properly installed specimens. However, when the prosthesis was mounted so that the flexion axis of the simulator was offset from that of the prosthesis, as might occur with improper implantation, discoloration and lipid absorption were observed. Modification of the design of the flexing hinge reduced or eliminated the absorption problem.[21] High failure rates are normally associated with progressive rheumatoid arthritis owing to the cutting effect of sharp thin bone edges.[31]

References

1. American Society for Testing and Materials (ASTM) F648-84: Standard Specification for Ultrahigh Molecular Weight Polyethylene Powder and Fabricated Forms for Surgical Implants. Philadelphia, ASTM Press, 1989.
2. Bartel, D. L., Bicknell, V. L., and Wright, T. M.: The effect of conformity, thickness, and material on stresses in ultrahigh molecular weight components for total joint replacement. J. Bone Joint Surg. 68A:1041–1051, 1986.
3. Bayley, J. C., Scott, R. D., Ewald, F. C., et al.: Failure of the metal-backed patellar component after total knee replacement. J. Bone Joint Surg. 70A:668–674, 1988.
4. Brown, S. A. and Bargar, W. L.: The influence on temperature and specimen size on the flexural properties of PMMA bone cement. J. Biomed. Mater. Res. 18:523–536, 1984.
5. Collins, D. N., Chetta, S. G., and Nelson, C. L.: Fracture of the acetabular cup: a case report. J. Bone Joint Surg. 64A:939–940, 1982.
6. Connelly, G. M., Rimnac, C. M., Wright, T. M., et al.: Fatigue crack propagation behavior of

ultrahigh molecular weight polyethylene. J. Orthop. Res. 2:119–125, 1984.

7. Charnley, J., Kamangar, A., and Longfield, M. D.: The optimum size of prosthetic heads in relation to the wear of plastic sockets in total replacement of the hip. Med. Biol. Eng. 7:31–39, 1969.
8. Davies, J. P., Jasty, M., O'Conner, D. O., et al.: The effects of centrifuging bone cement. J. Bone Joint Surg. 71B:39–42, 1989.
9. Eyerer, P., Kurth, M., McKellup, H. A., et al.: Characterization of UHMWPE hip cups run on joint simulators. J. Biomed. Mater. Res. 21:275–291, 1987.
10. Frisch, E. E.: Technology of Silicones in Biomedical Applications. Biomaterials in Reconstructive Surgery. Edited by L. R. Rubin. St. Louis, C. V. Mosby, pp. 73–90, 1983.
11. Gibbons, D. F., Anderson, J. M., Martin, R. L., et al.: Wear and Degradation of Retrieved Ultrahigh Molecular Weight Polyethylene and Other Polymeric Implants. Corrosion and Degradation of Implant Materials, ASTM, STP-684. Edited by B. C. Syrett and A. Acharya. Philadelphia, ASTM Press, pp. 20–40, 1979.
12. Haas, S. S., Brauer, G. M., and Dickson, G.: A characterization of polymethyl methacrylate bone cement. J. Bone Joint Surg. 57A:380–391, 1975.
13. Harley, J. M. and Boston, D. A.: Acetabular cup failure after total hip replacement. J. Bone Joint Surg. 67B:222–224, 1986.
14. Hood, R. W.: Retrieval Analysis of Total Joint Components from the University of Missouri-Kansas City School of Medicine Implant Retrieval Program. Corrosion and Degradation of Implant Materials, ASTM STP, 859. Edited by A. C. Fraker and C. D. Griffin. Philadelphia, ASTM Press, pp. 403–414, 1985.
15. Krause, W. R., Miller, J., and Ng, P.: The viscosity of acrylic bone cements. J. Biomed. Mater. Res. 16:219–243, 1982.
16. Krause, W. R., Krug, W., and Miller, J.: Strength of the cement-bone interface. Clin. Orthop. 163:290–299, 1982.
17. Lautenschlager, E. P., Stupp, S. I., and Keller, J. C.: Structure and Properties of Acrylic Bone Cement. Functional Behavior of Orthopaedic Biomaterials, Vol. II. Edited by P. Ducheyne and C. W. Hastings. Boca Raton, FL, CRC Press, 1984.
18. Lombardi, A. V. Jr., Engh, G. A., Volz, R. G., et al.: Fracture/dissociation of the polyethylene in metal-backed patellar components in total knee arthroplasty. J. Bone Joint Surg. 70A:675–679, 1988.
19. Nusbaum, H. J. and Rose, R. M.: The effects of radiation sterilization on the properties of ultrahigh molecular weight polyethylene. J. Biomed. Mater. Res. 13:557–576, 1979.
20. Rimnac, C. M., Wright, T. M., and Klein, R. W.: J integral measurements of ultrahigh molecular weight polyethylene. Poly. Eng. Sci. 28:1586–1589, 1988.
21. Rose, R. M., Paul, I. L., Weightman, B., et al.: The role of stress enhanced reactivity in failure of orthopaedic implants. J. Biomed. Mater. Res. Symp. 4:401–418, 1973.
22. Rose, R. M., Crugnola, A., Ries, M., et al.: On the origins of high *in vivo* wear rates in polyethylene components of total joint prostheses. Clin. Orthop. 145:277–286, 1979.
23. Rose, R. M., Nusbaum, H. J., Schneider, H., et al.: On the true wear rate of ultrahigh molecular weight polyethylene in the total hip prosthesis. J. Bone Joint Surg. 62A:537–549, 1980.
24. Rose, R. M., Goldfarb, E. V., Ellis, E., et al.: Radiation sterilization and the wear rate of polyethylene. J. Orthop. Res. 2:393–400, 1984.
25. Rostoker, W. and Galante, J. O.: Some new studies of the wear behavior of ultrahigh molecular weight polyethylene. J. Biomed. Mater. Res. 10:303–310, 1976.
26. Rostoker, W., Chao, E. Y. S., and Galante, J. O.: The appearances of wear on polyethylene—a comparison of *in vivo* and *in vitro* wear surfaces. J. Biomed. Mater. Res. 12:317–335, 1978.
27. Salvati, E. A., Wright, T. M., Burstein, A. H., et al.: Fracture of polyethylene acetabular cups. J. Bone Joint Surg. 61A:1239–1242, 1979.
28. Stulberg, S. D., Stulberg, B. N., Hamati, Y., et al.: Failure mechanisms of metal-backed patellar components. Clin. Orthop. 236:88–105, 1988.
29. Swanson, A. B., Meester, W. D., Swanson, G. G., et al.: Durability of silicone implants—an *in vivo* study. Orthop. Clin. North Am. 4:1097–1112, 1973.
30. Swanson, J. W. and Lebeau, J. E.: The effect of implantation on the physical properties of silicone rubber. J. Biomed. Mater. Res. 8:357–367, 1974.
31. Swanson, A. B., Poitevin, L. A., Swanson, G. G., et al.: Bone remodeling phenomena in flexible implant arthroplasty in the metacarpophalangeal joints. Clin. Orthop. 205:254–267, 1986.
32. Wright, T. M., Burstein, A. H., and Bartel, D. L.: Retrieval Analysis of Total Joint Replacement Components: A Six-year Experience. Corrosion and Degradation of Implant Materials, ASTM STP, 859. Edited by A. C. Fraker and C. D. Griffin. Philadelphia, ASTM Press, pp. 415–428, 1985.
33. Wright, T. M., Astion, D. J., Bansal, M., et al.: Failure of carbon fiber–reinforced polyethylene total knee–replacement components. J. Bone Joint Surg. 70A:926–932, 1988.

CHAPTER 4

Ceramics

STANLEY A. BROWN

The brittle character of ceramic materials affords some advantages over ductile materials, even though fracture can occur under sufficient stress.[27, 33] For example, the failure of ceramics is not dependent on the number of load cycles applied, i.e., the material does not fail because of cyclic fatigue as metallic material does. The effective strength of the material is a function of strain rate, i.e., the material acts stronger as the rate at which the load is applied increases. As a result, these brittle materials can be proof-tested.[27, 33] In proof-testing, a stress (load) is applied that exceeds the load expected in service. The ratio of the stress applied to the stress anticipated in service is used to predict how long the device will last. If the service load on a total hip replacement is expected to be 400 MegaPascals (MPa), proof-testing to a load of 1040 MPa—2.6 times that of the service load—would indicate that the device should last 50 years at the expected service load. Thus, ceramic devices can be tested individually to identify those with flaws. Those that survive testing can be used with relative confidence.

In this chapter, the following ceramic materials are discussed: alumina (aluminum oxide, or Al_2O_3); partially stabilized zirconia (zirconium oxide, or ZrO_2); calcium phosphate ceramics, i.e., tricalcium phosphate $[Ca_3(PO_4)_2]$ and hydroxylapatite $[Ca_{10}(PO_4)_6(OH)_2]$; and carbon and composites.

ALUMINA

Alumina (aluminum oxide, or Al_2O_3) is a ceramic material that has received much attention in the past 20 years as a potential material for total joint replacement because of its hardness and inertness.[7, 17] Alumina devices are made by sintering the powder at 1600°C. The material has a very high elastic modulus (380 GPa) and compressive strength (4500 MPa). When subjected to tensile stresses, however, its strength is comparatively low. In flexion, the tested strength is only 550 MPa. As a metal oxide (i.e., a compound that has already oxidized), alumina degrades very slowly in the challenging *in vivo* environment. This inertness results in a minimal biologic response *in vivo*.[17, 30] Despite its apparent inertness, evidence exists of slight deterioration in mechanical properties after exposure to simulated *in vivo* conditions.[33] Improper sintering, causing permeation of the test solution into the material, has been shown to result in environmental deterioration of mechanical properties.[26]

The mechanical failure of alumina, a brittle ceramic, is governed by the Griffith criterion, which states that failure is due to the propagation of preexisting cracks or flaws. When a ductile metal is strained, it deforms plastically; consequently, any crack tip is blunted and energy is absorbed. In other words, metals bend before they break. When brittle materials are strained, they do not deform plastically. The crack tip remains sharp and propagates. Elastic strain energy is converted to surface energy by the formation of new surfaces of the fracture, which means several things. Because no plastic deformation occurs, alumina implants show no warning signs of impending failure. Because all strain energy is converted to surface energy, as the amount of strain energy increases, the number of cracks and their associated surface energy increase. Therefore, the greater the impact, the more pieces are produced. When alumina devices fail, they usually break into many pieces.[31] The velocity of crack propagation is a function of the stress applied.

Alumina can be given a very high polish, resulting in an excellent bearing surface. Friction and wear studies have tested alumina against alumina and alumina against ultrahigh molecular weight polyethylene, as well as metal against polyethylene.[11, 34] The alumina-alumina combination has been found to have superior frictional forces and wear rates. Alumina-polyethylene is superior to metal-polyethylene (Fig. 4–1). Wear studies have also demonstrated the potential problem of three-body wear of alumina-alumina bearings (Fig. 4–2).[19]

When an alumina-polymer bearing has a heavy weight load, the plastic deforms elastically to conform to the sphericity of the harder ceramic component, resulting in load distribution over a wide area and comparatively low contact stress. However, when two hard materials are used in a bearing, elastic deformation is minimal. Any mismatch in the sphericity of alumina bearings can result in point contact and very high local stresses. If this causes localized wear, the wear products themselves will be subject to high contact stresses. The wear particles can act like grit or sandpaper, grinding up bearing surfaces and accelerating wear rapidly.[31, 32]

Clinical studies of alumina-bearing surfaces have demonstrated the potential problems. One is catastrophic fracture of alumina prosthetic components,[31] although as mentioned proof-testing can obviate this problem.[27] Careful matching of the taper of the metal stem to the ceramic ball and controlled impact during installation of the ball on the stem can also minimize the chances of fracture.[27, 31] In some of the early

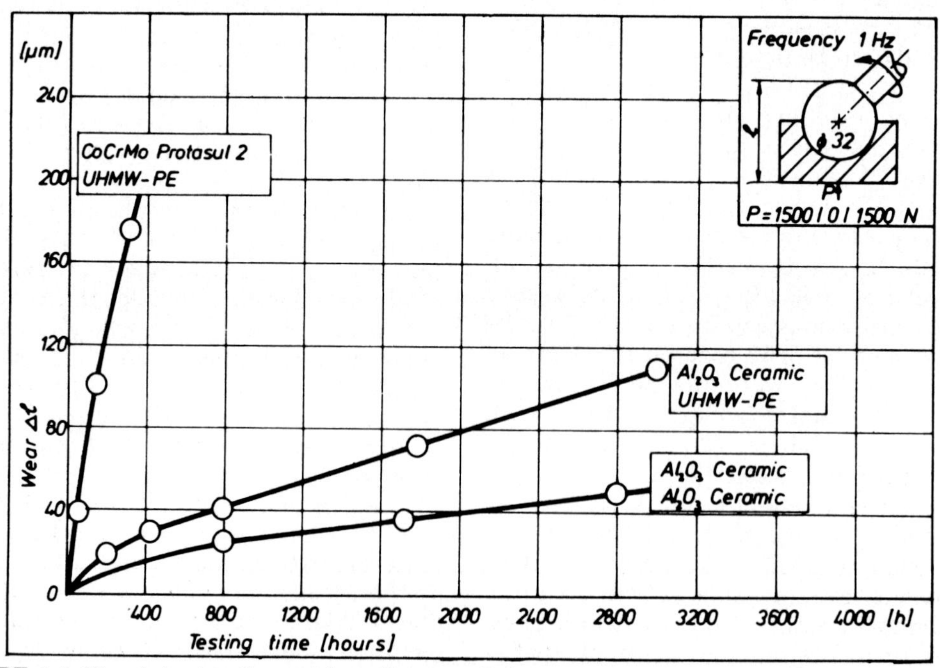

FIGURE 4–1. Wear behavior of material combinations for hip joint endoprostheses with load (P) cycling from 1500 to 0 Newtons. (CoCrMo Protasul 2 = cast CoCrMo alloy; UHMW-PE = ultra-high-molecular-weight polyethylene.) (Semlitsch, M., Lehmann, M., Weber, H., et al.: J. Biomed. Mater. Res. 11:537–552, 1977. By permission.)

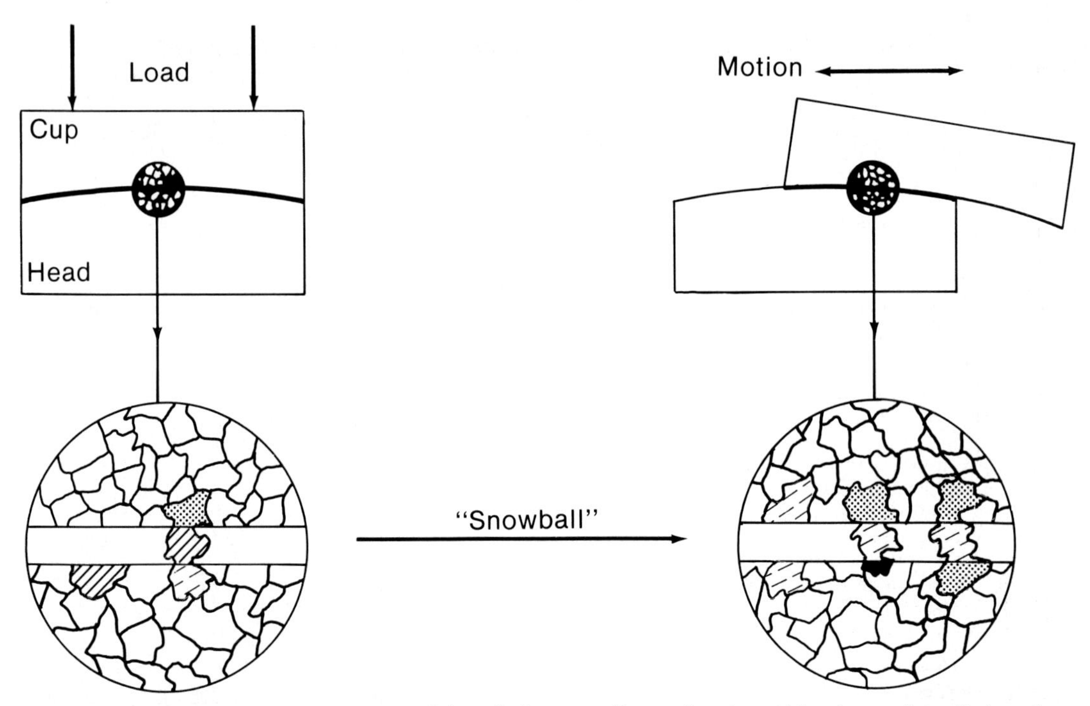

FIGURE 4–2. Schematic representation of three-body wear. Contaminant particles (e.g., polymethyl methacrylate, bone) get between articulating surfaces and result in increased wear. (From Plitz, W. and Griss, P.: National Bureau of Standards, SP-601.)

studies,[14, 31, 32] high wear rates were reported, apparently due to the grain excavation that was clearly seen in these devices. The individual particles utilized in the sintering process were plucked out of the surface and acted as abrasive particles, which caused rapid three-body wear.

Two improvements in processing techniques have drastically reduced the wear problem.[7] First, particle size is now kept below 3 μm to minimize the excavation problem. Grain excavation was seen only with large-grained materials. Second, matched pairs of alumina-alumina bearings are now employed. Because this practice demands a very high degree of match between components, to within 1 μm, the clinical wear rates are low.[7]

PARTIALLY STABILIZED ZIRCONIA

Zirconia (zirconium oxide, or ZrO_2) is another ceramic receiving attention as a potential bearing material.[7, 8, 15] Although zirconia is a brittle ceramic fabricated by sintering like alumina, it has a much finer grain structure (0.5 μm) and thus can be polished to a lower surface roughness than alumina. Therefore, its wear characteristics are superior. The other advantage of zirconia is that its mechanical properties can be improved by alloying.

Zirconia can be partially stabilized with 3 to 9 percent magnesia (MgO)[15] or with yttria (Y_2O_3).[7, 8] Crystal structures are produced, so that the material undergoes a localized phase transformation at a crack tip. The transformation is associated with volumetric expansion, resulting in compressive stresses at the crack front. Thus, the crack tip cannot propagate farther without extra energy and crack propagation is arrested. The hardening of zirconia due to phase transformation is somewhat analogous to metal ductility in which strain energy is absorbed by plastic deformation and work hardening. As shown in Table 4–1, zirconia is significantly stronger than alumina during bending. Sintering and HIPping (Hot Isostatic Pressing) further improve its strength.[8] Zirconia also has a lower elastic modulus than alumina. Biologic responses to zirconia are similar to those of alumina, as shown by short-term biocompatibility study results with magnesia-zirconia im-

Table 4–1. PHYSICAL PROPERTIES OF CERAMICS AND OTHER MATERIALS

	Yield (MPa)	Strength (MPa)	Elongation (%)	Modulus (GPa)
Ceramics				
Alumina		550		380
Partially stabilized zirconia HIPped		1200		200
Partially stabilized zirconia sintered		900		200
Metals				
Protosul-10 hot forged	1000	1200	10	200
Stainless steel-316L cold worked	750	1000	9	200
Stainless steel-316L annealed	170	400	45	200
Titanium-6 Aluminum-4 Vanadium	890	1000	12	105
Carbons and Composites				
Vapor-deposited		350 to >700	2 to >5	14 to 21
Vitreous carbon		70 to 200	0.8 to 1.3	24 to 31
Low-temperature isotropic carbon		275 to 550	1.6 to 2.1	17 to 28
Low-temperature isotropic carbon (+5 to 12% Si)		550 to 620	2.0	28 to 31
Polyacrylonitrile I fiber		1720	0.75	380
Polyacrylonitrile II fiber		2760	1.4	240
Carbon fiber–reinforced carbon 0°		1200		140
Carbon fiber–reinforced carbon 0° to 90°		500		60
PEEK APC-2 0°		2130	1.4	134
PEEK APC-2 ±45°		300	17	19
Biologic Tissues				
Hydroxylapatite		100	0.001	114, 130
Bone		80 to 150	1.5	18 to 20
Collagen		50		1.2
Polymers				
Polymethyl methacrylate cast (Lucite)		130	7.0	3.3
Polymethyl methacrylate bone cement		75	3.5	2.8
Ultrahigh molecular weight polyethylene		30	800	0.5
Silicone rubber		7	600	0.03

MPa = 10^6 N/m^2; GPa = 10^9 N/m^2; HIPped = Hot isostatic pressed; PEEK = polyetherketones.

planted in the paraspinal muscles of rabbits for up to 6 months[15] and with yttria-zirconia implanted in the lumbar muscles of rats for up to 12 weeks.[8]

CALCIUM PHOSPHATE

Calcium phosphate (CaP) ceramics have received much attention for their favorable biocompatibility. Because of their similarity to endogenous bone, no fibrous encapsulation occurs, inflammation and foreign body response are absent, no toxicity occurs, and the implant and bone remain in intimate contact.[22] Calcium phosphate ceramics interact with surrounding bone tissue, usually forming chemical bonds.[13, 16, 21] Two of the more popular synthetic ceramics are tricalcium phosphate [$Ca_3(PO_4)_2$] and hydroxylapatite [$Ca_{10}(PO_4)_6(OH)_2$]. Both are extremely bioactive and well accepted *in vivo*. The chemical and crystallographic structure of hydroxylapatite, particularly, closely resembles that of native bone.

The reaction of bone is not very sensitive to the form of calcium phosphate used. Within 1 month after implantation, both tricalcium phosphate and hydroxylaptite show direct bone apposition on the hydroxylapatite crystals on the implant surfaces.[21] Apposition has been observed as soon as 7 days after implantation.[25, 29] The two compounds differ markedly, however, in their rates of resorption and strength. In general, tricalcium phosphate resorbs considerably faster.[22, 25] In one study, a tricalcium phosphate ceramic dissolved 12.3 times faster in an acid medium and 22.3 times faster in a basic medium than did hydroxylapatite.[22] The porosity of a ceramic, an important determinant of strength, also plays a major role in resorption. Increasing porosity is associated with declining strength and increasing resorption.[12]

Because calcium phosphate ceramics

have limited strength in bulk form, interest has emerged lately in using them to coat stronger materials such as titanium for load-bearing applications. Of the two ceramics, hydroxylapatite is more desirable for this use; it interacts readily with host bone and dissolves slowly, assuring long-term intimate contact between the implant and surrounding tissue. Thus, bonding or anchoring of the implant to bone permits transfer of stress to the surrounding bone.[22, 23]

One technique employed to coat implants is plasma spraying—ionized gas or plasma is used to accelerate particles onto a surface. The powdered source material, carried in a stream of gas, is injected into a plasma flame. Having been melted by the flame, the liquid hydroxylapatite is propelled onto the target surface where it solidifies as a coating.

Titanium and the alloy of titanium, aluminum, and vanadium are currently the most appropriate choices for the substrate material under ceramic coatings. Titanium and hydroxylapatite bond together chemically at temperatures of 850°C to 1000°C, making the combination a good one. Unfortunately, the strength of bonding is still a critical problem.

Given the high temperature conditions of plasma spraying, the physical-chemical properties of the final coating may differ from those of the initial powder. Sintering and physical-chemical study findings have shown that hydroxylapatite undergoes phase transformation to tricalcium phosphate at 1400°C in the absence of water, as shown in the equation:[12]

$$Ca_{10}(PO_4)_6(OH)_2 = 2\ Ca_3(PO_4)_2 + Ca_4P_2O_9 + H_2O$$

For ceramic coatings to be effective, their thickness must optimize the mechanical properties of the ceramic as well as the properties necessary for adequate fixation of the implant. Although thinner coatings have better mechanical properties, between 10 and 15 μm may dissolve during the initial stages of interaction. In comparison, thicker coatings, although ensuring long-term implant fixation even if the exposed surfaces display slow continual dissolution over the long term, may fail under high tensile loads.[16] The best coating thickness thus appears to be 50 to 100 μm.

By regulating the conditions of plasma spraying carefully, it is possible to control the amount of each phase present in the coating, as well as the particle size, grain size, porosity, and substrate bond strength. All of these factors are critical to the development of a suitable surface for physical-chemical bonding with bone. Unfortunately, little information is available in the literature about the physical-chemical properties of powder sources, characterization of starting powder and final coating, and processing parameters. Most of what is known is proprietary information, held confidential by manufacturers. Without proper characterization of the coating, the possibility of implant failure due to unexpectedly high dissolution rates or unexpectedly low interfacial shear strengths exists.

CARBON AND COMPOSITES

Carbon and carbon composites, while not currently significant as material in total joint replacement, may receive more attention in the future. Carbon may be utilized in carbon-coated devices, as fibers alone, or as fibers in either a polymeric or carbon matrix. Many types of carbonaceous materials are available, with a wide variety of properties, and the terminology to describe them is often confusing. Graphitic carbon forms in planes, with carbon atoms arranged in hexagons. The carbon-carbon bond energy within the planes is high (114 kcal/mol), whereas the van der Waals bonding between layers is low (4 kcal/mol).[5] In graphite, the planes have a three-dimensional A-B-A-B order, and the crystals are quite large, on the order of 100 nm (1000 Å). The planes in the "turbostratic" structure have no three-dimensional relationship, and the grains are typically less than 10 nm. Because of the haphazard organization, the properties of turbostratic carbons are isotropic.

Turbostratic carbons can be created in several ways.[5] Controlled heating of a preformed polymeric block produces glassy or vitreous carbon. The pyrolysis drives off the volatile constituents leaving a glassy amorphous carbon residue. Typically, the residue has a low density owing to the release of by-products. Its crystallite size ranges from 1 to 4 nm, and its mechanical properties are comparatively poor (see Table 4–1). Vapor-deposited carbons are formed by the evaporation of carbon atoms from a heated source and deposition of a typically thin (<1 μm) and fine-grained (8–15Å) coating on a cool substrate. Vapor-deposited coatings confer the chemical characteristics of carbon to the underlying material without affecting its mechanical properties. Carbon coatings can also be produced by chemical vapor deposition when a gas such as methane is pyrolized to form a carbon coating.[9]

Carbon coatings that add to the mechanical properties of an underlying material ("pyrolytic" carbon coatings) are formed in a fluidized bed.[3, 5] It consists of a tube containing the bodies to be coated, typically graphitic, and other bodies, typically spheric zirconia. Fluidizing is accomplished by the flow of gases, such as methane or propane, to float the particles. When the chamber is heated to pyrolyze the gases, the coating forms. The resulting crystallites, consisting of sheets of atoms with no three-dimensional organization, are in the range of 3 to 4 nm. Because of the random orientation of the crystals, the coating has isotropic properties, i.e., invariant with respect to direction. The best coatings are produced at relatively low temperatures, in the 1500°C range. The coatings are referred to as "low-temperature isotropic (LTI) carbons." Coatings up to 1 mm thick can be achieved with high strength and a modulus close to that of bone. The low-temperature isotropic carbon can be alloyed with silicon by using a mixture of propane and methyltrichlorosilane (CH_3SiCl_3) for improved strength and wear resistance.[3]

Pyrolytic carbons do not fail owing to cyclic fatigue—one of their unique features. Their fatigue strength is equal to their single load strength.[36] Coatings of low-temperature isotropic carbon can be polished to produce a very smooth bearing surface with low friction.[35] The wear resistance of LTI carbon coatings improves greatly with increasing density and by alloying with silicon carbide. The wear of the LTI alloy articulating against itself and that of metal articulating with LTI carbon are low. However, the wear of LTI carbon against metal is much higher than that of LTI against LTI.

Carbon fibers are formed by pyrolyzing fibers of organic polymeric materials. The material used for most medical applications is polyacrylonitrile. In this process, fibers are stretched to maintain length. A multistage procedure is then performed to burn off noncarbon atoms and to develop a hexagonal structure. Two types of polyacrylonitrile fibers are generally used (see Table 4–1). Type I high-modulus fibers are produced utilizing a final pyrolysis temperature of 2000°C, which causes a significant amount of crystal orientation. Type II fibers, produced at 1500°C or below, have a lower modulus but higher strength.[28] Carbon fibers can be employed to repair ligaments or tendons or to reinforce polymeric or carbon matrix materials.

Polymeric composites reinforced with carbon fiber can be fabricated with continuous or short fibers in a polymeric matrix. Although short fibers do not provide the strength of long fibers, they can be processed by heating and then molding, using methods such as extrusion and injection molding.[6] Typically, long or continuous fiber composites are made from sheets of preimpregnated fibers ("prepregs"), with the fibers either parallel or woven into cloth.[20] In one method, carbon fibers are interwoven with polymer fibers. The prepreg sheets are then stacked with the fiber directions all parallel or with the fiber directions alternating relative to the long axis of the device (at 0° and 90° or at 45° in one direction and 45° in the other). The heating of the multilayer form melts the polymer and fuses the layers. Currently, matrices are made from thermoplastic materials such as polysulfones and the polyetherketones (PEEK or PEKEKK). Semicrystalline polyetherketones have greater chemical resistance than do amorphous polysulfones,[6] but their mechanical properties are similar. The mechanical properties and chemical stability are also influenced by the amount of "wet-out" or bonding between the carbon fibers and the polymer matrix materials.

Carbon fiber–reinforced carbon (CFRC) is made by first weaving fibers in a two- or three-dimensional array. The material is then impregnated with an organic material, such as an epoxy or phenolic resin, and pyrolyzed.[1, 10] The resulting vitreous or glassy carbon has low strength and a significant porosity due to shrinkage of the matrix during pyrolysis. Densification is accomplished by a multistage process of infiltrating the pores with methane, a methane-methyltrichlorosilane mixture, or resin, and subsequently pyrolyzing the material. The final product is carbon fiber in a carbon matrix. No actual bonding occurs between the fibers and carbon matrix. The strength of the material depends on the weave and the direction of testing (see Table 4–1), although it can be improved by alloying with silicon. The final process may involve vapor deposition of a carbon or silicon carbide alloy coating. The composite lacks the wear resistance necessary for joint-bearing surfaces; thus, an LTI carbon- or alumina-bearing[9] component might be added to the construct.

The biologic response to various forms of carbon has been found to be essentially independent of the method of fabrication. Typically, close apposition of bone to carbon without formation of fibrous tissue is seen by 8 to 12 weeks.[2, 5, 9, 10, 24] Bone has been observed growing into microporous (50 to 150 μm) carbon implants, but the phenomenon has not been seen with silicon carbide–coated specimens.[9]

Mechanical pushout data demonstrate that carbon confers higher interfacial shear strengths with bone than does smooth titanium (2.44 MPa versus 0.6 MPa at 20 weeks).[2] However, no bond seems to occur between carbon and bone. Rough carbon has greater pushout interfacial shear strength than does smooth carbon (e.g., 2.2 MPa for carbon fiber–reinforced carbon implants with 20 μm roughness versus 1.5 MPa for low-temperature isotropic carbon with 10 μm roughness). The pushout strength of carbon implants is much less than that of porous-coated titanium (1.9 MPa versus 22 MPa).[4] The rate of bone apposition formation is enhanced by coating with calcium phosphate ceramics.[9]

A potential problem with carbon materials is the release of particles due to abrasion. This phenomenon has been observed with carbon fiber–reinforced carbon implants.[1, 10] The problem can be minimized by final coatings with low-temperature isotropic carbon or silicon carbide.[9] However, the biologic response to carbon particles is minimal.[18]

References

1. Adams, D., Williams, D. F., and Hill, J.: Carbon fiber–reinforced carbon as a potential implant material. J. Biomed. Mater. Res. 12:35–42, 1978.
2. Adams, D. and Williams, D. F.: The response of bone to carbon-carbon composites. Biomaterials 5:59–64, 1984.
3. Akins, R. J. and Bokros, J. C.: The deposition of pure and alloyed isotropic carbons in steady-state fluidized beds. Carbon 12:439–452, 1974.
4. Anderson, R. C., Cook, S. D., Weinstein, A. M., and Haddad, R. J., Jr.: An evaluation of skeletal attachment to LTI pyrolytic carbon, porous titanium and carbon-coated porous titanium implants. Clin. Orthop. 182:242–257, 1984.
5. Bokros, J. C.: Carbon medical devices. Carbon 15:355–371, 1977.
6. Brown, S. A., Hastings, R. S., Mason, J. J., and Moet, A.: Characterization of short fiber reinforced thermoplastics for fracture fixation devices. Biomaterials (In press, 1990).
7. Christel, P., Meunier, A., Dorlot, J-M., et al.: Biomechanical compatibility and design of ceramic implants for orthopaedic surgery. Bioceramics: Material Characteristics Versus *In Vivo* Behavior. Edited by P. Ducheyne and J. E. Lemons. Ann. N. Y. Acad. Sci. 523:234–256, 1988.
8. Christel, P., Meunier, A., Heller, M., et al.: Mechanical properties and short-term *in vivo* evaluation of yttrium-oxide partially stabilized zirconia. J. Biomed. Mater. Res. 23:45–61, 1989.
9. Christel, P., Meunier, A., Leclercq, S., et al.: Development of carbon-carbon hip prosthesis. J. Biomed. Mater. Res. [Appl] 21A2:191–218, 1987.
10. Christel, P.: Carbon Reinforced Carbon. Biomechanics: Current Interdisciplinary Research. Edited by S. M. Perren and E. Schneider. Nijhoff, Dordrecht, 1985.
11. Dawson, D. and Linnett, I. W.: A Study of the Wear of Ultrahigh Molecular Weight Polyethylene against High Alumina Ceramic. Mechanical Properties of Biomaterials. Edited by G. W. Hastings and D. F. Williams. Chichester, Wiley, 1980.
12. de Groot, K.: Effect of Porosity and Physicochemical Properties on the Stability, Resorption, and Strength of Calcium Phosphate Ceramics. Bioceramics: Material Characteristics vs. *In Vivo* Behavior. Edited by P. Ducheyne and J. E. Lemons. New York, N. Y. Acad. Sci., 1988.
13. Denissen, G. T., de Groot, K., Makkes, P. Ch., et al.: Tissue response to dense apatite implants in rats. J. Biomed. Mater. Res. 14:713–721, 1980.
14. Dorlot, J-M., Christel, P., Sedel, L., et al.: Examination of Retrieved Hip Prostheses: Wear of Alumina/Alumina Components. Biological and Biomechanical Performance of Biomaterials. Edited by P. Christel, A. Meunier, and A. J. C. Lee. Amsterdam, Elsevier, 1986.
15. Garvie, R. C., Urbani, C., Kennedy, D. R., and McNeuer, J. C.: Biocompatibility of magnesia partially stabilized zirconia. J. Mater. Sci. 19:3224–3228, 1984.
16. Geesink, R. G., de Groot, K., and Klein, C. P. A.: Bonding of bone to apatite-coated implants. J. Bone Joint Surg. 70B:17–22, 1988.
17. Griss, P. and Heimke, G.: Biocompatibility of

High Density Alumina and Its Applications in Orthopaedic Surgery. Biocompatibility of Clinical Implant Materials, vol I. Edited by D. F. Williams. Boca Raton, CRC Press, 1981.
18. Helbing, G., Burri, C., Mohr, W., et al.: The Reaction of Tissue to Carbon Particles. Evaluation of Biomaterials. Edited by G. D. Winter, J. L. Leray, and K. de Groot. Chichester, Wiley, 1980.
19. Hinterberger, J., Ungethum, M., and Plitz, W.: Tribiological Properties of Aluminum Oxide Ceramics. Mechanical Properties of Biomaterials. Edited by G. W. Hastings and D. F. Williams. Chichester, Wiley, 1980.
20. Huttner, W. and Weiss, R.: High-performance Carbon Fiber Composites with Thermoplastic Matrices. Carbon, Fibers and Filaments. Edited by J. L. Figueiredo. Kluwer (In press).
21. Jarcho, M., Kay, J., Gunaer, K., et al.: Cellular and subcellular events at a bone ceramic hydroxylapatite interface. J. Bioengin. 1:79–92, 1977.
22. Jarcho, M.: Calcium phosphate ceramics as hard tissue prosthetics. Clin. Orthop. 157:259–278, 1981.
23. Kay, J.: A new concept for noncement fixation of orthopaedic devices. Techniq. Ortho. 2(1):1–6, 1987.
24. Kiefer, H., Claes, L., Burri, C., and Kuglmeier, K.: Biological Fixation of Various Titanium and Carbon Implants in Cancellous Bone: Biomechanical and Histomorphological Evaluation. Biological and Biomechanical Performance of Biomaterials. Edited by P. Christel, A. Meunier, and A. J. C. Lee. Amsterdam, Elsiever, 1986.
25. Klein, C. P. A., Driessen, A., and de Groot, K.: Biodegradation behavior of various CaP materials in bone tissue. J. Biomed. Mater. Res. 17:769–784, 1984.
26. Krainess, F. E. and Knapp, W. J.: Strength of a dense alumina ceramic after aging. J. Biomed. Mater. Res. 12:241–246, 1978.
27. Maier, H. R., Stark, N., and Krauth, A.: Reliability of Ceramic-metallic Hip Joints Based on Strength Analysis, Proof, and Structural Testing. Mechanical Properties of Biomaterials. Edited by G. W. Hastings and D. F. Williams. Chichester, Wiley, 1980.
28. McKee, D. W.: Carbon and graphite science. Ann. Rev. Mat. Sci. 3:195–232, 1973.
29. Ogiso, M., Kaneda, H., Arasaki, J., and Tabata, T.: Epithelial Attachment and Bone Tissue Formation on the Surface of Hydroxyapatite Ceramic Dental Implants. Biomaterials. Edited by G. D. Winter, D. F. Gibbons, and H. Plenk, Jr. Chichester, Wiley, pp. 59–64, 1982.
30. Plenk, H., Jr.: Biocompatibility of Ceramics in Joint Prostheses. Biocompatibility of Orthopaedic Implants, Vol I. Edited by D. F. Williams. Boca Raton, CRC Press, 1982.
31. Plitz, W. and Griss, P.: Clinical, Histomorphological and Material Related Observations on Removed Alumina-ceramic Hip Joint Components. Implant Retrieval: Material and Biological Analysis. Edited by Weinstein, A., Gibbons, D., Brown, S., and Ruff, W. Nat. Bureau of Stds. Washington, D.C., SP 601, 1981.
32. Plitz, W. and Hoss, H. U.: Wear of Alumina-ceramic Hip Joints: Some Clinical and Tribiological Aspects. Biomaterials, 1980. Edited by G. Winter, D. Gibbons, and H. Plenk, Jr. Chichester, Wiley, 1982.
33. Ritter, J. E., Greenspan, D. C., Palmer, R. A., and Hench, L. L.: Use of fracture mechanics theory in lifetime predictions for alumina and bioglass-coated alumina. J. Biomed. Mater. Res. 13:251–263, 1979.
34. Semlitsch, M., Lehmann, M., Weber, H., et al.: New prospects for a prolonged functional lifespan of artificial hip joints by using the materials combination of polyethylene/aluminum oxide ceramic/metal. J. Biomed. Mater. Res. 11:537–552, 1977.
35. Shim, H. S. and Schoen, F. J.: The wear resistance of pure and silicone-alloyed isotropic carbon. Biomat. Med. Dev. Art. Org. 2:103, 1974.
36. Shim, H. S.: The behavior of isotropic pyrolytic carbons under cyclic loading. Biomat. Med. Dev. Art. Org. 2:55–65, 1974.

CHAPTER 5

Allografts

NELSON SCARBOROUGH
ROBERT A. VANDER GRIEND

An important part of the history of orthopaedics has been the search for the ideal replacement for bones and joints. Bone transplantation has been one way to achieve these goals. Three types of bone transplants have been used: autografts from the patient's own body, allografts (homografts) from individuals other than the patient, and xenografts (heterografts) from other species.

Systematic use of bone transplants began in the mid-1800s, although a few earlier anecdotal reports were made.[6, 20] In 1878, the first successful allograft bone transplantation was reported.[6] In 1907, Axhausen presented the first extensive basic research in bone graft biology and introduced the term "creeping substitution" to describe the behavior of cancellous bone grafts.[6] Albee[1] subsequently reported his clinical results in more than 3000 patients who underwent bone transplantations. Lexer[25] reported a 50-percent success rate following 44 whole-joint and hemijoint allograft transplants. The failure rate with allografts remained high owing to problems with rejection, infection, fixation, and fracture of the grafts. These problems limited the usefulness of this method of bone transplantation until the 1950s.

In the 1950s and 1960s, Herndon and Chase,[20] Heiple and associates,[19] and Burwell and associates[8] reported a decreased immunologic reaction to allografts that had been prepared by deep freezing. Subsequent work by Ottolenghi,[31] Volkov,[39] Parrish,[32] Mankin and associates,[27] and others showed that allografts could be utilized successfully, although many of the previous problems remained. These grafts were generally chosen to reconstruct large skeletal defects resulting from limb salvage resections.

As joint replacement technology advanced, it became clear that some attempt to restore skeletal anatomy was needed when bone loss was severe. In cases of primary hip replacement, the femoral head was available; however, in complex reconstructions or prosthetic failure with loss of bone stock, additional sources of bone were needed.

Advances in immunology made transplantation of other tissues possible. This procedure led to the development of procurement networks and tissue banks, including bone banks. As a result of improvement in bone-bank technology, greater availability of graft material, and better understanding of allograft repair biology, the use of allografts has increased and the reported results have improved.

BIOLOGY OF ALLOGRAFT TRANSPLANTATION

An understanding of the biology of allograft incorporation depends on some knowledge of the repair process of autogenous bone grafts. The repair of autogenous

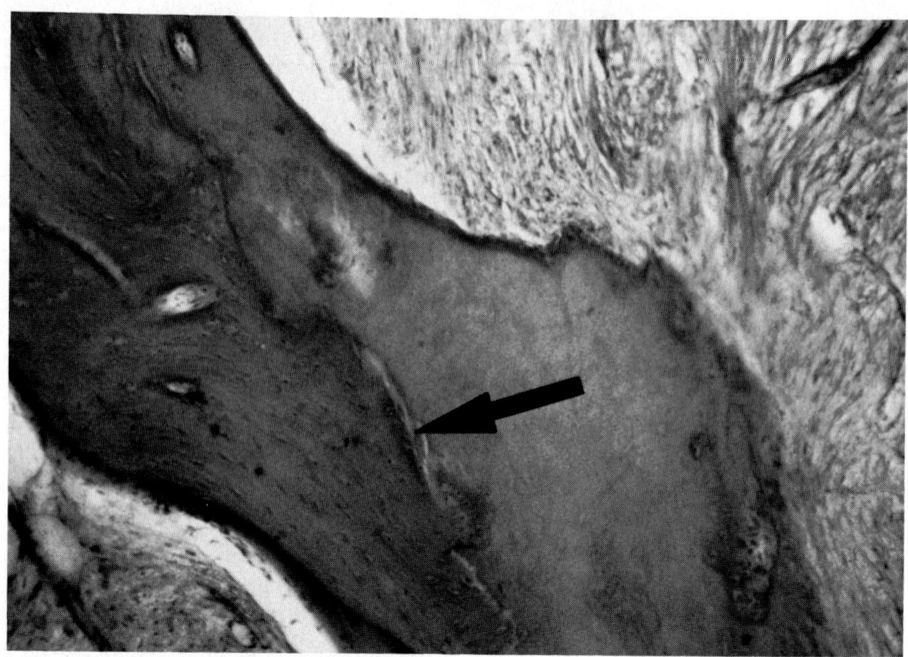

FIGURE 5–1. Cancellous allograft. Viable host bone is laid down on the surface (arrow) of the allograft trabeculae.

cancellous and cortical bone is similar in the first 2 weeks.[6, 10, 19] An initial inflammatory response occurs, followed by ingrowth of vascular tissue. Some of the transplanted cells on the graft surface may survive by diffusion. Cancellous bone then differs from cortical bone in the rate, mechanism, and completeness of repair. In cancellous bone grafts, revascularization is rapid and osteogenic cells form new bone on the necrotic trabeculae of the graft. These processes result in increased strength and density of the graft, which are visible radiographically. Remodeling then occurs, and eventually the graft is replaced by viable bone. This process, called "creeping substitution," represents an initial period of bone apposition followed by resorption and remodeling.

Autogenous cortical bone revascularizes slowly, beginning at the periphery of the graft.[6, 10, 19] Initially, resorption of bone occurs in the haversian system, increasing the porosity of the graft and decreasing its strength. New haversian systems are formed, with gradual return to normal density and strength of the graft. Because this repair process is incomplete, cortical grafts, unlike cancellous grafts, remain as a mixture of viable repaired bone and necrotic bone from the original graft. The repair of autogenous grafts is also influenced by a number of systemic and local factors (e.g., age, underlying illness, immunosuppression, vascularity, stability, infection).

Similarities exist between the repair of autogenous and allograft bone. Initially, an inflammatory response occurs, characterized by infiltration with lymphocytes.[6, 19] However, revascularization is limited and new blood vessels penetrate only a few millimeters into the allograft. These findings may be partly due to an immunologic response that impedes revascularization. A cancellous allograft heals as new bone from the host crosses the allograft-host junction and is laid down on the surface of the necrotic graft (Fig. 5–1). This increased bone density is visible radiographically as a thin, radiodense band on the allograft side of the junction. The process of incorporation and remodeling is generally slower and less complete than that in autogenous cancellous bone. Small pieces of cancellous allograft may also be more completely repaired than larger grafts. In allograft cortical bone, the extent of revascularization is limited. Blood vessels penetrate 2 to 3 mm into the bone, and a thin layer of periosteal new bone generally forms around the peripheral surface of the graft. Most of the interior of the graft remains avascular and unrepaired (Fig. 5–2). The allograft-host junction heals with a variable amount of periosteal and endosteal bone arising from the host side of the junction. Also, some limited, unilateral contact healing may occur, depending on the stability of the fixation. Because a large portion of the cortical allograft remains unrepaired, it cannot remodel in response to mechanical stresses; therefore, late fatigue failures may occur. The slow and incomplete revascularization may have some beneficial effect in decreasing the availability of antigens and slowing their release. In grafts that have demonstrated evidence of rapid revascularization, the immunologic reaction is often more profound and graft resorption may occur in many of these cases.

Allografts, particularly large, structural grafts, also appear to have a high rate of infection.[13, 26, 27] Lord and colleagues[26] reported a 12-percent infection rate, which was the principal complication in a large series of allografts in patients with neoplasms. These investigators suggested that immunologic factors, including some degree of rejection, may affect local host defenses and make allografts more prone to infections.

IMMUNOLOGY OF ALLOGRAFT TRANSPLANT

Although the underlying mechanisms of allograft and autograft repair are similar, a number of differences are imposed primarily by the immunologic response of the host to the allograft.[6, 8, 12, 13] Tissues of the musculoskeletal system (bone, cartilage, tendon, and ligament) have an immunologically privileged status compared with other organs. In allografts, the tissue antigens, recognized by the recipient as foreign, reside primarily on the surface of the cells in the bone and marrow.[6, 12] The bone matrix is less antigenic because the structure of collagen, glycoproteins, and other matrix components is similar among members of the same species. Xenografts have been unsuccessful because of differences between species in bone matrix composition resulting in significant antigen-antibody reaction.

Fresh allografts may elicit more antigen-antibody reaction, presumably because plasma and viable bone, marrow, and blood cells are present within the graft, each with tissue antigens.[6, 13, 15, 19, 24] Numerous methods have been investigated in attempt to block or minimize the immunologic re-

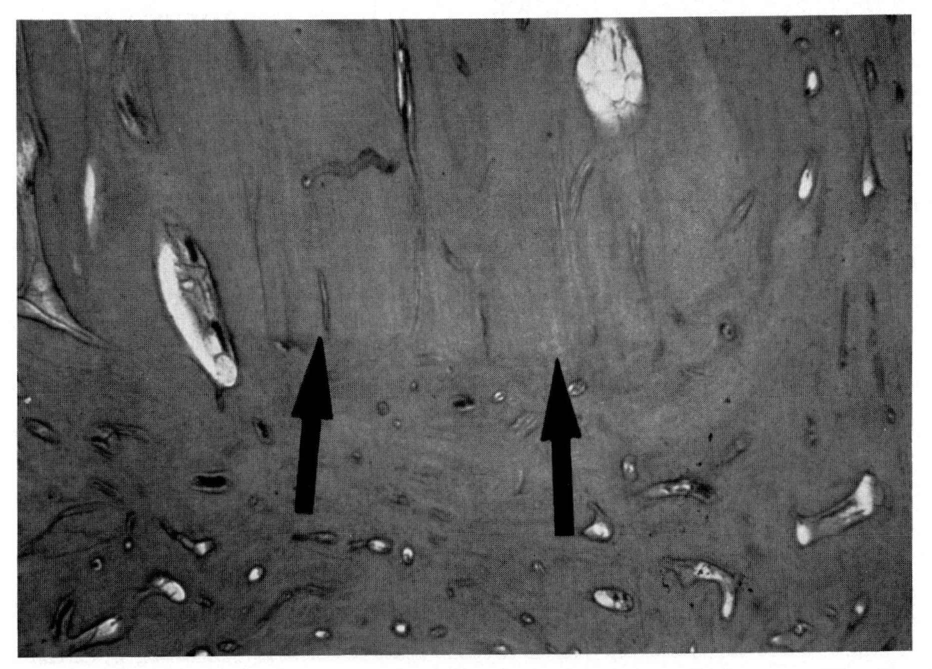

FIGURE 5–2. Cortical allograft. The host bone "heals" to the end (arrows) and adjacent peripheral surfaces of the allograft, whereas the remainder of the allograft is largely unrepaired.

sponse. These included various ways to treat the allograft and reduce its antigenicity and alter the host response to the allograft. Grafts have been boiled, decalcified, deproteinized, and treated with different topical agents. These techniques have had mixed effects on the immunology of allografts.[6] They may also adversely affect the repair process as well as the biomechanical properties of the allograft. Irradiation has been employed both as a sterilizing process and as a possible method for destroying antigens in the allograft. Sterilization generally requires approximately 2 to 3 megaRads.[6] This amount of radiation does not seem to appreciably affect the biomechanical properties of the graft, but the effects on the antigenicity and repair process are unclear, as are the long-term radiation effects.[4, 33, 38] The interest in irradiation and other sterilization techniques continues because of the risk of disease transmission by allograft transplantation.

Freezing and freeze-drying have been shown to decrease the antigen response to allografts. Experimental and clinical studies have demonstrated that reactions of the cellular-foreign body type can still occur when frozen allografts are used, but the response is less intense than with fresh allografts.[6, 15, 19, 24, 27] Freezing or freeze-drying also preserves bone and allows long-term storage. However, the biomechanical properties of allograft are affected by the method of preservation. Deep freezing appears to produce minimal effects, whereas freeze-drying diminishes the torsional and bending strength but does not significantly diminish the compressive and tensile strength.[6, 23, 33, 34, 38] Irradiation combined with freeze-drying reduces strength significantly in compression and torsion (Table 5–1).[38]

Other attempts to reduce graft rejection have included altering the host response and preventing the normal immunologic reaction, either by tissue-typing to carefully match the donor and host or by treating the host with immunosuppressive drugs. In studies that have evaluated tissue-typing, the degree of histocompatibility needed between donor and recipient for optimum incorporation of the graft has been unclear, although gross mismatching has resulted in a higher percentage of graft failures.[3, 15, 29] As a result, a difference of opinion continues regarding the practical application of human leukocyte antigen (HLA)–matching in bone transplantation.

The temporary administration of immunosuppressive drugs has been considered in an attempt to prevent or minimize an immunologic response until the allograft can be repaired with viable host bone and, as a result, the antigens in the allograft eliminated. Experimental studies indicate that immunosuppression affects the repair process and results in allograft incorporation similar to that of an autograft.[6, 7, 15] However, the toxicity and potential long-term side effects of these drugs are significant, and their effectiveness in clinical practice has not yet been demonstrated.

TISSUE BANKS

The use of allograft tissues, such as bone, cartilage, and ligaments, has undergone dramatic expansion since the 1970s. In response to the demand for musculoskeletal tissue, nearly 600 tissue banks have been established in the United States. They provide graft materials that are obtained surgically under aseptic conditions, often as part of multiple organ donation,

Table 5–1. EFFECT OF FREEZE-DRYING AND GAMMA IRRADIATION ON BIOMECHANICAL PROPERTIES OF BONE*

	Compression	Torsion	Bending
Freeze-Drying	120 percent[33] or no change[4]	39 percent[33]	55–90 percent[38]
Irradiated			
1 megaRad	No change[23]	90 percent[23]	No change[23]
3–4 megaRad	No change[4, 23]	90 percent[23]	90 percent,[23] 50–75 percent[38]
6 megaRad	80 percent[23]	65 percent[23]	70 percent[23]
Freeze-Dried and Irradiated	Significantly diminished[4] or no change[23]	70 percent[23]	80 percent,[23] 10–30 percent[38]

*Values reflect changes from control specimens according to each study protocol.

or under clean conditions (nonsterile procurement) and then sterilized. With the advent of the American Association of Tissue Banks in 1975 and the publication of donor screening criteria in 1980, the tissue banking industry has become increasingly sophisticated.[11, 36] In most states, the enactment of routine donor inquiry legislation has provided a mechanism for better donor availability. The availability of allograft material is limited by the number of suitable donors who, along with their families, are willing to grant consent for removal of these tissues. Although the efforts of tissue banking organizations have increased the number of donors, the demand for some types of tissues is still greater than the supply. This is particularly true with osteoarticular allografts. Large inventories must be maintained because precise size matching of the surface is needed to provide congruous articulation.

More important than the quantity of the allograft supplied is its quality and safety. Guidelines set by such organizations as the American Association of Tissue Banks have provided useful criteria for the assessment of donor acceptability and graft handling techniques.[11, 36] However, tissue banking remains a nonregulated field and it is incumbent on the users of these materials to be aware of the practices of their suppliers.

Tissue banks range in complexity from small freezers, where femoral heads are stored, to very comprehensive systems. These large banks may provide many types of tissue preparations from freeze-dried cancellous bone chips to entire bones with cryopreserved articular cartilage and intact ligamentous and capsular supporting structures.[11, 13, 36]

Successful bone banking requires meticulous quality control and standardized, reproducible methods of tissue processing. The effects of processing techniques and storage methods on the risk of infectious disease transmission as well as the immunologic, biologic, and biomechanical properties of bone are not clearly known. Grafts that are retrieved in a nonsterile setting require secondary sterilization. The two most common methods are irradiation and gas autoclaving with ethylene oxide. However, both methods may have some effect on the biologic properties of the graft. Further work is needed to find the optimum method of sterilization. Allograft musculoskeletal tissues are generally stored by either deep freezing or lyophilization (freeze-drying). The principal advantage of freeze-drying is the convenience of shelf storage, although this does affect the biomechanical properties of the graft. It is essential that users of allografts be aware of these differences in procurement, processing, and storage techniques and not assume that all allografts are uniformly the same.

RISK OF INFECTIOUS DISEASE BY TRANSPLANTATION

Concern over transmission of infectious disease by allograft transplantation is a particularly important issue—one that both physicians and patients must understand. A patient's decision to have an allograft procedure may be influenced by this very legitimate concern. Hepatitis of various types, human immunodeficiency virus (HIV), Creutzfeldt-Jakob disease, syphilis, and other diseases are known to be transmitted by many types of allograft transplants, including blood, tissue, and vital organs. Although the risk of disease transmission with allograft bone appears to be very low, routine follow-up testing of recipients has not been done. The escalating problem of HIV infections as well as the ongoing threat of hepatitis requires that all reasonable procedures be followed to eliminate infected donors from the donor pool.[5, 11]

JOINT RECONSTRUCTION

Bone stock is the crucial element in the reconstruction of failed, nonseptic, total joints.[17] Large bone defects have been filled with cements, implants, bone grafts, and combinations of all three materials. Because massive cement and implant constructs are often unsatisfactory in the presence of large skeletal defects, bone grafts have been employed in an attempt to restore skeletal anatomy. One of the goals of these difficult joint reconstructions is to have more bone stock at the end of the surgical procedure than was present at the beginning.

Two types of allografts are utilized in joint reconstruction: nonstructural and structural. Nonstructural grafts are selected to fill in small or cavitary defects. These grafts usually consist of corticocancellous chips or small wafers of cancellous bone. Graft material may be obtained from a bone bank or prepared by the surgeon from allograft femoral heads or other cancellous bone sources. These grafts are often placed without any specific internal fixation other than that normally supplied to support the implant. Freeze-dried grafts have less mechanical strength in torsion and should generally be used as nonstructural, defect-filling grafts rather than structural grafts.

Structural grafts are employed to reconstruct segmental defects. They are usually anchored with some type of internal fixation and may provide direct support for the implant.[2, 14, 16, 18, 21, 28, 30] In the acetabulum, deficiencies in the superior, anterior, or posterior rim may be reconstructed by contouring an allograft from the proximal femur, proximal tibia, or pelvis to fit in the defect; the graft is fixed securely, and an acetabular component is placed.[30, 37] Many types of acetabular components have been utilized. Jasty and Harris[21, 22] initially reported good results with cemented cups, but longer follow-up revealed a 32-percent failure rate. Failures were attributed partly to ongoing revascularization of the graft with some resorption and loss of fixation. Good short-term results have been reported with bipolar components, although migration has been noted when the graft provides the primary support.[40] Samuelson and colleagues[35] and Emerson[9] have reported initial good results with uncemented, ingrowth prostheses fixed with screws, but additional follow-up is needed. Structural allografts have also been combined with prosthetic implants to reconstruct the proximal femur, proximal humerus, and both sides of the knee and elbow.[14] Many different techniques are used with these composite allograft-prosthesis reconstructions. In one method, the allograft is fixed to the host bone with a plate, and the appropriate prosthesis is then placed on the opposite end of the allograft. In another method, a long-stem or custom implant replaces the joint surface and at the same time provides fixation across the allograft-host junction. Fixation has been obtained by press-fitting the components or cementing the components in allograft, host bone, or both. Healing of the allograft-host junction provides additional support to the prosthesis. The allograft surface provides points of attachment for muscles, periarticular soft tissues, and tendon-bone attachments (e.g., greater trochanter, tibial tubercle, humeral tuberosities, olecranon). Although the initial results of these reconstructions appear to be good, long-term follow-up is still needed.[14, 27]

Allografts have also been selected to reconstruct bone and the adjacent joint after resection for neoplasms. Both osteoarticular and composite allograft-prosthetic implant reconstructions have been used.[13, 14, 27] Osteoarticular allografts are fixed to the host bone with either a plate or an intramedullary fixation, and the periarticular soft tissues are reattached to the allograft. Good long-term function has been reported with these grafts. However, some degree of joint laxity almost always remains and the complication rate is not insignificant.[26, 27, 32] Bone stock is also restored, and the articular surface can be replaced later with a prosthesis if degenerative changes develop. Composite replacements are done in a manner similar to that for total joint revisions.

The ideal method of reconstruction with composites of an allograft and a prosthesis has not been determined. Clearly, the ultimate durability of the reconstruction requires some degree of healing and incorporation of the graft. Grafts require a vascular bed, ideally with a large contact area, from which union of the graft-host junction, revascularization, and incorporation, even though incomplete, can proceed. The presence of avascular tissue or cement or the unstable fixation of the allograft can impede healing and revascularization. Some amount of loading is needed because both stress-shielded and overstressed grafts tend to resorb. Resorption of the grafts, whether from mechanical, immunologic, or other causes, often results in failure. The prosthetic implant, particularly in the acetabulum, should receive some support from the host bone. Implants supported entirely by the allograft seem to have a higher failure rate.[21, 40] Protection of this construct is also needed during the period of healing and incorporation.

It may be difficult to determine when an allograft is healed or how much of it has been repaired. On plain radiographs, healing is suggested by bridging of trabeculae across the junction between the host and allograft bone and increased density in the cancellous portion of the allograft. A bone scan may show increased activity around the periphery of a structural graft as periosteal new bone is laid down on the graft surface. However, current imaging techniques, including bone scans, do not provide a totally accurate assessment of allograft repair.

Allografts continue to be options for reconstruction of bone and joints. Bone is replaced with bone with a potential for healing and incorporation of the allograft. Soft tissues can be reattached and will heal to the allograft. Osteoarticular allografts currently provide the only way to replace articular surfaces with articular cartilage. Both basic and clinical research have provided much information on the biology, immunology, biomechanics, and clinical applications of allograft bone transplants. However, additional work is needed to ensure that allografts can continue to be used safely and to address the many problems that remain.

References

1. Albee, F. H.: Fundamentals in bone transplantation. Experiences in three thousand bone graft operations. J.A.M.A. 81:1429–1432, 1923.
2. Borja, F. J. and Mnaymneh, W.: Bone allografts in salvage of difficult hip arthroplasties. Clin. Orthop. 197:123–130, 1985.
3. Bos, G. D., Goldberg, V. M., Powell, A. E., et al.: The effect of histocompatibility matching on canine frozen bone allografts. J. Bone Joint Surg. 65A:89–96, 1983.
4. Bright, R. and Burstein, A.: Material properties of preserved cortical bone. Trans. Orthop. Res. Soc. 3:210, 1968.
5. Buck, B. E., Malinin, T. I., and Brown, M. D.: Bone transplantation and human immunodeficiency virus. Clin. Orthop. 240:129–136, 1989.
6. Burchardt, H.: The biology of bone graft repair. Clin. Orthop. 174:28–42, 1983.
7. Burchardt, H., Glowczewski, F. P., and Enneking, W. F.: Short-term immunosuppression with fresh segmental fibular allografts in dogs. J. Bone Joint Surg. 63A:411–415, 1981.
8. Burwell, R. G., Gowland, G., and Dexter, F.: Studies in the transplantation of bone. VI. Further observations concerning the antigenicity of homologous cortical and cancellous bone. J. Bone Joint Surg. 45B:597–608, 1963.
9. Emerson, R. H., Jr.: Noncemented acetabular revision using allograft bone. Clin. Orthop. 249:30–43, 1989.
10. Enneking, W. F., Burchardt, H., Puhl, J. J., and Piotrowski, G.: Physical and biological aspects of repair in dog cortical-bone transplants. J. Bone Joint Surg. 57A:237–252, 1975.
11. Friedlaender, G. E.: Current concepts review. Bone banking. J. Bone Joint Surg. 64A:307–311, 1982.
12. Friedlaender, G. E.: Immune responses to osteochondral allografts. Clin. Orthop. 174:58–67, 1983.
13. Friedlaender, G. E., Mankin, H. J., and Sell, K. W. (eds.): Osteochondral Allografts: Biology, Banking and Clinical Applications. Boston, Little Brown & Co., 1983.
14. Gitelis, S., Heligman, D., Quill, G., and Piasecki, P.: Tumor reconstruction and salvage of failed total hip arthroplasty. Clin. Orthop. 231:62–70, 1988.
15. Goldberg, V. M., Bos, G. D., Heiple, K. G., et al.: Improved acceptance of frozen bone allografts in genetically mismatched dogs by immunosuppresion. J. Bone Joint Surg. 66A:937–950, 1984.
16. Gross, A. E.: The use of allograft bone in revision of total hip arthroplasty. Clin. Orthop. 197:115–122, 1985.
17. Harris, W. H.: Allografting in total hip replacement in adults with severe acetabular deficiency including a surgical technique for bolting the graft to the ilium. Clin. Orthop. 162:150–164, 1982.
18. Head, W. C.: Proximal femoral allografts in revision total hip arthroplasty. Clin. Orthop. 225:22–36, 1987.
19. Heiple, K. G., Chase, S. W., and Herndon, C. H.: A comparative study of the healing process following different types of bone transplantation. J. Bone Joint Surg. 45A:1593–1616, 1963.
20. Herndon, C. H. and Chase, S. W.: The fate of massive autogenous and homogenous bone grafts including articular surfaces. Surg. Gynecol. Obstet. 98:273–290, 1954.
21. Jasty, M. and Harris, W. H.: Salvage total hip reconstruction in patients with major acetabular bone deficiency using structural femoral head allografts. J. Bone Joint Surg. 72B:63–67, 1990.
22. Jasty, M. J. and Harris, W. H.: Total hip reconstruction using frozen femoral head allografts in patients with acetabular bone loss. Orthop. Clin. North Am. 18:291–299, 1987.
23. Komander, A.: Influence of preservation on some mechanical properties of human haversian bone. Mater. Med. Pol. 8:13–17, 1976.
24. Langer, F., Czitrom, A., Pritzker, K. P., and Gross, A. E.: The immunogenicity of fresh frozen allogeneic bone. J. Bone Joint Surg. 57A:216–220, 1975.
25. Lexer, E.: Joint transplantation and arthroplasty. Surg. Gynecol. Obstet. 40:782–809, 1925.
26. Lord, C. F., Gebhardt, M. C., Tomford, W. W., and Mankin, H. J.: Infection in bone allografts. J. Bone Joint Surg. 70A:369–376, 1988.
27. Mankin, H. J., Doppelt, S., and Tomford, W.: Clinical experience with allograft implantation.

The first ten years. Clin. Orthop. 174:69–86, 1983.
28. McGann, W., Mankin, H. J., and Harris, W. H.: Massive allografting for severe failed total hip replacement. J. Bone Joint Surg. 68A:4–12, 1986.
29. Muscolo, D. L., Caletti, E., Schajowicz, F., et al.: Tissue-typing in human massive allografts of frozen bone. J. Bone Joint Surg. 69A:583–595, 1987.
30. Oakeshott, R. D.: Revision total hip arthroplasty with osseous allograft reconstruction: A clinical and roentgenographic analysis. Clin. Orthop. 225:38–61, 1987.
31. Ottolenghi, C. E.: Massive osteoarticular bone grafts. Technic and results of 62 Cases. Clin. Orthop. 87:156–164, 1972.
32. Parrish, F. F.: Allograft replacement of part of the end of a long bone following excision of a tumor: Report of twenty-one cases. J. Bone Joint Surg. 55A:1–22, 1973.
33. Pelker, R. R., Friedlaender, G. E., and Markham, T. C.: Biomechanical properties of bone allografts. Clin. Orthop. 174:54–57, 1983.
34. Pelker, R. R., Friedlaender, G. E., and Marlham, T. C.: Effects of freezing and freeze-drying on the biomechanical properties of rat bone. J. Orthop. Res. 1:405–411, 1984.
35. Samuelson, K. M., Freeman, M. A. R., Levack, B., et al.: Homograft bone in revision acetabular arthroplasty. J. Bone Joint Surg. 70B:367–372, 1988.
36. Tomford, W. W., Doppelt, S. H., Mankin, H. J., and Friedlaender, G. E.: 1983 Bone banking procedures. Clin. Orthop. 174:15–21, 1983.
37. Trancik, T. M., Stulberg, B. N., Wilde, A. H., and Feiglin, D. H.: Allograft reconstruction of the acetabulum during revision total hip arthroplasty: clinical, radiographic, and scintigraphic assessment of the results. J. Bone Joint Surg. 68A:527–533, 1986.
38. Triantafyllou, N., Sotiorpoulos, E., and Triantafyllou, J.: The mechanical properties of lyophilized and irradiated bone grafts. Acta Orthop. Belg. 41:35–44, 1975.
39. Volkov, M.: Allotransplantation of joints. J. Bone Joint Surg. 52B:49–53, 1970.
40. Wilson, M. G., Nikpoor, N., Aliabadi, P., et al.: The fate of acetabular allografts after bipolar revision arthroplasty of the hip. A radiographic review. J. Bone Joint Surg. 71A:1469–1479, 1989.

CHAPTER 6

Biocompatibility

STANLEY A. BROWN
KATHARINE MERRITT

In the controlled environment of *in vitro* and *in vivo* laboratory research, the biologic responses to various metallic and polymeric materials can often be characterized and differences due to specimen shape and size can be identified. It is more difficult to pinpoint specific causes of cellular reactions and prosthetic failure in the clinical setting, as debris collects over time because of joint articulation and particles of bone and polymethyl methacrylate (PMMA) or because beads from porous coatings are released into tissue at the bone-prosthesis interface.

A standard biocompatibility study involves implantation of cylinders of test material in rabbits or dogs, either in the paravertebral muscle or as transcortical plugs in the femur.[3] The typical response to a "biocompatible" material includes an acute nonspecific inflammatory action, subsiding in a matter of days to weeks, and a benign fibrous tissue encapsulation.[28] This type of reaction has been observed with all the "surgical" alloys and polymers in current use.[14] If the implant has a rough or irregular shape with sharp edges, the inflammatory reaction is aggravated and the capsule is thicker.[55] If the same materials are implanted in a particulate form, however, a significant inflammatory granulomatous response is produced.[14] Smaller particles are phagocytized and larger pieces are surrounded by fibrous tissue and inflammatory cells.

The handling of metallic debris is initially the same as that for polymeric debris. The phagocytized debris is seen in macrophages or giant cells. The difference between the long-term response to the two materials relates to the ability of cells to destroy the debris. Debris remains in the cell until it can be processed and eliminated, that is, the particle is taken into the phagosome, processed, fused again with the cell membrane, and eliminated. If the phagosome cannot process the particle, a toxic reaction may occur in the cell, followed by cell damage, cell death, and further tissue toxicity. Polymeric debris usually produces this response, as phagocytes lack enzymes to degrade the polymer; it was most likely the observed cause of severe reactions in early Teflon total hip replacements.[8] In contrast, metallic debris is usually degraded by acidic enzyme conditions in the phagosome that hasten corrosion. Metals may also bind with available proteins and may be eliminated in this form by the cell or surrounding tissue compartments, reducing toxicity.

The reaction to most polymeric materials is assumed to be related to the size of the particles (i.e., whether they are small enough to be phagocytized) and is generally unrelated to chemical properties of the material. Large pieces are encapsulated; particles greater than 5 μm are phagocytized in giant cells; and those smaller than 5 μm are phagocytized in macrophages. However, PMMA monomer is known to evoke a sensitivity response,[18] and late laboratory data indicate that silicone oil elicits an IgE and type IV cell-mediated allergic response.[27] Sensitivity to metallic debris is discussed subsequently.

The following discussion focuses first on biologic responses to polymers and polymeric debris and second on responses to metals and metallic corrosion products.

BIOLOGIC RESPONSES TO POLYMERS

Animal Studies

A number of animal studies have been designed to model the clinical problem of prosthetic loosening due to bone resorption. Injection of PMMA particles into the medullary canal of rabbits produces a significant increase in phagocytic macrophages and giant cells. In a spinal fixation study in rats, macrophages and giant cells were seen at the cement interface with fibroblasts next to the bone.[10] These findings implicate the histiocytic secretion of collagenase as indicative of bone resorption in response to PMMA.

The heat of polymerization at the time of implantation of PMMA and the monomer that is released into surrounding tissue have been implicated as causes of local toxicity; they caused no significant local toxicity in studies of bone tissue following implantation of PMMA in the dough stage in the medullary canal of rabbits.[23]

The cellular response to ultrahigh molecular weight polyethylene particles has also been implicated as a direct cause of bone resorption at the bone-cement interface.[25] Whereas a shell of bone was observed around PMMA plugs inserted through the knee joint in the femoral canal of rats, injection of the joint with polyethylene powder resulted in active bone resorption around the plug. Cell culture studies indicate that the adherence of macrophages on polyethylene and PMMA surfaces can lead to PGE_2 release and bone resorption in a rat calvaria assay.[45] Resorption seems to increase with greater surface roughness of the materials. Injection of silicone elastomer in particulate form has also been shown to produce a foreign body reactive synovitis in rabbits.[63] The reaction to materials in particulate form is generally assumed to be associated with particle size, that is, it is not a specific immune response.

Clinical Studies

Clinical studies of the biocompatibility of total joint replacements fabricated from metal and polyethylene have focused primarily on the bone-cement interface and possible mediators of loosening. The early tissue response to cement is localized necrosis, perhaps due to the heat of polymerization; this process is followed by healing and new bone formation.[60] However, early necrosis could also be attributed to the heat and trauma of reaming, rasping, and broaching. The formation of a synovial-like membrane with cells capable of producing prostaglandin E_2 and causing bone resorption has been observed in the absence of inflammatory cells.[22] The tissue reaction to particles produced by wear has also been implicated in bone resorption at the interface. Possibly small amounts of debris are cleared by the lymphatic system, whereas large amounts produce granulation and tissue necrosis leading to loosening.[61]

Several methods are available to differentiate between particulate materials in tissue sections. Because PMMA is dissolved in many tissue fixation processes, its presence is identified by the empty spaces. Both polymethyl methacrylate and polyethylene are birefringent under crossed polarized light, and they must be heated to allow differentiation. When specimens are heated, PMMA loses its birefringence at 75°C, whereas polyethylene fades at 128°C. Also, PMMA does not regain birefringence upon cooling.[12] Particles of silicone elastomer are refractile but not birefringent.[2]

Mirra and coworkers[43] have proposed a cellular grading scheme based on their examination of tissue reactions at implant interfaces. The presence of significant numbers of polymorphonuclear leukocytes is considered an indicator of infection. Polyethylene particles produce a histiocytic response. Debris from PMMA is mostly phagocytized by giant cells. Although a correlation has been observed between the amount of PMMA debris and loosening,[43, 44] a direct cause-and-effect association has not been proven. Studies of the tissue interfaces of cemented tibial plateaus with screw fixation have demonstrated radiolucent lines and macrophages at the cement-bone interface but no lucency or cellular reaction at the screw-bone interface.[16] Conclusions were that a specific reaction to PMMA occurred and that macrophages could be osteoclastic precursors. However, this study did not differentiate between cellular reactions due to materials and reactions due to movement at the cement-bone interface, which could occur after loosening without motion at the screw-bone interface. It must also be kept in mind that wear and loosening are aggravated by increasing patient weight and activity.

Silicone elastomer joint prostheses require special consideration because of the surgical technique employed. The elastomer is placed directly in the medullary canal and thus is subjected to abrasion due to pistoning. Wear produces debris shards that can cause a local detritic synovitis.[2, 9, 26, 48, 63] Reactions are associated with macrophage and giant cell phagacytosis of small debris and with invasive synovitis and bone resorption.

Although most reports indicate a nonspecific inflammatory response to debris, Gordon and Bullough[24] have observed lymphocytes, plasma cells, and eosinophils in synovial tissues and bone marrow suggestive of an immunologically mediated response. Evidence of an immune response and hapten-like function of silicones has also been associated with soft tissue implants.[56] Lymphadenopathy from the accumulation of silicone debris in draining axillary[9] and inguinal nodes[26, 57] has also been reported. However, no evidence has been reported of a specific response to debris in lymph nodes. Although lymphadenopathy associated with polyethylene and PMMA debris has not been reported, there is nothing unique about the ability of silicone debris to be transported through the lymphatics.

BIOLOGIC RESPONSES TO METALS

Studies on the biocompatibility of metallic implants follow protocols similar to those previously described for polymeric materials. Fortunately, most of the metallic materials selected for joint replacement surgery are composed of metals that are also normal trace elements in humans. Many of the metals are components of enzymes or hormones vital for the functioning of the mammalian body. Problems arise when metallic corrosion or wear releases metal ions in abnormal locations or in quantities beyond what can be handled by the host. Under normal circumstances, trace metals are ingested in food or water, with a little acquired from inhaled air. Metallic ions that are released into the body from implants in deep tissues must be handled by different mechanisms until the metal ions are transferred to the site of normal utilization or elimination.

Protein-bound metals are thought to be transported rapidly from the site of binding and eventually eliminated with normal catabolism of the protein.[41] Cell-bound metals generally remain at the site or, if the cell is mobile (e.g., red blood cell), travel with it.[5, 41, 42] Membrane-bound metals may alter the function of the cells to which they are bound but probably have few additional effects. When metals enter cells, the concern is that they will bind to DNA or RNA, thus affecting the genetic code or translation of the genetic code and possibly altering the function of all future cell generations. Thus, studies on binding of metals to proteins, cells, and nucleic acids are important.

Metals are released from implants in one of three ways: dissolution, corrosion, or wear. Dissolution begins early, as the implant and body fluids equilibrate. It involves the release of metal atoms or ions. Corrosion of a metal component has three possible causes: fretting between the implant and another hard surface such as a metallic component or bone; crevice corrosion in constricted places; and electrolytic corrosion, although the last is unlikely in normal usage of orthopaedic implants. Wear often releases metallic debris as well as metal ions. The response to metallic debris is initially the same as that to the other debris. However, metals are usually eliminated without lasting cell damage because enzymes in the cell or cell environment catalyze continuing corrosion and dissolution.

In normal situations, the elements utilized in alloys are of minimal toxicity, but toxicity can occur in high doses or unusual circumstances. The metals of particular concern in joint replacement surgery are iron, nickel, cobalt, chromium, molybdenum, titanium, vanadium, and aluminum. The potential dangers are cellular toxicity, carcinogenicity, and hypersensitivity. For these reasons, careful *in vitro* and *in vivo* testing is important. *In vitro* studies are necessary for screening various metals and understanding how they interact but care must be taken in interpretation of results. These studies may indicate that a particular metal ion is toxic to a cell under certain culture conditions. However, the issue of level of toxicity of various metals cannot be addressed entirely by *in vitro* experiments; *in vivo* experiments are necessary to determine host toxicity when all the various organic carriers and cell types are present.[49, 50] Thus, a combination of various types of studies is needed.[40]

Cellular Toxicity

The capacity of a metal to damage and kill cells directly is generally due to its ability either to alter the cell membrane so that the protective and osmotic barrier is lost or to mask its receptor sites. This effect makes the interior of the cell vulnerable to compounds to which it would not normally be exposed, results in loss of some of the cellular contents, and deprives the cell of its ability to respond to outside influences. Thus, the cell no longer contributes to the overall functioning of the host. Eventually it dies, leaving debris for other cells and enzymes to clean up. The ultimate effect on the host also depends on whether the cell or tissue is labile, stable, or permanent.

Carcinogenicity

Potential carcinogenicity relates to the incorporation of metal into the nucleic acid of cells or the binding of metal onto sites of proteins or sugars in the nucleic acid to alter function. The resulting alteration of the genetic code can have sequelae ranging from simple toxicity and cell death to passage of the defect to succeeding generations of cells, altering control of cell multiplication and leading to benign or malignant tumors.

Hypersensitivity

When the immune system attempts to neutralize or destroy metal acting as an antigen, it may also inadvertently cause cell damage. There are four mechanisms or types of hypersensitivity reactions.[54] Metal-associated hypersensitivity is usually associated with types I and IV. For either mechanism to occur, the metal ion must bind to a protein or cell. In this way, the metal, a small molecular weight hapten, becomes a larger immunogenic antigen. The immune response begins with the processing of the organometallic complex by an antigen-processing cell. The antigen-processing cell presents the processed antigen to the T helper cell, which then sends the antigenic message either to the B cell (to initiate antibody formation, type I) or to the cytotoxic T cell (to initiate type IV cell-mediated immunity).

The hypersensitivity reaction from the humoral response occurs when the antibody produced is of the IgE class, which is responsible for type I hypersensitivity reactions. This skin-fixing, mast cell, and basophil-binding antibody produces the symptoms of atopic hypersensitivity so well known to patients with hay fever or penicillin allergy. The antigen-antibody reaction may cause local or systemic reactions. Local symptoms include wheal-and-flare reaction on skin contact and the runny nose and itchy eyes that accompany hay fever. Systemic reactions may include life-threatening anaphylaxis. Although type I reactions to metals are rare, the cell-mediated responses of mechanism IV are common. For example, dermatitis from contact with metal salts or corroding metals occurs in approximately 15 percent of the population. Most often it is seen in industrial workers and sensitive individuals wearing jewelry. The only treatment is elimination of contact with the metal ion. This is difficult with orthopaedic implants, of course, because contact with metal may be unavoidable. Fortunately, the incidence of metal sensitivity reactions to orthopaedic implants appears to be very low.[34, 35, 38]

RESPONSES TO INDIVIDUAL METALS

Iron

The human body has a high iron content. Iron is an essential component of hemoglobin, responsible for the transport of oxygen. Because iron stores are critical to life, additional iron is available as needed for the production of blood cells or myoglobin.[58] Iron is also martialed in host defense mechanisms against infection.[5, 59] Certain bacteria are harmed by increased levels of iron. Because other bacteria benefit from the presence of iron, the issue is very complex. The body has mechanisms in place for handling iron and excreting excess; therefore; the iron from corrosion of orthopaedic implants is unlikely to contribute much to the body's homeostasis, even in patients with iron overload diseases.

Nickel

A trace element required for the functioning of some enzymes, nickel is also a major cause of metal hypersensitivity. In fact, most patients who have metal sensitivity are actually reacting to nickel. Between 12 and 15 percent of the normal population has been estimated to be allergic to this metal,[34, 35] with hypersensitivity expressed as a contact dermatitis (type IV reaction). Nickel is rapidly transported from the blood and the organs, but it may not be rapidly transported from the dermis.[19, 20] When encountered as nickel subsulfide or nickel carbonyl, this metal is known to be carcinogenic. Fortunately, neither compound is likely to be formed as a consequence of corrosion of orthopaedic implants. Nickel chloride has been shown to be carcinogenic in rats under some unusual circumstances. Thus, the release of nickel from orthopaedic implants is of major concern.

Cobalt

Similar to nickel, cobalt is important for the activity of some enzymes. Interestingly, some diseases result from inadequate cobalt in the diet and some result from excess cobalt, due to either failure of elimination or excessive uptake. Hypersensitivity to cobalt appears to be similar to that of nickel.[36] Whether this similarity is due to immunologic cross-reactivity between the two metals or to simultaneous exposure to both metals remains unknown.[29, 30, 33] Cobalt is not generally considered carcinogenic, as cobalt ions are rapidly removed from the body. However, *in vitro* studies of metal salts and wear debris have indicated that cobalt produces more cellular toxicity than other elements. Because *in vivo* studies fail to confirm this finding, cobalt *in vivo* may be rapidly bound by proteins or other substances in the body that are not present in tissue culture media.

Chromium

Chromium is a trace element essential for glucose metabolism. Studies of chromium salts *in vitro* have shown little toxicity to Cr^{3+}. It is the chromium ion Cr^{6+} that is very biologically active. Because the Cr^{6+} ion binds to or enters cells, it is not eliminated from the body until the cell is.[39, 41, 42] Chromium hypersensitivity, while less prevalent than nickel and presumably cobalt hypersensitivity, occurs in 3 percent to 8 percent of the population. However, inhalation of industrial chromium salts is known to be carcinogenic, as are other types of industrial contact with chromium salts or corroding metal.[35] The metal ion released from orthopaedic implants could be biologically active in patients, depending on concentration, valence, and location of release.

Molybdenum

Toxicity studies of molybdenum are limited. This trace element is known to be essential for some enzyme functions and helps protect humans from a variety of diseases.[53] The amount of molybdenum in alloys utilized in prosthetic implants is very small and thus unlikely to cause problems.[15, 62] Nevertheless, studies are needed on the distribution, elimination, and toxicity of molybdenum.

Vanadium

Vanadium, another necessary trace element, is of some concern because elevated levels have been associated with cardiac toxicity. Because current orthopaedic implants contain 4 percent or less vanadium, the amount that could be released would not be expected to affect normal tissue levels significantly. Vanadium is rapidly transported and eliminated from the tissues and the body.[7, 31, 46]

Aluminum

Not only is aluminum a trace element in the body, it is also a common element in the environment. Although the amount of this element consumed in water each day would exceed that released from an implant, the location of the release may have a marked impact on homeostasis. Aluminum binds to bone and is associated with osteomalacia.[6] Aluminum deposits have also been found in the brains of healthy individuals; at one time, excess aluminum was thought to be associated with Alzheimer disease. Brain and bone accumulation of aluminum in patients who are undergoing chronic renal dialysis has been a major concern.[17, 47] Although it is unlikely that aluminum from implant corrosion would be sufficient to overburden the body, the possibility should be considered and the level of aluminum in the implant alloys kept low.

Titanium

The only metal in implant alloys not considered to be a trace element is titanium. However, the background level of titanium in tissue may be higher than previously thought. Titanium is a component of many household substances, including the white pigment in toothpaste, various ointments, and paint. However, the ability of titanium to bind to the cell and to protein is low because this metal does not generally exist as an ion at physiologic pH but rather as an oxide or hydroxide. For this reason, the physiologic response to titanium is quite different from that to the other metals discussed. The black precipitate that generally represents the wear debris or corrosion products of titanium in the tissue evokes no biologic reaction.

Unfortunately, little is known about the physiologic reaction to titanium in tissue. Although evidence to date indicates that the debris remains in the tissue without producing a cellular reaction, how long it will continue to stay there without causing toxic effects remains in question.[1, 7, 50] The metallic debris may eventually be treated as a foreign particle, much as polyethylene wear debris is, resulting in a tissue reaction involving a large monocyte, macrophage, and giant cell. Perhaps this factor contributes to the osteolysis seen in association with implantation of some titanium prostheses.

CONCLUSION

Most patients who have undergone total joint replacements have no troublesome biologic reactions to the devices or materials implanted. However, problems have been encountered. For example, osteolysis around total joint replacements has been associated with the presence of wear debris, generally from ultrahigh molecular weight polyethylene or particles from PMMA. Toxicity from metal corrosion appears to be no problem. The metal components of orthopaedic implants in use today have very low corrosion rates and are composed of normal trace elements; thus, the body handles the material well. Although transient local toxicity may occur, it apparently does not manifest itself in signs or symptoms.

The issue of carcinogenicity is of major concern, even though the evidence that prosthetic implants stimulate the growth of neoplasms is minimal. Considering the number of patients who have received total joint replacements, the number of local tumors is very small.[32] Often, devices are implanted in patients who have had previous partial or total tumor resections. Consequently, data from these patients must be considered as a separate base. The issue of tumors at distant sites is difficult to assess because of the age of the patient population. The incidence of lymphoma, leukemia, colon cancer, breast cancer, and lung cancer is already high in the patient population receiving total joint replacement. Prospective studies of large series of patients whose implants have been in place for long periods will be required to address this issue. One cannot deny that animal experiments have pointed to an association between tumor development and implants.[4, 5, 21] However, similar phenomena are unlikely over the remaining life span of most patients who undergo total joint replacements.

The dangers of hypersensitivity are also hard to evaluate. Although about 15 percent of the population is known to be sensitive to one or more of the metals used in stainless steel or cobalt-chromium alloy implants, it is known that far less than 15 percent of patients have observable reactions to implants made from these metals.[34, 35, 38] Although most reported cases of hypersensitivity involve cobalt-chromium or stainless steel, cases of suspected allergic reactions to titanium have been reported as well.[11] Patients who have shown hypersensitivity reactions to previous implants, orthopaedic devices, dental appliances, or other devices should not receive the same materials again, because reactions are likely. The possibility that a hypersensitivity reaction can lead to other problems, including an increased risk of infection or tumors, is suggested but unproved.[13, 37, 52]

Careful laboratory investigations are needed to evaluate the biocompatibility of various components of prostheses employed in total joint replacements. Although the incidence of adverse reactions appears to be low compared with the total number of implants, continued surveillance of this patient population is necessary.

References

1. Agins, H. J., Alcock, N. W., Bansal, M., et al.: Metal wear in failed titanium-alloy total hip replacements. J. Bone Joint Surg. 70A:347–356, 1988.
2. Aptekar, R. G., Davie, J. M., and Cattell, H. S.: Foreign body reaction to silicone rubber. Clin. Orthop. 98:231–232, 1974.
3. American Society for Testing and Materials F981: Assessment of Compatibility of Biomaterials (Nonporous) for Surgical Implants with Respect to Effect of Materials on Muscle and Bone. Philadelphia, ASTM Press, 1990.
4. Black, J.: Metallic Ion Release and Its Relationship to Oncogenesis. The Hip. Edited by R. H. Fitzgerald. St. Louis, C. V. Mosby Company, 1986.
5. Black, J.: Systemic effects of biomaterials. Biomaterials 5:11–18, 1984.
6. Blumenthal, N. C. and Posner, A. S.: *In vitro* model of aluminum-induced osteomalacia: inhibition of hydroxyapatite formation and growth. Calcif. Tissue Internat. 36:439–441, 1984.
7. Brown, S. A., Margevicius, R. W., and Merritt, K.: Fretting and accelerated fretting corosion of titanium *in vitro* and *in vivo*. Clinical Implant Materials. Edited by G. Heimke, U. Soltesz, A. J. C. Lee, Elsevier, Amsterdam, 1990.
8. Charnley, J.: Tissue Reactions to Implanted Plastics. Acrylic Cement in Orthopedic Surgery. Baltimore, Williams & Wilkins, 1970.
9. Christie, A. J., Weinberger, K. A., and Dietrich, M.: Silicone lymphadenopathy and synovitis, complications of silicone elastomer finger joint prosthesis. J.A.M.A. 237:1463–1464, 1977.
10. Coe, M. R., Fechner, R. E., Jeffrey, J. J., et al.: Characterization of tissue from the bone-polymethyl methacrylate interface in a rat experimental model. J. Bone Joint Surg. 71A:863–874, 1989.
11. Cook, S. D., McCluskey, L. C., Martin, P. C., et al.: Inflammatory response in retrieved noncemented porous coated implants. Clin. Orthop. (In press.)
12. Crugnola, A., Schiller, A., and Radin, E.: Polymeric debris in synovium after total joint replacement: histological identification. J. Bone Joint Surg. 59A:860–862, 1977.
13. Eisenbud, M.: Carcinogenicity and allergenicity. Science 236:1613, 1987.
14. Escalas, F., Galante, J., Rostoker, W., et al.: Biocompatibility of materials for joint replacement. J. Biomed. Mater. Res. 10:175–195, 1976.
15. Evans, E. J. and Thomas, I. T.: The *in vitro* toxicity of cobalt-chromium-molybdenum alloy and its constituent metals. Biomaterials 7:25–29, 1986.
16. Freeman, M. A. R., Bradley, G. W., and Revell, P. A.: Observations upon the interface between bone and polymethyl methacrylate cement. J. Bone Joint Surg. 64B:489–493, 1982.
17. Friedler, R. M.: Aluminum intoxication of bone in renal failure. Fact or fiction? Kidney Internat. [Suppl. 18]:70–73, 1986.
18. Fries, I. B., Fisher, A. A., and Salvati, E. A.: Contact dermatitis in surgeons from methyl methacrylate bone cement. J. Bone Joint Surg. 57A:547–549, 1975.
19. Fullerton, A., Andersen, J. R., Hoelgaard, A., et al.: Permeation of nickel through human skin *in vitro*: effect of vehicles. Br. J. Dermatol. 118:509–516, 1988.
20. Fullerton, A. and Hoelgaard, A.: Binding of nickel to human epidermis *in vitro*. Br. J. Dermatol. 119:675–682, 1988.

21. Gillespie, W. J., Frampton, C. M. A., Henderson, R. J., et al.: The incidence of cancer following total hip replacement. J. Bone Joint Surg. 70B:539–542, 1988.
22. Goldring, S. R., Schiller, A. L., Roelke, M., et al.: The synovial-like membrane at the bone-cement interface in loose total hip replacements and its proposed role in bone lysis. J. Bone Joint Surg. 65A:575–584, 1983.
23. Goodman, S. B., Fornasier, V. L., and Kei, J.: The effects of bulk versus particulate polymethyl methacrylate on bone. Clin. Orthop. 232:255–262, 1988.
24. Gordon, M. and Bullough, P. G.: Synovial and osseous inflammation in failed silicone-rubber prostheses. J. Bone Joint Surg. 64A:574–580, 1982.
25. Howie, D. W., Vernon-Roberts, B., Oakeshott, R., et al.: A rat model of resorption of bone at the cement-bone interface in the presence of polyethylene wear debris. J. Bone Joint Surg. 70A:257–263, 1988.
26. Jasim, K. A. and Weerasinghe, B. D.: Silicone lymphadenopathy, synovitis and osteitis complicating big toe Silastic prosthesis. J. Roy. Col. Surg. Edin. 32:29–33, 1987.
27. Kossovsky, N., Heggers, J. P., and Robson, M. C.: Experimental demonstration of the immunogenicity of silicone-protein complexes. J. Biomed. Mater. Res. 21:1125–1133, 1987.
28. Laing, P. G., Ferguson, A. B., Jr., and Hodge, E. S.: Tissue reaction in rabbit muscle exposed to metallic implants. J. Biomed. Mater. Res. 1:135–149, 1967.
29. Lammintausta, K. and Kalimo, K.: Do positive nickel reactions increase nonspecific patch test reactivity? Contact Dermatitis 16:160–163, 1987.
30. Lammintausta, K., Pitkanen, O-P., Kalimo, K., et al.: Interrelationships of nickel and cobalt contact sensitization. Contact Dermatitis 13:148–152, 1985.
31. Margevicius, R. M., Merritt, K., and Brown, S. A.: Storage and elimination of titanium, aluminum, and vanadium salts. J. Biomed. Mater. Res. (In press.)
32. Martin, A., Bauer, T. W., Manley, M. T., et al.: Osteosarcoma at the site of total hip replacement. J. Bone Joint Surg. 70A:1561–1567, 1988.
33. Menne, T.: Relationship between cobalt and nickel sensitization in females. Contact Dermatitis 6:337–340, 1980.
34. Merritt, K.: Role of medical materials both in implant and surface applications in immune response and resistance to infection. Biomaterials 5:47–53, 1984.
35. Merritt, K.: Biochemistry/Hypersensitivity/Clinical Reaction. International Workshop on Biocompatibility, Toxicity, and Hypersensitivity to Alloy Systems used in Dentistry. Ann Arbor, 1986.
36. Merritt, K.: Allergic reactions to materials used in prosthetic surgery. Biomaterials 7:711–716, 1987.
37. Merritt, K. and Brown, S. A.: Implant site infection in mice injected with metal chlorides. Trans. Soc. Biomat. III:122, 1979.
38. Merritt, K. and Brown, S. A.: Hypersensitivity to Metallic Biomaterials. Systemic Aspects of Biocompatibility, Vol. II. Edited by D. F. Williams. Boca Raton, FL, CRC Press, 1981.
39. Merritt, K. and Brown, S. A.: Effect of Valence of Chromium on Biological Responses. Biomaterials and Biomechanics 1983. Edited by P. Ducheyne, G. an der Perre, and A. E. Aubert. Amsterdam, Elsevier, 1984.
40. Merritt, K. and Brown, S. A.: Biological Effects of Corrosion Products from Metals. Corrosion and Degradation of Implant Materials: Second Symposium. ASTM STP, Vol. 859. Edited by A. Fraker and C. Griffin. Philadelphia, ASTM Press, 1985.
41. Merritt, K., Brown, S. A., and Sharkey, N. A.: Blood distribution of nickel, cobalt, and chromium following intramuscular injection into hamsters. J. Biomed. Mater. Res. 18:991–1004, 1984.
42. Merritt, K., Crowe, T. D., and Brown, S. A.: Elimination of nickel, cobalt and chromium following repeated injections of high dose metal salts. J. Biomed. Mater. Res. 23:845, 1989.
43. Mirra, J. M., Amstutz, H. C., Matos, M., et al.: The pathology of the joint tissues and its clinical relevance in prosthesis failure. Clin. Orthop. 117:221–240, 1976.
44. Mirra, J. M., Marder, R. A., and Amstutz, H. C.: The pathology of failed total joint arthroplasties. Clin. Orthop. 170:175–183, 1982.
45. Murray, D. W., Rae, T., and Rushton, N.: The influence of the surface energy and roughness of implants on bone resorption. J. Bone Joint Surg. 71B:632–637, 1989.
46. Nechay, B. R., Nanninga, L. B., Nechay, P. S. E., et al.: Role of vanadium in biology. Symposium of American Society for Pharmacology and Experimental Therapy, Federation of American Societies for Experimental Biology, 1985.
47. Oppenheim, W. L., Namba, R., Goodman, W. G., et al.: Aluminum toxicity complicating renal osteodystrophy. J. Bone Joint Surg. 71A:446–452, 1989.
48. Peimer, C. A.: Long-term complications of trapeziometacarpal silicone arthroplasty. Clin. Orthop. 220:86–98, 1987.
49. Rae, T.: A study of the effects of particulate metals on orthopaedic interest on murine macrophages *in vitro*. J. Bone Joint Surg. 57B:444–450, 1975.
50. Rae, T.: The biological response to titanium and titanium-aluminum-vanadium alloy particles. I. Tissue culture studies. Biomaterials 7:30–36, 1986.
51. Rae, T.: The biological response to titanium and titanium-aluminum-vanadium alloy particles. II. Long-term animal studies. Biomaterials 7:37–40, 1986.
52. Rae, T.: The action of cobalt, nickel and chromium on phagocytosis and bacterial killing by human polymorphonuclear leucocytes; its relevance to infection after joint arthroplasty. Biomaterials 4:175–180, 1983.
53. Rajagopalan, K. V.: Molybdenum: an essential trace element in human nutrition. Ann. Rev. Nutr. 8:401–427, 1988.
54. Roitt, I.: Essential Immunology. London, Blackwell Scientific Publications, 1987.
55. Salthouse, T. N. and Matlaga, B. F.: Effects of Implant Surface on Cellular Activity and Evaluation of Histocompatibility. Evaluation of Biomaterials. Edited by G. D. Winter, J. L. Leray,

and K. deGroot. New York, J. Wiley and Sons, 1980.

56. Sergott, T. J., Limoli, J. P., Baldwin, C. M., Jr., et al.: Human adjuvant disease, possible autoimmune disease after silicone implantation: a review of the literature, case studies and speculation for the future. Plast. Reconstr. Surg. 78:104–114, 1986.
57. Shiel, W. C., Jr., and Jason, M.: Granulomatous inguinal lymphadenopathy after bilateral metatarsophalangeal joint silicone arthroplasty. Foot Ankle 6(5):216–218, 1986.
58. Stevens, R. G., Jones, D. Y., Micozzi, M. S., et al.: Body iron stores and the risk of cancer. N. Engl. J. Med. 319:1047–1052, 1988.
59. Weinberg, E. D.: Iron and infection. Microbiol. Rev. 42:45–66, 1978.
60. Willert, H.-G., Ludwig, J., and Semlitsch, M.: Reaction of bone to methacrylate after hip arthroplasty. J. Bone Joint Surg. 56A:1368–1382, 1974.
61. Willert, H. G. and Semlitsch, M.: Reaction of articular capsule to wear products of artificial joint prostheses. J. Biomed. Mater. Res. 11:157–164, 1977.
62. Williams, D. F.: Biological Properties of Molybdenum. Systemic Aspects of Biocompatibility. Edited by D. F. Williams. Boca Raton, FL, CRC Press, 1981.
63. Worsing, R. A., Jr., Engber, W. D., and Lange, T. A.: Reactive synovitis from particulate silicone. J. Bone Joint Surg. 64A:581–585, 1982.

CHAPTER 7

Fixation Methods

WILLIAM PETTY

Three methods of fixation are used during implantation of joint prostheses: (1) fixation with bone cement, (2) porous fixation, and (3) press-fit fixation.

Fixation with bone cement, the most widely utilized method, was developed by Sir John Charnley in 1961.[11] Charnley has stated that the introduction of polymethyl methacrylate (PMMA) bone cement was one of three determinants of the procedure's success; the other two were the development of high molecular weight polyethylene socket replacements and the application of the low-friction principle.[12, 13] Previously, bone cement had been employed mainly by dental laboratories to manufacture artificial dentures and by neurosurgeons to repair skull defects. The chief innovations that orthopaedists introduced were *in vivo* polymerization and surgical application (total hip arthroplasty) involving extremely high mechanical stresses, i.e., those across the hip joint. The new mechanical demands placed on PMMA bone cement in joint replacement surgery stimulated a great deal of laboratory and clinical investigation, as researchers strove to characterize and refine the application of a bone cement that would produce the best possible long-term outcome.

The second method, porous fixation, actually had its beginnings in 1909, when Greenfield developed a system for bone ingrowth to stabilize an artificial tooth.[32] In the decades that followed, a few investigators reported the use of porous polymers to attach soft tissue or augment bone grafts, but it was over 50 years before Smith proposed a porous ceramic-plastic composite material for attachment of orthopaedic prostheses.[33, 57, 83, 88] As a result, in the late 1960s and early 1970s many basic experiments were designed in relation to manufacturing processes and characteristics of porous surfaces for biologic fixation. This research provided the basis for the introduction of porous materials into clinical applications for fixation of orthopaedic prostheses.

Press-fit fixation, the third method, was described by Moore and Bohlman in 1943[6a] after implantation of the first cementless hip prosthesis. Over the next 25 years, press-fit prostheses for insertion in the proximal femur were designed by Moore, Thompson, and others and utilized extensively for the treatment of both fractures and arthritic conditions.

FIXATION WITH BONE CEMENT

Bone cement consists primarily of PMMA, a self-curing acrylic resin (Fig. 7–1). It is supplied as a vial of liquid (20.0 ml) and a plastic bag of powder (40.0 gm) ready for mixing (Table 7–1). During manufacture, the liquid is sterilized by membrane filtration and the powder by gamma radiation. The chemical composition of the liquid is 97.5 percent methyl methacrylate, 2.5 percent dimethyl-*p*-toluidine, and 0.0076 percent hydroquinone. Dimethyl-*p*-toluidine promotes cold curing of the poly-

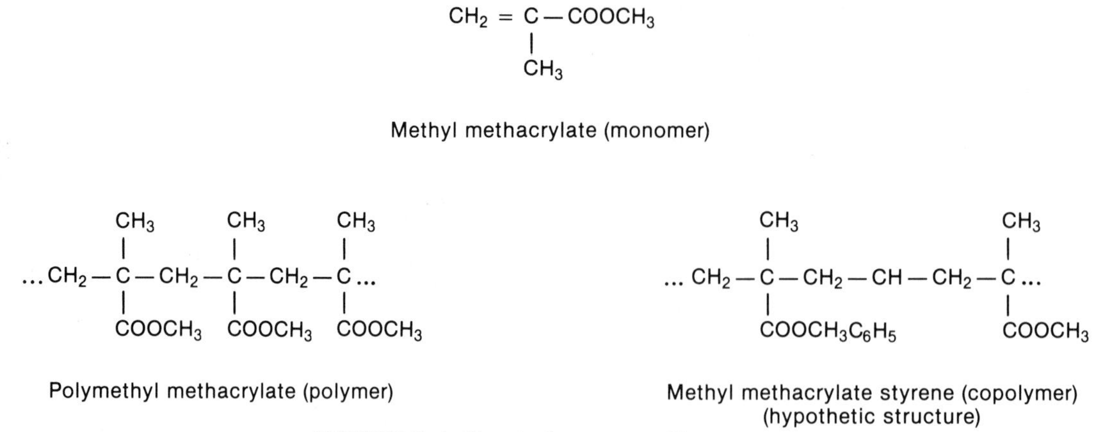

$$CH_2 = \underset{\displaystyle CH_3}{\underset{|}{C}} - COOCH_3$$

Methyl methacrylate (monomer)

$$\ldots CH_2 - \underset{COOCH_3}{\overset{CH_3}{C}} - CH_2 - \underset{COOCH_3}{\overset{CH_3}{C}} - CH_2 - \underset{COOCH_3}{\overset{CH_3}{C}} \ldots$$

Polymethyl methacrylate (polymer)

$$\ldots CH_2 - \underset{COOCH_3C_6H_5}{\overset{CH_3}{C}} - CH_2 - CH - CH_2 - \underset{COOCH_3}{\overset{CH_3}{C}} \ldots$$

Methyl methacrylate styrene (copolymer)
(hypothetic structure)

FIGURE 7–1. Chemical structure of bone cement.

mer, and hydroquinone inhibits polymerization of the monomer that might result from exposure to heat or light.

The powder comes in two forms—radiopaque and nonradiopaque. The radiopaque powder consists of 88 percent PMMA (mostly as a polystyrene copolymer), 10 percent barium sulfate, 2 percent benzoyl peroxide, and a small amount of residual monomer. The nonradiopaque form lacks barium sulfate and is 98 percent PMMA; the other ingredients remain the same.

Benzoyl peroxide initiates polymerization when the powder is mixed with the liquid. Polystyrene decreases the polymeric degradation from ionizing radiation during sterilization, may reduce the temperature rise during polymerization, and improves the working properties of the cement.[34]

Biologic Characteristics

When cured, bone cement has a composition similar to that of the commercially supplied powder, including a small amount of residual peroxide present as benzoyl peroxide or polymeric peroxide, both water insoluble. Although reducing agents in the tissues around the implanted cement might allow some decomposition of peroxide at the cement surface over time, it is unlikely that significant amounts would be released from cured material under clinical conditions.[34] Most of the release of monomer occurs during polymerization; it increases with more active stirring or hand kneading, two practices that are detrimental to the mechanical properties of cement.[48, 68] Immediately after polymerization, approximately 3 percent of residual monomer remains in the cement; this amount falls to 2 percent within a few hours and to 1.5 percent after 4 months (Fig. 7–2).[34] The local concentration of monomer is probably not high enough to contribute to the bone necrosis that occurs after total joint replacement.[16, 28, 40, 51–53, 55, 68, 81]

The amount of methyl methacrylate that reaches the systemic circulation during and shortly after polymerization causes no significant toxicity but does have an ob-

Table 7–1. BONE CEMENT COMPONENTS

Liquid		Powder			
		Radiopaque		*Nonradiopaque*	
Component	*(% wt)*	*Component*	*(% wt)*	*Component*	*(% wt)*
Methyl methacrylate	97.5	Polymethyl methacrylate*	88	Polymethyl methacrylate*	98
Dimethyl-*p*-toluidine	2.5	Barium sulfate	10	Benzoyl peroxide	2
Hydroquinone	0.0076	Benzoyl peroxide	2	Residual monomer	Trace
		Residual monomer	Trace		

*Polystyrene copolymer.

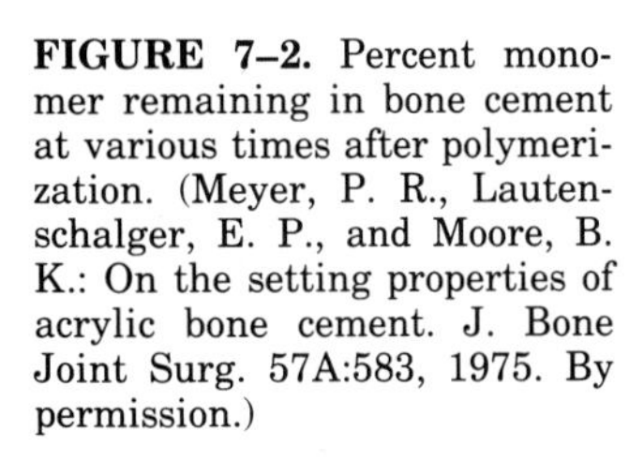

FIGURE 7–2. Percent monomer remaining in bone cement at various times after polymerization. (Meyer, P. R., Lautenschalger, E. P., and Moore, B. K.: On the setting properties of acrylic bone cement. J. Bone Joint Surg. 57A:583, 1975. By permission.)

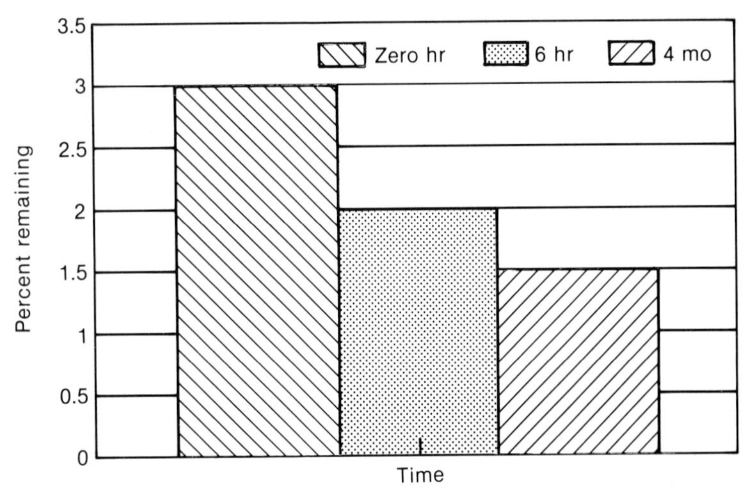

servable effect on several constituents of normal serum. The monomer inhibits the bacteriostatic factors in serum that act against *Staphylococcus epidermidis*, interferes with the production of the late-acting components of the complement sequence, impairs the production of active chemotactic factors of normal human serum, slows the migration of polymorphonuclear leukocytes, decreases phagocytosis by polymorphonuclear leukocytes, and slows the responses of human peripheral blood lymphocytes.[62, 64–69] The monomer has been shown to induce mutagenesis in bacteria, but experiments *in vivo* have demonstrated no evidence of carcinogenesis.[73, 76]

Setting Properties

The time period required for polymerization to take place ("setting") is defined in two ways. "Dough time" is the time that elapses between the first mixing of the powder and liquid and the time when the cement no longer adheres to a surgically gloved finger (an admittedly subjective measure). "Setting time" is the time between the start of mixing and the time when either the peak temperature or the temperature midway between ambient and peak is reached. Because the temperature rise is quite rapid, the difference between the two is negligible. "Working time" or "handling time" is the time between dough and setting times, although these terms are misleading because the cement can be neither worked nor handled when the prosthesis-cement composite is held in final position without movement (Fig. 7–3).[54]

The setting properties of bone cement may be altered significantly by changes in the composition of the cement. Composition, in turn, is affected by whether the cement is of standard or low viscosity and whether it contains barium sulfate. Setting properties also vary with the batch, manufacturer, temperature and humidity during storage and handling, mixing method,

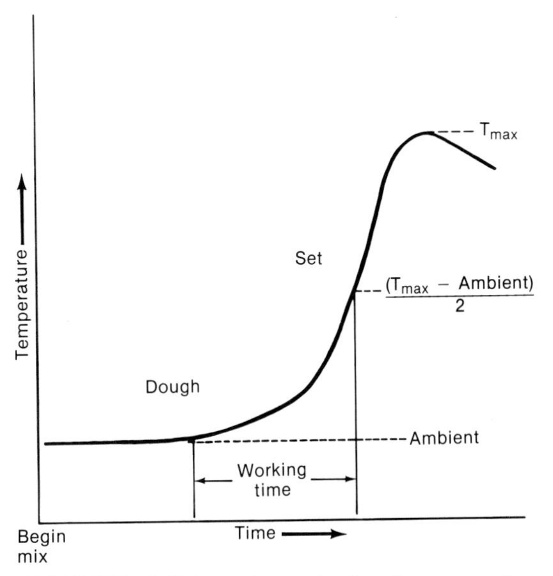

FIGURE 7–3. Schematic graph of setting properties of bone cement. (Modified from Haas, S. S., Brauer, G. M., and Dickson, G.: J. Bone Joint Surg. 57A:380–391, 1975. By permission.)

Table 7–2. EFFECT OF AMBIENT TEMPERATURE ON SETTING PROPERTIES OF ACRYLIC CEMENT

Ambient Temperature (°C)	Dough Time (min)	Set Time (min)	Working Time (min)	T_{max}* (°C)
4	34.0	60.0	26.0	53
15	10.5	21.5	11.0	89
20	4.5	13.0	8.5	101
25	3.0	8.0	5.0	107
30	2.0	5.0	3.0	111
37	1.0	3.0	2.0	125

*Measured in center of a specimen (10 mm thick, 36 gm); cement was mixed at powder:liquid ratio of 2:1 and placed in a Teflon mold 60 mm in diameter. Modified from Meyer, P. R., Lautenschlager, E. P., and Moore, B. K.: J Bone Joint Surg. 55A:149–156, 1973.

age of the cement components, and thickness of the cement. The time available to work with the cement is reduced by high room temperature, humid conditions, hand-kneading of the cement dough, increased powder-to-liquid ratio, increased age of cement, and thinner cement mantle. Cement containing barium sulfate has slightly longer dough, setting, and handling times. High ambient temperatures can shorten the setting time significantly (Table 7–2).[34, 54]

The amount of heat produced during polymerization is directly related to the amount of monomer polymerizing, but different conditions can modify the rise in temperature. Peak temperatures of polymerization are higher when the ratio of powder to monomer is lowered, when the mixing temperature is raised, and when the cement is thicker. When the standard ratio of powder to monomer is maintained at 2:1 and mixing takes place at standard room temperature, the temperature in the center of the cement may exceed 100°C when the mass is thick. However, the temperature at the surface of the cement mass in clinical situations is much lower (Table 7–3).[45] When bone cement is applied to an irregular bone surface over a large area, interface temperatures are generally only a few degrees above body temperature.[45]

Table 7–3. PEAK TEMPERATURE AT POLYMERIZATION (°C)

		Mean Peak Temperature at End Surface†		Mean Peak Temperature at Side Surface	
Cylinder Diameter* and Material	Mean Peak Temperature at Center	*Air Interphase at 20°C*	*Water Interphase at 37°C*	*20°C Interphase*	*37°C Interphase*
30 mm Teflon	122.25	100.5	41.3	45.0	58
20 mm Teflon	109.5	89.25	41.7	40.0	55
10 mm Teflon	79.5	62.5	41.5	33.0	51
5 mm Teflon	41.5	35.7	38.0	25.0	40
2.5 mm Teflon	No detectable rise	No detectable rise	No detectable rise	No detectable rise	No detectable rise
30 mm Aluminum	120.5	97.5	40.3	38.0	55
20 mm Aluminum	106.75	82.5	41.7	33.0	50
10 mm Aluminum	69.25	54.5	42.0	32.0	50
5 mm Aluminum	35.0	34.0	38.5	No detectable rise	41
2.5 mm Aluminum	No detectable rise	No detectable rise	No detectable rise	No detectable rise	No detectable rise

Note: Each figure is the mean of three readings.
*Constant ratio of diameter to length is 1:3.
†Surface thermocouples were in firm contact with the cement dough.
Modified from Jefferiss, C. D., Lee, A. J. C., and Ling, R. S. M.: J Bone Joint Surg. 57B: 511–518, 1975.

Mechanical Properties

The mechanical properties of polymers are related to their molecular weight. As molecular weight increases, tensile strength increases until a plateau is reached at approximately 242,000. At this point, mechanical properties remain constant. Commercially available bone cement powder has an average molecular weight of 198,000. When mixed and cured, the cement has a molecular weight of 242,000 because of the higher molecular weight of the monomer that polymerizes *in vivo*.

Bone cement reaches 90 percent of its maximum tensile strength within 4 hours and 100 percent within 24 hours. However, cooling of the prosthesis, the cement constituents, the mixing apparatus, or cooling by irrigation during polymerization may significantly prolong the time required for bone cement to reach its maximum strength.[34] Tensile strength is higher in commercially prepared PMMA than in bone cements utilized for joint replacement owing to the higher molecular weight of the commercially prepared products. The addition of barium sulfate results in a lower tensile strength (Table 7–4).[34, 48] Bone cement may shrink or expand slightly during the initial period after mixing, but it shrinks during rapid polymerization. This is not surprising; the volume occupied by methyl methacrylate monomer is reduced by 21 percent during the transformation to polymer. Because the cement mixture contains about 35 percent monomer, the overall shrinkage expected is 7 to 8 percent. In practice, shrinkage is considerably lower, probably about 2 to 4 percent, because of monomer evaporation and porosity in the cement.[34]

Porosity, a mechanical property that may result in significant weakening of bone cement, is produced in two ways: by air bubbles produced during the mixing process and by gas bubbles produced as some of the monomer evaporates at the high temperatures of polymerization. Porosity is always increased by air introduced during the hand mixing process, especially when stirring is vigorous. Porosity may reach 27 percent by volume as a result of open hand mixing; pore size has been found to exceed 300 μm in many specimens.[25, 34] Only under certain experimental conditions has cement expansion been demonstrated to be due to bubbles created by monomer vaporization during polymerization.[25, 34] For substantial vaporization to take place, the temperature must reach 100°C. This factor requires a large volume of cement with a low surface area, an unlikely situation in total joint replacement surgery.

A number of measures have been suggested to reduce porosity and to improve the mechanical properties of bone cement: centrifugation, mixing under vacuum, vibration or agitation during mixing, and pressurization of cement. Although centrifugation does decrease porosity, increase tensile strength, and increase fatigue life of bone cement, the effects vary with the conditions of centrifugation and the type of bone cement. The best results have been achieved with Simplex P. When centrifuged, this cement has the longest fatigue life of all cements tested, whether centrifuged or not. Even without special treatment, Simplex P has been shown to have

Table 7–4. COMPARISON OF MECHANICAL PROPERTIES OF VARIOUS TYPES OF BONE CEMENTS

	Radiopaque Cement	Radiolucent Cement	Commercial Acrylic Resin
Tensile strength, MPa	28.9 (1.6)	32.6 (1.2)	55–76
Compressive strength, MPa	91.7 (2.5)	93.1 (3.9)	76–131
Transverse breaking load, N	41.9 (3.1)	47.9 (1.3)	—
Modulus of rupture, MPa	51.1 (3.1)	56.9 (1.6)	83–117
Young's modulus			
From transverse loading data, MPa	2070 (90)	2200 (80)	2690–3280
From compressive loading data, MPa	2200 (60)	2300 (50)	2690–3280

Standard deviations are shown in parentheses. (MPa = MegaPascal; N = Newton.)
Modified from Haas, S. S., Brauer, G. M., and Dickson, G.: J Bone Joint Surg. 57A: 380–391, 1975.

a longer fatigue life than Palacos R, CMW, and Zimmer Regular or LVC under some experimental conditions. This cement is most easily handled and fatigue life is longest when mixing is done at room temperature and the cement is centrifuged for 30 seconds. If a lower viscosity is desired, the cement may be chilled to 0°C and centrifuged for 60 seconds. Centrifugation also prolongs the fatigue life of Zimmer Regular and LVC cements, although not quite as long. The porosity and fatigue life of CMW and Palacos R cements are unaffected by centrifugation, perhaps because they have a higher viscosity.[8, 19–24, 31, 75] Centrifugation does not alter the elastic modulus, setting time, or peak temperature of bone cement.[8]

Although centrifugation reduces porosity, it is a cumbersome process and requires careful planning and cooperation of the surgical team. Also, the problem of separation arises when bone cement contains barium sulfate, because barium sulfate is four times more dense than bone cement, making an inconsistent column or layer more likely.[82] Under some conditions of centrifugation, the top of the cement column is more porous than the rest; therefore, it may be a good practice to discard the upper 1 cm after centrifugation.[93] Careful and complete bone filling is especially important after centrifugation because polymerization shrinkage may be increased owing to a reduction in porosity.[36]

Porosity may also be reduced by mixing bone cement under a vacuum, a method that improves the other mechanical properties of bone cement as well. Vacuum mixing is considered more effective than centrifugation in reducing porosity; it lowers the volume occupied by air bubbles to less than 1 percent.[2, 20, 80, 96] Vacuum mixing improves the tensile and compressive strength markedly, increases the modulus of elasticity, and improves the hardness of bone cement; fatigue life is improved as much as tenfold.[2, 14, 49, 50, 80, 96] However, polymerization shrinkage is probably increased as a result of vacuum mixing owing to decreased porosity. It appears unlikely that mixing bone cement under vacuum results in layers in the various components, but no research data have been reported.

Pressurization of bone cement before polymerization also reduces its porosity and improves its mechanical properties, but the method has not been thoroughly studied or widely accepted in clinical practice.[14, 36, 94] Agitation, vibration, and exposure to sound waves have been proposed as other means to reduce the porosity and improve the mechanical properties of bone cement, but they have not been studied extensively or applied clinically.

If bone cement is mixed by an open manual method, the powder should be thoroughly wetted, but rapid, forceful mixing should be avoided. It is preferable to employ one of the centrifugation or vacuum mixing systems to improve the mechanical properties of bone cement for total joint arthroplasty (Fig. 7–4).

The addition of small amounts of antibiotic to commercially supplied bone cement does not alter the fatigue properties of cement significantly or change the effect of centrifugation on its mechanical prop-

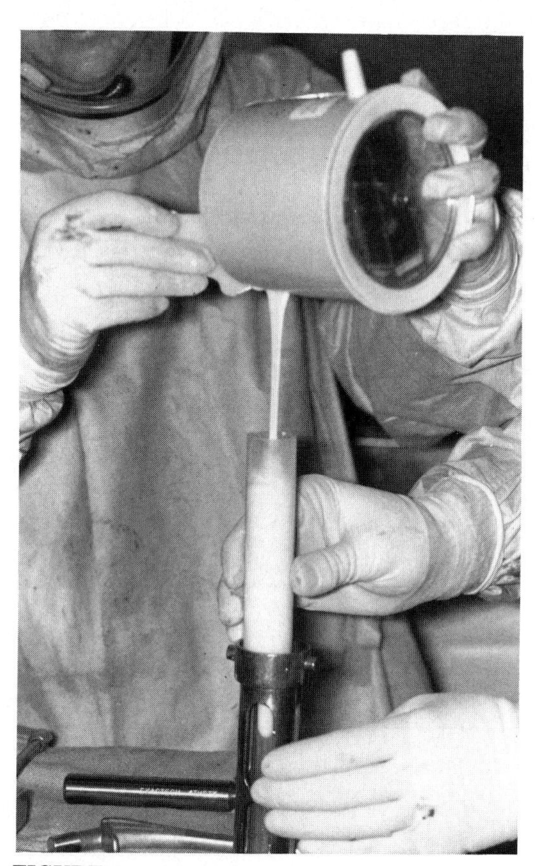

FIGURE 7–4. Uniform cement being poured into a syringe after vacuum mixing.

erties.[22] Centrifugation does not affect the distribution of antibiotic within the cement.[93] However, the addition of antibiotic powder to bone cement in the operating room affects the mechanical properties of the bone cement to a variable degree because of mixing inconsistency. The best technique for reducing this inconsistency is to combine an equivalent amount of bone cement powder with the predetermined amount of antibiotic powder, mixing thoroughly, and continue to combine equivalent amounts of the two powders, mixing thoroughly after each addition until all powder is mixed. Large amounts of antibiotic powder (i.e., 4 to 6 gm per 40 gm of bone cement powder) should be avoided. The mechanical strength of the cured cement may be reduced by as much as 25 percent. Also, the handling properties of the bone cement will be affected adversely. Liquid antibiotics should never be mixed with bone cement in total joint replacement; they weaken it markedly.[47]

Total Hip Arthroplasty

When bone cement was first introduced for the fixation of total hip prostheses, little effort was made to achieve a high degree of mechanical interdigitation of cement with irregular bone surface, especially on the acetabular side. Experienced orthopaedists are often surprised that the results from that era have remained as durable as they have.[12, 72, 74, 77, 87, 95, 97] Because bone cement is not an adhesive, the bone must be prepared for extensive mechanical interdigitation with the cement (Fig. 7–5). This mechanical interlock is provided by appropriate cutting, reaming, and broaching for the prosthesis being used; clearance of all soft tissue from bone where cement will be applied; clearance of hematoma and debris by brushing and vigorous washing; plugging of the femoral canal; cement application by syringe with pressure; and retrograde filling of the intramedullary canal.[3, 38, 58–61, 94]

POROUS FIXATION

The porous materials for biologic fixation of orthopaedic prostheses include metals, ceramics, and polymers singly or in combination. The most widely utilized are cobalt chrome alloy with a metallic bead coating and titanium alloy with a commercially pure titanium bead or wire coating or plasma spraying.[30, 35, 41, 89] Stainless steel porous systems allow for bone ingrowth, but the material probably corrodes too readily to be used in porous form.[63] Most commercially available prostheses consist of metal substrates with porous metallic coatings. Their mechanical properties are considered adequate, and the porous surface allows for tissue attachment. Porous systems made of nonmetallic materials include Teflon with graphite fibers (Pro-

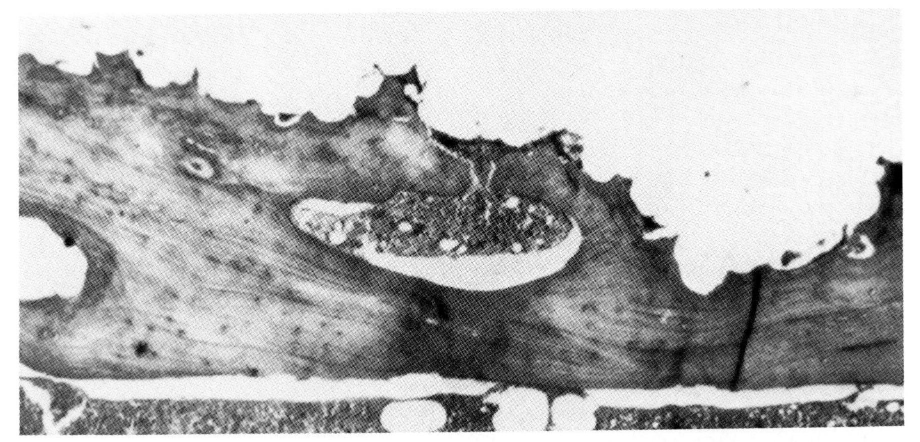

FIGURE 7–5. Interdigitation of bone cement with bone in a specimen of a clinically successful femoral stem 6 years after implantation. (Charnley, J: Low Friction Arthroplasty of the Hip. Berlin, Springer-Verlag, p. 30, 1979. By permission.)

Table 7–5. RELATIONSHIP OF PARTICLE SIZE OF MICROSPHERES TO PORE SIZE OF POROUS SURFACES*

Implant System Designation	Particle Size (μm)	Pore Size (μm)
A	25–45	20–50
B	45–150	50–200
C	150–300	200–400
D	300–840	400–800

*Modified from Bobyn, J. D., Pilliar, R. M., Cameron, H. U., et al.: Clin. Orthop. 150: 263–270, 1980. By permission.

plast), ceramics, polyethylene, polysulfone, and PMMA. None has been studied or used as widely as the metal-based systems.[46, 79, 84–86, 90–92]

For tissue ingrowth to occur, surface pores of the prosthesis must interconnect freely, and the surface must be thick enough to produce a three-dimensional lattice structure. As the layers of powder particles increase from one to three, interface strength increases. However, the addition of many more layers (7 to 12) weakens the interface bond.[6, 18] The pore size of metallic porous surfaces manufactured by powder metallurgic techniques is determined primarily by the size of the microspheres (Table 7–5).[4] Wire diameter and molding pressure determine the pore size in sintered fiber metal coatings; 0.19-mm titanium wire and a porosity of 50 percent result in a pore size ranging from 170 to 350 μm.[30] When the pore size is smaller than about 50 μm, fibrous rather than bone ingrowth occurs. If the pores are too large (probably >400 μm), interfacial strength declines. The optimum pore size for rapid attachment and maximum interfacial strength is 100 to 400 μm; maximum size may be somewhat larger.[4, 46, 83, 85]

Close contact between a porous surface and bone enhances the quality of bone ingrowth. In experimental studies in dogs, good bone apposition and ingrowth occur when the maximum distance between porous implant and endosteal bone surface is less than 2 mm. As the gap decreases, growth becomes more rapid. Even in humans, bone appears to fill in gaps between bone and a porous prosthesis in some instances, probably more commonly with femoral components of total knee replacements and acetabular components of hip replacements (Fig. 7–6).[43] At distances greater than 2 mm, bone apposition and ingrowth are decreased. Maximum incorporation requires 12 weeks in the dog; with the acetabular component, gaps as small as 0.5 mm may not fill with bone.[5, 37, 70, 78]

In humans, closer contact between porous surface and endosteal bone is thought to result in faster, more complete attachment and ingrowth. Micromotion affects the type and quality of ingrowth into porous surfaces. If the degree of motion at the tissue-implant interface approaches or exceeds the pore diameter, bone ingrowth probably cannot occur. Even fibrous ingrowth is better organized if interface motion is minimal. Experimentally, bone ingrowth occurs with movement up to about 28 μm; movement of 150 μm or more results in fibrous attachment.[10, 15, 26, 39, 42, 71] Although bone ingrowth occurs consistently in many experimental models, it appears less predictable in humans but does occur (Fig. 7–7).[27] In the femoral component of hips, up to one third of retrieved specimens exhibit no bone ingrowth. The remainder show a maximum of 2 to 10 percent of available porous surface covered with bone growth. Both the surface amount and depth of bone ingrowth are better in distal regions of the porous coating where cortical bone predominates over metaphyseal bone.[17] In one study of retrieved prosthetic acetabular components, extensive bone ingrowth was found; in another study, less bone ingrowth was found in acetabular components than in femoral components.[17, 44] As with femoral components of total hips, up to one third of retrieved total knee components exhibit no bone ingrowth, whereas the remainder show a maximum of 2 to 10 percent of available porous surface covered with bone ingrowth. Little difference exists in the amount of ingrowth in tibial, femoral, and patellar components of total knee replacements. Ingrowth was generally better around screws or pegs of acetabular and total knee components. In specimens retrieved from humans, the pore structure contains mostly fibrous tissue.[17, 37, 44]

PRESS-FIT FIXATION

Modern designs of cementless prostheses without porous coatings continue to be developed, keeping pace with improvements

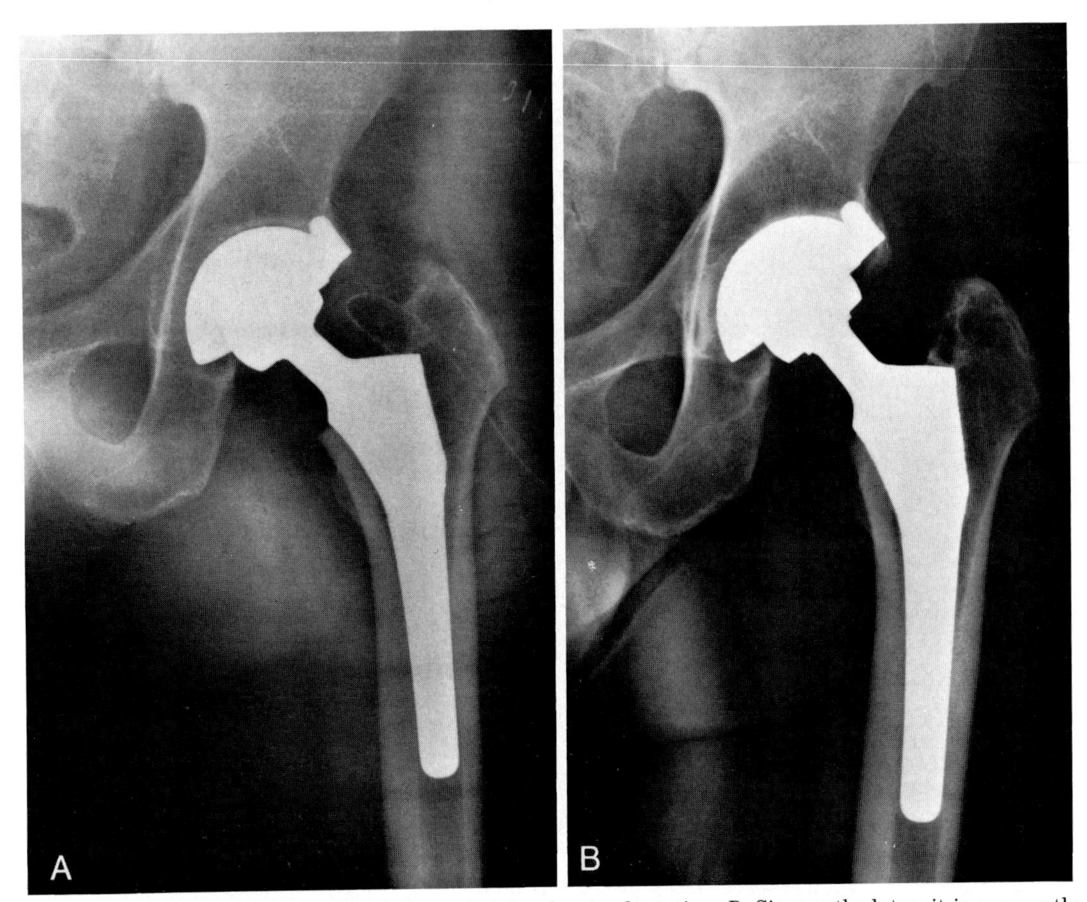

FIGURE 7–6. Bone-prosthesis gap. *A*, Immediately after implantation. *B*, Six months later, it is apparently filled in.

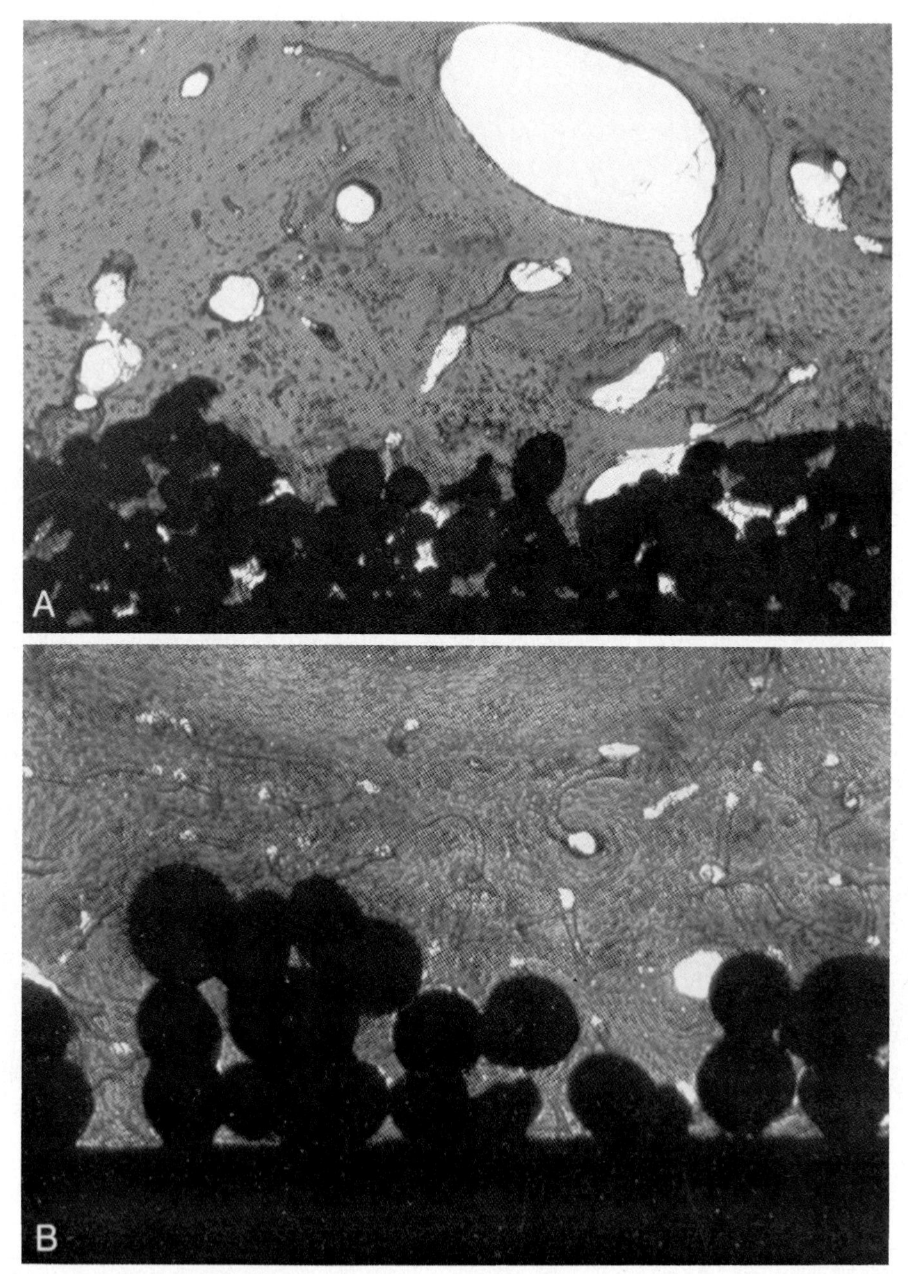

FIGURE 7–7. Bone ingrowth in femoral specimens retrieved after 3 to 7 years of implantation. *A*, Proximal femoral metaphyseal specimen retrieved after 7 years. *B*, Diaphyseal cortical specimen retrieved after 3 years. (Engh, C. A., Bobyn, J. D., and Glassmen, A. H.: J. Bone Joint Surg. 69B:45–55, 1987. By permission.)

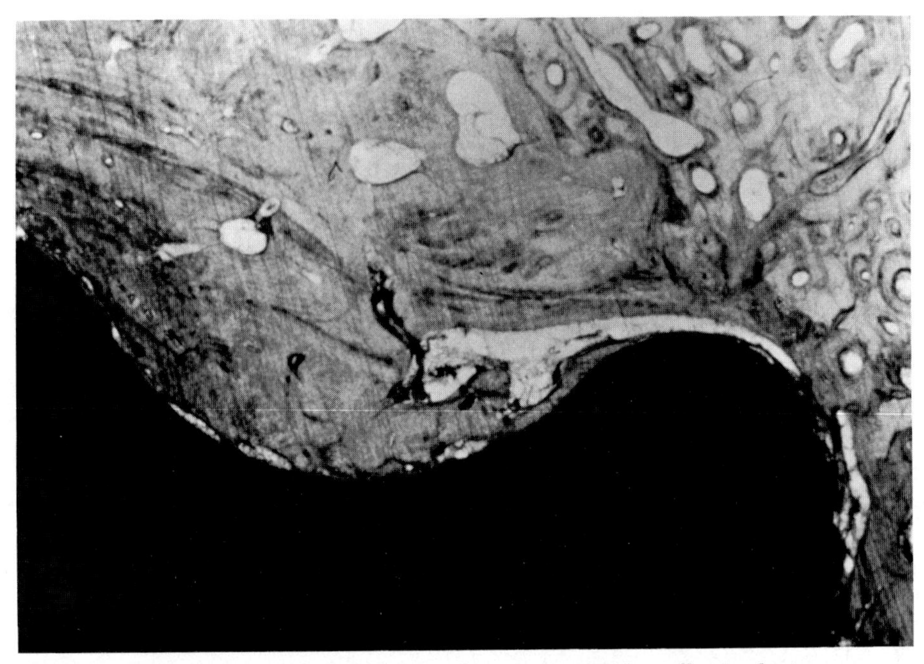

FIGURE 7–8. Osseointegration of nonporous titanium alloy implant.

in cemented prostheses and porous-coated devices. Some press-fit prostheses have provision for macrointerlock with bone, some have roughened surfaces, and others have smooth surfaces. Usually these devices are constructed from cobalt chrome and titanium alloys and polyethylene. Titanium alloys have demonstrated excellent osseointegration in joint replacement in some instances, similar to that seen in dental applications (Fig. 7–8).[1, 7, 98] The problems of loosening and extensive membrane formation that occurred with earlier designs of press-fit prostheses have been reduced by the availability of a wide range of sizes, improved materials, and better instrumentation that permits greater surgical precision.[29, 56]

References

1. Albrektsson, T., Branemark, P. I., Hansson, H. A., et al.: Osseointegrated titanium implants. Requirements for ensuring a long-lasting, direct bone-to-implant anchorage in man. Acta Orthop. Scand. 52:155, 1981.
2. Alkire, M. J., Dabezies, E. J., and Hastings, P. R.: High vacuum as a method of reducing porosity of polymethyl methacrylate. Orthopedics 10(11):1533–1539, 1987.
3. Amstutz, H. C., Markolf, K. L., and McNeice, G. M.: Loosening of Total Hip Components: Cause and Prevention. The Hip. St. Louis, C. V. Mosby Company, 1976.
4. Bobyn, J. D., Pilliar, R. M., Cameron, H. U., et al.: The optimum pore size for the fixation of porous-surfaced metal implants by the ingrowth of bone. Clin. Orthop. 150:263–270, 1980.
5. Bobyn, J. D., Pilliar, R. M., Cameron, H. U., et al.: Osteogenic phenomena across bone-implant spaces with porous surfaced intramedullary implants. Acta Orthop. Scand. 52:145–153, 1981.
6. Bobyn, J. D., Pilliar, R. M., Cameron, H. U., et al.: The effect of porous surface configuration on the tensile strength of fixation of implants by bone ingrowth. Clin. Orthop. 149:291–298, 1980.

6a. Bohlman, H. R. and Moore, A. T.: Metal hip joint: A case report. J. Bone Joint Surg. 25:688, 1943.

7. Branemark, P. I., Hansson, B. O., Adell, R., et al.: Osseointegrated implants in the treatment of the edentulous jaw. Experience from a ten-year period. Scand. J. Plast. Reconstr. Surg. 16:1, 1977.
8. Burke, D. W., Gates, E. I., and Harris, W. H.: Centrifugation as a method of improving tensile and fatigue properties of acrylic bone cement. J. Bone Joint Surg [Am.] 66(8):1265–1273, 1984.
9. Cameron, H. U.: Six-year results with a microporous-coated metal hip prosthesis. Clin. Orthop. 208:81–83, 1986.
10. Cameron, H. U., Pilliar, R. M., and McNab, I.: The effect of movement on the bonding of porous metal to bone. J. Biomed. Mater. Res. 7:301, 1973.
11. Charnley, J.: Arthroplasty of the hip. A new operation. Lancet 1:1129, 1961.
12. Charnley, J.: Acrylic Cement in Orthopaedic Surgery. Edinburgh, Churchill Livingstone, 1970.

13. Charnley, J.: The long-term results of low-friction arthroplasty of the hip performed as a primary intervention. J Bone Joint Surg. 54B:61–76, 1972.
14. Chee, W. W., Donovan, T. E., Daftary, F., and Siu, T. M.: The effect of vacuum-mixed autopolymerizing acrylic resins on porosity and transverse strength. J. Prosthet. Dent. 60(4):517–519, 1988.
15. Collier, J. P., Colligan, G. A., and Brown, S. A.: Bone ingrowth into dynamically loaded porous coated intramedullary nails. J. Biomed. Mater. Res. 7:485, 1976.
16. Convery, F. R., Gunn, D. R., Hughes, J. D., and Martin, W. E.: The relative safety of polymethyl methacrylate. J. Bone Joint Surg. 57A:57–64, 1975.
17. Cook, S. D., Thomas, K. A., and Haddad, R. J.: Histological analysis of retrieved human porous coated total joint components. Clin. Orthop. 234:90–101, 1988.
18. Cook, S. D., Walsh, K. A., and Haddad, R. J., Jr.: Interface mechanics and bone growth into porous Co-Cr-Mo alloy implants. Clin. Orthop. 193:271–280, 1985.
19. Davies, J. P., Burke, D. W., O'Connor, D. O., and Harris, W. H.: Comparison of the fatigue characteristics of centrifuged and uncentrifuged Simplex P bone cement. J. Orthop. Res. 5(3):366–371, 1987.
20. Davies, J. P., Jasty, M., O'Connor, D. O., et al.: The effect of centrifuging bone cement. J. Bone Joint Surg. [Br.] 71(1):39–42, 1989.
21. Davies, J. P., O'Connor, D. O., Burke, D. W., et al.: Comparison and optimization of three centrifugation systems for reducing porosity of Simplex P bone cement. J. Arthroplasty 4(1):15–20, 1989.
22. Davies, J. P., O'Connor, D. O., Burke, D. W., et al.: Influence of antibiotic impregnation on the fatigue life of Simplex P and Palacos R acrylic bone cements, with and without centrifugation. J. Biomed. Mater. Res. 23(4):379–397, 1989.
23. Davies, J. P., O'Connor, D. O., Burke, D. W., et al.: The effect of centrifugation on the fatigue life of bone cement in the presence of surface irregularities. Clin. Orthop. 229:156–161, 1988.
24. Davies, J. P., O'Connor, D. O., Greer, J. A., and Harris, W. H.: Comparison of the mechanical properties of Simplex P, Zimmer Regular, and LVC bone cements. J. Biomed. Mater. Res. 21:719–730, 1987.
25. Debrunner, H. U.: The porosity of bone cement. Arch. Orthop. Unfallchir. 86(3):261–278, 1976.
26. Ducheyne, P., Demeester, P., Aernoudt, E., et al.: Influence of a functional dynamic loading on bone ingrowth into surface pores of orthopaedic implants. J. Biomed. Mater. Res. 11:811–838, 1977.
27. Engh, C. A., Bobyn, J. D., and Glassmen, A. H.: Porous-coated hip replacement. J. Bone Joint Surg. 69B:45–55, 1987.
28. Feith, R.: Side-effects of acrylic cement implanted into bone. Acta Orthop. Scand. [Suppl.] 161, 1975.
29. Freeman, M. A. R., McLeod, H. C., and Levai, J.: Cementless fixation of prosthetic components in total arthroplasty of the knee and hip. Clin. Orthop. 176:88–94, 1983.
30. Galante, J., Rostoker, W., Lueck, R., and Ray, R. D.: Sintered fiber metal composites as a basis for attachment of implants to bone. J. Bone Joint Surg. 53A:101–114, 1971.
31. Gates, E. I., Carter, D. R., and Harris, W. H.: Comparative fatigue behavior of different bone cements. Clin. Orthop. 189:294–299, 1984.
32. Greenfield, E. J.: Mounting for Artificial Teeth. U.S. Patent No. 478360, 1909.
33. Grindlay, J. H. and Waugh, J. M.: Plastic sponge which acts as a framework for living tissue. Arch. Surg. 63:288, 1951.
34. Haas, S. S., Brauer, G. M., and Dickson, G.: A characterization of polymethyl methacrylate bone cement. J. Bone Joint Surg. 57A:380–391, 1975.
35. Hahn, H. and Palich, W.: Preliminary evaluation of porous metal surfaced titanium for orthopaedic implants. J. Biomed. Mater. Res. 4:571, 1970.
36. Hamilton, H. W., Cooper, D. F., and Fels, M.: Shrinkage of centrifuged cement. Orthop. Rev. 17(1):48–54, 1988.
37. Harris, W. H. and Jasty, M.: Bone Ingrowth into Porous Coated Canine Acetabular Replacements: The Effect of Pore Size, Apposition, and Dislocation. The Hip. St. Louis, C. V. Mosby Company, 1985.
38. Harris, W. H. and McGann, W. A.: Loosening of the femoral component after use of the medullary-plug cementing technique. Follow-up note with a minimum five-year follow-up. J. Bone Joint Surg. [Am.] 68(7):1064–1066, 1986.
39. Heck, D. A., Nakajima, I., Chao, E. Y., and Kelly, P. J.: The Effect of Immobilization on Biologic Ingrowth into Porous Titanium Fibermetal Prostheses. Proceedings of the 30th Annual Meeting of the Orthopaedic Research Society, Atlanta, p. 178, 1984.
40. Herndon, J. H., Morrison, W. A., and Pilcher, F. J.: Effects of methyl methacrylate on liver function in patients undergoing total hip or total knee replacement. Surg. Gynecol. Obstet. 150(2):177–183, 1980.
41. Hirschhorn, J. and Reynolds, J.: Powder Metallurgy Fabrication of Cobalt-Base Alloy Surgical Implants. Research in Dental and Medical Materials. Edited by E. Korostoff. New York, Plenum Publishing Co., 1969.
42. Hulbert, S. F., Matthews, J. R., and Klawitter, J. J.: Effect of stress on tissue ingrowth into porous aluminum oxide. J. Biomed. Mater. Res. 5:85, 1974.
43. Hungerford, D. S.: Clinical Experience with an Acetabular Cup for Cementless Use. The Hip. St. Louis, C. V. Mosby Company, 1985.
44. Jasty, M., Sumner, R., Galante, J. O., et al.: Bone Ingrowth into Porous-Surfaced Harris/Galante Prosthesis Acetabular Components Retrieved from Human Patients. American Academy of Orthopaedic Surgeon's Annual Meeting. Atlanta, p. 102, 1988.
45. Jefferiss, C. D., Lee, A. J. C., and Ling, R. S. M.: Thermal aspects of self-curing polymethyl methacrylate. J. Bone Joint Surg. 57B:511–518, 1975.
46. Klawitter, J. J.: Application of porous ceramics for the attachment of bearing internal orthopaedic applications. J. Biomed. Mater. Res. 2:161, 1971.
47. Lee, A. J. and Ling, R. S.: Improved cementing techniques. Instr. Course Lect. 30:407–413, 1981.

48. Lee, A. J. C., Ling, R. S. M., and Wrighton, J. D.: Some properties of polymethyl methacrylate with reference to its use in orthopaedic surgery. Clin. Orthop. 95:281–287, 1973.
49. Lidgren, L., Bodelind, B., and Moller, J.: Bone cement improved by vacuum mixing and chilling. Acta Orthop. Scand. 58(1):27–32, 1987.
50. Lidgren, L., Drar, H., and Moller, J.: Strength of polymethyl methacrylate increased by vacuum mixing. Acta Orthop. Scand. 55(5):536–541, 1984.
51. Linder, L.: Reaction of bone to the acute chemical trauma of bone cement. J. Bone Joint Surg. 59A:82–87, 1977.
52. Linder, L., and Romanus, M.: Acute local tissue effects of polymerizing acrylic bone cement. Clin. Orthop. 115:303–312, 1976.
53. McLaughlin, R. E., DiFazio, C. A., Hakala, M., et al.: Blood clearance and acute pulmonary toxicity of methylmethacrylate in dogs after simulated arthroplasty and intravenous injection. J. Bone Joint Surg. 55A:1621–1628, 1973.
54. Meyer, P. R., Lautenschlager, E. P., and Moore, B. K.: On the setting properties of acrylic bone cement. J. Bone Joint Surg. 55A:149–156, 1973.
55. Modig, J., Busch, C., and Olerud, S.: The importance of intravascular coagulation, fat embolism, and acrylic monomers for respiratory and circulatory dysfunctions during intramedullary endoprosthetic surgery. Proceedings Orthopaedic Research Society. J. Bone Joint Surg. 57A:583, 1975.
56. Morscher, E. W. and Dick, W.: Cementless fixation of "isoelastic" hip endoprostheses manufactured from plastic materials. Clin. Orthop. 176:77–87, 1983.
57. Newman, Z.: The use of the non-absorbable polyethylene sponge, "Polystan Sponge" as a subcutaneous prosthesis. Br. J. Plast. Surg. 9:195, 1952.
58. Oh, I., Bourne, R. B., and Harris, W. H.: The femoral cement compactor. An improvement in cementing technique in total hip replacement. J. Bone Joint Surg. [Am.] 65(9):1335–1338, 1983.
59. Oh, I., Carlson, C. E., Tomford, W. W., and Harris, W. H.: Improved fixation of the femoral component after total hip replacement using a methacrylate intramedullary plug. J. Bone Joint Surg. [Am.] 60(5):608–613, 1978.
60. Oh, I. and Harris, W. H.: A cement fixation system for total hip arthroplasty. Clin. Orthop. 164:221–229, 1982.
61. Oh, I., Merckx, D. B., and Harris, W. H.: Acetabular cement compactor. An experimental study of pressurization of cement in the acetabulum in total hip arthroplasty. Clin. Orthop. 177:289–293, 1983.
62. Panush, R. S. and Petty, W.: The effect of methyl methacrylate on normal human peripheral blood lymphocytes. Clin. Orthop. 128:354–360, 1978.
63. Peterson, C. D., Miles, J. S., and Solomans, C.: Union between bone and implants of open pore ceramic and stainless steel: a histologic study. J. Bone Joint Surg. 51A:805, 1969.
64. Petty, W.: The effect of methyl methacrylate on the bacterial inhibiting properties of normal human serum. Clin. Orthop. 132:266–278, 1978.
65. Petty, W.: The effect of methyl methacrylate on bacterial phagocytosis and killing by human polymorphonuclear leucocytes. J. Bone Joint Surg. 65A:752–757, 1978.
66. Petty, W.: The effect of methyl methacrylate on chemotaxis of polymorphonuclear leucocytes. J. Bone Joint Surg. 60A:492–498, 1978.
67. Petty, W.: The effect of methyl methacrylate on quantitative gel diffusion assay of immunoglobulins. J. Biomed. Mater. Res. 13:645–656, 1979.
68. Petty, W.: Methyl methacrylate concentration in tissues adjacent to bone cement. J. Biomed. Mater. Res. 14:427–434, 1980.
69. Petty, W. and Calldwell, J. R.: The effect of methyl methacrylate on complement activity. Clin. Orthop. 128:354–360, 1977.
70. Pilliar, R. M.: Porous-surfaced metallic implants for orthopedic applications. J. Biomed. Mater. Res. 21[Suppl. A1]:1–33, 1987.
71. Pilliar, R. M., Lee, J. M., and Maniatopoulos, C.: Observations on the effect of movement on bone ingrowth into porous-surfaced implants. Clin. Orthop. 208:108–113, 1986.
72. Poss, R., Brick, G. W., Wright, R. J., et al.: The effects of modern cementing techniques on the longevity of total hip arthroplasty. Orthop. Clin. North Am., 19(3):591–598, 1988.
73. Poss, R., Thilly, W. G., and Kaden, D. A.: Methyl methacrylate is a mutagen for *Salmonella typhimurium*. J. Bone Joint Surg. 61A:1203, 1979.
74. Ranawat, C. S., Rawlins, B. A., and Harju, V. T.: Effect of modern cement technique on acetabular fixation total hip arthroplasty. A retrospective study in matched pairs. Orthop. Clin. North Am. 19(3):599–603, 1988.
75. Rimnac, C. M., Wright, T. M., and McGill, D. L.: The effect of centrifugation on the fracture properties of acrylic bone cements. J. Bone Joint Surg. [Am.] 68(2):281–287, 1986.
76. Ritts, R. E.: Mutagenesis versus carcinogenesis of plastic implants. J. Bone Joint Surg. 61A:1201, 1979.
77. Salvati, E. A., Wilson, P. D., Jr., Jolley, M. N., et al.: A ten-year follow-up study of our first one hundred consecutive Charnley total hip replacements. J. Bone Joint Surg. 63A:753–767, 1981.
78. Sandborn, P. M., Cook, S. D., Spires, W. P., and Kester, M. A.: Tissue response to porous-coated implants lacking initial bone apposition. J. Arthroplasty 3(4):337–346, 1988.
79. Sauer, B. W., Weinstein, A. M., and Klawitter, J. J.: The role of porous polymeric materials in prosthesis attachment. J. Biomed. Mater. Res. 5:145, 1974.
80. Schreurs, B. W., Spierings, P. T., Huiskes, R., and Slooff, T. J.: Effects of preparation techniques on the porosity of acrylic cements. Acta Orthop. Scand. 59(4):403–409, 1988.
81. Sherman, R. M., Byrick, R. J., Kay, J. C., et al.: The role of lavage in preventing hemodynamic and blood-gas changes during cemented arthroplasty. J. Bone Joint Surg. [Am.] 65(4):500–506, 1983.
82. Skinner, H. B. and Murray, W. R.: Variations in the density of bone cement after centrifugation. Clin. Orthop. 207:263–269, 1986.
83. Smith, L.: Ceramic-plastic material as a bone substitute. Arch. Surg. 87:137, 1963.
84. Spector, M., Flemming, W. R., Kreutner, A., et al.: Bone growth into porous high-density polyethylene. J. Biomed. Mater. Res. 7:595, 1976.

85. Spector, M., Harmon, S. L., and Kreutner, A.: Characteristics of tissue growth into Proplast and porous polyethylene implants in bone. J. Biomed. Mater. Res. 13:667, 1979.
86. Spector, M., Michno, M. J., Smarook, W. H., and Kwiatkonski, G. T.: A high-modulus polymer for porous orthopaedic implants: biomechanical compatibility of porous implants. J. Biomed. Mater. Res. 12:665, 1978.
87. Stauffer, R. N.: Ten-year follow-up study of total hip replacement, with particular reference to roentgenographic loosening of the components. J. Bone Joint Surg. 64A:983–990, 1982.
88. Struthers, A. M.: An experimental study of Polyvinyl Sponge as a substitute for bone. Plast. Reconstr. Surg. 15:274, 1955.
89. Stulberg, S. D.: Design Rationale and Clinical Results of a Titanium Porous Coated Total Knee Replacement: The Microloc Total Knee System. Uncemented Total Joint Replacement. Edited by A. M. Weinstein and A. K. Hedley. Phoenix, Harrington Arthritis Research Center, 1984.
90. Taylor, D. R. and Smith, F. B.: Porous methyl methacrylate as an implant material. J. Biomed. Mater. Res. 2:467, 1971.
91. Tullos, H. S., McCaskill, B. L., Dickey, R., and Davidson, J.: Total hip arthroplasty with a low-modulus porous coated femoral component. J. Bone Joint Surg. 66A:888, 1984.
92. Van Mullem, P. J., De Wijn, J. R., and Vaandrager, J. M.: Porous acrylic cement: evaluation of a novel implant material. Ann. Plast. Surg. 21(6):576–582, 1988.
93. Walker, J. L., Gustke, K., Toney, J., et al.: Centrifugation of antibiotic impregnated bone cement. Orthopedics 11(6):891–893, 1988.
94. Weinstein, A. M., Bingham, D. M., Sauer, B. W., et al.: The effect of high pressure insertion and antibiotic inclusions upon the mechanical properties of polymethylmethacrylate. Clin. Orthop. 121:67–73, 1976.
95. Welch, R. B., McGann, W. A., and Picetti, G. D.: Charnley low-friction arthroplasty. A fifteen-to seventeen-year follow-up study. Orthop. Clin. North Am. 19:551–555, 1988.
96. Wixson, R. L., Lautenschlager, E. P., and Novak, M. A.: Vacuum mixing of acrylic bone cement. J. Arthroplasty 2(2):141–149, 1987.
97. Wroblewski, B. M.: Fifteen- to twenty-one-year results of the Charnley low-friction arthroplasty. Clin. Orthop. 211:30–35, 1986.
98. Zweymuller, K. A., Lintner, F. K., and Semlitsch, M. F.: Biologic fixation of a press-fit titanium hip joint endoprosthesis. Clin. Orthop. 235:195–206, 1988.

SECTION III

SYSTEMIC COMPLICATIONS FOR TOTAL JOINT REPLACEMENT

CHAPTER 8

Prevention of Postoperative Infections

J. PHILLIP NELSON

The most serious cause of postoperative morbidity following total joint arthroplasty is deep infection. Although the incidence of this complication has declined significantly during the past 20 years from 8.9 percent to less than 1 percent,[8, 23, 29] infection continues to be a persistent threat to the success of surgery. Infection usually requires removal of all foreign materials, administration of intravenous antibiotics for several weeks, insertion of antibiotic-impregnated cement beads or spacers, and later revision arthroplasty. As a result, the patient experiences prolonged suffering, disability, and further risk of morbidity, as well as the additional hospitalization and expense. For these reasons, surgeons must continue to direct their efforts toward prevention of postoperative infections.

HOST DEFENSE MECHANISMS

Host defense mechanisms are classified as mechanical, cellular, and humoral.[1] Mechanical defenses are the skin and mucous membranes whose actions are enhanced by secretions such as oils, tears, and mucus. Cellular defenses are provided early by phagocytic leukocytes and later by tissue macrophages. Phagocytosis is initiated by tissue injury or invasion of tissue by foreign substances and is dependent on activation by serum complement. Humoral defenses are antibodies produced by lymphocytes and plasma cells that react with specific antigens, such as bacteria, resulting in direct bacteriolysis or phagocytosis enhancement.

Inflammation is the mediator of cellular and humoral defenses because vasodilatation allows increased delivery of white blood cells and serum factors, whereas greater capillary permeability allows local delivery to the affected tissues. Amoeba-like mobility of phagocytic cells permits them to actively pursue and engulf bacteria. The intrinsic vascularity of tissues and their potential for a rapid inflammatory response to injury are therefore of prime importance to the effectiveness of host defenses. Clearly, the presence of devascularized tissue isolated from cellular and humoral defenses predisposes a patient to unbridled bacterial replication and invasion.

Foreign bodies potentiate the virulence of bacteria, i.e., it takes fewer bacteria of almost any type to produce clinical infection in the presence of foreign substances.[3] The exact mechanism for this enhancement of virulence is unknown but it may be related to decrease in local vascularity or direct inhibition of host defenses. Petty[32, 33] has demonstrated that methyl methacrylate monomer inhibits the activity of complement, polymorphonuclear leukocytes, and lymphocytes. Gristina and Costerton[15] have shown that many bacteria produce a slime-like glycocalyx that protects the bacteria from humoral and cellular defenses (Fig. 8–1).

PATHOGENESIS

The response of the body to a surgical wound infection usually includes pain, loss of function, swelling, redness, and increased production of cells and fluid. When surgery violates the mechanical barriers that are part of the host defense system, e.g., the skin and mucous membranes, internal defense barriers become most important—specifically, the nonimmune, nonspecific defense and the immune, specific defense. Nonimmune defense consists of (1) the various antibacterial proteins, such as complement and lysozyme; (2) the vascular responses such as vasodilatation, increased blood flow, and increased vessel permeability; and (3) the production of phagocytes, such as polymorphonuclear leukocytes. The specific immune defense consists of immunoglobulins (antibodies), B lymphocytes, and plasma cells that produce antibodies, and the cellular immunity provided by T lymphocytes. Immune defense is most important for the clearing of established infection, but some components such as the so-called natural or normal antibodies may be important for eradicating bacteria from the tissues before infection is established.

Many factors determine whether an infection occurs in association with surgery: the competency of host defense mechanisms; the type, virulence, and number of implanted bacteria; the presence or absence of foreign body or necrotic tissue; the body region in which surgery is performed; the violation of a contaminated viscus; and the duration and extent of the surgical procedure.

A surgical wound (operation) may be classified as ultraclean, clean, clean-contaminated, contaminated, or dirty, depending on the amount of intrinsic or extrinsic bacterial contamination occurring at the time of wounding or surgery. An example of an ultraclean operation is total joint replacement; laminectomy is a clean operation; hysterectomy is clean-contaminated; colon resection is contaminated; and a mutilating barnyard wound is dirty. The incidence of infection rises with greater amounts of wound contamination.[11, 19] Most, if not all, ultraclean and clean surgical wounds are contaminated with bacteria by the conclusion of the procedure.[6] Postoperative wound infections may be classified as superficial or deep, depending on the relationship to the deep fascia, and early or late, depending on the relationship of the expected time to per primam healing.

Whether infection occurs depends on the type and size of the bacterial inoculum and the competency of host defenses. Krizek and Robson[22] have shown that bacterial invasion and replication in healthy tissue develop only when the concentration of bacteria exceeds 1×10^5 per gram of tissue. However, some types of bacteria are more virulent and therefore fewer are required to establish infection.[38] For example, *Staphylococcus aureus* is more virulent than *S. epidermidis*, and a *Proteus* species is more virulent than *Bacillus subtilis*.

Wound contamination may occur from the patient (endogenous) or from environmental sources (exogenous). Examples of endogenous contamination that may lead to postoperative sepsis include unrecognized preexisting local infection, seeding from intraoperative or postoperative bacteremia, and skin-edge contamination during the operative procedure. Exogenous wound contamination may result from direct inoculation of the wound due to nonsterile technique or from deposition of airborne bacteria on sterile surfaces and into the wound. Airborne exogenous contamination had been relatively neglected as a source of wound infection until the advent of total hip arthroplasty and the attention called to its importance by Charnley.[8, 9]

Traditional antiseptic and sterile technique was primarily concerned with prevention of endogenous and exogenous contact contamination. However, airborne bacteria may abound in an enclosed space such as the operating room. They originate almost exclusively from the bodies of the persons in the room. In an unoccupied conventional operating room, air bacterial sampling shows about one bacterium per cubic foot of air; when several persons enter the operating room, counts increase by at least sixfold.[13] Humans shed microorganisms into the environment at rates up to 5000 colony-forming units per min-

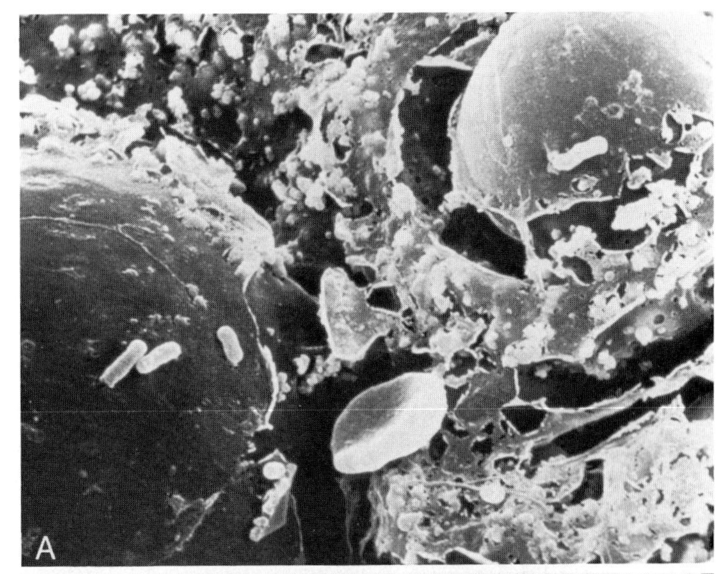

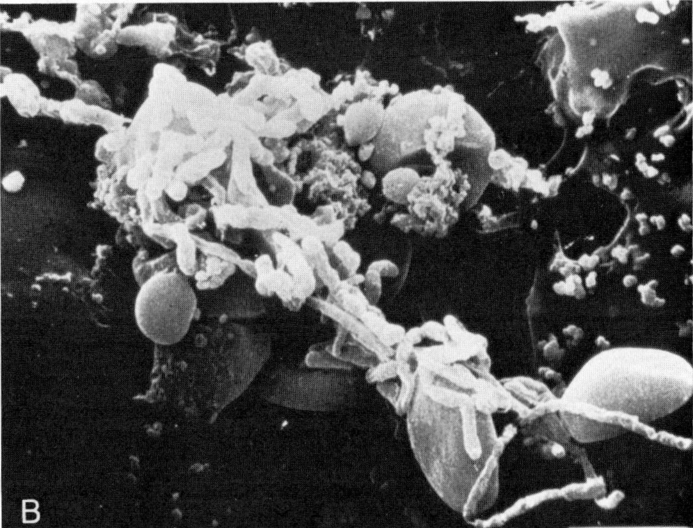

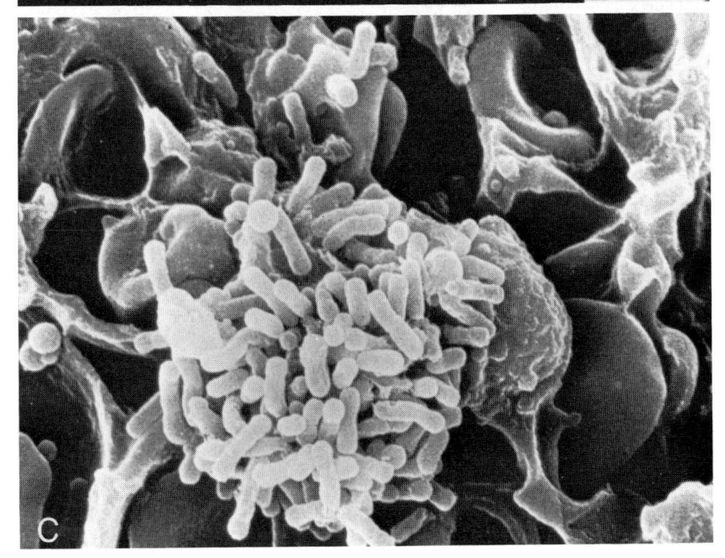

FIGURE 8–1. Biofilm protecting bacteria. *A*, Scanning electron micrograph of intramedullary bone cement from infected and loosened total hip prosthesis showing rod-shaped bacteria in association with and partly buried in extensive biofilm of the cement's surface. *Pseudomonas aeruginosa* was isolated from this specimen. *B*, Biofilm is incompletely formed in this area. Individual adherent bacterial microcolonies can be seen. *C*, Surface of bone from infected total hip joint showing development of discrete adherent microcolonies in which bacteria of a single morphotype are partly surrounded by amorphous condensed material. (Gristina, A. G. and Costerton, J. W.: J. Bone Joint Surg. 67A:264–273, 1985. By permission.)

ute.[34] The rate of shedding depends on a number of factors; some individuals shed more microorganisms than others, and some anatomic areas shed more than others. For instance, the perineum is the area of greatest shedding.[18] When an individual sheds unusually large numbers of bacteria into the air, the person is called a "disperser." Dispersers of pathogenic bacteria have been associated with increased rates of infection.[12, 16, 39, 40] Their presence in the operating room is readily detected with serial airborne bacteria sampling.[13] Shedding is aggravated by increases in personal activity. It decreases when garment barriers are worn. Airborne bacteria are primarily gram-positive aerobes; they reside on particulate matter larger than 2 μm in diameter.[31]

Methods that have proved effective in reducing the concentration of airborne bacteria include increasing air turnover rates, improving air filtration, improving personnel barriers, using positive pressure ventilation, and reducing personnel movement.

PREVENTION

The prevention of postoperative infection is predicated on the reduction of bacterial contamination in the surgical wound and the enhancement of host defenses. Factors that contribute to the occurrence of postoperative infection and methods of controlling or eliminating these factors in the patient, the wound, and the operating room environment are discussed.

Patient Factors

Obesity predisposes a patient to infection for several reasons: (1) fat has a relatively scant blood supply, (2) it interferes with the technical performance of surgery and prolongs operating time, and (3) it creates technical problems in wound closure. Although weight reduction prior to surgery is often not feasible, it may be helpful in the prevention of infection. However, if the patient loses substantial weight, the surgeon must be sure that nutritional status is not compromised or, if it is, that nutritional health is restored before surgery.

Hospitalization for more than a few days preoperatively is associated with a higher incidence of infection. This finding may reflect the fact that a patient who requires hospitalization has seriously impaired general health or it may reflect colonization with more virulent, resistant bacteria from the hospital environment.[10] Because of the possibility that exposure to more virulent bacteria is the cause, preoperative hospitalization should be minimized.

Patients with infections at a distance from the operative sites may have a higher risk of clean wound infection. Examples of sites where such distant infections may occur are the teeth, upper respiratory tract, skin, and urinary tract. Infection in these sites must be diagnosed and eradicated before elective surgery. Patients who carry more virulent strains of so-called pathogenic bacteria in the upper respiratory tract or on the skin may be at risk for postoperative sepsis from these organisms. However, the incidence of this type of endogenous contamination is very low and may be eliminated with proper skin preparation, barrier technique, and preventive antibiotics.

Immunologic deficiency of significant degree always predisposes a patient to postoperative sepsis. The deficiency may be due to physiologic incompetence, such as that associated with the extremes of age, or it may be due to a pathologic cause, such as malnutrition; immunosuppression, resulting from antimetabolite or corticosteroid administration; various forms of malignancy; or a variety of systemic illnesses, such as diabetes and collagen disease. Furthermore, a number of congenital or acquired defects in white blood cell function and antibody production are known that may predispose a patient to infection.[25] A careful history usually elicits clues to these problems. It is important that such conditions be diagnosed precisely and corrected preoperatively, if possible.

Wound Factors

Patients who have undergone previous surgery, those who have had previous infection in the operative site, and those who have coexisting local infection at the time of surgery all have an increased risk of sepsis after total joint arthroplasty. Before proceeding with definitive surgery, examinations and tests may be indicated to rule out subclinical infection, including physical examination and thorough history, erythrocyte sedimentation rate, radiographic and radionuclide scanning studies, aspiration with culture, and even open biopsy.

Shortly before surgery, the skin in the operative area should be examined for lacerations, abrasions, blisters, and established dermatitis. Such lesions may provide an excellent culture medium, providing the inoculum for wound contamination. Shaving of the operative site before surgery should be limited to a small area around the incision and should be done in the operating room just before skin washing. Shaving the operative site several hours earlier stimulates bacterial multiplication and increases the likelihood of infection.[11] Local surface skin bacteria may be reduced at least 90 percent by having operating room personnel wash their hands and the operative site immediately before surgery with povidone-iodine, hexachlorophene, or chlorhexidine. Ritter[36] has demonstrated equally effective reductions in skin bacteria utilizing a hexachlorophene-alcohol surgical hand scrub and an iodophor-solution spray at the surgical site. Gilliam and Nelson[14] have shown that painting the operative site with an iodophor in alcohol solution without any other type of preoperative skin washing reduces surface skin bacteria 88 percent—the same reduction achieved by washing for 5 minutes with an aqueous iodophor scrub. The wound may be further protected from contact contamination by adhesive plastic sheets, which also serve to stabilize drapes. Antibacterial adhesive drapes applied after cleansing the operative site with alcohol solution provide excellent immediate kill of surface bacteria and prolonged bacteriostatic action during the operative procedure.

Patients with poor local vascularity due to extensive scarring from previous injury or surgery are at increased risk for sepsis, presumably because of impaired host defense delivery. Therefore, the scar should be excised when possible. The location, extent, and length of surgery all influence infection rates. For instance, patients who undergo clean knee meniscectomy and hand surgery have low rates of infection; those with hip and back operations have higher rates. Patients whose operations last more than 2 hours have higher infection rates; incidence rises with time.[11] It is therefore important to maximize surgical efficiency.

Some surgeons have lower rates of postoperative infections than others. All other factors being equal, the difference appears to be related to surgical skill, which, in turn, is governed by the principles of surgical technique. The basic tenets of surgical technique are careful retraction and sharp dissection to avoid necrotic tissue, careful hemostasis to avoid hematoma, minimization of dead space to avoid hematoma and seroma, debridement of necrotic tissue, meticulous but nontense wound closure, and suction drainage with small tubes through separate stab incisions. Wounds should be irrigated frequently to prevent wound drying and to wash out necrotic debris and bacteria.

Incontrovertible evidence exists that preventive antibiotics reduce the incidence of deep postoperative infection following clean implant surgery.[37] Miles and associates[26] and Burke[7] showed that antibiotics must be present in tissues in therapeutic levels at the time of wounding to be effective. Because all antibiotics rapidly achieve therapeutic levels in bone, they should be given within 1 hour before surgery is started. Schurman and Goodman[38] recommend that antibiotics be administered in the operating theater when anesthesia is induced. Some controversy exists about how long intravenous antibiotics should be given after surgery, but current recommendations are for no more than 72 hours[38]; many believe that 24 hours or less may be sufficient.[28, 41] A first-generation cephalosporin such as cefazolin is recommended unless the patient has a penicillin allergy or the institutional incidence of methicillin-resistant *Staphylococcus* infections is high; in these cases, vancomycin or clindamycin should be given.[38, 41] The initial bolus may be up to 2 gm because higher bone levels are achieved. This dose may be followed by 1 gm administered every 8 hours for the duration of treatment. Recommended manufacturer's dose schedules and precautions should be followed. Cephalosporins are bactericidal, effective against the most common postoperative pathogens (*Staphylococcus aureus* and *S. epidermidis*), and produce minimal allergic and systemic toxic side effects. If the patient is allergic to the antibiotic, this complication is more easily controlled under general anesthesia. The 1- to 3-day regimen minimizes the development of resistant organisms.

Topical antibiotic irrigations of neomycin, kanamycin, and polymyxin, either singly or in combination, during the operative procedure have not been definitely proven to reduce postoperative infections. Copious irrigations with any physiologic fluid remove loose foreign and necrotic debris and probably reduce superficial surface bacterial contamination if the fluid is sterile. However, Halarj[17] believed, in a literature survey, that topical antibiotics were effective. Benjamin and Volz[4] showed that topical antibiotic irrigations are very effective *in vitro* when compared with saline and that therapeutic tissue concentrations of neomycin are achieved *in vivo* via irrigations. Pulsatile lavage further enhances the clearance of detritus from the wound. If an intraoperative autotransfusion system is employed, care must be taken to avoid mixing topical antibiotic irrigant with blood. Liquid irrigant must be completely removed from blood salvaged for autotransfusion because of the potential systemic toxicity of neomycin, kanamycin, and polymyxin.

The addition of antibiotics to cement for the prevention of postoperative sepsis has achieved wide acceptance, particularly in Europe, where the work of Buchholz and Gartmann[5] and that of Josefsson, Lindberg, and Wiklander[21] have demonstrated the effectiveness of prophylactic gentamicin in polymethyl methacrylate. Gentamicin and other heat-stable antibiotics elute from cement, initially in very high local concentration, falling to a low concentration within a few days. However, preventive antibiotics in bone cement have not been widely utilized in the United States for several reasons: the possibility of allergy, the impairment in the strength of the cement caused by addition of the antibiotic, and the lack of uniform mixing of the antibiotic in cement. Also, rates of infection in the United States are already low because of the use of preventive antibiotics, improved air control, and barrier techniques. In patients at an increased risk of postoperative infection, it does seem reasonable and prudent to include antibiotics in the cement. Examples are patients undergoing revision arthroplasty for aseptic loosening, those undergoing reconstruction after previous deep implant infection, and those undergoing revision in which cement is used. Tobramycin is the aminoglycoside of choice in the United States because gentamicin is not available in powder form. No allergies have been reported. No reports have appeared of premature cement decay or of loosening associated with the inclusion of up to 2 gm of powdered antibiotic per 40 gm of polymethyl methacrylate.[27]

Factors in the immediate postoperative period that do not appear to influence the incidence of infection include the type of skin closure, the type of dressings and how long they are left in place, the amount and timing of patient mobility, and the short-term (2 days or less) use of suction drains.

The major cause of deep wound infection in the postoperative period is a draining hematoma. When it occurs, retrograde contamination and infection with gram-negative microorganisms can be expected. Expanding tense hematomas should be drained in the operating room employing full surgical and antiseptic precautions.

Operating Room Environment

Wound or sterile surface contamination by the exogenous contact route always results from a violation of the principles of sterile technique. A glove hole or a torn drape or gown may be the cause. Soaked cotton drapes and gowns rapidly transfer bacteria from unsterile to sterile surfaces by capillary action.[9] Instruments and implants contaminated because of sterilization failure are another source of contact contamination. To counteract these sources of contamination and potential wound sepsis, the operating team must be constantly alert for violation of sterile and antiseptic procedures. Double gloves are suggested for all but the most delicate procedures. Drape and gown materials such as finely woven cotton, plastic-backed paper, and woven polymers should supplant regular cotton.[35]

Airborne contamination of wounds and

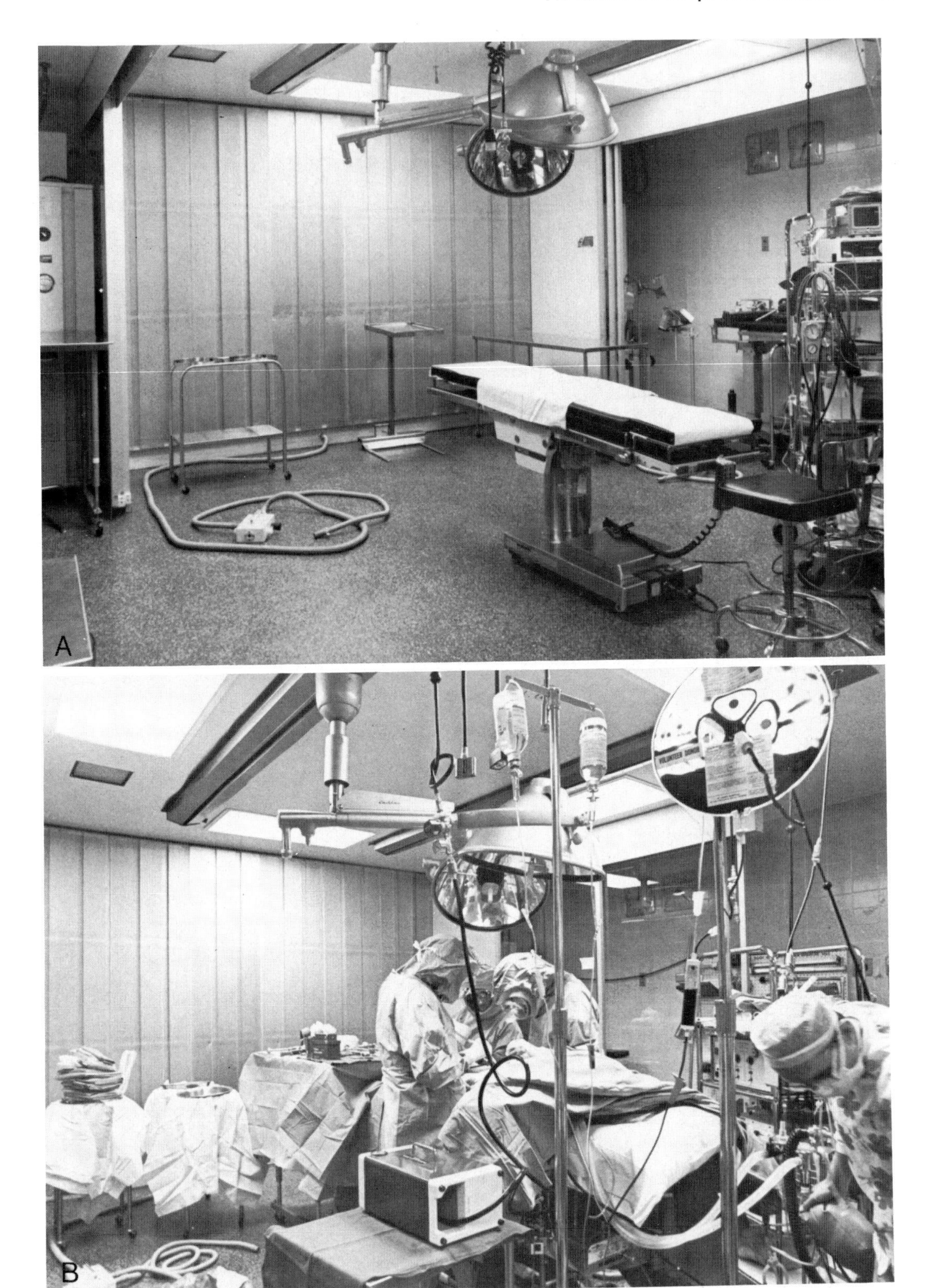

FIGURE 8–2. Horizontal laminar airflow. *A*, Unoccupied, horizontal, laminar-flow clean room that is 12 ft wide with retractable side walls installed in the existing operating room. *B*, The same operating room with personal isolator system in use during total hip arthroplasty operation.

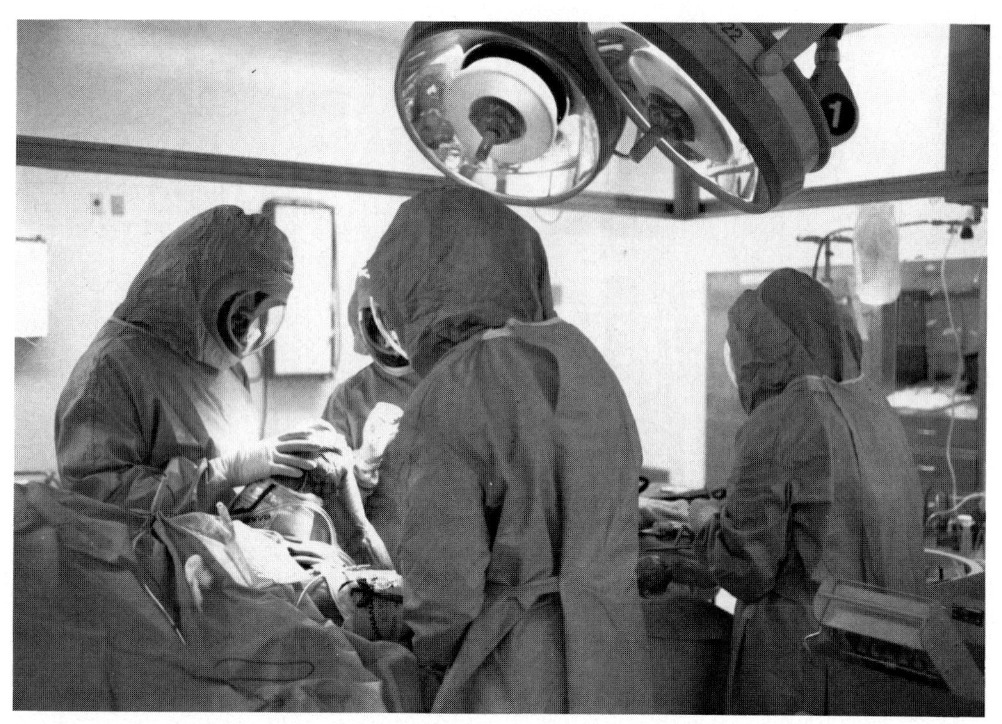

FIGURE 8–3. Vertical laminar flow with personal isolator system.

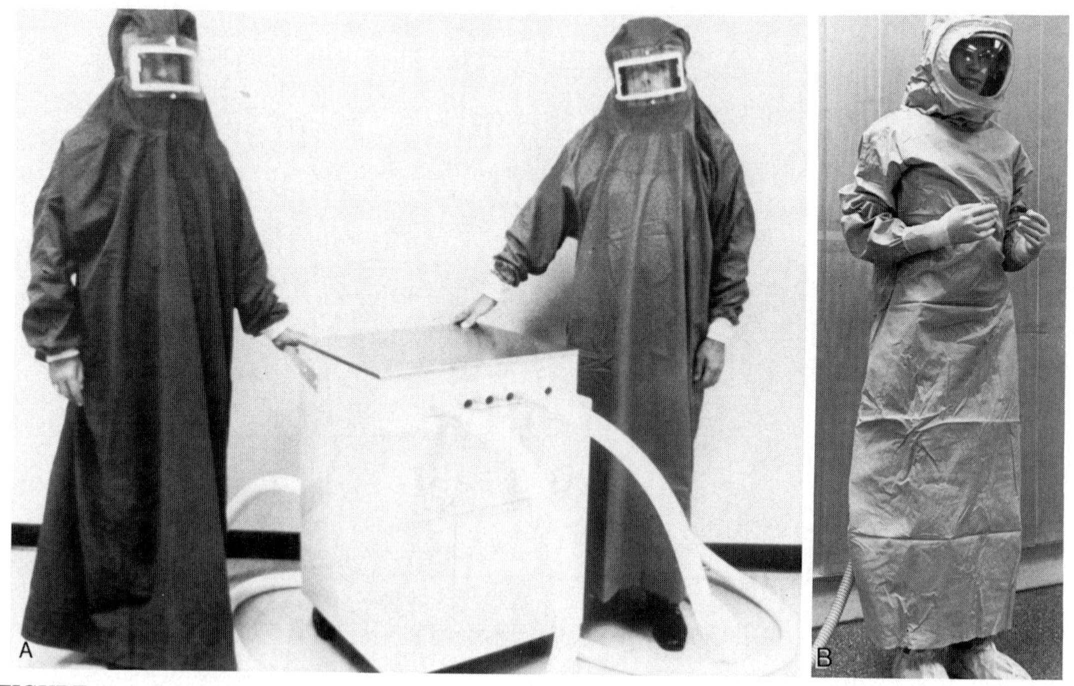

FIGURE 8–4. Personal isolation system. *A*, Original Charnley design of the personal isolator system. *B*, Disposable personal isolator system.

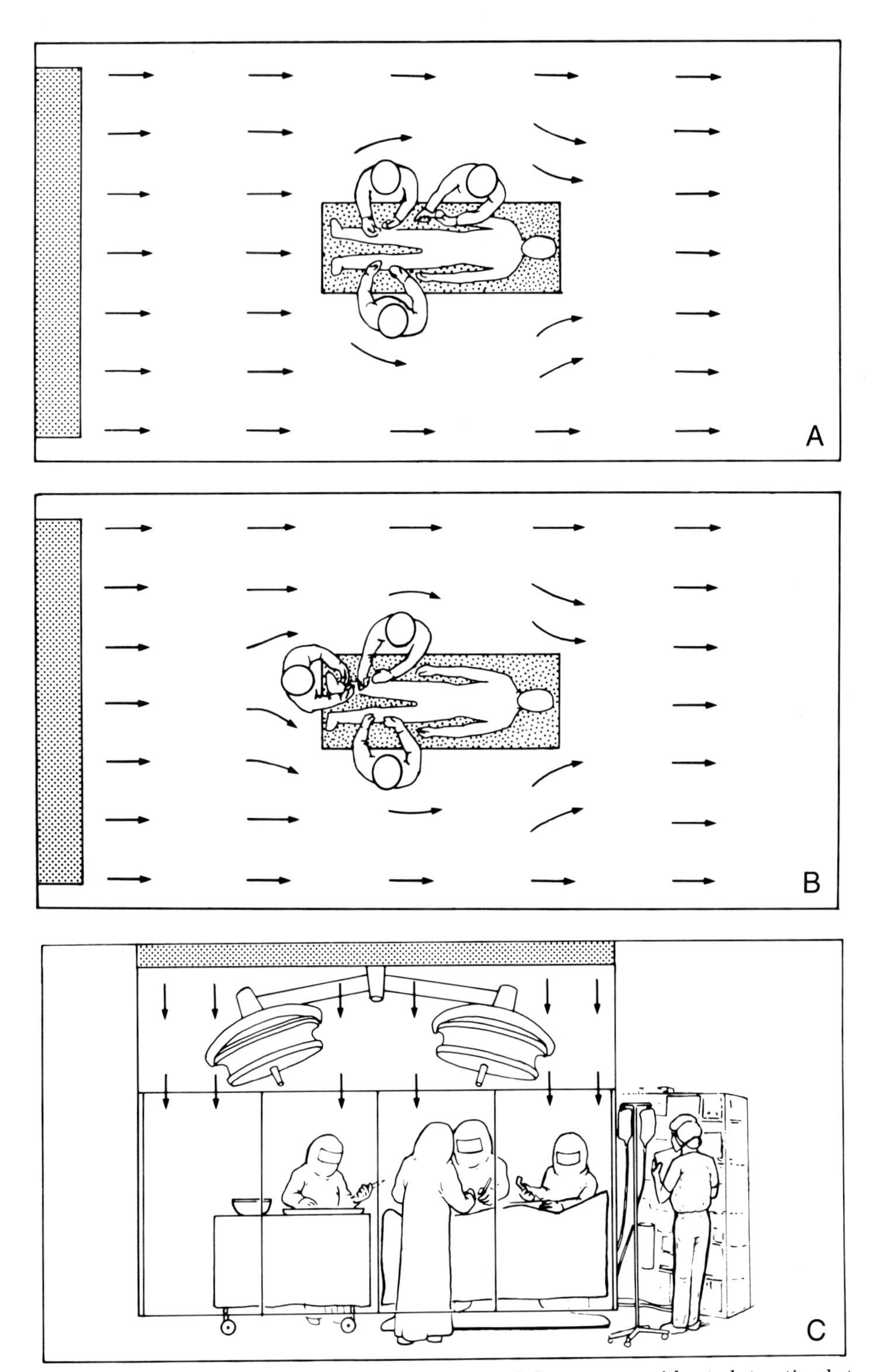

FIGURE 8–5. Ultraclean air-handling systems. *A*, Horizontal flow system, without obstruction between air source and operative wound. *B*, Obstruction of air source by operating room personnel, with the potentially increased risk of infection. *C*, Vertical system combined with body exhaust apparatus providing excellent operative environment. Body exhaust systems with either horizontal or vertical system free the surgical team from concern about coming between air source and operative wound.

sterile surfaces is a major hazard in clean implant surgery; the source is always microorganisms shed by the individuals in the operating room.[8, 29] Relatively high airborne bacterial concentrations (over five viable particles per cubic foot) are the result of inadequate exchange rates of operating room air and poor control of personnel shedding. Standard air filters should be replaced periodically in order to reduce the possibility of introducing microorganisms from the general hospital environment or even from the exterior environment. In some older operating rooms, air is exchanged less than 12 times hourly, contributing to high concentrations of airborne bacteria shed by active operating room staff. Airflow patterns in standard operating rooms are turbulent. They may be checked with smoke tests to determine whether clearance is relatively rapid in the area of surgery. Air pressure should be greater in the operating room than in the corridor to create a positive pressure gradient toward the corridor. Temperature should be 70°F and humidity as close to 50 percent as possible.[2]

Convincing evidence has been published that airborne bacteria are associated with the majority of postoperative implant infections.[8, 19, 23] For this reason, the use of a clean room or ultraviolet light[19] should be seriously considered, because both reduce the concentrations of airborne bacteria markedly. The clean room alone reduces at-wound airborne bacterial concentration and sterile surface contamination by 80 percent. When helmet aspirator systems are also worn, the reduction is at least 95 percent. Our data showed a reduction in deep total hip arthroplasty infection rates from 5.8 percent in a regular operating room to 0.6 percent in a clean room.[29] Lidwell[23] showed a 50-percent reduction in the clean room and an additional 25-percent reduction when helmet aspirator systems were used in total hip and knee arthroplasties (Figs. 8–2, 8–3, 8–4, and 8–5).

Late Hematogenous Infection

The occurrence of late deep total joint infection caused by bacteremia from a distant site of infection is well known. If an infection at a distant site develops in a patient with a total joint implant, the infection should be vigorously and promptly treated with the appropriate antibiotics as determined by culture and sensitivity results or empirically, if cultures cannot be obtained.

Antibiotic prophylaxis against bacteremic seeding of a total joint replacement in a patient who is planning to undergo a dental procedure, genitourinary tract operation, or gastrointestinal surgery is more controversial. Some surgeons would argue that the morbidity and cost associated with prophylaxis for these patients outweigh the preventive benefits, because the incidence of deep implant infection is very low. However, most surgeons in the United States are strong advocates of this type of prophylactic measure. For patients who plan to undergo dental procedures in which the risk of streptococcal infection is high, penicillin V is recommended, 2 gm, 1 hour before the procedure and 1 gm, 6 hours later.[30] A cephalosporin may be used. If penicillin is contraindicated, erythromycin may be substituted. For other procedures in areas with different indigenous microflora, antibiotic prophylaxis must be individualized and directed against the local bacterial population. The advice of an infectious disease specialist may be helpful in any difficult situation.

References

1. Alexander, J. W.: Host defense mechanisms against infection. Surg. Clin. North Am. 52:1367–1378, 1972.
2. Altemier, W. A., Burke, J. F., Pruitt, B. A., and Sandusky, W. R.: Manual on Control of Infection in Surgical Patients. Philadelphia, J. B. Lippincott Company, 1976.
3. Altemier, W. A. and Furste, W. L.: Studies in the virulence of *Clostridium welchii*. Surgery 25:12–19, 1949.
4. Benjamin, J. B. and Volz, R. G.: Efficacy of topical antibiotic irrigant in decreasing or eliminating bacterial contamination in surgical wounds. Clin. Orthop. 184:114–117, 1984.
5. Buchholz, H. W. and Gartmann, H. D.: Infektions Prophylaxe und Operative Behandlund der Schleichen tiefen Infektion beider Totalen Endoprosthese. Chirurg 43:453, 1972.
6. Burke, J. F.: Identification of the sources of staphylococci contaminating the surgical wound during operations. Ann. Surg. 158:898, 1963.
7. Burke, J. F.: The effective period of preventative antibiotic action in experimental incisions and dermal lesions. Surgery 50:161, 1961.

8. Charnley, J.: Postoperative infection after total hip replacement with special reference to air contamination in the operating room. Clin. Orthop. 87:167–187, 1972.
9. Charnley, J. and Eftekhar, N.: Penetration of gown material by organisms from the surgeon's body. Lancet 1:172, 1969.
10. Cruse, P. J. E. and Foord, R.: A five-year prospective study of 23,649 surgical wounds. Arch. Surg. 107:206–210, 1973.
11. Cruse, P. J. E. and Foord, R.: The epidemiology of wound infections. Surg. Clin. North Am. 60:27, 1980.
12. Dineen, P.: Influence of operating room conduct on wound infections. Surg. Clin. North Am. 55:1283, 1975.
13. Fitzgerald, R. H., Jr. and Peterson, L. F. A.: Wound Contamination and Deep Wound Sepsis. Infection in Joint Replacement Surgery. Edited by N. Eftekhar. St. Louis, C. V. Mosby, 1984.
14. Gilliam, D. L. and Nelson, C. L.: Comparison of a one-step iodophor skin preparation versus traditional preparation in total joint surgery. Clin. Orthop. 250:258–260, 1990.
15. Gristina, A. G. and Costerton, J. W.: Bacterial adherence and the glycocalyx and their role in musculoskeletal infection. Orthop. Clin. North Am. 15:517, 1984.
16. Gryska, P. F. and O'Dea, A. E.: Postoperative streptococcal wound infections: The anatomy of an epidemic. J.A.M.A. 213:1189, 1970.
17. Halarj, N. A.: Wound infection and topical antibiotics. Arch. Surg. 112:1240–1244, 1977.
18. Hill, J., et al.: Effects of clothing on dispersal of *Staphylococcus aureus* by males and females. Lancet 2:1131, 1974.
19. Howard, J. M., et al.: Postoperative wound infections: The influence of ultraviolet irradiation of the operating room and of various other factors. Am. Surg. 160[Suppl]:1, 1964.
20. Jaspers, M. T. and Little, J. W.: Prophylactic antibiotic coverage in patients with total arthroplasty: Current practice. J. Am. Dent. Assn. 111:943–948, 1985.
21. Josefsson, G., Lindberg, L., and Wiklander, B.: Systemic antibiotics and gentamicin-containing bone cement in the prophylaxis of postoperative infections in total hip arthroplasty. Clin. Orthop. 159:194, 1981.
22. Krizek, T. J. and Robson, M. C.: Biology of surgical infection. Surg. Clin. North Am. 55:1261, 1975.
23. Lidwell, O. M.: Infection following orthopaedic surgery in conventional and unidirectional airflow operating theatres: The results of a prospective randomized study. Br. Med. J. 285:10, 1982.
24. Lowell, J. D.: Use of Ultraviolet Radiation in Total Joint Replacement Surgery. Infections in Total Joint Replacement. Edited by N. Eftekhar. St. Louis, C. V. Mosby, 1984.
25. Manicol, M. F.: Osseous Infections and Immunodeficiency. Musculoskeletal Infections. Edited by S. P. F. Hughes and R. H. Fitzgerald, Jr. Chicago, Year Book Medical Publishers, Inc., 1986.
26. Miles, A. A., Miles, E. M., and Burke, J.: The value and duration of defense reactions of the skin to primary lodgement of bacteria. Br. J. Exp. Path. 38:79, 1959.
27. Nelson, C. L. and Bergman, B.: Antibiotic Impregnated Acrylic Composites. Infection in Joint Replacement Surgery. Edited by N. Eftekhar. St. Louis, C. V. Mosby, 1984.
28. Nelson, C. L., Green, T. G., Porter, K. A., and Warren, R. D.: One day versus seven days of preventative antibiotic therapy in orthopaedic surgery. Clin. Orthop. 176:258–263, 1983.
29. Nelson, J. P.: The Operating Room Environment and Its Influence on Deep Wound Infections. The Hip: Proceedings of the Fifth Open Scientific Meeting of the Hip Society. St. Louis, C. V. Mosby, 1977.
30. Nelson, J. P., Fitzgerald, R. H., Jr., Jaspers, M. T., and Little, J. W.: Prophylactic antimicrobial coverage in arthroplasty patients. J. Bone Joint Surgery 72A:1, 1990.
31. Noble, W. C., Lidwell, O. M., and Kingston, D.: The size distribution of airborne particles carrying microorganisms. J. Hyg. (Camb.) 61:358, 1963.
32. Petty, W.: The effect of methyl methacrylate on bacterial phagocytosis and killing by human polymorphonuclear leukocytes. J. Bone Joint Surg. 60A:752–757, 1978.
33. Petty, W.: The effect of methyl methacrylate on chemotaxis of polymorphonuclear leucocytes. J. Bone Joint Surg. 60A:492–498, 1978.
34. Riemensnider, D. K.: Human Bacterial Shedding in Workshop on Control of Operating Room Airborne Bacteria. Washington, D.C., National Academy of Sciences, 1976.
35. Ritter, M. A.: Ecology of the Operating Room, pp. 138–139. Infection in Joint Replacement Surgery. Edited by N. Eftekhar. St. Louis, C. V. Mosby, 1984.
36. Ritter, M. A.: Ecology of the Operating Room, pp. 144–146. Infection in Joint Replacement Surgery. Edited by N. Eftekhar. St. Louis, C. V. Mosby, 1984.
37. Schurman, D. J.: Use of Systemic Antibiotics in Total Joint Replacement. Infection in Joint Replacement Surgery. Edited by N. Eftekhar. St. Louis, C. V. Mosby, 1984.
38. Schurman, D. J. and Goodman, J. B.: Surgical Prophylaxis. Orthopaedic Infections. Edited by R. D. D'Ambrosia and R. L. Morier. Thorofare, New Jersey, Slack, 1989.
39. Walter, C. W. and Kundsin, R. B.: The airborne component of wound contamination and infection. Arch. Surg. 107:588, 1973.
40. Walter, C. W., Kundsin, R. B., and Brubaker, M. M.: The incidence of airborne wound infections during operations. J.A.M.A. 186:903, 1963.
41. Williams, D. N.: Antibiotic Prophylaxis in Bone and Joint Surgery. Orthopaedic Infections. Edited by R. B. Gustilo. Philadelphia, W. B. Saunders Company, 1989.

CHAPTER 9

Thromboembolic Disease

WILLIAM PETTY
C. McCOLLISTER EVARTS

Thromboembolism is a major complication of certain medical conditions, elective surgery, and trauma. Deep venous thrombosis may develop as the result of vessel wall injury, local venous stasis, and release of factors that activate the coagulation system. All of these events are prominent following a major operation, such as total hip or knee arthroplasty, accounting for the high incidence of both venous thrombosis and pulmonary embolism in the unprotected patient.

Although venous thrombosis of the lower extremity may lead to continuing symptoms, such as leg edema and even leg ulcer, the major concern is development of pulmonary embolism.[29] Between 10 and 20 percent of thrombi associated with hip or knee surgery occur in the femoral and popliteal veins—the locations from which a pulmonary embolus is most likely to arise.[13, 15]

Venous thrombosis is the most common complication after lower extremity surgery in adults, occurring in 40 to 60 percent of patients over age 40 years who are undergoing surgery about the hip or knee. Pulmonary embolism is the most common fatal complication following lower extremity trauma or surgery: 1 to 3 percent of patients having total hip replacements without prophylactic measures experience fatal pulmonary emboli.[14, 24] It is estimated that 150,000 to 200,000 fatalities per year in the United States are the result of pulmonary embolisms. Many of these deaths occur in individuals with conditions that are otherwise not fatal.

Major risk factors for development of thromboembolic disease include advanced age, immobility, prior thromboembolic disease or vein surgery, obesity, malignancy, leg edema, and operation on the trunk or lower extremities (Table 9–1).[17, 30] Deep

Table 9–1. RISK FACTORS PREDISPOSING A PATIENT TO THROMBOEMBOLIC DISEASE*

Risk factors
Inherited risk factors
Antithrombin III deficiency
Protein C deficiency
Protein S deficiency
Dysfibrinogenemia
Disorders of plasminogen and plasminogen activation
Acquired risk factors
Lupus anticoagulant
Nephrotic syndrome
Paroxysmal nocturnal hemoglobinuria
Cancer
Stasis—congestive heart failure, myocardial infarction, cardiomyopathy, constrictive pericarditis, anasarca
Advancing age
Estrogen therapy
Sepsis
Immobilization
Stroke
Polycythemia rubra vera
Inflammatory bowel disease
Obesity
Prior thromboembolic disease
Prior vein surgery
Trunk or lower extremity surgery

*Modified from Prevention of Venous Thrombosis and Pulmonary Embolism. National Institutes of Health Consensus Development Conference Statement. Vol. 6, No. 2, 1986.

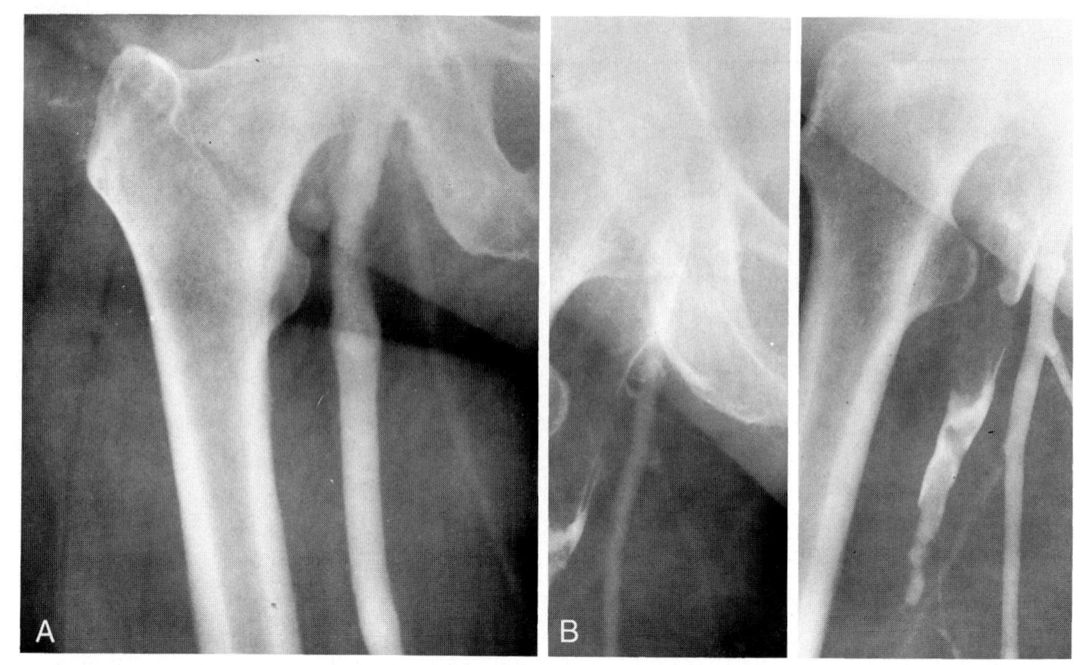

FIGURE 9–1. Venography of lower extremity. *A*, Normal examination findings. *B*, Multiple thrombi.

vein thrombosis and fatal pulmonary embolism are relatively uncommon in Orientals.[17] Among elderly patients with hip fractures that require surgical fixation and among patients with total hip or knee replacements, thromboembolic disease is less likely with spinal anesthesia than with general anesthesia, possibly because of the vasodilation and increased blood flow resulting from the effect of spinal anesthesia on vascular tone.[21, 27] Thromboembolism may be less likely with cementless than with cemented total hip or total knee replacement,[9, 20] perhaps because less debris is introduced into the venous system without cement. A study in dogs that had cemented hip replacements demonstrated venous endothelial damage, which might serve as a nidus for the initiation of a venous thrombus.[28]

DIAGNOSIS

Venous Thrombosis

Evaluation of patients at risk for thromboembolic disease includes physical examination, venography, radioactive scanning, and measurement of outflow obstruction. Relying exclusively on history and physical examination, including complaints of pain, swelling, tenderness, Homans sign, fever, and leukocytosis, leads to the marked underdiagnosis of thromboembolic disease. Only 5 to 30 percent of venous thromboses will be detected by physical examination alone. Conversely, 50 percent of all patients suspected by physical examination to have venous thromboses in fact do not.

Venography is the most accurate evaluation technique for diagnosing venous thrombosis (Fig. 9–1). This technique has many disadvantages: it is painful, it cannot be repeated frequently, it must be performed by experienced personnel, and it may cause venous thrombosis. Allergic reaction to the dye occurs in approximately 1 in 5000 cases and has resulted occasionally in fatalities. Despite these disadvantages, phlebography is consistently accurate in the calf and femoral veins and approximately 70 percent accurate in the iliac veins. This accuracy has made venography the test by which other evaluation methods are assessed. Venography has been especially valuable in clinical research on thromboembolic disease.

Radioactive fibrinogen (^{125}I) scanning is 90 percent accurate in detecting venous thromboses in the absence of recent trauma or surgery in the area being evaluated. Trauma or recent surgery will cause increased uptake on scanning. Therefore, this examination would not be helpful, for example, in the proximal thigh following hip surgery. Radioactive scanning causes little discomfort for the patient and may be repeated as often as required.

Measurements of outflow obstruction include pneumatic plethysmography, cuff-impedance phlebography, and Doppler ultrasound techniques. Most accurate for thrombi in major veins, these methods may complement radioactive fibrinogen studies. Advances such as real-time B-mode ultrasound have led to continued improvement in accuracy and sensitivity, even in smaller veins. Preliminary studies suggest that these improved techniques may be equal or even superior to venography (Figs. 9–2 and 9–3). Unlike venography, ultrasound venous imaging is noninvasive and is not painful, and it will not cause deep venous thrombosis.[10, 31, 32] Because of these advantages, real-time B-mode ultrasound is being utilized increasingly for diagnosis of deep venous thrombosis, both clinically and experimentally.

Another diagnostic method under study is coagulolysis assay. In this technique, the coagulation and fibrinolysis processes are assessed by evaluating products in the serum. This method shows some promise but will require considerable improvement and verification of accuracy before it can be considered for routine clinical use.[19]

Pulmonary Embolism

Although venous thrombosis is common in patients with major risk factors, occurring in about 50 percent of such patients, pulmonary embolism is not nearly as common. The incidence of pulmonary embolism is only about 10 percent but is a very serious complication. Physical signs and symptoms of pulmonary embolism may be misleading. Hence, they should not be con-

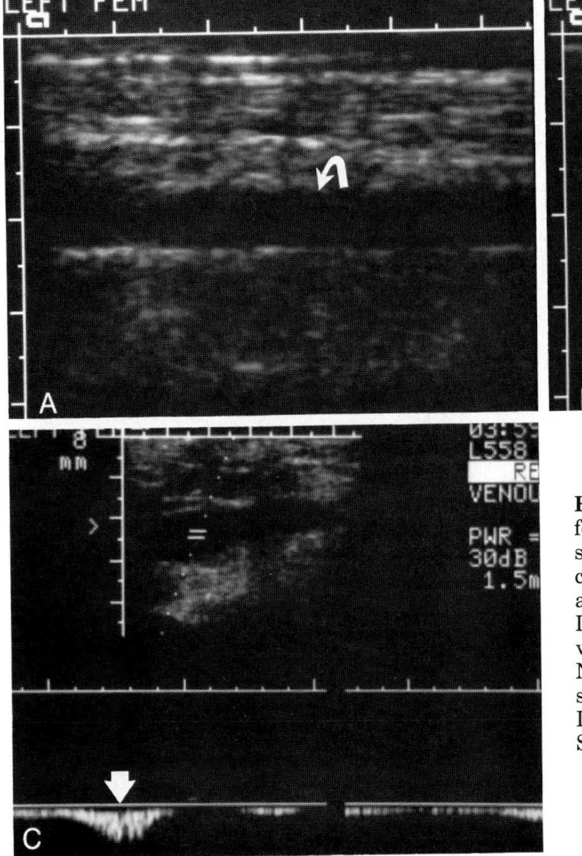

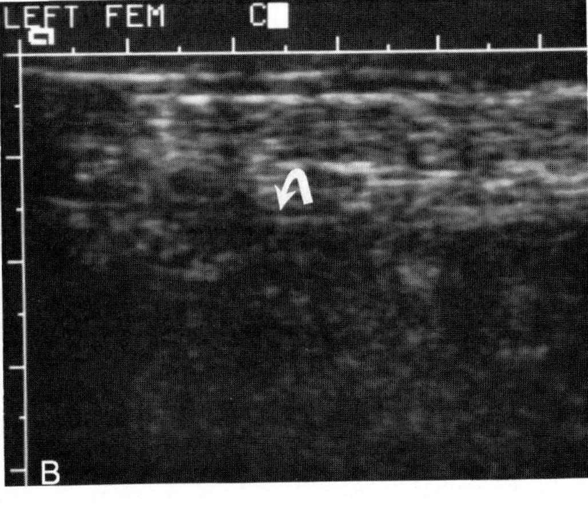

FIGURE 9–2. Ultrasonograms of the superficial femoral vein. *A*, Longitudinal ultrasonogram of the superficial femoral vein (curved arrow), without compression. *B*, Longitudinal ultrasonogram made at the same location as *A* but with compression. *C*, Doppler ultrasonogram demonstrating spontaneous venous flow and respiratory variation or plasticity. Normal augmentation of flow occurs after compression of the calf (large arrow). (Froehlich, J. A., Dorfman, G. S., Cronan, J. J., et al.: J. Bone Joint Surg. 71A:249–256, 1989. By permission.)

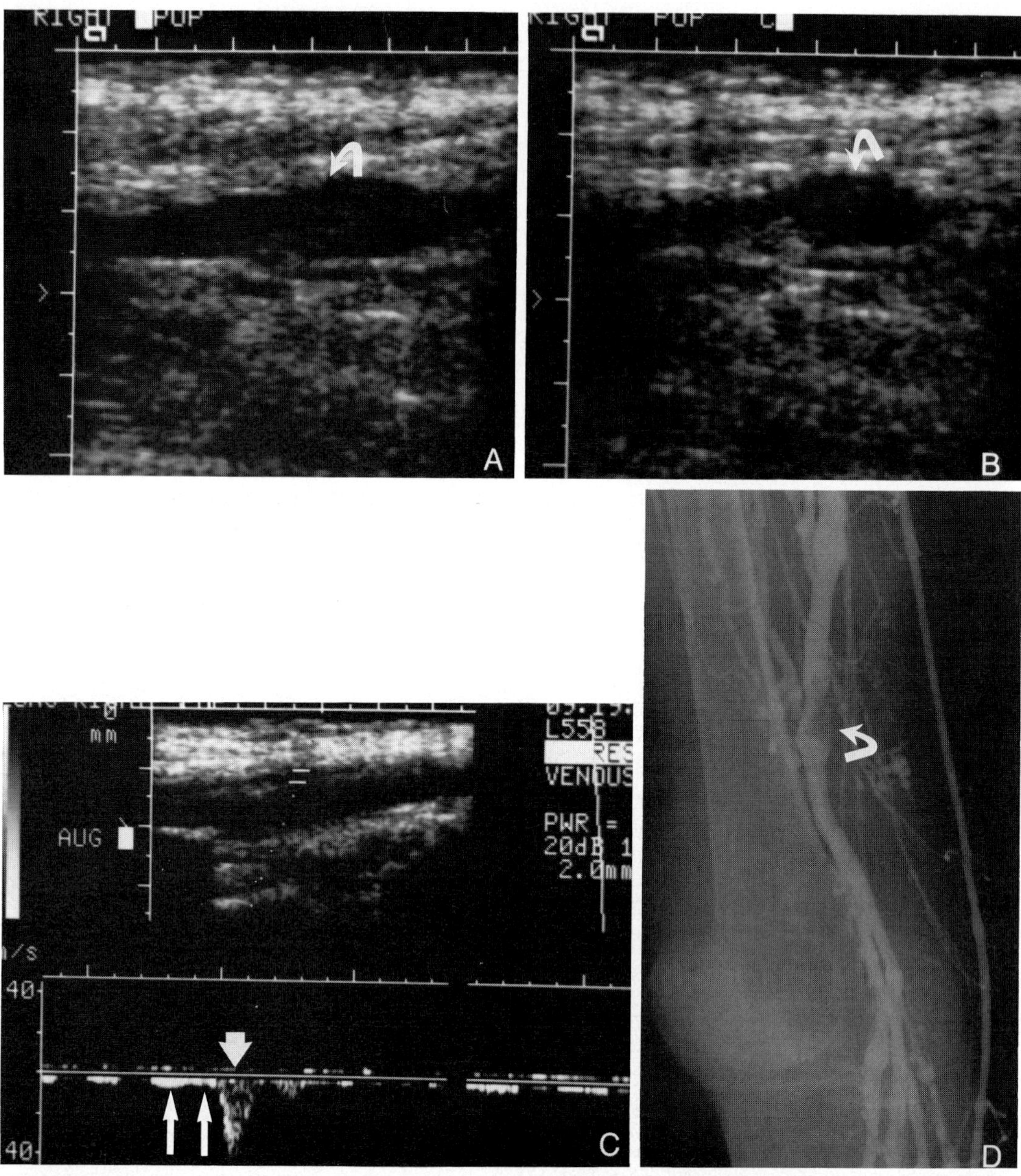

FIGURE 9–3. Ultrasonograms of the popliteal vein. *A*, Longitudinal ultrasonogram of the popliteal vein (curved arrow) at the adductor hiatus. Note the focal area of dilation. *B*, Longitudinal ultrasonogram made at the same location as in *A* but with compression. The focal area of noncompressibility (curved arrow) is indicative of an intraluminal thrombus. *C*, Doppler ultrasonogram made at the same location as *A* demonstrating spontaneous phasic flow (small arrows) and augmentation (large arrow) with compression of the calf. This finding is indicative of a nonocclusive thrombus. *D*, Control contrast venogram demonstrating a focal nonocclusive thrombus (curved arrow) at the location that was predicted by compression ultrasonography in *C*. (Froehlich, J. A., Dorfman, G. S., Cronan, J. J., et al.: J. Bone Joint Surg. 71A:249–256, 1989. By permission.)

sidered diagnostic but should lead to further evaluation.

Arterial oxygenation has been suggested as a screening test for pulmonary embolism. Although the partial pressure of oxygen (Po_2) will seldom be higher than 80 to 90 mmHg with significant pulmonary embolism, this thromboembolic event has been documented with a Po_2 as high as 84 mmHg. Furthermore, some patients without pulmonary embolisms will have a Po_2 of less than 80 to 90 mmHg following major surgery, such as total hip arthroplasty.[4] The arterial puncture for blood gas evaluation should be made before the patient undergoes anticoagulation, to avoid the possibility of severe sequelae. Arterial puncture while anticoagulation is evidenced may lead to substantial hematoma and result in skin slough, neuropathy, and muscle ischemia. Once a patient is receiving full anticoagulation therapy, the response should be followed by some means other than blood gas evaluation through arterial puncture.

When pulmonary embolism is suspected clinically, the patient should undergo a ventilation and perfusion scan (Figs. 9–4 and 9–5). If this examination is consistent with pulmonary embolism, appropriate therapy can be started. When the diagnosis remains in question, pulmonary angiography may be necessary (Fig. 9–6). These objective tests may also be necessary if recurrent pulmonary embolism is suspected while the patient is receiving adequate anticoagulation therapy, in which case vena cava interruption may be indicated.

Because venous thrombosis is common but does not in itself usually lead to serious sequelae, it would be best if pulmonary embolism were treated only when it occurred. Unfortunately, this is not practical. About 80 percent of pulmonary emboli are not suspected, and about 60 percent of patients with fatal pulmonary embolism die within 30 minutes of the first symptoms. Once pulmonary embolism is diagnosed, treatment is full anticoagulation, which may lead to significant bleeding complications in the operative wound as well as in other sites.

Because it is not possible to predict which patients are going to develop pulmonary embolism following a deep venous clot, the consensus is that all high-risk patients should be treated to prevent the onset of thromboembolic disease.

PROPHYLACTIC TREATMENT

Two methods have been recommended for the prevention of thromboembolic disease: (1) anticoagulants and antithrombotics and (2) physical and mechanical measures. The ideal treatment would be highly effective in preventing thromboembolic disease and would have few if any potential complications.

Anticoagulants and Antithrombotics

Drugs that have an anticoagulant or antithrombotic effect are the most thoroughly studied means of preventing thromboembolic disease. Because of their action, however, these drugs are associated with the risk of bleeding complications.

Warfarin

Sodium warfarin has been demonstrated to reduce the occurrence of both venous thrombosis and pulmonary embolism.[1, 5, 8, 11, 19, 23] Warfarin is probably most effective if begun prior to elective surgery, but it can prevent pulmonary embolism, especially fatal pulmonary embolism, if begun 1 to 5 days following elective surgery.

The warfarin dose is adjusted according to the prothrombin time. Classically, the warfarin dose has been adjusted to alter prothrombin activity such that the prothrombin test is 1.5 to 2 times normal. However, this high level causes bleeding in the postoperative patient. Prophylaxis has been shown to be just as effective when the prothrombin time is maintained in the range of 1.3 to 1.5 times control. At this level, bleeding complications are lessened. Thus, 1.5 times control is the maximum that the prothrombin time should reach; 3 or 4 seconds over control is sufficient.[1, 8]

The most common complication of warfarin therapy is bleeding, usually from the operative wound. Bleeding complications also occur in other sites, especially the gastrointestinal tract. Significant hematoma formation occurs in approximately 5 to 15 percent of patients treated with warfarin. This complication may be reduced to 1 percent with the low-dose regimen in patients having cemented arthroplasty. As mentioned, the risk of bleeding seems to be somewhat higher with cementless arthroplasty, probably because there is no tamponade of intraosseous bleeding from the cement.[1] As many as 5 percent of wound hematomas will require aspiration or surgical evacuation or will drain spon-

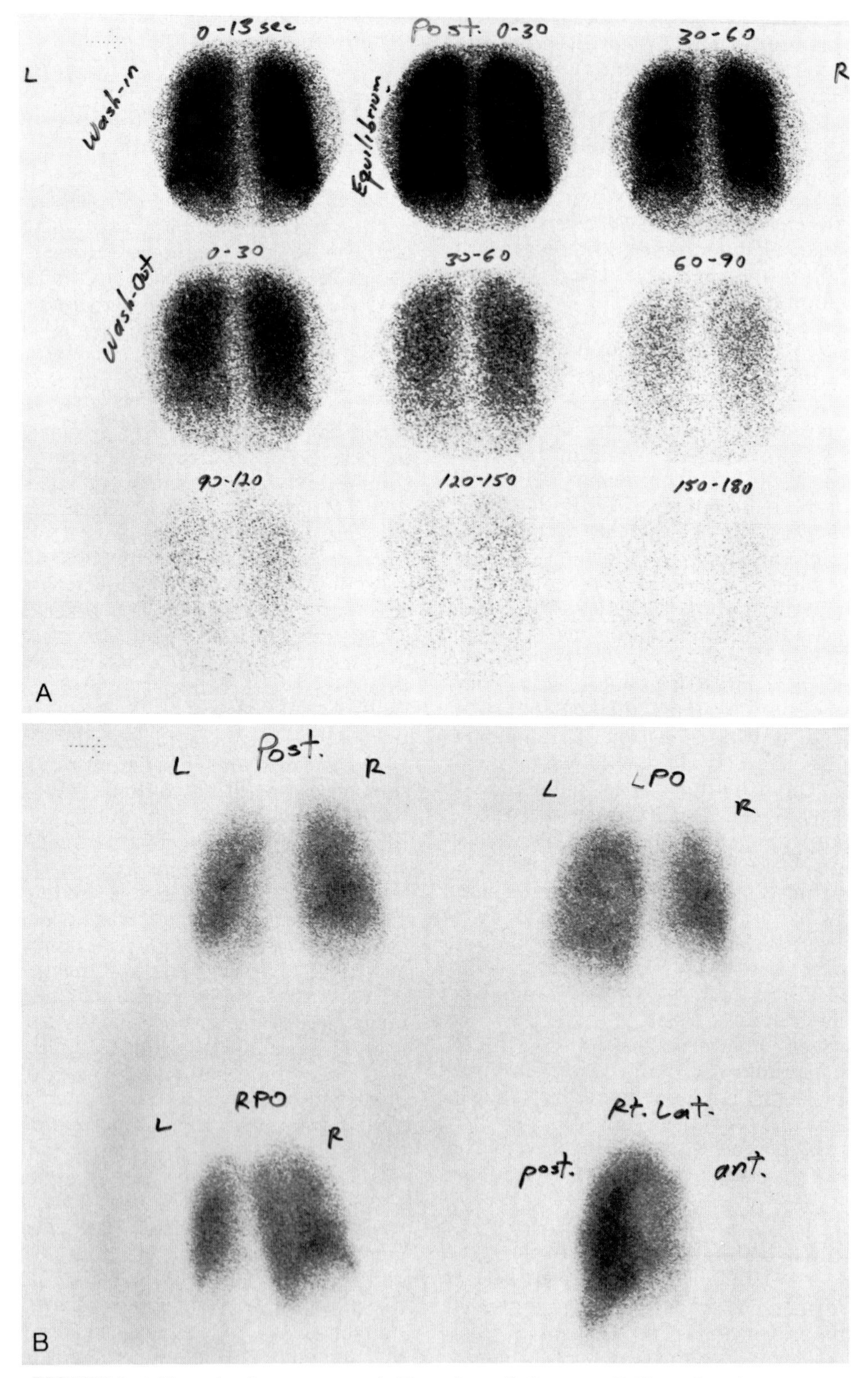

FIGURE 9–4. Normal pulmonary scan. *A*, Normal ventilation scan. *B*, Normal perfusion scan.

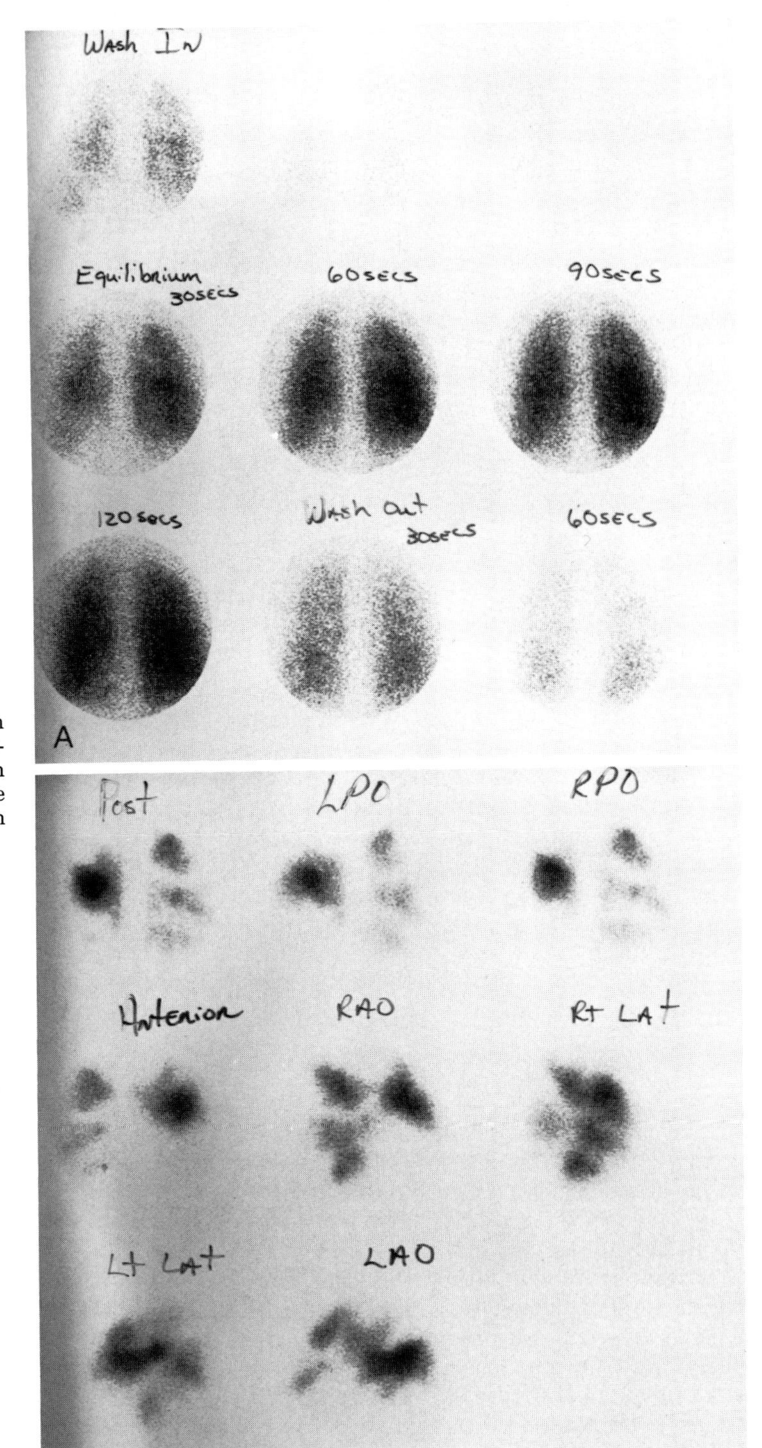

FIGURE 9–5. Pulmonary scan in a patient with pulmonary embolism. *A*, No defects are evident on the ventilation scan. *B*, Multiple defects are seen on the perfusion scan.

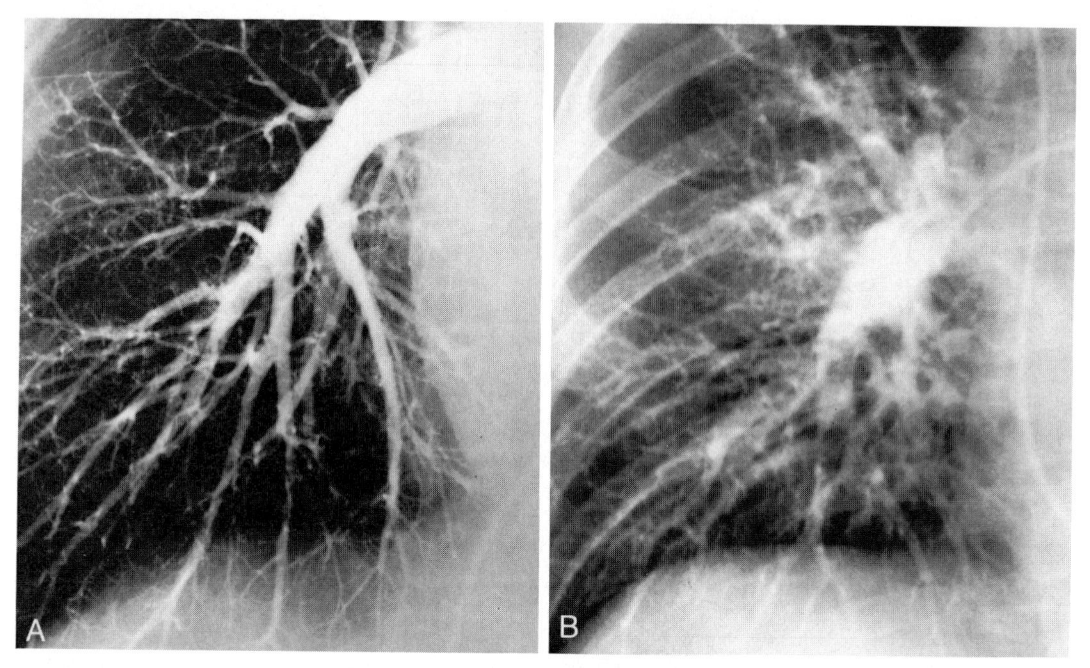

FIGURE 9–6. Pulmonary angiogram. *A*, Normal study revealing excellent filling of pulmonary arteries. *B*, Study showing numerous pulmonary emboli.

taneously. The incidence of infection may be increased in association with hematomas. Another serious sequela of hematoma formation is nerve paralysis.

Despite these potential complications, warfarin remains one of the most conclusively proven, effective methods for preventing serious thromboembolism. With low-dose warfarin schedules that maintain prothrombin time at no greater than 3 to 4 seconds above control, bleeding complications are much less.

Heparin

In thoracic, abdominal, and pelvic surgical procedures, heparin has been shown to be effective in preventing thromboembolic disease when administered subcutaneously in doses of 5000 units every 8 to 12 hours. However, although some investigators report low-dose heparin to be effective in preventing thromboembolic disease following major surgery of the lower extremity, most studies have revealed little or no decrease in the incidence of lower extremity thromboembolic disease. In addition, the incidence of wound hematoma is increased with low-dose heparin therapy.[12, 13, 19, 22, 26]

The mechanism of action of low-dose heparin therapy involves an increase in the rate at which antithrombin III inhibits activated factor X and thrombin. During a major surgical procedure, such as total hip arthroplasty, activation of the coagulation system may be so intense that thrombin generation exceeds the rate at which it can be inhibited, even in the presence of small amounts of heparin. Thrombin generation also releases platelet factor IV, which has antiheparin activity.

In those series in which heparin has been found to be effective in the prevention of thromboembolic disease in the lower extremity, the doses of heparin have been somewhat higher than those recommended for abdominal procedures. Heparin is started with a fixed dose of 3500 units and then adjusted to maintain the partial thromboplastin time between 31 and 36 seconds. Most patients exhibit a state of significant hypercoagulability 5 to 7 days following surgery; therefore, heparin probably should be continued well beyond this time. Progressively higher doses than those given in low-dose regimens will be necessary for up to 8 days after surgery. Bleeding complications are not increased and may be decreased, with the adjusted dose compared with the fixed low-dose regimen.[18]

A potentially serious complication of heparin for prophylaxis of thromboembolism is the paradoxical effect of arterial embolism. Clinically apparent arterial embolism may occur 7 to 15 days after heparin therapy is initiated. Most patients who develop clinically apparent embolisms have premonitory symptoms of the gastrointestinal tract and musculoskeletal system a day or two before. Surgery must be performed immediately to remove the embolus, and heparin therapy must be discontinued.[19] The mortality rate in patients who have major embolisms while on heparin therapy is 60 percent.

The most common embolization site is the aortic bifurcation, but embolism may also occur in other major arteries, including the iliac and femoral. The embolus consists of platelet-rich fibrin with a few red blood cells. A suggested cause of this embolism is aggregation of platelets, which may be associated with prolonged administration of heparin. Possibly, an antiheparin antibody may become active, leading to platelet aggregation. Heparin-induced thrombocytopenia often results in a platelet count less than 100,000, sometimes as low as 30,000 to 40,000.

Dextran

Dextran is a glucose polymer introduced as a volume expander but subsequently used as an antithrombotic agent. It has been administered clinically in a molecular weight of either 40,000 or 70,000. Both forms have been shown to be effective in reducing the incidence of venous thrombosis following hip surgery.[6, 13, 19, 25] Dextran lowers blood viscosity, reduces platelet aggregation, and alters fibrin stability, thus reducing the growth rate of thrombi. Similar to heparin, dextran increases the rate at which antithrombin III inhibits activated factor X and thrombin; dextran is 40 to 50 times less effective than heparin in this action.[19]

Dextran 70 is administered just before or at the time of surgery and continued on a daily basis for several days. Administration of low doses of dextran 40, 250 mL during surgery and 500 mL on postoperative days 2 and 4, was found to be effective in reducing thromboembolism associated with total hip replacement.[25]

Care must be taken to avoid fluid retention in patients who are receiving dextran, especially in those with histories of congestive heart failure. Increased bleeding has been reported by some investigators but is not usually a major problem. Bleeding complications can be lessened by not administering more than 500 mL of dextran during surgery.

Aspirin

If effective in the prevention of thromboembolic disease, aspirin would have significant advantages. It is inexpensive, simple to administer, and associated with a low complication rate when given in low doses.

The antithrombotic action of aspirin is related to its inhibition of prostaglandins (PGs). Aspirin blocks the activity of prostaglandin cyclooxygenase by irreversible acetylation, thus preventing the formation of active prostaglandins. Platelet prostaglandin cyclooxygenase converts platelet arachidonic acid to PGH_2, which is then converted to thromboxane, a potent stimulus to platelet aggregation. The prostaglandin prostacyclin (PG_{12}) is a vasodilator and an inhibitor of platelet aggregation that is synthesized by human endothelial cells. By inhibiting PG formation, aspirin has both a thrombotic and an antithrombotic effect.

Because platelet aggregation probably is not involved primarily in the initiation of venous thrombosis, aspirin would not be expected to be effective in preventing thromboembolic disease. Several clinical investigations have evaluated low-dose aspirin in this regard. Most studies have not included very high-risk patients, such as those who have had previous thromboembolic diseases. The general consensus among most investigators is that aspirin is not an effective prophylactic agent against thromboembolic disease associated with total arthroplasty of the lower extremity.[2, 11, 19, 24]

Hydroxychloroquine and Sulfinpyrazone

Two other drugs with antithrombotic activity that have been suggested for prevention of thromboembolic disease are hydroxychloroquine and sulfinpyrazone. The results in orthopaedic surgery have been somewhat controversial. Less evidence of effectiveness has accumulated for sulfinpyrazone than for hydroxychloroquine.

Hydroxychloroquine inhibits platelet adhesiveness and, to a lesser extent, platelet aggregation. The most common dose has been 200 mg three times daily. Reversible eye changes occur occasionally in the ciliary body and cornea, and permanent retinitis may occur after prolonged high-dose hydroxychloroquine administration, i.e., a total dose of 100 gm or more. Doses in this range should never be given for thromboembolic prophylaxis. The incidence of bleeding complications has been low.[16, 19]

Combination Drugs

Numerous studies have investigated various combinations of anticoagulant and antithrombotic medications. Most drug combinations have not been found to be more effective than one of the more effective single agents alone. In many instances combination therapy has resulted in increased complications, particularly bleeding.

In a study comparing dextran 40 with a combination of low-dose heparin and antithrombin III, the incidence of venous thrombosis was 4.9 percent with the combination and 28.6 percent with the dextran 40. At the present time, antithrombin III is not commercially available.[9]

Physical and Mechanical Measures

Most clinicians have employed physical and mechanical means of preventing thromboembolic disease. Physical measures should continue to be investigated because they have low complication rates.

Fewer thrombi occur in the calves of patients in whom tourniquets are applied, probably because of increased systemic fibrinolytic activity following release. This finding may in part explain the lower incidence of thromboembolism with knee surgery compared with hip surgery.[7] Early mobilization of patients after surgery, wearing of antithromboembolism stockings, and early initiation of muscle exercises and motion in the lower extremity are important adjunctive antithromboembolic methods.

More sophisticated mechanical means that have been investigated include passive motion and mechanical compression devices to improve venous outflow from the lower extremities. Both of these measures can be applied during as well as after surgical procedures. No pulmonary emboli occurred in a study that evaluated the effect of continuous passive motion after total knee arthroplasty. However, venous thrombosis occurred in 40 percent of patients, whether or not they had continuous passive motion.[20] Gradient elastic stockings and external pneumatic compression reduce the incidence of deep venous thrombosis when employed alone or in combination with each other or with heparin, dihydroergotamine, or low-dose warfarin.[24]

In some cases, anticoagulant or antithrombotic medication may be contraindicated. If the patient is at very high risk for pulmonary embolism, prophylactic placement of a vena cava filter may be considered. A Greenfield filter has been utilized to prevent fatal pulmonary embolism in a patient who underwent total hip and knee arthroplasty who had a history of thromboembolism but in whom anticoagulation was contraindicated as well as in patients who had complications associated with anticoagulation.[3]

SUMMARY

Thromboembolic disease is one of the most common complications in patients who are having total hip or knee replacements. The disease cannot be ignored, because it may result in death. All patients with major risk factors should have prophylaxis against thromboembolic disease. High-risk patients are those who are over 40 years old, are obese, have a malignancy, have a history of previous thromboembolic disease, or have any of the other risk factors listed in Table 9–1.

Until further information is gathered, most patients undergoing elective hip surgery or knee replacement who have major risk factors should be treated with one of the agents conclusively demonstrated to be effective—low-dose warfarin, dextran, or adjusted-dose heparin. The 1986 National Institutes of Health Consensus Development Conference recommended this treatment for 7 days or longer if the patient is bedridden. At a minimum, a patient who does not have major risk factors but who has a lower risk for developing thromboembolic disease should be carefully monitored by history and physical examination. Early mobilization, exercise, and compression stockings, if used appropriately, are helpful adjuncts for both high-risk and low-risk patients.

References

1. Amstutz, H. C., Friscia, D. A., Dorey, F., and Carney, B. T.: Warfarin prophylaxis to prevent mortality from pulmonary embolism after total hip replacement. J. Bone Joint Surg. 71A:321–326, 1989.
2. Butterfield, W. J. H., Hicks, B. H., and Ambler, A. R.: Effect of aspirin on postoperative venous thrombosis. Report of the steering committee of a trial sponsored by the Medical Research Council. Lancet 2:441–445, 1972.
3. Collins, D. N., Barnes, C. L., McAndrew, M. P., et al.: Vena Caval Filter Use in Orthopaedic Patients with Recognized Preoperative Deep Venous Thrombosis. Presented at the Annual Meeting of the American Academy of Orthopaedic Surgeons. New Orleans, 1990.
4. Dorr, L. D., Sakimuri, I., and Mohler, J. G.: Pulmonary embolus following total hip arthroplasty: Incidence study. J. Bone Joint Surg. 61A:1083–1087, 1979.
5. Eskeland, G., Solheim, K., and Skjorten, F.: Anticoagulant prophylaxis. Thrombolism and mortality in elderly patients with hip fractures. A controlled clinical trial. Acta Chir. Scand. 131:16–29, 1966.
6. Evarts, C. M. and Feil, E. J.: Prevention of thromboembolic disease after elective surgery of the hip. J. Bone Joint Surg. 53A:1271–1280, 1971.
7. Fahmy, N. R. and Patel, D. G.: Hemostatic changes in postoperative deep vein thrombosis associated with use of a pneumatic tourniquet. J. Bone Joint Surg. 63A:461–465, 1981.
8. Francis, C. W., Marder, V. J., Evarts, C. M., and Yaukoolbodi, S.: Two-step warfarin therapy. Prevention of postoperative venous thrombosis without excessive bleeding. J.A.M.A. 249:374–378, 1983.
9. Francis, C. W., Pellegrini, V. D., Marder, V. J., et al.: Prevention of venous thrombosis after total hip arthroplasty. J. Bone Joint Surg. 71A:327–335, 1989.
10. Froehlich, J. A., Dorfman, G. S., Cronan, J. J., et al.: Compression ultrasonography for the detection of deep venous thrombosis in patients who have a fracture of the hip. J. Bone Joint Surg. 71A:249–256, 1989.
11. Guyer, R. D., Booth, R. E., Jr., and Rothman, R. H.: The detection and prevention of pulmonary embolism in total hip replacement. A study comparing aspirin and low-dose warfarin. J. Bone Joint Surg. 64(7):1040–1044, 1982.
12. Hampson, W. G. J., Harris, F. C., and Lucas, H. K.: Failure of low-dose heparin to prevent deep-vein thrombosis after hip-replacement arthroplasty. Lancet 2:795–797, 1974.
13. Harris, W. H., Athanasoulis, C., Waltman, A. C., and Salzman, E. W.: Cuff-impedance phlebography and ^{125}I-fibrinogen scanning versus roentgenographic phlebography for diagnosis of thrombophlebitis following hip surgery. J. Bone Joint Surg. 58A:939–944, 1976.
14. Hirsh, J. and Salzman, E.: Prevention of Venous Thrombolism. Hemostasis and Thrombosis: Basic Principles and Practice. Edited by R. W. Colemen, J. Hirsh, and J. W. Marder. Philadelphia, J. B. Lippincott Company, 1982.
15. Hull, R., Hirsh, J., Sackett, D. L., et al.: The value of adding impedence plethysmography to ^{125}I-fibrinogen leg scanning for the detection of deep vein thrombosis in high-risk surgical patients. A comparative study between patients undergoing general surgery and hip surgery. Thromb. Res. 15:227–234, 1979.
16. Johnson, R. and Charnley, J.: Hydroxychloroquine in prophylaxis of pulmonary embolism following hip arthroplasty. Clin. Orthop. 144:174–177, 1979.
17. Kim, Y. and Suh, J.: Low incidence of deep-vein thrombosis after cementless total hip replacement. J. Bone Joint Surg. 70A:878–882, 1988.
18. Leyvraz, P. F., Richard, J., Bachmann, F., et al.: Adjusted versus fixed-dose subcutaneous heparin in the prevention of deep-vein thrombosis after total hip replacement. N. Engl. J. Med. 309:954–958, 1983.
19. Lowe, L. W.: Venous thrombosis and embolism. J. Bone Joint Surg. 63B:155–167, 1981.
20. Lynch, A. F., Bourne, R. B., Rorabeck, C. H., et al.: Deep-vein thrombosis and continuous passive motion after total knee arthroplasty. J. Bone Joint Surg. 70A:11–14, 1988.
21. Modig, J., Hjelmstedt, A., Sahlstedt, B., and Maripuu, E.: Comparative influences of epidural and general anaesthesia on deep venous thrombosis and pulmonary embolism after total hip replacement. Acta Chir. Scand. 147(2):125–130, 1981.
22. Morris, G. K., Henry, A. P. J., and Preston, B. J.: Prevention of deep-vein thrombosis by low-dose heparin in patients undergoing total hip replacement. Lancet 2:797–800, 1974.
23. Morris, G. K. and Mitchell, J. R. A.: Warfarin sodium in the prevention of deep venous thrombosis and pulmonary embolism in patients with fractured neck of femur. Lancet 2:869–872, 1976.
24. National Institutes of Health Consensus Development Conference: Prevention of Venous Thrombosis and Pulmonary Embolism. Volume 6, Number 2, 1986.
25. Roberts, T. S., Nelson, C. L., Barnes, C. L., et al.: Low-dose dextran 40 in reconstructive hip surgery patients. Orthopedics 12(6):797–801, 1989.
26. Salzman, E. W.: Progress in preventing thrombolism. (Letter.) N. Engl. J. Med. 309:980–982, 1983.
27. Sharrock, N. E., Hargett, M. J., Urquhart, B., et al.: Effects of Epidural Anesthesia on Deep Vein

Thrombosis Following Total Knee Arthroplasty. Presented at the Annual Meeting of the American Academy of Orthopaedic Surgeons. New Orleans, 1990.
28. Stewart, G. J., Alburger, P. D., Jr., Stone, E. A., Soszka, T. W.: Total hip replacement induces injury to remote veins in a canine model. J. Bone Joint Surg. 65(1):97–102, 1983.
29. Strandness, D. E., Jr., Langlois, Y., Cramer, M., et al.: Long-term sequelae of acute venous thrombosis. J.A.M.A. 250:1289–1292, 1983.
30. Terayama, K.: Experience with Charnley low-friction arthroplasty in Japan. Clin. Orthop. 211:79–84, 1986.
31. Tremaine, M. D., Choroszy, C. J., Gordon, G., and Sheldon, D. A.: Duplex Venous Venography in the Total Joint Patient: Which is the Gold Standard? Presented at the Annual Meeting of the American Academy of Orthopaedic Surgeons. New Orleans, 1990.
32. White, R. E., Helpenstell, T., and Jacob, T. P.: Accuracy of Evaluation of Deep Venous Thrombosis in the Calf Following Total Hip Replacement by Use of Real-Time B-Mode Ultrasound Venous Imaging. Presented at the Annual Meeting of the American Academy of Orthopaedic Surgeons. New Orleans, 1990.

SECTION IV

PREOPERATIVE CONCERNS FOR TOTAL JOINT REPLACEMENT

CHAPTER 10

Anesthesia for Joint Replacement Surgery

NIKOLAUS GRAVENSTEIN

Joint replacement surgery focuses on joint replacement operations from the perspective of interactions between patient, anesthesiologist, and surgeon. These interactions may predict the occasional postponement of elective cases; guide preoperative evaluations; on occasion, suggest a preferred anesthetic technique; and provide insight into perioperative pain management options.

MEDICAL CONTRAINDICATIONS

Medical contraindications to major elective surgery and accompanying anesthesia include recent myocardial infarction, inadequately treated coexisting disease, and significant electrolyte abnormality. The preoperative evaluation of the patient by both surgeon and anesthesiologist is an integral component of any anesthetic plan, as they cooperate to identify and evaluate any coexisting disease. This is done with the understanding that joint replacement operations are elective in nature, and therefore coexisting disease should be optimally managed. When it is not, the anesthesiologist will recommend case postponement.

Recent Myocardial Infarction

Most anesthesiologists view a myocardial infarction within the last 6 months as a contraindication to elective surgery. The patients so affected have been found to have a higher incidence of recurrent perioperative myocardial infarction.[51, 63] In 1978, Steen and associates[63] described reinfarction rates of 37 percent, 16 percent, and 5 percent in patients who were undergoing anesthesia and operation who were within 0 to 3, 4 to 6, and more than 6 months of a previous myocardial infarction, respectively.[63] The incidence was less than 0.5 percent in patients without previous myocardial infarctions. Because the risk of reinfarction does not decrease further after 6 months, this is the typically cited cut-off period.

Further data (1977 to 1982) showed an encouraging drop in reinfarction rates to 5.8 percent, 2.3 percent, and about 1.5 percent at postinfarct intervals of 0 to 3, 4 to 6, and more than 6 months (Table 10–1),[51] with no further decrease thereafter. Later data are sobering, however, because even with the institution of more modern medical management and monitoring, the mortality associated with perioperative reinfarctions in patients who do have them remains over 30 percent.[51] For this reason, elective surgery is still delayed for at least 6 months after a myocardial infarction.

Coexisting Disease

Among the most common coexisting diseases in patients presenting for joint re-

Table 10–1. RELATIONSHIP OF INTERVAL BETWEEN PREVIOUS MYOCARDIAL INFARCTION AND ANESTHESIA WITH INCIDENCE OF REINFARCTION*

Months between Myocardial Infarction and Anesthesia	Postanesthetic Reinfarctions (%)	
	1973–1976 (%)	*1977–1982 (%)*
0–3	36	5.8
4–6	26	2.3
7–12	5	1
13–24	5	1.6
>25	5	1.7

*Modified from Rao, T., Jacobs, K. H., El-Etr, A. A., et al.: Anesthesiology 59:499–505, 1983.

placement are angina, congestive heart failure, hypertension, diabetes, asthma, and rheumatoid arthritis.

Angina

Any patient with chest pain should be questioned in detail. If angina appears to be the cause, preoperative evaluation must ascertain whether the condition is chronic or recent and whether the symptoms are stable. The interviewer must determine whether the patient has received optimal medical management and whether coronary artery bypass is possible or indicated before joint replacement. Patients with incompletely defined or managed heart disease should be evaluated by a cardiologist before surgery is scheduled.

Angina of recent onset implies progression of previously asymptomatic coronary artery disease. Symptomatic disease is thought to predispose patients to perioperative cardiac complications. The cardiologist's evaluation may be as simple as taking a history and doing a physical examination, or it may include stress testing and coronary angiography. Three different outcomes are possible: (1) the patient will be considered a safe candidate for surgery, (2) the patient will require medical therapy, and (3) the patient will require surgical correction of occluded coronary arteries before elective joint replacement.

Patients with stable preexisting angina have pain of a characteristic frequency and duration, predictably following certain activities, which vary among patients. Unstable angina occurs at rest or has been present for less than 2 months. The condition is considered to be a signal of impending myocardial infarction. By definition, angina represents symptomatic myocardial ischemia; in contrast, the majority of myocardial ischemia cases are asymptomatic ("silent ischemia") (Fig. 10–1).[15] Typically, the endpoint of medical therapy is control of angina, i.e., symptomatic improvement without any monitoring to verify that no ischemia is present. Consequently, even patients treated for angina remain at increased risk for perioperative ischemia and myocardial infarction.[59] Perioperative myocardial ischemia and infarction sometimes occur, often in the absence

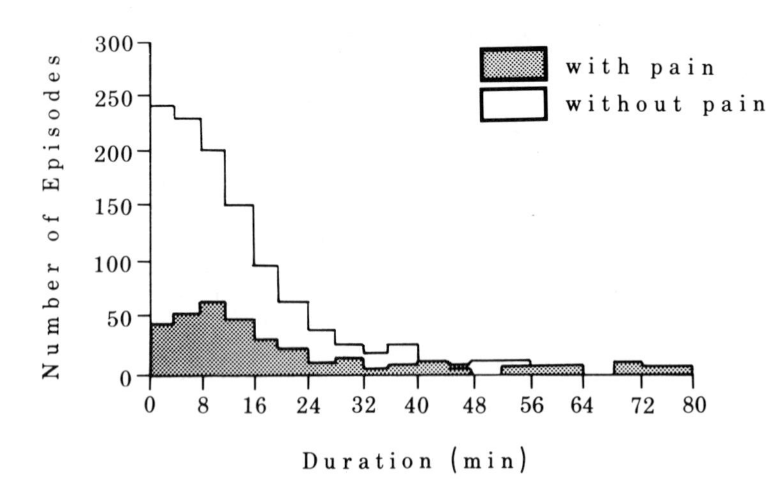

FIGURE 10–1. Duration and frequency of symptomatic and asymptomatic episodes of ST depression in patients with stable angina. (Deanfield, J. E., Selwyn, A. P., Maseri, A., et al: Lancet 2:755, 1983. By permission.)

of significant hemodynamic change and despite everyone's best efforts.

Congestive Heart Failure

The presence of heart failure is suggested by symptoms of orthopnea, dyspnea and paroxysmal nocturnal dyspnea and by physical findings of rales, S_3 gallop, and jugular vein distention. They indicate inadequate cardiac function and therefore little or no cardiac reserve. Of all the predictors of perioperative cardiac morbidity, preexisting congestive heart failure is perhaps the most important.[25] Before joint replacement is performed, congestive heart failure should be corrected by such methods as administration of an inotropic or a diuretic agent and afterload reduction therapy.

Hypertension

High blood pressure is likely the most common medical abnormality in candidates for joint replacement. Clinicians vary in what they consider the upper limit of blood pressure before elective operations; no standard exists. No reliable findings suggest that moderately elevated diastolic pressures (90 to 110 mmHg) predispose the patient to perioperative cardiac complications.[24] However, hypertensive patients do undergo greater changes in blood pressure intraoperatively than normotensive patients. Those most prone to develop severe hypertension following endotracheal intubation appear to have significant blood pressure fluctuations preoperatively, such as the increases associated with the stress of hospital admission.[2] Several patients with this hemodynamic profile have been shown to require therapy for myocardial ischemia associated with postintubation hypertension.[2] In general, all patients with sustained diastolic blood pressure above 90 mmHg should at some point be treated on a long-term basis. Those with sustained diastolic blood pressures above 110 mmHg are best served with preoperative therapy to correct hypertension.

Diabetes

Diabetes affects many organ systems, each with potential influence on the patient's perioperative course. Preoperative evaluation should confirm adequate medical control of the disease, with no evidence of a recent hyperglycemic or hypoglycemic crisis or glucosuria. If preoperative blood glucose levels exceed 300 mg/dl, the joint replacement procedure should be postponed. Good control of blood glucose levels preoperatively facilitates perioperative insulin management; euglycemia or only mild hyperglycemia may also facilitate wound healing.[26]

Asthma

Patients with asthma have a marked predisposition to bronchospasm with airway manipulation and tracheal intubation. Therefore, the perioperative evaluation of asthmatic patients should determine whether significant respiratory dysfunction is present and whether current therapy is effective. An appropriate preoperative treatment plan should be devised, if needed, as well as an anesthetic plan.[36]

If a patient has wheezing, a trial of bronchodilator therapy is suggested with inhaled or oral agents. Successful management is evidenced by symptomatic improvement and resolution of wheezing. If wheezing persists despite combination beta agonist (albuterol) and phosphodiesterase inhibitor (aminophylline) therapy, with the latter documented to be at a therapeutic level, complete resolution may be impossible. In such a case, regional anesthesia should be considered.

Patients who take theophylline regularly should have the serum level determined preoperatively to document that a therapeutic concentration has been reached (10 to 20 μg/ml). If the serum level is below 10 μg/ml, the supplemental dose required to bring the value up to a therapeutic concentration can be easily calculated.

Asthmatic patients who take steroids on a continuing basis should have the medication continued perioperatively. They should also be considered at risk for perioperative adrenal insufficiency.

Rheumatoid Arthritis

Of patients presenting for total hip joint replacement, a modest percentage have rheumatoid arthritis, with 7 percent reported at one medical center.[47] The incidence of course may be substantially higher in those centers specializing in the management of rheumatoid disease. Preoperative evaluation should address the systemic nature of the disease, cervical spine involvement, and current or recent steroid medication. Patients with systemic involvement have a higher incidence of heart disease (pericardial effusions, congestive heart failure, and angina), pulmonary involvement (lowered lung compliance), and arthritic/degenerative involvement of other joints.

The rheumatoid patient with symptoms of congestive heart failure may have pericardial effusion or restriction with resulting cardiac tamponade. Transthoracic echocardiography is a simple, noninvasive way to make the diagnosis. In patients with pulmonary symptoms, a chest radiograph is useful to identify significant rheumatoid pleural effusions. Although pulmonary fibrosis is not treatable, pulmonary function studies will reveal the extent of fibrosis in symptomatic patients. This information may help predict intraoperative difficulties with oxygenation and the need for postoperative ventilation.

Perhaps the most significant preoperative problem is involvement of structures other than the joint being replaced. Of particular concern are the cervical spine, temporomandibular joint, and larynx. Rheumatoid involvement of the cervical spine may be manifest as decreased range of motion, perhaps hampering intubation, or it may be manifest as atlantoaxial instability, making possible spinal cord injury during intubation and positioning unless they are done while the patient is awake.[61] When general anesthesia is planned, radiographic films of the neck in lateral flexion and extension will identify the rheumatoid patient at risk for spinal cord injury.[54] Radiographs will reveal instability, i.e., motion of the odontoid proc-

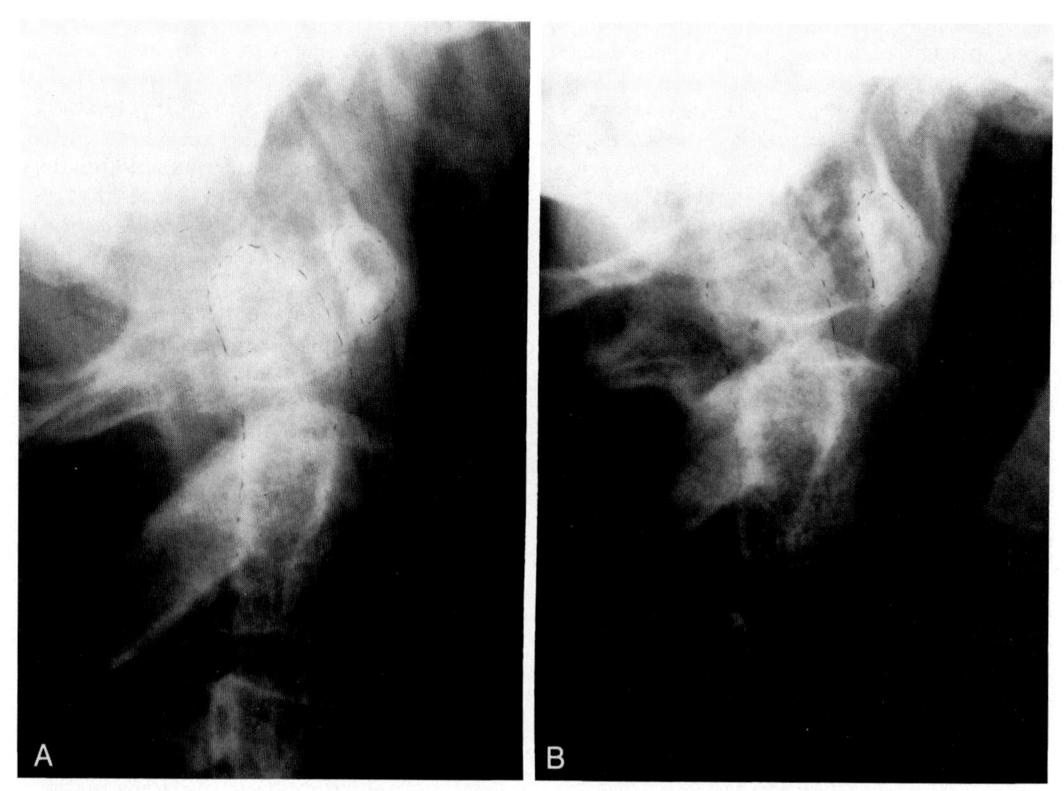

FIGURE 10–2. Lateral flexion and extension views of the neck in a patient with rheumatoid arthritis and no symptoms of cervical instability. *A*, The lateral view of the upper cervical spine in extension shows an atlantodental interval of 3 mm, within normal limits. *B*, With flexion, the atlantodental interval increased to 6 mm, indicating instability (i.e., >2 mm movement).

ess in relation to the atlas exceeding 3 mm between flexion and extension. Even an asymptomatic patient may show considerable instability (Fig. 10–2). The airway may be involved at the temporomandibular joints, preventing adequate mouth opening (<3 fingerbreadths) for routine oral intubation. Involvement may occur at the cricoarytenoid joints, preventing adequate exposure of the larynx or placement of the customary sized endotracheal tube.

Hoarseness suggests cricoarytenoid involvement. Cervical instability and involvement of the temporomandibular joint, cricoarytenoid, or both can be effectively and safely managed when general anesthesia is planned. However, fiberoptic intubation must be performed with the patient awake and the patient positioned carefully before anesthetic induction.

COEXISTING MEDICAL THERAPIES

Steroid Therapy

Any patient who has taken steroid medication for 5 days or more within 12 months before surgery must be considered for perioperative steroid coverage.[49] The small, but real, risk of an adrenal insufficiency crisis makes glucocorticoid coverage a common practice. Dose and regimen are individualized because the cortisol response to stress depends on the degree of surgical stress.[7] Potential adrenal suppression requires that replacement therapy at least equal the normal daily cortisol output in adults (25 mg/day), as well as any anticipated increased perioperative cortisol requirement (up to 300 mg/day).

Deep anesthesia suppresses the usual glucocorticoid surge that occurs intraoperatively. Consequently, acute adrenal insufficiency usually develops after, not during, surgery. In studies of adrenally deficient primates that underwent cholecystectomy, Udelsman and associates[72] found that those with steroid replacement therapy at 1/10 the normal cortisol level were hemodynamically unstable and had a significantly higher mortality than those with either physiologic cortisol levels or 10 times normal levels. Wound healing was not different between the physiologic and supraphysiologic groups. Several conclusions are logical: (1) steroids should be replaced, (2) amounts should at least equal normal daily steroid production or intake plus the anticipated increase associated with surgical stress, and (3) excess amounts carry no significant risk. One of many proposed steroid coverage schedules is given in Table 10–2, and it will have the desired effect on plasma cortisol levels (Fig. 10–3).[67]

Diuretic and Digoxin Therapy

Patients taking diuretics should have serum potassium levels measured preoperatively, whether they take potassium supplements or not. The same is true of patients taking digitalis. Many anesthesiologists believe that preoperative hypokalemia predisposes patients to intraoperative arrhythmias,[64] despite reports to the contrary.[30, 76] Little controversy exists,

Table 10–2. REGIMEN FOR PERIOPERATIVE STEROID REPLACEMENT/SUPPLEMENT*

Minor Surgery	Morning of surgery, 1.5 to 2 times the usual prednisone dose. Next day, normal dose or parenteral equivalent. During prolonged or extensive surgery, extraparenteral steroids kept ready, as the patient is glucocorticoid dependent.
Moderate Surgery	Morning of surgery, 2 times the usual glucocorticoid dosage orally if possible and/or 25 mg IV† hydrocortisone preoperatively; intraoperatively, 75 mg IV. Postoperatively, 50 mg IV, rapidly tapering over 48 hr to usual dose, if postoperative course is uneventful.
Major Surgery	Morning of surgery, 2 times the usual glucocorticoid dosage orally if possible and/or 50 mg IV hydrocortisone preoperatively; intraoperatively, 100 mg IV. Postoperatively, 100 mg IV every 8 hr for 24 hr, rapidly tapering over the next 48 to 72 hr to usual dose, if postoperative course is uneventful.

*Modified from Chernow, B., Alexander, H. R., Smallridge, R. C., et al: Arch. Intern. Med. 147:1273–1278, 1987.
†IV = intravenously.

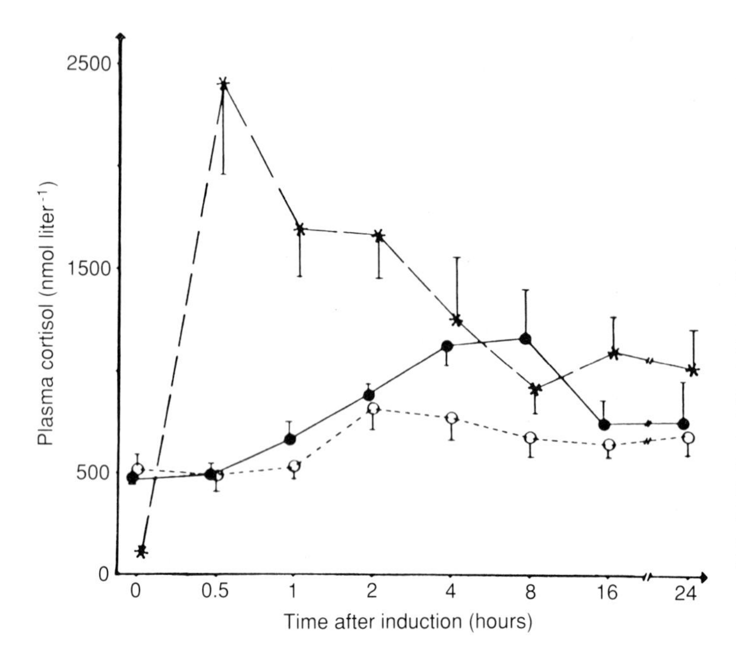

FIGURE 10–3. Plasma cortisol concentrations before and after induction of anesthesia (mean ± SEM). Filled circles indicate control patients without prior steroid therapy. Open circles indicate patients on prior steroid therapy but with normal cortisol response to adrenocorticotropic hormone (ACTH) (i.e., not adrenally suppressed). The asterisks represent patients on corticosteroid therapy with abnormal ACTH response (i.e., adrenally suppressed) who were treated with low-dose cortisol substitution (25 mg) at induction, followed by 100 mg during the next 24 hours. (Symreng, T., Karlberg, B. E., Kagedal, B., et al: Br. J. Anaesth. 53:951, 1981. By permission.)

however, regarding the need for preoperative potassium supplementation in patients with serum potassium levels below 3 mEq/L. Replacement should take place over several days.

Antidepressant Drug Therapy

Considerable controversy exists regarding the preoperative management of patients taking antidepressant medications—either tricyclic antidepressants or monoamine oxidase inhibitors (Tables 10–3 and 10–4). Tricyclic agents are also used to induce sleep and control pain. Monoamine oxidase inhibitors are sometimes prescribed to treat high blood pressure. Concern about these preparations arises from their association with intraoperative arrhythmias and hemodynamic instability. The administration of monoamine oxidase inhibitors has also been associated with a syndrome of hyperpyrexia, cardiovascular instability, rigidity, and coma following narcotic administration.[11] Meperidine (Demerol), which has been the most strongly implicated, should not be administered to patients taking monoamine oxidase inhibitors.

Tricyclic antidepressants (see Table 10–3) have a relatively short serum half-life. Their effect on catecholamine clearance is reversible; clearance is 70 percent by 72 hours. Discontinuation of tricyclic antidepressants 72 hours preoperatively is considered an adequate preventive measure. The combination of halothane and pancuronium (Pavulon) has been shown to provoke arrhythmias in a patient who is taking tricyclic drugs and therefore should be avoided.[17] If concern exists that tricyclic discontinuation might precipitate depression severe enough to result in a suicide attempt, the anesthesiologist can be consulted to help plan appropriate intraoperative management.

When patients take monoamine oxidase

Table 10–3. TRICYCLIC ANTIDEPRESSANTS

Amitryptyline (Elavil)
Desipramine (Norpramin)
Doxepin (Sinequan)
Imipramine (Tofranil)
Nortriptyline (Aventyl)
Protriptyline (Vivactil)

Table 10–4. MONOAMINE OXIDASE INHIBITORS

Hydrazines
Phenelzine (Nardil)
Isocarboxazid (Marplan)
Nonhydrazines
Tranylcypromine (Parnate)
Pargyline (Eutonyl, Eutron)

inhibitors (see Table 10–4) of either the hydrazine or nonhydrazine type, a concern is raised for the anesthesiologist. The hydrazine type irreversibly reacts with the enzyme monoamine oxidase, with effects persisting for 2 to 3 weeks after discontinuation of the drug, until the enzyme is regenerated. The nonhydrazine type interacts reversibly with monoamine oxidase and, therefore, needs to be discontinued for only 2 to 3 days prior to anesthesia.[40] To prevent confusion and avoid errors, however, the general recommendation is that monoamine oxidase inhibitors be stopped at least 2 weeks before elective surgery.[75] Some reports suggest that this conservative approach may not be necessary in patients treated for a month or more.[19, 40] If a patient's depression might be seriously worsened by preoperative cessation of monoamine oxidase inhibitor therapy, a safe anesthetic is still possible, but prior consultation with the anesthesiologist is necessary. Also, the patient should probably be identified as allergic to Demerol. Any narcotic that is required should be given in doses 1/4 to 1/5 the usual amount initially because the patient may have an increased narcotic sensitivity.[34] Morphine is the narcotic of choice, in this case.

CHOICES OF ANESTHETICS

Effective and safe anesthesia for joint replacement operations can be provided by general anesthesia or regional anesthesia—two very different techniques (Table 10–5).

A general anesthetic, which renders the patient unconscious, requires protection of the airway. Selective administration of sedatives during regional anesthesia may make the patient sleep, but consciousness and the airway are maintained. The onset of general anesthesia is rapid, requiring only one circulation time after intravenous administration. In contrast, regional anesthesia requires from 5 to 30 minutes to take full effect. The patient usually emerges from general anesthesia before leaving the operating area. After regional anesthesia, return of sensation in the extremity may require several hours. The exception is intravenous regional anesthesia (Bier block), which resolves within minutes of tourniquet deflation.

Table 10–5. ANESTHETIC CHARACTERISTICS

	General	Regional
	Unconscious	*Conscious/ Sedated*
Onset	Fast	Slow
Recovery	Fast	Slow
Postoperative analgesia	No	Yes
Failure rate	None	≤10%
Myocardial depression	Yes	No
Depressed ventilation	Yes	No
Sympathectomy	No	Yes
Muscle relaxation	Yes	Yes
Intraoperative blood loss (hip)	—	Reduced
Thromboembolism (hip)	—	Reduced (?)
Complications	Yes	Yes

Unfortunately, the failure rate of regional anesthesia is much higher than that of general anesthesia. In the absence of complications, general anesthesia is uniformly successful, whereas regional anesthesia has a failure rate approaching 10 percent. A failed block may be either converted to a general anesthetic or repeated if the total administered dose does not exceed the toxic limit.

The physiologic effects of general and regional anesthesia also differ. General anesthetics typically cause myocardial depression and inhibit respiration but have little effect on the sympathetic nervous system. Regional anesthetics do not depress myocardial contractility (in the absence of a toxic reaction) or inhibit respiration, except for changes that may occur attendant to coadministered sedatives. They also cause a regional sympathectomy. Both types of anesthesia provide excellent muscle relaxation. Regional anesthetics are associated with less intraoperative bleeding during hip replacement[42] and a lower incidence of deep venous thrombosis (13 percent versus 67 percent with general anesthesia).[44] Still, both types of anesthesia are associated with complications. Problems attending general anesthesia are usually related to airway management, positioning, and cardiovascular effects of both the operation and anesthesia. Complications of regional anesthesia are most commonly inadequate analgesia and less

Table 10–6. OPERATIVE SITE AND ANESTHETIC TECHNIQUE

Operative Site	Anesthetic Technique
Ankle	General Spinal block
Knee, hip	General Spinal block Epidural block
Shoulder	General Interscalene block
Elbow	General Interscalene block Axillary block Bier block
Hand/wrist	General Axillary block Bier block

commonly local anesthetic toxicity and hypotension.

The choice of anesthetic technique for individual patients depends on a combination of factors, including the patient's preference, coexisting disease, anatomy, absence of contraindications, operative site (Table 10–6), length of procedure, and position.

The following discussion focuses on specific regional techniques rather than the more familiar general anesthesia techniques.

Contraindications to Regional Anesthesia

Although all joint replacement operations can be performed with the patient under regional anesthesia, not all patients are candidates for this method. Contraindications include patient refusal, coagulopathy (except for Bier block), block site that precludes adequate skin preparation, inaccessible block site, and unpredictable duration of surgery unless a continuous technique is used.

Although coagulopathy is an absolute contraindication to regional anesthesia, the patient receiving minidose heparin may still be considered a candidate. This drug rarely renders the patient coagulopathic as evidenced by clotting studies. However, it is prudent to verify that coagulation parameters are normal. In a patient who is taking aspirin, a history of normal coagulation is adequate. When the history is unclear, bleeding time should be checked before a spinal or an epidural block is administered. In a patient who is receiving nonsteroidal anti-inflammatory agents, discontinuation the night before surgery is sufficient. No significant effect on platelet function should remain the next morning, and a regional block is acceptable.

Epidural Anesthesia

In epidural anesthesia, a local anesthetic solution is injected into the epidural space. This space between the two layers of the dura runs from the foramen magnum to the sacrococcygeal ligament (Fig. 10–4) and contains epidural veins, segmental nerves, and fat. Either a lumbar intervertebral (epidural) space or the sacral (caudal) hiatus provides access for a single injection or continuous infusion. When a

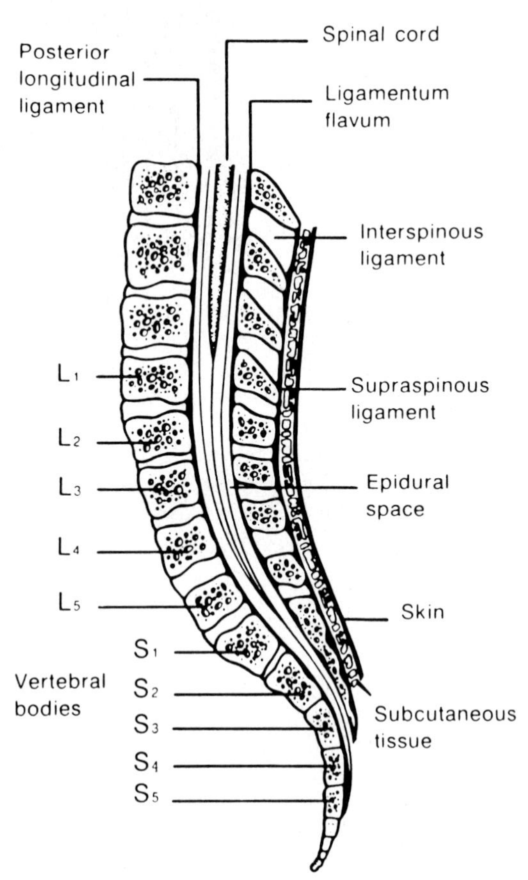

FIGURE 10–4. Sagittal view of the lumbar and sacral epidural space. (Ostheimer, G. W.: Regional Anesthetic Techniques in Obstetrics. Breon Laboratories, 1980. By permission.)

continuous infusion is given, supplemental anesthetic can be periodically injected through a catheter threaded into the epidural space. In most patients who are undergoing hip or knee replacement, a 2-percent lidocaine or 0.5-percent bupivacaine solution will produce an adequate sensory and motor block, with onset of surgical anesthesia occurring within 15 minutes. However, nerve roots L_4 through S_2 (especially S_1), are reportedly the most difficult to block, with failure rates up to 18 percent (Fig. 10–5).[23] The large diameter of these spinal nerve roots may be one explanation. Another explanation for inadequate or asymmetric block is the presence of a dorsal median fold of the dura[4]—a connective-tissue fold that attaches the dura against the dorsal portion of the epidural space, dividing it into two dorsal lateral compartments. The fold sometimes extends over several spinal segments in the lower lumbar and upper sacral region. Failed or unilateral epidural block has been reported in obese patients in obstetrics, i.e., those with greater distances from the skin to the epidural space.[46] The postulated reason is that the epidural needle tip tends to deviate from the midline further as it is inserted more deeply, resulting in more lateral needle placement and restricted or uneven spread of the anesthetic agent.

Caudal instillation of a local anesthetic agent can provide anesthesia for the sacral and lumbar dermatomes. The overall success rate and ability to predict necessary dose are less than those for lumbar epidural anesthesia, especially in adults, partly because the caudal epidural space has more unpredictable volume and patency. Most anesthesiologists consider caudal anesthesia in adults technically more difficult and less successful than lumbar epidural anesthesia. However, the caudal route does provide access to the epidural space when the lumbar epidural route is unavailable. DeBoard and colleagues[16] reported three patients in whom lumbar epidural placement was impossible owing to ossification of the interspinous ligaments and bony bridges between vertebrae in association with ankylosing spondylitis. In each case, hip replacement was performed successfully with caudal anesthesia after patency of the caudal canal had been verified with spot lateral and angulated anteroposterior view radiographs. They recommend this as the regional technique of choice in such patients.

Spinal Anesthesia

In spinal anesthesia (subarachnoid block) local anesthetics are injected into

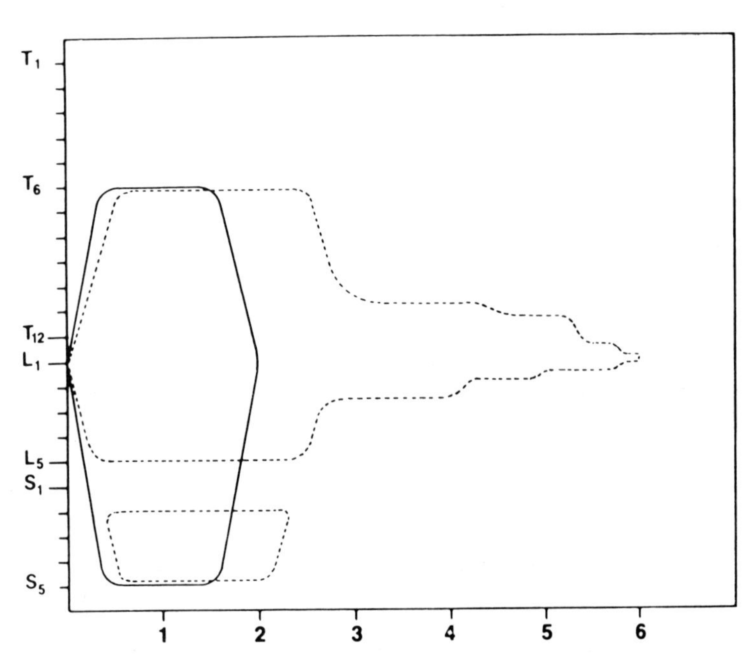

FIGURE 10–5. Spreading characteristics of epidural block after injection into the epidural space at L_1. The vertical axis represents the spinal level V and the horizontal axis, the time in hours. Lidocaine anesthesia is shown by the area within the solid line and bupivacaine, the area within the dotted line. Onset for both drugs is fastest and lasts longest at the injection site. Note the sacral sparing effect seen with bupivacaine, whereby L_5-S_1 may remain unblocked. (Murphy, T. M.: Spinal, epidural, and caudal anesthesia. Anesthesia, 2nd ed. Edited by R. D. Miller. New York, Churchill Livingstone, p. 1095, 1986. By permission.)

the subarachnoid space, which contains the spinal fluid, spinal cord, and nerve roots. A very dense sensory and motor block of the hip, knee, and foot can be achieved by manipulation of dose and specific gravity of the solution. Onset of anesthesia is normally rapid, occurring within 5 minutes of instillation. Anesthesia of the foot and knee is much more reliable with spinal than epidural anesthesia. Spinal anesthesia also has a higher success rate (>95 percent) than epidural. However, unless a catheter is placed for repeat injections of anesthetic, spinal anesthesia has a finite duration, the extent of which is dependent on the coadministration of a vasoconstrictor and the local anesthetic injected. The more rapid onset of spinal anesthesia makes the hypotensive sequelae of the accompanying sympathectomy more prominent. The sympathectomy that accompanies spinal and epidural techniques is used to advantage in the patient with abnormal myocardial contractility and mitral or aortic valvular insufficiency. The lowered systemic vascular resistance enhances cardiac output and decreases regurgitant valvular flow. Prophylactic enhancement of preload (10 to 15 ml/kg) with a balanced salt solution just prior to spinal or epidural anesthesia diminishes the likelihood of significant hypotension.

An important debilitating complication of spinal anesthetic is postoperative headache—characterized by its postural nature. Characteristically, the headache worsens on sitting or standing and is relieved by lying down. The incidence is higher in younger patients (Table 10–7) and in women. It is also more frequent following the use of larger-gauge spinal needles (Table 10–8). Since anesthesiologists began utilizing 25-gauge or smaller needles, the incidence has been observed to be less than 1 percent. Nevertheless, to avoid this complication, in the absence of a specific indication for a spinal anesthetic, many anesthesiologists recommend an alternative technique for patients under 50 years of age. When a postlumbar puncture headache occurs, initial therapy consists of hydration, bedrest, and analgesics. If the headache persists more than 24 hours, intravenous caffeine and especially epidural blood patch may be given. Both have been found effective.

Table 10–7. RELATION OF AGE TO INCIDENCE OF SPINAL HEADACHE*

Age (year)	Number of Anesthetics	Headache	
		Number	*Percent*
10–19	537	51	10
20–29	1994	321	16
30–39	1833	261	14
40–49	1759	192	11
50–59	1736	133	8
60–69	1094	45	4
70–79	297	7	2
80–89	27	1	3
Total	9277	1011	11

*Modified from Vandam, L. D. and Dripps, R. D. J.A.M.A. 161: 586, 1956.

Table 10–8. RELATIONSHIP OF GAUGE OF NEEDLE FOR LUMBAR PUNCTURE AND INCIDENCE OF HEADACHE*

Gauge	Number of Anesthetics	Headache	
		Number	*Percent*
16	839	151	18
19	154	16	10
20	2698	377	14
22	4952	430	9
24	634	37	6
Total	9277	1011	

*Vandam, L. D. and Dripps, R. D.: J.A.M.A. 161: 586, 1956. By permission.

Axillary Block

The axillary block is accomplished by the perivascular infiltration of local anesthetic into the axillary sheath. This blocks the distal brachial plexus (ulnar, median, and radial nerves), i.e., the sensory and motor innervation of the hand, wrist, forearm, and elbow. The medial aspect of the extremity is blocked more reliably than the lateral aspect (Fig. 10–6). For this reason, the technique is not adequate for shoulder operations, and its reliability in elbow procedures that require circumferential anesthesia of the joint is unpredictable. Onset of anesthesia after injection is variable, but 20 to 30 minutes may be required to achieve surgical anesthesia. It is important that an adequate volume of anesthetic be injected; generally, in an adult patient, the volume of the axillary sheath in milliliters is approximately

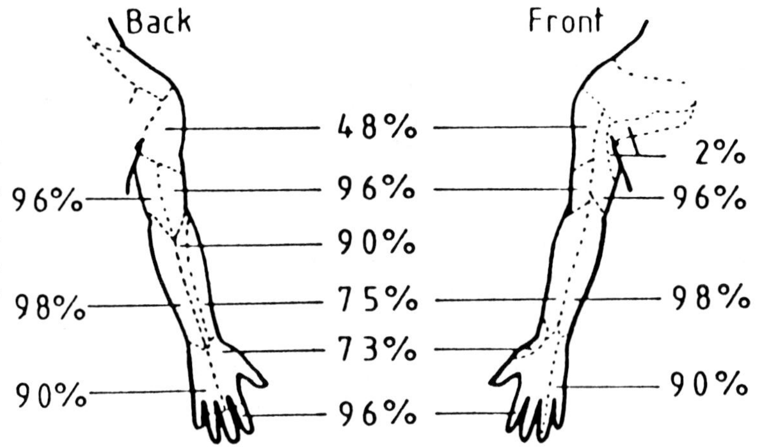

FIGURE 10–6. Areas of analgesia after perivascular axillary block using 40 ml mepivacaine with epinephrine 1:200,000. (Vester-Andersen, T., Christiansen, C., Sorensen, M., et al: Acta Anaesthesiol. Scand. 27:96, 1983. By permission.)

equal to one-half the patient's height in inches. Despite administration of large volumes and application of a tourniquet just distal to the injection site, not all nerves are reliably blocked, most notably the musculocutaneous nerve that leaves the axillary sheath proximally (Fig. 10–7). Winnie and coworkers[80] have observed that one can enhance cephalad spread of the injected solution to the proximal sheath where the musculocutaneous nerves exit by pressing firmly on the axillary artery and axillary sheath during injection. The fingers should press just distal to the injection site. Immediately adducting the patient's arm after injection also helps, relieving the pressure of the humeral head on the axillary sheath and improving cephalad spread of the injected solution. An alternative or supplemental technique is to make a separate injection into the proximal coracobrachialis muscle through which the musculocutaneous nerve travels, blocking it at that level.

The axillary block can be accomplished in one of two ways: (1) by an injection

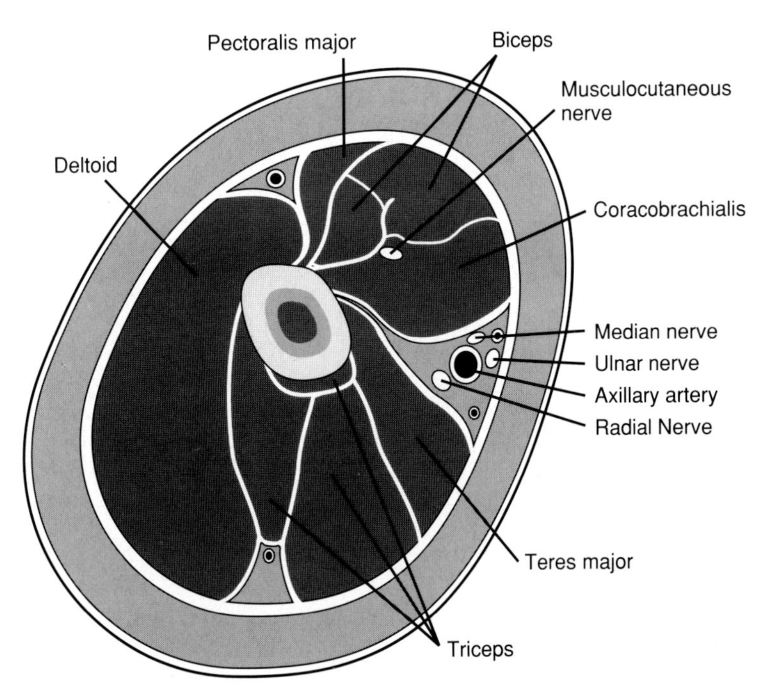

FIGURE 10–7. Cross-section of the upper arm at approximately the level where the axillary block is performed. Note the position of the musculocutaneous nerve, discrete from the axillary neurovascular bundle. (Redrawn from Moore, D. C.: Regional Block, 4th ed. Springfield, IL, Charles C Thomas, p. 246, 1981.)

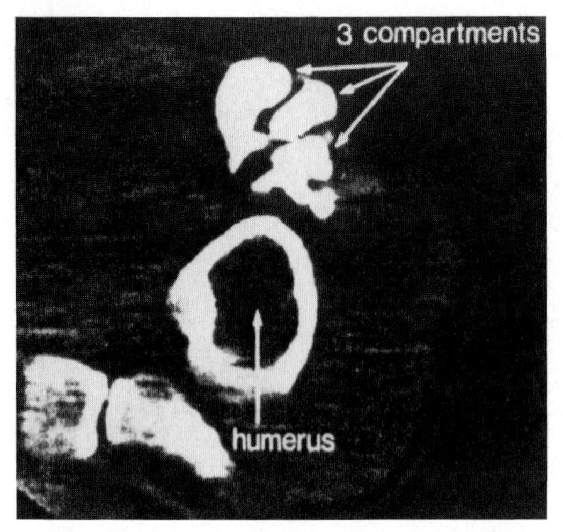

FIGURE 10–8. Computerized tomographic scan of the proximal arm after injection of 30 ml contrast medium containing local anesthetic solution during an axillary block. Note that the solution is confined to three compartments. (Thompson, G. E. and Rorie, D. K.: Anesthesiology 59:120, 1983. By permission.)

following elicitation of paresthesias of each major nerve (radial, ulnar, and median) plus a field block of the musculocutaneous nerve and (2) by a single transarterial injection via the axillary artery. The second approach is based on the fact that the sheath encloses the neurovascular bundle; thus, an injection just beyond the axillary arterial wall should bathe the associated nerves. Thompson and Rorie[69] have shown that the axillary sheath is separated into compartments, interfering with uniform longitudinal spread of local anesthetic agents (Fig. 10–8). This finding suggests that relocation of the needle during the injection may help limit the occurrence of spotty blocks.

Axillary blocks are successful in 90 to 95 percent of cases. However, tourniquet pain and neuropathies may occur. Up to two out of three patients are estimated to experience pain within 60 minutes of tourniquet inflation. In the patient under general anesthesia, tourniquet pain is often manifested only by hypertension.[73] The patient receiving a regional block not only becomes hypertensive but also complains of a dull, deep ache that becomes more intense over time. Without anesthesia, the ache usually begins after 30 minutes; a regional block tends to delay onset in most patients to 60 to 90 minutes.[27, 35] Therapy for tourniquet pain is aimed at symptom relief, with tourniquet release the most effective measure (Fig. 10–9). When symptomatic therapy is insufficient and tourniquet release not an option, a general anesthetic must be considered. Not all forms of anesthesia or regional block appear to have equal incidences of tourniquet pain and hypertension; brachial plexus block has a much lower incidence of this phenomenon than does general anesthesia (Table 10–9).[73]

In 1979, Selander and colleagues[57] reported that 2 percent of patients who undergo axillary block develop paresthesias. Symptoms may be mild, lasting only a few weeks, or severe paresthesias may occur, lasting more than a year. These investigators found a 2.8-percent incidence of postoperative neuropathy in patients

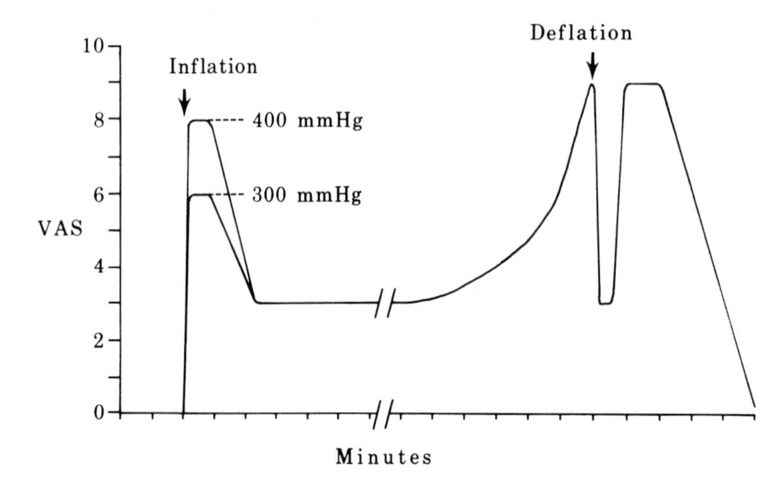

FIGURE 10–9. Typical visual analog pain score (VAS). Note the difference with thigh tourniquet inflation to 300 and 400 mmHg. After a variable time, the pain again increases up to the moment of deflation. Deflation initially provides only temporary relief, after which the pain, although different in nature, usually peaks again. It then recedes within minutes to about zero. (Hagenouw, R. R. P. M., Bridenbaugh, P. O., Van-Egmond, J., et al: Anesth. Analg. 65:1177, 1986. By permission.)

Table 10–9. OCCURRENCE OF HYPERTENSION IN THE VARIOUS TYPES OF ANESTHESIA*

		Hypertension	
Type of Anesthesia	Number of Patients	*Number of Cases*	*Percent*
General	240	160	66.7
Spinal	335	9	2.7
Plexus block	40	1	2.5
Bier block	59	11	18.6
Combination	25	4	16.0
Total	699	185	26.5

*Valli, H., Rosenberg, P. H., Kytta, J., et al: Acta Anaesthesiol. Scand. 31: 279–283, 1987. By permission.

with paresthesias induced by axillary block, whether induced intentionally or not, compared with a 0.8-percent incidence in patients without paresthesias. The incidence of unintentional paresthesias was high (40 percent) even when a transarterial method of block placement was selected. In an earlier study of needle-induced nerve lesions in a rabbit model, Selander and other coworkers[56] found a much higher incidence of nerve injury when sharp, long-beveled (14 degrees) needles were employed for intraneural injection than when blunter, short-beveled (45 degrees) needles were employed (Fig. 10–10). Whether the needle bevel was perpendicular or parallel to the nerve axis had no effect on lesion frequency, although nerve injury was generally more severe when the needle bevel was perpendicular to the nerve axis. The observations of Selander's group support a method to localize nerves without causing paresthesias. This can be done with a peripheral nerve stimulator, in which even an unshielded needle can localize nerves. However, shielded, short-beveled "block" needles are better; they decrease the risk of neural injury, offer improved nerve localization, and are readily available.[1, 20]

Interscalene Block

The interscalene block, a regional block of the proximal brachial plexus, has two advantages over the axillary block: (1) the shoulder and upper arm are anesthetized and (2) the block can be performed with the arm in any position.[10] The second advantage is especially helpful in patients who are undergoing joint replacements, as the joint disease often affects other joints of the arm or shoulder for which the block is being placed.

The anesthetic agent is injected in the interscalene groove, between the anterior and middle scalene muscles at the level of the sixth cervical vertebra. For a reliable block of the brachial plexus by the interscalene approach, either elicitation of paresthesias or nerve stimulation to localize the brachial plexus in the interscalene groove is thought to be essential.[79] This is not true with axillary block. The lower trunk of the brachial plexus is the most difficult to block reliably by this route unless large volumes (40 ml) of local anesthetic are administered. The interscalene block is also the slowest to set up.[74, 79] The percentage of each dermatome blocked by this technique is shown in Figure 10–11. Thus, most clinicians who choose a regional technique prefer axillary or intravenous regional anesthesia for hand and wrist surgery; axillary or interscalene block for elbow procedures; and interscalene block for shoulder procedures. In hand or wrist surgery, an interscalene block may have to be supplemented by local infiltration or peripheral block of the ulnar nerve at the elbow.

The patient's respiratory status should be evaluated prior to interscalene block. A patient with chronic obstructive pulmo-

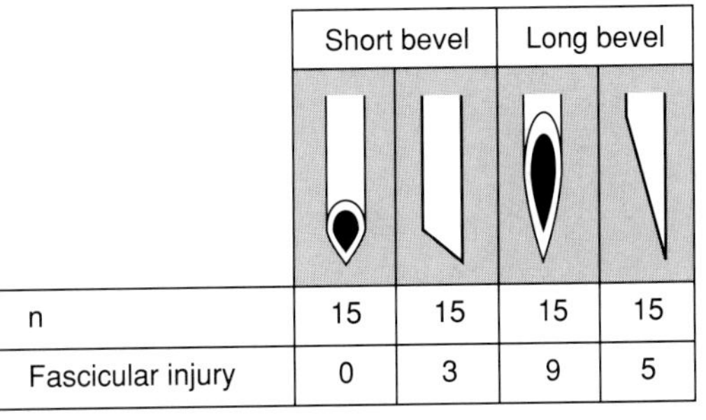

FIGURE 10–10. Fascicular injury after injecting isolated nerve preparations from rabbits with transverse or parallel orientation of the needle bevel to the nerve. (Redrawn from Selander, D., Dhunér, K. G., and Lundborg, G.: Acta Anaesth. Scand. 21:185, 1977.)

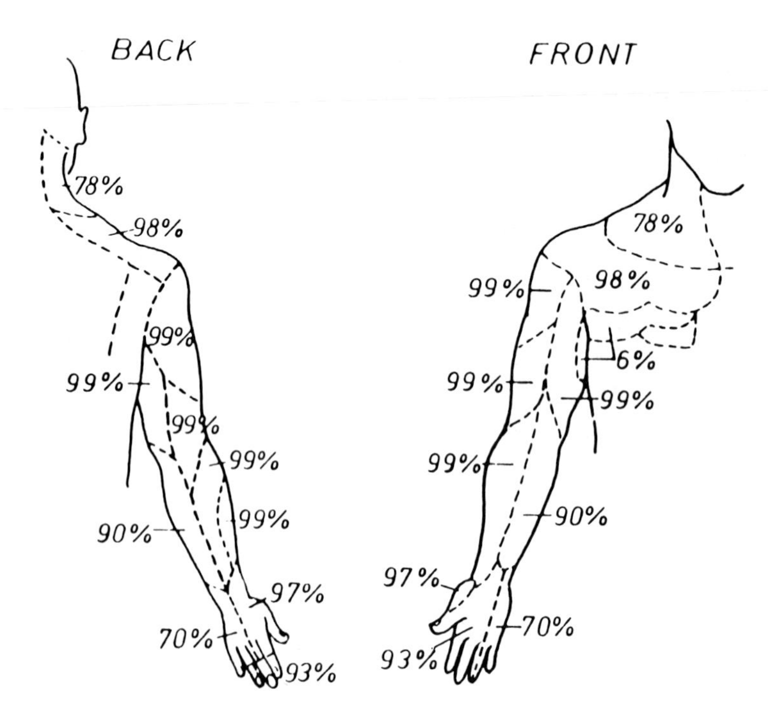

FIGURE 10–11. Areas of analgesia in 100 interscalene blocks. Numbers indicate success rate with which each cutaneous nerve was blocked. (Vester-Andersen, T., Christiansen, C., Hansen, A., et al: Acta Anaesth. Scand. 25:82, 1981. By permission.)

nary disease or other respiratory insufficiency may have the symptoms aggravated if the block is complicated by a pneumothorax or phrenic nerve block. The reported incidence of phrenic nerve block following interscalene block has ranged from 5 to 35 percent.[74, 79] The ideal application for interscalene block in joint arthroplasty is during shoulder replacement procedures.

Intravenous Regional Anesthesia (Bier Block)

In 1908, Bier described the intravenous injection of local anesthetic between two tourniquets. The technique that bears his name is thought to produce anesthesia by several mechanisms, including those unrelated to the anesthetic properties of the drug. Exsanguination and tourniquet inflation probably provide some of the anesthetic effect by producing ischemia and direct pressure on the nerves.[41] Over the years, the technique has been modified: currently, a double tourniquet is applied proximal to the operative site. After limb exsanguination, the tourniquet is inflated to 100 to 150 mmHg above systolic blood pressure; a lidocaine or prilocaine solution (0.5 percent) without epinephrine is then slowly injected intravenously.[8] The volume of drug is based on the mass of the extremity to be anesthetized and the toxic dose of the drug. The toxic dose is especially important, because premature tourniquet release, a common complication, causes acute release of instilled local anesthetic into the systemic circulation. Toxic drug levels produce central nervous system excitation, with sequelae ranging from dizziness and tinnitus to seizures and myocardial depression. The severity of myocardial depression ranges from bradycardia to cardiac arrest. Bupivacaine, once popular, is no longer recommended for Bier block because the central nervous system/cardiac toxicity ratio is much lower than that for lidocaine or prilocaine. Also, resuscitation after bupivacaine-induced cardiovascular collapse is extremely difficult. It has been demonstrated that, even with the tourniquet inflated, local anesthetic enters the systemic circulation (Fig. 10–12).[53] The agent is thought to escape beyond the cuff owing to high pressure created during injection, especially when the injection cannula is in the forearm rather than the hand, or the tourniquet is too small and fails to occlude all vascular channels.[37]

Bier block is a simple but highly effec-

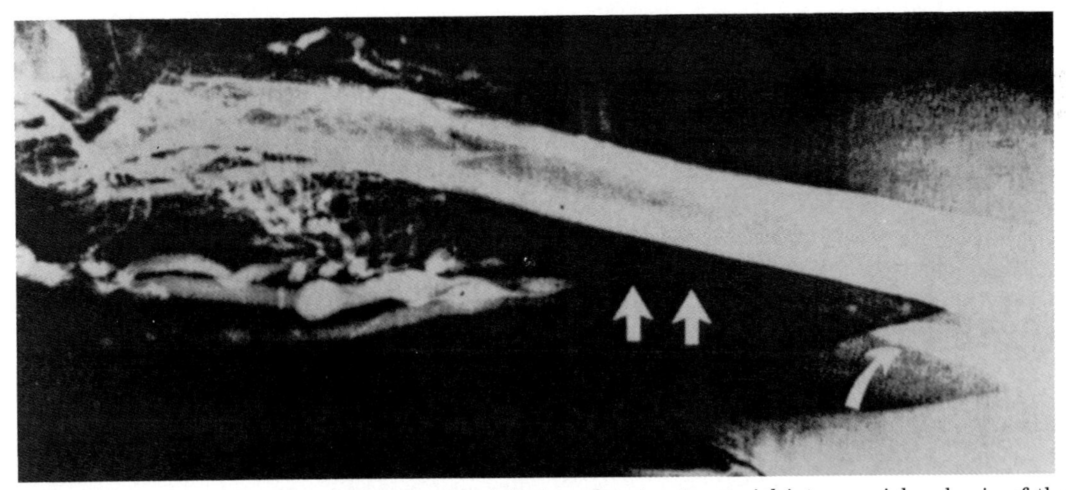

FIGURE 10–12. Phlebography of the arm after injection of contrast material into a peripheral vein of the exsanguinated arm. Tourniquet cuff (double arrow) was 300 mmHg. Note the filled axillary vein at the proximal side of the cuff area (curved arrow) and a continuous narrow streak of contrast under the cuff on the medial side of the humerus. (Rosenberg, P. H., Kalso, E. A., Tuominen, M. K., et al: Anesthesiology 58:96, 1983. By permission.)

tive method for obtaining rapid analgesia of the forearm and hand. The area of slowest onset is the distribution of the radial nerve, possibly because the nerve courses through the forearm discrete from any vascular channels (Fig. 10–13). When a Penrose tourniquet is also applied to the forearm during anesthetic instillation, the time of onset to surgical anesthesia has been shown to decrease from 8 to 4 minutes; this method causes the distal vasculature to fill first instead of last. Peak local anesthetic plasma levels following Bier block tourniquet release are inversely proportional to the duration of tourniquet inflation.[71] To prevent toxic reactions, the tourniquet should never be released until at least 20 minutes after block placement; the release should then be cycled—10 seconds of deflation followed by 1 minute of reinflation.[31, 65]

Although Bier block can provide anesthesia for 60 to 90 minutes, most patients start complaining of tourniquet pain within 60 minutes. A double cuff may provide 30 to 40 minutes more of analgesia. The distal cuff is inflated, underneath which the tissue is anesthetized, and the proximal cuff is released. Because of the time limitation, the Bier block is not recommended for procedures expected to last more than 1 hour. It is also not generally recommended for lower extremity procedures because of the large volumes of local anesthetic required when the tourniquet is placed over the thigh. In addition, if the tourniquet is placed over the calf, it is difficult to obtain and maintain adequate exsanguination and the patient is more uncomfortable. Bier block is most effective for brief procedures of the hand or wrist.

TECHNIQUES FOR SPECIFIC PROCEDURES

Foot and Ankle Joint Replacement

Similar to other joint replacement procedures, arthroplasty of the foot and ankle joint can be performed with the patient under general or regional anesthesia. If a regional technique is chosen, a spinal block is more reliable than an epidural block, in which commonly missed dermatomes cause problems (see Fig. 10–5).[23] The Bier block is not popular among most clinicians because adequate vascular isolation is difficult to obtain with application of a calf tourniquet, increasing the likelihood of local anesthetic toxicity, inadequate block, and bloody operative site. In addition, most patients do not tolerate calf tourniquets as well as thigh tourniquets.

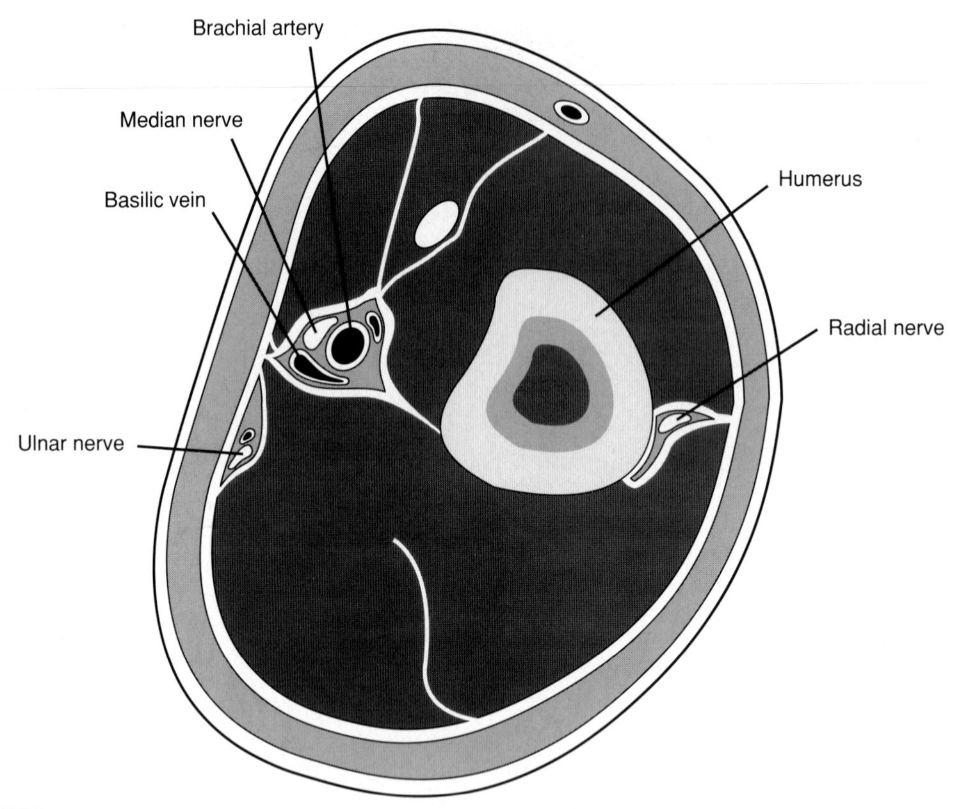

FIGURE 10–13. A cross-section of the arm at the elbow. Nearby the median and ulnar nerves on the anteromedial aspect are rich vascular channels. The radial nerve has less vascularity in its vicinity, possibly explaining the later onset of analgesia after Bier block in the radial nerve distribution. (Redrawn from Holmes, C. McK.: Intravenous regional neural blockade. Neural Blockade, 2nd ed. Edited by M. J. Cousins and P. O. Bridenbaugh. Philadelphia, JB Lippincott Company, p. 456, 1988.)

Total Knee Replacement

Total knee replacement can be successfully performed with the patient under general, epidural, or spinal anesthesia. However, the incidence of inadequate block for the L_4-S_2 dermatomes is high.[23] Because tourniquets are always utilized during total knee replacement, tourniquet pain is common. During general anesthesia, symptomatic improvement is readily obtained with vasodilator and narcotic therapy. However, the patient under spinal anesthesia wants complete resolution of the tourniquet pain but tolerates less narcotic. Because therapy is rarely satisfactory in the awake patient, the emphasis is on prevention.

Concepcion and associates[9] have found that bupivacaine spinal anesthesia reduces the incidence of tourniquet pain to 25 percent compared with 60 percent with tetracaine, despite longer sensory blockade in tetracaine-treated patients. Tourniquet pain also begins later in the bupivacaine group (106 versus 78 minutes). Because tourniquet pain is such a frequent complication during an otherwise satisfactory spinal anesthetic, the findings of Concepcion's group suggest that bupivacaine may be the spinal anesthetic of choice for total knee replacement. Others have found that the addition of clonidine (150 mcg) to a bupivacaine spinal further reduces the incidence of tourniquet pain. Of 15 patients treated with bupivacaine alone, three had tourniquet pain, whereas none of 15 patients treated with bupivacaine and clonidine had pain.[3]

Total Hip Replacement

Effective options for the patient who is undergoing total hip replacement are general, caudal, epidural, and spinal anesthesia. More has been written about the choice and effect of anesthetic technique for this joint replacement operation than any other because of the considerable differences that can occur in patient comfort, intraoperative physiology, perioperative blood loss, and perioperative thrombosis and thromboembolism. These are discussed next.

Patient Comfort

When the lateral decubitus position is employed for surgery, the patient under general anesthesia is more comfortable and stationary. However, the patient is also more vulnerable to position-related injuries of the cervical spine and upper extremity. Also, the endotracheal tube may become dislodged during positioning, because anesthesia is induced with the patient supine. When a regional anesthetic is given, the patient can help in the positioning process by identifying pressure points and supporting the head, chest, and arm until appropriate padding is placed. However, the patient must also be able and willing to lie relatively still throughout the procedure. Many patients with significant arthritic pain in other joints cannot lie motionless on their sides long enough for even a primary arthroplasty to be completed using a regional anesthetic technique.

Intraoperative Physiology

Type of anesthesia, position of patient, and mode of ventilation affect the normal ventilation-perfusion relationships of the lungs.[29] When anesthesia is induced with the patient supine, a cephalad shift of the diaphragm occurs.[21] With the patient in the decubitus position, the dependent lung is further compressed by the weight of the mediastinal and abdominal contents. During spontaneous ventilation, ventilation-perfusion relations are well maintained, but the situation changes as soon as systemic muscle relaxants are administered and mechanical ventilation is begun. At this time, the nondependent lung is better ventilated because compliance is better in this position, whereas most of the perfusion goes to the dependent lung. This effect produces a shunt of 20 to 30 percent, predisposing the patient to intraoperative and postoperative hypoxemia.[6, 81] Reduced ventilation in the dependent lung postoperatively persists for an unknown amount of time despite restored spontaneous ventilation, presumably secondary to the vascular congestion and atelectasis that occur during mechanical ventilation. Continuous monitoring of the patient in the lateral position by pulse oximetry makes it simpler to identify and correct any hypoxemia associated with positioning. During regional anesthesia with spontaneous ventilation, ventilation-perfusion relationships are well maintained, and atelectasis of the dependent lung is less common.

Anesthetic technique also affects the neuroendocrine response to surgical stress. The response is significantly lower with regional than with general anesthesia[12, 66] as demonstrated by comparisons of serial serum cortisol and glucose levels, which change less during regional anesthesia. However, clinical outcomes are comparable. A study of mental recovery following total hip replacement in patients receiving different types of anesthesia showed no difference among general anesthesia, epidural anesthesia, and their combination (Fig. 10–14).[52]

Perioperative Blood Loss

Intraoperative blood loss is 30 to 40 percent less with regional anesthesia than with general anesthesia during hip replacement surgery (Fig. 10–15A).[42] If local epidural analgesia is continued postoperatively, blood loss is 25 to 35 percent less than that with parenteral analgesia (Fig. 10–15B).[42] These observations are attributed to lower arterial and venous blood pressures with regional anesthesia. General anesthesia with mechanical ventilation interferes with venous drainage from the operative site by increasing intrathoracic pressure. In contrast, spontaneous ventilation reduces intrathoracic pressure. Regional anesthesia also causes a sympathectomy of the anesthetized region, reducing arterial and venous resistance and thereby improving venous drainage—less

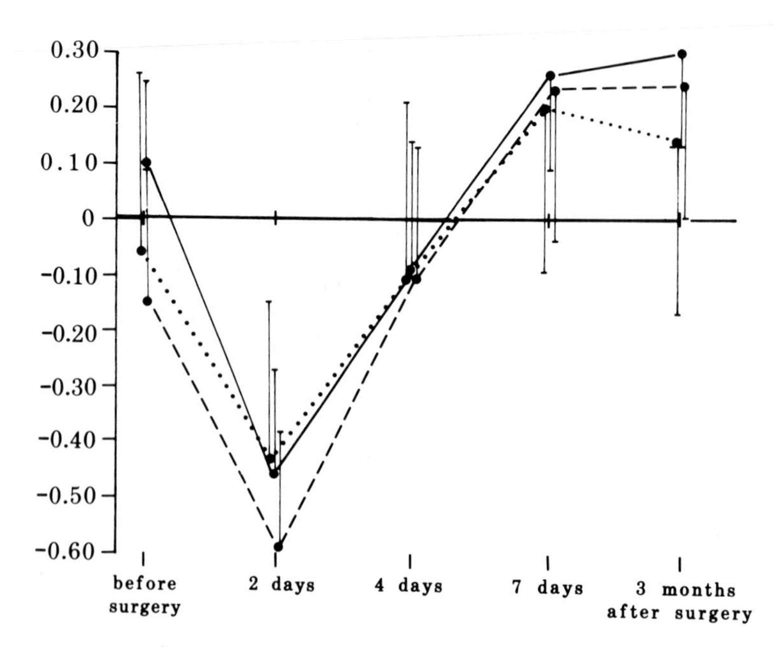

FIGURE 10–14. Comparison of attention test scores before and after hip replacement arthroplasty performed while utilizing general anesthesia (solid line, n = 9), epidural analgesia (dotted line, n = 10), and general anesthesia plus epidural analgesia (dashed line, n = 9) (mean ± SEM). (Riis, J., Lomholt, B., Haxholdt, D., et al: Acta Anaesthesiol. Scand. 27:44, 1983. By permission.)

venous bleeding is observed. Modig[42] noted a strong correlation between peripheral venous pressure measured in the wound and intraoperative blood loss (Fig. 10–16). Several investigators have reported prospective studies demonstrating that hypotensive anesthesia, whether general or regional, does not lessen intraoperative blood loss.[68, 78] Previously, it was believed that systolic blood pressure influenced blood loss during hip replacement. Because hypotensive anesthesia offers no benefit in elderly patients, potential complications with this technique make it hard to justify.

Perioperative Thrombosis and Thromboembolism

One of the most serious complications after hip replacement surgery is perioperative thrombosis with thromboembolism. One reviewer estimates the incidence of pulmonary embolism at 6 percent, with deep vein thrombosis occurring in about 50 percent of patients who are undergoing hip replacement.[60] Factors that are thought to predispose a patient to thrombosis and embolism include old age, female gender, degenerative arthropathy, lateral operative approach, undertransfusion, and immobility.[60] Anesthesia may also affect the incidence.[43, 44, 70] When Modig compared the incidence of peripheral thrombosis in popliteal and femoral veins of patients who were undergoing epidural and general anesthesia, it was over five times higher in the general anesthesia group. Thrombosis in calf and thigh veins was almost twice as high; pulmonary embolism was more than three times as high (Table 10–10). However, these dramatic data must be viewed with caution, as the epidural group received local anesthesia (i.e., sympathectomy), with its attendant benefits, for 24 hours postoperatively. The reasons for the differences are unclear. Effects on the hemostatic response to surgery, venous im-

Table 10–10. INCIDENCE OF VENOUS THROMBOSIS AND PULMONARY EMBOLISM

	Epidural Anesthesia (%)	General Anesthesia (%)
Popliteal and femoral veins	13	67
Calf and thigh veins	40	70
Pulmonary embolism	10	33

Modig, J.: Acta Chir. Scand. 151:589–594, 1985. By permission.

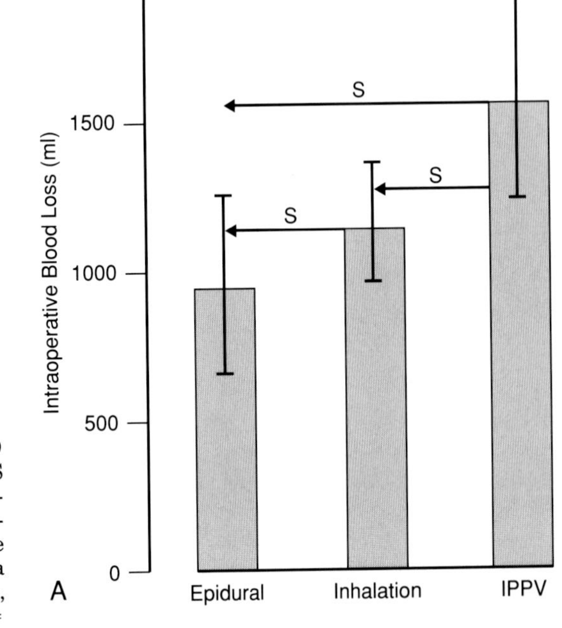

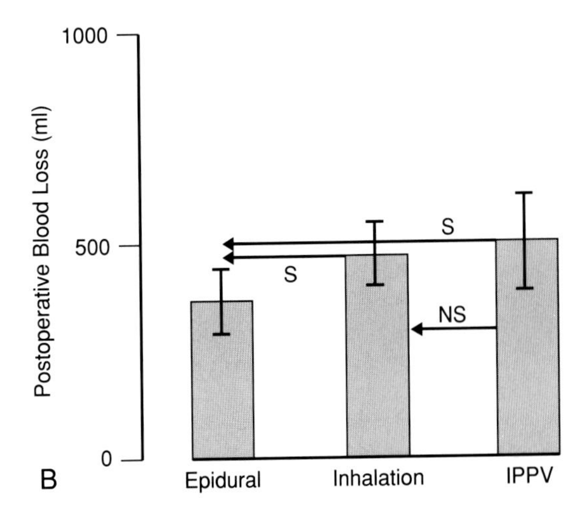

FIGURE 10–15. Intraoperative blood loss (ml) *(A)* and postoperative blood loss *(B)* (mean ± SD). S indicates significant differences between groups. Inhalation represents general anesthesia with spontaneous ventilation, and intermittent positive-pressure ventilation (IPPV) represents general anesthesia with mechanical ventilation. (Redrawn from Modig, J.: Acta Anaesthesiol. Scand. 32:45–46, 1988.) (ns = not significant.)

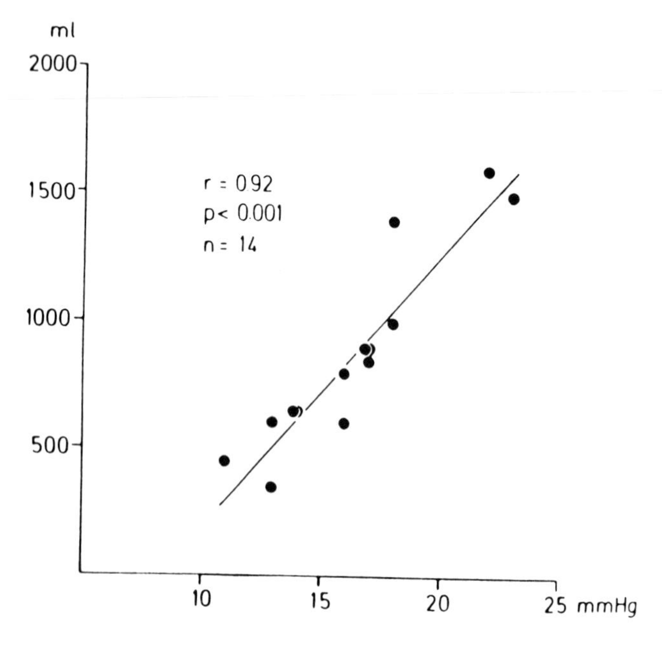

FIGURE 10–16. Relationship between mean peripheral venous blood pressure measured in the operative wound (averaged five intraoperative phases) and the intraoperative blood loss. (Modig, J.: Acta Anaesthesiol. Scand. 32:46, 1988. By permission.)

pedance, and leg blood flow could be implicated (Fig. 10–17).[13, 14, 43, 44, 70] However, even when one parameter such as calf blood flow clearly differs, the relationship between this finding and the incidence of deep vein thrombosis is not always apparent.[13]

Because many clinicians consider these data to be only suggestive, rather than compelling, anesthetic approaches continue to vary. In some series, no benefit has been demonstrated, even in the most at-risk patients, i.e., the elderly.[33] The data should be considered thoughtfully, however, in the interests of lowering the incidence of thrombosis and embolism in patients (see Chapter 9, *Thromboembolic Disease*).

Total Shoulder Replacement

Either general or regional anesthesia may be administered for total shoulder replacement. However, interscalene block is the only reasonably successful regional technique. The benefits of early mobilization and prolonged postoperative analgesia must be weighed against the failure rate. In a series of 100 patients who were undergoing major shoulder surgery, the success rate was 82 percent for blocks placed in standard fashion (i.e., surgical anesthesia achieved within 30 minutes).[74] Of the patients in this series, 4 percent had significant side effects, consisting of loss of consciousness, respiratory depression, and seizure. The complications were attributed to high serum levels of local anesthetic, which occurred despite the usual safeguards. Of the patients in the series, 91 percent were satisfied with interscalene anesthesia and 2 percent had neuropraxis lasting longer than 6 months.[10] The experience of Vester-Andersen and colleagues emphasizes the need for a risk-benefit assessment before recommending a specific anesthetic technique.

Elbow Replacement

Anesthetic options for patients who are undergoing elbow replacement include general anesthesia, axillary or interscalene anesthesia, and Bier block. However, neither axillary nor interscalene block are completely reliable (Figs. 10–6 and 10–11). Use of the Bier block may be limited by the length of the procedure and the interference caused by the bulkier double tourniquet at the operative site.

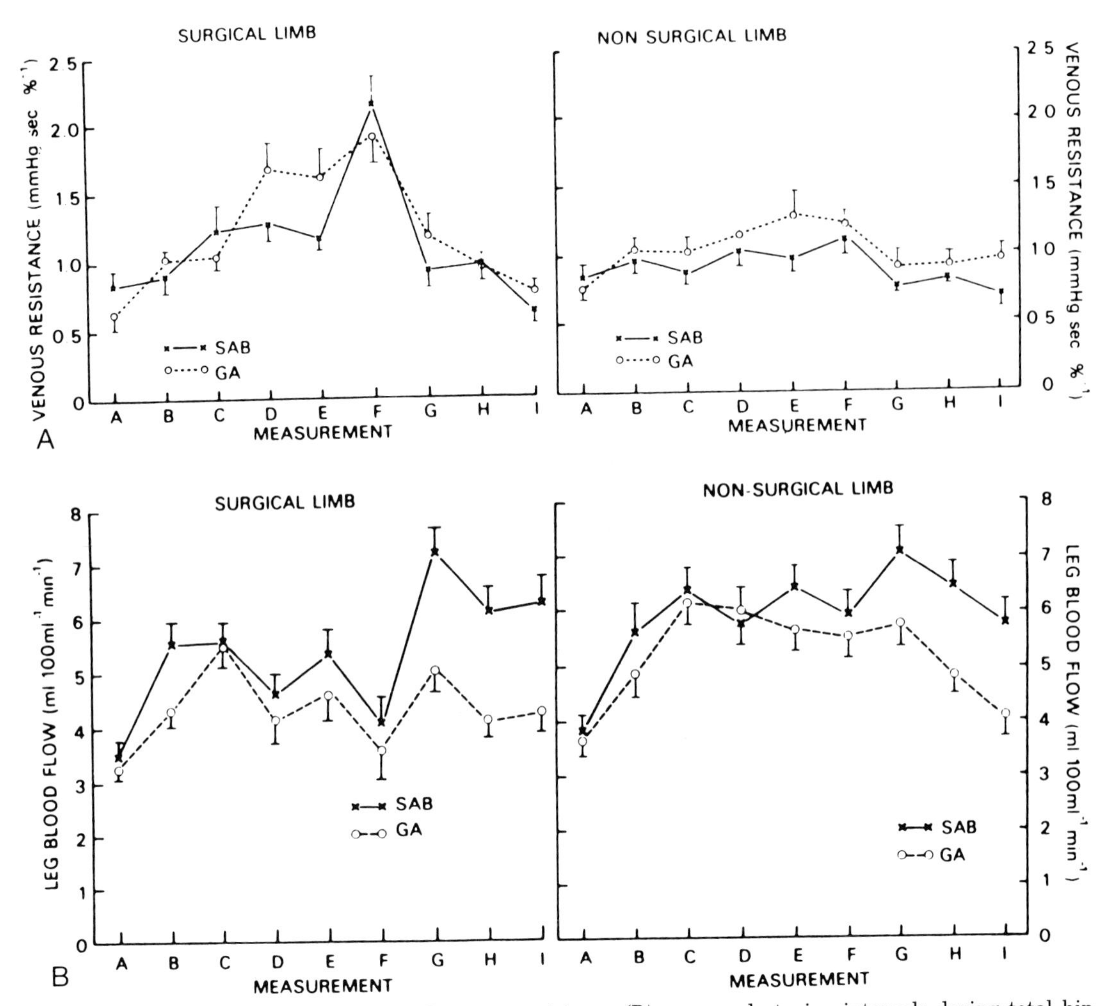

FIGURE 10–17. Leg blood flow *(A)* and venous resistance *(B)* measured at nine intervals during total hip replacement in 140 patients. **A** = Supine (preinduction) with legs elevated 20 degrees. **B** = Lateral 10 minutes after induction. **C** = Before joint dislocation. **D** = Immediately after dislocation, femoral head removed. **E** = During setting of cement, acetabular component. **F** = During setting of cement, femoral component. **G** = Within 5 minutes of relocation of prosthetic joint. **H** = End of surgery. **I** = Supine 20 minutes postoperatively, legs elevated 20 degrees. (Davis, F. M., Laurenson, V. G., Gillespie, W. J., et al: Anaesth. Intens. Care 17:138–139, 1989. By permission.) (SAB = spinal anesthesia; GA = general anesthesia.)

Hand and Wrist Replacement

General anesthesia, axillary block, Bier block, and occasionally local anesthetic block are effective options for hand and wrist replacement procedures. Regional techniques have the advantage of allowing outpatient surgery and avoiding the unpleasant side effects of general anesthesia (nausea, vomiting, and general malaise). Also, outpatients without access to parenteral pain medications may benefit from the longer-lasting analgesia offered by a local or axillary block.

BLOOD REPLACEMENT

Although blood loss occurs during any operation, blood replacement in arthroplastic procedures is normally an issue only in knee, hip, and possibly shoulder operations. Suction and sponges remove blood intraoperatively, and drains postoperatively. Less obvious blood loss occurs by extravasation into adjacent tissues and by sequestration in hematomas. When the circulating red blood cells can no longer meet tissue oxygen requirements, blood replacement becomes necessary. This concept is in keeping with the principle that transfusion is not normally used to treat hypovolemia. In fact, most patients tolerate normovolemic anemia well.[48] For anemia to be manageable, it must occur in a normovolemic patient, i.e., the patient capable of a compensatory increase in cardiac output to maintain adequate oxygen delivery. No standard minimum hematocrit exists for normovolemic patients. Coexisting diseases must be taken into consideration. A patient with significant coronary artery disease may experience myocardial ischemia with hemodilution to a hematocrit of 30 percent, whereas a healthy patient may tolerate a hematocrit of 20 percent.[22, 50] The observations for patients with heart disease parallel those for patients with compromised cerebral or other organ blood flow.

Called the "transfusion trigger," the threshold maximum blood loss or minimum serum hematocrit value is based on preoperative evaluation of coexisting diseases and both anticipated and actual blood loss. A method for calculating allowable blood loss is described in Table 10–11.

Table 10–11. CALCULATION FOR ALLOWABLE BLOOD LOSS*

$$ABL = EBV \times (H_I - H_F) \div 100 \times [3 - (H_I + H_F) \div 200]$$

or, less accurately

$$[ABL = EBV \times (H_I + H_F) \div H_I]$$

Where ABL = allowable blood loss (L)
EBV = estimated blood volume (L)
H_I = initial hematocrit (%)
H_F = final lowest acceptable hematocrit (%)

*Bourke, D. L. and Smith, T. C.: Anesthesiology 41:609, 1974. By permission.

Blood may be replaced by reinfusion of washed autologous red blood cells collected from the operative site, autologous blood donated by the patient preoperatively, or random cross-matched donor red blood cells from the blood bank. The first two methods avoid the risk and expense of dealing with unknown donors. Although the risk of transfusion reaction and acquired immune deficiency syndrome (AIDS) are both very low, the incidence of post-transfusion viral hepatitis is approximately one in 200 units transfused.[77] The current trend is toward preoperative autologous donations. Patients appreciate the enhanced safety, and blood banks accommodate such special arrangements better than they did a few years ago. The expense of transfusion varies from one hospital to another.

PERIOPERATIVE PAIN MANAGEMENT

The management of perioperative pain is divided into three phases: preoperative, acute postoperative, and late postoperative. Preoperatively, the clinician may wish to stop nonsteroidal anti-inflammatory agents when the patient is no longer permitted anything by mouth. This practice is sufficient to ensure normal intraoperative platelet function. However, salicylate preparations should be discontinued at least 1 week before surgery to ensure normal platelet function, if this is the goal.

The management of acute postoperative pain begins in the operating room. If a general anesthetic is being administered, careful titration of intravenous narcotics allows the patient to wake up in relative comfort, providing analgesia for up to several hours. At some point, supplemental analgesics will have to be provided. Current options include intramuscular, intravenous, and epidural narcotics with or without local anesthesia and nerve block.

In 1968, Sechzer first described what is now called "patient-controlled analgesia."[55] It has become popular among both physicians and patients. The chief advantage to patients is that it provides better pain relief than intramuscular injection. Other advantages are that it is available on demand and controlled by the patient, is conveniently located at the bedside, offers rapid onset of action, and is administered painlessly. Spetzler and Anderson[62] found that the method provided excellent analgesia in patients who had undergone total hip and knee replacement procedures. About one in three patients requires an adjustment of the delivery setting.[62] To provide optimal analgesia, the method should be instituted in the recovery room after analgesia has been established by intravenous narcotic administration. In this way, a therapeutic level is maintained by the patient, rather than having to achieve it slowly postoperatively. In the latter case, incremental doses can be delivered only after the prescribed "lock-out" time has elapsed. Thus, adequate analgesia may take a long time.

Once a patient is taking liquids, the narcotic agent can be supplemented by an oral nonsteroidal anti-inflammatory agent, such as piroxicam. In one study, this drug reduced the postoperative morphine requirement by 50 percent after total hip arthroplasty.[58] The investigators postulated that much postoperative pain is musculoskeletal in origin and is caused by the patient's position and prolonged immobility. A new nonsteroidal agent with potent analgesic action is ketorolac;[5] it has the advantage of being available for intramuscular administration. The drug has been found to be as effective as morphine or meperidine and has fewer side effects.

Epidural narcotics with or without admixed bupivacaine have found greater use in the postoperative management of orthopedic patients, although their efficacy is limited to lower extremity procedures. The resulting analgesia is better than that achieved by either intramuscular or patient-controlled analgesia (Table 10–12).[18, 28, 38] However, a small but increased risk of respiratory depression occurs, requiring that the patient be monitored frequently. Still, the technique is so successful that the anesthesiology departments of many medical centers provide this service. Some investigators have reported earlier mobilization and recovery of range of motion, without a significant increase in side effects.[38, 39] Caution must be exercised if a local anesthetic is coadministered or administered alone by this route, because approximately 20 percent of patients manifest some motor block of the lower extremities. The patient should be assessed before being allowed out of bed. If motor block is present, it can be readily resolved by removing the anesthetic agent from the infusion or lowering the concentration. Partial analgesia via femoral nerve block after knee arthroplasty has been found to bring initially improved analgesia, with 80-degree flexion achieved postoperatively on day 5 versus day 7 in those treated with patient-controlled analgesia.[32] Parenteral narcotics are usually discontinued between 48 and 96 hours postoperatively, as the transition is made to an oral narcotic, nonsteroidal preparation, or both.

The options for analgesia after upper extremity procedures are similar to those after lower extremity procedures with regard to administration of narcotic or nonsteroidal agents. The residual postoperative analgesia that follows an interscalene or axillary block may be extended by providing a long-acting local anesthetic combination initially or by leaving a catheter in place through which additional anesthetic may be infused. This technique is useful when early mobilization of the operated joint is important. Peripheral nerve block also offers effective postoperative analgesia after hand and finger arthroplasty.

Table 10–12. EFFICACY OF EPIDURAL BLOCK, PATIENT-CONTROLLED ANALGESIA, AND INTRAMUSCULAR MORPHINE

Route of Administration	Percent of Patients with Good Analgesia		
	I[18]	II[28]	III[38]
Intramuscular	25	45	—
Intravenous and patient controlled	40	60	50
Epidural	65	85	95

What does the future hold in terms of anesthetic options for patients who will undergo joint replacement surgery and for the physicians who treat them? Just as patients today expect to have complete intraoperative analgesia, by the end of this century it will be reasonable for them to expect the same in the postoperative period. Rapid growth in the field of anesthesia, and particularly in the subspecialty area of acute pain management, will make this an achievable goal.

References

1. Bashein, G., Haschke, R. H., and Ready, L. B.: Electrical nerve location: Numerical and electrophoretic comparison of insulated vs. uninsulated needles. Anesth. Analg. 63:919–924, 1984.
2. Bedford, R. F. and Feinstein, B.: Hospital admission blood pressure: A predictor for hypertension following endotracheal intubation. Anesth. Analg. 59:367–370, 1980.
3. Bennet, F., Drallo, A., Saada, M., et al.: Prevention of tourniquet pain by spinal isobaric bupivacaine with clonidine. Br. J. Anaesth. 63:93–96, 1989.
4. Blomberg, R. G. and Olsson, S. S.: The lumbar epidural space in patients examined with epiduroscopy. Anesth. Analg. 68:157, 1989.
5. Buckley, M. M. T. and Brogden, R. N.: Ketorolac: A review of its pharmacodynamic and pharmacokinetic properties and therapeutic potential. Drugs 39:86–109, 1990.
6. Capan, L. M., Turndorf, H., Patel, C., et al.: Optimization of arterial oxygenation during one-lung anesthesia. Anesth. Analg. 59:847–851, 1980.
7. Chernow, B., Alexander, H. R., Smallridge, R. C., et al.: Hormonal responses to graded surgical stress. Arch. Intern. Med. 147:1273–1278, 1987.
8. Colbern, E. C.: The Bier block for intravenous regional anesthesia. Anesth. Analg. 49:935, 1970.
9. Concepcion, M. A., Lambert, D. H., Welch, K. A., et al.: Tourniquet pain during spinal anesthesia: A comparison of plain solutions of tetracaine and bupivacaine. Anesth. Analg. 67:828–832, 1988.
10. Conn, R. M., Cofield, R. H., Byer, D. E., et al.: Interscalene block anesthesia for shoulder surgery. Clin. Orthop. 216:94–98, 1987.
11. Cullen, B. F. and Miller, M. G.: Drug interactions and anesthesia: A review. Anesth. Analg. 58:413, 1979.
12. Davis, F. M., Laurenson, G., and Lewis, J.: Metabolic response to total hip arthroplasty under hypobaric subarachnoid or general anaesthesia. Br. J. Anaesth. 59:725, 1987.
13. Davis, F. M., Laurenson, V. G., Gillespiem, W. J., et al.: Leg blood flow during total hip replacement under spinal or general anaesthesia. Anaesth. Intens. Care 17:136–143, 1989.
14. Davis, F. M., McDermott, E., Hickton, C., et al.: Influence of spinal and general anaesthesia on haemostasis during total hip arthroplasty. Br. J. Anaesth. 59:561–571, 1987.
15. Deanfield, J. A., Selwyn, A. P., Chierchia, S., et al.: Myocardial ischaemia during daily life in patients with stable angina. Its relation to symptoms and heart rate changes. Lancet 1:753–758, 1983.
16. DeBoard, J. W., Ghia, J. N., and Guildford, N. B.: Caudal anaesthesia in a patient with ankylosing spondylitis for hip surgery. Anesthesiology 54:164–166, 1981.
17. Edwards, R. P., Miller, R. D., Roizen, M. F., et al.: Cardiac responses to imipramine and pancuronium during anesthesia with halothane or enflurane. Anesthesiology 50:421, 1979.
18. Eisenbach, J. C., Grice, S. C., and Dewan, D. M.: Patient-controlled analgesia following cesarean section: A comparison with epidural and intramuscular narcotics. Anesthesiology 68:444, 1988.
19. El-Ganzouri, A. R., Ivankovich, A. D., Braverman, R., et al.: Monoamine oxidase inhibitors: Should they be discontinued preoperatively? Anesth. Analg. 64:592–596, 1985.
20. Ford, D. J., Pither, C., and Raj, P. P.: Comparison of insulated and uninsulated needles for locating peripheral nerves with a peripheral nerve stimulator. Anesth. Analg. 63:925, 1984.
21. Froese, A. B. and Bryan, A. C.: Effects of anesthesia and paralysis on diaphragmatic mechanics in man. Anesthesiology 41:242, 1973.
22. Gaehtgens, P., Benner, K. U., and Schickendantz, S.: Effect of hemodilution on blood flow, O_2 consumption and performance of skeletal muscle during exercise. Bibl. Haematol. 41:54, 1975.
23. Galindo, A., Hernandez, J., Benavides, S., et al.: Quality of spinal extradural anesthesia: The influence of spinal nerve root diameter. Br. J. Anaesth. 47:41, 1975.
24. Goldman, L. and Caldera, D. L.: Risks of general anesthesia and elective operation in the hypertensive patient. Anesthesiology 50:285, 1979.
25. Goldman, L., Caldera, D. L., Nussbaum, S. R., et al.: Multifactorial index of cardiac risk in noncardiac surgical procedures. N. Engl. J. Med. 297:845–850, 1977.
26. Goodson, W. H. and Hunt, T. K.: Studies of wound healing in experimental diabetes mellitus. J. Surg. Res. 22:221, 1977.
27. Hagenouw, R. R. P. M., Bridenbaugh, P. O., van Egmond, J., et al.: Tourniquet pain: A volunteer study. Anesth. Analg. 65:1175, 1986.
28. Harrison, D. H., Sinatra, R., Morgesel, L., et al.: Epidural narcotic and patient-controlled analgesia for post-cesarean section pain relief. Anesthesiology 68:454, 1988.
29. Hedenstierna, G. and Löfström, J.: Effect of anaesthesia on respiratory function after major lower extremity surgery: A comparison between bupivacaine spinal analgesia with low-dose morphine and general anaesthesia. Acta Anaesthesiol. Scand. 29:55–60, 1985.
30. Hirsch, I. A., Tomlinson, D. L., Slogoff, S., et al.: The overstated risk of preoperative hypokalemia. Anesth. Analg. 67:131–136, 1988.
31. Holmes, C. McK.: Intravenous Regional Neural Blockade. Neural Blockade. Edited by M. J. Cousins and P. O. Bridenbaugh. Philadelphia, J. B. Lippincott Company, 1988.

32. Hord, A. H., Roberson, J. R., Thompson, W. F., et al.: Evaluation of continuous femoral nerve analgesia after primary total knee arthroplasty. Anesth. Analg. 70:S164, 1990.
33. Hosking, M. P., Lobdell, C. M., and Warner, M. A.: Anaesthesia for patients over 90 years of age. Outcomes after regional and general anaesthetic techniques for two common surgical procedures. Anaesthesia 44:142–147, 1989.
34. Janowsky, E. C., Risch, C., and Janowsky, D. S.: Effect of anesthesia on patients taking psychotropic drugs. J. Clin. Psychopharmacol. 1:14–20, 1981.
35. Kaufman, R. D. and Walts, L. F.: Tourniquet-induced hypertension. Br. J. Anaesth. 54:333–336, 1982.
36. Kingston, H. G. G. and Hirschman, C. A.: Perioperative management of the patient with asthma. Anesth. Analg. 63:844–855, 1984.
37. Lawes, E. G.: Venous pressures during simulated Bier's block. Anaesthesia 39:147–149, 1984.
38. Loper, K. A. and Ready, L. B.: Epidural morphine after anterior cruciate ligament repair: A comparison with patient-controlled intravenous morphine. Anesth. Analg. 68:350–352, 1989.
39. Lubenow, T. R., McCarthy, R. J., Grande, S., et al.: Comparison of continuous epidural narcotic bupivacaine mixtures to patient-controlled analgesia after major orthopedic surgery. Anesth. Analg. 70:S250, 1990.
40. Michaels, I., Serrins, M., Shier, N. Q., et al.: Anesthesia for cardiac surgery in patients receiving monoamine oxidase inhibitors. Anesth. Analg. 63:1041–1044, 1984.
41. Miles, D. W., James, J. L., Clark, D. E., et al.: Site of action of intravenous regional anaesthesia. J. Neurol. Neurosurg. Psychiatry 27:574, 1964.
42. Modig, J.: Regional anaesthesia and blood loss. Acta Anaesthesiol. Scand. 32[Suppl 89]:44–48, 1988.
43. Modig, J.: The role of lumbar epidural anaesthesia as antithrombotic prophylaxis in total hip replacement. Acta Chir. Scand. 151:589–594, 1985.
44. Modig, J., Borg, T., Karlström, G., et al.: Thromboembolism after total hip replacement: Role of epidural and general anesthesia. Anesth. Analg. 62:174–180, 1983.
45. Montgomery, S. J., Raj, P. R., Nettles, D., et al.: The use of the nerve stimulator with standard unsheathed needles in nerve blockade. Anesth. Analg. 52:827–831, 1973.
46. Narang, V. P. S. and Linter, S. P. K.: Failure of epidural blockade in obstetrics. Br. J. Anaesth. 60:402, 1988.
47. National Institutes of Health Consensus Development Conference: Total Hip Joint Replacement. Bethesda, Maryland, March 1982.
48. National Institutes of Health Consensus Conference: Office of Medical Applications of Research. Perioperative red blood cell transfusion. J.A.M.A. 260:2700, 1988.
49. Plorn, G. W.: Clinical considerations in the use of corticosteroids. N. Engl. J. Med. 274:775–781, 1966.
50. Rao, T. L. K., El-Etr, A. A., and Montoya, A.: Hemodynamic changes due to normovolemic anemia in coronary artery disease patients. Anesthesiology 51:S164, 1979.
51. Rao, T. L. K., Jacobs, K. H., El-Etr, A. A.: Reinfarction following anesthesia in patients with myocardial infarction. Anesthesiology 59:499–505, 1983.
52. Riis, J., Lomholt, B., Haxholdt, D., et al.: Immediate and long-term mental recovery from general vs. epidural anesthesia in elderly patients. Acta Anaesthesiol. Scand. 27:44, 1983.
53. Rosenberg, P. H., Kalso, E. A., Tuominen, M. K., et al.: Acute bupivacaine cardiotoxicity as a result of venous leakage under the tourniquet cuff during Bier block. Anesthesiology 58:95–98, 1983.
54. Rothman, R. H.: Operative Technique for Primary Total Hip Arthroplasty. Total Hip Arthroplasty. Edited by R. E. Booth, R. A. Balderston, and R. H. Rothman. Philadelphia, W. B. Saunders Company, 1988.
55. Sechzer, P. H.: Objective measurement of pain. Anesthesiology 29:209–210, 1968.
56. Selander, D., Dhunér, K. G., and Lundborg, G.: Peripheral nerve injury due to injection needles used for regional anesthesia. Acta Anaesth. Scand. 21:182–188, 1977.
57. Selander, D., Edshage, S., and Wolff, T.: Paresthesiae or no paresthesiae? Nerve lesions after axillary blocks. Acta Anaesth. Scand. 23:27, 1979.
58. Serpell, M. G. and Thompson, M. F.: Comparison of piroxicam with placebo in the management of pain after total hip replacement. Br. J. Anaesth. 63:354, 1989.
59. Shah, K. B., Kleinman, B. S., Rao, T. L. K., et al.: Angina and other risk factors in patients with cardiac disease undergoing noncardiac operations. Anesth. Analg. 70:240–247, 1990.
60. Sikorski, J. M.: Thromboembolic Complications. Complications of Total Hip Replacement. Current Problems in Orthopedics. New York, Churchill Livingstone, 1984.
61. Smith, P. H., Sharp, J., and Kellgren, J. H.: Natural history of rheumatoid cervical subluxations. Ann. Rheum. Dis. 31:222–223, 1972.
62. Spetzler, B. and Anderson, L.: Patient-controlled analgesia in the total joint arthroplasty patient. Clin. Orthop. 215:122–125, 1987.
63. Steen, P. A., Tinker, J. H., and Tarhan, S.: Myocardial reinfarction after anesthesia and surgery. J.A.M.A. 239:2566–2570, 1978.
64. Stewart, D. E., Ikram, H., and Espiner, E. A.: Arrhythmogenic potential of diuretic-induced hypokalaemia in patients with mild hypertension and ischaemic heart disease. Br. Heart J. 54:290–297, 1985.
65. Sukhari, R.: Lidocaine disposition following intravenous regional anesthesia with different tourniquet deflation techniques. Anesth. Analg. 68:633–637, 1989.
66. Svartling, N., Lehtinen, A. M., and Tarkkan, N. L.: The effect of anaesthesia on changes in blood pressure and plasma cortisol levels induced by cementation with methyl methacrylate. Acta Anaesthesiol. Scand. 30:247, 1986.
67. Symreng, T., Karlberg, B. E., Kågedal, B., et al.: Physiological cortisol substitution of long-term steroid-treated patients undergoing major surgery. Br. J. Anaesth. 53:549, 1981.
68. Thoburn, J.: Subarachnoid block and total hip replacement: Effect of ephedrine on intraoperative blood loss. Br. J. Anaesth. 57:290–293, 1985.

69. Thompson, G. E. and Rorie, D. K.: Functional anatomy of the brachial plexus sheaths. Anesthesiology 59:117–122, 1983.
70. Thorburn, T., Louden, J. R., and Vallance, R.: Spinal and general anaesthesia in total hip replacement: Frequency of deep vein thrombosis. Br. J. Anaesth. 52:1117–1121, 1980.
71. Tucker, G. T. and Boas, R. A.: Pharmacokinetic aspects of intravenous regional anesthesia. Anesthesiology 34:538, 1971.
72. Udelsman, R., Ramp, J., Galluci, W. T., et al.: Adaptation during surgical stress: A reevaluation of the role of glucocorticoids. J. Clin. Invest. 77:1377–1381, 1986.
73. Valli, H., Rosenberg, P. H., Kytta, J., et al.: Arterial hypertension associated with the use of a tourniquet with either general or regional anaesthesia. Acta Anaesthesiol. Scand. 31:279–283, 1987.
74. Vester-Andersen, T., Christiansen, C., Hansen, A., et al.: Interscalene brachial plexus block: Area of analgesia, complications, and blood concentrations of local anesthetics. Acta Anaesth. Scand. 25:81–84, 1981.
75. Viegas, O. J.: Psychiatric Illness. Anesthesia and Coexisting Disease. Edited by R. K. Stoelting and S. F. Dierdorf. New York, Churchill Livingstone, 1983.
76. Vitez, T. S., Soper, L. E., Wong, K. C., et al.: Chronic hypokalemia and intraoperative dysrhythmias. Anesthesiology 63:127–129, 1985.
77. Walker, R. H.: Special report: Transfusion risks. Am. J. Clin. Pathol. 88:374, 1987.
78. Wittmann, F. W.: Blood loss associated with uncemented total hip replacement: Hypotension does not affect blood loss. J. Roy. Soc. Med. 80:213–215, 1987.
79. Winnie, A. P.: Interscalene brachial plexus block. Anesth. Analg. 49:455, 1970.
80. Winnie, A. P., Radonjic, R., Akkineni, S. R., et al.: Factors influencing distribution of local anesthetic injected into the brachial plexus sheath. Anesth. Analg. 58:225–234, 1979.
81. Wulff, K. and Aulin, I.: The regional lung function in the lateral decubitus position during anesthesia and operation. Acta Anaesthesiol. Scand. 16:195–205, 1972.

CHAPTER 11

Imaging of Total Joint Replacement

MARJ M. HEARE
WILLIAM J. MONTGOMERY

Total joint replacement is a mainstay of treatment for many types of arthropathy, most notably degenerative joint disease and rheumatoid arthritis. After implantation, imaging is done to detect complications. This chapter begins with descriptions of imaging modalities that are generally useful in patients with joint prostheses: plain radiography, aspiration arthrography, radioisotope scanning, computerized tomography, magnetic resonance imaging, and ultrasound. Imaging of problems particular to each joint (the hip, knee, ankle, shoulder, elbow, and wrist and hand) are then individually addressed. The chapter concludes with a brief synopsis of how to image common postarthroplasty problems.

MODALITIES

Plain Radiography

Plain radiography constitutes the backbone of radiographic evaluation of any patient with total joint arthroplasty. Basic radiographs include anteroposterior (AP) and lateral views of the involved articulation with the patient in the supine position and with the x-ray beam centered on and parallel to the joint line. Additional radiographs of specific joints, such as the tangential view of the patella and the axillary view of the shoulder, are certainly appropriate. A baseline set of radiographs should be made shortly after implantation to rule out intraoperative fracture or gross malposition (Fig. 11–1) and to provide a basis for comparison of follow-up radiographs.[95]

Because serial films are frequently made with different radiographic techniques meaningful comparison is precluded, and therefore subtle changes may be missed. The specific radiographic technique is not as important as taking the radiograph in the same way at every clinic visit.[2, 34, 70] Film size, tube-to-film distance, patient-to-film distance, and positioning of the patient and x-ray beam should be specified for each type of total joint arthroplasty radiographed.

Two studies reported excellent reproducibility using chariot and grid devices. With these devices the patient can be positioned and the x-ray beam centered in a reproducible fashion every time a radiograph is taken.[2, 63] Serial films therefore can be precisely superimposed allowing detection of even minimal changes in prosthetic position. However, such positioning devices have not been widely accepted. Some sources have suggested manipulating the extremity under fluoroscopic guidance to

We wish to acknowledge and thank Dr. Travis Heare and Miss Heather Ward for their patient assistance in the preparation of this manuscript.

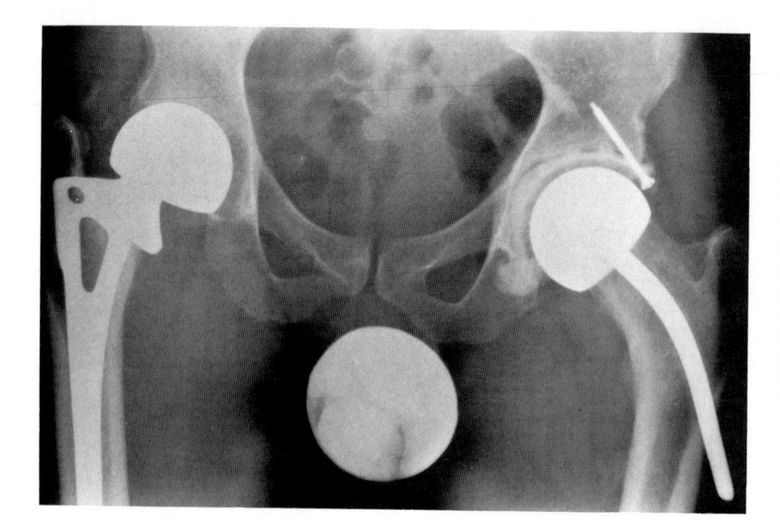

FIGURE 11–1. Component malposition. This anteroposterior film of the pelvis reveals an uncemented right bipolar hemiarthroplasty and a left surface replacement arthroplasty. The stem of the left femoral prosthesis projects through the lateral cortex of the femur. (Courtesy of T. Gillespy III, M.D., Seattle, WA.)

optimize positioning for overhead films.[49] This method is time-consuming and probably does not enhance comparability of serial films better than standard radiography done according to strict protocols.

Stereophotogrammetry is an even more elaborate method for obtaining comparable radiographs and determining prosthesis position. Metallic beads must be placed in the femur and acetabulum adjacent to the prosthesis at the time of total hip arthroplasty[52] or, later, percutaneously.[74] When making follow-up films, the radiologic technologist uses a system of external film markers and a specially designed cage film holder with fixed opaque markers. A pair of stereoscopic radiographs is generated by angling the x-ray beam slightly differently on each AP film. One pair of stereoscopic views is made with weightbearing and the other without. The x,y coordinates of certain points on the prosthesis, the metallic beads in the bone, and the metal markers on the cage are entered into a computer. A software program locates the precise position of the markers and, therefore, the prosthesis in the patient. Any motion that may have occurred between weightbearing and nonweightbearing films, as well as any differences between serial films, can be detected by stereophotogrammetry to 0.8 mm in linear measurement at the 95 percent confidence level.[52] Although this procedure appears to be the most sensitive radiographic technique to document migration, it has not been widely incorporated into routine follow-up procedures because of time, technology, and cost-benefit constraints.

For the hip, knee, and ankle, weightbearing views may add important information about ligamentous integrity and the orientation of the prosthetic components compared with the weightbearing axis of the extremity. Stress views may demonstrate motion of the prosthesis relative to bone as well as joint laxity not shown on routine radiographs.

Standard radiographs demonstrate the prosthetic components and their interfaces with bone. Adding barium to bone cement makes it radiopaque and enables evaluation of the cement-bone interface. However, only the portion of this interface parallel to the x-ray beam is seen in profile on routine views, whereas the prosthesis articulates with bone or cement in three dimensions.

Component motion found at revision surgery is probably the gold standard for loosening, but some radiographic signs are suggestive of loosening. Radiographic signs of loosening are similar whether the patient has an unconstrained, semiconstrained, or constrained prosthesis, but they are more frequently seen with a constrained prosthesis. Any progressive change in the position of prosthetic components, such as subsidence, migration, or tilting, constitutes loosening.[96] Unless sequential films are carefully compared, new bone formation at the cut edges of bone may create the illusion that the prosthesis is subsiding into the bone.[97] Also highly suggestive of loosening are cement-bone lucencies ≥2 mm surrounding the prosthesis or lucencies that progress on serial films.[96, 108] Most components that have loosened to the point where revision is required have such a radiographic appearance.[95, 97] However, clinical symptoms requiring revision do not uniformly accompany radiolucent lines about the prosthesis.[96]

Small (≤2 mm) cement-bone lucencies, or prosthesis-bone lucencies with uncemented components, are common the first postoperative year in asymptomatic patients.[95] Radiodense lines may outline the uncemented prostheses, with or without radiolucent lines.[61, 70] If these do not progress, they usually do not signify a problem.[96] However, because of the relatively short follow-up available, definitive radiographic signs of loosening of uncemented prostheses are not known with certainty.

Wide zones of lucency may surround components of a revision arthroplasty. They may reflect fibrous or synovial tissue around the previous prosthesis that was not completely removed. These do not indicate loosening unless they progress.[97]

Plain radiography also can demonstrate dislocation and instability; fracture of the bone, prosthesis, or cement; heterotopic bone (Fig. 11–2); and ectopic cement. Ectopic cement fragments may act as loose bodies in the joint or may impinge upon adjacent nerves or blood vessels.[95] Tendon ruptures in patients with total joint arthroplasties may occasionally be evident radiographically as focal soft tissue swelling, which represents the retracted tendon stump.[108] Periosteal reaction in the absence of fracture may signify infection, with or without loosening.[96]

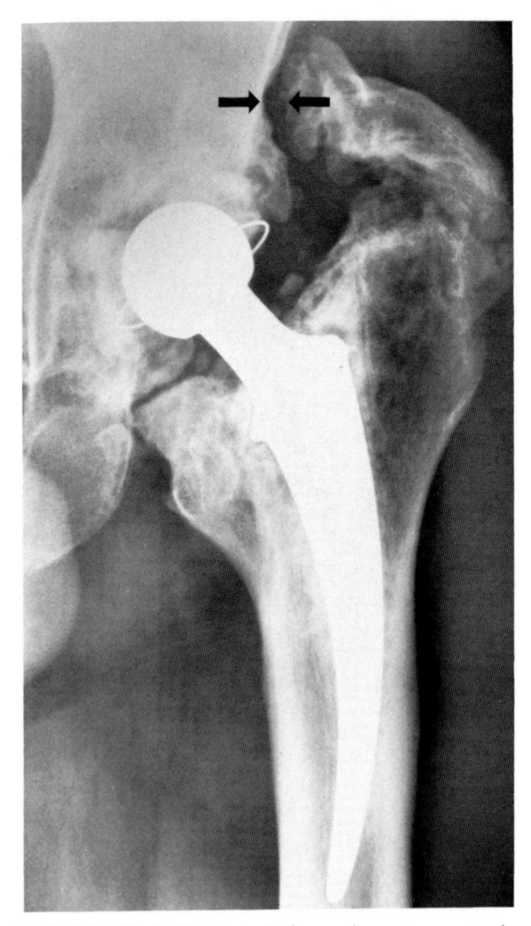

FIGURE 11–2. Heterotopic bone. An anteroposterior film of the left hip demonstrates a cemented total hip replacement with heterotopic bone extending from the greater trochanter to within 1 cm of the ilium (arrows), making it class III.[15] (Courtesy of T. Gillespy III, M.D., Seattle, WA.)

Aspiration Arthrography

Although painful loosening of a prosthesis is frequently accompanied by radiographic changes, acute infection without loosening usually is not.[96, 97] When pain is present without radiographic changes, puncture of the joint for culture and determination of antibiotic sensitivities may be warranted. Joint culture is also indicated when the patient has a history, physical signs, or laboratory findings suggestive of infection, whether or not the radiographs indicate loosening.

It cannot be emphasized too strongly that puncture of prosthetic joints must be carried out with strict aseptic technique to avoid contaminating the sample and, more importantly, the arthroplasty. The radiologist punctures the joint under fluoroscopic guidance. After aspirating fluid through a needle in the patient, the radiologist must prove the needle was in the joint by injecting "x-ray dye" through the same needle. Contrast has not been shown to hinder bacterial growth *in vitro*.[71] Local anesthetic is usually bottled with a bacteriostatic agent; therefore, the anesthetic should not be injected into a joint prior to aspiration

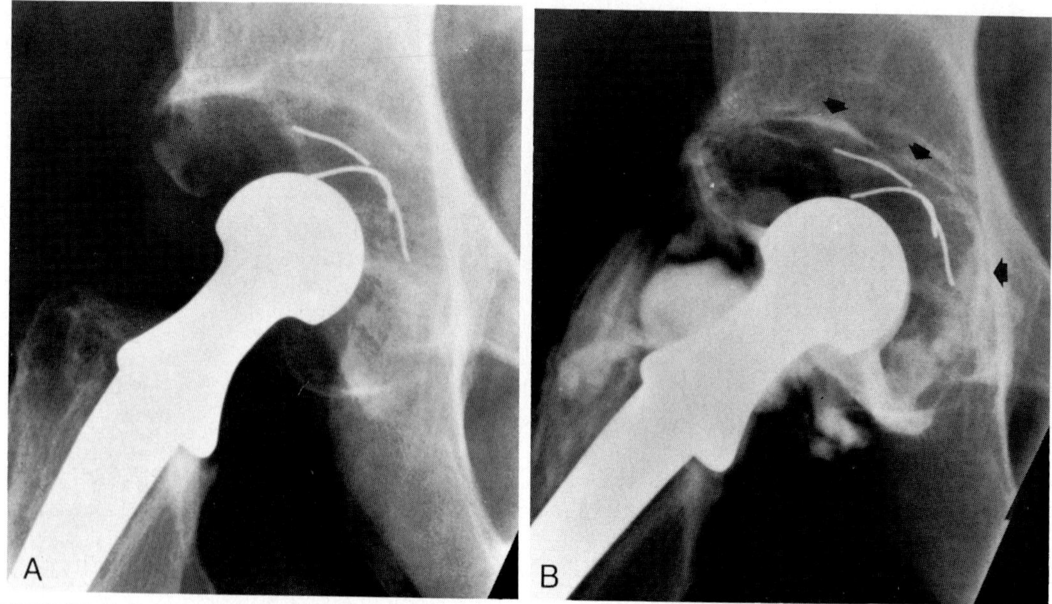

FIGURE 11–3. False-positive arthrogram for acetabular loosening. *A*, On this plain film anteroposterior view of the right hip, the cement-bone interface cannot be evaluated because the cement is radiolucent. The acetabular component of the total hip arthroplasty was cemented using cement that did not contain barium. *B*, After injection of contrast within the pseudocapsule, the cement-bone interface in all zones about the acetabular component is surrounded by a thin rim of contrast (arrows). However, at surgery, the socket was found to be solidly fixed. (Courtesy of T. Gillespy III, M.D., Seattle, WA.)

of the sample.[94, 95] In a patient with known allergy to radiographic contrast material, air alone may be injected to confirm intra-articular positioning of the needle.

Radiologists are commonly called upon to aspirate hip arthroplasties in cases of suspected infections, because fluoroscopy simplifies puncture of this deep joint. Knee joints can be punctured reliably without fluoroscopic guidance.[97] Compared with intraoperatively obtained cultures, percutaneous joint sampling cultures detect only up to 74 percent of prosthetic infections and sometimes yield different organisms.[67, 96] However, aspiration can be quite helpful in preoperative planning and treatment.

Arthrography can demonstrate loosening if the contrast material dissects between the prosthesis (or cement) and bone, but lack of contrast material around the components does not rule out loosening. Radiographic contrast material is a fairly viscous liquid and may be unable to penetrate the space around loose components.[86] This interface contains radiolucent substances, such as synovial, fibrous, and granulation tissue, which could occlude passage of the contrast medium.[42, 43, 102] Also, contrast material may flow around the prosthesis in a plane not tangential to the x-ray beam and therefore not be visible on any of the films. Contrast agents may occasionally track around components that are found to be solid at surgery; presumably, fixation in these cases is sufficient in planes not demonstrated by the radiographs (Fig. 11–3). In any case, findings at arthrography should be interpreted in correlation with the patient's history, physical signs, plain film findings, and isotope scan findings, if any.

Visualization of contrast medium tracking adjacent to a metal prosthesis or cement of similar density may be improved with subtraction radiography.[3, 76, 85] With this technique, even small amounts of contrast material next to metal or cement can be detected. To produce a subtraction arthrogram, the preinjection radiograph is reversed to a negative by copying it with subtraction film. This negative is called the mask. When the mask is superimposed over a postinjection image, densities present on both, such as bone, metal, and cement, cancel each other, leaving contrast material as the only visible density. In standard subtraction radiography, the mask and postinjection films are physically superimposed over one another and viewed. In digital subtraction radiography, a computer mathematically subtracts the mask from the postinjection image. A major disadvantage of subtraction arthrography is that the patient positioning for the preinjection and postinjection images must be identical, otherwise radiodense objects will misregister, making interpretation difficult (Fig. 11–4). If standard subtraction is used, the radiologic technologist must position the patient and the x-ray beam exactly the same way for the preinjection and postinjection films, a difficult task to accomplish. For successful digital subtraction arthrography, the patient must remain motionless throughout the injection. Postexercise imaging is not possible with this technique.

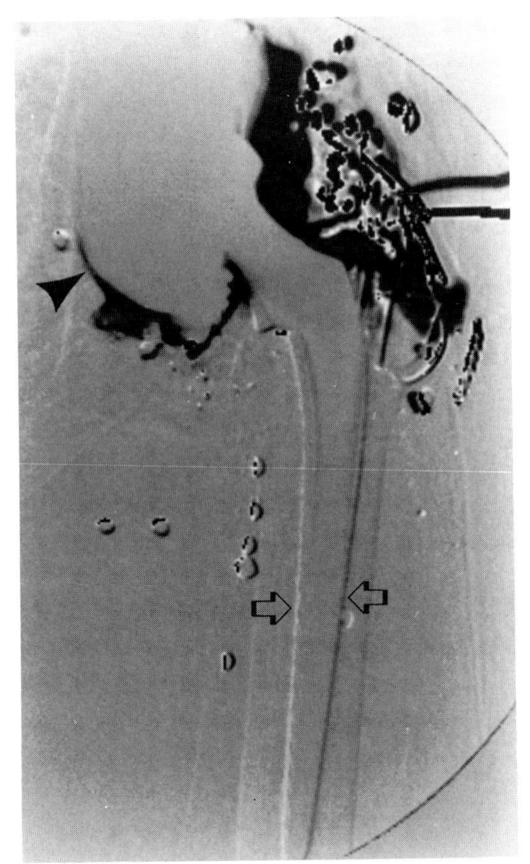

FIGURE 11–4. Misregistration artifact in a digital subtraction arthrogram. This digital subtraction arthrogram of a left total hip arthroplasty shows contrast material filling the pseudocapsule and tracking along the inferomedial surface of the acetabular component (arrowhead). The socket did not prove to be loose, but the nearly vertical angle places the patient at risk for dislocation. The black line along the lateral aspect of the femoral stem has a white counterpart on the medial surface (open arrows). These constitute a misregistration artifact due to slight patient motion, rather than to contrast material tracking along the prosthesis.

Arthrography usually demonstrates any communicating bursae or abscesses that have developed about the joint. Separate puncture of these cavities is often required to recover organisms, if present. Sinus tracts emanating from prosthetic joints are probably best visualized by injection of contrast into the joint, rather than into the tract.[96]

For some patients with hip pain after arthroplasty with no obvious cause, aspiration arthrography may be followed by intra-articular injection of local anesthetic, with or without steroid. If this relieves the pain, the source probably lies within the joint. If not, an extra-articular source of the pain, such as nerve root impingement or stress fracture, should be sought. (See the discussion of *Problem-Oriented Imaging: Pain* at the end of this chapter.)

Radioisotope Scanning

Bone scans with phosphate analogs, most commonly technetium-99m methylene diphosphonate (^{99m}Tc-MDP), are quite sensitive and show many complications of arthroplasty, such as loosening, infection (Fig. 11–5), fracture, and heterotopic bone. Bone scans usually are done in three phases: flow, pool, and static images. Flow and pool images correlate with blood flow to the area. The flow phase is essentially a nuclear arteriogram; images are made every 3 to 6 seconds during intravenous injection of radionuclide (Fig. 11–5C). The blood pool scan is made right after the flow series and reveals the radioisotope in the extravascular space (Fig. 11–5D). The static images are made 2 to 4 hours after radionuclide injection and represent blood flow and osteoblastic activity (Fig. 11–5E).[97]

A positive bone scan finding is rather nonspecific unless it is correlated with the history, physical examination, laboratory findings, plain films, and any other radioisotope scans.[96] Increased uptake of radio-

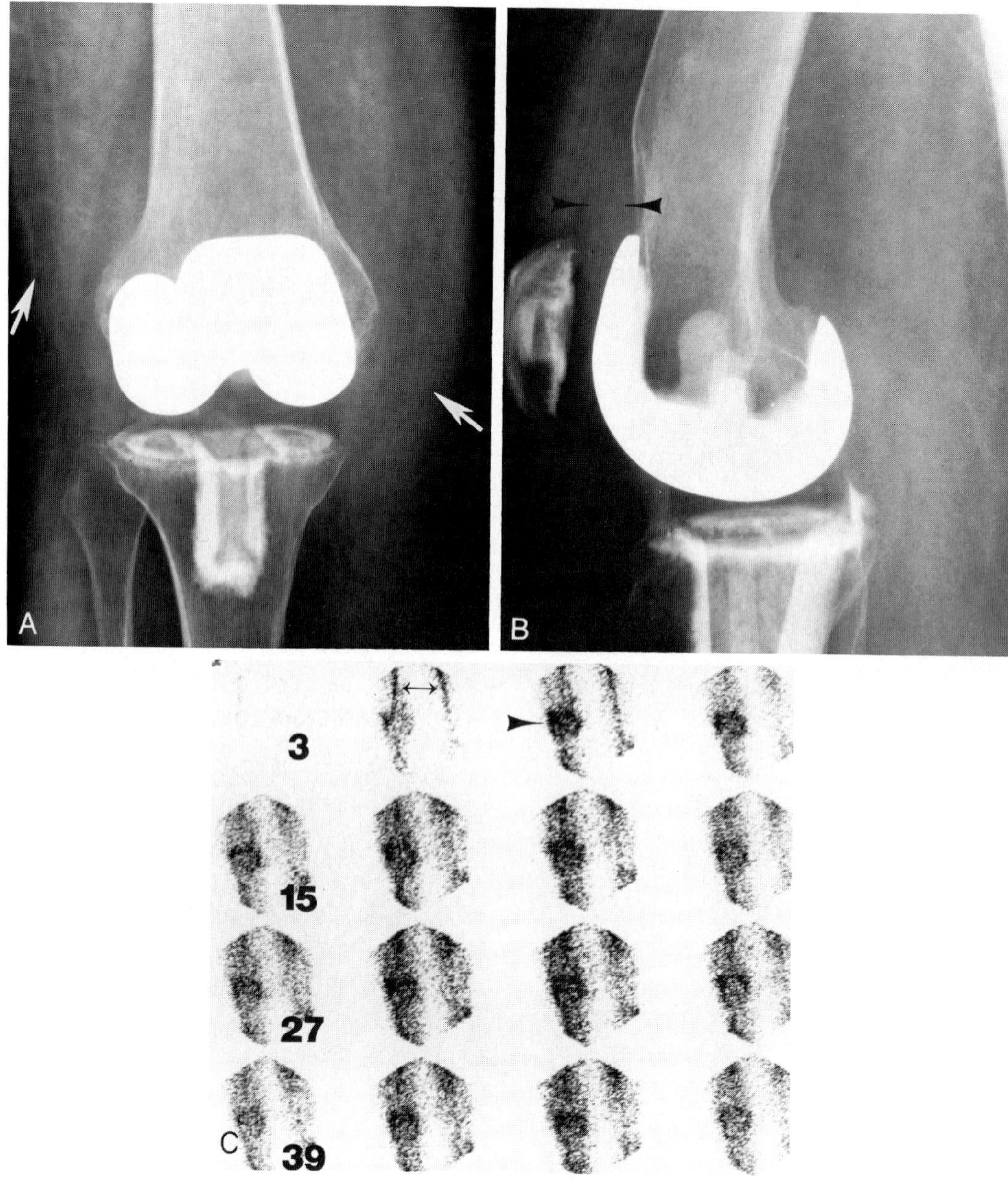

FIGURE 11–5. Prosthetic infection. *A*, The anteroposterior film of a patient with a painful cemented total knee replacement demonstrates swelling and reticulation of the subcutaneous fat (arrows) consistent with edema. *B*, The lateral view reveals a joint effusion in the suprapatellar bursa (arrowheads), a frequent finding even in patients with asymptomatic knee replacements. *C*, Scintigrams from the flow phase of a technetium-99m methylene diphosphonate (^{99m}Tc-MDP) bone scan were made at 3-second intervals. The numbers indicate seconds postinjection. Images progress from left to right. The 6-second image demonstrates radiotracer in the superficial femoral arteries bilaterally (double-headed arrow). On the 9-second scan, radiotracer is already accumulating in the right knee (arrowhead). Some washout occurs by the end of the flow phase.

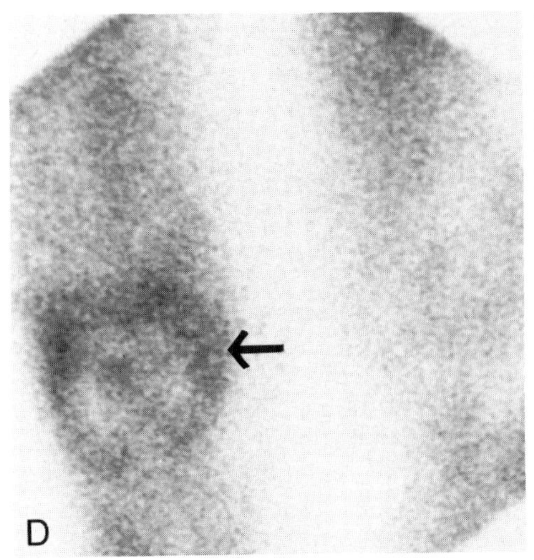

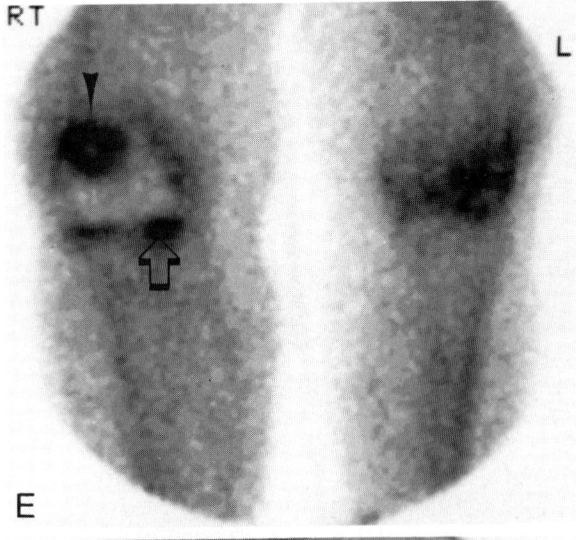

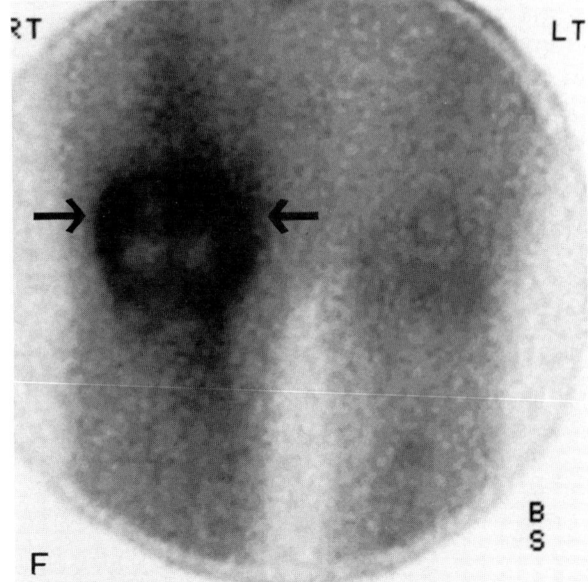

FIGURE 11–5 *Continued D*, The blood pool image made right after completion of the flow phase shows increased uptake around the margins of the femoral (arrow) and tibial prostheses. *E*, The static or delayed bone scan demonstrates more limited increased concentration of ^{99m}Tc-MDP, especially along the medial aspect of the tibial component (open arrow) and in the patella (arrowhead). *F*, The gallium-67 citrate ^{67}Ga scan reveals a dramatically increased concentration about the entire right knee (arrows). Uptake is much more marked than that seen on the static ^{99m}Tc-MDP bone scan. This incongruent uptake was interpreted as infection, and intraoperative cultures yielded *Staphylococcus aureus*. (Courtesy of W. Drane, M.D., Gainesville, FL.)

nuclide around the prosthesis is normal in the first postoperative year.[90, 95] However, a bone scan without evidence of increased uptake around the prosthetic joint makes the presence of loosening or infection highly unlikely.[96]

A stress fracture will accumulate variable amounts of radionuclide, depending on the size and chronicity of the lesion.[112] Decreased sensitivity of bone scans after fracture has been shown in rabbits on high doses of hydrocortisone for 6 weeks prior to scanning as well as in rabbits on low doses when scanning was done within 48 hours after fracture.[98] This study has important implications for patients with total joint replacements, because steroids are often given for treatment of conditions that require arthroplasty.

Bone scanning may also be utilized to stage heterotopic bone. In a study of para-articular ossification in paralyzed patients, increased uptake on bone scans disclosed formation of heterotopic bone before it was visible on radiographs. When the uptake decreased to a steady state on serial scans, the heterotopic ossification was mature and less likely to recur if excised. Tanaka and associates[101] pointed out that a single bone scan viewed in isolation was inadequate to judge maturity of heterotopic bone. Sequential scans need to be compared with uptake standardized to that of normal bone.[101]

Gallium-67 citrate (^{67}Ga) was first employed as a bone scanning agent but is now employed most often in imaging of inflammatory and neoplastic processes. Although not very helpful on its own, the ^{67}Ga scan interpreted in concert with the ^{99m}Tc-MDP bone scan may yield fairly high sensitivity, specificity, and accuracy for infection of prostheses.[90] If the ^{67}Ga scan shows no increased uptake or increased uptake in a pattern that coincides with the ^{99m}Tc-MDP scan, the likelihood of infection is slight. In contrast, if the ^{67}Ga scan demonstrates greater uptake in a pattern that does not match the ^{99m}Tc-MDP scan or is markedly more intense, then infection is likely (Figs. 11–5E and 11–5F).[90, 97] Because interpretation of scans is subjective to some degree, giving rise to false-positive and false-negative results, and because matching patterns of uptake on the two scans are inconclusive,[96] correlation with clinical circumstances and with plain radiographs is important.

White blood cells labeled with indium-111 oxine or tropolonate (^{111}In-WBC) concentrate in inflammatory foci, making this radioisotope study useful in cases of suspected prosthetic infection. Significantly greater uptake in the region of a prosthesis, a joint space, or an adjacent soft tissue is considered a positive finding for infection. Scans showing increased uptake but less uptake than that of normal marrow are indeterminate.[67] Studies of ^{111}In-WBC scanning in orthopaedics have reported the following results: sensitivity, 83 to 100 percent; specificity, 73 to 89.5 percent; and accuracy, 58 to 93.3 percent.[20, 67, 72, 82] In some studies, the ^{111}In-WBC scan has been more sensitive than percutaneous aspiration (sensitivity, 12 to 74 percent)[20, 67] and more sensitive and accurate than combined ^{99m}Tc-MDP and ^{67}Ga scans (sensitivity, 48 percent; accuracy, 57 percent).[72] Whereas the ^{99m}Tc-MDP bone scan is more sensitive (sensitivity, 100 percent), it is much less specific (specificity, 18 percent).[67] Some investigators recommend sequential ^{111}In-WBC and ^{99m}Tc-MDP scans to increase specificity. As with interpretation of combined ^{99m}Tc-MDP and ^{67}Ga scans, markedly higher or incongruent uptake on the ^{111}In-WBC compared with the ^{99m}Tc-MDP scan is considered positive for infection.[20]

Although the sensitivity of ^{111}In-WBC scans in chronic infections has been questioned, further studies have found no significant difference in sensitivity for patients with symptoms for 2 weeks or less and patients with symptoms for more than 2 weeks.[26, 67] Leukocytes are normally associated with acute infection, but these cells continue to migrate in significant numbers into chronically infected foci. Also, during the process of labeling the leukocytes with indium-111 oxine, some lymphocytes may become tagged as well, and these cells can carry the radionuclide to sites of chronic infection. Significant decreases in sensitivity of ^{111}In-WBC scans have not been found in patients on antibiotics[25] or steroids.[67]

Nuclear medicine scanning may be sensitive for detection of an infected prosthesis, but the organism must still be identified for appropriate treatment. For this reason, isotope imaging may be bypassed in favor of aspiration arthrography. In patients in whom puncture-induced infection of the arthroplasty would be especially disastrous, such as in immunocompromised patients, radionuclide scanning may be a prudent first step, as negative findings might obviate percutaneous aspiration.

Several groups have reported on radioisotope arthrography for detection of prosthetic loosening. Technetium-99m sulfur colloid (^{99m}Tc-SC) is injected into the joint under fluoroscopic guidance, usually at the time of standard aspiration arthrography.[1, 86, 105] The patient may then exercise freely, facilitating radioisotope tracking around the prosthesis, and the joint is imaged with an ordinary gamma camera. Because the intra-articular radioisotope is "hot" and the prosthesis and cement are "cold," no need exists for subtraction arthrography or limited patient motion. The risk of sensitivity to radiographic contrast material is obviated with intra-articular radioisotope scans.[86] The major disadvantage is inability to evaluate the acetabular component. Radionuclide normally flows around the head of the femoral component, and this accumulation can easily be mistaken for dissection between the socket and bone on scintigrams.

Computerized Tomography

Computerized tomography (CT) has revolutionized visualization of the complex anatomy of the pelvis and hip joints. Before arthroplasty, CT can demonstrate not only the abnormality for which joint replacement is required, but also the available bone stock in the acetabular walls and femur. Many CT scanners have software to generate reformatted images in the sagittal or coronal plane. Some imaging centers have three-dimensional work stations that are capable of generating images reformatted in multiple planes as well as three-dimensional images that show the topographic anatomy of bones. Three-dimensional images displayed in an interactive format may be rotated in any direction, which might be helpful to display a point of anatomy and assist in surgical planning. Images on the screen can be copied for later reference.

The digital data from CT scans can be utilized to generate resin anatomic models of the joints (Fig. 11–6). This technique can be the key to successful planning in complicated cases, as the surgery may be practiced on the model preoperatively. Data from CT scanning may also be employed in the manufacture of custom prostheses for special cases.[4, 53]

When an implant is already in place in or near the joint to be imaged, artifacts generated by a metallic implant could obscure diagnostic details of both the contralateral joint and the one containing the implant. In practice, this problem rarely renders the CT study nondiagnostic (Fig. 11–7).[4, 12] Metals are not equal in their propensity to generate artifacts on CT

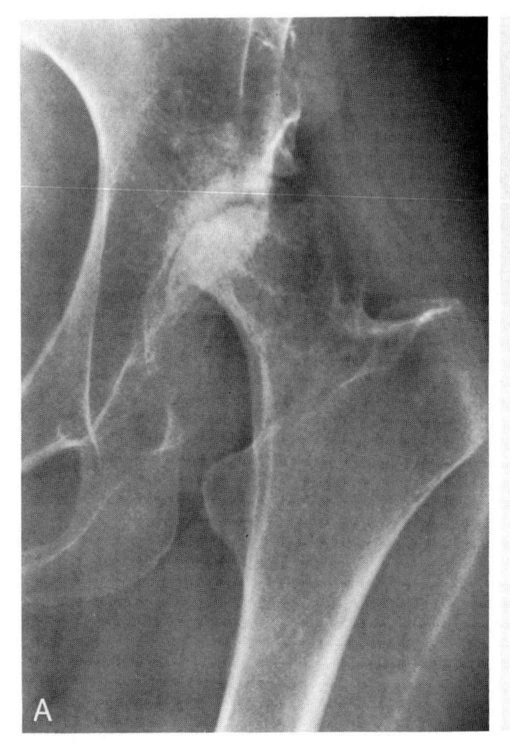

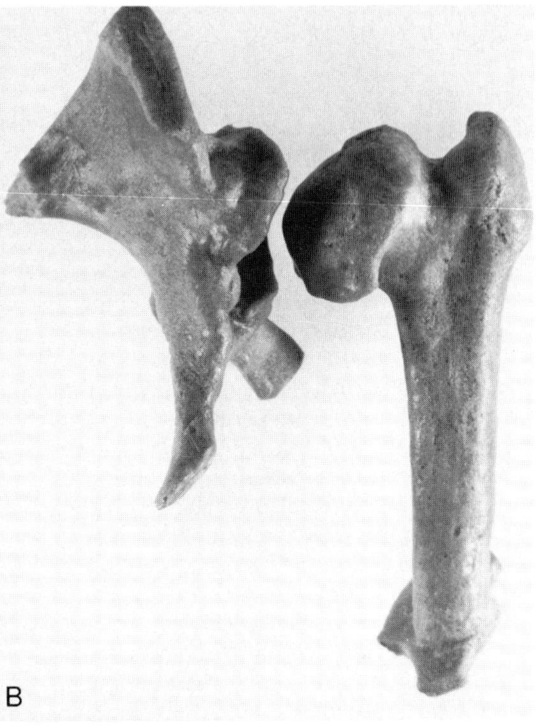

FIGURE 11–6. Computerized tomography (CT) data for preoperative planning. *A*, This radiograph of a 37-year-old woman with a history of congenital hip dysplasia and pain aggravated by a recent pregnancy demonstrates a flattened femoral head articulating superolaterally with a shallow acetabulum. The lesser trochanter lies more cephalad than the ischial tuberosity, indicating shortening of the left lower extremity. *B*, Utilizing CT scan data, these resin models were generated for preoperative planning (Techmedica, Camarillo, CA.).

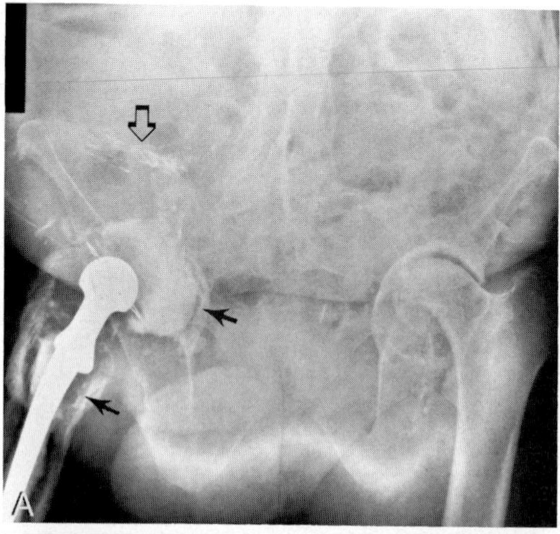

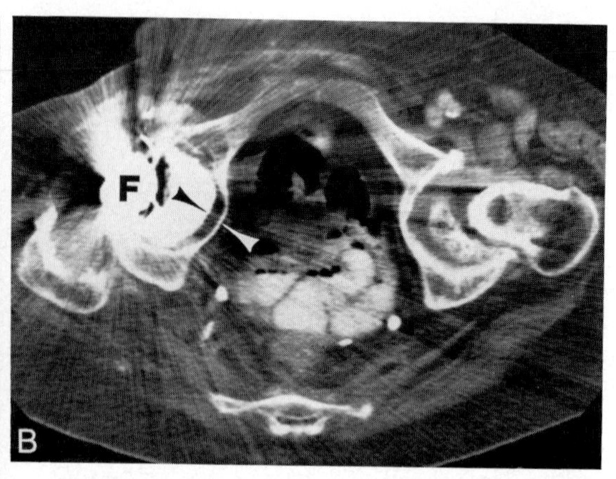

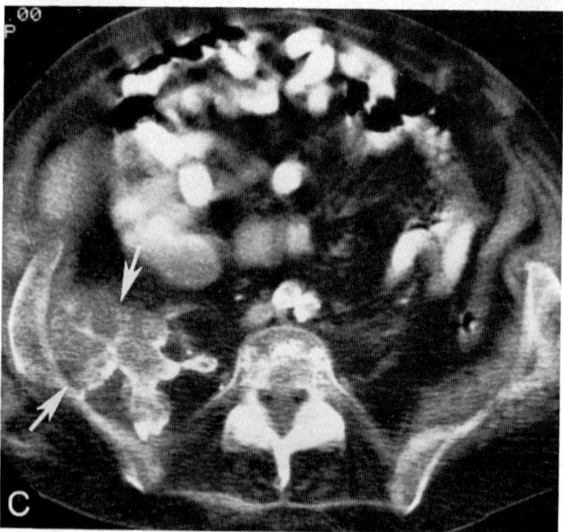

FIGURE 11–7. Infected, loose total hip arthroplasty communicating with an abscess. *A*, This anteroposterior film of the pelvis of an elderly man with a history of ankylosing spondylitis and Crohn's disease was deliberately underexposed to better demonstrate the right hip arthroplasty. The black arrows point to wide cement-bone lucencies surrounding the acetabular and femoral components of a total hip replacement. The open arrow indicates calcifications nearby in the right pelvis. Note the left hip arthropathy and the fused sacroiliac joints and lumbar spine. *B*, A computerized tomography scan of the pelvis demonstrates streaks of metal artifact radiating from the head of the femoral prosthesis (F). The arrowheads indicate the lucency between cement and bone of the acetabulum. *C*, In another image from the same study made more cephalad at the level of the iliac wings, the calcifications seen on the plain film outline a mass (arrows). An arthrogram of the right hip done later demonstrated communication with this retroperitoneal mass, which proved to be an abscess, probably consequent to Crohn's disease.

scans. The following substances commonly used in prostheses are listed in order of decreasing x-ray attenuation and artifact production: chromium-cobalt, stainless steel, titanium, and plastic.[38] Software for CT scanners is available to smooth out metal artifacts, but application of these programs can be time-consuming and may still not improve the diagnostic quality of the images, particularly with bulky metal implants, such as joint prostheses.[60, 88] One group of investigators has salvaged scans of diagnostic quality from axial images marred by metal artifacts by first reformatting them into the coronal plane and then into the sagittal plane.[38] This technique may be useful in planning a contralateral arthroplasty or a revision of the side already containing an implant.

Magnetic Resonance Imaging

Magnetic resonance imaging (MRI) frequently offers key diagnostic information for many conditions in which arthroplasty is part of the treatment. This imaging modality is sensitive and interpreted without much difficulty for osteonecrosis of the femoral head[73] and perhaps of other anatomic locations. Unlike CT, MR scans can be obtained directly in any plane. This capability allows for accurate measurement of the intramedullary extent of bone tumors,[40] which is critical to achieve adequate resection. In the current era of limb salvage, custom arthroplasty, replacing segments of bone, and composite arthroplasty, combining cadaveric grafts with prostheses, often follow these tumor resections. Radiologists are currently exploring the efficacy of MRI in imaging various types of arthritis, especially with the aid of gadolinium, an MRI contrast agent.

Although useful for diagnosis and preoperative planning, MRI has little if any place in the postoperative evaluation of joints with prostheses already in place. The metal causes local distortion of the magnetic field, and the extent and severity of the resulting artifact increase in proportion to the strength of the magnetic field. Most musculoskeletal MRI devices incorporate magnets with mid (0.5–1.0 tesla) or high (1.5–2.0 tesla) field strength. We have obtained some scans of marginal diagnostic quality for tissues near metallic prostheses and other hardware utilizing a low field strength (0.1–0.3 tesla) magnet. These scans were performed when a mass relatively close to the metallic device was suspected, and CT would almost surely have been nondiagnostic.

The radius of distortion does not extend into the contralateral joint, enabling successful diagnostic MRI scans of the side opposite the arthroplasty. Although MRI can clearly demonstrate rupture of the patellar, Achilles,[10, 68, 83] and rotator cuff[18, 33, 64, 111] tendons, it remains to be seen how successfully these structures can be imaged near metallic prostheses. Such imaging may be superfluous, however, when tendon rupture is obvious upon physical examination.

Significant heating or motion of the prosthetic components in these strong magnetic fields has proved to be no more than a theoretic risk.[17] Preliminary screening for contraindications by orthopaedic personnel will prevent the scheduling of a study that cannot take place. Patients who have certain metallic devices in place may be imaged safely; these include total joint prostheses, dental devices, intrauterine devices, surgical clips other than intracranial aneurysm clips, coronary bypass clips, cardiac valves, and cerebral ventricular shunts. Contraindications to MRI include the presence of cardiac pacemakers, ferromagnetic intracranial aneurysm clips, some vena cava embolism filters, cochlear implants, and spinal cord stimulators. Some patients with intracranial clips can be imaged safely,[8] and the metal artifact may be less than that on CT.[51] Even stainless steel clips with a nickel content of 10 to 14 percent have shown no significant deflection, torque, or artifact production in low- or high-field strength magnets.[75] If the exact metallic composition of a patient's intracranial clip is unknown, another clip of the same brand and model can be tested in the magnet to determine whether deflection or torque is induced.[75] A relative contraindication is a history of metal fragments in the eye.

Ultrasound

Although transmission of the ultrasound beam would abruptly stop at a metallic implant, this would not pose an obstacle to ultrasound evaluation of tendons that lie superficial to the prosthesis. Ultrasound has been reported useful in imaging tenosynovitis and tendon rupture in the rotator cuff; long head of the biceps; and Achilles, patellar, and wrist tendons.[39, 46]

Ultrasound may also be helpful when a mass is palpable adjacent to a joint replacement. In such cases, CT and MRI could be nondiagnostic because of metal artifact. Ultrasound can demonstrate abscess cavities, bursae, and neoplasms.[106] This imaging modality may also be employed to guide aspiration or biopsy.[21, 46]

IMAGING OF THE HIP

Routine Evaluation

Immediately after implantation of a hip replacement, an AP radiograph should be obtained to exclude intraoperative fracture or malposition of the components (see Fig. 11–1). As soon after surgery as possible, an AP view of the pelvis and a true lateral film of the operated hip should be obtained as baselines for follow-up. In many institutions the standard AP pelvis study is modified by caudad centering of the x-ray beam, which results in complete visualization of the prosthesis and omits the iliac wings.

For standardized description of radiographic findings, seven zones around femoral prostheses[45] and three zones around sockets[27] have been designated for the AP view. A committee of the Hip Society

(1990) suggested that signs on lateral radiographs are also important, especially for uncemented prostheses. Their study incorporated the zones already described for the socket and stem on AP films and proposed seven more zones visible on lateral films (Fig. 11–8).[59] Findings possible on films of joint prostheses, whether cemented or uncemented, include migrations, radiolucencies about the prostheses, hardware failures, bony resorptions, and heterotopic bone formations. In addition, radiographic studies can confirm the location of the center of hip rotation, the status of the greater trochanter, and the positioning of the components.

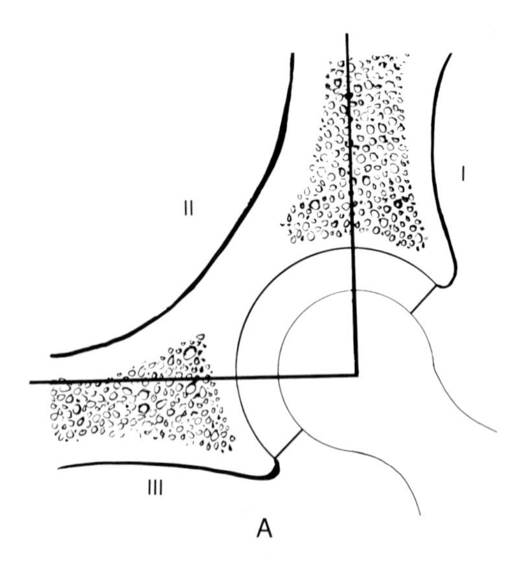

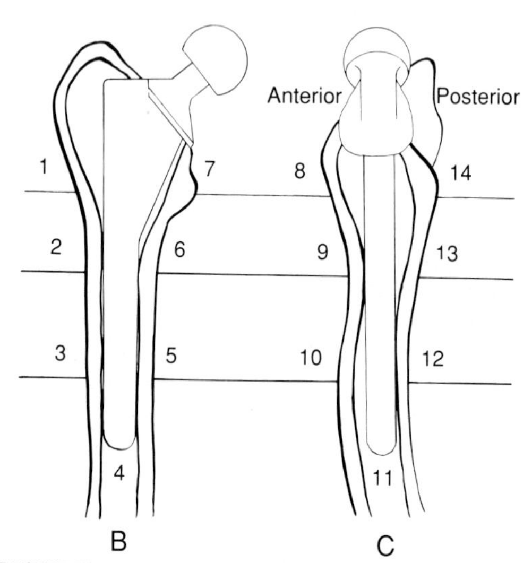

FIGURE 11–8. Zones to be evaluated in total hip arthroplasty. *A*, Anteroposterior (AP) view shows zones of the acetabular component. (Redrawn from DeLee, J. G. and Charnley, J.: Clin. Orthop. 121:20–32, 1976.) *B*, The AP view of the femoral prosthesis. (Redrawn from Gruen, T. A., et al: Clin. Orthop. 141:17–27, 1979.) *C*, Lateral view includes the zones added by Johnston and coworkers.[59]

The angle of the acetabular component of a total hip replacement is measured on the AP film in the following manner. A line is drawn connecting the most superolateral and most inferomedial edges of the socket or its marker wire. The angle that this line makes with a horizontal reference line drawn tangential to either the ischial tuberosities or the inferior margins of the acetabular teardrops describes the angle of the component.[109, 110] The true lateral projection demonstrates the degree of anteversion of the acetabular component. The AP film should reveal acetabular angles ranging from 30 to 50 degrees, and the lateral view should show sockets that are slightly anteverted. Guidelines for normal positioning of the socket of a surface replacement arthroplasty are similar.[6] Whereas limits of normal for the acetabular portion of a bipolar hemiarthroplasty are much broader because movement in relation to the native acetabulum is allowed, the angle often approximates that of a fixed acetabular component.

On the frontal view, the femoral component of a total hip replacement or bipolar hemiarthroplasty should be positioned with the stem centered in the medullary space. The center of the femoral head should be even with the top of the greater trochanter.[109] Varus and valgus of the prosthesis are determined by measuring the angle between the long axis of the metal stem and the long axis of the femur. If the distal end of the femoral stem angles medially, the prosthesis is in valgus; if it points laterally, the prosthesis is in varus. Some femoral surface replacements resemble the older cup arthroplasties on radiographs. The angle of the femoral component of a surface arthroplasty is determined by two lines, one being perpendicular to the collar of the prosthesis and the other being the long axis of the femoral neck.[6] Neutral or slight valgus constitutes normal positioning.

Although not routinely used, a CT scan can be performed and the component position, especially the angle of the acetabular prosthesis, measured.[53]

Revision arthroplasties present widely variable radiographic appearances. Frequently, only the component found to be loose will be replaced if a prosthesis that can articulate with the remaining solidly attached component is available. Revision femoral prostheses usually have stems considerably longer than their predecessors. Cemented primary components do not necessarily dictate that the revision will also be cemented. Total hip replacements may be revised with bipolar prostheses. The acetabulum is augmented with autograft or allograft in the patient with insufficient acetabular bone stock to affix a socket.[87] Allograft segments may be utilized for severe proximal femoral deficiency.

Loosening

The definition of loosening of total hip replacements varies from one report to another[13] and, therefore, so do the rates. Some studies describe radiographic evidence alone, regardless of whether the symptoms dictate revision. Other studies report that only motion of components demonstrated at surgery constitutes true loosening. If serial studies are available, comparison with previous films may reveal migration, the most reliable radiographic proof of loosening.[44, 77, 102] This motion may be between cement mantle and bone or between prosthesis and cement. However, loosening may exist in the absence of obvious migration.

Other evidence suggesting loosening is lucency at the cement-bone interface. Most investigators consider loosening to be present if (a) a bone-cement lucency of at least 2 mm is seen in the projected circumference of the prosthesis or if (b) a prosthesis-cement lucency that is not present on the immediate postoperative film is detected (Fig. 11–9).[77, 93, 95] However, disagreement as to whether such lucencies are present is common, especially with regard to the socket.[14] Moreover, radiographs of cemented prostheses (acetabular and femoral components) often show lucencies at the cement-bone interface, but these prostheses are not necessarily loose.[30, 84] Cement fractures reliably indicate loosening and component failure, even in the absence of immediate symptoms (Fig. 11–10).

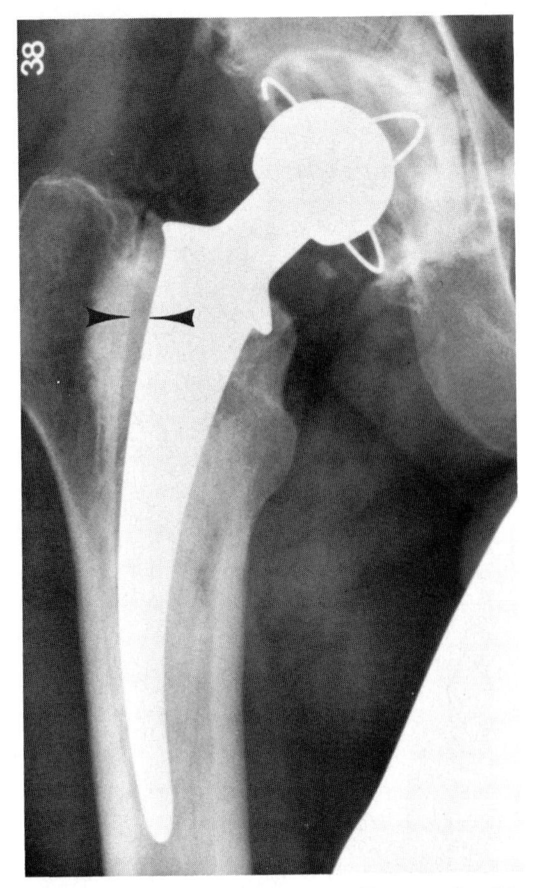

FIGURE 11–9. Prosthesis-cement lucency. In this patient with hip pain, wide prosthesis-cement lucency along the lateral aspect of the proximal femoral stem (arrowheads) suggests loosening. (Courtesy of T. Gillespy III, M.D., Seattle, WA.)

Plain films are especially unreliable in determining whether acetabular components have loosened.[102] Cement-bone lucencies ≥2 mm may be seen around prostheses that are found to be solidly fixed at surgery. Radiographs show the cement-bone interface only in planes tangential to the x-ray beam, and other segments of the interface may be solidly bonded in those cases. Likewise, some sockets that prove to be loose have no suggestive radiographic findings. Radiolucencies <2 mm commonly develop around the socket in the first postoperative year and they do not signify loosening unless they progress. Cement-bone lucencies at the inferomedial aspect of the acetabular prosthesis correlate more

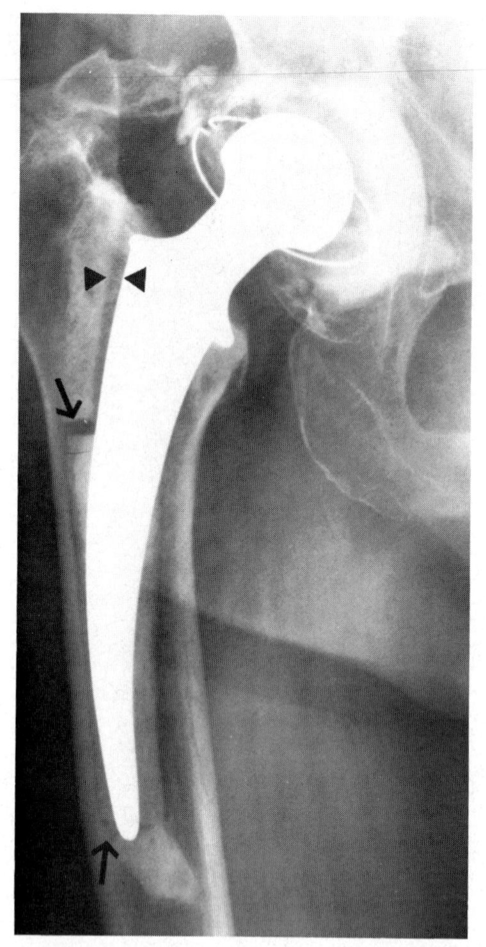

FIGURE 11–10. Cement fracture. This anteroposterior view of a cemented total hip replacement demonstrates fracture of the cement around the femoral stem in two places (arrows). This finding alone is diagnostic of loosening. Note the prosthesis-cement lucency proximally along the lateral aspect of the stem (arrowheads), an example of medial midstem pivot as described by Gruen and associates.[45] (Courtesy of T. Gillespy III, M.D., Seattle, WA.)

with loosening than do superolateral lucencies.[95]

When cement is rendered radiopaque by the addition of barium, chronic loosening of femoral stems is reliably demonstrated on radiographs by wide or progressive cement-bone lucencies.[102] Loosening of a femoral prosthesis may correlate with young age, heavy weight, male sex, unilateral hip disease, wide femoral canal, and varus position of the prosthesis.[100]

Gruen and associates[45] analyzed a nonhomogeneous population of cemented stem-type femoral components and classified them into four modes of failure: (1) pistoning behavior (stem-cement as well as cement-bone); (2) medial midstem pivot caused by weak calcar support plus poor distal cement support; (3) calcar pivot caused by poor distal cement support with secondary bone reaction, producing medial-lateral toggle of the distal end of the stem; and (4) bending cantilever fatigue, secondary to partial or complete loss of the proximal support, which leads to medial migration of the proximal stem with adequate fixation of the distal end (Fig. 11–11). Calcar pivot was least frequently noted, followed by medial midstem pivot. Pistoning occurred most frequently, with stem-cement pistoning behavior noted less frequently than cement-bone pistoning behavior.[45]

Some investigators have observed a relationship between acetabular component placement and femoral stem loosening with cemented prostheses. Inferomedial positioning of the acetabular component

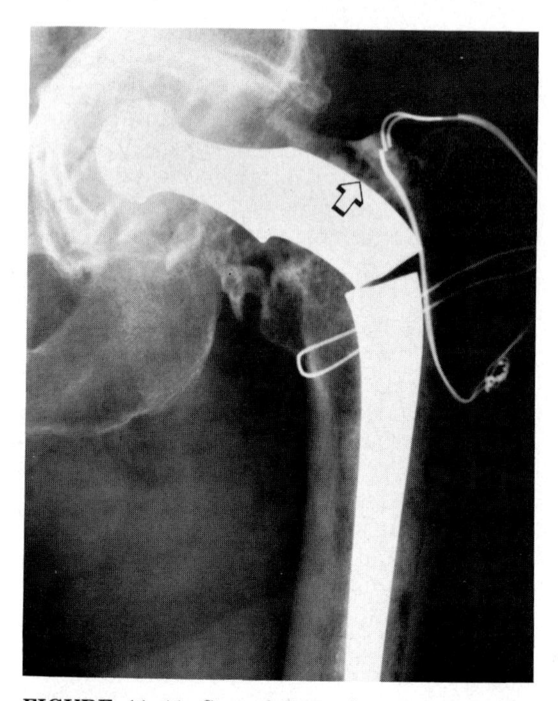

FIGURE 11–11. Stem failure. An anteroposterior radiograph of the left hip demonstrates fracture of the femoral stem of the cemented total hip replacement. A wide prosthesis-cement lucency is seen laterally (open arrow). The failure of this arthroplasty fits into the category of bending cantilever fatigue described by Gruen and associates.[45] (Courtesy of T. Gillespy III, M.D., Seattle, WA.)

appears to produce fewer radiographic changes of loosening.[58, 110] The femoral component of a surface replacement arthroplasty obscures the underlying cement-bone or prosthesis-bone interface. Radiographic evidence of loosening of these prostheses consists of a change in position. Bone scans may reveal increased uptake along the collar of a loose prosthesis.[6]

Early postoperative migration of a cementless femoral prosthesis may be detected after the patient's first attempt at weightbearing if the stem acutely subsides into the femoral shaft. This migration is most easily observed when the relationship of the prosthesis to the calcar region of the femur changes or when it is accompanied by fracture.[9, 45]

Long-term follow-up data on cementless prostheses remain to be reported. Initial (necessarily short) follow-up studies have revealed several radiographic changes: remodeling of the proximal femoral neck (calcar), linear lucency with a thin sclerotic margin at the prosthesis-bone interface, endosteal sclerosis at the prosthetic tip, heterotopic bone, cortical thickening, prosthetic subsidence, intraoperative fracture, and periosteal reaction. These findings do not necessarily indicate clinical failure (Fig. 11–12).[61] Femoral subsidence that continues for more than 12 months or ex-

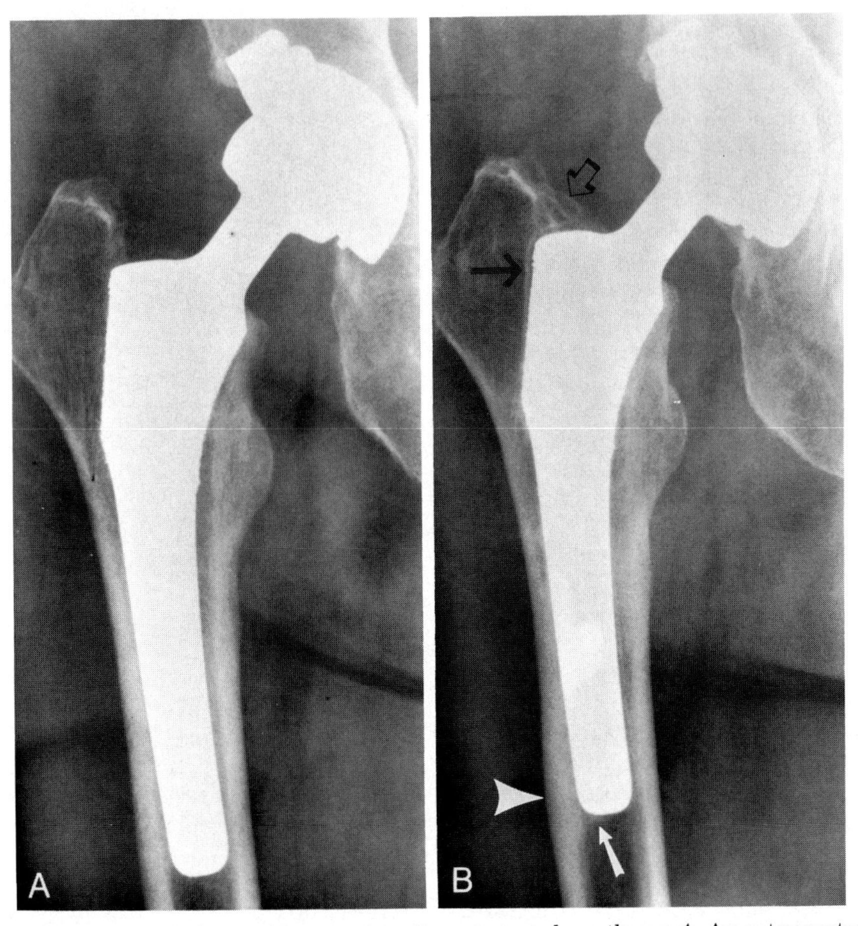

FIGURE 11–12. Common findings with asymptomatic uncemented prostheses. *A*, An anteroposterior view of the right hip, made immediately after implantation of a porous-coated, uncemented total hip arthroplasty, demonstrates acceptable anatomic placement of the components. *B*, After 16 months, endosteal (white arrow) and periosteal (arrowhead) reactive bone have formed adjacent to the tip of the femoral stem. A thin rim of lucency lined by sclerosis surrounds the lateral portion of the stem proximally (black arrow). All of these findings are commonly seen in radiographs of patients with uncemented prostheses and do not signify loosening. Reactive bone forming over the proximal portion of the stem (open arrow) creates the illusion of subsidence. (Courtesy of T. Gillespy III, M.D., Seattle, WA.)

tends more than 10 mm may be associated with a relatively high incidence of clinical failure.[62]

When failed cemented total hip replacements are revised with uncemented components, subsidence of as much as 5 mm is common. The subsidence tends to stabilize between 6 and 12 months postrevision.[47] Cementless acetabular components have been found to migrate superomedially, but they stabilize by 12 months. Despite this motion, acetabular bone graft, if used, remains intact. Radiography and CT are helpful in assessing union or complication of these grafts.

Arthrography may add significant evidence of loosening in sockets but is of little help in detecting loose stems except when aspiration is performed for suspected concurrent infection.[80, 102] Nevertheless, arthrography has yielded numerous false-positive reports of loosening of sockets (see Fig. 11–3) and false-negative reports of loosening of both components (Fig. 11–13).[48, 80, 102] Most investigators agree that arthrographic sensitivity for loosening of any component increases when contrast agent is injected to the patient's tolerance,[24, 48] when postexercise images are obtained,[77, 108] and when some type of subtraction technique is utilized (Fig. 11–14).[3, 76, 85]

Arthroscintigraphy has been reported to be a sensitive method for detecting loosening of the femoral component.[1, 86, 105] To perform arthroscintigraphy, 0.5 to 1.0 millicuries (MCi) of nonabsorbable technetium-99m Tc-SC mixed with 1 to 2 ml of saline is injected into the joint at the time of conventional arthrography. Imaging is performed after exercise, within the next 1 to 2 hours. Any isotope activity along the shaft of the femoral component indicates loosening. The acetabular component cannot be evaluated by arthroscintigraphy because the superimposed activity of the isotope in the joint cavity overlies the acetabulum.[86] Another disadvantage is that studies become nondiagnostic if the tracer extravasates along the needle tract or accumulates within communicating fluid pockets. Correlation with conventional arthrograms should be helpful in this situation.

In a study correlating surgical outcome with radiologic examinations,[86] arthroscintigraphy was performed in 19 patients and the sensitivity was 93 percent, specificity 75 percent, and overall accuracy 89 percent. Conventional arthrography, performed in 18 of these patients, demonstrated a sensitivity of 93 percent, a specificity of 100 percent, and an accuracy of 94 percent. When interpreted together, sensitivity, specificity, and accuracy all increased to 100 percent, suggesting that arthroscintigraphy is best employed as a complement to conventional arthrography. Another study noted four false-negative conventional arthrogram findings that were positive for loosening on radionuclide arthrography and at surgery.[105]

Accurate information regarding loosening may not be available from CT.[4, 12]

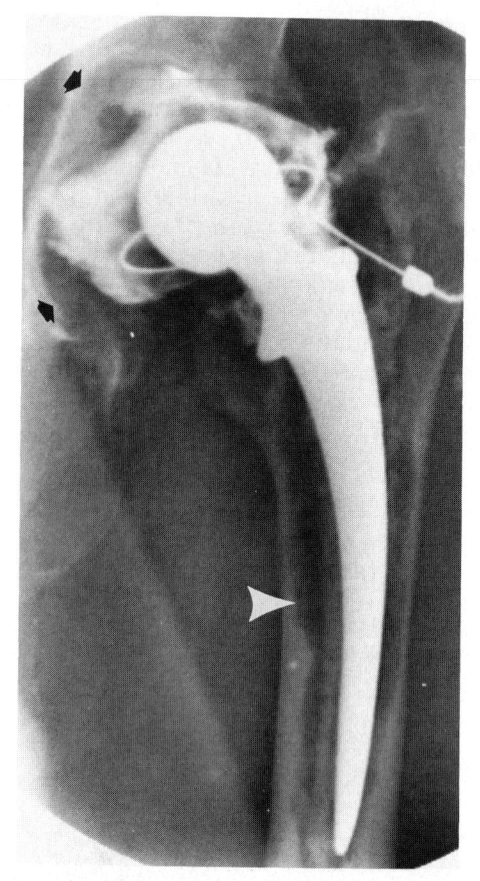

FIGURE 11–13. False-negative arthrogram for loosening in a total hip replacement. Despite markedly wide cement-bone lucencies about the acetabular (black arrows) and femoral (white arrowhead) components of this loose arthroplasty, contrast material injected during the arthrogram fails to fill these areas, probably because they contain radiolucent soft tissue. This radiographic appearance suggests the presence of granulomatous pseudotumor.

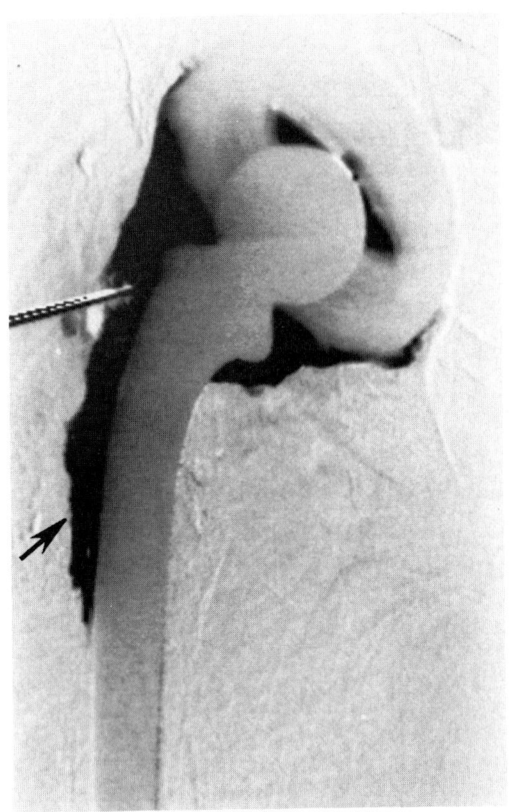

FIGURE 11–14. Loosening of the femoral stem. This digital subtraction arthrogram of a right total hip arthroplasty shows a wide track of contrast (arrow) along the lateral aspect of the femoral stem, suggesting loosening.

Infection

Radiographic evidence of loosening may or may not accompany prosthetic infection.[102] With unipolar hemiarthroplasties, acute narrowing of the acetabular cartilage in the immediate postoperative period, accompanied by groin pain, probably indicates infection.[109] Although cultures obtained at percutaneous aspiration of hip joints are less sensitive than cultures obtained at surgery, positive results of aspiration are helpful. For puncture of prosthesis-containing joints, the needle may have to be repositioned slightly several times before fluid can be freely aspirated. When aspiration is performed in the radiology department, contrast material can be injected concurrently. Injection of contrast material enables visualization of bursae and abscess cavities that communicate with the hip joint. Communicating bursae or abscesses may yield extensive fluid. Consequently, injected contrast material decompresses itself into the cavity, and large volumes must be instilled before intra-articular pressure rises enough to push contrast material into the prosthesis-cement-bone interface.[48] Arthrographic demonstration of a communicating cavity with irregular margins or a sinus tract is virtually diagnostic of infection. Noncommunicating fluid collections must be punctured directly to obtain fluid for culture. Ultrasound or CT may help in locating and aspirating such collections (see Fig. 11–7).[99]

The pseudocapsules of patients with resection arthroplasties may be successfully aspirated, even though no steadfast landmarks are evident in these patients. We have obtained fluid by inserting the needle between the resected margin of the femur and the acetabular orifice. Contrast material filling an irregular but well-delimited pseudocapsule indicates intracapsular positioning of the needle. This procedure is often done prior to implantation of the new prosthesis in a two-stage revision arthroplasty.

Because the sensitivity of preoperative aspiration alone is low, methods of scanning with a bone-seeking agent and an inflammation/infection–seeking agent may prove desirable for preoperative assessment of infection. Elaborate techniques have been employed with ^{67}Ga and ^{99m}Tc-MDP imaging in cases of complicated total hip arthroplasties. The ^{67}Ga imaging has some propensity to localize in normal bone as well as in foci of inflammation. If the normal accumulation could be subtracted from the total, the remaining concentration presumably would be due to inflammation.[90] Some investigators have imaged with ^{67}Ga and ^{99m}Tc-MDP simultaneously, providing the gallium 48 hours and the technetium 4 hours prior to imaging.[20] Because the two radionuclides emit photons of different energies, the gamma camera can be adjusted to "see" the photons of one substance and then the photons of the other, and isotope activity of the two studies can then be digitally subtracted. If significant ^{67}Ga uptake remains after the ^{99m}Tc-MDP uptake has been subtracted, the prosthesis presumably is inflamed and probably is infected. Although this technique offers the advantage of simultaneous acquisition of data from two scans, the literature suggests that the results may not be any better than the information gained by simply comparing ^{99m}Tc-MDP and ^{67}Ga scans visually.[20]

Performed alone, ^{111}In-WBC imaging may have high sensitivity for infected total hip arthroplasty, but the specificity is unacceptably low. Combined with technetium ^{99m}Tc-MDP, however, the specificity of the imaging procedure rises to 95 percent and the sensitivity remains high.[56]

Periprosthetic soft tissue abscess collections may be revealed on CT,[99] as associated metal artifact is rarely sufficient to render the study nondiagnostic. Ultrasound may be used as well. Either CT or ultrasound may provide guidance for puncture and aspiration of periarticular fluid collections.

Fracture

Cement in the soft tissues about the femoral shaft on radiographs taken immediately postimplantation suggests fracture.[109] Later fractures associated with total hip replacement most often occur adjacent to the tip of the femoral prosthesis[95] and may be related to inadequate thickness of the cement about the tip (Fig. 11–15).[69] Femoral fractures in patients with surface replacements are more likely when the prostheses are in varus. Stress fractures usually involve the pubic rami.[69, 109]

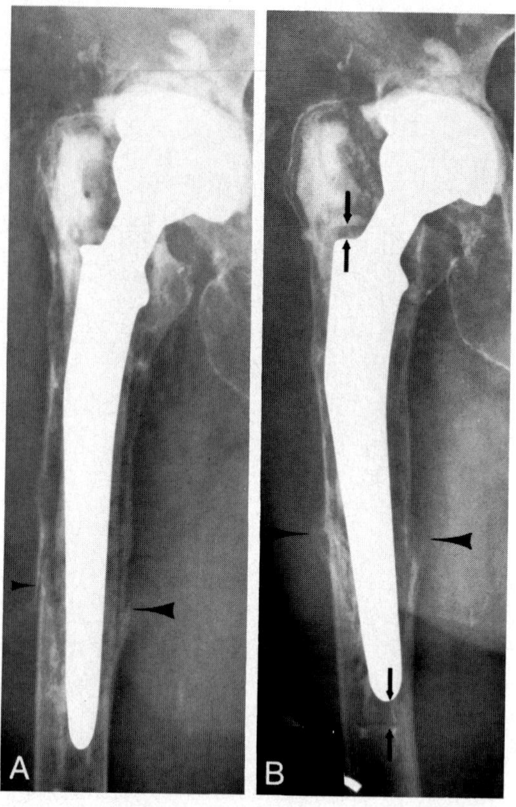

FIGURE 11–15. Femoral fracture and subsidence. *A*, This radiograph of a cemented total hip replacement demonstrates wide cement-bone lucencies around the femoral stem and endosteal bone destruction. Cortical disruption (arrowheads) adjacent to the distal part of the stem indicates fracture. *B*, After 2 months, callus (arrowheads) has developed at the fracture. This film also reveals subsidence, as the distance between the stem and the adjacent cement (arrows) has changed compared with the previous film.

Risk factors for fracture of the metallic femoral stem include the following: cement-bone or prosthesis-cement lucencies $\geq$2 mm, cement thickness $<$2 mm, cement fracture, varus positioning of the stem, resorption of bone from the calcar region, and early breakage of the trochanter wires.[95, 109]

Dislocation

Prostheses dislocate in 1 to 5 percent of total hip arthroplasties or hemiarthroplasties (Fig. 11–16).[95, 108, 109] Risk factors for dislocation include detachment of the greater trochanter, leading to loss of the abductor mechanism, and shortening of the limb due to a short femoral neck or high socket. Component malpositions that may lead to dislocation include a vertically oriented socket, a retroverted socket, a retroverted femoral prosthesis, and a socket anteverted more than 30 degrees.[95, 109]

Bone, cement, or wire fragments may prevent reduction of the dislocation.[108] (See Chapter 19, *Total Hip Arthroplasty: Complications*.)

Heterotopic Bone

Heterotopic bone formation in the soft tissues adjacent to the hip is common, occurring in 39 percent of patients.[109] It is of variable functional significance. If resection is contemplated, bone scanning may help confirm whether the mass is mature bone.[101]

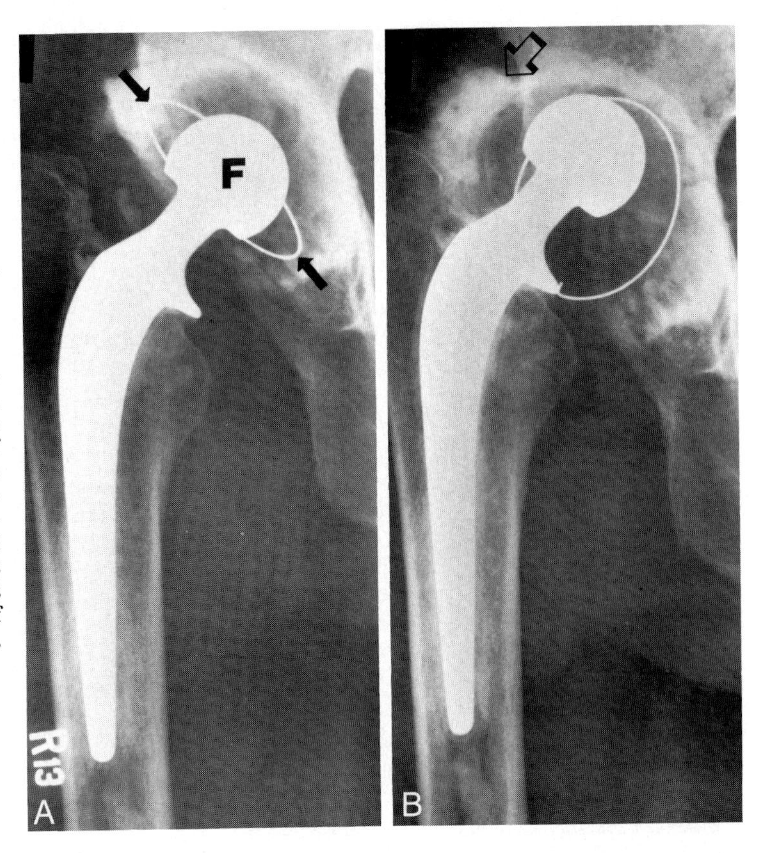

FIGURE 11–16. Dislocation of a total hip arthroplasty. *A*, This right total hip replacement has a poorly cemented femoral stem and a cemented socket. The head of the femoral prosthesis (F) lies equidistant from the superolateral and inferomedial edges (arrows) of the marker wire in the acetabular component, a normal "Saturn-ring" sign. *B*, A follow-up film made after the acute onset of hip pain shows dislocation of the prosthetic joint and of the acetabular component. Some of the superolateral cement has fractured and dislocated with the prosthesis (arrow). The inferomedial cement remains unchanged. (Courtesy of T. Gillespy III, M.D., Seattle, WA.)

Brooker and colleagues[15] noted ectopic bone formation in the periprosthetic soft tissues in 21 percent of total hip arthroplasties at 6 months.[15] They classified this phenomenon into four categories: class I involves islands of bone within the soft tissues about the hip; class II involves bone spurs forming from the pelvis or proximal end of the femur, leaving at least 1 cm between opposing bone margins; class III is similar to class II, except the bone margins are separated by less than 1 cm (see Fig. 11–2); and class IV involves bony ankylosis of the hip. In this review the hip function was not affected unless ankylosis was present. (See Chapter 19, *Total Hip Arthroplasty: Complications.*)

Planning for Revision

Many revisions of hip replacements are carried out on the bases of plain radiographs alone. However, CT certainly can assist in preoperative planning. This is the imaging modality of choice for demonstrating bone detail, such as acetabular and femoral bone stock, intra-articular bone or cement fragments, and occult fracture. The metal artifact produced by the prosthesis is usually not enough to preclude a diagnostic study,[4, 12] especially if reformatted images are added.[38, 88]

Granulomatous Pseudotumor

Granulomatous pseudotumor is thought to be a foreign body reaction of bone to either bone cement or prosthesis. Griffiths and coworkers[43] have proposed that micromovement of the prosthesis leads to debris formation, which causes a giant cell response and the production of prostaglandin E_2. Histologic samples from areas of lysis contain histiocytes and multinucleated giant cells resembling foreign body cells. Foreign material, including polymethyl methacrylate, barium sulfate, polyethylene, and metal debris, can sometimes be seen within or among the giant cells. A prominent fibrous tissue response may also be evident. (See Chapter 12, *Histology and Pathology in Total Joint Replacement.*)

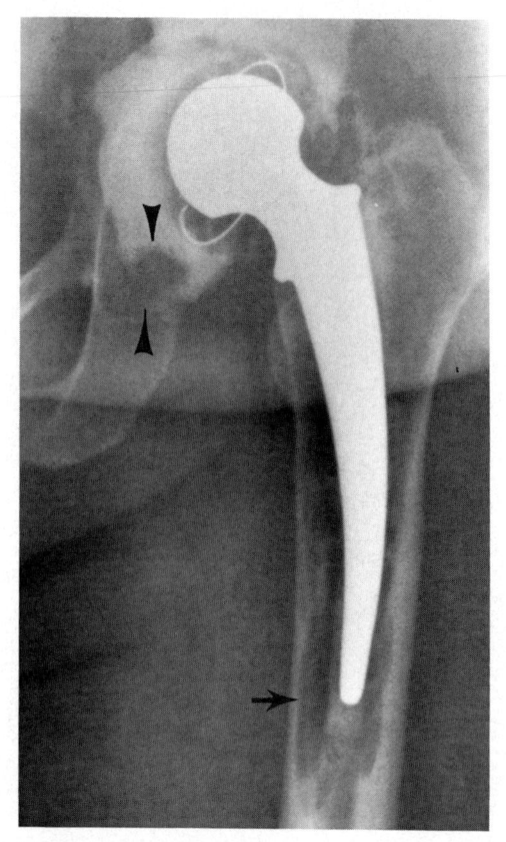

FIGURE 11–17. Granulomatous pseudotumor. An anteroposterior view of the left hip demonstrates wide somewhat lobulated cement-bone lucencies around the femoral stem distally (arrow). At the inferomedial aspect of the acetabular component, a rounded lucency encompasses both bone and cement (arrowheads), suggesting a diagnosis of granulomatous pseudotumor.

Radiographically, granulomatous pseudotumor produces focal ovoid or rounded radiolucencies. They are seen most commonly about the cortex surrounding the femoral component, but the radiolucencies can be seen about the acetabular component as well (see Fig. 11–13). The focal areas enlarge and, if multiple, begin to coalesce (Fig. 11–17).[43] Both bone and cement are destroyed. Granulomatous pseudotumor has also been reported in noncemented prostheses.[16]

Goldring and colleagues[42] have noted tissue with histologic and histochemical characteristics of a synovial-like membrane occurring at the cement-bone interface in loose total hip arthroplasties. They proposed that this membrane may be responsible for the bone destruction accompanying granulomatous pseudotumor. The membrane, which may originate secondary to motion of the prosthesis, is capable of producing significant amounts of prostaglandin E_2 and collagenase. (See Chapter 12, *Histology and Pathology in Total Joint Replacement.*)

Other Complications

Proximal migration of >2 cm of the osteotomized greater trochanter may be associated with abductor weakness and diminished function.[11] Pain, limp, and possibly adductor contracture may occur.[32]

Polymethyl methacrylate cement that has extruded into the pelvis usually causes no symptoms, but it may impinge on adjacent nerves and blood vessels. Symptoms of impingement on the bowel, bladder, uterus, and vagina may occur.[109] To delineate the relationship of cement collections to nearby structures, CT may be helpful.

IMAGING OF THE KNEE

Routine Evaluation

Both AP and lateral films of a total knee arthroplasty should be obtained immediately after implantation to rule out malposition and intraoperative fracture. As soon as the patient can bear weight, standing AP and lateral films, with the x-ray beam centered on the joint line,[34] plus a sunrise view are made as a baseline set.[96] The identical technique should be used when radiographs are obtained for follow-up or assessing complications. Films at least 17 inches long assure that enough of the femoral and tibial shafts is included to determine their long axes.

On behalf of the Knee Society, Ewald[34] divided the area around total knee prostheses into zones to enable uniform description of lucencies. He described seven tibial component zones on the AP views, seven femoral and three tibial zones on the lateral views, and three or five patellar zones on the sunrise views (Fig. 11–18). He also suggested that component angles and subluxation be measured on all three views.[34]

Ideally, the femoral component lies in 7 degrees ±3 degrees of valgus on the AP

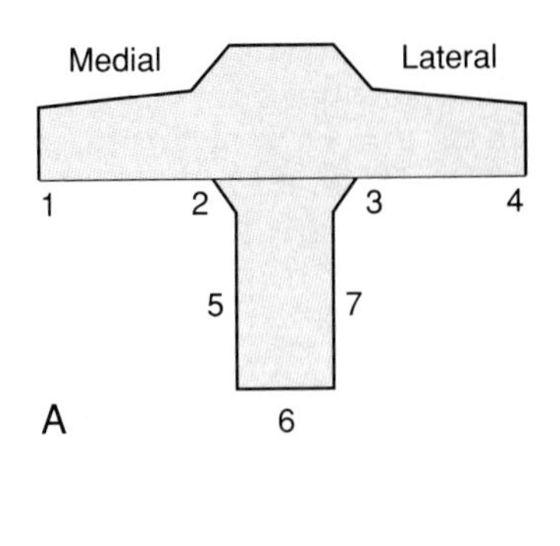

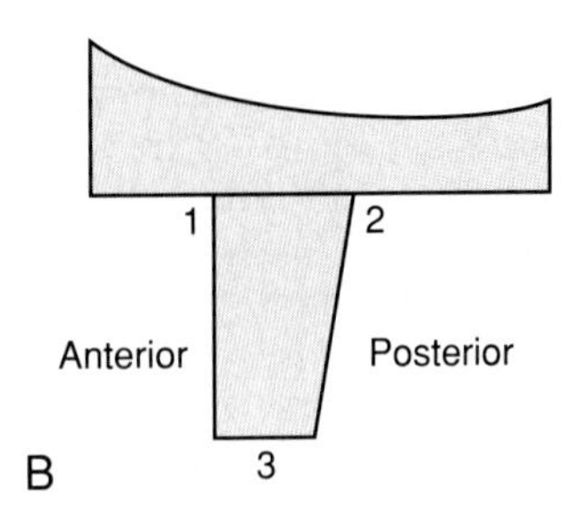

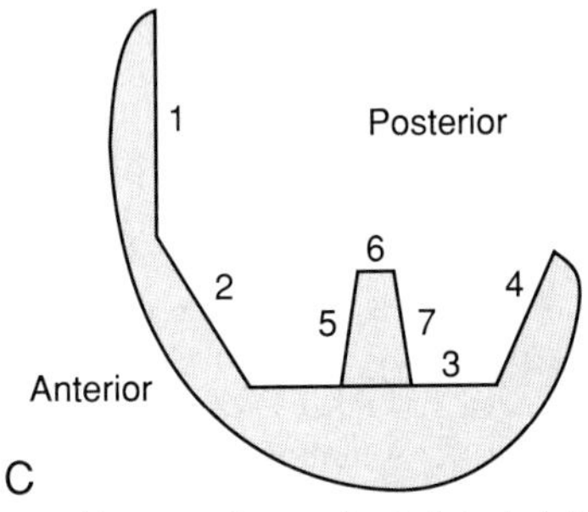

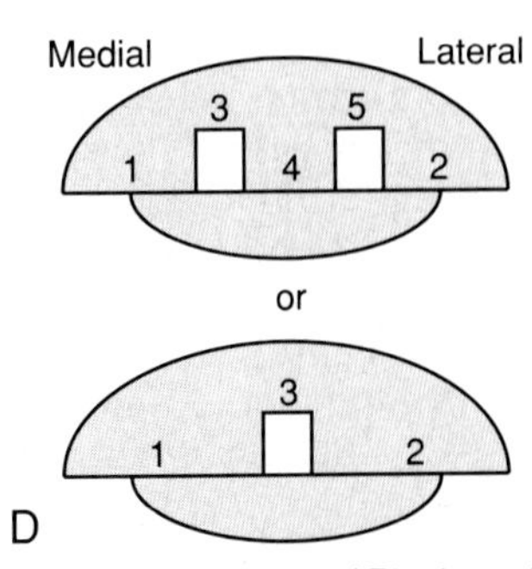

FIGURE 11–18. Zones to be evaluated in total knee arthroplasty. *A*, Anteroposterior (AP) view of the tibial component. *B*, Lateral view of the tibial component. *C*, Lateral view of the femoral prosthesis. The prosthesis-bone interface of the femoral component of a knee replacement cannot be seen on the AP view. *D*, "Sunrise" view of the patellar component. (Redrawn from Ewald, F. C.: Clin. Orthop. 248:9–12, 1989.)

views and at an angle of 90 degrees ±5 degrees in relation to the long axis of the femur on the lateral views. The plane of the tibial component of an unconstrained knee arthroplasty should be 90 degrees ±3 degrees in relation to the long axis of the tibia on the AP view. On the lateral view, no anterior tilt should be seen and with some prosthesis designs up to 10 degrees posterior tilt should be seen. Overall alignment of the long axes of the femur and tibia should be 7 degrees ±3 degrees of valgus.[55] The femoral and tibial prostheses should articulate congruently on AP and lateral views as should the femoral and patellar components on lateral and sunrise views. With constrained prostheses, the hinge should be parallel to the ground on weightbearing views.[108]

In unicompartmental knee arthroplasty, the femoral component should be centered in the involved condyle on the AP view and the tibial component should be centered under the femoral implant and perpendicular to the long axis of the tibia. Lateral views show the tibial prosthesis perpendicular to the long axis of the tibia, or the posterior portion may tilt caudad as much as 10 degrees. On this film, the femoral prosthesis covers the posterior part of the condyle and extends far enough anteriorly to articulate with the tibial prosthesis in full extension.[108]

Standing hip-to-ankle views or long knee views should be done prior to operation and soon after implantation. A line drawn from the center of the femoral head to the center of the tibiotalar joint should pass through the center of the knee. The joint line of the knee arthroplasty should be at a 90-degree angle to this line.[96]

For evaluation of the knee, CT is most useful prior to implantation of the arthroplasty. This imaging modality can also be helpful in the design of custom arthroplasties and quantification of bone stock.

Loosening

Cement-bone lucencies <2 mm are common in total knee arthroplasties, but only a small percentage of prostheses surrounded by radiolucencies are actually loose or symptomatic.[66, 84, 91, 104] Moderately increased uptake on the ^{99m}Tc-MDP bone scan frequently is associated with these thin cement-bone radiolucencies. Neither of these findings, alone or in concert, necessarily signifies loosening or infection.[91] The significance of prosthesis-bone lucencies around uncemented components is even less clear. Probably, if such lucencies appear within the first 2 to 3 years after arthroplasty, if they do not progress, and if the patient is asymptomatic, they do not indicate loosening. Radiolucencies that are ≥2 mm wide or progressive are highly suggestive of loosening in the presence of pain. Most total knee arthroplasties that fail because of loosening have such radiographic findings.[97] The femoral or tibial component, or both, may be involved.

Any shift of component position detected on serial films indicates loosening. Loosening of unconstrained total knee prostheses, whether bicondylar or unicondylar,[65] most commonly involves the tibial component (Fig. 11–19).[5, 96] Loosening of femoral and patellar components occurs less frequently.[97] Several workers have noted that even slight variations in radiographic technique can make the components look very different.[34, 96] Thus, true migration may be obscured and solid components may appear to shift if strict guidelines are not followed by the radiologic technologist.

The AP view may reveal the tibial component sinking into the underlying cancellous bone, which is especially likely for a replacement without a metal tray and in a patient with underlying osteopenia. The intercondylar eminences, if present in these cases, may impact upon the femur and prevent normal articulation of the femoral and tibial components.[104] Lateral views may show anterior or posterior tilting of components.[104]

Eccentric loading of the tibial prosthesis frequently leads to deformation[104] and fragmentation of the polyethylene plateau and crushing of the cancellous bone beneath.[5] Deformation of the polyethylene plateau correlates closely with loosening.[97] Displacement or breakage of wire markers in polyethylene components indicates prosthetic disintegration and loosening.

Loosening of constrained total knee arthroplasty is even more common because of the increased stress transmitted to the prosthesis-bone interface.[55] Reactive bone forming along the edge of the bone-cement or prosthesis-cement surfaces of hinged replacements is a normal finding.[108]

The ^{99m}Tc-MDP scan alone is not specific for loosening. More than other prosthetic joints, the knee is particularly prone to mildly or moderately increased uptake of ^{99m}Tc-MDP for years after implantation surgery, in the absence of any complications.[96] This finding holds true for both cemented and uncemented prostheses, and uptake is particularly prevalent around the tibial component.[50] Because of the normal increased uptake, loosening or infection can only be suggested by a marked elevation in the concentration of radioisotope.[50] Negative scan findings make these complications highly unlikely.[91] Lateral scintigrams are mandatory for the knee because uptake in the patella obscures accumulation in the femur behind it.

Although arthrography can show loosening if contrast material tracks around the prostheses, arthrography of the prosthetic knee is rarely performed.[66] Contrast agent outlining the arthroplasty components can be detected only tangentially to the x-ray beam. The opacified suprapatellar bursa precludes evaluation of the femoral prosthesis on the AP view.

Infection

If infection is allowed to go untreated, prostheses will eventually loosen. The difficulty is that acute infection may or may not be accompanied by radiographic evidence of loosening (see Figs. 11–5A and 11–5B).[97] The presence of a knee joint effusion, although fairly and reliably ascertained from plain films,[109] is a nonspecific finding by itself.

Combined ^{99m}Tc-MDP bone scans and ^{67}Ga scans may be quite sensitive for detecting infection in total knee arthroplasty (see Figs. 11–5C to 11–5F).[96] If the two scans show incongruent patterns of abnormal uptake, infection is fairly likely. The ^{111}In-WBC scans are perhaps more specific for infection.[97]

Percutaneous aspiration of the knee may yield a fair number of false-negative results compared with intraoperative sampling, but positive culture results are of great assistance. Radiologists are rarely

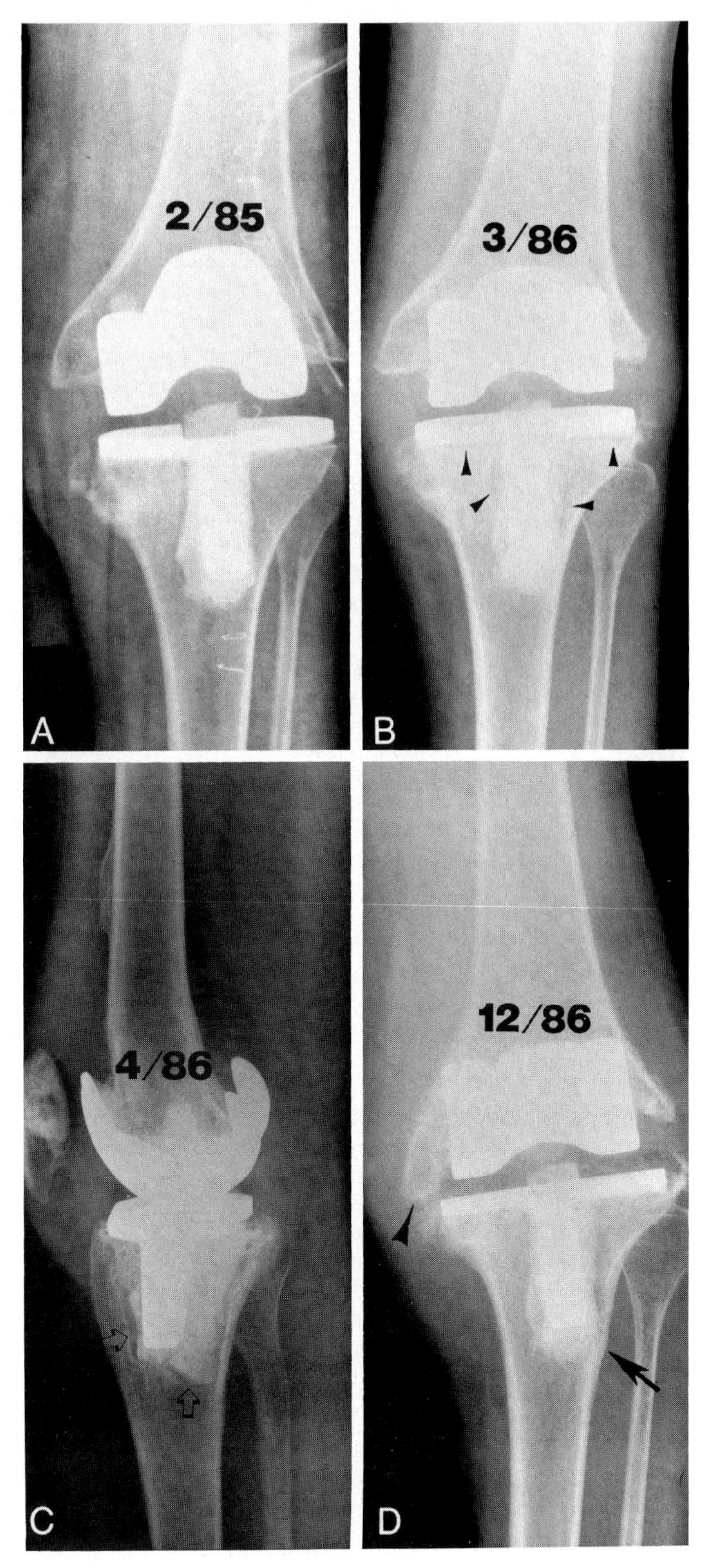

FIGURE 11–19. Prosthetic migration in a total knee arthroplasty. *A*, An anteroposterior film of the left knee of a 39-year-old man, who underwent total knee replacement for arthropathy related to hemophilia, made immediately after implantation shows the cemented tibial component tilted in slight varus. *B*, At 13 months, the medial portion of the tibial tray has subsided into the underlying cancellous bone, resulting in more varus. A thin radiolucent line (arrowheads) surrounds the prosthesis. The inferolateral cement at the tip of the tibial stem now approaches the lateral tibial cortex. *C*, A lateral view made 1 month later demonstrates an even wider cement-bone lucency (open arrows). Reactive bone forming along the anterior aspect of the femur was thought to be a result of periosteal disruption during the implantation procedure. *D*, At 22 months after implantation, the tibial component has subsided even farther into varus. Now the distal tip of the tibial cement impinges upon the lateral cortex of the tibia, inciting reactive bone formation (arrow). The femoral prosthesis has also subsided into the femur, causing the medial corner of the femur to abut the tibia (arrowhead). Genu vara is present.

called upon to aspirate knee joints, because these joints are easily punctured without fluoroscopic guidance.[97]

Arthrography is commonly used to image Baker cysts, which may be a source of pain in patients with total knee replacement.[66] Ultrasound can also demonstrate these cysts and other periarticular fluid collections and can guide aspiration if infection is suspected.[21, 46] Metal artifacts might preclude CT or MRI of fluid collections about prosthetic knees.

Malalignment

Abnormal angulation and subluxation are mostly problems of unconstrained and semiconstrained prostheses. Such malalignment may be seen in 3 to 18 percent of patients with total knee arthroplasties.[66, 104] The AP radiographs should be examined for genu varus or valgus, especially if such deformities were present prior to arthroplasty. When varus or valgus is due to ligamentous or capsular laxity, the opening of the space between the femoral and tibial components is asymmetric, and the components retain the previous position within the bone. If varus or valgus is present and the articulation between the components is symmetric, the components are malpositioned (Fig. 11–20). The cause may be either loosening or imprecise insertion. Alignment in the AP direction, as determined by the lateral views, is more difficult to evaluate unless obvious subluxation or dislocation occurs (Fig. 11–21).[96]

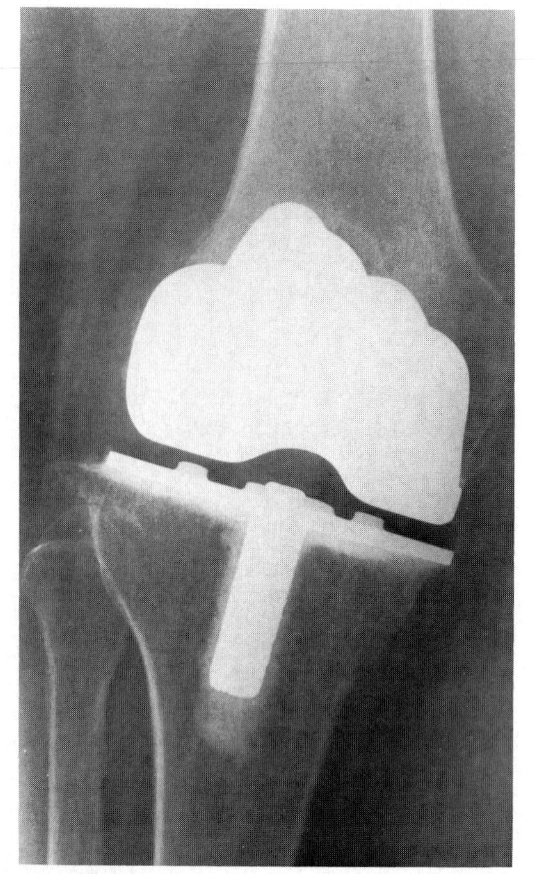

FIGURE 11–20. Component malposition in knee arthroplasty. An anteroposterior film of a right total knee replacement demonstrates a varus tilt of the cemented tibial component and a valgus tilt of the femoral component.

Alignment and tracking of the patella, whether resurfaced or not, should be sought on the patellar (sunrise) view, as malposition is a significant source of pain in a patient with total knee arthroplasty. Patellar subluxation has been reported in 1 to 2 percent of patients, with or without a patellar button.[23, 66] In general, postoperative malalignments tend to mimic those that occur preoperatively, and they may occur without prosthetic loosening.[66, 104]

Fracture

The patella is the bone about the knee most commonly fractured after arthroplasty, occurring in 5 percent or less of patients.[23, 55] Factors contributing to patellar fracture include resection of too thick a portion of the surface; overzealous drilling of holes for placement of the prosthesis; osteonecrosis, which may be due to thermal damage by bone cement; devascularization during the surgical approach; resection of the patellar fat pad; and lateral release.[23] Fractures of the femur, tibia, and fibula occur occasionally and do not necessarily doom the arthroplasty to failure, even when they extend to the prosthesis.

Stress fractures may complicate total knee arthroplasty. They most commonly occur in the proximal medial tibia or the pelvis.[104] Plain films may show focal cortical lucency or focal periosteal reaction. If located primarily in cancellous bone, stress fractures appear as focal areas of increased

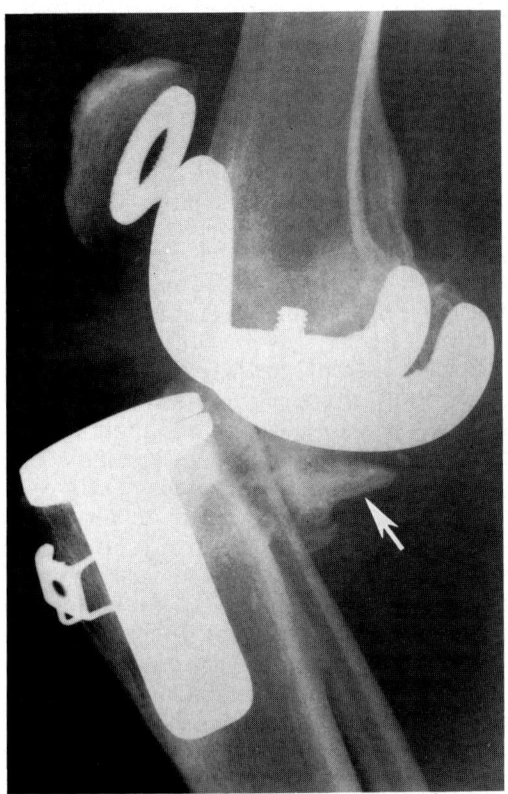

FIGURE 11–21. Dislocation of a total knee arthroplasty. A lateral film of a patient with a total knee arthroplasty demonstrates anterior dislocation of the tibia. The femoral component has fractured a fragment from the posterior tibial plateau (arrow).

density.[96] However, radiographs are frequently nonspecific or provide negative findings, especially with early stress fractures. In this situation, ^{99m}Tc-MDP bone scanning reveals focal uptake.[112]

Fracture of the metallic components is rare with unconstrained arthroplasties but has been reported with metallic tibial trays and constrained prostheses.[95]

Associated Arthritis

If the patella is not resurfaced during total knee arthroplasty, progressive arthritis may ensue. One group reported patellar arthritis in 11 percent of 224 total knee arthroplasties.[66] Another study described patellofemoral radiographic findings in 49 of 52 knees; in only two of them were patients symptomatic.[104] Radiographic findings include cartilage loss, reactive bone formation, and fragmentation. Similar problems may be found in the unoperated compartment of a patient with unicondylar knee replacement.[65]

Other Complications

Plain films show heterotopic bone about the knee in 10 percent of cases, but it is rarely symptomatic.[66] Mature heterotopic bone concentrates radioisotope at a constant rate on serial scans. If the amount of uptake continues to change on sequential studies, the mass is not yet mature.[101] Loose cement bodies in the joint or in Baker cysts[66] can be symptomatic.

Rarely, patients with total knee arthroplasties sustain rupture of the patellar tendons.[23, 108] This source of knee pain or functional loss may be obvious on physical examination. Ultrasound probably is the modality of choice if imaging is desired.[46] Whether MRI scans of diagnostic quality could be obtained in the presence of metal components is uncertain.

IMAGING OF THE ANKLE

Routine Evaluation

Standard AP, mortise, and lateral views, plus AP and lateral weightbearing views of the ankle with the x-ray beam centered on the joint line, suffice for follow-up of total ankle arthroplasty. One study recommended fluoroscopic guidance to obtain views tangential to the components.[49] If properly aligned, the flat surface of the tibial component is perpendicular to the long axis of the tibia on AP and lateral weightbearing views, and the flat surface of the talar component is parallel to the floor.[28] When AP films are made with varus and valgus stress, no medial or lateral opening of the joint should be seen.[49] Lateral radiographs in active flexion and extension allow for measurement of range of motion in the AP direction.[28, 49] The subtalar and intertarsal joints should be studied serially to detect progressive degenerative joint disease.

Loosening

Total ankle replacements loosen in 10 to 24 percent of cases.[28, 31, 49] Radiolucent zones almost always surround loose tibial components, whereas loose talar components tend to sink into the underlying cancellous bone. Migration of either prosthesis indicates loosening.[28] Stress views may show motion between the prostheses and bone.[49]

Infection

As for other joints, infection of the ankle arthroplasty may or may not be accompanied by radiographic evidence of loosening. Joint effusion can be seen on lateral views but is nonspecific.[109] Periosteal reaction without fracture suggests infection under the appropriate clinical circumstances.

Instability

Instability will be indicated on AP views of the ankle by medial or lateral opening of the joint with varus and valgus stress. The significance of this finding must be judged in the context of the clinical picture.

IMAGING OF THE SHOULDER

Routine Evaluation

Follow-up radiographs of a patient with shoulder hemiarthroplasty or total shoulder arthroplasty may include AP, axillary, 45-degree posterior oblique,[108] and transscapular views. It is virtually impossible for the radiologic technologist to reproduce comparable views at each clinic visit because of differences in the patient's range of motion during rehabilitation and in the inherent instability of the shoulder.[70] Even so, radiology personnel should establish strict guidelines for obtaining these films.

The inferior aspect of the head of the humeral prosthesis should rest on the cut edge of the humerus and align with the inferior edge of the glenoid fossa or glenoid component on AP and posterior oblique views.[108] The axillary and transscapular views should show anatomic articulation of the humeral prosthesis and the glenoid.

In patients with irreparable rotator cuff tears, a polyethylene subacromial spacer may be inserted to prevent acromiohumeral impingement. The Neer spacer is radiolucent but contains a marker wire.[22]

Loosening

Radiolucent and radiodense lines may be seen around uncemented shoulder prostheses and their anchoring screws without clinical evidence of loosening.[70] Although not necessarily indicative of loosening, proximal medial cortical resorption and remodeling of the humerus has been described when an uncemented humeral component does not rest on the cut edge of the humerus, especially in a more active patient. Migration of components correlates with loosening but is difficult to document with shoulder arthroplasties because of positioning differences on follow-up films, especially with humeral components.[70]

As for other joints, loosening is more common in constrained shoulder arthroplasties. When plain films of a constrained total shoulder arthroplasty show excessive resection of glenoid bone the patient should be followed closely, as this finding correlates highly with loosening of the glenoid component.[81]

Infection

Imaging options for suspected infections of shoulder arthroplasties parallel those described for the hip and knee. Arthrography is not commonly done for this indication, but when it is done, aspiration of the shoulder under fluoroscopic guidance may assist the surgeon, as this joint is rather difficult to puncture blindly. Few descriptions of radioisotope imaging in shoulder arthroplasty have appeared in the literature,[67] yet such imaging may be helpful in certain cases.

Malalignment

Alignment of unconstrained shoulder arthroplasties depends to a large extent upon the integrity of surrounding soft tissues, especially the rotator cuff. Because these tissues are frequently deficient in patients requiring shoulder arthroplasty, most no-

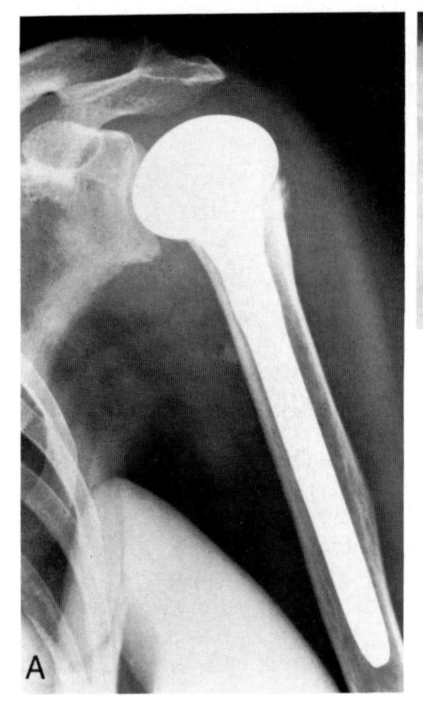

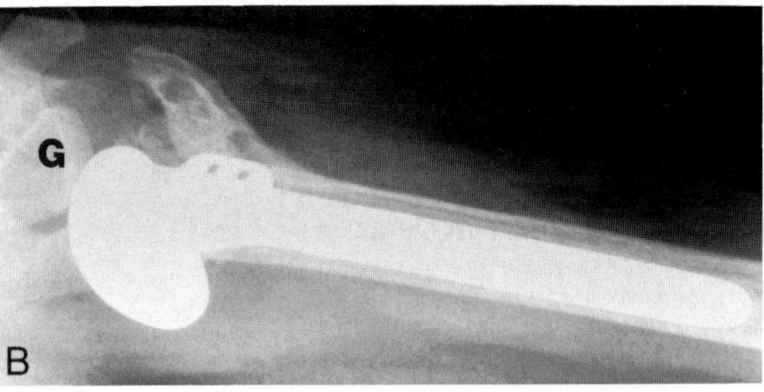

FIGURE 11–22. Subluxation of a shoulder hemiarthroplasty. *A*, In the anteroposterior film of a patient with an uncemented shoulder hemiarthroplasty, the head of the prosthesis is well seated against cortical bone and seems to articulate normally with the glenoid. *B*, The axillary view reveals posterior subluxation of the humeral prosthesis from the glenoid (G).

tably in those with rheumatoid arthritis, subluxation is common. Both AP and posterior oblique views that show superior displacement of the humeral prosthesis in relation to the glenoid correlate with deficient rotator cuff musculature.[70] Displacements in the AP direction are best demonstrated on axillary or transscapular views (Fig. 11–22). Subacromial spacers also may become displaced.[22]

Other Complications

With shoulder hemiarthroplasties, articulation of the metal humeral prostheses on the native glenoids may result in slow, progressive loss of cartilage.[22]

Plain radiography is well suited to revealing heterotopic bone and bony and prosthetic fractures in patients with shoulder arthroplasties.[108] Fracture of metallic components is much more common with constrained arthroplasty.[81]

The status of the rotator cuff usually is addressed during the implantation procedure. If the cuff is suspected of tearing postoperatively and if repair is contemplated, arthrography could be employed for diagnosis. Proximity of the bulky humeral prosthesis to the rotator cuff would undoubtedly generate too much artifact on MRI to enable diagnosis of rotator cuff tears. A few investigators have found ultrasound quite accurate for detecting tears of the rotator cuff and long head of the biceps tendon.[46] The presence of total shoulder replacement should not preclude this examination. However, in most radiologists' experience, ultrasound studies have not yielded the accuracy reported in the literature or obtained with arthrography.[18]

IMAGING OF THE ELBOW

Routine Evaluation

Standard AP and lateral views of the elbow constitute appropriate follow-up films. The shafts of the prosthesis should parallel the shafts of the humerus and ulna.[41] Some surgeons find the axial view of the flexed elbow helpful in evaluating the articulation of the olecranon with the humerus.

Loosening

Radiographic signs suggestive of loosening consist of wide or progressive lucencies and migration.[92] Lucencies around elbow prostheses may not be symptomatic enough to warrant revision.[35, 54, 57] In one study, in which average follow-up was 6 years, radiographs of nine of 44 hinged elbow prostheses showed radiolucencies around the components, but only two of these patients were symptomatic and none required revision.[57] Rates of loosening of hinged elbow arthroplasties have been higher than rates of loosening of unconstrained models, but further reports show little difference, with rates of 1 to 3 percent for both types.[41]

Infection

Infection may occur in 1 to 3 percent of elbow arthroplasties.[41] The contribution of imaging to the diagnosis of infection is minimal, as this joint is easily punctured without fluoroscopy.

Elevation of the anterior and posterior fat pads on the lateral view signifies elbow joint effusion.[109] This may be seen in an asymptomatic arthroplasty as well as in an infected arthroplasty.

Malalignment

To achieve a balance of the soft tissues and therefore stability, insertion of unconstrained elbow arthroplasties is technically demanding. Frequently, the soft tissues are deficient, and some incongruence of the components is common.[92] Frank dislocation occurs at a rate of 3 to 9 percent.[35, 41]

Other Complications

Excessive anterior and proximal placement of the ulnar prosthesis in hinged replacements may result in triceps rupture and ulnar neuropathy.[41] In the absence of gross malposition, suboptimal placement may be difficult to detect radiographically. Ultrasound shows muscle tears well[46, 106] and would probably be superior to MRI in the imaging of triceps ruptures adjacent to elbow replacements.

Fractures of the olecranon and humerus may occur.[108] Fractured prosthetic components are uncommon and generally involve constrained prostheses. Loose cement bodies in the elbow may cause pain and require removal.[54]

IMAGING OF THE WRIST AND HAND

Routine Evaluation

Unlike the metallic prostheses utilized for other joints, silicone rubber (Silastic) implants are similar in density to soft tissue and somewhat difficult to distinguish from adjacent structures.[29] Nevertheless, AP, lateral, and oblique views of the hand and wrist usually suffice for follow-up of wrist, metacarpophalangeal, and interphalangeal interpositional arthroplasties. Radiographs made with traction on the digits have not proven helpful.[29]

The proximal rim of the collar of a Silastic prosthesis is tangential to the x-ray beam in anatomic alignment and may appear as a dense line on the AP film.[19] The collar of a Silastic prosthesis may rest against the cut edges of the bones or may lie 1 to 2 mm away, allowing for pistoning action during joint motion. In contrast, the mesh on Dacron-covered Silastic implants is meant to encourage bony ingrowth, and motion of these types of stems within bone is undesirable. The stems should otherwise lie within the intramedullary canal of the articulating bones. If an ulnar cap has been applied, the patient should be followed for migration or fragmentation of the cap.

Metal or metal-and-plastic resurfacing arthroplasties of the wrist should articulate congruently on all views. The stems of the implants should be parallel to the long axes of the radius and metacarpal.

Complications

Silicone interpositional joint replacements usually are performed to relieve pain due to rheumatoid arthritis,[29, 36] which is frequently accompanied by subluxation. The propensity for malalignment to recur with time, even if initially reduced by implantation of the arthroplasty has often been noted.[29, 37] Accordingly, the most frequent early complication of silicone arthroplasty is instability.[78] Because the implants are relatively radiolucent, it is usually difficult to determine by radiographs whether recurrent subluxation is due to fracture of the prosthesis or to loosening of the implant because of destruction of the bony bed. Interpositional silicone prostheses fracture fairly commonly,[78] most often at the junction of the distal stem and the collar.[19, 36] In one study, fractures were identified in 15 of 162 implants by loss in continuity of the outline of the prosthesis or by a definite radiolucent line.[37]

A pseudocapsule forms postoperatively to keep the stems of a silicone joint replacement within the intramedullary canal.[19] On all views on plain radiography, stems that have separated from the intramedullary canal are outlined by soft tissue and are not within the confines of the cortex (Fig. 11–23). The radiographic findings may not be very striking, and comparison with previous films assists greatly in detection of this abnormality. Serial radiographs may also show progressive sinking of the collar of the prosthesis into adjacent bone. Silicone synovitis may result from fragmentation of carpal bone replacements and interpositional Silastic implants.[79, 89, 103] This process may be similar to the granulomatous pseudotumor described in patients with hip replacements. Radiographs in these cases demonstrate wide zones of endosteal scalloping about the stems of the interpositional prostheses. Microscopic examination reveals proliferative synovitis with accompanying osteoclastic resorption of bone, not unlike that seen in pigmented villonodular synovitis.[78, 79] A study of patients with Dacron-reinforced silicone metacarpophalangeal arthroplasties found bony destruction in 87 percent of the prostheses, but the investigators declined to attribute this to silicone synovitis.[29]

Although resurfacing total wrist arthroplasties are subject to loosening and infection, a series of 41 total wrist replacements followed as long as 34 months revealed that no components had loosened or become infected.[107] The most common complication in this study was recurrent ulnar drift of the wrist. Immediate postoperative subluxations and dislocations were seen in two of the 41 arthroplasties (Fig. 11–24),

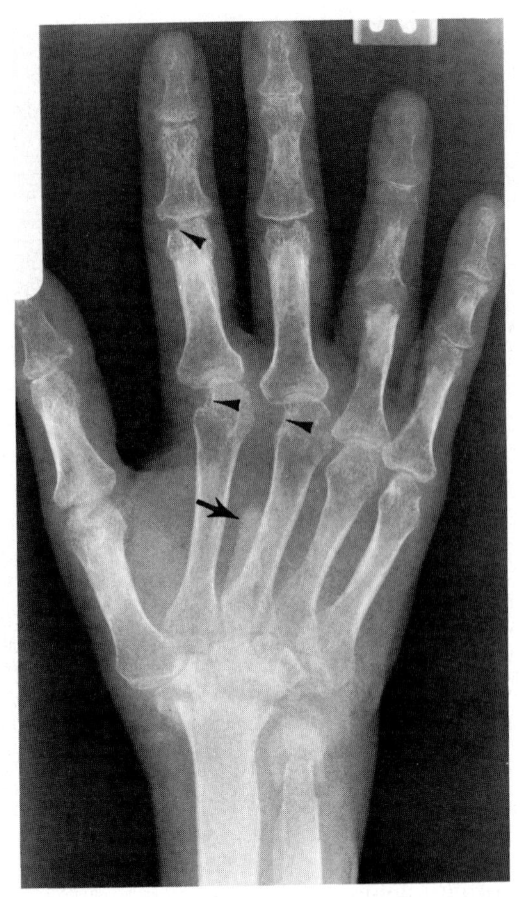

FIGURE 11–23. Displacement of a Silastic stem from the intramedullary canal. An anteroposterior view of the right hand shows typical rheumatoid erosions in the metacarpal heads and index proximal phalanx (arrowheads). The patient received Silastic interpositional arthroplasties of the first metacarpophalangeal, fourth proximal interphalangeal, and wrist joints. The distal stem of the wrist implant lies outside the third metacarpal (arrow). Despite this position, the wrist remained functional.

but these did not recur after initial reduction.[107]

PROBLEM-ORIENTED IMAGING

Pain

Nearly all total joint replacements accomplish the goal of pain relief for some time after implantation, unless early infection, intraoperative fracture, or malposition occurs. Loosening or infection is the most common cause of subsequent painful total joint arthroplasty. If routine radio-

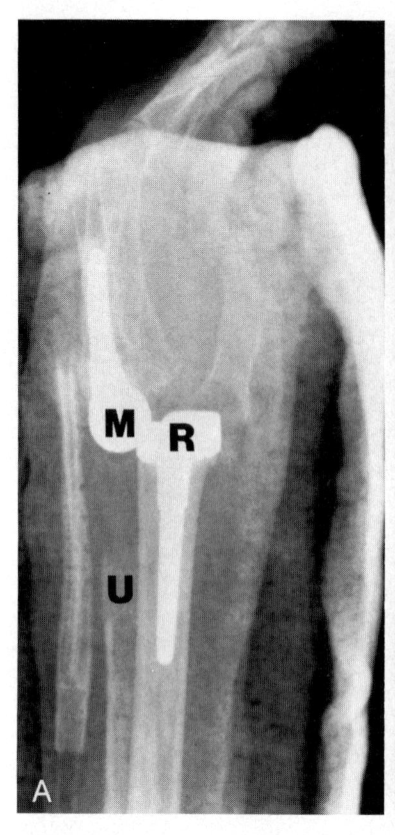

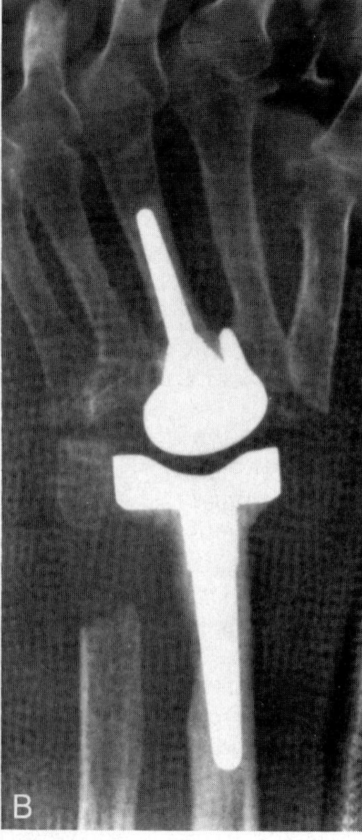

FIGURE 11–24. Dislocation of a total wrist arthroplasty. *A*, Radiograph of a patient with rheumatoid arthritis who had had a painful dorsal subluxation of the wrist and underwent a total wrist arthroplasty with resection of the distal ulna (U). This film, made through a cast immediately after implantation, shows recurrence of the preoperative deformity, with dorsal dislocation of the metacarpal component (M) in relation to the radial component (R). *B*, A later anteroposterior film made after reduction and removal of the drain demonstrates congruent articulation of the porous-coated components.

graphs demonstrate loosening, obvious fracture of bone or prosthesis, stress fracture, dislocation, or instability, no further imaging studies are required, unless concurrent infection is suspected as well. When infection is suspected, the surgeon may proceed directly to percutaneous aspiration or open culture and debridement. If the joint is difficult to puncture blindly, aspiration arthrography can be done. Some surgeons perform combined ^{99m}Tc-MDP and ^{67}Ga scans or ^{111}In-WBC scans prior to aspiration to avoid puncturing a sterile joint. Loosening requiring revision is usually but not always accompanied by radiographic changes. When routine radiographs are normal, ^{99m}Tc-MDP bone scan may reveal abnormal increased uptake about the prosthesis in cases of loosening or infection. When the bone scan findings are positive and infection is suspected, ^{67}Ga or ^{111}In-WBC scans should be performed and interpreted in concert with ^{99m}Tc-MDP bone scans. Loosening and infection are unlikely when bone scan findings are negative; therefore, another source of pain should be sought. Uptake of radionuclide also is seen within heterotopic bone or stress fracture.

When radiographs and bone scans are normal and no signs of infection are present, pain may be caused by a juxta-articular fluid collection or instability, or it may originate from another source outside the joint. Stress views can demonstrate instability not apparent on routine radiographs. Instillation of local anesthetic into the joint can clarify the source of pain. Standard aspiration arthrography confirms that the anesthetic was indeed placed inside the joint. If pain is allayed by intra-articular anesthetic, other causes of pain within the joint itself, such as intra-articular ectopic cement, should be considered. Persistent pain with intra-articular anesthetic on board suggests that the source of pain is probably outside the joint and may be due to a herniated disc or a noncommunicating, inflamed bursa. Even though arthrography reveals no bursa, CT or ultrasound may yet demonstrate a fluid collection.[46, 99]

Planning for Revision

In many cases, the only imaging study required for revision arthroplasty is plain radiography. However, CT scanning with or without multiplanar reconstructions provides useful information about available bone stock. Metal artifact would probably degrade three-dimensional images so that they would add no information. But in cases in which the prostheses were resected as separate procedures prior to revision and no metals are in the joints, CT with three-dimensional interactive images can be of help. A resin model may be generated if the radiologist is informed that the CT is being done for revision planning and sets up the scan according to the appropriate protocol.

Masses

A mass palpated adjacent to a joint replacement probably represents a bursa or an abscess related to the arthroplasty, especially if the patient has pain. In this situation, arthrography is indicated to aspirate fluid for culture and to opacify the bursa. If contrast material does not fill the bursa, the mass may nonetheless represent a fluid collection relating to the prosthesis, or it may be a neoplasm. At this point, CT or ultrasound could be done to localize the mass and characterize it as solid or cystic.[46, 99, 106] Mixed echogenic and hypoechoic patterns can be seen on ultrasound studies of abscesses and neoplasms. Aspiration of fluid-filled masses can be done under CT or ultrasound guidance.[21, 99] A mass that is clearly solid on ultrasound studies may represent neoplasm and should be approached as such.

References

1. Abdel-Dayem, H. M., Bardowala, Y. M., Papademitrio, T., et al.: Loose hip prosthesis appearance in radionuclide arthrography. Clin. Nucl. Med. 11:713–715, 1986.
2. Amstutz, H. C., Ouzounian, T., Grauer, D., et al.: The grid radiograph. J. Bone Joint Surg. 68A:1052–1056, 1986.
3. Apple, J. S., Roberts, R. Jr., Gamba, J., et al.: Digital subtraction arthrography of the prosthetic hip. South. Med. J. 79:808–810, 1986.
4. Barmeir, E., Dubowitz, B., and Roffman, M.: Computed tomography in the assessment and planning of complicated total hip replacement. Acta Orthop. Scand. 53:597–604, 1982.
5. Bartel, D. L., Burstein, A. H., Santavicca, E. A., and Insall, J. N.: Performance of the tibial component in total knee replacement. J. Bone Joint Surg. 64A:1026–1033, 1982.
6. Bassett, L. W., Gold, R. H., and Hedley, A. K.: Radiology of failed surface-replacement total-hip arthroplasty. Am. J. Radiol. 139:1083–1088, 1982.
7. Beabout, J. W.: Radiology of total hip arthroplasty. Radiol. Clin. North Am. 13:3–19, 1975.
8. Becker, R. L., Norfray, J. F., Teitelbaum, G. P., et al.: MR imaging in patients with intracranial aneurysm clips. A.J.N.R. 9:885–889, 1988.
9. Bechtol, C. O.: Failure of femoral implant components in total hip replacement operations. Orthop. Rev. 4:23–29, 1974.
10. Beltran, J., Noto, A. M., Herman, L. J., and Lubbers, L. M.: Tendons: High field–strength, surface-coil MR imaging. Radiology 162:735–740, 1987.
11. Bergström, B., Lindberg, L., Persson, B. M., and Önnerfält, R.: Complications after total hip arthroplasty according to Charnley in a Swedish series of cases. Clin. Orthop. 95:91–95, 1973.
12. Berman, A. T., McGovern, K. M., Paret, R. S., and Tanicko, D. R.: The use of preoperative computed tomography scanning in total hip arthroplasty. Clin. Orthop. 222:190–196, 1987.
13. Brand, R. A., Pedersen, D. R., and Yoder, S. A.: How definition of "loosening" affects the incidence of loose total hip reconstructions. Clin. Orthop. 210:185–191, 1986.
14. Brand, R. A., Yoder, S. A., and Pedersen, D. R.: Interobserver variability in interpreting radiographic lucencies about total hip reconstructions. Clin. Orthop. 192:237–239, 1985.
15. Brooker, A. F., Bowerman, J. W., Robinson, R. A., and Riley, L. H.: Ectopic ossification following total hip replacement. Incidence and a method of classification. J. Bone Joint Surg. 55A:1629–1632, 1973.
16. Brown, I. W. and Ring, P. A.: Osteolytic changes in the upper femoral shaft following porous-coated hip replacement. J. Bone Joint Surg. 67B:218–221, 1985.
17. Buchli, R., Boesiger, P., and Meier D.: Heating effects of metallic implants by MRI examinations. Magn. Reson. Med. 7:255–261, 1988.
18. Burk, D. L. Jr., Karasick, D., Krutz, A. B., et al.: Rotator cuff tears: Prospective comparison of MR imaging with arthrography, sonography, and surgery. Am. J. Radiol. 153:87–92, 1989.
19. Calenoff, L. and Stromberg, W. B.: Silicone rubber arthroplasties of the hand. Radiology 107:29–34, 1973.
20. Chafetz, N., Hattner, R. S., Ruarke, W. C., et al.: Multinuclide digital subtraction imaging in symptomatic prosthetic joints. Am. J. Radiol. 144:1255–1258, 1985.
21. Christensen, R. A., Van Sonnenberg, E., Casola, G., and Wittich, G. R.: Interventional ultrasound in the musculoskeletal system. Radiol. Clin. North Am. 26:145–155, 1988.
22. Clayton, M. L., Ferlic, D. C., and Jeffers, P. D.:

Prosthetic arthroplasties of the shoulder. Clin. Orthop. 164:184–191, 1982.
23. Clayton, M. L. and Thirpathi, R.: Patellar complications after total condylar arthroplasty. Clin. Orthop. 170:152–155, 1982.
24. Cone, R. O., Taru, N., Resnick, D., et al.: Intracapsular pressure monitoring during arthrographic evaluation of painful hip prostheses. Am. J. Radiol. 141:885–889, 1983.
25. Datz, F. L. and Thorne, D. A.: Effect of antibiotic therapy on the sensitivity of indium-111–labeled leukocyte scans. J. Nucl. Med. 27:1849–1853, 1986.
26. Datz, F. L. and Thorne, D. A.: Effect of chronicity of infection on the sensitivity of the In-111–labeled leukocyte scan. Am. J. Radiol. 147:809–812, 1986.
27. DeLee, J. G. and Charnley, J.: Radiological demarcation of cemented sockets in total hip replacement. Clin. Orthop. 121:20–32, 1976.
28. Demottaz, J. D., Mazur, J. M., Thomas, W. H., et al.: Clinical study of total ankle replacement with gait analysis. A preliminary report. J. Bone Joint Surg. 61A:976–988, 1979.
29. Derkash, R. S., Niebauer, J. J., and Lane, C. S.: Long-term follow-up of metacarpal phalangeal arthroplasty with silicone Dacron prostheses. J. Hand Surg. 11A:553–558, 1986.
30. DeSmet, A. A., Kramer, D., and Martel, W.: The metal-cement interface in total hip prostheses. Am. J. Radiol. 129:279–282, 1977.
31. Dini, A. A. and Bassett III, F. H.: Evaluation of the early results of Smith total ankle replacement. Clin. Orthop. 146:228–230, 1980.
32. Dolinskas, C., Campbell, R. E., and Rothman, R. H.: The painful Charnley total hip replacement. Am. J. Radiol. 121:61–68, 1974.
33. Evancho, A. M., Stiles, R. G., Fajman, W. A., et al.: MR imaging diagnosis of rotator cuff tears. Am. J. Radiol. 151:751–754, 1988.
34. Ewald, F. C.: The Knee Society total knee arthroplasty roentgenographic evaluation and scoring system. Clin. Orthop. 248:9–12, 1989.
35. Ewald, F. C., Scheinberg, R. D., Poss, R., et al.: Capitellocondylar total elbow arthroplasty. J. Bone Joint Surg. 62A:1259–1263, 1980.
36. Fatti, J. F., Palmer, A. K., and Mosher, J. F.: The long-term results of Swanson silicone rubber interpositional wrist arthroplasty. J. Hand Surg. 11A:166–175, 1986.
37. Ferlic, D. C., Clayton, M. L., and Holloway, M.: Complications of silicone implant surgery in the metacarpophalangeal joint. J. Bone Joint Surg. 57A:991–994, 1975.
38. Fishman E. K., Magid, D., Robertson, D. D., et al.: Metallic hip implants: CT with multiplanar reconstruction. Radiology 160:675–681, 1986.
39. Fornage, B. D.: Soft-tissue changes in the hand in rheumatoid arthritis: Evaluation with US. Radiology 173:735–737, 1989.
40. Gillespy III, T., Manfrini, M., Ruggieri, P., et al.: Staging of intraosseous extent of osteosarcoma: Correlation of preoperative CT and MR imaging with pathologic macroslides. Radiology 167:765–767, 1988.
41. Goldberg, V. M., Figgie III, H. E., Inglis, A. E., and Figgie, M. P.: Current concepts review. Total elbow arthroplasty. J. Bone Joint Surg. 70A:778–783, 1988.
42. Goldring, S. R., Schiller, A. L., Roelke, M., et al.: The synovial-like membrane at the bone-cement interface in loose total hip replacements and its proposed role in bone lysis. J. Bone Joint Surg. 65A:575–584, 1983.
43. Griffiths, H. J., Burke, J., and Bonfiglio, T. A.: Granulomatous pseudotumors in total joint replacement. Skeletal Radiol. 16:146–152, 1987.
44. Griffiths, H. J., Lovelock, J. E., Evarts, C. M., and Geyer, D.: The radiology of total hip replacement. Skeletal Radiol. 12:1–11, 1984.
45. Gruen, T. A., McNeice, G. M., and Amstutz, H. C.: "Modes of failure" of cemented stem-type femoral components. A radiographic analysis of loosening. Clin. Orthop. 141:17–27, 1979.
46. Harcke, H. T., Grissom, L. E., and Finkelstein M. S.: Evaluation of the musculoskeletal system with sonography. Am. J. Radiol. 150:1253–1261, 1988.
47. Hedley, A. K., Gruen, T. A., and Ruoff, D. P.: Revision of failed total hip arthroplasties with uncemented porous-coated anatomic components. Clin. Orthop. 235:75–90, 1988.
48. Hendrix, R. W., Wixson, R. L., Rana, N. A., and Rogers, L. F.: Arthrography after total hip arthroplasty: A modified technique used in the diagnosis of pain. Radiology 148:647–652, 1983.
49. Herberts, P., Goldie, I. F., Körner, L., et al.: Endoprosthetic arthroplasty of the ankle joint. A clinical and radiological follow-up. Acta Orthop. Scand. 53:687–696, 1982.
50. Hofmann, A. A., Wyatt, R. W. B., Daniels, A. U., et al.: Bone scans after total knee arthroplasty in asymptomatic patients. Clin. Orthop. 251:183–188, 1990.
51. Holtås, S., Olsson, M., Romner, B., et al.: Comparison of MR imaging and CT in patients with intracranial aneurysm clips. A.J.N.R. 9:891–897, 1988.
52. Hunter, J. C., Baumrind, S., Genant, H. K., et al.: The detection of loosening in total hip arthroplasty: Description of a stereophotogrammetric computer assisted method. Invest. Radiol. 14:323–329, 1979.
53. Iida, H., Tamamuro, T., Okumura, H., et al.: Socket location in total hip replacement. Preoperative computed tomography and computer simulation. Acta Orthop. Scand. 59:1–5, 1988.
54. Inglis, A. E. and Pellicci, P. M.: Total elbow replacement. J. Bone Joint Surg. 62A:1252–1258, 1980.
55. Insall, J., Scott, N., and Ranawat, C. S.: The total condylar knee prosthesis. J. Bone Joint Surg. 61A:173–180, 1979.
56. Johnson, J. A., Christie, M. J., Sandler, M. P., et al.: Detection of occult infection following total joint arthroplasty using sequential technetium-99m HDP bone scintigraphy and indium-111 WBC imaging. J. Nucl. Med. 29:1347–1353, 1988.
57. Johnson, J. R., Getty, C. J. M., Lettin A. W. F., and Glasgow, M. M. S.: The Stanmore total elbow replacement for rheumatoid arthritis. J. Bone Joint Surg. 66B:732–736, 1984.
58. Johnston, R. C., Brand, R. A., and Crowninshield, R. D.: Reconstruction of the hip. A mathematical approach to determine optimum geometric relationships. J. Bone Joint Surg. 61A:639–652, 1979.

59. Johnston, R. C., Fitzgerald, R. H., Harris, W. H., et al.: Clinical and radiographic evaluation of total hip replacement. A standard system of terminology for reporting results. J. Bone Joint Surg. 72A:161–168, 1990.
60. Kalender, W. A., Hebel, R., and Ebersberger, J.: Reduction of CT artifacts caused by metallic implants. Radiology 164:576–577, 1987.
61. Kaplan, P. A., Montesi, S. A., Jardon, O. M., and Gregory, P. R.: Bone ingrowth hip prostheses in asymptomatic patients: Radiographic features. Radiology 169:221–227, 1988.
62. Kattapuram, S. V., Lodwick, G. S., Chandler, H., et al.: Porous-coated anatomic total hip prostheses: Radiographic analysis and clinical correlation. Radiology 174:861–864, 1990.
63. Kirkpatrick, J. S., Clarke, I. C., Amstutz, H. C., and Jinnah, R. H.: Radiographic techniques for consistent visualization of total hip arthroplasties. Clin. Orthop. 174:158–163, 1983.
64. Kneeland, J. B., Middleton, W. D., Carrera, G. F., et al.: MR imaging of the shoulder: Diagnosis of rotator cuff tears. Am. J. Radiol. 149:333–337, 1987.
65. Larsson, S., Larsson, S., and Lundkvist, S.: Unicompartmental knee arthroplasty. Clin. Orthop. 232:174–181, 1988.
66. Lovelock, J. E., Griffiths, H. J., Silverstein, A. M., and Anson, P. S.: Complications of total knee replacement. Am. J. Radiol. 141:985–992, 1984.
67. Magnuson, J. E., Brown, M. L., Hauser, H. E., et al.: In-111–labeled leukocyte scintigraphy in suspected orthopedic prosthesis infection: Comparison with other imaging modalities. Radiology 168:235–239, 1988.
68. Marcus, D. S., Reicher, M. A., and Kellerhouse, L. E.: Achilles tendon injuries: The role of MR imaging. J. Comput. Assist. Tomogr. 13:480–486, 1989.
69. McElfresh, E. C. and Coventry, M. B.: Femoral and pelvis fractures after total hip arthroplasty. J. Bone Joint Surg. 56A:483–492, 1974.
70. McElwain, J. P. and English, E.: The early results of porous-coated total shoulder arthroplasty. Clin. Orthop. 218:217–224, 1987.
71. Melson, G. L., McDaniel, R. C., Southern, P. M., and Staple, T. W.: *In vitro* effects of iodinated arthrographic contrast media on bacterial growth. Radiology 112:593–595, 1974.
72. Merkel, K. D., Brown, M. L., Dewanjee, M. K., and Fitzgerald, R. H.: Comparison of indium-labeled–leukocyte imaging with sequential technetium-gallium scanning in the diagnosis of low-grade musculoskeletal sepsis. A prospective study. J. Bone Joint Surg. 67A:465–475, 1985.
73. Mitchell, D. G., Rao, V. M., Dalinka, M. K., et al.: Femoral head avascular necrosis: Correlation of MR imaging, radiographic staging, radionuclide imaging, and clinical findings. Radiology 162:709–715, 1987.
74. Mjöberg, B., Hansson, L. I., and Selvik, G.: Instability, migration and laxity of total hip prostheses. A roentgen stereophotogrammetric study. Acta Orthop. Scand. 55:141–145, 1984.
75. New, P. F. J., Rosen, B. R., Brady, T. J., et al.: Potential hazards and artifacts of ferromagnetic and nonferromagnetic surgical and dental materials and devices in nuclear magnetic resonance imaging. Radiology 147:139–148, 1983.
76. Newberg, A. H. and Wetzner, S. M.: Digital subtraction arthrography. Radiology 154:238–239, 1985.
77. O'Neill, D. A. and Harris, W. H.: Failed total hip replacement: Assessment by plain radiographs, arthrograms, and aspiration of the hip joint. J. Bone Joint Surg. 66A:540–546, 1984.
78. Peimer, C. A.: Arthroplasty of the hand and wrist: Complications and failures. Instr. Course Lect. 38:15–30, 1989.
79. Peimer, C. A., Medige, J., Eckert, B. S., et al.: Original communications. Reactive synovitis after silicone arthroplasty. J. Hand Surg. 11A:624–638, 1986.
80. Phillips, W. C. and Kattapuram, S. V.: Prosthetic hip replacements: Plain films and arthrography for component loosening. Am. J. Radiol. 138:677–682, 1982.
81. Post, M.: Constrained arthroplasty of shoulder. Orthop. Clin. North Am. 18:455–462, 1987.
82. Pring, D. J., Henderson, R. G., Keshavarzian, A., et al.: Indium-granulocyte scanning in the painful prosthetic joint. Am. J. Radiol. 146:167–172, 1986.
83. Quinn, S. F., Murray, W. T., Clark, R. A., and Cochran, C. F.: Achilles tendon: MR imaging at 1.5 T. Radiology 164:767–770, 1987.
84. Reckling, F. W., Asher, M. A., and Dillon, W. L.: A longitudinal study of the radiolucent line at the bone-cement interface following total joint-replacement procedures. J. Bone Joint Surg. 59A:355–358, 1977.
85. Resnick, D., Derr, R., Andre, M., et al.: Digital arthrography in the evaluation of painful joint prostheses. Invest. Radiol. 19:432–437, 1984.
86. Resnik, C. S., Fratkin, M. J., and Cardea, J. A.: Arthroscintigraphic evaluation of the painful total hip prosthesis. Clin. Nucl. Med. 11:242–244, 1986.
87. Roberson, J. R. and Cohen, D.: Bipolar components for severe periacetabular bone loss around the failed total hip arthroplasty. Clin. Orthop. 251:113–118, 1990.
88. Robertson, D. D., Weiss, P. J., Fishman, E. K., et al.: Evaluation of CT techniques for reducing artifacts in the presence of metallic orthopedic implants. J. Comput. Assist. Tomogr. 12:236–241, 1988.
89. Rosenthal, D. I., Rosenberg, A. E., Schiller, A. L., and Smith, R. J.: Destructive arthritis due to silicone: A foreign-body reaction. Radiology 149:69–72, 1983.
90. Rosenthall, L., Lisbona, R., Hernandez, M., and Hadjipavlou, A.: ^{99m}Tc-PP and ^{67}Ga imaging following insertion of orthopedic devices. Radiology 133:717–721, 1979.
91. Rozing, P. M., Bohne, W. H., and Insall, J.: Bone scanning for the evaluation of knee prosthesis. Acta Orthop. Scand. 53:291–294, 1982.
92. Rydholm, U., Tjörnstrand, B., Pettersson, H., and Lidgren, L.: Surface replacement of the elbow in rheumatoid arthritis. Early results with the Wadsworth prosthesis. J. Bone Joint Surg. 66B:737–741, 1984.
93. Salvati, E. A., Wilson, P. D., Jr., Jolley, M. N.,

et al.: A ten-year follow-up study of our first one hundred consecutive Charnley total hip replacements. J. Bone Joint Surg. 63A:753–767, 1981.
94. Schmidt, R. M. and Rosenkranz, H. S.: Antimicrobial activity of local anesthetics lidocaine and procaine. J. Infect. Dis. 121:597–607, 1970.
95. Schneider, R., Freiberger, R. H., Ghelman, B., and Ranawat, C. S.: Radiologic evaluation of painful joint prostheses. Clin. Orthop. 170:156–168, 1982.
96. Schneider, R., Hood, R. W., and Ranawat, C. S.: Radiologic evaluation of knee arthroplasty. Orthop. Clin. North Am. 13:225–244, 1982.
97. Schneider, R. and Soudry, M.: Radiographic and scintigraphic evaluation of total knee arthroplasty. Clin. Orthop. 205:108–120, 1986.
98. Scott, S. M., Manaster, B. J., Alazraki, N., et al.: Technetium-99m imaging of bone trauma: Reduced sensitivity caused by hydrocortisone in rabbits. Am. J. Radiol. 148:1175–1178, 1987.
99. Steinbach, L. S., Schneider, R., Goldman, A. B., et al.: Bursae and abscess cavities communicating with the hip. Diagnosis using arthrography and CT. Radiology 156:303–307, 1985.
100. Sutherland, C. J., Wilde, A. H., Borden L. S., and Marks, K. E.: A ten-year follow-up of one hundred consecutive Müller curved-stem total hip-replacement arthroplasties. J. Bone Joint Surg. 64A:970–982, 1982.
101. Tanaka, T., Rossier, A. V., and Hussey, R. W.: Quantitative assessment of para-osteoarthropathy and its maturation on serial radionuclide bone images. Radiology 123:217–221, 1977.
102. Tehranzadeh, J., Schneider, R., and Freiberger, R. H.: Radiological evaluation of painful total hip replacement. Radiology 141:355–362, 1981.
103. Telaranta, T., Solonen, K. A., Tallroth, K., and Nickels, J.: Bone cysts containing silicone particles in bones adjacent to a carpal Silastic implant. Skeletal Radiolol. 10:247–249, 1983.
104. Torisu, T. and Morita, H.: Roentgenographic evaluation of geometric total knee arthroplasty with a six-year average follow-up period. Clin. Orthop. 202:125–134, 1986.
105. Uri, G., Wellman, H., Capello, W., et al.: Scintigraphic and x-ray arthrographic diagnosis of femoral prosthesis loosening: Concise communication. J. Nucl. Med. 25:661–663, 1984.
106. Vincent, L. M.: Ultrasound of soft tissue abnormalities of the extremities. Radiol. Clin. North Am. 26:131–144, 1988.
107. Volz, R. G.: Total wrist arthroplasty. A new approach to wrist disability. Clin. Orthop. 128:180–189, 1977.
108. Weissman, B. N.: The radiology of total joint replacement. Orthop. Clin. North Am. 14:171–191, 1983.
109. Weissman, B. N. and Sledge, C. B.: Orthopedic Radiology. Philadelphia, W. B. Saunders, 1986.
110. Yoder, S. A., Brand, R. A., Pedersen, D. R., and O'Gorman, T. W.: Total hip acetabular component position affects component loosening rates. Clin. Orthop. 228:79–87, 1988.
111. Zlatkin, M. B., Iannotti, J. P., Roberts, M. C., et al.: Diagnostic performance of MR imaging. Radiology 172:223–229, 1989.
112. Zwas, S. T., Elkanovitch, R., and Frank, G.: Interpretation and classification of bone scintigraphic findings in stress fractures. J. Nucl. Med. 28:452–457, 1987.

SECTION V

HISTOLOGIC AND PATHOLOGIC CONSIDERATIONS

CHAPTER 12

Histology and Pathology of Total Joint Replacement

SUZANNE SPANIER

Materials for prosthetic replacements are selected for biocompatibility, but they are nonetheless foreign to the body. Their introduction always results in some type of response, which may range from acceptance by the local tissues to necrosis of the tissues or rejection of the foreign material. Wear debris derived from the articulating interfaces elicits a host reaction, which varies both in kind and degree. This wear debris, per se, as well as the tissue response, may contribute to implant failure. Knowledge of what happens when a prosthesis fails is vital if the goal of a durable, trouble-free joint replacement is to be achieved. This chapter explores pathologic alterations beginning with what happens when foreign bodies are introduced into the tissues. Histologic responses to various materials and types of joint replacement components are also described.

TISSUE RESPONSES TO FOREIGN BODIES

In 1959, Cohen[18] pointed out that "inertness is relative" and that even materials considered chemically inert may provoke appreciable tissue reaction. The type and extent of the tissue responses are influenced by certain characteristics of the implant material. The most important of these are particle size and chemical composition. The size or surface area of a given material may determine not only whether it is biologically inert or gives rise to a major tissue response but also what type of cellular response will occur.[18, 34, 46]

For example, large, intact pieces of high molecular weight polyethylene typically will become encased in a layer of fibrous tissue, which sequesters it from surrounding tissues. However, the finely divided products of polyethylene wear are among the most provocative stimulants of a granulomatous response.[82, 84] Large flakes of up to 1 mm are rimmed by a syncytium of foreign body giant cells. As the fragments of polyethylene become smaller, they are engulfed by single, multinucleated giant cells. Very small particles of less than 1 to 2 μm, as well as fine, 2 to 5 μm splinters and fibrils of up to 40 μm, generally elicit a mononuclear histiocytic response. The histiocyte cytoplasm becomes acidophilic and granular. With polarized light, tiny particles of birefringent polyethylene can be seen (Fig. 12–1).[34, 82] At the ultrastructural level, this material is shown to accumulate within lysosomes.[12]

The biologic effects of metals are based on their chemical composition and particle size.[12, 18] Implant surfaces are subjected to degradation by mechanical wear and may also be corroded by ionizing salts in body fluids. The complex corrosion products are then shed. Microscopic examination of the gray and blackened tissue around metallic

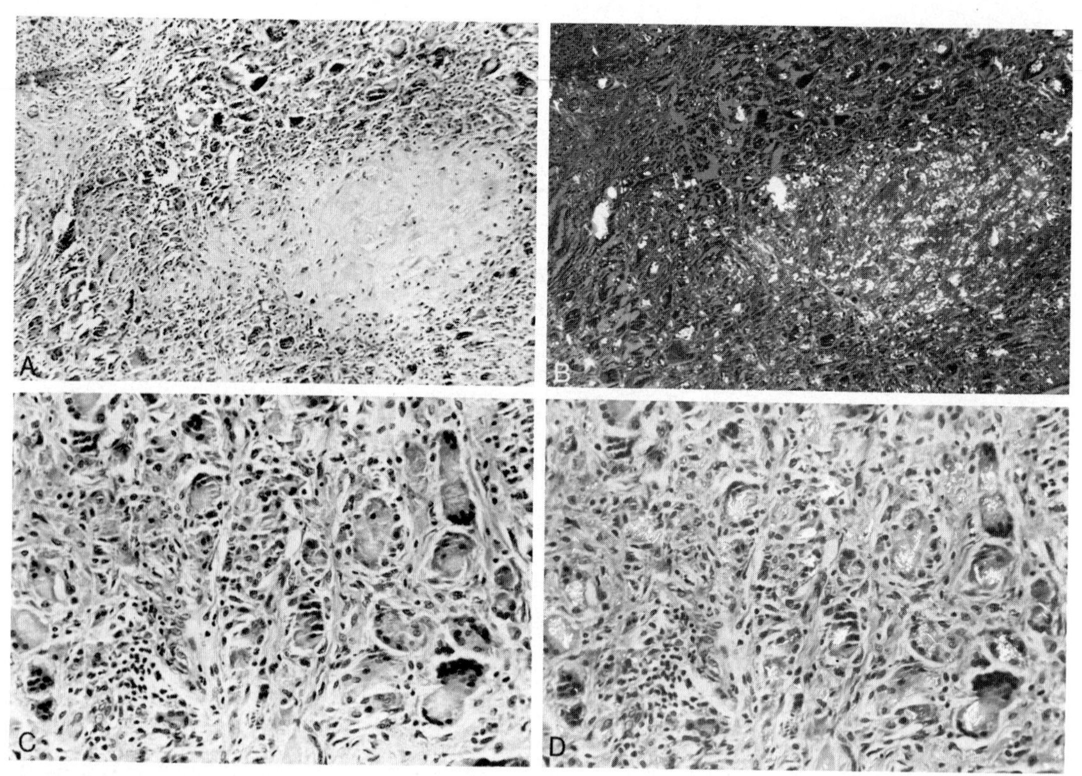

FIGURE 12–1. Florid granulomatous synovitis secondary to polyethylene debris from failed total knee replacement. *A*, The synovium is filled with mononuclear and multinucleated histiocytes. Just to the right of center is an area of necrosis (100×). *B*, Polarized light reveals large amounts of brightly birefringent polyethylene concentrated in the necrotic tissues. In the center and to the left, larger fragments of polyethylene can be seen. *C*, A higher power view of the tissue from about the edge of the necrotic area reveals a sea of mononuclear and multinucleated histiocytes with a ragged appearance. The few small, round, dark nuclei in the bottom left corner are lymphocytes (450×). *D*, With polarized light the frayed appearance of the giant cells is caused by the packing of cytoplasm with polyethylene debris. Smaller particles can also be found within the mononuclear cell cytoplasm (450×).

implants reveals small spheres, irregular fragments, and metallic debris splinters measuring 1 to 4 μm. These particles are seen within mononuclear histiocytes or in the extracellular fibrous matrix. Ultrastructural studies demonstrate that most of the engulfed metal particles are in phagolysosomes and many are less than 0.5 μm in diameter, which is below the resolution of light microscopy.[12] Although metals are not birefringent, their detection in tissues is aided by polarized light because of diffraction at the edge of the particle.[1, 12, 82]

In addition to their effects on the host tissues, metallic salts and ions formed by corrosion can influence the integrity of other prosthetic components. For example, vanadium significantly accelerates the chemical degradation of polyethylene.[12] A less common effect is interaction with proteins to induce an immunologic or a hypersensitivity response.[12, 38, 61]

The acrylic cement often used to bond both the polyethylene and the metallic components to the underlying bone is formed when the liquid monomer is mixed with 10- to 30-μm spherules of polymethyl methacrylate (PMMA). Although numerous noxious effects have been attributed to the monomeric form,[12, 41, 88–91] it is the polymerized form that is of the greatest importance in foreign body tissue reactions. Because PMMA is soluble in the xylene routinely employed to process histologic sections, its location in the tissues must be determined by other means. The 1- to 2-μm barium sulfate particles that are added to give opacity to the radiolucent cement do survive the processing, and they mark the otherwise optically clear spaces as the previous location of the cement. These spaces, often referred to as "pearls," may be circular and similar in size to the spherules, or they may occur as aggregates of 100 μm to 1 mm or more.

When the acrylic cement abuts soft tissues, it is usually surrounded by one or more layers of multinucleate giant cells or fibroblasts or a thin pseudomembrane forms as the advancing edge of the cement compresses the marrow elements.[15, 34, 82, 96] Charnley[15, 17] was the first to describe that the profile that the cement surface imprints on a tissue in contact with the surface of the cured acrylic has an irregular convex contour caused by protrusion of the polymer spherules. This effect explains the characteristic scalloped outline of concavities in the soft tissues in contact with the cement.

SUCCESSFUL CEMENTED TOTAL JOINT REPLACEMENT

Repair Process

If all or most of the joint capsule is removed during arthroplasty, a new capsule develops in the wound bed about the prosthesis. After a time, the joint surface of this new capsule acquires the appearance and function of synovium.

Although the capsular tissues about an implant may share many of the characteristics of the interface membrane (to be discussed), the two should not be confused.

One of the most important of synovial-type functions is the removal of foreign materials. Wear debris accumulating within the joint cavity mixes with a fibrinous exudate or is ingested by macrophages and incorporated into the capsule. Once in the capsule, the debris particles may stimulate further histiocytic reaction, necrosis, formation of granulation tissue, and fibrosis. As with normal synovium, particles may be carried from the joint by the lymphatics to distant sites, particularly the regional lymph nodes.[12, 52, 109] Polyethylene debris has even been found in the alveolar lining of the lung.[12]

A consistent histologic finding following implantation of acrylic dough is a rim of necrosis extending 0.5 to 5 mm from the cement surface into the adjacent bone and marrow.[12, 15, 107] The distribution and constancy of this zone suggested to early investigators that it was caused by a combination of reaming, heat generated by polymerization of the cement, and monomer toxicity.[3, 15, 107] Further studies suggest that neither the local concentration of monomer[46, 66] nor the heat of polymerization[7, 46, 60, 78] is likely to be great enough to contribute to the necrosis. However, surgical interference with the vascular supply is a likely cause.[60]

The repair process begins postoperatively with a nonspecific inflammatory phase, consisting of reactive hyperemia and exudation of inflammatory cells. This phase is followed by invasion of granulation tissue, accompanied by macrophages, osteoclasts, and osteoblasts. Within the first few weeks, repair of the necrotic bone occurs by apposition of living bone onto necrotic bone (buttressing), creeping substitution, and replacement by metaplastic bone and fibrocartilage. Stability and load transmission between the cement and underlying bone are achieved by ossification of the deeper layers of metaplastic fibrocartilage that develop in the tissues at the bone-host interface as well as bridging adjacent trabeculae.[15, 34] After about 2 years, a period of stabilization ensues and any further repair proceeds at a considerably slower rate.

By about 5 years, remnants of dead bone are covered by a layer of lamellar bone. Some fibrocartilage appears to be replaced by lamellar bone. Trabeculae initially orientated perpendicularly to the cement surface may remodel to a parallel orientation.[34] Any soft tissue between bone and cement persists as discontinuous foci varying from layers of delicate areolar tissue up to 300 μm thick to narrow layers of dense fibrous tissue up to 20 μm.[15] The number of foreign body giant cells on the surface of fibrous tissue in contact with cement is diminished. Charnley[15] observed that the metaplastic fibrocartilage in direct contact with the cement was molded to the contour of the acrylic spheres. Because polarized light revealed that it was structurally similar to bone, Charnley believed that this fibrocartilage was mechanically effective for weight transmission.

Long-Term Bone-Cement Interface in Total Hip Replacement

The histologic appearance of the successful permanent implant bed was a matter of controversy for almost two decades. Many investigators, on the basis of clinically nonloose surgical specimens, held that a fibrous membrane of variable thickness was in immediate contact with the cement everywhere, separating it from the living host tissues.[12, 53, 107] Charnley's studies did not support this observation. He stated: "The discouraging histology illustrated in the literature probably results from the specimens having been derived from secondary operations on replacements already in failure or from cadaveric material from senile patients with sparse clinical and radiologic records to supplement the study."[17]

Comparison with long-term successful implants forms the basis for recognizing and assessing failed implants. It is therefore crucial that only specimens obtained postmortem from those with long-term, successful clinical results be included in an analysis. The largest series of such cases is that of Charnley,[17] who studied 41 femoral shafts and 26 acetabula from low friction arthroplasties an average 7.3 years (range, 5 to 11.75 years) after operation. Of these, 13 specimens were of implants with over 9 years of success.

In the 41 "perfect" femoral shaft specimens radiographic signs suggesting demarcation between cement and bone were rarely seen, and all prostheses were solidly anchored.

No thick, continuous layer of fibrous tissue separated the cement from the cancellous bone. Instead, any fibrous tissue lining the medullary cavity was fine, delicate, and discontinuous. No tissue of any kind intervened between the cement surface and the "caps of changed bone," and the cement at these sites appeared to be completely accepted by the host tissue. "Caps" were described as pale pink zones of fibrous tissue on the end of a trabecula, which were less cellular than the underlying bone. The shape and distribution of the cells were reminiscent of chondrocytes, and in polarized light their collagen lamellae were continuous with those of the underlying bone. Charnley referred to these caps as "changed bone," "de-mineralized bone," or "fibrocartilage" in his later works.[17] I believe that these caps are identical to or are derived from fibrocartilage, as depicted and described in his earlier studies.[15] Charnley believed that these capped trabeculae were the sites of load transmission to the underlying bone—even though only six to 20 capped trabeculae might be found in a complete transverse section of the shaft.[17]

The scalloped impressions produced on the endosteal surface by spherules of the cured cement were clear and free of debris. From these impressions, Charnley deduced that no relative motion had occurred at the interface during cyclic loading and unloading. Nonweightbearing intertrabecular marrow in contact with the cement was usually separated from it by an extremely thin membrane. When a layer of fibrocytes could be distinguished, it was only two to three cells thick. Thicker layers of fibrocytes were associated with the impressions of cement spherules. A layer of inactive-appearing macrophages, foreign body giant cells, or both lined the surface in contact with the cement. Fat and hematopoietic marrow only a short distance from the cement surface were healthy. No evidence was seen of macrophage reactions progressing to caseous necrosis. Charnley attributed these findings in successful femoral diaphyses to sound mechanical fixation resulting from a good cementing technique.[17]

Unlike the femoral shaft samples, which rarely demonstrated radiographic signs of demarcation, about 60 percent of the "perfect" acetabular specimens demonstrated demarcation of the bone-cement interfaces. The acetabular component was easily ruptured in 50 percent of cases and was frankly loose in two of the 26 samples.[17] In none of the 26 acetabular sockets was direct contact seen between cement and bone. The tissue lining the acetabulum adjacent to the cement frequently was covered with a layer of amorphous, caseous debris containing particles of polyethylene.

In most acetabular specimens, a 0.5 to 1.5-mm thick band of fibrous tissue, oriented parallel to the bone surface, interrupted the cement-bone interface. In some instances, layers of histiocytes were trapped within the fibrous tissue. Well-differentiated cartilaginous tissue, often resembling hyaline cartilage, sometimes developed in the fibrous layer at the bone-cement interface. Cartilage in these zones bore the scalloped imprint of the cement spherules. The histologic appearance of the acetabular interface led Charnley to urge more sophisticated methods of handling cement in the acetabulum. He was able to balance the discomforting histologic picture with the observation that the scalloped outline of the cartilage indicated contact with the cement. Charnley concluded: "The cartilage zone obviously transmitted load directly to the underlying bone."[17]

These observations were independently confirmed by Eftekhar and colleagues.[34] Linder and Hansson's[67] ultrastructural study of femoral-cement interfaces corroborated close contact between living bone and cement. In that study the cement was always separated from the bone by a thin layer of uncalcified proteoglycans, probably corresponding to Charnley's bone caps.[15, 17, 67] Macrophages found in the soft tissue adjacent to the cement contained little or no phagocytized material within their lysosomes. The macrophages were separated from the cement by a proteoglycan layer and gave no sign of resorptive activity.[67] These findings suggest that macrophages are not necessarily associated with bone resorption.

LOOSE CEMENTED TOTAL JOINT REPLACEMENT

The usual cause of failure of cemented implants is aseptic loosening of the components.[12, 45–47, 56, 68] Loosening has been attributed to such things as prosthetic design; defective materials[98]; malalignment and malpositioning; surgical preparation of the bone[3, 80, 96]; cementing technique[17, 53]; tissue reaction to the procedure,[15, 34, 96] to the cement,[15, 17, 34] or to the products of wear debris[12, 34, 46, 47, 72, 82, 109]; hypersensitivity reaction to metal[10, 26, 38, 61]; proteolytic enzymes in the interface membrane[34, 45, 47, 68]; and toxicity to the metals or trapped monomer.[61] Although the precise etiology is still unknown, research focusing on the formation and function of the interface membrane implicates mechanical instability, micromotion, or both as the important etiologic factors in most instances.

Whatever the reason for failure, a final common result is the formation of a fibrous membrane up to several millimeters thick. The membrane separates bone from the cement-prosthesis complex and causes loss of fixation.[12, 45, 47, 68] Eftekhar and colleagues[34] coined the term "prosthetic synovitis" to refer to the development of reactive changes resulting from formation of the synovial-like membrane at the interface of a noninfected, failed, cemented hip prosthesis.

Histologically, four features are consistently present to variable degrees: fibrosis, histiocytosis, necrosis, and particulate foreign body debris.[12, 34, 68] Fibrosis is usually most prominent on the osseous side of the membrane,[12, 45] but it may also occur as a middle layer.[68] The prevalent cells are acidophilic mononuclear histiocytes, which tend to accumulate adjacent to the cement surface. They may appear as sheets phagocytizing bits of polyethylene or as palisades resembling synovium.[45, 46] Phagocytic foreign body giant cells are also abundant, and they may be seen surrounding acrylic spherules and particles of polyethylene.[45, 46] Chronic inflammatory cells are uncommon in this membrane, and neutrophils are rare. Necrosis may occur throughout the membrane or may be confined to the surface next to the cement. In addition, PMMA, polyethylene, or metal debris is almost always present.[12, 34, 68] Whether occurring as spherules or large fragments, acrylic cement always seems to be associated with giant cells.[34]

Charnley and his associates were the first to recognize that acrylic cement elicits a macrophage reaction. It evokes histiocytes in nonweightbearing areas, such as areas where soft tissues bridge intertrabecular spaces. Although Charnley[17] expressed concern that their presence might portend eventual failure of fixation, he also observed that under some circumstances the histiocytes appeared to be inactive. Independently performed histochemical analyses have confirmed that histiocytes are not uniformly active. Rather, they exhibit foci of activity. Their activity is associated with phagocytized wear products and is especially pronounced in cells with phagocytized PMMA or high-density polyethylene. Connective tissue cells walling off large fragments of PMMA do not have increased activity.[34, 45, 47, 68] This membrane has also been shown to contain high levels of prostaglandin E_2, especially with uncemented, loose components.[45, 47] These studies provide strong evidence that wear products can induce lysosomal and proteolytic activity within the histiocyte population. Either the macrophages do not respond uniformly or constantly to the presence of prosthetic debris or periods of quiescence occur. Linder and associates[68] found that living, rather than dead, bone was resorbed by the membrane, and new bone was formed in these same areas. This finding was interpreted as the body's attempt to stabilize an unstable prosthesis with new bone, which fails because of implant movement.

Goldring and coworkers[45] demonstrated a number of synovial-like properties in membranes obtained from clinically loose prostheses reminiscent of the familiar synovial-like bursae over bony points subjected to the motion of overlying tendons. The implication that motion is required for the development of synovial tissue is supported by the observation of Drachman and Sokoloff,[31] regarding the absence of joint cavitation in the paralyzed limbs of chick embryos. This suggested that the presence of a bursa-like membrane over a long time might create a communication between the joint cavity and the bone-cement interface, allowing wear products to travel long distances from the joint. In this scheme, mechanical instability leading to micromotion is the initiating event, and ensuing wear products continue or accelerate the loosening process.

Based on clinical, radiologic, and histologic observations, Eftekhar and colleagues[34] advanced the theory that the first step in loosening is micromotion between cement and bone due to failure of cement fixation. Surgical removal of the weightbearing subchondral plate of the acetabulum causes loss of stiffness in the bone. This effect results in fatigue of the exposed trabeculae and micromotion at the bone-cement interface. The necrotic bone is replaced by a fibrous membrane, which may or may not develop into a strong, fibrocartilaginous, weightbearing structure. If it does not, further motion breaks down the cement creating more micromotion. In the attempt to degrade particles of PMMA and polyethylene, macrophages increase in number, and quiescent ones may become activated. The activated macrophages release proteolytic enzymes and prostaglandin E_2, stimulating bone lysis and further undermining the bone support. More instability and more motion ensue in a self-perpetuating cycle that eventually results in destruction of the joint.

This theory is supported by Hedley and associates.[53] They reported a relationship between osteoclastic removal of trabecular bone and membrane thickness that, in turn, was related to the adequacy of cement fixation. Their data suggest that motion caused by mechanical instability of the implant provokes osteoclastic activity within the fibrous membrane and leads to further bone loss and motion.

OSTEOLYSIS FOLLOWING TOTAL JOINT ARTHROPLASTY

In 1975, Charnley reported peculiar radiographic abnormalities resembling infection in six noninfected patients following total hip replacements. Three patients with fractured femoral components had radiographs showing cavities that invaded cortical bone from the endosteal surface, and the other three had localized cavities at points in contact with cement but no evidence of mechanical failure. In the patients with fractures, the caseous debris was dominated by giant cells that were attributed to the movement of acrylic cement on bone. In the mechanically sound group, the predominant finding was accumulations of foamy histiocytes, similar to those seen in the tissues adjacent to the Judet prosthesis, which were filled with submicroscopic particles of acrylic. Charnley[16] attributed the diverse histologic appearances to the difference in PMMA particle size.

In 1976, Harris and coworkers[49] reported four similar cases of extensive bone resorption associated with loose femoral components. The histologic picture featured sheets of mononuclear histiocytes, a few giant cells, and a plethora of birefringent particulate matter. Neither acute nor chronic inflammatory cells were present. These investigators speculated that the lysis was caused by loosening and fragmentation of the methacrylate. All four patients underwent revision arthroplasties with good results.

As further reports accumulated, the disorder appeared to be a disease of cement, as the common link was failure of fixation and fragmentation of the cement surface.[45, 49, 68, 72, 86] Hence, the osteolysis was attributed to highly localized stresses; micromotion between cement and bone[16, 34, 49, 68, 72]; abrasion particles from the artificial joint surfaces[86]; and fragmentation of cement.[40, 49, 59]

In 1986, extensive osteolysis was reported in four patients with rigidly fixed implants. These cases displayed a similar histologic pattern: aggressive infiltration of the marrow and cortical destruction by histiocytes and foreign body giant cells containing traces of barium.[59] This report raised the possibility that invasive macrophage-mediated reactions to acrylic cement could occur without loosening. Further reports have indicated that cement may not be a prerequisite to the development of this mysterious disorder.[54] Lombardi and coworkers[70] reported osteolysis in two patients with nonionimplanted titanium alloy modular femoral heads. Cement was not used in one of these cases, and the cause was believed to be metallic debris from wear of the femoral head. Both patients had a dense, fibrous, blackened membrane containing metallic fragments and histiocytes filled with metallic debris.

Several features distinguish osteolysis from the usual loose prosthesis. Although typical loosening affects men and women about equally, Huddleston[54] found a 4:1 preponderance of osteolysis in men. The time to onset is variable, but an interval of 5 to 15 years after joint replacement is frequent.

The proximal femur is by far the most common site of osteolysis, followed by the acetabulum. The proximal tibia has also been affected.[48] In patients who have had bilateral total hip replacements, both hips can be affected, but usually only one is.[48, 54, 59] Most patients, but not all, experience increasing pain and have radiographic evidence of typical loosening prior to the onset of osteolysis.[48, 59, 86] In Huddleston's series of 51 patients, 26 percent had associated acetabular loosening.

The clinical progression is usually torpid, but it can be alarmingly rapid. Bone destruction may be massive. Pathologic fracture of the bone is not infrequent. Once initiated, the process is inexorable and always culminates in loosening of the implant.[54] Therefore, as soon as the diagnosis is made, most surgeons proceed with revision to take advantage of sufficient remaining bone stock.

The radiographic pattern marking the onset of osteolysis is characterized by the appearance of one or more localized, discrete, oval or rounded "cookie-cutter" lucencies on the endosteal side of the bone-cement or bone-metal surface. The radiolucencies frequently begin at sites where metal abuts bone or where cement is deficient or fractured.[57] The calcar and medial aspects of the stem are favored sites. Multiple, independent lucencies may appear almost simultaneously about the perimeter of the implant and then coalesce into large areas of endosteal destruction. The cortex may be completely destroyed, with only a thin subperiosteal layer of bone remaining. Periosteal elevation and bulging and intraosseous extension far beyond the implant have been described by Pazzaglia and Byers,[86] but penetration of the periosteum has not been reported.[54] In this process, both bone and cement are actually destroyed.[48, 54]

Although most specimens contain membranous tissue grossly indistinguishable from the thick fibrous tissue typically found between cement and bone in loose arthroplasties, many of the larger areas of destruction are filled with a dry, yellow, pultaceous or caseous material.[54] The histologic picture has no distinguishing features. It consists of uniform fields and sheets of mononuclear histiocytes, variable numbers of giant cells, and different sized particles of foreign debris. Osteolysis differs from conventional loosening only because of the aggressive destruction of bone and infiltration of the marrow spaces.[48, 49, 54, 68, 70] The pathologist would be unlikely to make the correct diagnosis based solely on the tissue examination, without radiographs and knowledge of the clinical course.

We have seen three patients with radiographic features similar to those of lysis (Figs. 12–2, 12–3, and 12–4). However, two patients had no radiographic evidence of loosening, and no loosening was found in the one patient who underwent surgery.

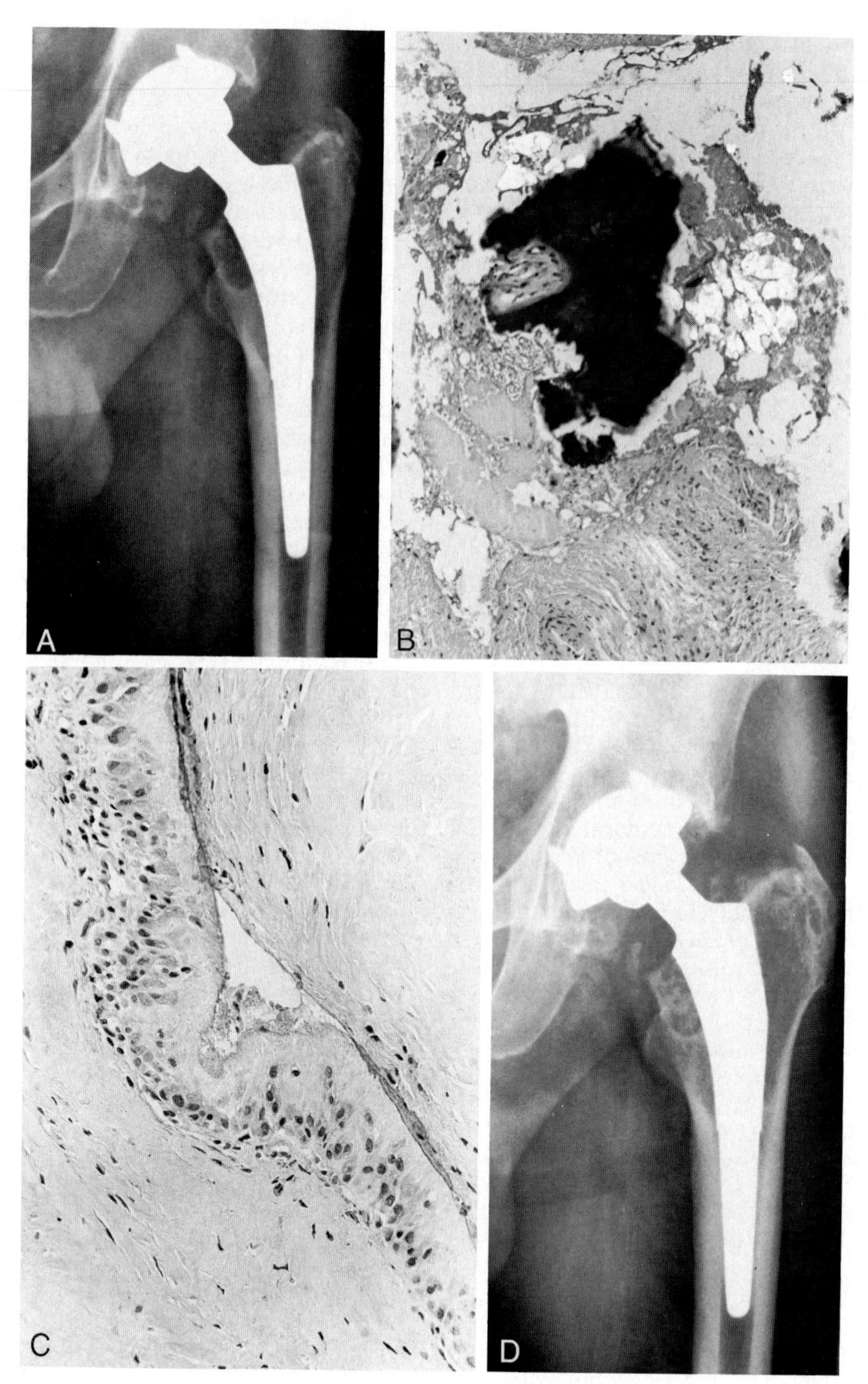

FIGURE 12–2 *See legend on opposite page*

Neither patient had pain. Cement was not used in either case. The metallic composition of the acetabular and femoral components differed: titanium in one case and cobalt-chromium alloy in the other. The third case is unusual because of the presence of a carbon-fiber cup (see Fig. 12–4). The common denominator in these three cases was polyethylene.

POROUS INGROWTH PROSTHESES

For some patients, many surgeons have abandoned the use of acrylic cement in favor of other methods of fixation. One of the newer methods of fixation is coating of the implant surface with metal particles of various diameters or with wire mesh.[43, 62] The increased porosity is expected to allow ingrowth of bone, thus providing a more biologic fixation than cement. Although ingrowth has been demonstrated in dogs[50, 99] and the short-term clinical results have been favorable,[36, 37, 56, 62] long-term clinical performance is unknown.[50] The extent to which bone ingrowth actually occurs and its relation to clinical success are still unsettled issues. Moreover, inconsistencies between radiographic and anatomic observations are troublesome.

Engh and colleagues[37] examined 11 uncemented femoral stems made of cast cobalt-chromium alloy and coated with a powder-made, sintered porous surface. The implants were retrieved 4 weeks to 7 years after insertion (average 28 months). Ten protheses were recovered at autopsy, and one at revision due to failure of the acetabular component. Bone ingrowth was seen in nine of the 11 stems and fibrous ingrowth in two. Histologically, the bone ingrowth did not occur uniformly over the entire coated surface. Rather it arose from regions where the implant was either in contact or close to the endosteum, and the bone ingrowth formed discrete bridges between the porous coating and the endosteum. Ingrowth went deeply into the coating, sometimes all the way to the substrate. Mild cortical osteoporosis, believed to be caused by stress shielding, was noted in a few cases and seemingly was related to large stem size and rigidity.[36] The corresponding radiographs demonstrated new endosteal bone with an increase in density at points of contact with the prosthesis, as well as osteopenia in areas most distant from the stem. In the two cases in which bone ingrowth did not occur, a prominent radiopaque line was seen around most of the implant length. Histologically, this corresponded to a thin shell of bone around the implant surface that was separated by a layer of fibrous tissue.

Cook and associates[20] performed histologic and microradiographic analyses on 90 noncemented, porous-coated total joint implants recovered from 58 patients treated at a number of institutions. The ten types of implants were from several different manufacturers. The 62 total knee components were retrieved 2 weeks to 31

FIGURE 12–2. Proximal femoral osteolysis associated with cementless total hip arthroplasty. A 71-year-old man with severe osteoarthritis had total hip replacement with a cementless titanium alloy stem and an acetabular cup with nonremovable polyethylene liner. Routine follow-up radiographs after 36 months of a clinically successful result revealed an area of radiolucency in the medial cortex that had not been present on previous examinations. Radiographs 4 months later showed slight enlargement of the radiolucency, and biopsy was advised. *A*, Plain anteroposterior radiograph 43 months after implantation shows well-placed components with excellent apposition of bone and remodeling of bone in relation to the titanium acetabular shell. No evidence of loosening exists. An area of localized destruction appears in the proximal medial femoral neck. *B*, At surgery, no evidence existed of loosening, capsular tissue discoloration, or gross abnormalities of the polyethylene liner. A cavity, filled with soft, gray-white, caseous, amorphous, fibrous material was encountered. It extended distally approximately 1.5 to 2 cm and around the circumference of the medial femur approximately 40 percent. This material was curetted, and the defect was packed with autogenous iliac crest bone graft. Histologic examination of the curetted specimen revealed extensive necrosis with occasional foci of mononuclear histiocytes. Despite the excellent appearance of the polyethylene liner, polyethylene debris was found by examination of the tissues with polarized light. Just below and to the right of the black bone fragment in the center of the field are large birefringent flakes of polyethylene (250 ×). *C*, A synovial-like lining was present focally, overlying dense fibrous and necrotic tissue (450 ×). *D*, At 3 months postgrafting, early consolidation of the graft occurred.

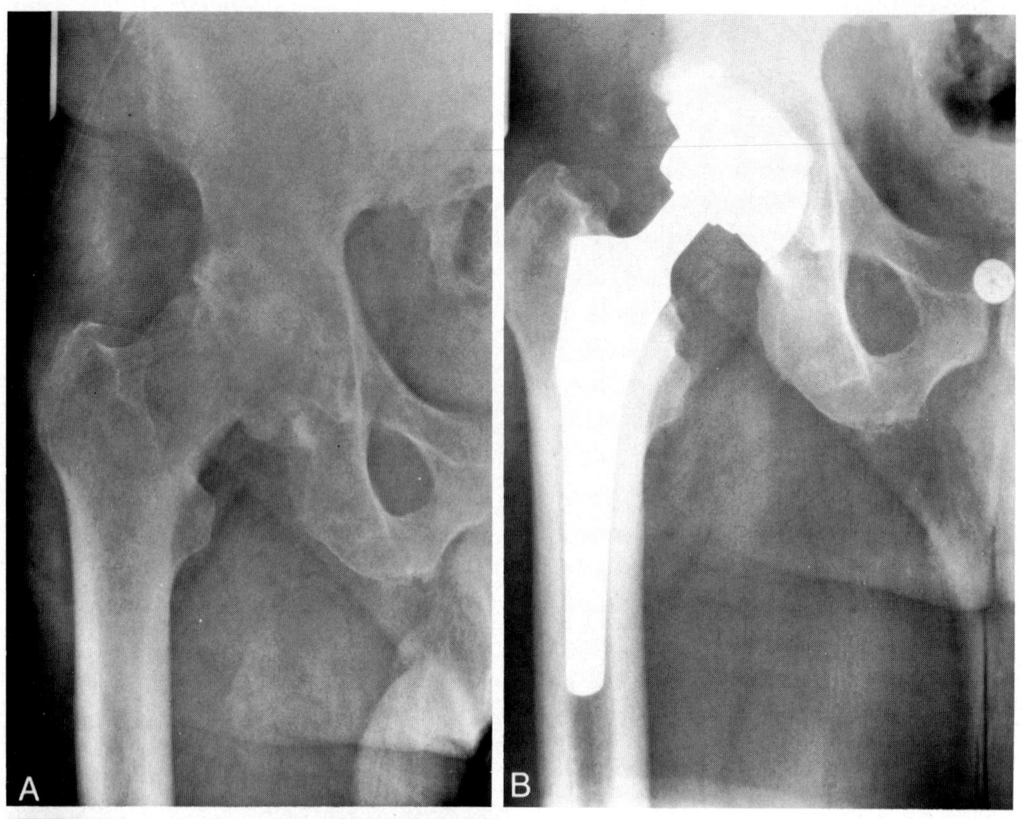

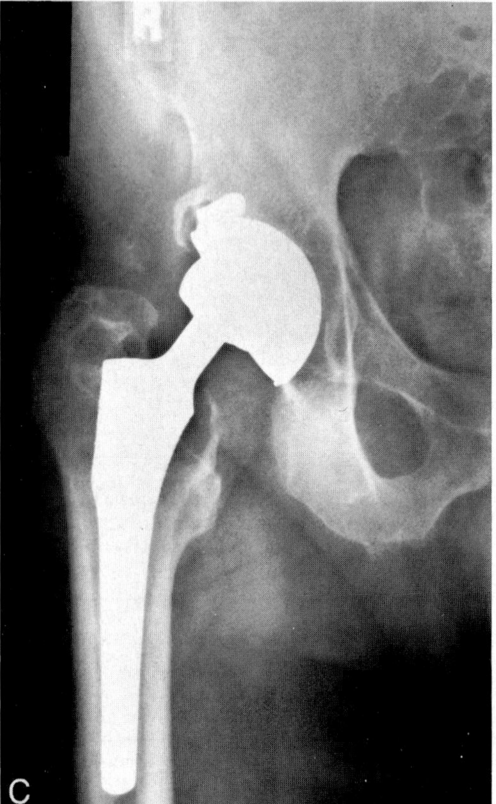

FIGURE 12–3. Proximal femoral lysis with cementless porous coated cobalt-chromium alloy prosthesis. *A*, The preoperative radiograph of a 73-year-old man with severe osteoarthritis shows loss of articular cartilage and osteophyte formation. *B*, Total hip arthroplasty was performed using cementless porous coated cobalt-chromium alloy stem and an acetabular shell with polyethylene liner. This radiograph taken 3 months postoperatively shows the prosthesis in satisfactory alignment with good bone stock. *C*, Radiograph taken 5 years and 4 months after replacement shows a large area of geographic destruction involving the medial femoral neck. The patient remains asymptomatic and has refused further surgery.

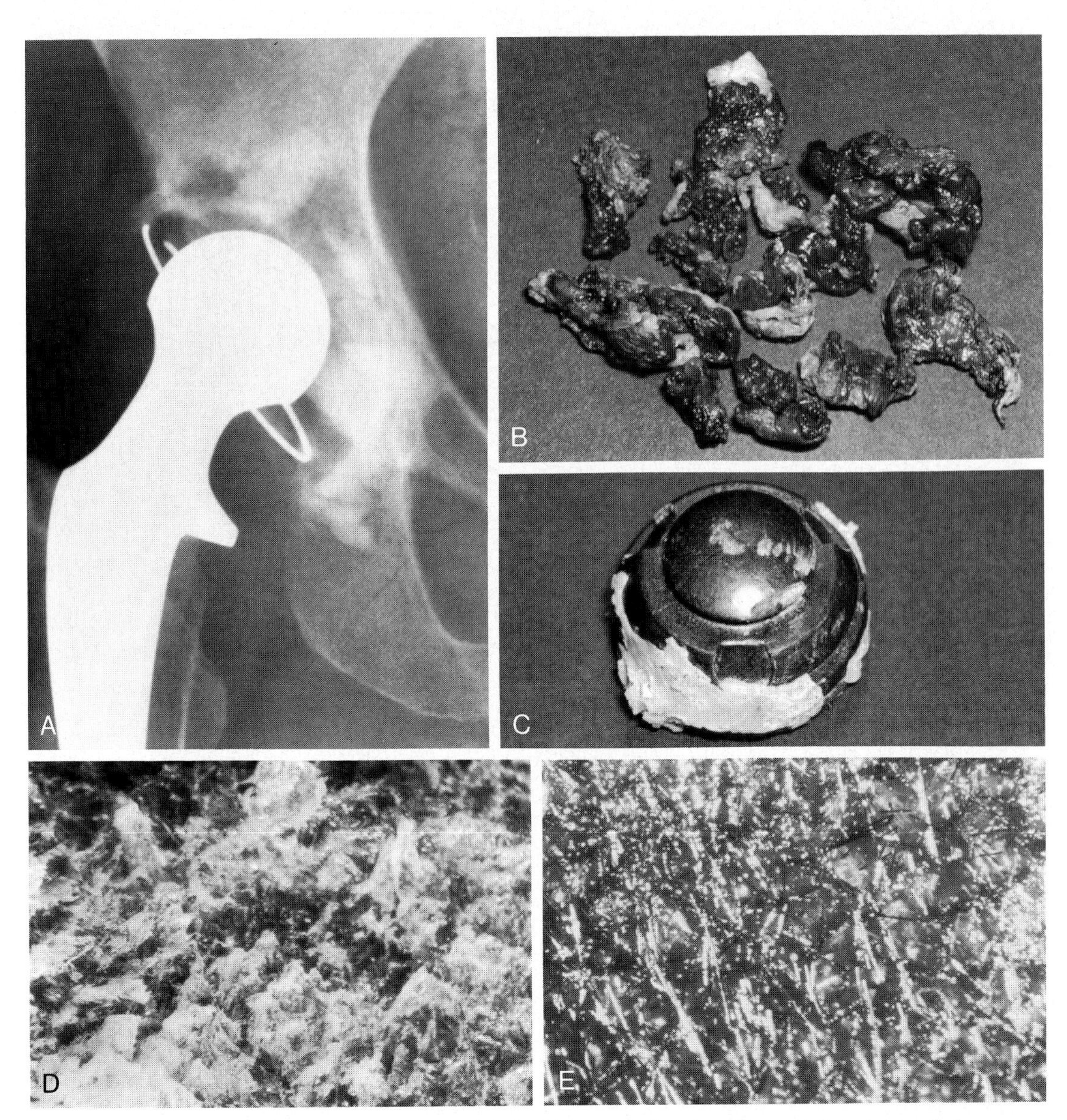

FIGURE 12–4. Loosening with osteolysis associated with cemented carbon fiber–reinforced polyethylene cup. *A*, Preoperative radiograph of a 69-year-old woman, who had total hip arthroplasty 7.5 years prior to recent onset of pain, reveals a grossly loose acetabular component. The cup has migrated. Reactive bone is seen about both the cup and the cement fixation pegs. In addition to the lucencies associated with loosening are discontinuous areas of bone destruction with poorly defined, irregular borders and lack of reactive bone. These findings are radiographically aggressive. *B*, At the time of acetabular revision, the capsular tissues and the interface membrane are blue-black. Tissue with the same discoloration invades the bone. *C*, The polyethylene cup is black because of impregnation with carbon fibers. A few fragments of cement cling to the rim. The white, scruffy markings on the dome were probably caused by cement abrasion. *D*, The scruffy area on the dome is frayed polyethylene (16 ×). *E*, Smooth areas of the cup reveal randomly oriented carbon-fiber filaments embedded in polyethylene. Most of the filaments are highly refractile and appear white in incident light. With very close inspection, a few black fibers can be distinguished (40 ×).

Illustration continued on following page

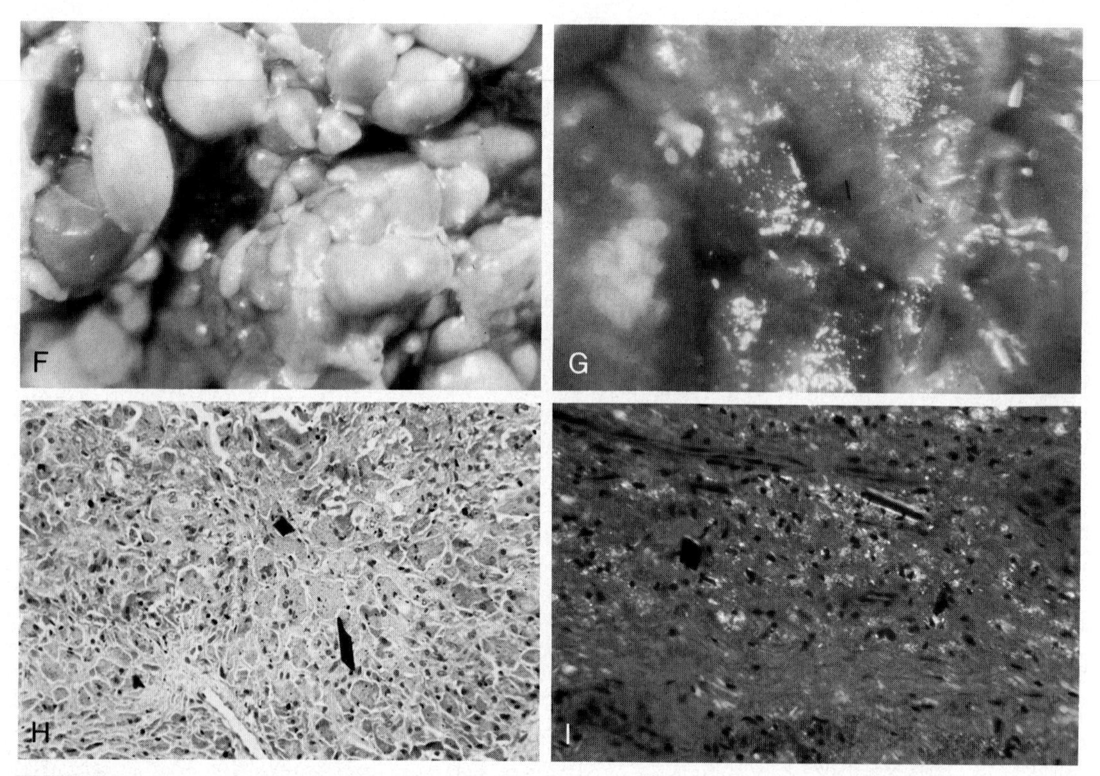

FIGURE 12–4 *Continued F,* The formalin-fixed blackened tissue removed at the time of revision consists of a papillary labyrinth of convoluted, synovial-like proliferation (10×). *G,* At higher magnification, a black splinter of the carbon filament can be seen penetrating the dusky surface of the "synovium" (40×). *H,* Routinely processed surgical pathology sections reveal an intense, largely mononuclear, histiocytic infiltrate with dusky gray cytoplasm. The jet-black particles with straight edges are shards of carbon fiber (250×). *I,* When viewed with polarized light (a different field than in Fig. 12–4*H*), faint specks of bright birefringence caused by polyethylene can be seen as well as the orange and pink birefringence of collagen. However, the refractile black carbon filaments do not polarize light.

months (average 12 months) after implantation, and the 28 total hip components were retrieved 3 weeks to 24 months (average 10 months). All but seven implants were removed during revision procedures most commonly performed owing to malposition or unexplained pain. None of the patients had clinical or radiographic signs of loosening.

One third of the specimens had neither bone ingrowth nor apposition; one third had ingrowth into less than 2 percent of the porous surface; the remaining third had ingrowth or apposition involving 2 to 10 percent of the available porous surface. In no component was more than 10 percent of the available porous material ingrown with bone. The radiographic appearance, the adherence of bony tissue at removal, and the time of implantation did not correlate with bone ingrowth. Pain did not indicate lack of bone ingrowth.

A fibrous layer ranging from a few cell layers to 2 mm in thickness separated most of the implant surfaces from the underlying bone. In areas with some bone ingrowth, the orientation of the fiber bundles often became perpendicular to the implant surface, indicating load-transmission capability. The bone at the fibrous tissue interface often showed active osteoclastic resorption. Fibrous tissue containing macrophages and multinucleated foreign body giant cells was uncommon and encountered primarily in implants with no evidence of bone ingrowth.

In a similar study of 85 nonloose knee components removed from 45 patients at intervals ranging from 2 weeks to 53 months (average 12 months), no bone ingrowth whatsoever was detected in 52 percent. Minimal ingrowth (less than 2 percent of available porous volume) was observed in 29 percent, moderate ingrowth (2 to 5 percent) in 12 percent, and extensive ingrowth (5 to 10 percent of the porous volume) in 7 percent.[21] As noted by Cook and associates,[20] no more than 10 percent of the available porous surface ever demonstrated osseous ingrowth. The anatomic sites of ingrowth were consistent for each type of component and were similar to those observed with total hip components: around pegs and in areas where the implant was in direct contact with the endosteal surface. No significant differences were found in the incidence or extent of bone ingrowth among femoral, tibial, or patellar components. Similarly, no differences were seen among manufacturers, implant designs, materials, or coating types.

These investigators[20, 21] concluded that extensive bone ingrowth was unlikely with total knee components. The paltry ingrowth suggested that some combination of bone and fibrous ingrowth may be sufficient for stability in this system. This view is interesting considering how few "capped" trabeculae were found in Charnley's long-term successful femoral components.[17] Furthermore, Cook's group suggested micromotion as a possible cause for the poor bone ingrowth in the tibial component, even though neither clinical nor radiographic evidence of loosening was found.

These studies have provided much valuable information. Nevertheless, we urge caution in extrapolating the histologic findings. Only patients having excellent clinical results and good clinical evidence of weightbearing and range of motion should be included when defining the "gold standard." The almost exclusive use of surgical specimens in these studies and the reasons for their removal are cause for concern. As these workers recognize, implants that are malpositioned or unstable almost certainly cannot be subjected to the same biomechanical considerations as those that are properly aligned and stable. Considering the thousands of patients who have not had implants removed, something in these retrieved component systems obviously went awry. For whatever reason, these studies deal with failed implants.

PRESS-FIT NONPOROUS DEVICES

Very little has been published at this time about the tissue response to nonporous press-fit devices. This discussion is therefore limited to the experience of Zweymuller[110] and Zweymuller and associates.[111]

The modular press-fit system consists of a forged titanium alloy femoral stem (Ti-6Al-4V or Ti-6Al-7Nb). The femoral component design incorporates a conically tapered straight stem with a rectangular cross-section that directly fixes to both cortical and cancellous bone in the metaphysis and to cortex in the diaphysis. This design ensures a firm, rotationally stable primary fixation, without completely filling the medullary cavity. Hence, the endosteal blood supply is preserved, and circumferential necrosis of the inner cortex is not expected. The implant bed is prepared by rasps rather than reamers, so that thermal damage to the bone bed is minimal. The surface area of the stem is increased by fine (3 to 5 μm) roughening.

Histologic studies were conducted on implants retrieved at autopsy 3 weeks to 5 years after implantations. The prostheses had remained stable in the two individuals who died of pulmonary embolism 3 weeks postoperatively. Bone and metal were in contact throughout the prosthetic bed. Trabeculae that had been bluntly shortened by rasping were in immediate contact with the metal. From areas of amputated trabeculae not in contact with metal, new bone was forming in the direction of and along the surface of the metal.

In the other cases, from the third month after surgery and for the next 2 to 3 years, newly forming osseous tissues spread along the surface of the implant, forming bony processes resembling elephant feet. The foot-like processes then gradually merged, leading to bony incorporation of the implant. The newly formed bone exactly traced the surface roughness of the implant without any interposition of connective tissue. Foreign-body giant cells were not observed. Gradually, the newly formed osseous tissue changed into lamellar, normally mineralized bone.

INFECTION

Historically, deep infection was not only the most common reason for early failure of implanted joints but also the most devastating, in terms of both functional recovery and survival.[24, 57, 93] Nowadays, the incidence of infection with almost all types of joint replacement has become quite low, < 1 to 1.5 percent, and tremendous progress has been made in salvaging those arthroplasties that do become infected.[11] Nonetheless, because of the potential for catastrophic sequelae, deep infection remains a serious complication.

Etiology

A number of factors associated with the implantation of a prosthesis make the bed an inviting environment for bacterial habitation. Surgical preparation of the implant bed always disrupts the blood supply to some extent, resulting in at least some bone necrosis and cutting off the route of normal host defenses, such as antibodies and inflammatory cells, or exogenous aids, such as antibiotics. The medullary canal is packed tightly with cement, a prosthesis, or both further thwarting any attempts to revascularize dead endosteal bone. In this compromised environment, even small numbers of bacteria may produce infection.

Foreign bodies profoundly alter the environment, another reason for assiduous attempts to reduce the number of bacteria in the wound through such measures as clean air and antibiotics. In a classic experiment, Elek and Conen[35] demonstrated that placing a single silk suture in the area of bacterial inoculation reduced by 10,000-fold the number of *Staphylococcus aureus* organisms required to establish infection.

In an *in vitro* system using murine macrophages, Rae[95] demonstrated the effect on phagocytosis of variously sized particulate cobalt, nickel, and cobalt-chromium alloys. In addition to causing cytoplasmic damage to the macrophage, lactic dehydrogenase, an indicator of damage to the cell membrane, was released. Decreased intracellular levels of glucose-6-phosphate dehydrogenase activity suggested deficient phagocytic capacity in these cells. In contrast, particles of titanium, chromium, and molybdenum did not produce these effects. Because it takes some time for the production of wear particles, this phenomenon, if operative in humans, would be expected to influence primarily late infections.

Cement was targeted early as an important factor in the establishment of infection, and it has been extensively studied. In a series of *in vitro* investigations, Petty and associates and other investigators demonstrated a multitude of ways in which methyl methacrylate might interfere with various aspects of the immune system. Small quantities of methyl methacrylate monomer had a detrimental effect on the following: (1) factors in normal human serum that are effective against *Staphylococcus epidermidis*[89]; (2) late-acting components of the complement sequence[88]; (3) production of zymosan-induced chemotactic factors in normal human serum[90]; (4) migration of polymorphonuclear leukocytes (PMNs)[90]; (5) phagocytosis and killing of bacteria by PMNs[91]; and (6) responses of human peripheral blood lymphocytes.[85] Further studies indicated that for a brief period methyl methacrylate monomer is present in tissues bordering implanted cement in sufficient concentration to adversely affect immune function.[92]

A study in a canine model compared the effect of commonly employed implant materials on the rates of infection with common pathogens *(Staphylococcus epidermidis, Staphylococcus aureus,* and *Escherichia coli)*. All the implant materials studied—stainless steel, cobalt-chromium alloys, high-density polyethylene, prepolymerized PMMA, and PMMA polymerized *in vivo*—significantly increased the likelihood of infection with *S. aureus*. However, PMMA polymerized *in vivo* was the only implant material associated with infection when contaminated with less than 1000 colony-forming units and the only material to have a significantly increased incidence of infection with *S. epidermidis* or *E. coli*.[94] These results suggest not only that the tested materials make infection with some bacteria more likely but also that for some bacteria the method of implantation influences the incidence of infection.

The immensely increased surface area of porous-coated implants, together with alterations in the microenvironment caused by the release of metal ions or corrosion products, might be expected to affect the development and severity of infection. Cooper and colleagues[22] compared the effect of satin-finished with porous-coated cobalt-chromium implants on the incidence and severity of infection with *S. aureus* in rabbits. In this model, the addition of a porous coating had no demonstrable effect. This study substantiated previous work implicating the presence of an implant in the development of osteomyelitis.[94]

Diagnosis

Infections are usually classified as early or delayed. From the viewpoint of pathology, i.e., thinking of infections in terms of their likely cause, the categories early, delayed, and hematogenous are more serviceable.

Early infections usually become evident within the first 3 months of the wound-healing period and are easily related to the operation.[82] Delayed infections become symptomatic or diagnosed months (or, uncommonly, years) after the joint implantation. They still can be related to the operation. The course of delayed infections is insidious. Patients may have slowly progressive pain but lack systemic symptoms. The sole laboratory abnormality finding may be a persistently elevated erythrocyte sedimentation rate (ESR).[2] Plain radiographs eventually display abnormalities, and isotopic bone imaging may display increased uptake about the components. The incidence of delayed infections has decreased since the introduction of clean-air enclosures, perioperative antibiotic prophylaxis, and antibiotic-impregnated cement, providing presumptive evidence that these infections are caused by delayed growth of bacteria that were implanted at the time of operation.[2, 24]

Hematogenous infections are relatively less common. They may arise at any time and are not related to the operation. Almost always, the patient has been well, with no symptoms to suggest wound infection. The clinical presentation of hematogenous infections resembles that of acute osteomyelitis. In contrast to the delayed type, these infections are associated with systemic symptoms and, often, clinically identifiable sources. As with acute osteomyelitis, the initial radiographs and isotopic imaging scans may lag behind the developing pathologic processes. Culture of the same strain of bacteria from the joint, the blood, and the primary focus establishes the diagnosis.[2, 24, 30, 57]

When a prosthesis fails because of late loosening, the differential diagnosis includes lysis and infection. Definitive diagnosis is usually established by the clinical, laboratory, and radiographic findings. One of the most helpful laboratory signs is elevation of the ESR. Although the ESR becomes higher following joint replacement and remains high for several months, persistent or late elevations to > 35 mm/hr and up to 50 mm/hr are consistent with infection.[30, 34, 57] Elevation of C-reactive protein level is also consistent with infection. Most investigators agree on the importance of positive culture results of a specific organism from the joint aspirate or immediately adjacent tissue.[34] When the clinical, laboratory, and radiographic data do not clearly establish the diagnosis, an experienced surgical pathologist may be able to help, provided representative tissue is supplied.[94] In studies to analyze the reaction in the periprosthetic tissues of failed joint arthroplasties, Mirra and colleagues[82, 84] performed extensive semiquantitative estimations of debris (metal, polyethylene, and cement), acute and chronic inflammatory cell infiltration, and histiocytic reaction. These findings were then correlated with the clinical and radiographic findings.

The single most reliable histologic parameter of infection was focal or diffuse infiltration, or both, of the synovial, subsynovial, or capsular tissues by more than 5 PMNs/high-power field (hpf). Twenty one of 22 patients with more than 5 PMNs/hpf had both clinical evidence of infection and positive culture findings. The remaining case had negative culture findings but clinical evidence of infection.[84] The joint was revised in five patients who did not have significant PMN responses but did have positive cultures findings (four with *Corynebacterium* and one with *Micrococcus*, consistent with low virulent or contaminant organisms). Clinical follow-up revealed no evidence of infection, loosening, or developing pain. No PMNs were observed in the biopsy specimens of joints without clinical or culture evidence of infection, even though variable quantities of metal and polyethylene or acrylic debris were present.[82]

The second most important indicator of

infection identified by Mirra was focal, diffuse, or focal and diffuse accumulation of chronic inflammatory cells. In 36 cases, lymphocytes or plasma cells exceeded 10/hpf or lymphoid follicles exceeded 2/hpf. Infections occurred in 23 of those 36 cases. In 13 with negative culture results, the inflammation was associated with large quantities of polyethylene or acrylic debris, or both, or was related to rheumatoid arthritis.

Interpretation of tissue specimens occasionally is made difficult by the presence of inflammatory cells unrelated to infection. Agins and coworkers[1] found numerous plasma cells in the tissues of two of nine patients with failed titanium alloy prostheses who also had high tissue levels of aluminum and vanadium. As Willert and Semlitsch[109] and Mirra and associates[82, 84] noted, the substantial lymphocytic and plasma cell infiltration occasionally observed in the absence of bacterial inflammation may be related to hypersensitivity or to chronic irritation in conjunction with the foreign-body reaction to wear particles. Whereas numerous foamy histiocytes associated with PMNs, chronic inflammatory cells, and edematous granulation tissue are indicators of infection, spindle-shaped histiocytes and those with granular cytoplasm are usually related to polyethylene or acrylic debris.[82]

Interpretation of the synovial tissues of patients with rheumatoid arthritis can present special problems. Up to 10 PMNs/hpf may be found in these cases without bacterial infections. Mirra and colleagues[82, 84] could usually discriminate those tissues on the bases of other histologic features of rheumatoid arthritis: papillary and synoviocytic hyperplasia with masses of lymphocytes and plasma cells in the absence of massive granulation tissue, abscesses, and foamy histiocytes.

Gram stain for bacteria has limited value. In more than 200 consecutive revision arthroplasties, Eftekhar and associates[34] found only one instance in which the Gram stain and culture findings from the same specimen were reported as positive. Three false-positive results were reported.

Many experienced pathologists look for increased numbers of neutrophils as the most reliable index for infection. Eftekhar and associates[34] prefer the use of touch imprints, in which the clustering of neutrophils can be observed in almost pure colonies. Our own preference is the use of frozen sections. The pathologist's familiarity with the clinical course and the radiographic studies of the patient enhances the accuracy of interpretation of the frozen section.

SARCOMA

It is well-established that a variety of plastics, including PMMA and polyethylene, in a host of different physical forms, can induce soft tissue sarcomas in rodents.[13, 103] Carter and Roe[13] described two patients with tuberculosis treated with pulmonary plombage, utilizing polyethylene balls, who developed tumors. Many of the alloys employed in human orthopaedic implants contain a variety of metals that are carcinogenic in rats in their pure forms (cobalt and nickel), salts (chromates), corrosion products, or as wear particles (cobalt-chromium alloy).[55] Although pure forms of chromium and molybdenum have not elicited tumors in rats, wear particles from the McKee total hip prostheses and from the Walldius hinged total knee prostheses have induced sarcomas of varied histologic types.[55, 105]

The obvious question is whether these observations have any relevance in humans. Despite the known hazards to experimental animals, extrapolation to humans has been difficult because of the significant differences in species susceptibility.

Veterinary Medicine and Biochemical Evidence

The most compelling evidence that certain metallic implants might in some way participate in the oncogenic process comes from veterinary medicine. Between 1975 and 1977, 13 malignant tumors were reported arising from sites of metal implants used for fixation of fractures in 12 dogs and a cat.[6, 51, 71, 100]

The veterinary experience clearly indicates a high incidence of an uncommon histologic type (osteosarcoma in ten of the 13 cases), occurring in the wrong bone (the femur in six of the 12 canine tumors) and in the wrong place (the shaft in 11 cases).[9, 69] All of these tumors were intimately associated with metallic corrosion, mostly of stainless steel. Of these animals, seven were treated with the Jonas splint that was widely used in veterinary medicine. The Jonas splint consisted of three components of varying metallic composition and characteristics and was notably subject to corrosion.

Of 20 osteosarcomas seen by Harrison and colleagues[51] during a 5-year period, two were associated with metallic fixation devices. One occurred in a dog that also had mammary carcinoma and had experienced two episodes of trauma. None of the other 18 dogs with osteosarcomas had fractures, and only one had a history of recent trauma to the tumor site. During this 5-year period, 1959 of 4000 fractures in 3300 dogs were fixed with some type of metallic implant. Sinbaldi and associates[100] reported eight malignancies, five of them osteosarcomas, from a pool of 2600 fractures treated by internal fixations during the period from 1968 to 1974. These investigators noted that the two undifferentiated sarcomas histologically resembled malignant histiocytomas, which had recently been described in humans.[100] The experience with dogs may have implications for humans.

When implanted into the physiologic milieu, all types of metallic alloys ionize and form corrosion products. These occur no matter how resistant to corrosion the metal may seem. For example, titanium, which is markedly resistant to corrosion in industrial chloride solutions, has been shown to be present in high concentrations in the tissues.[39] The rate of corrosion depends on a number of factors, including particle size, metal solubility, and chemical character of the environment. Metals of dissimilar chemical composition in close contact will generate electrolytic potentials, which promote corrosion.

Nickel salts and corrosion products bind to serum albumin, cobalt binds to blood cells and proteins, and dichromates bind to blood cells.[77] Hence, these metallic substances may be transported far from the implant site. This may explain the demonstration of increased levels of cobalt and chromium in the blood and urine of patients after total hip replacements with cast cobalt chromium alloy by Coleman and associates.[19]

Clinical Evidence

Since 1956, 17 isolated reports of sarcomas in patients with orthopaedic implants have appeared in the medical literature published in the English language.[4, 5, 14, 25, 27, 32, 55, 64, 65, 73, 75, 76, 87, 97, 104, 106, 108] Although these events seem to be exceedingly rare, speculation has been raised about whether the association is coincidental or causal. All but three cases were sarcomas of bone, although one case reported as a soft tissue sarcoma radiographically appears to have come from bone.[97] Of the sarcomas, eight occurred at the site of the metallic device used for fixation of fractures or osteotomies; nine were associated with total joint replacements (eight hips and one knee); and one was in a patient having both internal fixation and a Moore prosthesis. The interval between implantation and clinical recognition of the sarcoma ranged from 14 months to over 30 years. Stainless steel and cobalt-chromium-molybdenum alloys figured prominently in the cases involving metallic implants for fracture fixation. Most investigators have stressed corrosion of dissimilar metals with loosening of the implant and have described discoloration of the adjacent tissues.

The histologic types have varied. Malignant fibrous histiocytoma has been seen frequently, definitely in four patients and possibly in six. Osteosarcoma occurred in four patients and Ewing's tumor and non-Hodgkin's lymphoma each in two patients. In most patients the anatomic site (metaphyseal or diaphyseal), although related to the implant, also coincided with the expected site for the corresponding histologic type. For example, Tayton described a 3 1/2-year-old child who underwent bilateral osteotomies with fixation by Sherman plates that were removed a year later when the osteotomies had healed. At age 11 years, Ewing's sarcoma appeared at the exact site of one of the Sherman plates.[106] Both the location of the tumor in the femoral shaft and the age of the patient are expected for this neoplasm. In contrast, Berry and colleagues[8] reported an osteosarcoma occurring after 7 1/2 years at the site of a fracture in which internal fixation had not been used. The diaphyseal location was unusual.

Castleman and McNeely[14] diagnosed a case as "giant-cell tumor (probably malignant)," which was associated with metallic fixation of the proximal femur followed by implantation of a Moore prosthesis.[14] This case is important for several reasons. It is now known that the histologic diagnosis of malignant giant cell tumor of bone correlates poorly with clinical malignancy. Some pathologists today would classify the tumor as a giant cell variant of malignant fibrous histiocytoma. The tumor was associated with profound osteomalacia. Retrospective review of radiographs suggested that the tumor was present, but overlooked, when the femoral head was removed and the Moore prosthesis inserted.

Weber's case was described as "epithelioid sarcoma, possibly malignant fibrous histiocytoma or fibrosarcoma."[108] Epithelioid sarcoma is not currently recognized as arising in bone, and the photomicrographs presented do not support this diagnosis. During the 1970s, many fibrosarcomas and osteosarcomas were retrospectively reclassified as malignant fibrous histiocytomas. Weber's tumor almost surely represents malignant fibrous histiocytoma arising in either an enchondroma or a bone infarct.[55] Malignant fibrous histiocytoma and, less commonly, osteosarcoma are known to arise in areas of bone infarction.[29, 42, 79, 81, 102] Increasing evidence exists of a direct relationship between the infarction and the subsequent development of bone sarcoma, the prevalent type being malignant fibrous histiocytoma.[33, 44, 74, 79, 81, 83] This bone tumor is notorious for its association with non-neoplastic conditions in which a higher than normal level of mesenchymal activity is associated with turnover and repair.[23, 58, 63, 81, 83, 101, 102]

Some investigators have suggested that the chronicity of the repair process or foreign body reaction provides an active environment in which malignancy may develop. The situation is analogous to the well-known phenomenon of carcinoma arising in scars, chronic ulcers, and osteomyelitis.[29, 83] The potential link between sarcoma and joint replacement is intriguing because of the inevitable bone necrosis and repair associated with joint replacement.

The few reports of implant-associated sarcoma compared with the large number of implants means one of three things: (a) implant-associated sarcomas are not being reported, (b) the relationship is coincidental, or (c) the risk is minimal. Most of the sarcomas in humans, as in canine osteosarcomas, have been associated with corrosion products arising from implants of dissimilar metals that have been abandoned in modern orthopaedic practice. Further, most of the tumors occurred many years after the implant insertions. Thus, even if a causal relationship is eventually shown, the risk that an elderly patient would develop a sarcoma is exceedingly small. Because of the increasing application of noncemented prostheses that have a much larger metallic surface area and the trend to replace joints in younger patients, the potential for carcinogenicity nonetheless will require continuing investigation.

References

1. Agins, H. J., Alcock, N. W., Bansal, M., et al. Metallic wear in failed titanium-alloy total hip replacements. J. Bone Joint Surg. 70A:347–356, 1988.
2. Ahlberg, A., Carlsson, A. S., and Lindberg, L.: Hematogenous infection in total joint replacement. Clin. Orthop. 137:69–75, 1978.
3. Andersson, G. B. J., Freeman, M. A. R., and Swanson, S. A. V.: Loosening of the cemented acetabular cup in total hip replacement. J. Bone Joint Surg. 54B:590–599, 1972.
4. Arden, G. P. and Bywaters, E. G. L.: Tissue Reaction. Surgical Management of Juvenile Chronic Polyarthritis. Edited by G. P. Arden and B. M. Ansell. London, Academic Press, 1978.
5. Bago-Granell, J., Aguirre-Canyadell, M., Nardi, J., and Tallada, N.: Malignant fibrous histiocytoma of bone at the site of a total hip arthroplasty. J. Bone Joint Surg. 66B:38–40, 1984.
6. Banks, W. C., Morris, E., Herron, M. R., and Green, R. W.: Osteogenic sarcoma associated with internal fracture fixation in two dogs. J. Am. Vet. Assoc. 167:166–167, 1975.
7. Berman, A. T., Reid, J. S., Yanicko, Jr., D. R., et al: Thermally induced bone necrosis in rabbits. Clin. Orthop. 186:284–292, 1984.
8. Berry, M. P., Jenkin, D. T., Fornasier, V. L., and Rideout, D. F.: Osteosarcoma at the site of previous fracture. J. Bone Joint Surg. 62A:1216–1218, 1980.
9. Brodey, R. S. and Riser, W. H.: Canine osteosar-

coma. A clinicopathologic study of 194 Cases. Clin. Orthop. 62:54–64, 1969.
10. Brown, G. C., Lockshin, M. D., Salvati, E. A., and Bullough, P. G.: Sensitivity to metal as a possible cause of sterile loosening after cobalt-chromium total hip-replacement arthroplasty. J. Bone Joint Surg. 59A:164–168, 1977.
11. Buchholz, H. W., Elson, R. A., Engelbrecht, E., et al: Management of deep infection of total hip replacement. J. Bone Joint Surg. 63B:342–353, 1981.
12. Bullough, P. G., DiCarlo, E. F., Hansraj, K. K., and Neves, M. C.: Pathologic studies of total joint replacement. Orthop. Clin. North Am. 19:611–625, 1988.
13. Carter, R. L. and Roe, F. J. C.: Induction of sarcomas in rats by solid and fragmented polyethylene: Experimental observations and clinical implications. Br. J. Cancer 23:401–407, 1969.
14. Castleman, B. and McNeely, B. U.: Case 38-1965. Case Records of the Massachusetts General Hospital. N. Engl. J. Med. 273:494–504, 1965.
15. Charnley, J.: The reaction of bone to self-curing acrylic cement. A long-term histological study in man. J. Bone Joint Surg. 52B:340–353, 1970.
16. Charnley, J.: Proceedings and reports of universities, colleges, councils and associations. J. Bone Joint Surg. 57B:245, 1975.
17. Charnley, J.: Low Friction Arthroplasty of the Hip. New York, Springer-Verlag, 1979.
18. Cohen, J.: Assay of foreign-body reaction. J. Bone Joint Surg. 41A:152–166, 1959.
19. Coleman, R. F., Herrington, J., and Scales, J. T.: Concentration of wear products in hair, blood, and urine after total hip replacement. Br. Med. J. 1:527–529, 1973.
20. Cook, S. D., Thomas, K. A., and Haddad, Jr., R. J.: Histologic analysis of retrieved human porous-coated total joint components. Clin. Orthop. 234:90–101, 1988.
21. Cook, S. D., Barrack, R. L., Thomas, K. A., and Haddad, Jr., R. J.: Quantative histologic analysis of tissue growth into porous total knee components. J. Arthroplasty 4:[Suppl]:S33–S43, 1989.
22. Cooper, R. A., Petty, R. W., Miller, G. J., and Spanier, S.: Comparison of the incidence and severity of infection between porous-coated and smooth cobalt-chrome implants in a rabbit model. Captiva, Florida, Florida Orthopaedic Society, 1990 Annual Meeting, April 20, 1990. (In preparation.)
23. Dahlin, D. C., Unni, K. K., and Matsuno, T.: Malignant (fibrous) histiocytoma of bone—Fact or fancy? Cancer 39:1508–1516, 1977.
24. D'Ambrosia, R. D., Shoji, H., and Heater, R.: Secondarily infected total joint replacements by hematogenous spread. J. Bone Joint Surg. 450–453, 1976.
25. Delgado, E. R.: Sarcoma following a surgically treated fractured tibia. Clin. Orthop. 12:315–318, 1958.
26. Deutman, R., Mulder, Th. J., Brian, R., and Nater, J. P.: Metal sensitivity before and after total hip arthroplasty. J. Bone Joint Surg. 59A:862–865, 1977.
27. Dodion, P., Putz, P., Amiri-Lamraski, M. H., et al: Immunoblastic lymphoma at the site of an infected vitallium bone plate. Histopathology 6:807–813, 1982.
28. Doll, R.: Cancer of the lung and nose in nickel workers. Br. J. Industr. Med. 15:217–223, 1958.
29. Dorfman, H. D., Norman, A., and Wolff, H.: Fibrosarcoma complicating bone infarction in a caisson worker. J. Bone Joint Surg. 48A:528–532, 1966.
30. Downes, E. M.: Late infection after total hip replacement. J. Bone Joint Surg. 59B:42–44, 1977.
31. Drachman, D. B. and Sokoloff, L.: The role of movement in embryonic joint development. Devel. Biol. 14:401–420, 1966.
32. Dube, V. E. and Fisher, D. E.: Hemangioendothelioma of the leg following metallic fixation of the tibia. Cancer 30:1260–1266, 1972.
33. Dunham, W. K. and Wilborn, W. H.: Malignant fibrous histiocytoma of bone. J. Bone Joint Surg. 61A:939–942, 1979.
34. Eftekhar, N. S., Doty, S. B., Johnston, A. D., and Parisien, M. V.: Prosthetic Synovitis. The Hip: Proceedings of the 13th Open Scientific Meeting of the Hip Society. St. Louis, C. V. Mosby Company, 1985.
35. Elek, S. D. and Conen, P. E.: The virulence of *Staphylococcus pyogenes* for man: A study of problems of wound infection. Br. J. Exp. Pathol. 38:573–586, 1957.
36. Engh, C. A. and Bobyn, J. D.: Principles, Techniques, Results, and Complications with a Porous-coated Sintered Metal System. Edited by Lewis D. Anderson. American Academy of Orthopaedic Surgeons Instructional Course Lectures 35:169–183, 1986.
37. Engh, C. A., Bobyn, J. D., and Glassman, A. H.: Porous-coated hip replacement. The factors governing bone ingrowth, stress shielding, and clinical results. J. Bone J. Surg. 69B:45–55, 1987.
38. Evans, E. M., Freeman, M. A. R., Miller, A. J., and Vernon-Roberts, B.: Metal sensitivity as a cause of bone necrosis and loosening of the prosthesis in total joint replacement. J. Bone Joint Surg. 56B:626–642, 1974.
39. Ferguson, Jr., A. B., Laing, P. G., and Hodge, E. S.: The ionization of metal implants in living tissues. J. Bone Joint Surg. 42A:77–90, 1960.
40. Freeman, M. A. R., Bradley, G. W., and Revel, P. A.: Observations upon the interface between bone and polymethyl methacrylate cement. J. Bone Joint Surg. 64B:489–493, 1982.
41. Fries, I. B., Fisher, A. A., and Salvati, E. A.: Contact dermatitis in surgeons from methyl methacrylate bone cement. J. Bone Joint Surg. 57A:547–549, 1975.
42. Furey, J. G., Ferrer-Torells, M., and Reagan, J. W.: Fibrosarcoma arising at the site of bone infarcts. J. Bone Joint Surg. 42A:802–810, 1960.
43. Galante, J., Rostoker, W., Lueck, R., and Ray, R. D.: Sintered fiber metal composites as a basis for attachment of implants to bone. J. Bone Joint Surg. 53A:101–114, 1971.
44. Galli, S. J., Weintraub, H. P., and Proppe, K. H.: Malignant fibrous histiocytoma and pleomorphic sarcoma in association with medullary bone infarcts. Cancer 41:607–619, 1978.
45. Goldring, S. R., Schiller, A. L., Roelke, M., et al: The synovial-like membrane at the bone-

cement interface in loose total hip replacements and its proposed role in bone lysis. J. Bone Joint Surg. 65A:575–584, 1983.
46. Goodman, S. B., Fornasier, V. L., and Kei, J.: The effects of bulk versus particulate polymethyl methacrylate on bone. Clin. Orthop. 232:255–262, 1988.
47. Goodman, S. B., Chin, R. C., Chiou, S. S., et al: A clinical-pathologic-biochemical study of the membrane surrounding loosened and nonloosened total hip arthroplasties. Clin. Orthop. 244:182–187, 1989.
48. Griffiths, H. J., Burke, J., and Bonfiglio, T. A.: Granulomatous pseudotumors in total joint replacement. Skeletal Radiol. 16:146–152, 1987.
49. Harris, W. H., Schiller, A. L., Scholler, J-M., et al: Extensive localized bone resorption in the femur following total hip replacement. J. Bone Joint Surg. 58A:612–618, 1976.
50. Harris, W. H., White, Jr., R. E., McCarthy, J. C., et al: Bony ingrowth fixation of the acetabular component in canine hip joint arthroplasty. Clin. Orthop. 176:7–11, 1983.
51. Harrison, J. W., McLain, D. L., Hohn, R. B., et al: Osteosarcoma associated with metallic implants (Report of two cases in dogs). Clin. Orthop. 116:253–257, 1976.
52. Heath, J. C., Freeman, M. A. R., and Swanson, S. A. V.: Carcinogenic properties of wear particles from prostheses made in cobalt-chromium alloy. Lancet 1:564–566, 1971.
53. Hedley, A. K., Clarke, I. C., Bloebaum, R. D., et al: Viability and Cement Fixation of the Femoral Head in Canine Hip Surface Replacement. The Hip: Proceedings of the Seventh Open Scientific Meeting of The Hip Society. St. Louis, C. V. Mosby Company, 1979.
54. Huddleston, H. D.: Femoral lysis after cemented hip arthroplasty. J. Arthroplasty 3:285–297, 1988.
55. Hughes, A. W., Sherlock, D. A., Hamblen, D. L., and Reid, R.: Sarcoma at the site of a single hip screw. J. Bone Joint Surg. 69B:470–472, 1987.
56. Hungerford, D. S. and Kenna, R. V.: Preliminary experience with a total knee prosthesis with porous coating used without cement. Clin. Orthop. 176:95–107, 1983.
57. Hunter, G. and Dandy, D.: The natural history of the patient with an infected total hip replacement. J. Bone Joint Surg. 59B:293–297, 1977.
58. Huvos, A. G., Woodard, H. Q., and Heilweil, M.: Postradiation malignant fibrous histiocytoma of bone (a clinicopathologic study of 20 patients). Am. J. Surg. Pathol. 10:9–18, 1986.
59. Jasty, M. J., Floyd, W. E., Schiller, A. L., et al: Localized osteolysis in stable, non-septic total hip replacement. J. Bone Joint Surg. 68A:912–919, 1986.
60. Jefferiss, C. D., Lee, A. J. C., and Ling, R. S. M.: Thermal aspects of self-curing polymethyl methacrylate. J. Bone Joint Surg. 57B:511–518, 1975.
61. Jones, D. A., Lucas, H. K., O'Driscoll, M., et al: Cobalt toxicity after McKee hip arthroplasty. J. Bone Joint Surg. 57B:289–296, 1975.
62. Judet, R., Siguier, M., Brumpt, B., and Judet, T.: A noncemented total hip prosthesis. Clin. Orthop. 137:76–84, 1978.
63. Kahn, L. B., Webber, B., Mills, E., et al: Malignant fibrous histiocytoma (malignant fibrous xanthoma: xanthosarcoma) of bone. Cancer 42:640–651, 1978.
64. Lamovec J., Zidar, A., and Cucek-Plenicar, M.: Synovial sarcoma associated with total hip replacement. J. Bone Joint Surg. 70A:1558–1560, 1988.
65. Lee, Y. S., Pho, R. W. H., and Nather, A.: Malignant fibrous histiocytoma at site of metal implant. Cancer 54:2286–2289, 1984.
66. Linder, L.: Reaction of bone to the acute chemical trauma of bone cement J. Bone Joint Surg. 59A:82–87, 1977.
67. Linder, L. and Hansson, H.: Ultrastructural aspects of the interface between bone and cement in man. J. Bone Joint Surg. 65B:646–649, 1983.
68. Linder, L., Lindberg, L., and Carlsson, A.: Aseptic loosening of hip prostheses. A histologic and enzyme histochemical study. Clin. Orthop. 175:93–104, 1983.
69. Ling, G. V., Morgan, J. P., and Pool, R. R.: Primary bone tumors in the dog: A combined clinical, radiographic, and histologic approach to early diagnosis. J. Am. Vet. Med. Assoc. 165:55–67, 1974.
70. Lombardi, A. V., Mallory, T. H., Vaughn, B. K., and Drouillard, P.: Aseptic loosening in total hip arthroplasty secondary to osteolysis induced by wear debris from titanium-alloy modular femoral heads. J. Bone Joint Surg. 71A:1337–1342, 1989.
71. Madewell, B. R., Pool, R. R., and Leighton, R. L.: Osteogenic sarcoma at the site of a chronic nonunion fracture and internal fixation device in a dog. J. Am. Vet. Assoc. 171:187–189, 1977.
72. Maguire, J. K., Jr., Coscia, M. F., and Lynch, M. H.: Foreign body reaction to polymeric debris following total hip arthroplasty. Clin. Orthop. 216:213–223, 1987.
73. Martin, A., Bauer, T. W., Manley, M. T., and Marks, K. E.: Osteosarcoma at the site of total hip replacement. J. Bone Joint Surg. 70A:1561–1567, 1988.
74. McCarthy, E. F., Matsuno, T., and Dorfman, H. D.: Malignant fibrous histiocytoma of bone: A study of 35 cases. Human Pathol. 10:57–70, 1979.
75. McDonald, I.: Malignant lymphoma associated with internal fixation of a fractured tibia. Cancer 48:1009–1011, 1981.
76. McDougall, A.: Malignant tumour at site of bone plating. J. Bone Joint Surg. 38B:709–713, 1956.
77. Merritt, K., Brown, S. A., and Sharkey, N. A.: The binding of metal salts and corrosion products to cells and proteins *in vitro*. J. Biomed. Mater. Res. 18:1005–1015, 1984.
78. Meyer, P. R., Lautenschlager, E. P., and Moore, B. K.: On the setting properties of acrylic bone cement. J. Bone Joint Surg. 55A:149–156, 1973.
79. Michael, R. H. and Dorfman, H. D.: Malignant fibrous histiocytoma associated with bone infarcts. Clin. Orthop. 118:180–183, 1976.
80. Miller, J., Burke, D. L., Stachiewicz, J. W., et al: Pathophysiology of Loosening of Femoral Components in Total Hip Arthroplasty. The Hip: Proceedings of the Sixth Open Scientific Meeting of the Hip Society. St. Louis, C. V. Mosby Company, 1978.

81. Mirra, J. M., Bullough, P. G., Marcove, R. C., et al: Malignant fibrous histiocytoma and osteosarcoma in association with bone infarcts. J. Bone Joint Surg. 56A:932–940, 1974.
82. Mirra, J. M., Amstutz, H. C., Matos, M., and Gold, R.: The pathology of the joint tissues and its clinical relevance in prosthesis failure. Clin. Orthop. 117:221–240, 1976.
83. Mirra, J. M.: Bone Tumors, Diagnosis and Treatment. Philadelphia, J. B. Lippincott Company, 1980.
84. Mirra, J. M., Marder, R. A., and Amstutz, H. C.: The pathology of failed total joint arthroplasty. Clin. Orthop. 170:175–183, 1982.
85. Panush, R. S. and Petty, R. W.: Inhibition of human lymphocyte responses by methyl methacrylate. Clin. Orthop. 134:356–363, 1978.
86. Pazzaglia, U. and Byers, P. D.: Fractured femoral shaft through an osteolytic lesion resulting from the reaction to a prosthesis. J. Bone Joint Surg. 66B:337–339, 1984.
87. Penman, H. G. and Ring, P. A.: Osteosarcoma in association with total hip replacement. J. Bone Joint Surg. 66B:632–634, 1984.
88. Petty, W. and Caldwell, J. R.: The effect of methyl methacrylate on complement activity. Clin. Orthop. 128:354–360, 1977.
89. Petty, W.: The effect of methyl methacrylate on the bacterial inhibiting properties of normal human serum. Clin. Orthop. 132:266–278, 1978.
90. Petty, W.: The effect of methyl methacrylate on chemotaxis of polymorphonuclear leukocytes. J. Bone Joint Surg. 60A:492–498, 1978.
91. Petty, W.: The effect of methyl methacrylate on bacterial phagocytosis and killing by human polymorphonuclear leukocytes. J. Bone Joint Surg. 60A:752–756, 1978.
92. Petty, W.: Methyl methacrylate concentrations in tissues adjacent to bone cement. J. Biomed. Mater. Res. 14:427–434, 1980.
93. Petty, W. and Goldsmith, S.: Resection arthroplasty following infected total hip arthroplasty. J. Bone Joint Surg. 62A:889–896, 1980.
94. Petty, W., Spanier, S. S., Shuster, J. J., and Silverthorne, C.: The influence of skeletal implants on incidence of infection. Experiments in a canine model. J. Bone Joint Surg. 67A:1236–1244, 1985.
95. Rae, T.: A study on the effects of particulate metals of orthopaedic interest on murine macrophages *in vitro*. J. Bone Joint Surg. 57B:444–450, 1975.
96. Rhinelander, F. W., Nelson, C. L., Stewart, R. D., and Stewart, C. L.: Experimental Reaming of the Proximal Femur and Acrylic Cement Implantation: Vascular and Histologic Effects. The Hip: Proceedings of the Seventh Open Scientific Meeting of the Hip Society. St. Louis, C. V. Mosby Company, 1979.
97. Ryu, R. K. N., Bovill, Jr., E. G., Skinner, H. B., and Murray, W. R.: Soft tissue sarcoma associated with aluminum oxide ceramic total hip arthroplasty. Clin. Orthop. 216:207–212, 1987.
98. Salvati, E. A., Wright, T. M., Burstein, A. H., and Jacobs, B.: Fracture of polyethylene acetabular cups, report of two cases. J. Bone Joint Surg. 61A:1239–1242, 1979.
99. Sandborn, P. M., Cook, S. D., Spires, W. P., and Kester, M. A.: Tissue response to porous-coated implants lacking initial bone apposition. J. Arthroplasty 3:337–346, 1988.
100. Sinibaldi, K., Rosen, H., Liu, S. K., and DeAngelis, M.: Tumors associated with metallic implants in animals. Clin. Orthop. 118:257–266, 1976.
101. Spanier, S. S., Enneking, W. F., and Enriquez, P.: Primary malignant fibrous histiocytoma of bone. Cancer 36:2084–2098, 1975.
102. Spanier, S. S.: Malignant fibrous histiocytoma of bone. Orthop. Clin. North Am. 8:947–961, 1977.
103. Stinson, N. E.: Tissue reaction induced in guinea pigs by particulate polymethyl methacrylate, polythene, and nylon of the same size range. Br. J. Exp. Pathol. 46:135–146, 1965.
104. Swann, M.: Malignant soft-tissue tumour at the site of a total hip replacement. J. Bone Joint Surg. 66B:629–631, 1984.
105. Swanson, S. A. V., Freeman, M. A. R., and Heath, J. C.: Laboratory tests on total joint replacement prostheses. J. Bone Joint Surg. 55B:759–773, 1973.
106. Tayton, K. J. J.: Ewing's sarcoma at the site of a metal plate. Cancer 45:413–415, 1980.
107. Vernon-Roberts, B. and Freeman, M. A. R.: Morphological and Analytical Studies of the Tissues Adjacent to Joint Prostheses: Investigations into the Causes of Loosening of Prostheses. Advances in Artificial Hip and Knee Joint Technology. International Symposium on Advances in Artificial Hip and Knee Joint Technology, Erlangen, 1975. New York, Springer-Verlag, 1976.
108. Weber, P. C.: Epithelioid sarcoma in association with total knee replacement. J. Bone Joint Surg. 68B:824–826, 1986.
109. Willert, H. G. and Semlitsch, M.: Reactions of the articular capsule to wear products of artificial joint prostheses. J. Biomed. Mater. Res. 11:157–164, 1977.
110. Zweymuller, K.: A cementless titanium hip endoprosthesis system based on press-fit fixation: Basic research and clinical results. Edited by Lewis D. Anderson. American Academy of Orthopaedic Surgeons Instructional Course Lectures 35:203–225, 1986.
111. Zweymuller, K. A., Lintner, F. K., and Semlitsch, M. F.: Biologic fixation of a press-fit titanium hip joint endoprosthesis. Clin. Orthop. 235:195–206, 1988.

SECTION VI

LOWER EXTREMITY REPLACEMENT: THE HIP

CHAPTER 13

Biomechanics and Design

GARY J. MILLER

Successful total hip arthroplasty depends on an understanding of the anatomy of the hip and of the biomechanics of the normal joint during walking (gait) and other daily activities. The normal human hip is a ball and socket, which provide inherent stability while allowing considerable mobility and low frictional forces under substantial load.

A detailed anatomic discussion of the intact joint is beyond the scope of this chapter, but knowledge of the range of motion and of the forces encountered during daily activity is imperative to gain insight into the design of prostheses for reconstruction of the diseased hip joint.

BIOMECHANICS OF THE HIP

Range of Motion

The hip is a complex structure that allows motion in three anatomic planes: coronal, sagittal, and transverse. When viewed in the sagittal plane, the hip exhibits flexion from neutral to 140 degrees and allows extension from neutral to 15 degrees. In the coronal plane, abduction from neutral to 30 degrees and adduction from neutral to 25 degrees are observed. Along the femoral long axis, internal rotation from neutral to 70 degrees occurs, with external rotation of up to 90 degrees.[67] Thus, the range of motion in the normal hip circumscribes a large global area on the spheric articulating surface.

Because of soft tissue restraints, however, extremes of motion may be seen only in certain positions. Maximum flexion and extension are achieved when the hip is slightly abducted and in the neutral rotation position. Abduction-adduction is maximized when the hip is slightly flexed and externally rotated. Maximum internal-external rotation is achieved in the slightly flexed position.

Early investigations of range of motion concentrated on analysis of the normal gait cycle. Fischer was one of the first to describe the biomechanics of the hip during normal gait.[30, 31] His work was limited to discrete positions during the gait cycle, which consisted of 11 positions for assessing human ambulation on a flat surface. Further investigations using more sophisticated techniques have refined our understanding of motion during ambulation.[47, 65, 73, 92]

The motions of ambulation represent only part of the requirements for mobility and activities of daily life. As can be seen in Table 13–1, most daily activities require considerable motion in the sagittal plane as well as large portions of motion in the coronal and transverse planes.[52] The dynamics of motion during these activities and the ground reaction forces necessary to maintain equilibrium create significant loads on the hip joint.

These ranges of motion form the bases for the design of total hip replacements intended to provide near-normal activity after reconstruction of diseased hips.

Table 13–1. MEAN VALUES FOR MAXIMUM HIP MOTION IN THREE PLANES DURING COMMON ACTIVITIES

Activity	Plane of Motion	Recorded Value (Degrees)
Tying shoe with foot on floor	Sagittal	124
	Coronal	19
	Transverse	15
Tying shoe with foot across opposite thigh	Saggital	110
	Coronal	23
	Transverse	33
Sitting down on chair and rising from sitting	Sagittal	104
	Coronal	20
	Transverse	17
Stooping to obtain object from floor	Sagittal	117
	Coronal	21
	Transverse	18
Squatting	Sagittal	122
	Coronal	28
	Transverse	26
Ascending stairs	Sagittal	67
	Coronal	16
	Transverse	18
Descending stairs	Sagittal	36

Mean for 33 normal men.
Data from Johnson, R. C., and Smidt, G. L.: J. Bone Joint Surg. 51A:1083–1094, 1969.

Forces

Equilibrium considerations and force analyses help in estimating the forces seen in the hip during gait. Bombelli[9] consolidated and refined the analyses presented by Fischer to describe the loading during the various phases of gait. He reinforced the concept, often overlooked, that the joint undergoes loading in a three-dimensional fashion and not in the idealized two-dimensional representation often shown in basic biomechanics texts. Loads are present not only in the coronal plane but in the sagittal plane as well.

The results of two-dimensional analysis, illustrated in Figure 13–1, predict joint reaction forces during single limb stance of two to three times body weight. Often forgotten are the assumptions made in deriving this analysis—the most pertinent being that all forces are in the plane of analysis only. Whereas this assumption may be correct for single limb stance, loading is more complex throughout the gait cycle, because of inertia and muscular activity.

To elucidate this point, Figure 13–1 shows the free body diagram of the stance phase of gait in the frontal plane. The position of the joint reaction force at 16 degrees is seen without difficulty and relates to the abductor loading needed to stabilize the hip under load. However, a more complete three-dimensional assessment of this phase of the cycle reveals that loads are not planar. The load vector in the sagittal plane inclines −30 degrees to 20 degrees, as shown in Figure 13–2. The resulting load vector circumscribes an area with varying angles in the frontal and sagittal planes, allowing for both bending and torsion of the femur and, therefore, of the replacement prosthesis. Various investigators have emphasized the need to consider both bending and torsion in designs and implantations of hip reconstruction components.[21, 59, 85]

Daily activity makes additional demands on an arthroplasty. Climbing stairs, rising from a chair, and other important daily living activities alter the forces on the hip. Burke and associates[12] and Harris and associates[42] have detailed these motions in relation to loading of the hip and have shown the considerable torsional loads. These findings are supported by the teams of Collier[17] and Hodge,[44] who have documented considerable force generation during these important, nonambulating, activities. The predicted torsion loads make demands on the inherent stability of cemented and press-fit implants. For these reasons, three-dimensional loads must be addressed in the design of hip joint replacement components.

PROSTHESES INTENDED FOR CEMENTED USE

Femoral Component Design

Based on clinical observations of failures, many investigators have proposed that the key to prevention of stem fracture is prevention of stem loosening.[5, 34, 35] Many of the biologic and mechanical problems that led to loosening and early implant failure have been lessened, but late failures are still observed. In an attempt to prevent these late problems, the design of hip prostheses has evolved over the years since Charnley first introduced his prosthesis. However, the rationale for many of these changes is difficult to discern.

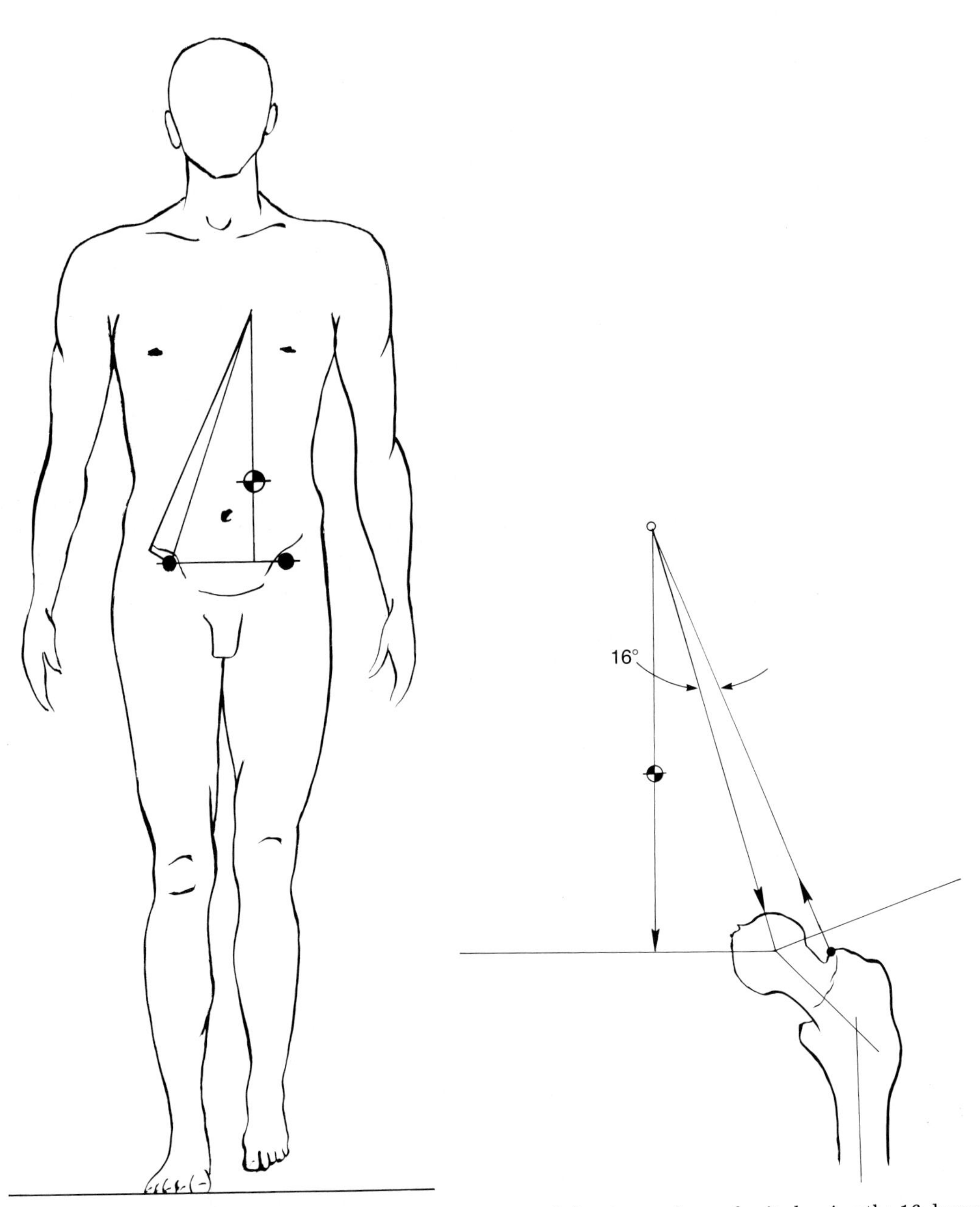

FIGURE 13–1. Frontal plane view of the free body diagram of the stance phase of gait showing the 16-degree incline of the resultant load vector. (Redrawn from Bombelli, R.: Osteoarthritis of the Hip. Berlin, Springer-Verlag, 1976.)

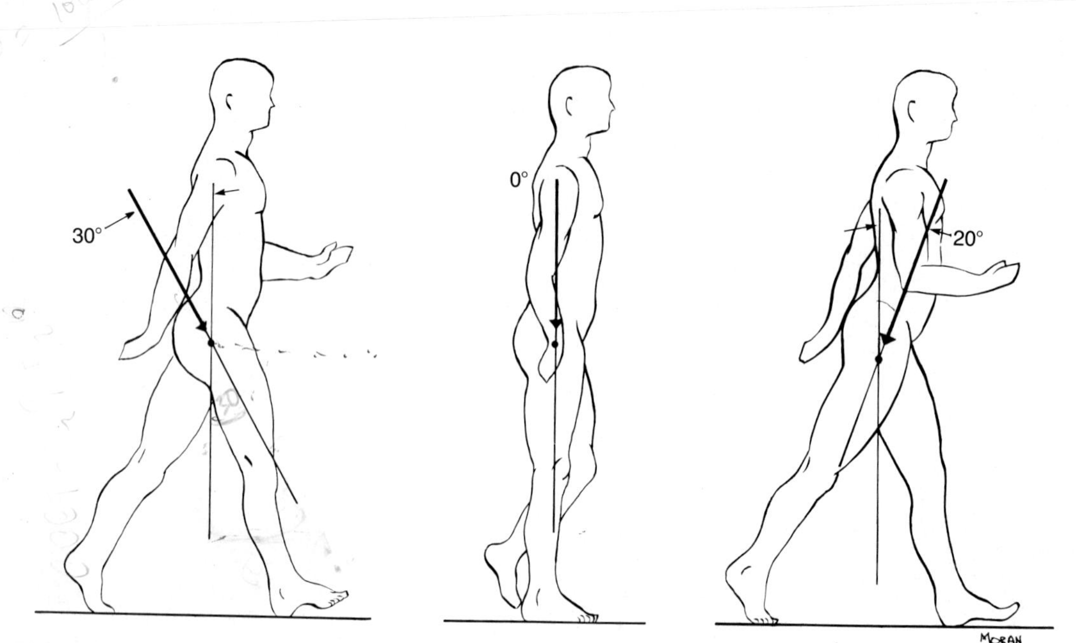

FIGURE 13–2. The sagittal plane view of the same stride depicted in Figure 13–1 shows inclination of the load vector at −30 degrees to 20 degrees. (Redrawn from Bombelli, R.: Osteoarthritis of the Hip. Berlin, Springer-Verlag, 1976.)

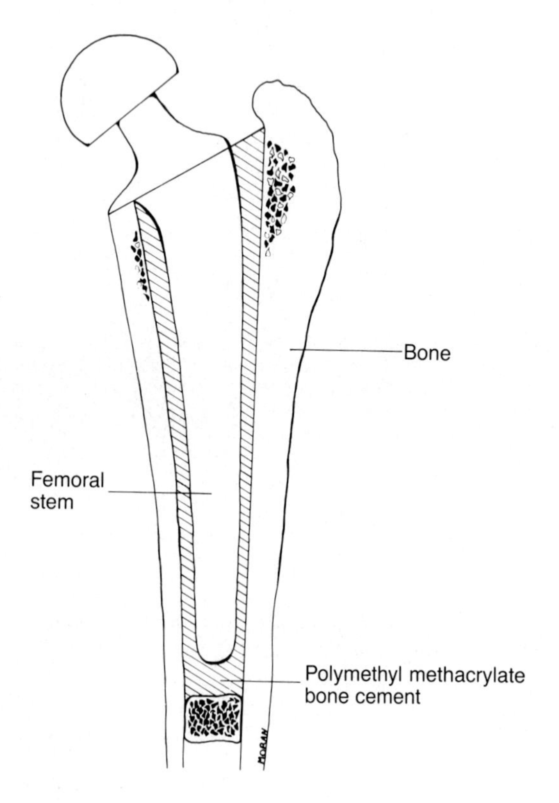

FIGURE 13–3. Composite structure of the total joint arthroplasty including the implant, bone cement, and bone.

Cemented total hip arthroplasty results in a composite structure, with the implant, bone cement, and bone interacting under load (Fig. 13–3). Each of these factors must be considered in evaluating the overall effect of changes in individual parts of the construct.

Hip prosthesis design is dependent on many implant characteristics (Fig. 13–4). These include geometric configuration, e.g., shape; adjuncts, e.g., collars; surface characteristics; material properties of alloys, e.g., their biocompatibility, fatigue, and ultimate strength; manufacturing method; and implantation instrumentation.

Femoral Component Geometry

The inherent differences in available components have been analyzed to determine design criteria that might improve implant performance.[20, 72] Using finite element modeling analysis, Crowninshield and associates[20] compared the basic design characteristics of cemented femoral components in relation to both stem and cement stresses. When the stem cross-section size (the area moment of inertia) was increased, stem, cement, and calcar bone stresses were reduced (Fig. 13–5). Increases in the stem length led to increases in stem stress and decreases in cement and calcar stresses (Fig. 13–6). Changes in the material properties of the stem also had pronounced effects (Fig. 13–7). Reducing the modulus of elasticity of the stem material reduced the stem stresses at the expense of increased cement stresses proximally and decreased cement stresses distally. Increasing the modulus of the polymethyl methacrylate (PMMA) cement led to stem stress decreases and cement stress increases (Fig. 13–8). These results corroborate clinical observations regarding commercially available designs and indicate that the proximal cement region is critical in maintaining implant stability.

Martens and colleagues,[61] in their clinical review of failure of Charnley-Mueller stems, found that the stem cross-section shape appeared to contribute to cement failure and implant breakage. Finite element modeling provides insights into this question.[19] Analysis of various cross-section shapes shows that prostheses with relatively small anteroposterior medial dimensions (those with a sharp medial surface, such as the Charnley-Mueller prosthesis) are associated with high cement compressive stresses, whereas prostheses with more blunt medial profiles are associated with lower, more manageable stresses. When sharp medial edges are compared with blunt medial edges, a 69 percent increase in compressive stresses is seen (Fig. 13–9). Similar effects of shape can be seen also in tensile cement stresses (Fig. 13–10).

The mode or distribution of dominant cement loading—compression or tension—may be controlled by geometric design (Fig. 13–11). The cement mantle may be generally divided, with tension on the lateral side and compression on the medial side. Computer modeling shows that stems with broadened anteroposterior lateral dimensions, e.g., those with lateral flanges, create larger regions of compressive stress and less tensile stress. Additionally, the flange has been shown to reduce subsidence (Fig. 13–12).[56] Geometric features, such as the lateral flange, blunt medial edge, and midstem recess or cement groove, can reduce the stresses in the cement and provide more optimal compressive loading.[10, 68]

A high area moment of inertia, and thus a more rigid implant, leads to lower tensile and compressive stresses in the cement. Modification of the modulus of elasticity of the material can also influence stem stiffness. Stem stiffness can be reduced by incorporating lower modulus alloys such as titanium rather than stainless steel or cobalt-chromium. Reduction in stem stiffness can lead to marked increases in strain in the cement mantle with a noncollared, cemented stem.[4] The lower modulus material leads to reduction in stem stresses and small improvements in calcar bone stresses (30 versus 16 percent of normal). However, these effects occur at the expense of greater (38 percent) cement stresses proximally. Distal cement stresses are reduced somewhat at the same time. Inclusion of a calcar collar changes these results, as discussed subsequently. Nonetheless, a titanium stem with a calcar collar still results in 20 percent more cement stress.

The analytic and clinical data make a strong case for designs that include a rel-

Text continued on page 198

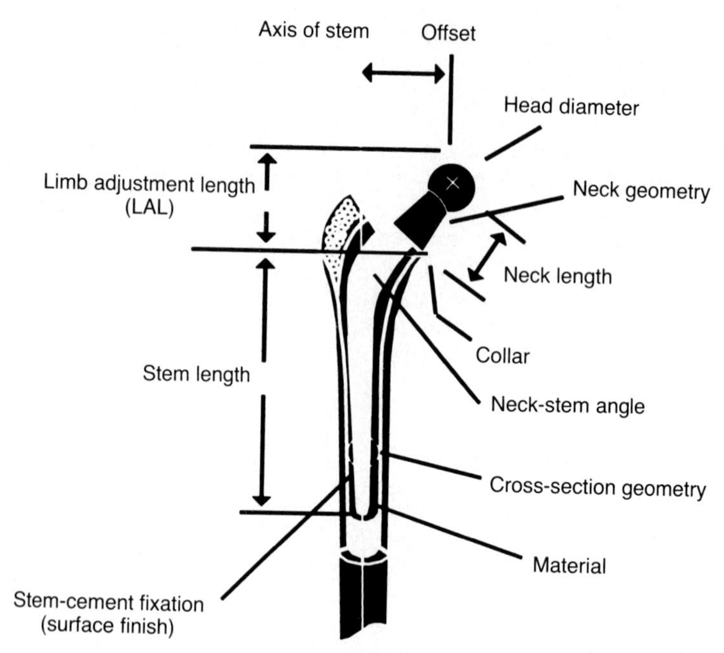

FIGURE 13–4. The many variables in the design of the modern femoral component of the total hip replacement.

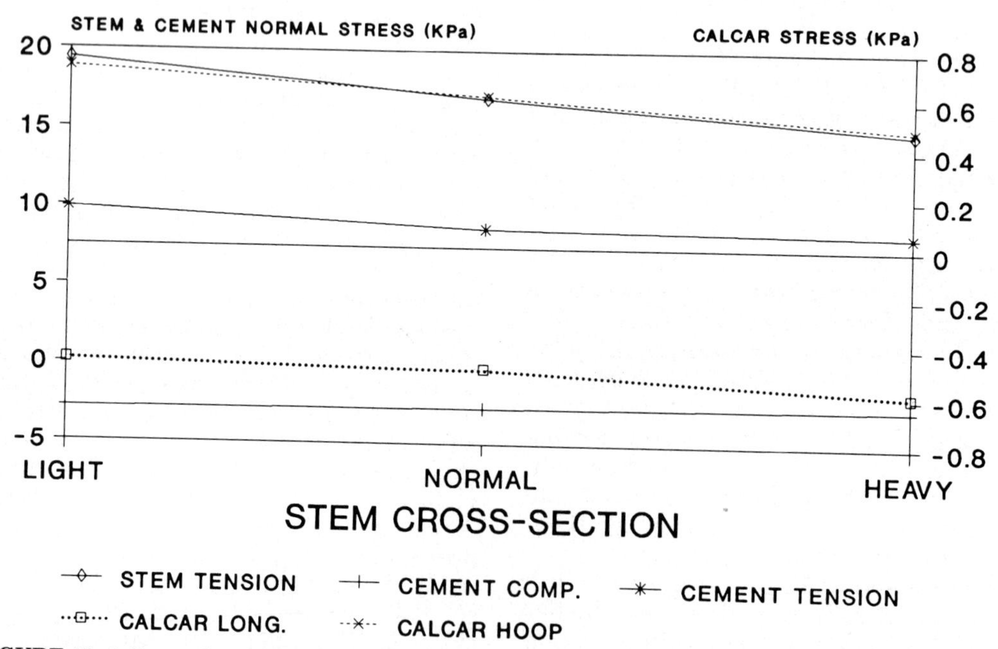

FIGURE 13–5. Femoral stem and cement normal stresses and calcar stress as a function of stem cross-section. (Adapted from Crowninshield, R.D., Brand, R.A., Johnston, R.C., and Milroy, J.C.: J. Bone Joint Surg. 62-A: 68–78, 1980.)

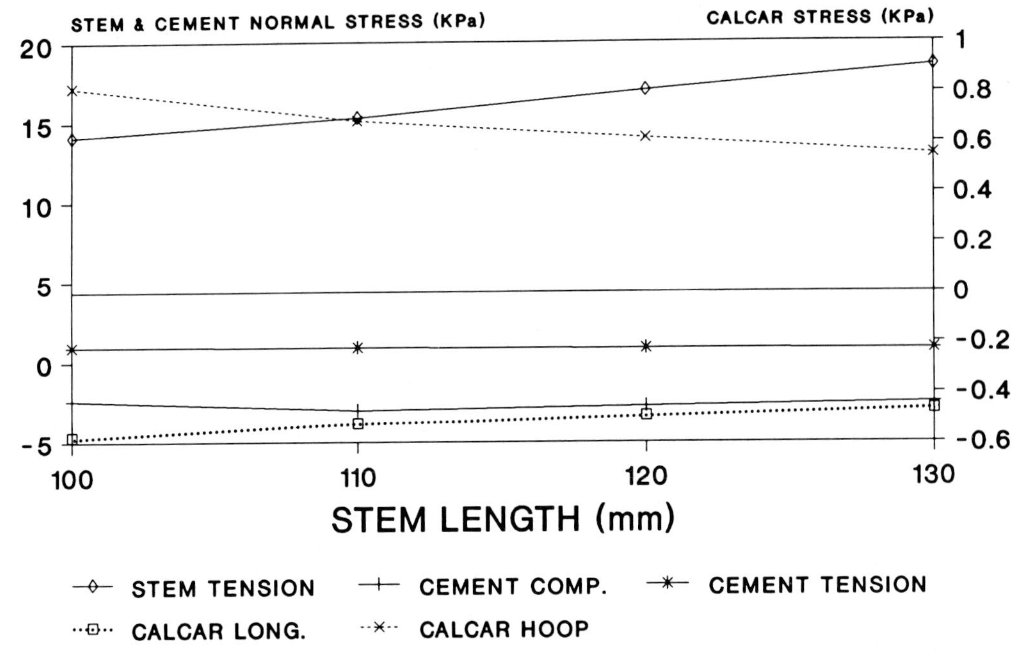

FIGURE 13–6. Stem and cement normal stresses and calcar stress as a function of stem length from 100 to 130 mm. (Adapted from Crowninshield, R.D., Brand, R.A., Johnston, R.C., and Milroy, J.C.: J. Bone Joint Surg. 62-A: 68–78, 1980.)

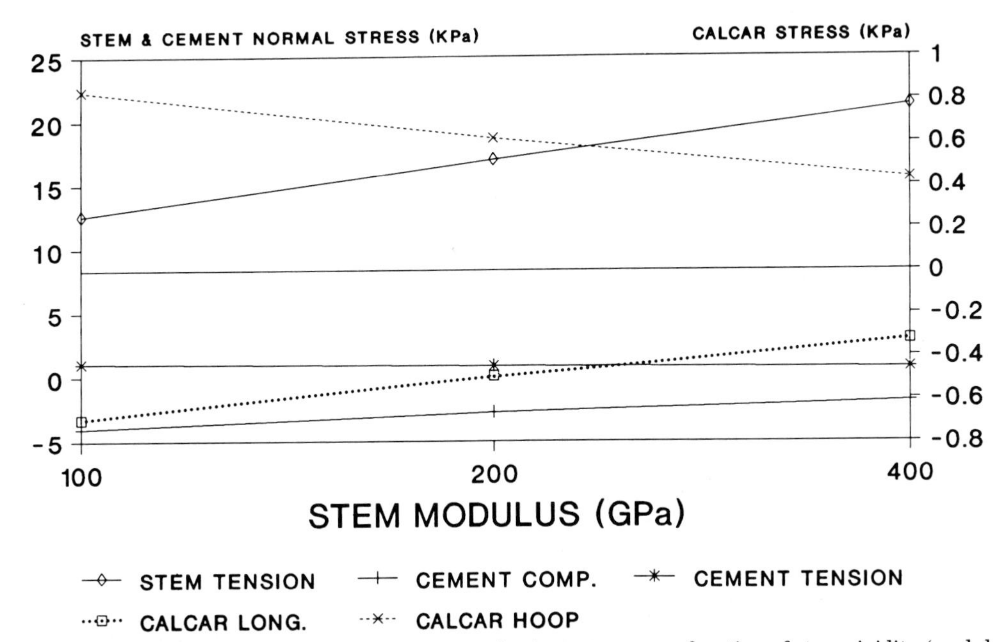

FIGURE 13–7. Stem and cement normal stresses and calcar stress as a function of stem rigidity (modulus of elasticity). (Adapted from Crowninshield, R.D., Brand, R.A., Johnston, R.C., and Milroy, J.C.: J. Bone Joint Surg. 62-A: 68–78, 1980.)

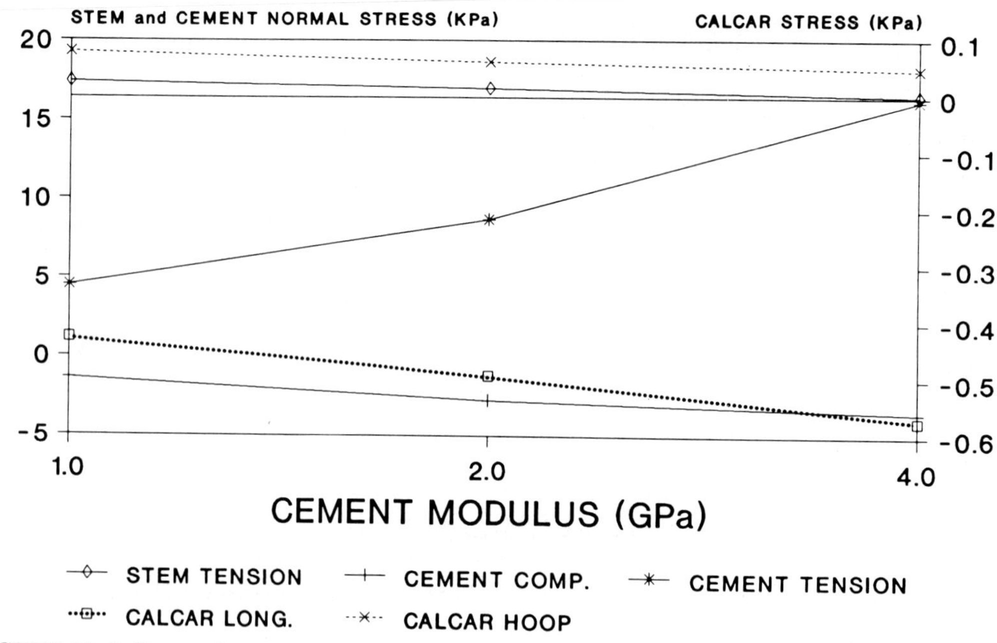

FIGURE 13–8. Stem and cement normal stresses and calcar stress as a function of the modulus of elasticity of polymethyl methacrylate bone cement. (Adapted from Crowninshield, R.D., Brand, R.A., Johnston, R.C., and Milroy, J.C.: J. Bone Joint Surg. 62-A: 68–78, 1980.)

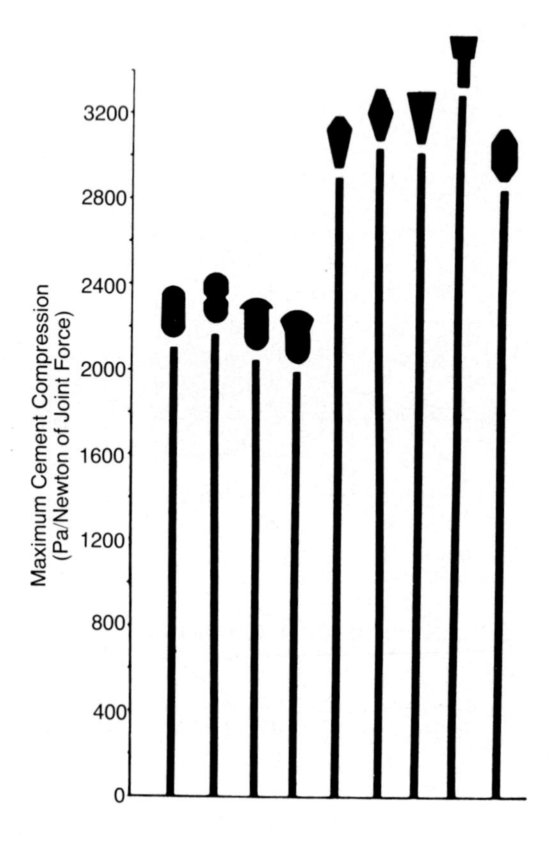

FIGURE 13–9. The effect of shape on maximum compressive stresses seen in bone cement (stress per unit joint force). (Crowninshield, R. D., Brand, R. A., Johnston, R. C., and Milroy, B. S.: Clin. Orthop. 146: 71–77, 1980. By permission.)

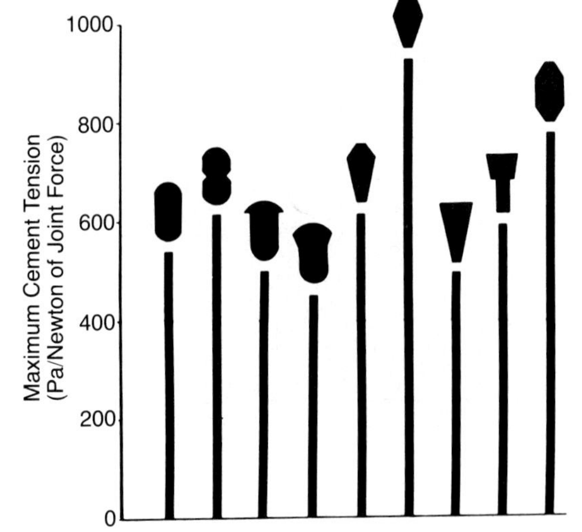

FIGURE 13–10. The effect of shape on maximum tensile stresses seen in bone cement (stress per unit joint force). (Redrawn from Crowninshield, R. D., Brand, R. A., Johnston, R. C., and Milroy, B. S.: Clin. Orthop. 146: 71–77, 1980.)

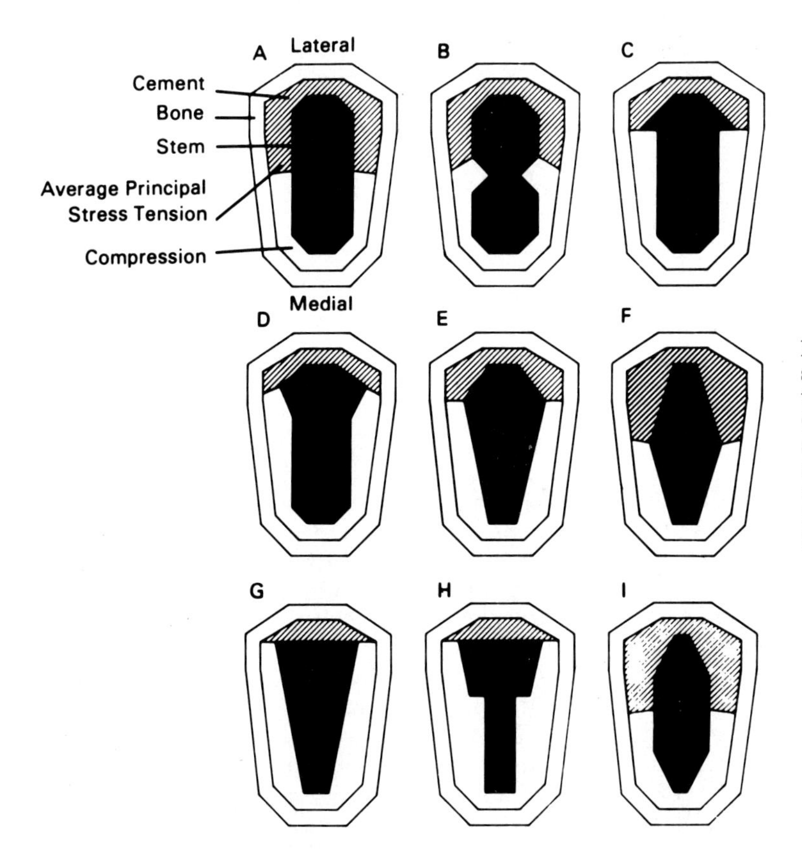

FIGURE 13–11. The effect of stem shape on distribution of tensile bone cement stress (cross-hatch) and compressive stress (unshaded). (Crowninshield, R. D., Brand, R. A., Johnston, R. C., and Milroy, B. S.: Clin. Orthop. 146: 71–77, 1980. By permission.)

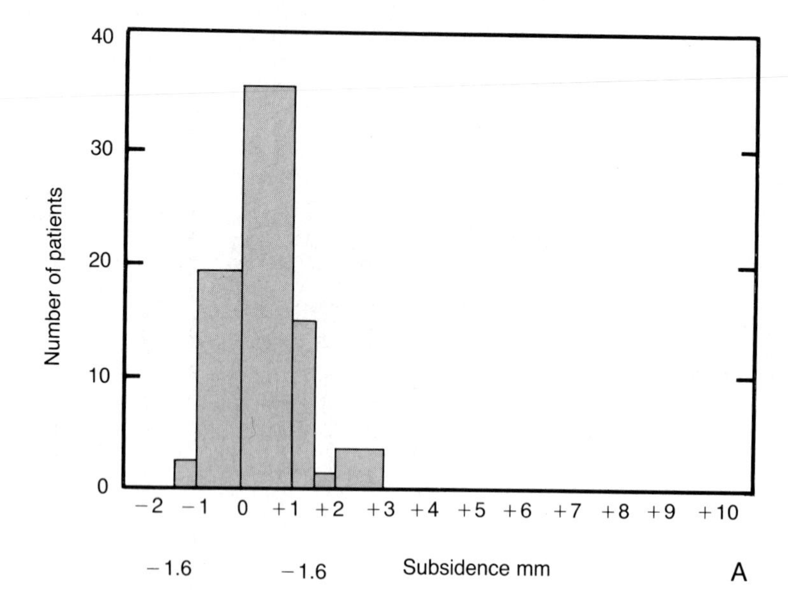

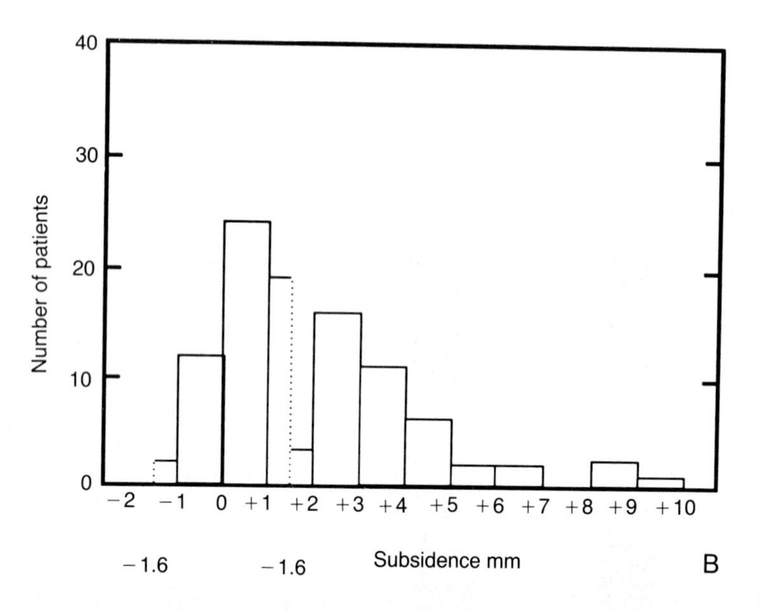

FIGURE 13–12. The effect of a lateral flange on subsidence. *A,* The majority of patients with a prosthesis with a lateral flange have subsidence ranging from −1.5 mm to +1.5 mm. *B,* Most of those without a flange have subsidence ranging from −1.5 mm to +5 mm. (Redrawn from Loudon, J. R. and Charnley, J.: J. Bone Joint Surg. 62-B: 450–453, 1980.)

atively rigid stem based on both geometry and material. Also favored are a lateral ridge or flange, a cement groove along the center of the proximal stem, and a relatively soft or blunt edge. Designs that maintain proximal cement integrity perform best. The size of the medullary canal imposes limits on the overall size of the cement-stem complex. Implants of sufficient size are necessary to maintain strength, yet as stem size gets larger, the cement mantle must be sacrificed. Decreasing the thickness of the PMMA allows more bony support and thus less stem stress with better bone stress distribution, but this thickness must be adequate to create a uniform mantle that maintains the cement's mechanical integrity.[2, 71] A 2- to 4-mm mantle of cement is necessary to prevent cement fragmentation under load while balancing stem stresses. This mantle is especially needed in the critical middle third of the stem.[2, 54]

Thinner cement mantles lead to significantly higher cement stresses, although stem stresses decrease somewhat. Cement thickness also affects prosthesis-cement interfacial stresses. Thin cement layers (2 mm or less) and excessively thick layers (greater than 4 mm) lead to high interfa-

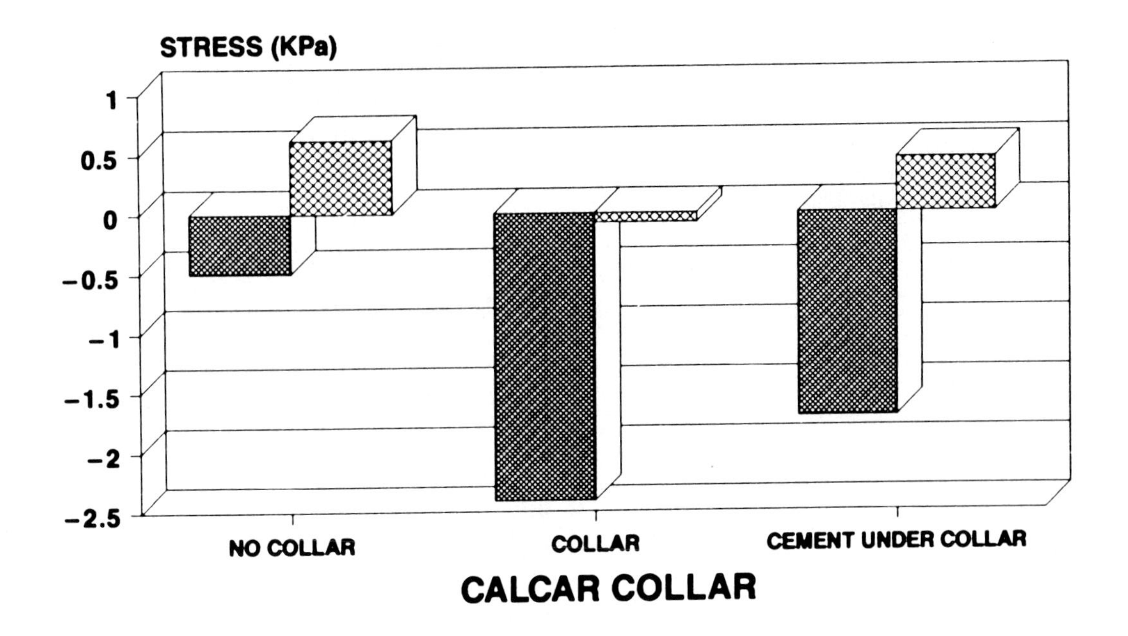

FIGURE 13–13. The effect of a calcar prosthetic collar on both calcar longitudinal and calcar hoop stresses. (Adapted from Crowninshield, R.D., Brand, R.A., Johnston, R.C., and Milroy, J.C.: J. Bone Joint Surg. 62-A: 68–78, 1980.)

cial stresses, which could cause debonding and cement fractures and thus stem loosening. Thus, a 2- to 4-mm cement mantle would appear to balance stem size and cement thickness and to create a reliable reconstruction for hip arthroplasty. Various clinical reports confirm these analytic findings.[26]

Polymethyl methacrylate is a relatively brittle material that performs better in compression than in tension. When cement is not loaded above its ultimate tensile or compressive strength, fatigue may be the dominant mode of failure. The fatigue properties of PMMA are poor, and cement failure occurs if applied cyclic stresses are not minimized.

Calcar Collar

A calcar collar to decrease stresses in the cement and stem and to return the femur to a more normal strain pattern has been the subject of considerable debate. Rand and Ilstrup,[77] in their clinical study of 80 patients with and without collared prostheses, found no advantage to the collar on a T–28 prosthesis in terms of resorption or subsidence. However, the groups of both Collier[16] and Oh[72] showed that a collar restored 30 to 40 percent of the normal calcar strain and shifted the strain pattern toward a more normal distribution. Additionally, larger and stiffer collared stems did not adversely affect strains in proximal femurs.

Design features cannot be considered independently. Stresses are affected by the collar, but these effects are highly dependent on overall implant design. Both the magnitude and direction of stresses are important. Normal medial proximal femoral stresses are longitudinal. In those stems without medial collars, stresses in the proximal femurs are predominantly hoop or circumferential—only small longitudinal stresses are present (Fig. 13–13). These compressive longitudinal stresses are greater with decreases in stem length or with increases in stem cross-section or cement modulus.[20] When a collar is added, longitudinal stresses on the bone are increased greatly, but they still remain below those predicted for the intact femur. The hoop stresses that result from wedging of the uncollared prosthesis are reduced with the addition of a calcar collar (Fig. 13–13).

Decreases in stem subsidence and prevention of cement fracture are advantages of stems with collars.[58] Collar size is important. Should the collar be too narrow or too small, contact is difficult to achieve and contact stresses are high. Broader collars provide more contact area and greater support, thereby reducing subsidence. It is often difficult to achieve and maintain good surface-to-surface contact.[60] Manufacturers have begun to provide calcar planers as part of the implantation instrumentation. With these tools, the surfaces can be prepared to achieve better appositions.

Surface Finish

Maintaining the integrity of the interfaces in the bone-cement-implant construct is important to achieve good load-carrying capabilities and to prevent failures. Enhancement of cement bonding to the stem can reduce cement failure. Manley and coworkers[58] found a sixfold increase in subsidence when a smooth stem surface was utilized instead of a roughened surface. *In vitro* experiments by Bundy and Penn[11] confirm these findings and indicate that grit-blasted or highly polished and cleaned surfaces result in much improved load-carrying capacity. These very clean surfaces are difficult to maintain in the operating room environment, however. Some manufacturers have placed a coating of PMMA on the surface of the component, which may help the cement bond. Titanium generally is less able to sustain interfacial loading than the cobalt-chromium alloys and stainless steels.[11] Porous-coated (beaded) and flame-sprayed surfaces exhibit much improved interfacial load-carrying capacity.[18] Interfacial shear strength may rise more than fourfold when cement is bonded to porous surfaces compared with the strength of satin-finished samples. A larger pore size further enhances the strength of the bond.

For these aforementioned coating methods, the stem must be heated or thermally cycled. When these coatings are placed on forged cobalt-chromium prostheses, mechanical properties of the substrate may be lost, negating the advantages of coating. Titanium alloys are not only affected by the heating but are also susceptible to changes in surface texture (notch sensitivity) when treated with coatings. Thus, a grit-blasted surface would appear to be the most appropriate method of enhancement to improve cement adhesion.

Cemented Acetabular Components

Acetabular Component Design

The original ultrahigh molecular weight polyethylene acetabular component conceived by Charnley for cemented use has evolved in an attempt to reduce the late-onset loosening. Several design elements bear scrutiny in relation to the wear, the plastic flow or creep of the component, the fixation of the component employing PMMA, and the component failure.

Historically, Charnley's employment of the 22-mm diameter prosthetic head was predicated on two issues: reduction in the frictional torques generated under load and adequate polyethylene thickness so that sufficient material would be available if wear should occur.[14] Wear has not been a problem, except with components constructed of polyethylene of insufficient molecular weight (Fig. 13–14) and with devices that have additional debris in the articulating surfaces, which leads to "third-body" wear of the polymer.[25, 39, 82, 87] It is important to note, however, that total hip arthroplasty has been performed in a relatively old population. With more treatment of younger individuals, who are more active and have greater life expectancies, long-term wear may become more problematic.

Surface finish of both the head and polyethylene contributes to the low wear rates. Highly polished femoral head components are requisite and may be achieved with both cobalt-chromium and titanium alloy heads, although other problems with the latter could make its use as an articulating surface questionable.[30] The ability to polish high-density aluminum oxide to a very fine surface finish and congruity makes it a candidate for femoral head application. This topic is discussed further in this chapter.

Because PMMA is not an adhesive but a grouting material dependent on mechanical interlock, the surface configuration of the acetabular component must be relied on to improve the cement bond. Grooves and spacer pods enhance fixation. No statistical differences in fixation integrity are seen with variations of groove depth, although undercutting of the groove itself may improve performance.[70] Deep grooves are unnecessary and may be detrimental. With deeply grooved polyethylene components, the wall thickness of the component decreases and a stress riser is created in the polyethylene. Both conditions add to stress in the polyethylene. The result may be increased creep of the material, leading to loss of congruity, loosening, or frank failure of the polyethylene.[83, 93] Integral pods at the surface further improve the torque-carrying capability of the acebabular component and aid in centralization, thus creating a more uniform cement mantle. However, these protrusions are not incorporated into the cement and so may create a cement void, which would be interpreted as a stress concentration in the cement mantle. This problem is alleviated by PMMA spacers, which are mounted to the surface of the component and incorporated directly into the cement mantle during polymerization.

Achievement of a uniform mantle of cement is of great importance for maintaining appropriate stress levels in the cement, at the interface, and within the bone.[69, 71, 75, 76] The creation of a flange equal in size to the diameter of the reamed hole and the included diameter of the pods or spacers helps achieve this centralization. The flange also helps pressurize the cement, making for better cement penetration.[70]

Finite element analysis has been used to assess the importance of polyethylene thickness in relation to stresses.[74] Thin walls increase maximum stresses in the polyethylene and in the cement-bone composites. Conversely, thicker polyethylene reduces the stresses.

Metal Backing

A major advance in design of cemented acetabular components has been the addition of metal backing to the polyethylene acetabular component. Several *in vivo* and *in vitro* reports detail the advantages of metal backing for improving the cement and bone stress distribution.[13, 41, 62, 69, 74, 89, 90] Finite element analyses and strain gauge investigations of pelves *in vitro* have shown that the stress distribution is significantly altered after reaming of the subchondral bone and insertion of a standard polyethylene acetabular component. Additionally, high peak stresses are observed in both the cement and the component itself. Thickening the components eases these problems somewhat, but metal backing on the polyethylene is the most expeditious way to return the medial pelvic wall to a more normal stress state while decreasing cement stresses. The metal-backed component-cement construct must not be excessively rigid, as this may dis-

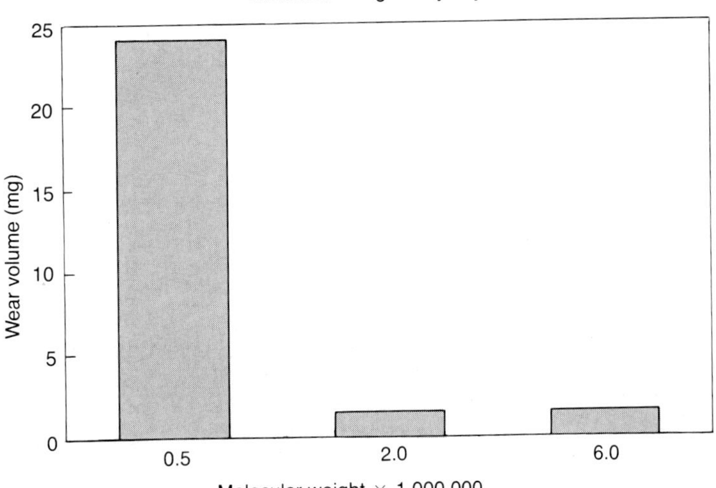

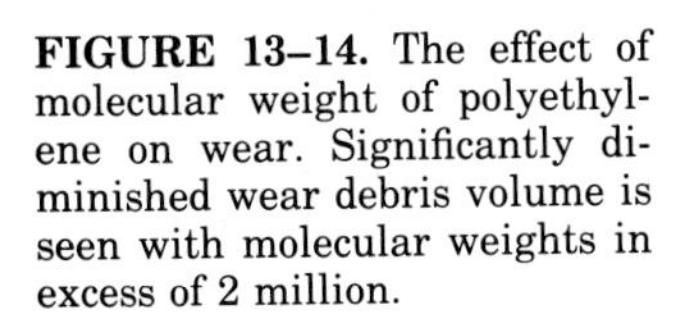
FIGURE 13–14. The effect of molecular weight of polyethylene on wear. Significantly diminished wear debris volume is seen with molecular weights in excess of 2 million.

turb the return to more normal strain patterns.[62] If the metal backing is too thin, e.g., thin titanium, an overly compliant cup will lead to a situation not unlike an unbacked polyethylene component with its large pelvic strain increase.

Many reports point out the importance of concentric component placement to minimize cement stress and appropriately distribute bone stress. The use of PMMA spacers on the surface of the component can help achieve these goals. Concentric placement and 3 to 4 mm of cement achieve adequate fixation and stress distribution while maintaining reconstruction (Fig. 13–15).[71]

The surface texture of the metal-backed acetabular component is important as well. The addition of grit blasting or porous coating, as noted in the discussion of the femoral stem, enhances cement-component bonding. Flame-sprayed surfaces have been shown to improve the interfacial bonding of the cement.[24] Addition of circumferential ridges to the metal shell also improves fixation.

PROSTHESES INTENDED FOR NONCEMENTED USE

Femoral Component Design

Design of noncemented femoral components, although similar in some ways to design of cemented components, must meet requirements for biologic ingrowth and stabilization. These constructs depend heavily on the biologic activity of the host bone and highly stable initial fixation to allow maturation of osseous integration.

Femoral Component Geometry

The geometric properties of the femoral stem design have been evaluated extensively.[66] The exact femoral geometry is probably impossible to predict, and the surgeon should expect line-to-line or surface-to-surface contact only at discrete locations.

Cement reduces the number of sizes and shapes required because of its space-filling character. This is not the case for press-fit biologic ingrowth. Noble and associates[66] and Kamaric and associates[53] maintain that a proportional relationship between the shape and size of the medullary canal does not exist. Design based on an average canal size, proportionally scaled for larger or smaller canals in the anatomic range, is therefore not possible. Optimal proximal canal fit, important for successful press-fit arthroplasty, should be based on the proximal canal geometry not on the isthmus diameter. Compared with cemented devices, press-fit components must be relatively wider proximally for a given distal isthmus diameter. Thus, a stem designed for a cemented application would not be expected to function well in a noncemented application.

The goal in press-fit arthroplasty is to achieve large areas of contact between implant and bone. This can be accomplished either through exact reproduction of the existing canal or through instrumentation to prepare the proximal femur and canal so that they adequately and accurately match the stem to be inserted. Although the exact extent of implant-bone contact required to maintain stable fixation remains unsettled, the need for accurate fit has been well-documented. Jasty and coworkers[48–51] found that with accurate fit, 70 to 90 percent of normal proximal strains could be regained. Loss of fit, however, can lead to excessive stresses in both the bone and stem. Tightness of fit and accuracy of fit are not to be confused.[35, 50] An initially tight prosthesis may have a poor fit with little contact area.

Instrumentation and bone preparation are critical to the success of noncemented components. Although fit can in theory be improved significantly through custom prostheses based on computerized tomographic imaging, much of the advantage may be lost when preparing the canal for insertion of the stem.[81] The creation of a more standardized set of stems carefully matched to instrumentation may obviate the problem.

Currently, femoral components have either a curved stem or a straight stem configuration. The goal of the curved design is to match the anatomy of the proximal femur, thereby maximizing surface contact. A straight-stemmed component requires instrumentation to prepare the cavity to yield several points or areas of contact. Although each stem design has theoretic advantages, neither has been

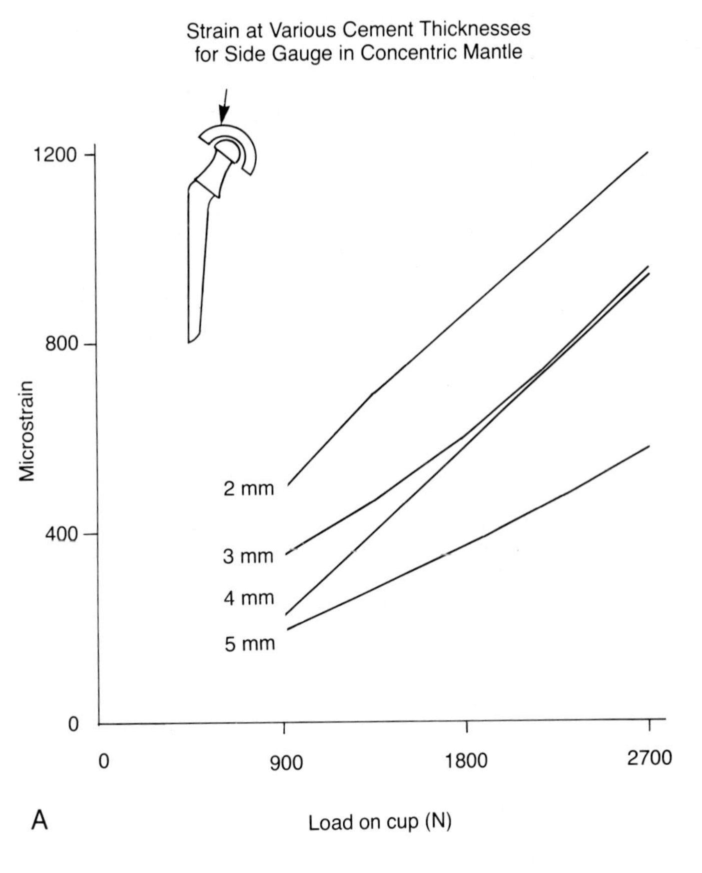

FIGURE 13–15. Strain comparisons as a function of cement thickness and concentricity of implant placement. *A*, Increases in concentric cement thickness lead to decreases in stress. *B*, Nonconcentric placement negates the improvement seen at the side.

Illustration continued on following page

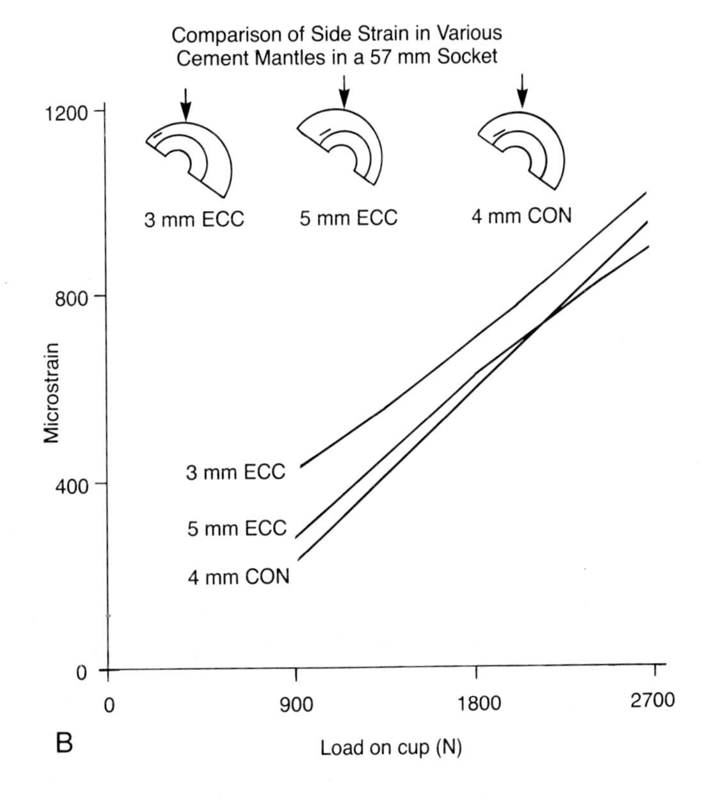

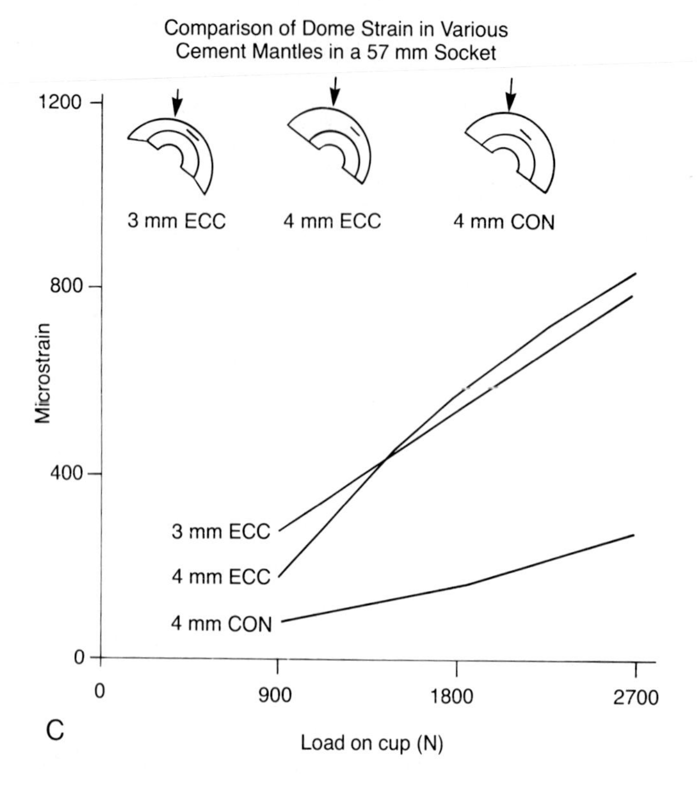

FIGURE 13–15 *Continued C,* Eccentric placement also negates improvement at the dome. (ECC = eccentric placement; CON = concentric placement.) (Oh, I., Treharne, R. W., Sanders, T. W.: Trans. Biomat. 6:95, 1983. By permission.)

shown to be superior with regard to quality of fit, reinforcing the difficulty of matching this complex geometry. The straight stem does have one advantage: right and left stems do not need to be manufactured if the neck is not anteverted.

Jasty and colleagues[49] have shown that excessive hoop stresses are produced during insertion of noncemented stems when geometry is not appropriately matched. Poor performance and excessive subsidence attributable to mismatch in implant sizes have been found.[27, 40, 66, 84] In addition to longitudinal subsidence or micromotion, rotation due to torsional loads has been found to be a problem with noncemented components. Burke and colleagues[12] reported a tenfold increase in motion in noncemented components due to out-of-plane torques. Stem design must include features to inhibit rotation.[42] Stems that engage the cortex (e.g., those with rectangular or trapezoidal cross-sections) would be more suitable for noncemented application because they block rotation. Stems with more circular designs may cause problems unless additional design features block rotation.

Calcar Collar

In proximally coated stems without calcar collars, simulated ingrowth results in little change in bone strain. The proximal shape creates a "wedging" effect, and transverse hoop stresses are then generated to help maintain stable fixation. The inclusion of a collar in the design causes load bearing on the medial bone, resulting in more longitudinal stress in this region. When ingrowth and collar are simulated in a computer model, stresses approach normal.[91] Without a collar, motion of 100 μm or more may be seen, which may inhibit ingrowth. This motion can be reduced with a well-fitting collared device.

The research of Whiteside and associates[94] indicated that collared devices have less subsidence and increased load to failure. They argued further that collarless implants cannot be relied on to tighten under load and that "Improved rigidity of fixation and increased strength achieved by seating on the collar are distinct advantages for pain control and biological fixation of non-cemented femoral components."

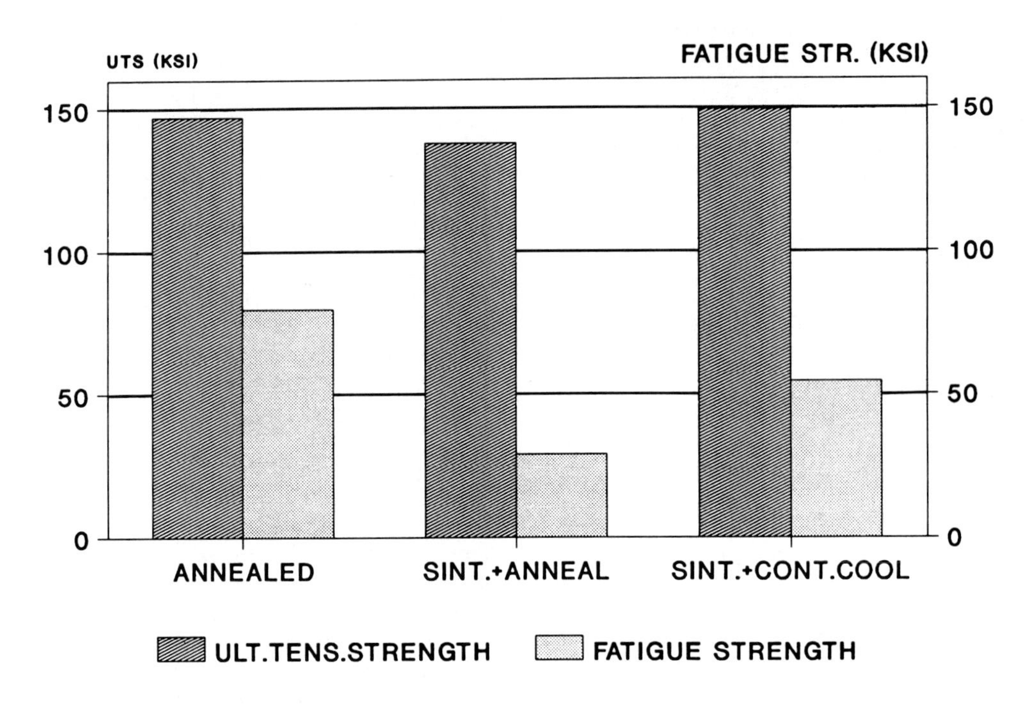

FIGURE 13–16. The effect of heat treatment of Ti-6Al-4V alloy and application of porous coating on ultimate strength and fatigue strength.

Materials for Noncemented Stems

Material selection is important to the design of the noncemented stem. The biocompatability and strength of cobalt-chromium and titanium suggest these materials as candidates for noncemented applications. Unfortunately, the heat treatment process for applying porous surfaces has a pronounced effect on the mechanical properties of these materials, which can have serious consequences, especially in femoral stems with high applied loads. With titanium alloys, a 34 percent decrease in fatigue strength occurs from heat treatment alone, and a 77 percent decrease in strength occurs from application of the porous material, owing to notch sensitivity (Fig. 13–16).[36, 78] Reduction in strength is seen with cobalt-chromium alloys as well, although they are not as notch sensitive as the titanium alloys (Fig. 13–17). Postsintering heat treatments have been suggested, which improve the positive properties somewhat due to subtle changes in the microstructure.[1, 36, 78]

The optimal structure of the porous coating has received considerable attention.[7, 27, 46] Much of the *in vivo* work related to biologic ingrowth into cobalt-chromium surfaces shows that bone responds similarly to pore sizes ranging from 50 μm to 400 μm when ingrowth rate, tissue maturity, and interfacial strength are considered. A layer two to three beads thick has proved to be best for overall coating integrity and ingrowth.[8] Maintenance of the mechanical integrity of the porous-coated surface itself is of great importance.[57] Implant surface contour or bead recess pockets lead to substantial increases—54 percent—in the fatigue strength of the coating. Crimped titanium fiber mesh has also been successful as a porous surface for biologic ingrowth.[51] Animal studies show excellent ingrowth of bone into these structures.[32, 33, 88]

In its early use, porous coating was placed on the entire stem surface, and problems ensued. In Engh and Bobyn's[28] review of their first 411 cases, significant femoral resorption took place in fully coated stems. With rigid cobalt-chromium components, stems greater than or equal to 13.5 mm in diameter have a fivefold increase in resorption compared with stems 12.5 mm or less in diameter. Resorption is increased two to four times in stems with two-thirds and full coating, owing to more distal load transfers. These findings suggest that less rigid devices with one-third proximal coating would result in a stable construct that would supply sufficient ingrowth.

Resorption in the area of the coating still occurs with stems with one-third proximal coating, but it appears to be nonprogressive. These results also suggest that flexural rigidity of the stem is important to the performance of these devices. Lower modulus materials, such as titanium alloys that make a more flexible stem, may have advantages for biologic ingrowth prostheses.

Another consideration in porous coating is the stem stability immediately after implantation. The design must provide a stable reconstruction in the immediate postoperative phase for ingrowth to occur.

Noncemented Acetabular Components

Noncemented metal-backed acetabular components, both with and without porous surfaces, have gained great popularity. These include components that are threaded directly into the reamed acetabulum and those press-fit or fixed with bone screws.

Threaded-cup acetabuloplasty is associated with a high incidence of loosening and problems in maintaining fixation. Disadvantages of these components appear to negate potential advantages.[3, 29] *In vivo* and *in vitro* investigations show these devices to be very rigid, to develop very high stresses at the thread-bone interface, and to create high medial wall strains during insertion.[29, 38, 45, 80]

Press-fit and screw-fixed metal-backed shells have performed well over the short term.[86] Geometries that achieve good bone apposition have been shown to be important in *in vivo* animal studies.[15] Jasty and colleagues[48] reported that to achieve adequate bone ingrowth, the design must allow intimate bone-implant contact—12.5 percent bone ingrowth was observed with intimate contact and 7 percent without.[48] Utilization of an oversized shell to achieve intimate contact may be a problem, based on evidence of high pelvic stresses following insertion of screw-in acetabular com-

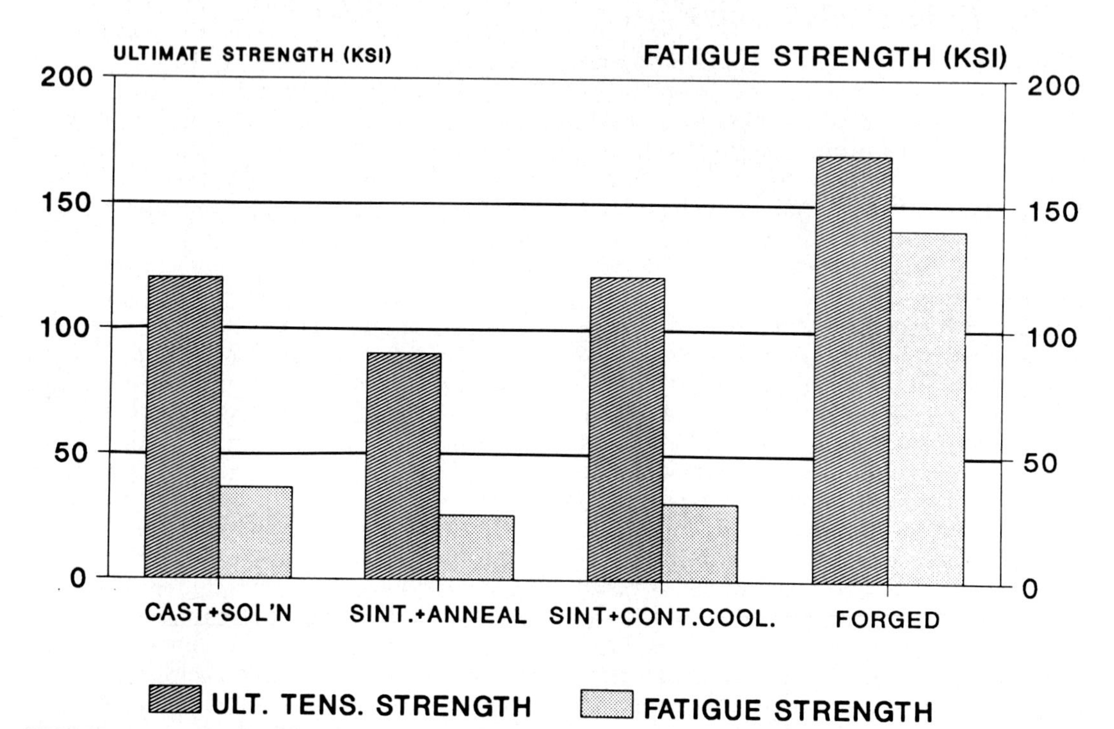

FIGURE 13–17. The effect of heat treatment of Co-Cr-Mo alloy and application of porous coating on ultimate strength and fatigue strength. (Cast + sol'n = as cast with solution annealing; sint. + anneal = sintered plus solution anneal; sint + cont.cool. = sintered plus controlled cooling.)

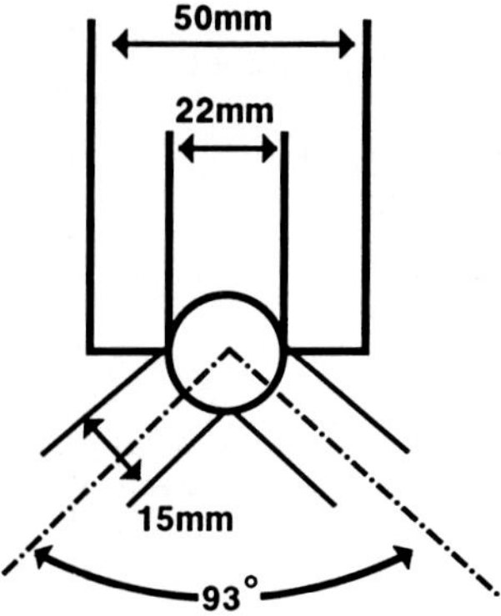

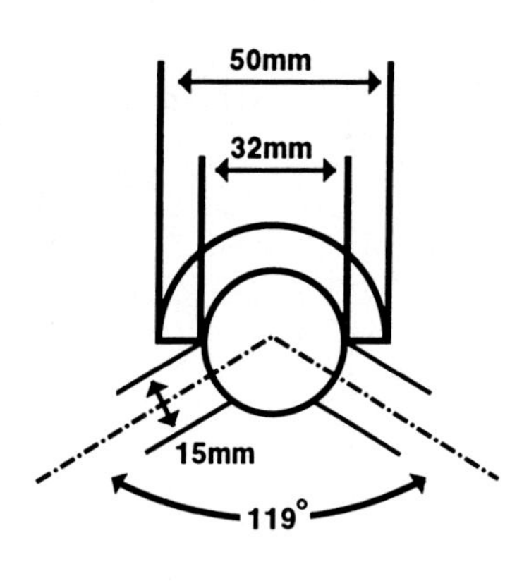

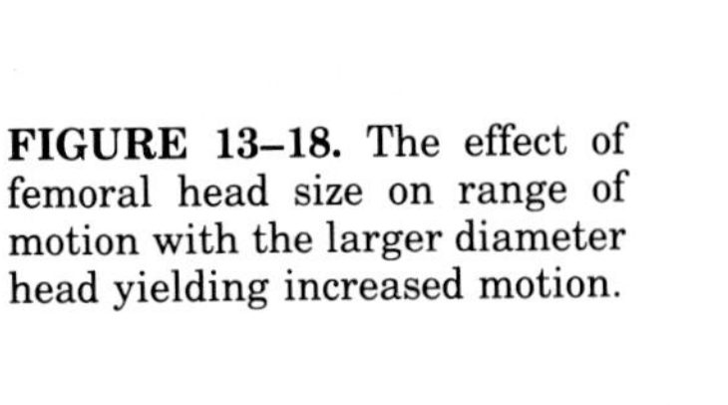
FIGURE 13–18. The effect of femoral head size on range of motion with the larger diameter head yielding increased motion.

ponents. Addition of either peripheral or central bone screws to achieve initial fixation appears to be a more sound choice.[40] Those acetabular devices with recesses for bead placement are less prone to bead loss during implant placement.

FEMORAL HEAD

Although total hip arthroplasty is billed as low friction, a reciprocating frictional torque or moment occurs when the femoral head articulates with the ultrahigh molecular weight polyethylene of the acetabular component. This torque and ensuing wear are governed by the geometry and the material of the femoral head as well as the acetabular component.

Geometry

In his early work, Charnley[14] placed the utmost importance on minimizing the attendant frictional torque. His concerns have been championed by others who believe that larger-diameter femoral heads lead to increased loosening due to higher friction.[15, 64] Thus, the earliest femoral heads were of small diameter, 22 mm, to create a device with minimum friction.[22, 37] When these femoral heads were coupled with the large external diameters of the acetabular components, the torque necessary to maintain stability at the bone-cement interface would be minimized, although still appreciable. A larger femoral head reduces contact stresses and also minimizes the problems with dislocation and increased range of motion (Fig. 13–18). Some researchers believe, however, that wear debris might be the major cause of loosening.[63, 79] Development of the total hip arthroplasty has come to a compromise in an attempt to minimize the friction and wear phonomena. Not only are 22-mm and 32-mm femoral heads available, but so are intermediate 26-mm and 28-mm heads.

Material Properties

Several materials are available for femoral head components. They include the cobalt-chromium alloys, titanium alloys, and ceramics. The majority of the implants currently being employed have cobalt-chromium prosthetic heads of either forged or cast material and Morse taper attachments to the stems.

Figure 13–19 details the effects of the head material and size in relation to the frictional moment or torque. The cobalt-chrome head yields lower torque values than all the other metals cited. However, the ceramic material—aluminum oxide and zirconium oxide—lead to even lower frictional moments and, therefore, lower wear rates. These ceramic materials are currently receiving considerable attention for orthopaedic applications. Caution must be exercised in controlling the Morse taper configuration, purity, and overall quality so that this extremely brittle material does not fail prematurely because of mechanical or material factors.

Titanium has proved to be a poor performer as an articulating surface. At the present time, titanium should be reserved for structural elements but not for a head-bearing surface against ultrahigh molecular weight polyethylene.[6, 43, 55] Ion implantation has been suggested to protect the

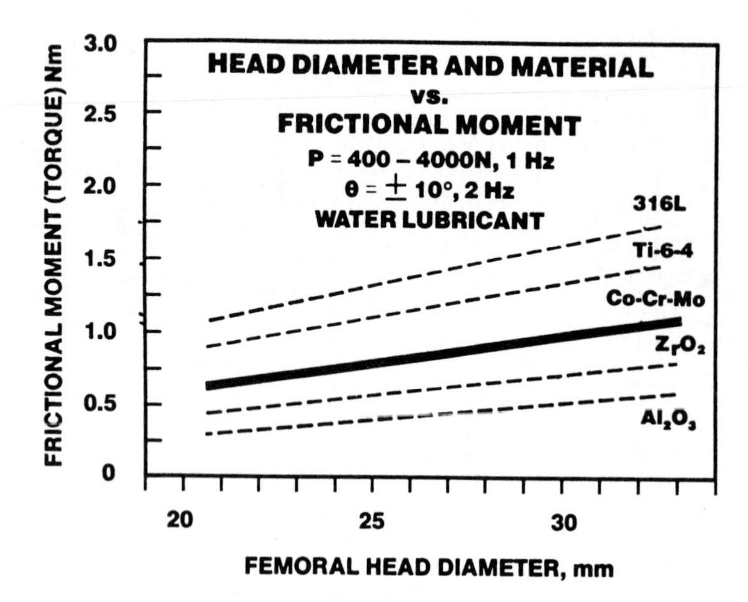

FIGURE 13–19. The effects of femoral head diameter and material on the frictional moment or torque (Davidson, J. A. and Brasher, T.: Technical Memo OR–90–13: Smith and Nephew Richards, Inc., Memphis, Feb., 1990. By permission.)

titanium-articulating surface, but such surface treatment may not provide sufficient long-term protection.[23] The adequate performances of cobalt-chromium, which may be mated with a titanium stem, and of ceramic appear to make them the materials of choice for the femoral head.

THE FUTURE

Materials and designs of components of total hip arthroplasties will continue to evolve. Major thrusts for the coming decade will involve optimization of the noncemented, press-fit prosthesis, with or without porous coating, for orthopaedic reconstruction. New designs will attempt to model the inherent rigidity of the proximal femur more adequately so that bone resorption will not be a problem. These are already being seen in devices being developed in Europe, in which the geometry significantly reduces the flexural rigidity of the femoral stem components. The development of bioactive coatings is focusing on rapid and long-term incorporation or fixation of the devices so that they may perform harmoniously with survival times greater than 25 years. Development of ultrahigh molecular weight polyethylene is also continuing in an attempt to further enhance mechanical properties and, therefore, reduce wear rates.

References

1. Anderson, R. C., Cook, S. D., Thongpreda, N., and Haddad, R. J.: Post-sintering heat treatments to improve the mechanical properties of Ti–6A1–4V alloy. Trans. Biomat. 12:39, 1986.
2. Andriacchi, T. P., Galante, J. O., Belytschko, T. B., and Hampton, S.: A stress analysis of the femoral stem in total hip prostheses. J. Bone Joint Surg. 58A:618–624, 1976.
3. Apel, D. M., Smith D. G., Schwartz, C. M., and Paprosky, W. G.: Threaded cup acetabuloplasty. Clin. Orthop. 241:183–189, 1989.
4. Beals, N B., Davidson, J. A., and Maddox, R. L.: Influence of stem stiffness on cement mantle strains. Trans. Biomat. 15:213, 1989.
5. Beckenbaugh, R. D. and Ilstrup, D. M.: Total hip arthroplasty. J. Bone Joint Surg. 60A:306–312, 1978.
6. Black, J., Sherk, H., Bonini, J., et al: Metallosis associated with a stable titanium-alloy femoral component in total hip replacement. J. Bone Joint Surg. 72A:126–130, 1990.
7. Bobyn, J. D., Pilliar, R. M., Cameron, H. U., and Weatherly, G. C.: The optimum pore size for the fixation of porous-surfaced metal implants by the ingrowth of bone. Clin. Orthop. 150:263–270, 1980.
8. Bobyn, J. D., Pilliar, R. M., Cameron, H. U., et al: The effect of porous surface configuration on the tensile strength of fixation of implants by bone ingrowth. Clin. Orthop. 149:291–298, 1980.
9. Bombelli, R.: Osteoarthritis of the Hip. Berlin, Springer-Verlag, 1976.
10. Bourne, R. B., Oh, I., and Harris, W. H.: Femoral cement pressurization during total hip arthroplasty. Clin. Orthop. 183:12–16, 1984.
11. Bundy, K. J. and Penn, R. W.: The influence of surface preparation on the strength of the metal/bone cement interface. Trans. Biomat. 9:124, 1983.
12. Burke, D. W., O'Conner, D. O., Zalenski, E. B., et al: Biomechanics of femoral total hip compo-

nents in simulated stair climbing. Trans. O.R.S. 34:345, 1988.
13. Carter, D. R., Vasu, R., and Harris, W. H.: Stress distribution in the acetabular region. II. Effects of cement thickness and metal backing of the total hip acetabular component. J. Biomechanics 15:165–170, 1982.
14. Charnley, J.: Arthroplasty of the hip, a new operation. Lancet 1:1129, 1961.
15. Clarke, I. D.: Advances in Biomaterials. Edited by S. M. Lee, Lancaster, PA, Technomic Publ., 1987.
16. Collier, J. P., Kennedy, F., Mayor, M., et al: The importance of stem geometry, porous coating, and collar angle of femoral hip prostheses on the stress distribution in the human femur. Trans. Biomat. 9:96, 1983.
17. Collier, J. P., Orr, T., and Kennedy, F.: Saggital plane strain-gauge analysis of the femur before and after prosthetic hip implantation. Trans. Biomat. 10:317, 1984.
18. Cook, S. D., Thongpreda, N., Anderson, R. C., et al: Optimum pore size for bone cement fixation. Clin. Orthop. 223:296–302, 1987.
19. Crowninshield, R. D., Brand, R. A., Johnston, R. C., and Milroy, B. S.: The effect of femoral stem cross-sectional geometry on cement stresses in total hip reconstruction. Clin. Orthop. 146:71–77, 1980.
20. Crowninshield, R. D., Brand, R. A., Johnston, R. C., and Milroy, J. C.: An analysis of femoral component stem design in total hip arthroplasty. J. Bone Joint Surg. 62A:68–78, 1980.
21. Crowninshield, R. D., Brand, R. A., and Pedersen, D. R.: A stress analysis of acetabular reconstruction in protrusio acetabuli. J. Bone Joint Surg. 65A:495–499, 1983.
22. Davidson, J. A. and Brasher, T.: The effect of femoral head size and material on the frictional moment during articulation. Technical Memo OR–90–13: Smith and Nephew Richards, Inc., Memphis, Feb., 1990.
23. Davidson, J. A. and Kovacs, P.: Evaluation of metal ion release during articulation of metal and ceramic femoral heads. Proc. Eighth S. Biomed. Eng. Conf. 33–37, 1989.
24. DelliSanti, G. T., Fox, M. A., and Crowninshield, R. D.: Fixation of metal-backed acetabular components by a plasma spray textured surface. Trans. Biomat. 9:125, 1983.
25. Dowling, J. M., Atkinson, J. R., Dowson, D., and Charnley, J.: The characteristics of acetabular cups worn in the human body. J. Bone Joint Surg. 60B:375–382, 1978.
26. Ebramzadeh, E., Gogan, W., McKellop, H., and Sarmiento, A.: Correlation of stem size and positioning with radiographic performance of cemented total hip prostheses. Trans. O.R.S. 36:455, 1990.
27. Engh, C. A. and Bobyn, J. D.: Biological Fixation in Total Hip Arthroplasty. Thorofare, NJ, Slack, 1985.
28. Engh, C. A. and Bobyn, J. D.: The influence of stem size and extent of porous coating on femoral bone resorption after primary cementless hip arthroplasty. Clin. Orthop. 231:7–28, 1988.
29. Engh, C. A., Griffin, W. L., and Marx, C. L.: Cementless acetabular components. J. Bone Joint Surg. 72B:53–59, 1989.
30. Fischer, O.: Uber den Schwerpunkt des menschlichen Korpers. Leipzig, Hirzel, 1889.
31. Fischer, O.: Der Gang des Menschen. Leipzig, Teubner, 1899.
32. Galante, J. and Rostoker, W.: Fiber metal composites in the fixation of skeletal prosthesis. J. Biomed. Mat. Res. 4:43–61, 1973.
33. Galante, J., Rostoker, W., Lueck, R., and Ray, R. D.: Sintered fiber metal composites as a basis for attachment of implants to bone. J. Bone Joint Surg. 53A:101–114, 1971.
34. Galante, J. O.: Causes of fractures of the femoral component in total hip replacement. J. Bone Joint Surg. 62A:670–673, 1980.
35. Galante, J. O., Rostoker, W., and Doyle, J. M.: Failed femoral stems in total hip prostheses. A report of six cases. J. Bone Joint Surg. 57A:230–236, 1975.
36. Georgette, F. S., Cook, S. D., Skinner, H. B., et al: Fatigue behavior of coated and uncoated Ti–6A1–4V implant material. Trans. Biomat. 9:6, 1983.
37. Gold, B. L. and Walker, P. S.: Variables affecting the friction and wear of metal-on-plastic total hip joints. Clin. Orthop. 100:270–278, 1974.
38. Goto, H., Bobyn, J. D., Usui, T., et al: Effect of femoral implant stiffness and threaded acetabular cup design on non-cemented fixation and bone remodeling: A canine total hip model. Trans. Biomat. 15:70, 1989.
39. Griffith, M. J., Seidenstein, M. K., Williams, D., and Charnley, J.: Socket wear in Charnley low friction arthroplasty of the hip. Clin. Orthop. 137:37–47, 1978.
40. Haddad, R. J., Cook, S. D., and Brinker, M. R.: A comparison of three varieties of noncemented porous-coated hip replacement. J. Bone Joint Surg. 72B:2–8, 1990.
41. Harris, W. H.: Advances in total hip arthroplasty. Clin. Orthop. 183:4–11, 1983.
42. Harris, W. H., Zalenski, E. B., and Jasty, M.: Rotatory instability: The crucial failure in cementless femoral components of total hip replacement. Trans. Biomat. 15:60, 1989.
43. Harwin, C., McKellop, H., and Ebramzadeh, E.: *In vivo* wear of titanium alloy-polyethylene hip prostheses. Trans. O.R.S. 33:505, 1987.
44. Hodge, W. A., Zimmerman, S., Schutzer, S. F., et al: Hip dynamics for stair climbing and rising from a chair. Trans. O.R.S. 33:398, 1987.
45. Huiskes, R., Peeters, H., and Sloof, T. J.: Biomechanical analysis of. Trans. O.R.S. 33:507, 1987.
46. Hulbert, S. F., Cooke, F. W., Klawitter, J. J., et al: Attachment of prostheses to the musculoskeletal system by tissue ingrowth and mechanical interlock. J. Biomed. Mat. Res. 4:1–23, 1973.
47. Inman, V. T., Ralston, H. J., and Todd, F.: Human Walking. Baltimore, Williams & Wilkins, 1981.
48. Jasty, M., Jensen, N. F., Weinberg, E. H., et al: The effect of bone implant apposition on bone ingrowth into canine acetabular porous metal implants. Trans. Biomat. 10:165, 1984.
49. Jasty, M., Harrigan, T. P., Henshaw, R. M., et al: Residual strains produced in the proximal femur during rasping and during the insertion of uncemented metal femoral components. Trans. O.R.S. 33:399, 1987.
50. Jasty, M., Henshaw, R. M., O'Connor, D. O., et al: Strain alterations in the proximal femur with

an uncemented femoral prosthesis, emphasizing the effect of component fit. An experimental *in vitro* strain study. Trans. O.R.S. 34:335, 1988.
51. Jasty, M., McGann, H. E., Rubash, H. E., et al: Comparison of bone ingrowth into cobalt chrome spheres vs. titanium fiber mesh coatings on canine cementless acetabular components. Trans. O.R.S. 33:433, 1987.
52. Johnson, R. C. and Smidt, G. L.: Measurement of hip joint motion during walking. Evaluation of an electrogoniometric method. J. Bone Joint Surg. 51A:1083–1094, 1969.
53. Kamaric, E., Noble, P. C., Alexander, J. W., and Tullos, H. S.: Distal stem centralization critically affecting the acute fixation of cementless femoral components. Trans. Biomat. 15:58, 1989.
54. Kwak, B. M., Lim, O. K., and Rim, K.: An investigation of the effect of cement on an implant by finite element stress analysis. Int. Orthop. 2:315–319, 1979.
55. Lombardi, A. V., Mallory, T. H., Vaughn, B. K., and Drouillard, P.: Aseptic loosening in total hip arthroplasty secondary to osteolysis induced by wear debris from titanium alloy modular femoral heads. J. Bone Joint Surg. 71A:1337–1342, 1989.
56. Loudon, J. R. and Charnley, J.: Subsidence of the femoral prosthesis in total hip replacement in relation to the design of the stem. J. Bone Joint Surg. 62B:450–453, 1980.
57. Manley, M. T., Kotzar, G., Stern, L. S., and Wilde, A.: Effects of repetitive loading on the integrity of porous coatings. Clin. Orthop. 217:293–301, 1987.
58. Manley, M. T., Stern, L. S., Averill, R., and Serekian, P.: Load carrying and fatigue properties of the stem-cement interface with smooth and porous coated femoral components. Trans. Biomat. 10:333, 1984.
59. Maquet, P. G. J.: Biomechanics of the Hip. Berlin, Springer-Verlag, 1985.
60. Markolf, K. L., Amstutz, H. C., and Hirschowitz, D. L.: The effect of calcar contact on femoral component micromovement. J. Bone Joint Surg. 62A:1315–1323, 1980.
61. Martens, M., Aernoudt, E., de Meester, P., et al: Factors in mechanical failure of the femoral component in total hip prosthesis. Acta Orthop. Scand. 45:693–710, 1974.
62. Miller, G. J., Petty, R. W., and Piotrowski, G.: A comparison of acetabular strain changes following Ti6A14V and CoCr metal-backed component implantation. Trans. O.R.S. 32:469, 1986.
63. Mirra, M., Amstutz, H. C., and Matos, M.: The pathology of the joint and joint tissues and its clinical relevance in prosthesis failure. Clin. Orthop. 117:221–240, 1976.
64. Morrey, B. and Ilstrup, D.: Size of the femoral head and acetabular revision in total hip replacement arthroplasty. J. Bone Joint Surg. 71A:50–55, 1989.
65. Murray, P., Drought, A. B., and Kory, R. C.: Walking patterns of normal men. J. Bone Joint Surg. 46A:335–360, 1964.
66. Noble, P. C., Alexander, J. W., Lindahl, L. J., et al: The anatomic basis of femoral component design. Clin. Orthop. 235:148–165, 1988.
67. Nordin, M. and Frankel, V. H.: Basic Biomechanics of the Musculoskeletal System, 2nd ed. Philadelphia, Lea & Febiger, 1989.
68. Oh, I.: Effect of femoral stem design on the cement stress in total hip arthroplasty. Trans. Biomat. 9:94, 1983.
69. Oh, I., Bushelow, M., Sander, T. W., and Treharne, R. W.: An *In vitro* strain gauge study of metal-backed acetabular cups. Trans. Biomat. 10:148, 1984.
70. Oh., I., Sanders, T. W., and Treharne, R. W.: Acetabular cup groove and pod design and its effect on cement fixation in total hip arthroplasty. Clin. Orthop. 189:308–312, 1984.
71. Oh, I., Treharne, R. W., and Sanders, T. W.: Acetabular cement strain for different cement thicknesses and shapes of the cement mantle: *In vitro* strain gauge study. Trans. Biomat. 9:95, 1983.
72. Oh, I. and Harris, W. H.: Proximal strain distribution in the loaded femur. J. Bone Joint Surg. 60A:75–85, 1978.
73. Pauwels, F.: Biomechanics of the Normal and Diseased Hip. New York, Springer-Verlag, 1976.
74. Pedersen, D. R., Crowninshield, R. D., Brand, R. A., and Johnston, R. C.: An axisymmetric model of acetabular components in total hip arthroplasty. J. Biomechanics 15:305–315, 1982.
75. Petty, W., Miller, G. J., and Piotrowski, G.: *In vitro* evaluation of the effect of acetabular prosthesis implantation on human cadaver pelves. Bull. Prosth. Res. 17:80–89, 1980.
76. Petty, W., Piotrowski, G., and Miller, G. J.: *In vitro* evaluation of the effect of acetabular prosthesis implantation on human cadaver pelves. Trans. O.R.S. 27:73, 1981.
77. Rand, J. A. and Ilstrup, D. M.: Comparison of Charnley and T–28 total hip arthroplasty. Clin. Orthop. 180:201–205, 1983.
78. Renz, E. A., Cook, S. D., Collins, C. L., and Haddad, R. J.: Heat treatment for porous-coated Ti–6A1–4V alloy. Trans. Biomat. 10:109, 1984.
79. Revell, P. A., Weightman, B., Freeman, M., and Roberts, B.: The production and biology of polyethylene wear debris. Arch. Orth. Trauma Surg. 91:167–181, 1978.
80. Ries, M., Pugh, J., Au, J., Gurtowski, J., and Dee, R.: Pelvic strains in normal and protrusio with hemiarthroplasty and screw in acetabular components. Trans. O.R.S. 33:508, 1987.
81. Robertson, D. D., Walker, P. S., Hirano, S. K., et al: Improving the fit of press-fit hip stems. Clin. Orthop. 228:134–140, 1988.
82. Rose, R. M., Nusbaum, H. J., Schneider, S. B., et al: On the true wear rate of ultrahigh molecular weight polyethylene in the total hip prosthesis. J. Bone Joint Surg. 62A:537–549, 1980.
83. Salvati, E. A., Wright, T. M., Burstein, A. H., and Jacobs, B.: Fracture of polyethylene acetabular cups. J. Bone Joint Surg. 61A:1239–1242, 1979.
84. Salzer, M., Knahr, K., and Frank, P.: Radiologic and Clinical Follow-ups of Uncemented Femoral Endoprostheses with and without Collars. The Cementless Fixation of Hip Endoprostheses. Edited by E. Morscher. New York, Springer-Verlag, 1984.
85. Seireg, A. and Arvikar, R. J.: The prediction of muscular load sharing and joint forces in the lower extremities during walking. J. Biomechanics 8:89–102, 1975.
86. Sumner, D. R., Jasty, M., Turner, T. M., et al:

Bone ingrowth in porous-coated cementless acetabular components retrieved from human patients. Trans. O.R.S. 33:509, 1987.
87. Thirupathi, R. G. and Husted, M. D.: Failure of polyethylene acetabular cups. Clin. Orthop. 179:209–213, 1983.
88. Turner, T. M., Sumner, D. R., Urban, R. M., et al: A comparative study of porous coatings in a weight-bearing total hip arthroplasty model. J. Bone Joint Surg. 68A:1398–1409, 1986.
89. Van Syckle, P. B. and Walker, P. S.: Parametric analysis of design criteria for acetabular components of surface replacement hip devices. Trans. O.R.S. 26:292, 1980.
90. Vasu, R., Carter, D. R., and Harris, W. H.: Stress distributions in the acetabular region. I. Before and after total joint replacement. J. Biomechanics 15:155–164, 1982.
91. Walker, P. S. and Robertson, D. D.: Design and fabrication of cementless hip stems. Clin. Orthop. 235:25–34, 1988.
92. Weber, W. and Weber, E.: Mechanik der menschlichen Gehwerkzeuge. Berlin, Springer, 1895.
93. Weightman, B., Isherwood, D. P., and Swanson, S. A. V.: The fracture of ultrahigh molecular weight polyethylene in the human body. J. Biomed. Mat. Res. 13:669, 1979.
94. Whiteside, L. A., Amador, D., and Russell, K.: The effects of the collar on total hip femoral component subsidence. Clin. Orthop. 231:120–126, 1988.

CHAPTER 14

Surgical Approaches for Total Hip Replacement

BERNARD STULBERG
TIMOTHY HUPFER

To perform a satisfactory total hip arthroplasty, adequate surgical exposure must be achieved. An unobstructed view of the acetabulum and proximal femur is essential to the proper placement of arthroplasty components. Without it, component placement can become erratic and the long-term success of the arthroplasty jeopardized.

Many descriptions of surgical approaches to the hip joint have appeared in the orthopaedic literature.[10, 17] The purpose of this chapter is to focus on the approaches to the hip most commonly used at this time: the anterolateral, direct lateral, transtrochanteric, and posterolateral. (For a more extensive discussion of surgical approaches, the reader is referred to several excellent reviews.[1, 10])

In general, the best way to characterize a surgical approach to the hip joint is by assessing the deep muscle interval through which the surgeon must proceed to reach the hip joint. In the anterolateral approach, the surgeon reaches the hip joint in the muscle interval between the tensor fascia latae and the anterior fibers of the gluteus medius. The lateral approaches include the direct lateral and the transtrochanteric. The former divides the substance of the gluteus medius and minimus, whereas the latter elevates the gluteus medius and minimus with a bone fragment of the greater trochanter. The posterolateral approach involves splitting fibers of the gluteus maximus and identifying the posterior edge of the gluteus medius, thus defining an interval between the gluteus maximus and gluteus medius. Approaches that proceed more anteriorly or more posteriorly than these four approaches have been thoroughly described elsewhere and are selected for other types of hip surgery.[20, 27] They are less useful in total hip arthroplasty.

Another important consideration in selecting a surgical approach is its relationship to the preoperative plan (see Chapter 15, *Indications and Preoperative Planning*). The ease with which an arthroplasty is carried out is related to many factors, surgical approach being one. Primary arthroplasty in a hip with normal anatomic features may be performed accurately and expeditiously through any of the four approaches discussed here when the surgeon is familiar with the one chosen. However, when the anatomy is complex or when revision arthroplasty is being performed, accuracy and ease of insertion (or extraction if necessary) can be strongly influenced by the surgical approach. Admittedly, skilled and experienced surgeons can make any approach work, but in our ex-

Table 14–1. FOUR COMMONLY USED SURGICAL APPROACHES IN TOTAL HIP ARTHROPLASTY (THA)

Approach	Intervals	Advantages	Limitations
Anterolateral	Tensor fascia latae Gluteus medius	Excellent acetabular exposure Minimizes abductor muscle disruption Less prone to dislocation Adequate femoral exposure	Potential for compromised femoral exposure Risks varus placement of component Risks femoral fracture in revision cases
Direct lateral	Through anterior one third of fibers of gluteus medius and minimus	Excellent acetabular exposure in primary and revision procedures Minimizes disruption of trochanteric bed in uncemented fixation Adequate femoral exposure for many revision THAs Less prone to dislocation	Disrupts abductors and can lead to prolonged lurch if repair is unsatisfactory May compromise exposure for distal femoral cement removal in revision cases Puts limits on limb lengthening ability in complex THA Limited posterior acetabular exposure for complex revision THA
Transtrochanteric	Elevates portion of greater trochanter with gluteus medius and minimus	Excellent exposure of acetabulum and femur for both primary and revision THA Best approach for complex anatomy Allows unrestricted visualization of anterior and posterior columns of acetabulum for complex reconstruction Allows proper muscle tension after limb length restoration	Occasionally difficult to obtain and maintain secure fixation May increase length of operative procedure and blood loss Greater risk of muscle/tissue tension problems if fixation is lost
Posterolateral	Posterior aspect of gluteus medius and maximus	Minimal disruption of abductor musculature Allows early rehabilitation without abductor compromise Excellent femoral exposure in primary THA Adequate acetabular exposure for primary and some revision THA	Greater risk of inaccurate placement of acetabular component Risks femoral fracture in tight hip if insufficiently released Limited visualization of distal femoral cement in revision cases Higher incidence of dislocation

perience certain approaches make exposure less difficult and therefore facilitate the arthroplasty procedure (Table 14–1).

One other consideration in selecting the surgical approach is the influence of prior hip procedures. Preexisting skin incisions about the hip often cause the surgeon undertaking primary or revision arthroplasty to select from a number of choices: If enough skin and subcutaneous tissue are present we excise prior incisions as appropriate; if incision scars are less than 6 months old, we reuse or excise these incisions rather than cross them with new ones; and if they are older than 6 months, we can proceed safely with the desired line of approach. In addition to prior skin incisions, surgical hardware, other than hip arthroplasty components, may have been placed. The surgeon may need to remove these in order to proceed with total hip arthroplasty.

In each of the following descriptions, we briefly discuss the anatomic structures that allow accurate identification of the interval as well as the critical structures that must be carefully retracted to minimize damage—with emphasis on the essential steps of each approach.

FOUR BASIC APPROACHES FOR TOTAL HIP ARTHROPLASTY

Anterolateral Approach

(Figure 14–1)

In 1936 Watson-Jones[29] described and popularized the anterolateral approach to the hip joint. Slight modification of this

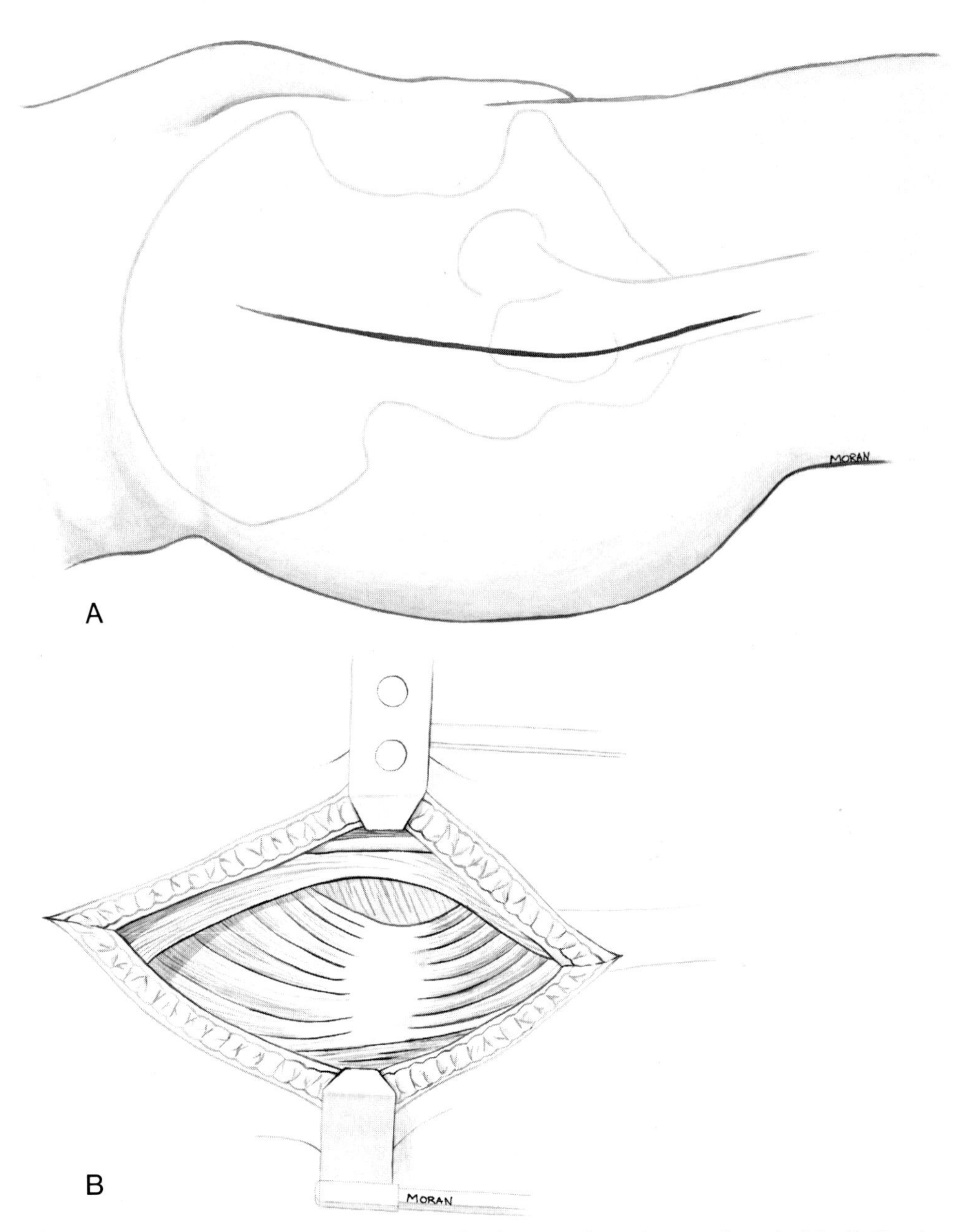

FIGURE 14–1. Anterolateral approach. *A,* Incision for the anterolateral approach to the hip. *B,* Development of the interval between the tensor fascia lata and gluteus medius muscles.

Illustration continued on following page

basic approach with release of a portion of the anterior fibers of the gluteus medius or gluteus minimus, or both, is often employed to allow its application to total hip arthroplasty. The anterolateral approach exposes the hip through the interval of the tensor fascia latae and gluteus medius muscles. The inferior branch of the superior gluteal nerve, which supplies the tensor fascia latae, is located approximately 4.5 cm above the tip of trochanter.[13, 16] It should be protected, but occasional demands of exposure may require its sacrifice. Care must be taken when placing retractors anteriorly to the acetabulum to avoid damage of the femoral nerve and blood vessels. Careful separation of anterior capsular fibers from the iliopsoas and gluteus minimus fibers is important in protecting these structures. This exposure

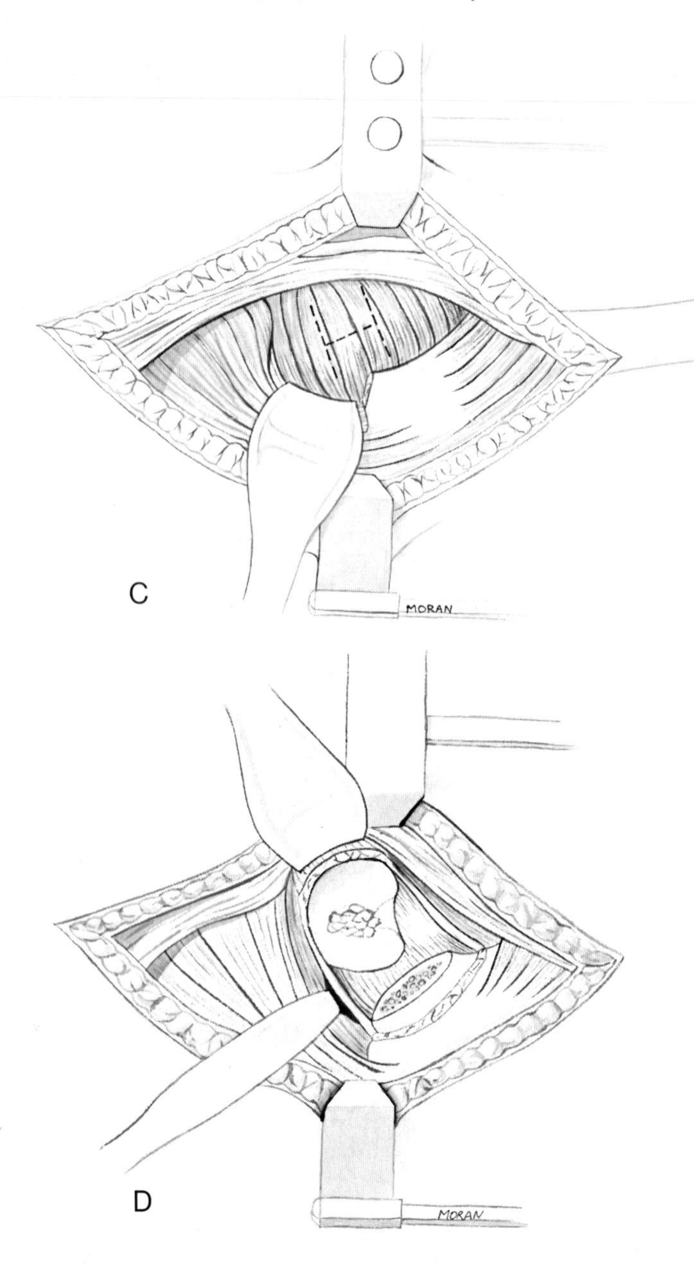

FIGURE 14–1 *Continued C,* Exposure of the anterior hip joint capsule and capsulotomy. *D,* Placement of retractors after joint dislocation, femoral neck osteotomy, and removal of the femoral head to expose the acetabulum.

should allow excellent visualization of the acetabulum and the anterior column of the acetabulum and acceptable exposure of the proximal femur and femoral canal.

Technique

The incision is started 2.5 cm distally and laterally to the anterior superior iliac spine and curved distally and posteriorly over the greater trochanter. The interval between the gluteus medius and tensor fasciae latae is identified. A blunt Hohmann retractor is placed distally along the base of the femoral neck superior to the iliopsoas insertion. Another is placed superiorly along the femoral neck to retract the abductors. Cautery is utilized to detach anterior fibers of the gluteus medius or minimus tendon. A periosteal elevator is employed to remove the fat overlying the capsule and to carefully reflect the iliopsoas tendon. The reflected head of the rectus femoris may be released from its capsular insertion to improve exposure. Special care is taken in placing anterior retractors. An H-shaped capsulotomy is performed, followed by a complete capsulectomy. The hip is dislocated by applying flexion with adduction and external rotation. Following femoral neck osteotomy, a curved and pointed Hohmann retractor is carefully placed posteriorly to retract the proximal femur and to expose the posterior acetabulum. For acetabular preparation, it is often preferable to have the limb in extension. For proximal femoral exposure, flexion and external rotation of the femur are needed. We accomplish these by crossing the leg and placing it in a sterile bag anteriorly.

Limitations

Although the anterolateral approach provides excellent exposure for primary hip arthroplasty, visualization of the proximal femur may be inadequate. In primary arthroplasty this inadequacy can lead the surgeon to place the femoral component in varus, as femoral reaming may impinge upon the lateral cortex or may be limited by the tip of the greater trochanter. Attention to these potential sources of impingement is necessary. The situation may be particularly troublesome in revision total hip arthroplasty when cement removal requires excellent visualization of the distal portion of the femoral cement column.

Direct Lateral Approach

(Figure 14–2)

A direct lateral approach was described by Kocher[19] in 1903 and later modified by McFarland and Osborne[22] in 1954. It has undergone several subsequent modifications.[14, 18] The approach has proved useful in cases in which preservation of the bony bed of the trochanter is important, such as cementless arthroplasty. Exposure is gained by dividing the anterior insertions of the gluteus medius and minimus muscles. Because of the extensive nature of exposure, visualization of the acetabulum and proximal femur is better than that obtained through an anterolateral approach. Thus, it can be selected for some revision procedures in which exposure through an anterolateral approach would be insufficient. We have found it useful in revisions in which the femoral components remain well fixed. The major structures at risk are the inferior branch of the superior gluteal nerve and the femoral nerve and vessels. To protect these structures we advise precautions similar to those recommended for the anterolateral approach. Anatomically accurate and secure repair is required to ensure healing of the divided tendon.

Technique

The incision begins approximately 5 cm distal to the base of the greater trochanter along the lateral femoral shaft. It continues proximally to the greater trochanter, then curves slightly posteriorly. The underlying fascia is split in line with the skin incision. A Charnley retractor is placed deep to the fascia. Cautery is utilized to incise the gluteus medius beginning 4 cm cephalad to the greater trochanter and well anterior to the thick tendinous portion of the gluteus medius. The incision continues along the anterior aspect of the greater trochanter. Special care is taken to incise within the tendon itself, so that viable tendon is present on both sides of the incision. The curved portion of a Hibbs retractor is employed to retract the gluteus medius fibers. The gluteus minimus insertion can then be identified without difficulty and divided in line with its fibers. Cobra retractors are placed in extracapsular fashion around the superior and inferior neck, and the capsule is exposed. A T-shaped capsulotomy is performed. The hip is then dislocated by flexion, adduction, and external rotation of the femur. Femoral neck osteotomy is followed by capsulotomy along the medial base of the neck. This maneuver releases the capsule and frees the femur. Posterior capsular release may be necessary before placement of retractors.

Exposure of the proximal femur is similar to that of the anterolateral approach with special attention paid to placement of a retractor beneath the greater trochanter. This exposure should be done by gently pulling up on the greater trochanter and placing a smooth Hohmann retractor posteriorly to avoid injury to the sciatic nerve.

At closure, the gluteus minimus tendon is repaired with sutures through drill holes

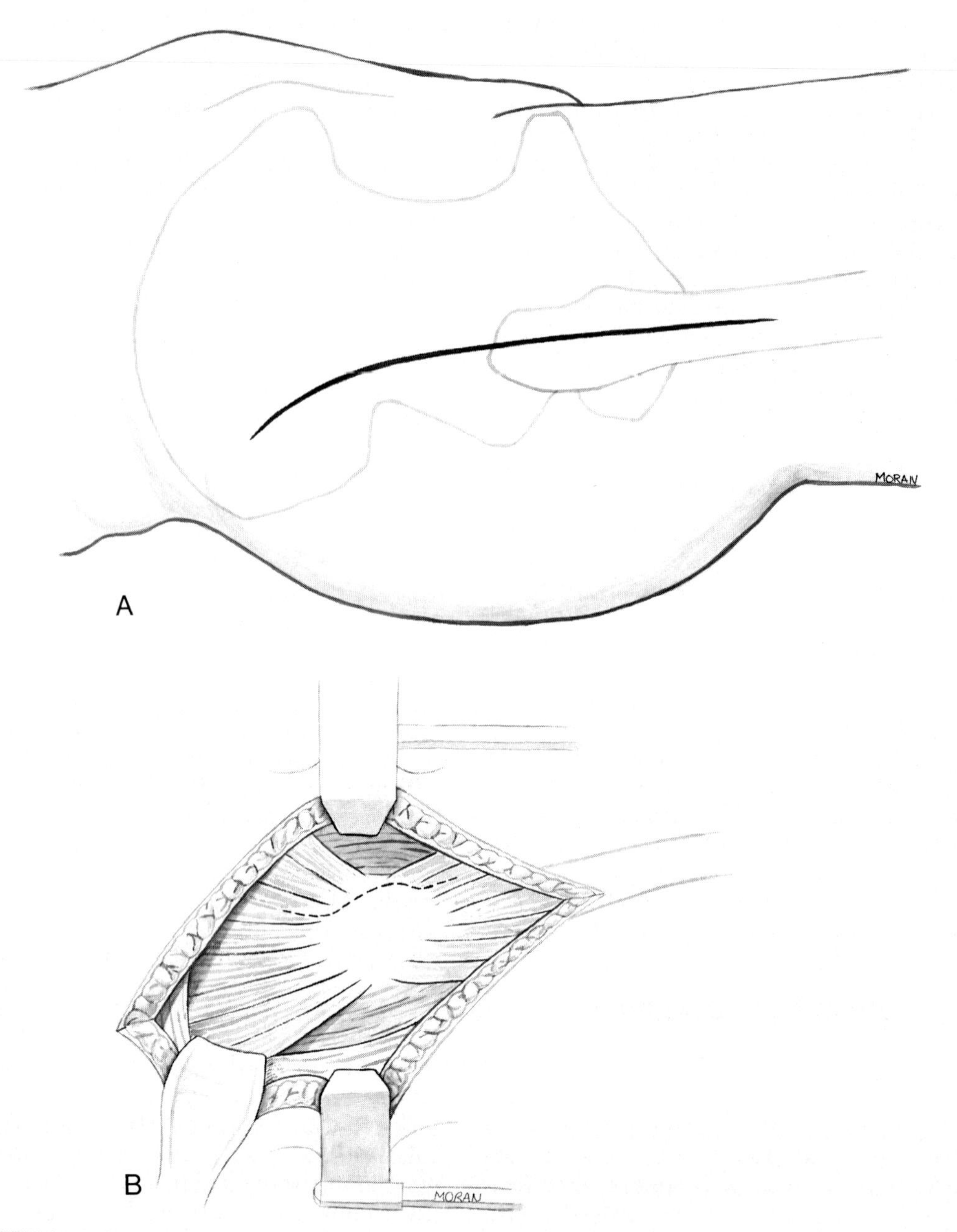

FIGURE 14–2. Direct lateral approach. *A,* Skin incision for the direct lateral approach. *B,* Incision line in the fibrous gluteus medius muscle and along the insertion of the muscle into the greater trochanter. Tendinous tissue must be left on the greater trochanter to improve later repair.

in the proximal aspect of the anterior greater trochanter. In addition, the minimus should be sutured to remaining posterior fibers as completely as possible to protect against dehiscence. The gluteus medius tendon is then repaired. Every attempt should be made to restore the gluteus medius and minimus tendons to their anatomic insertions.

Modifications

Several workers have suggested modifications that may be of benefit. Hardinge[14] recommends division of the vastus lateralis muscle and tendon in line with the incision in the gluteus medius. Others have voiced concern that a bowstring-like effect can result, leading to loss of repair at the

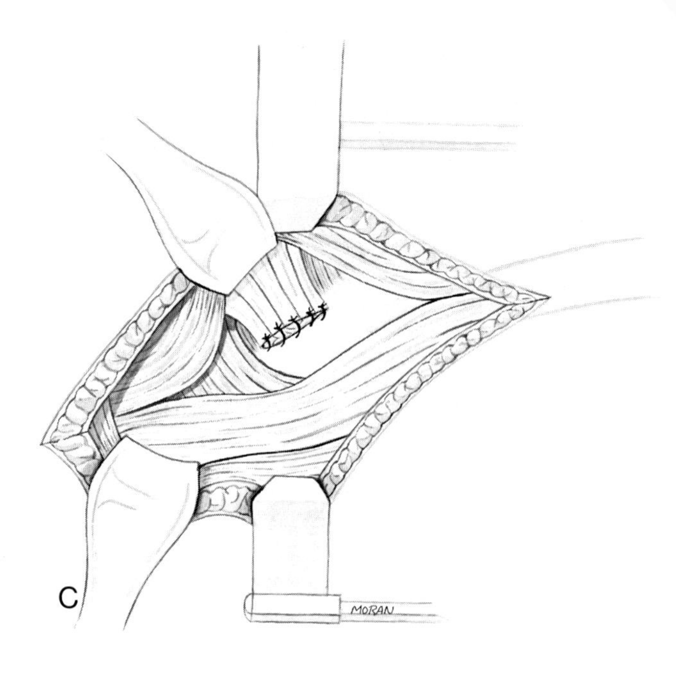

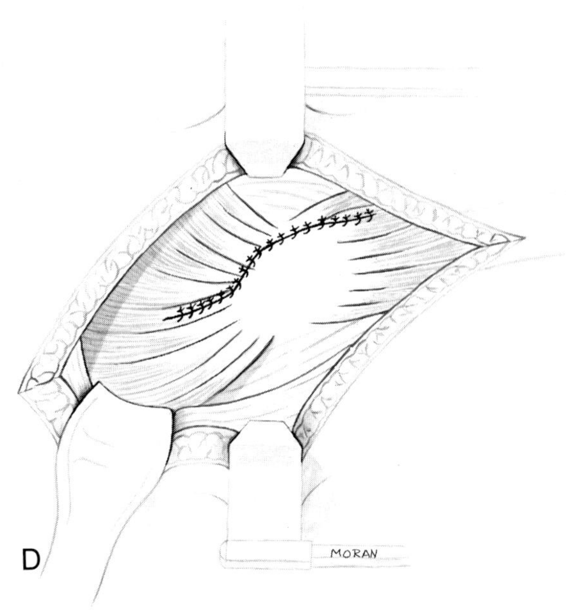

FIGURE 14–2 *Continued C,* Repair of the gluteus minimus tendon after completion of arthroplasty with sutures placed through drill holes in the proximal aspect of the anterior greater trochanter. *D,* The gluteus medius is then securely repaired.

insertion of the gluteus medius. We have had this experience on two occasions, when inadvertent trauma led to avulsion of the bone segment that had been "perforated" by the drill holes. In some patients, an anterior trochanteric osteotomy, with removal of the tendinous insertions with trochanteric bone and subsequent bone-to-bone fixation at closure, may be of value.

For more extensive exposure of the proximal femur during revision total hip arthroplasty, Head and colleagues[16] have recommended a modification of this exposure. In their approach, the vastus lateralis is elevated off the posterior intermuscular septum. It is reflected anteriorly by dividing a portion of the vastus lateralis 1 cm below the vastus tubercle, proceeding proximally through the fibers of the gluteus medius and minimus. An anterior trochanteric osteotomy can be utilized, if the soft tissues on the anterior aspect of the trochanter have been previously compromised.

Limitations

Although many investigators have found this a useful approach to the hip joint, two major concerns have led to its limited application on a routine basis. The first concern is the muscle disruption and subsequent compromise of repair that can occur with this approach. Anatomic and secure repair is critical to the return of normal function. If not possible, or if repair is lost in the early postoperative period, an abductor lurch can persist that is not remedied by exercises. The second concern relates to complex revision surgery in which visualization of the femoral shaft can be limited, and inadequate removal of acrylic debris, fracture, or inaccurate placement of components can result. If new methods for improving trochanteric healing following osteotomy prove successful the transtrochanteric approach would seem a preferable alternative.

Transtrochanteric Approach

(Figure 14–3)

The transtrochanteric approach was developed by Charnley[8] and has been thoroughly described. It remains the single most versatile approach for all arthroplasty surgery of the hip joint and is the best approach for dealing with complex problems of acetabular and femoral reconstructions, whether in primary or revision situations. However, the transtrochanteric approach is less popular than other standard approaches for primary hip arthroplasty because of the complications related to exposure and subsequent fixation of the trochanteric fragment as well as the greater potential for morbidity.[3, 4, 7, 9, 11, 15, 21, 23, 28]

The transtrochanteric approach is most appropriate for extensive acetabular reconstruction, in which substantial grafting requires excellent visualization of both the anterior and posterior columns of the acetabulum. This approach is excellent when substantial leg lengthening is anticipated, as it provides the safest means of visualization and protection of the neurovascular structures. Also, the transtrochanteric approach allows for repositioning of the abductor mechanism in such a manner that proper muscle tension and hip mechanics can be restored. For femoral arthroplasty, the approach provides the most universal exposure of the proximal femur and offers optimal visualization for removal of acrylic from the medullary canal.

The major structures at risk for injury in this exposure are the sciatic nerve posteriorly; the inferior branch of the superior gluteal artery, if the muscle fibers are dissected too proximally; and the femoral nerve and vessels anteriorly. Inadvertent stretching of the sciatic nerve can occur if the limb is allowed to fall anteriorly. This situation can occur when extensive work is being performed on the femur, while the patient is in the lateral decubitus position and the femur is held in flexion, adduction, and external rotation. A small roll under the knee, counter-pressure on the knee applied by the surgical assistant, or support of the limb with a stool is recommended.

Our experience with the Dall-Miles (TM) cable system for trochanteric fixation has been positive. This system addresses many of the problems related to trochanteric fixation, as subsequently discussed. Should it prove to be of substantial benefit and find simple application, it will add to the surgeon's confidence in resuming a more frequent use of this approach in more complex arthroplasties.

Technique

A straight lateral skin incision is centered over the greater trochanter. The iliotibial band is then divided in line with the skin. A Charnley retractor is placed deep to the fascia. The short external rotators, including the piriformis, superior gemellus, obturator externus, and inferior gemellus, are identified and released. The interval between the gluteus medius and tensor fasciae latae is identified and divided. The vastus lateralis is divided 1 cm below the vastus tubercle. Utilizing a periosteal elevator, the anterior capsule of the hip joint is visualized. The greater trochanter is osteotomized with a curved gouge, saw, or broad straight osteotome. Osteotomy of a chevron or hemispheric nature may provide some additional bony stability at the time of reattachment and is recommended.[6] For conventional total hip arthroplasty, a large trochanteric fragment

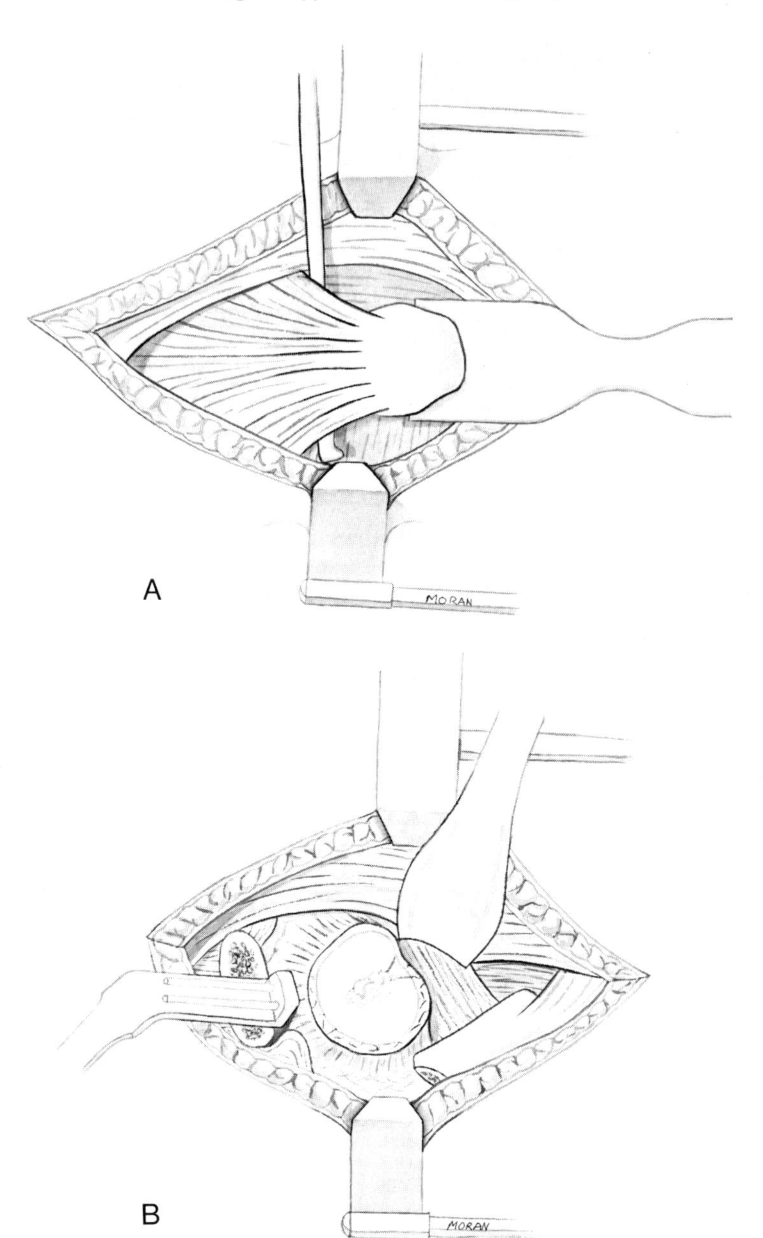

FIGURE 14–3. Transtrochanteric approach. *A*, Osteotomy of the greater trochanter for conventional total hip arthroplasty. The osteotomy may extend in an intracapsular direction. For surface replacement arthroplasty, the osteotomy should be extracapsular. *B*, Retraction of greater trochanter superiorly. It is helpful to use a self-retaining retractor. Additional retractors are placed. Exposure is excellent for the acetabulum and for both the anterior and posterior columns.
Illustration continued on following page

that is extended in intracapsular fashion is appropriate. However, for double-cup arthroplasty, the osteotomy may be extracapsular.[5] The greater trochanter is retracted superiorly and the capsule exposed. Circumferential capsulectomy is performed. The hip is dislocated by flexion, adduction, and external rotation. Neck osteotomy is then performed. The proximal femur may be retracted anteriorly or posteriorly as needed to provide visualization of both the anterior and posterior columns of the acetabulum. For femoral preparation, the hip is held in flexion, adduction, and external rotation and the leg is placed in a sterile leg bag anteriorly.

The greater trochanter is repaired using the Dall-Miles trochanteric clamp with the largest cables appropriate for the patient. The 2.0-mm cables are preferred. The cables are placed through drill holes in the lesser trochanter.[11]

Modifications

Engh[12] has suggested a trochanteric osteotomy that is performed moving the trochanter anteriorly, leaving the muscle en-

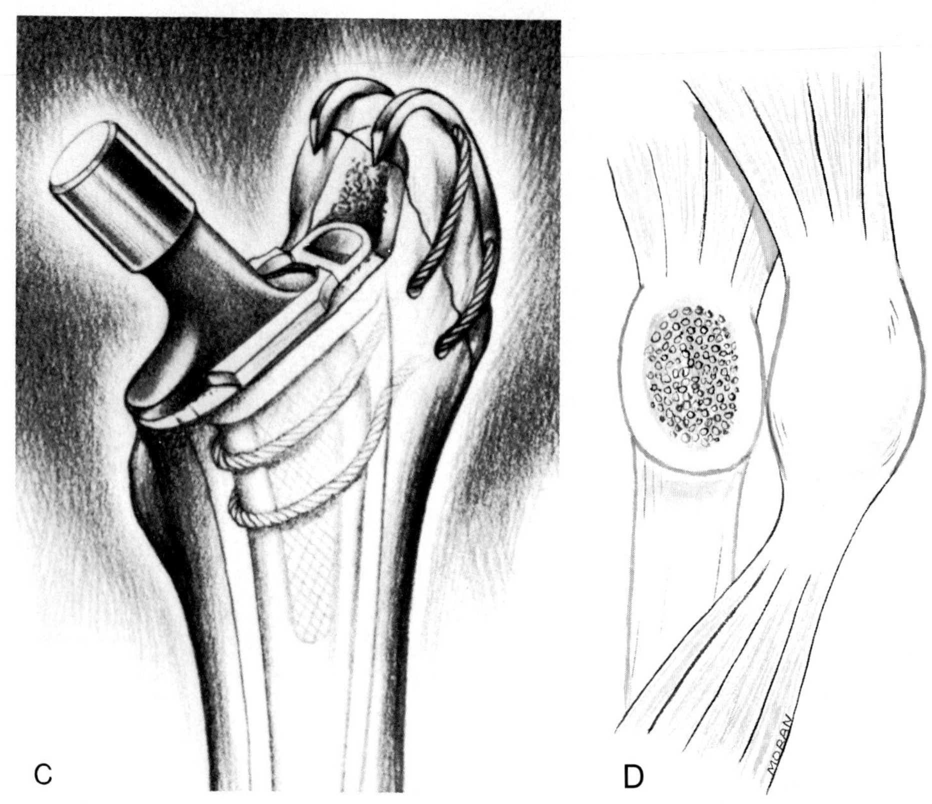

FIGURE 14–3 *Continued C,* Trochanteric repair with the Dall-Miles trochanteric clamp and cables. (Courtesy of Howmedica, Inc.) *D,* Modification of the transtrochanteric approach leaving the vastus lateralis attached to the greater trochanter distally.

velope of abductors and vastus lateralis intact. This approach has been advocated for removal of proximal femoral cement but may be less advantageous when full acetabular exposure is required.[12]

Several methods of trochanteric fixation are described in the literature.[3, 4, 7–9, 11, 15, 21, 23, 28] Some workers frequently express a disparaging attitude toward predictable reattachment and express disappointment about loss of fixation. We believe that the Dall-Miles (TM) cable system is substantially superior to other methods. For alternative approaches to trochanteric fixation, should they be needed, refer to the aforementioned sources.

Limitations

The greatest limitations of the transtrochanteric approach relate to problems encountered with obtaining and maintaining adequate trochanteric fixation. Fixation problems have been reported in 2.3% of primary total hip arthroplasties and 7% of revision arthroplasties.[3] Problems include trochanteric bursitis, wire breakage, loss of fixation, and heterotopic ossification. Other major limitations are related to the potential increases in operative time and postoperative morbidity that accompany this approach when primary arthroplasty is performed, especially in the hands of surgeons with limited experience. New attachment systems should lessen problems associated with the procedure and make it less compromising to the surrounding tissues.

Posterolateral Approach

(Figure 14–4)

In the posterolateral approach, the hip joint is visualized through the interval of the posterior aspect of the gluteus medius and gluteus maximus. It differs from the southern approach of Moore, which goes directly through the gluteus maximus fibers and divides the short external rotators

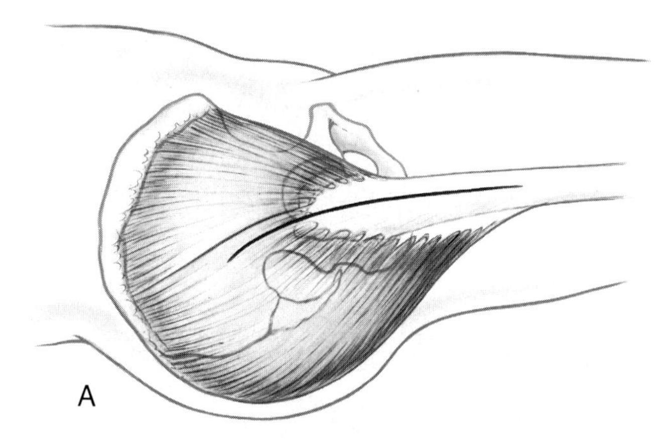

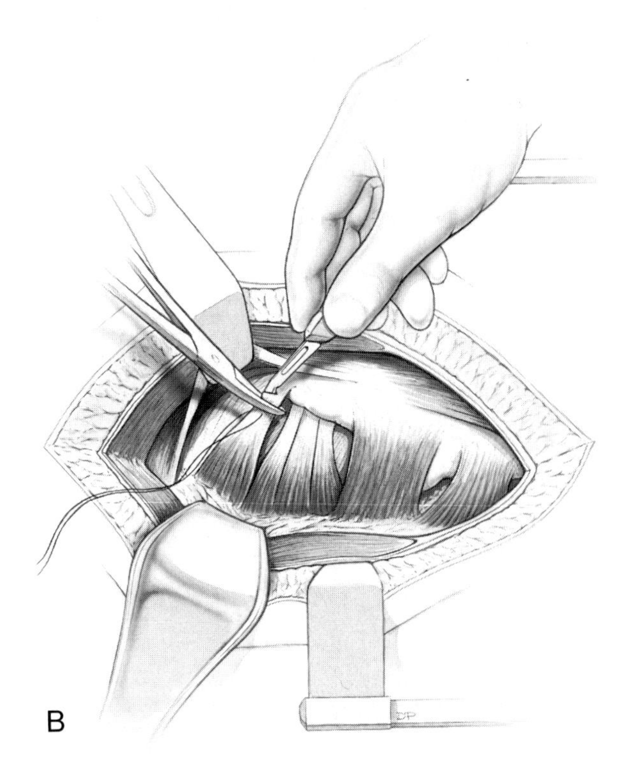

FIGURE 14–4. Posterolateral approach. *A,* Skin incision. *B,* Incision of short external rotators near their insertions to the greater trochanter. If the piriformis is located and incised first, the hip joint capsule can be identified immediately beneath the piriformis tendon. Appropriate incision of the remaining short external rotators is then more easily obtained.

Illustration continued on following page

more directly.[6, 10, 20] The posterolateral approach has proved popular for arthroplasty because it involves minimal compromise of the abductor musculature, allows early rehabilitation with minimal limitation, and provides excellent visualization of the proximal femur. The major structure at risk is the sciatic nerve, which is best protected by reflecting the short external rotators and carefully placing the retractors posteriorly. The approach is useful for primary total hip arthroplasty and hemiarthroplasty but may have limited application in more complex arthroplasty, including revision, in which other approaches provide greater exposure of the acetabulum and femur.

Technique

The incision is made laterally along the shaft of the femur and continued proximally to the level of the greater trochanter, where it is curved gently posteriorly. The incision is carried down through the subcutaneous tissue to the level of the fascia. After the fascia is split in line with the incision, blunt dissection of the gluteus maximus muscle fibers allows exposure of the posterior aspect of the hip joint with

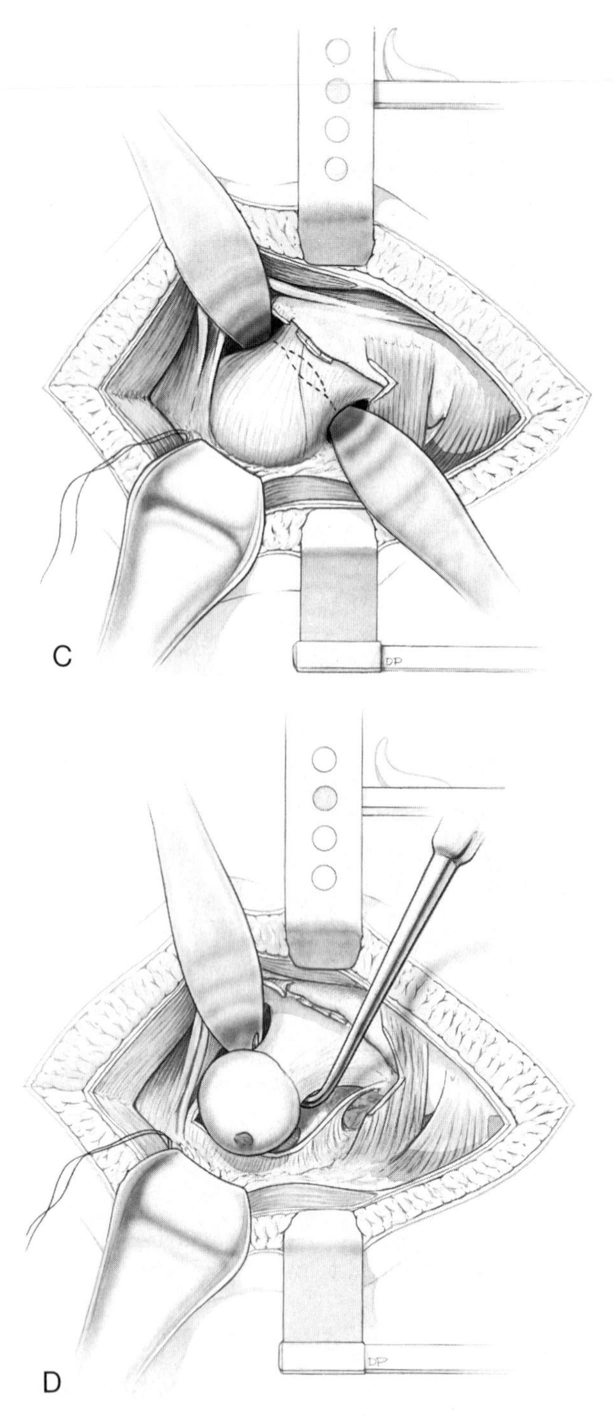

FIGURE 14–4 *Continued C,* Placement of retractors superiorly beneath the gluteus medius and minimus and inferiorly below the femoral neck, followed by hip joint capsulotomy. *D,* Dislocation of the hip joint posteriorly by flexion, adduction, and internal rotation. A bone hook may be helpful in completing the dislocation.

minimal bleeding. The hip is rotated internally, and the posterior edge of the gluteus medius is identified. By careful dissection, either bluntly or with electrocautery, the medius is retracted anteriorly and the piriformis tendon is identified. The tendon is then released from its insertion from the piriformis fossa. The superior gemellus, obturator internus, inferior gemellus, and quadratus femoris muscles are then released near their insertions.

Additional exposure without undue tension can be achieved by dividing the gluteus maximus tendinous insertion at the

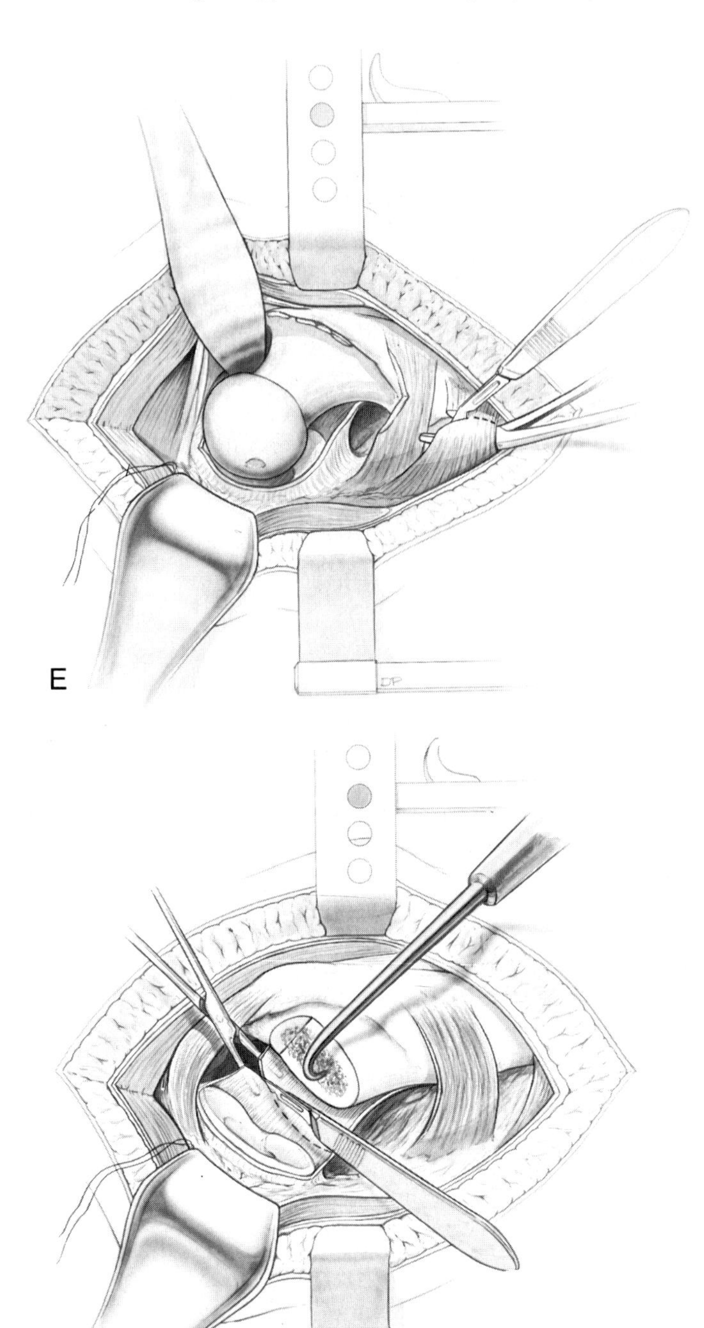

FIGURE 14–4 *Continued E,* Improved exposure of tight tissues by release of the gluteus maximus tendon. Release should be performed as close to tendon-bone insertion as possible. *F,* Improved exposure of both the acetabulum and proximal femur by complete anterior capsulotomy.

Illustration continued on following page

femur. A smooth retractor is then placed deep to the gluteus minimus and anterior to the femoral neck, and a curved cobra retractor is placed inferiorly. This maneuver exposes the hip capsule. We prefer the capsulotomy method suggested by Sculco,[26] with a superior capsulotomy above and in line with the superior border of the piriformis and an inferior capsulotomy that provides a broad-based flap. The retractors are then placed around the femoral neck. The hip is flexed, adducted, and internally rotated to allow gentle dislocation of the femoral head.

Femoral neck osteotomy is then performed; anterior and inferior capsulotomy

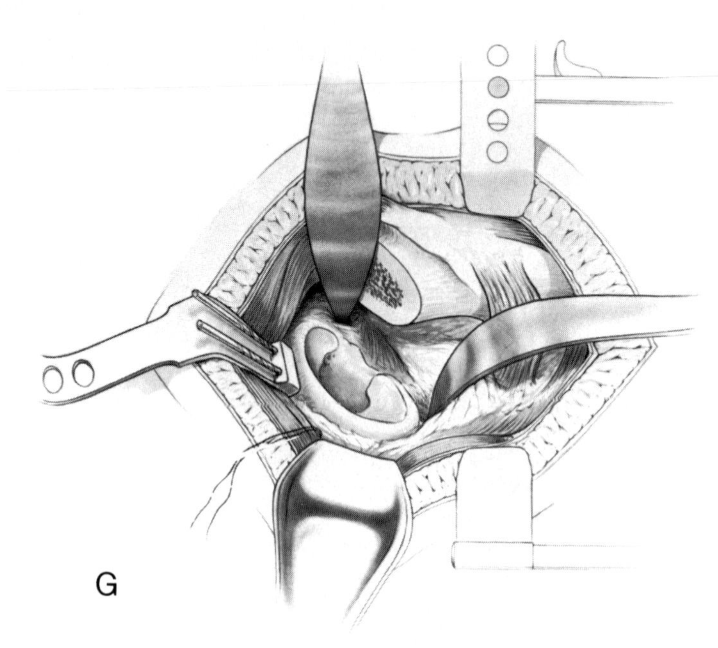

FIGURE 14–4 *Continued G,* Placement of retractors in four quadrants around the acetabulum providing excellent exposure.

can then be performed as needed. Retractors are positioned to displace the femoral shaft anteriorly. Femoral rotation is adjusted to allow maximum exposure of the acetabulum. Improper release or tight exposure can force the acetabular reamers into inadequate anteversion and results in improper acetabular reaming. After completion of placement of the acetabular component, the proximal femur is brought into flexion and 90-degrees internal rotation. Retractors are placed under the femoral neck or at the level of the lesser trochanter displacing the neck laterally from the wound to allow improved visibility during femoral preparation.

After careful reduction of the hip, the short external rotators and posterior capsule are reattached in near anatomic position, as described by Sculco. This maneuver involves tying two double-limbed #2-sutures through drill holes in the trochanter, one at the level of the piriformis fossa and one at the level of the femoral neck. The hip is held in flexion, abduction, and external rotation as the suture is tied.

Limitations

If the femur is difficult to position anteriorly to the pelvis, it can be difficult to obtain satisfactory acetabular exposure with the posterolateral approach, especially in an obese patient or in a patient during a revision procedure. When a problem of exposure is encountered intraoperatively, the surgeon can proceed to a transtrochanteric approach without compromise. If the problem is identified preoperatively, the surgeon should select an alternative approach.

A widespread concern regarding this approach is the reportedly greater incidence of postoperative dislocation.[24, 25] Proper surgical placement of components and appropriate rehabilitation and patient education in the postoperative period can minimize this problem. The capsular/muscle repair suggested here is one surgical technique that may prove of benefit.

References

1. Acton, R. K.: Surgical Approaches to the Hip. Surgery of the Hip Joint. Edited by R. G. Tronzo. Philadelphia, Lea & Febiger, 1973.
2. Amstutz, H. C., Clarke, I. C., Christie, J., and Graff-Radford, A.: Total hip articular replacement by internal eccentric shells. Clin. Orthop. 128:261–284, 1977.
3. Amstutz, H. C., Mai, L. L., and Schmidt, I.: Results of interlocking wire trochanteric reattachment and technique refinement to prevent complications following total hip arthroplasty. Clin. Orthop. 183:82–89, 1984.
4. Amstutz, H. C. and Maki, S.: Complications of trochanteric osteotomy in total hip replacement. J. Bone Joint Surg. 60A:214–216, 1978.

5. Askew, M. J., Shybut, G. T., Hori, R. Y., and Stulberg, S. D.: Theoretical and experimental studies of femoral stresses following surface replacement hip arthroplasty. Trans. Orthop. Res. Soc. 1980.
6. Aufranc, St. George Tucker: The Transtrochanteric Approach. The Art of Total Hip Arthroplasty. Edited by W. T. Stillwell. Orlando, Grune & Stratton, 1987.
7. Clarke, Jr., R. P., Shea, W. D., and Bierbaum, B. E.: Trochanteric osteotomy: Analysis of pattern of wire fixation failure and complications. Clin. Orthop. 141:102–110, 1979.
8. Charnley, J.: Low Fixation Arthroplasty of the Hip. New York, Springer-Verlag, 1979.
9. Charnley, J. and Ferreira, A. de S. D.: Transplantation of the greater trochanter in arthroplasty of the hip, J. Bone Joint Surg. 46B:191–197, 1964.
10. Crenshaw, A. H.: Surgical Approaches. Campbell's Operative Orthopaedics. St. Louis, C. V. Mosby Company, 1987.
11. Dall, D. M. and Miles, A. W.: Reattachment of the greater trochanter. J. Bone Joint Surg. 65B:55–59, 1983.
12. Engh, C. A.: Technique for Revision Surgery. Biological Fixation in Total Hip Arthroplasty. Thorofare, NJ, Slack, 1985.
13. Foster, D. E. and Hynter, J. R.: The direct lateral approach to the hip for arthroplasty: Advantages and complications. Orthopaedics 10:274, 1987.
14. Hardinge, K.: Direct lateral approach to the hip. J. Bone Joint Surg. 64B:17, 1982.
15. Harris, W. H.: Advances in surgical technique for total hip replacement: Without and with osteotomy of the greater trochanter. Clin. Orthop. 146:188–204, 1980.
16. Head, W. C., Mallory, T. H., Berklacich, F. M., et al.: Extensile exposure of the hip for revision arthroplasty. J. Arthroplasty 2:(4)265–273, 1987.
17. Hoppenfeld, S.: The Hip. Surgical Exposures in Orthopaedics. Philadelphia, J. B. Lippincott Co., 1984.
18. Hungerford, D., Hedley, A., Habermann, E., et al: Total hip arthroplasty: A new approach, Baltimore, University Park Press, 1984.
19. Kocher, T.: Textbook of Operative Surgery. London, Adam and Charles Black, 1903.
20. Moore, A. T.: The self-locking metal hip prosthesis. J. Bone Joint Surg. 39A:811, 1957.
21. Markolf, K. L., Hirschowitz, D. L., and Amstutz, H. C.: Mechanical stability of the greater trochanter following osteotomy and reattachment by wiring. Clin. Orthop. 141:111–121, 1979.
22. McFarland, B. and Osbourne, G.: Approach to the hip: A suggested improvement on Kocher's method. J. Bone Joint Surg. 36B:364, 1954.
23. Parker, H. G., Wiesman, H. G., Ewald, F. C., et al: Comparison of preoperative, intraoperative, and early postoperative total hip replacements with and without trochanteric osteotomy. Clin. Orthop. 121:44–49, 1976.
24. Roberts, J. M., Fu, F. H., McClain, E. J., and Ferguson, Jr., A. B.: A comparison of the posterolateral and anterolateral approaches to total hip arthroplasty. Clin. Orthop. 187:205–210, 1984.
25. Robinson, R. P., Robinson, Jr., H. J., and Salvati, E. A.: Comparison of the transtrochanteric and posterior approaches for total hip replacement. Clin. Orthop. 147:143–147, 1980.
26. Sculco, T. P.: The Lower Extremity. Orthopaedic Care of the Geriatric Patient. St. Louis, C. V. Mosby Company, 1985.
27. Smith-Peterson, M. N.: A new supra-articular subperiosteal approach to the hip joint. Am. J. Orthop. Surg. 15:592, 1917.
28. Thompson, Jr., R. C. and Culver, J. E.: The role of trochanteric osteotomy in total hip replacement. Clin. Orthop. 106:102–106, 1975.
29. Watson-Jones, R.: Fractures of the neck of the femur. Br. J. Surg. 23:787, 1936.

CHAPTER 15

Indications and Preoperative Planning for Total Hip Arthroplasty

BERNARD STULBERG
TIMOTHY HUPFER

Since the advent of predictable arthroplasty results in the 1960s, the indications for total hip arthroplasty have been controversial because the procedure has been applied to patients who were not originally considered candidates for this approach.[9] The dramatic pain relief and return to function that follow successful total hip arthroplasty have created expectations in both surgeons and patients for results of a highly reproducible nature. Persistent efforts to expand indications have led to improvements in surgical technique, instrumentation, and implant technology. The success of these efforts has made it possible for surgeons to continue to push the limits of prosthetic devices. At the same time, surgeons must be guided by the limitations of technology, realizing that no joint replacement procedure has yet proved to last 20 years.[4] Surgeons must continue to assess alternative methods of management and to make ongoing commitments to acquire the surgical skills needed to produce good long-term results in their patients. Only then can the role of new technologies and their effects on the indications for total hip arthroplasty be judged accurately.

With this caveat in mind, we attempt here to define the indications for total hip arthroplasty that we believe to be appropriate. The general indications for arthroplasty are discussed followed by suggestions on how these indications are tempered in young patients with advanced hip disease. Guidelines for preoperative planning are given regarding primary or revision arthroplasty to help the surgeon reach appropriate decisions in making it a safe, expeditious, and effective procedure for the patient.

INDICATIONS

As a general rule, arthroplasty of the hip is indicated for end-stage arthritic involvement of the hip in a patient with pain severe enough to cause disability and require pain medication. Usually, the patient also has loss of joint mobility. Frequent features of such end-stage disease are functional loss due to pain, decreased mobility, and accommodation of activities to lessen symptoms. Causes of end-stage disease include, but are not limited to, primary and secondary osteoarthritis, osteonecrosis, rheumatoid arthritis, gouty arthropathy, calcium pyrophosphate deposition, ochronosis, failed prior hip procedures, and post-traumatic conditions. Hemiarthroplasty and total hip arthroplasty are frequently utilized as primary treatments for displaced fractures of the femoral neck in elderly individuals.[13, 15, 34] They are used for other pathologic conditions, including primary and secondary tumors involving the hip. Metabolic conditions of bone, such as Paget's disease,[25, 35] may lead to advanced arthritis. The previously fused hip or the resected hip may be another indication for total hip arthroplasty.[37] It may also be indicated for the hip destroyed by remote sepsis. In the "hip-spine syndrome," in which spine symptoms predominate but are severely aggravated by an arthritic stiff hip, total hip arthroplasty is often the preferred first operative step to providing relief.[2]

First, the surgeon determines whether total hip arthroplasty is the best operation for the particular diseased hip. Second, the surgeon must decide if the operation is indicated for that particular individual. The surgeon must then help the patient weigh the risks against the benefits of undergoing intervention. Factors such as the patient's physical status, general medical condition, level of pain and disability, response to conservative therapy, and desired lifestyle must be considered.

For revision total hip arthroplasty, indications may be more difficult to define. Pain and loosening usually occur together with failed arthroplasty, but pain without obvious loosening is quite possible as is obvious loosening without pain. In such a situation, the decision to revise a hip arthroplasty must be individualized. The patient should be evaluated thoroughly to exclude infection as a source of loosening. Serial clinical and radiographic follow-up findings are helpful in determining the right timing for revision arthroplasty. Although significant pain is one justification, revision may also be indicated in a patient with progressive loosening or osteolysis severe enough to compromise the bony integrity of the proximal femur or acetabulum. In the case of osteolysis, the major compromise of the clinical result is related to insufficient local bone stock.[6, 21, 22]

End-stage hip disease in young patients poses a complex problem for the experienced surgeon. Although we now have a better understanding of the diseases leading to such compromises, have improved surgical techniques at our disposal, and have new technologies that may increase the longevity of arthroplasties, the fact remains that few devices of a mechanical nature have survived within the human body for more than 20 years. The physiologic and biologic effects of such devices are unknown. Even if the mechanical problems that plague implant longevity can be solved, the biologic consequences must be more thoroughly assessed and understood.

Armed with this perspective, one approaches arthroplasty procedures for the young adult with concern. Alternative interventions must be carefully considered, and an informed patient should be a partner in the decision to proceed with arthroplasty. It is our bias that these procedures are, by their very nature, experimental for a young patient and that the patient and surgeon should approach them as such. For the patient with unilateral arthropathy, under the age of 40, other surgical procedures should be considered when extensive medical management has been unsuccessful. These procedures are briefly discussed next.

ALTERNATIVE PROCEDURES

Pelvic Osteotomy

Several types of osteotomy of the pelvis have been recommended for the young adult with hip dysplasia. Osteotomies, such as those of Chiari,[10, 18] Salter,[31] and Dial,[12] are designed to improve acetabular coverage in patients with hip disability but with well-preserved passive range of motion. Clear signs of mechanical overload should be identified. Various methods are available to determine acetabular insufficiency, including measurement of plain radiographs,[38] fluoroscopic evaluation of acetabular coverage with varying femoral head position, arthrography, and computerized axial tomography (CAT) scanning with three-dimensional reconstruction.[1] Bone models can be employed when anatomic disruption is severe.[40] These procedures are useful even when arthritic changes are present, as pain relief and joint preservation are predictable in properly selected patients (Fig. 15–1).

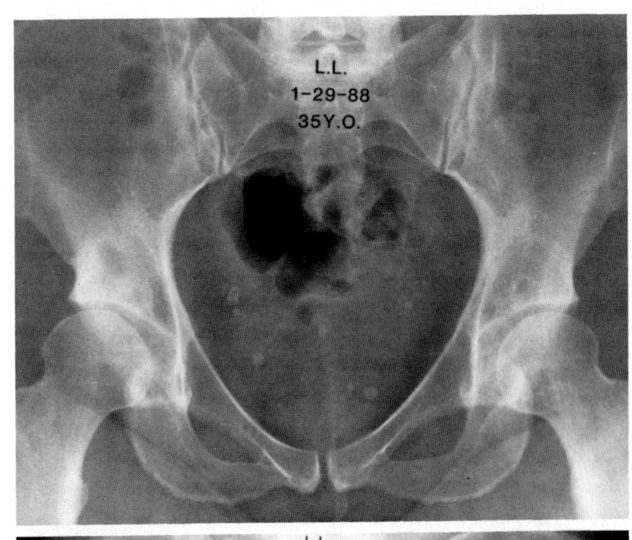

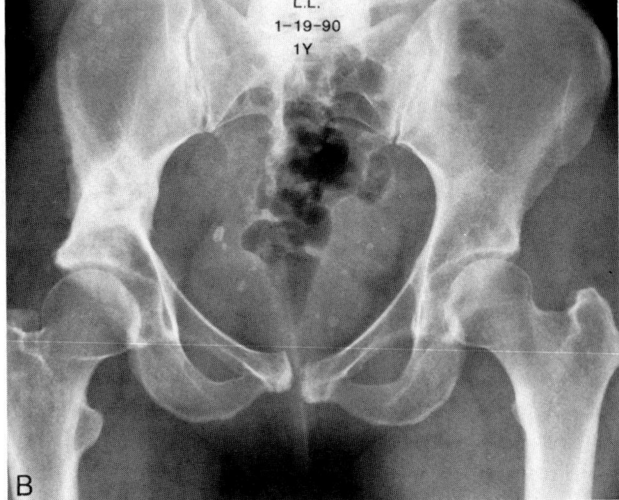

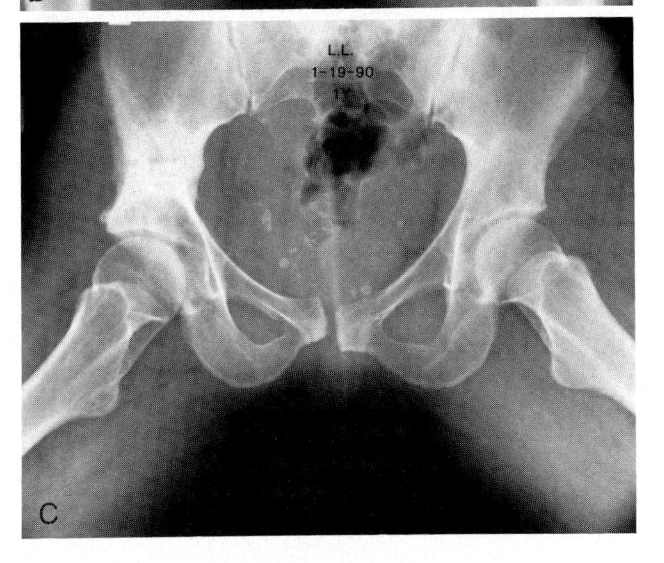

FIGURE 15–1. Osteotomy for painful dysplastic hip in a young woman. *A,* Preoperative film shows bilateral congenital dysplasia with secondary degenerative change, which is worse on the right side. *B,* Pelvic osteotomy (anteroposterior view) was done to improve femoral head coverage and distribution of contact force. *C,* Lateral view. Patient became asymptomatic postoperatively.

Femoral Osteotomy

Osteotomy of the proximal femur should be considered for the young adult with unilateral hip disease, in whom passive joint mobility is nearly complete, clear signs of mechanical overload are present, and enough articular surface is preserved to allow for redistribution of joint forces.[1, 24] Preoperative assessment is similar to that for pelvic osteotomy—it should be extensive enough to permit accurate diagnosis of the disease state and to allow for careful preoperative planning. In properly selected patients, osteotomy offers excellent pain relief while preserving the joint (Fig. 15–2). Unlike pelvic osteotomies, however, femoral osteotomies can alter proximal femoral anatomy significantly. This alteration may affect any future arthroplasty procedures that are needed. We believe that such procedures are clearly warranted for young adults, especially as the patients are provided with long-term function with minimal restrictions. With advancing technology, particularly newer techniques for custom arthroplasty, it should be possible to address altered proximal femoral geometry with predictable results.

Hip Arthrodesis

Although not a joint-preserving procedure, hip arthrodesis should remain in the surgeon's armamentarium. Hip fusion is an appropriate procedure for the young patient who has unilateral end-stage ar-

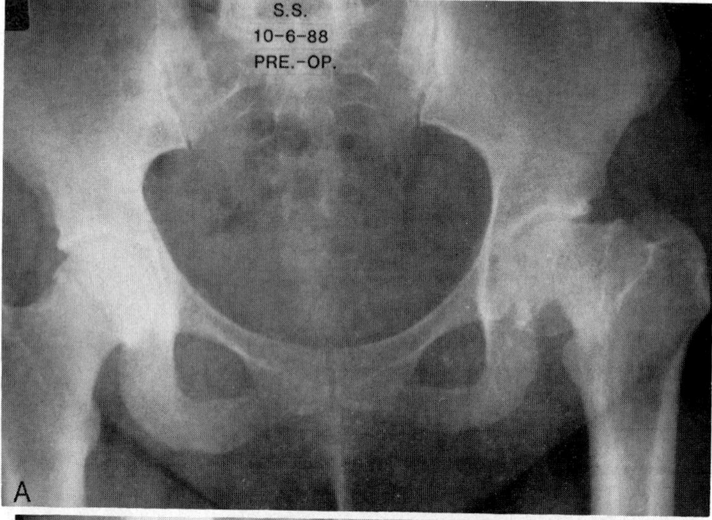

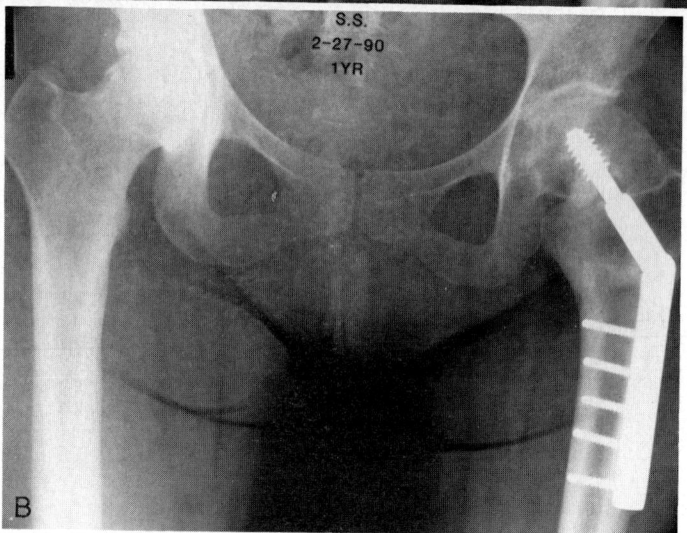

FIGURE 15–2. Young woman treated by femoral osteotomy for disabling hip pain. *A*, Preoperative film shows varus deformity and degenerative arthrosis. *B*, Valgus osteotomy provided excellent pain relief.

thritis and a vigorous lifestyle and who has anatomically and functionally normal lumbar spine and knee joints.[30, 37]

CONTRAINDICATIONS

Because of the excellent pain relief and functional improvement associated with total hip arthroplasty, few absolute contraindications exist. The contraindications include hip sepsis, any neurologic or mental disorder that precludes the patient's ability to rehabilitate to a reasonable degree; and multiple prior surgical procedures that have severely compromised the soft tissues about the hip, making functional arthroplasty impossible without extensive bracing.

Sepsis

Clearly, artificial devices should not be placed into acutely infected joints. Although great progress is being made in applying arthroplasty techniques to the joint that has been infected and treated, this practice remains an area of controversy and development. Patients with such hips are probably best treated in medical centers that have surgeons who are specialists in hip procedures, infectious disease specialists, and support personnel with substantial experience with these problems.

At this time, two-stage reimplantation for infection is an accepted practice, given appropriate preparations.[14, 32, 39] In some areas outside the United States, one-stage removal, debridement, and reimplantation are performed commonly; however, the practice remains controversial.[3] Treatment for this patient population should be highly individualized (see Chapter 23, *Revision Total Hip Arthroplasty*).

Neurologic Disorders

Little reason exists to proceed with total hip arthroplasty in the mentally or neurologically compromised patient who cannot exercise voluntary control over hip mobility and function. Complications in this patient population can be significant and overshadow what could be the limited benefits of the procedure.[5]

Multiple Surgical Procedures

In this era of high technology and availability of devices and bone allografts, it is tempting for the surgeon to attempt reconstruction of any hip. However, for the patient who has undergone multiple operations with substantial soft tissue and bone loss, a time may come for both surgeon and patient to look for other forms of management. Issues of tissue viability, patient nutrition, patient cooperation, and low-grade sepsis all enter into evaluation of these complex cases.[5, 19] Careful judgment must be exercised before proceeding further with surgical intervention.

CEMENTED VERSUS CEMENTLESS FIXATION

It is our belief that the decision to proceed with hip arthroplasty should be separated from the decision regarding fixation techniques. As new technologies become available, it is tempting to believe that they will last longer, and thus can be applied to younger patients, or that they can be applied in more difficult reconstruction problems.[11] These technologies and their benefits are controversial and require careful and thoughtful study in prospective fashion to prove their application. Until long-term outcomes are known, the patients' best interests are served by individualizing treatment on the basis of their goals, characteristics, and expectations. This treatment is best done once a decision to proceed with total hip arthroplasty is made. (A thorough discussion of the present role of cemented, cementless, and hybrid total hip arthroplasty can be found in Chapters 17, 20, 23, and 24.)

PREOPERATIVE PLANNING

The surgeon should be familiar with planning issues that relate to the style of the implant and the method of fixation (cemented or cementless). For preoperative planning that relates to the device selected, the surgeon is referred to the manuals and articles available from the implant designers and manufacturers.[27, 28]

Guidelines for preoperative evaluation of orthopaedic patients appear in several excellent reviews and elsewhere in this text (see Chapter 16, *Preoperative Evaluation* and Chapter 10, *Anesthesia for Joint Replacement Surgery*). We agree with Sculco that the orthopaedic surgeon must be fully conversant with the details of each patient's preoperative evaluation.[33] As more elderly patients undergo total hip arthroplasty, the surgeon's challenges become more complex. Particular attention to hematologic parameters, pulmonary function, and coronary vessel integrity is important to avoid perioperative complications.[20, 36] The nutritional status of the patient must receive greater attention.[16]

Communication between the patient, surgeon, anesthesiologist, and the patient's medical specialist must receive high priority. Surgeons will find that patients who stay involved in their care tend to have better outcomes. Fortunately, many educational aids are available to help a patient understand the reasons for surgical intervention, the goals and the expected outcome, and what must be done to achieve that outcome. Some patients choose to participate in autotransfusion programs to lessen that risk of surgery. In patients who refuse blood transfusions for religious or other reasons,[26] planning must be especially careful to avoid the need for transfusions. A history of good communication with the patient and family is the surgeon's best guarantee of continued amicable collaboration, even if problems arise.

Preoperative Radiographic Assessment

The goal of preoperative radiographic assessment is to confirm the diagnosis leading to surgical intervention, to determine the anatomic relationships of the femur and pelvis, and to allow for the accurate restoration of joint anatomy and biomechanics. Factors that influence the ease of insertion of the implants may suggest the need for special techniques or special equipment or for bone grafting materials to make up for anticipated deficits. Additional studies may be necessary.

The surgeon has a number of options for radiographic assessment preoperatively. For the primary total hip arthroplasty of a routine nature, in which a cemented prosthesis will be used, only the standard anteroposterior and lateral radiographs may be necessary. With cementless arthroplasty, however, significant miscalculation may result from the use of these radiographs alone. The surgeon should be aware of their limitations. Other studies that may be desirable include the following:

1. Anteroposterior and lateral radiographs with magnification markers
2. Oblique radiographs of the pelvis
3. Bone scans (technetium, gallium, indium)
4. Aspiration/arthrograms
5. Computer-assisted tomographic scans
6. Computer-assisted scans with bone models
7. Angiograms/venograms for severe intrapelvic protrusions
8. Intravenous pyelograms for severe intrapelvic protrusions.

The manner in which the radiographs are taken must be given specific attention if templating is to be of value. Correct judgment regarding acetabular and femoral component sizing depends upon the standardized positioning of the patient and limb to assure a neutral position of the acetabulum, the standardized view of the femur either internally rotated or neutral,[7, 8, 11] and the magnification of the radiographs. Oblique radiographs and tomograms allow for additional assessment of available bone support for the implants. Computer-assisted tomographic scans with three-dimensional reconstructions or models aid in the design of custom implants and allow the surgeon to visualize abnormal architecture as it will be encountered during surgery. When reconstructions are expected to be complex, these scans facilitate an understanding of spatial relationships and make it simpler to plan the steps needed to correct problems. This knowledge can reduce intraoperative guesswork substantially and can avoid the need to delay or abandon a surgical procedure because of the absence of the correct equipment or devices.[7] Preoperative vascular

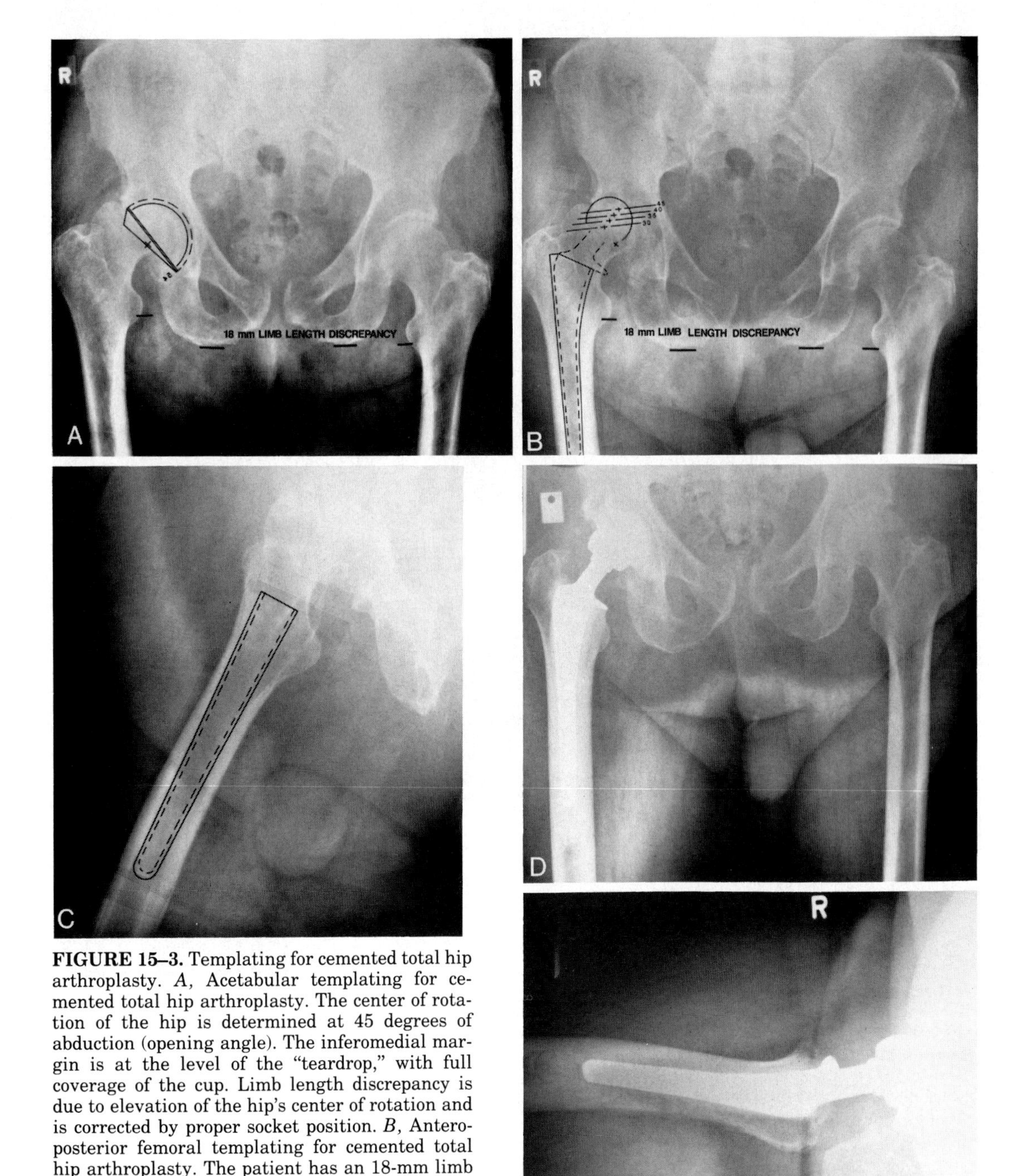

FIGURE 15–3. Templating for cemented total hip arthroplasty. *A,* Acetabular templating for cemented total hip arthroplasty. The center of rotation of the hip is determined at 45 degrees of abduction (opening angle). The inferomedial margin is at the level of the "teardrop," with full coverage of the cup. Limb length discrepancy is due to elevation of the hip's center of rotation and is corrected by proper socket position. *B,* Anteroposterior femoral templating for cemented total hip arthroplasty. The patient has an 18-mm limb length discrepancy; therefore, measurement is made 18 mm superior to the center of rotation determined from acetabular templating. The selected neck length is placed in that position for femoral templating. Operative reconstruction provides proper placement of the center of rotation of the hip joint and correction of the limb length discrepancy. *C,* Lateral femoral templating. This template assures adequate sizing. *D,* Postoperative anteroposterior view of cemented total hip reconstruction shows proper placement of center of rotation of the hip joint and correction of the limb length discrepancy. *E,* Postoperative lateral film shows excellent fit of the prosthesis within the bone and cement mantle.

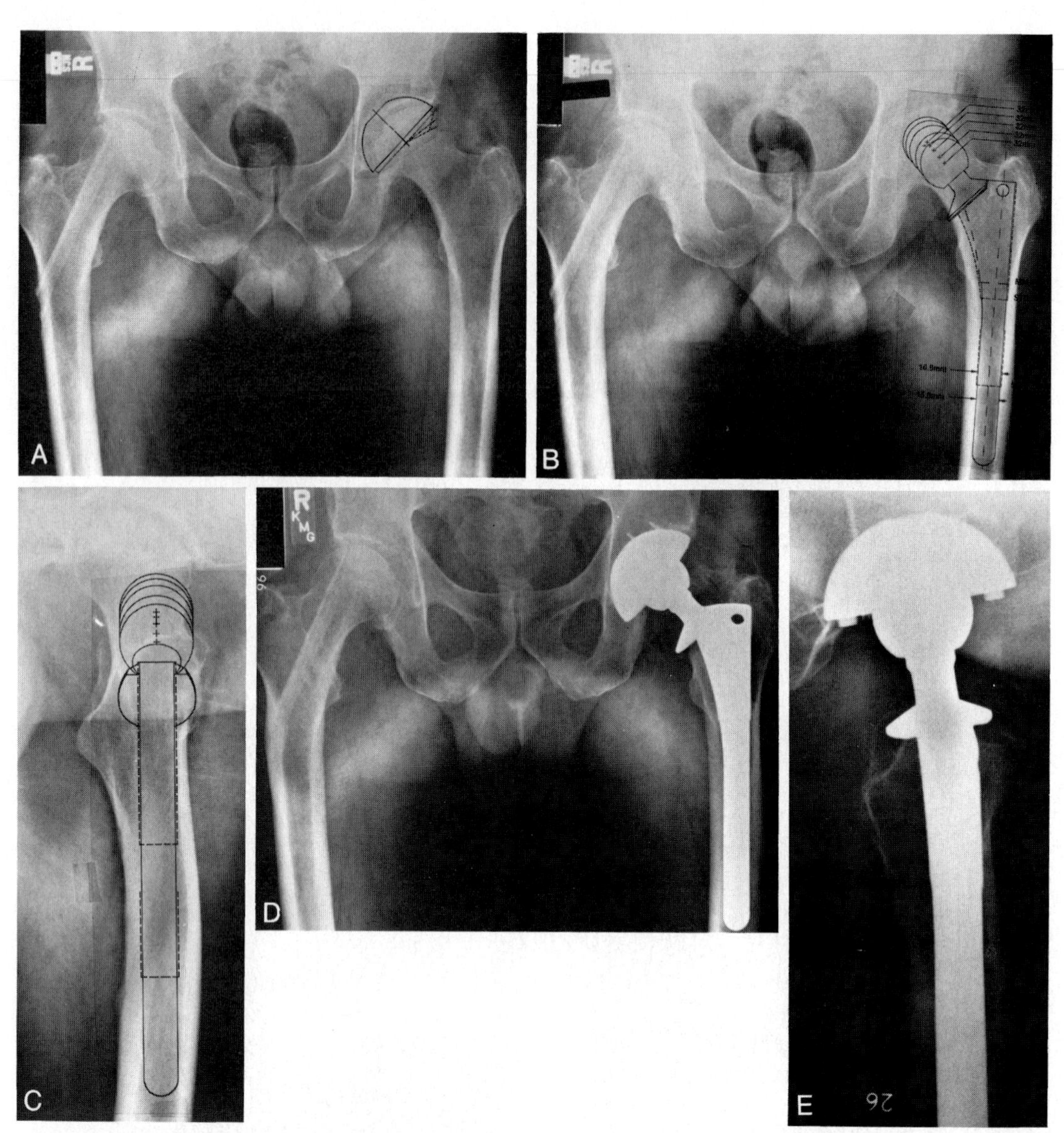

FIGURE 15–4. Templating for cementless total hip arthroplasty. *A*, Acetabular templating for cementless total hip arthroplasty. The center of rotation of the hip is determined at 45 degrees of abduction (opening angle). The inferomedial margin is at the level of the "teardrop," with full coverage of the cup. *B*, Anteroposterior femoral templating for cementless total hip arthroplasty. Operative reconstruction provides proper placement of the center of rotation of the hip joint. *C*, Lateral femoral templating. This template assures adequate sizing. *D*, Postoperative anteroposterior view of cementless total hip reconstruction. *E*, Postoperative lateral film shows excellent fit of the prosthesis within the bone.

and pyelographic studies are needed only when substantial intrapelvic protrusion by a previously implanted device suggests encroachment on critical structures or when intrapelvic dissection is required to augment pelvic support of an acetabular component.[17]

The general goals of preoperative templating are to determine the correct positioning of the implants within the bone to restore limb length, to place the hip center at its proper anatomic and biomechanical center, and to restore appropriate muscle relationships about the hip. The measurements are done by establishing reference points about the pelvis and comparing the operative hip to the contralateral hip. If neither hip is normal, an alternative method of determining the hip center should be used. In these circumstances we use the method of Ranawat[29] (see Chapter 23, *Revision Total Hip Arthroplasty*). When the contralateral hip is normal, many surgeons prefer to template this hip first. This template identifies the "normal" hip center and allows the surgeon to estimate how closely the femoral device matches the upper femoral anatomy of the patient. The information helps the surgeon determine the needed neck length and neck offset for the patient. Once visualized, the template should be applied to the involved side to determine the degree to which the anatomy has been altered by the disease process or by any previous intervention. The surgeon may then judge the fit of the implant within the available bone structure. The necessary steps are demonstrated in Figures 15–3 and 15–4. An estimate of the size of the femoral stem to be implanted is desirable, especially when the hip is very small or very large and when "off-the-shelf" devices might be of the incorrect dimensions.

Preoperative radiographic planning is particularly important in the revision of previously failed hip arthroplasties. Before a procedure is undertaken, the surgeon must assess the component fixation, the status with regard to infection, the degree of anatomic disruption, and the degree of available bone support after removal of the device. Moreover, the appropriate surgical approach must be determined to achieve exposure for safe removal and implantation and the need established for special equipment, implants, and bone grafts. Assessment of appropriate implant positioning is more difficult, and special techniques such as those of Ranawat[29] for acetabular component positioning and scanograms or computer-assisted tomographic scans may be needed (see Chapter 23, *Revision Total Hip Arthroplasty*).

Proposed Surgical Intervention

After the preoperative radiographic studies have been reviewed, the surgeon should have a clear idea of the goals to be accomplished intraoperatively and the steps required to reach these goals. If the anatomic relationships appear to be minimally disrupted and routine approaches and implant inventory are likely to be satisfactory, little additional planning may be needed. If not, however, both the surgeon and the operating room staff must be prepared for the atypical features of the procedure, such as the need for bone grafts (autografts or allografts), special implants, or internal fixation devices (plates and screws to affix bone grafts). Special equipment may be required, such as cement-removal instruments, high-speed drills or burrs, and cerclage wires or cables. Thorough planning may suggest surgical positions and approaches that are not standard. The entire operative team, including the surgeon, benefits from minimization of intraoperative guesswork.[7] So, of course, does the patient.

References

1. Bombelli, R., Santore, R.F., and Poss, R.: Mechanics of the normal and osteoarthritic hip: A new perspective. Clin. Orthop. 182:69–78, 1984.
2. Boumphrey, F., Borden, L.S., MacNab, I., and Stulberg, B.N.: Hip-spine syndrome. American Academy of Orthopaedic Surgeons Annual Meeting, Anaheim, CA, 1983.
3. Buchholz, H.W., Elson, R.A., Engelbrecht, E., et al.: Management of deep infection of total hip replacement. J. Bone Joint Surg. 63B:342, 1981.
4. Burstein, A.H.: Critical analysis of today's knee implants. American Academy of Orthopaedic Surgeons Annual Meeting, New Orleans, LA, 1990.
5. Calandruccio, R.A.: Arthroplasty of the Hip. Campbell's Operative Orthopaedics. St. Louis, C. V. Mosby Company, 1987.
6. Callaghan, J.J., Salvati, E.A., Pellicci, P.M., et al.: Results of revision for mechanical failure after cemented total hip replacement, 1979 to 1982. J. Bone Joint Surg. 67A:1074, 1985.
7. Capello, W.N.: Preoperative planning of total hip arthroplasty. AAOS Instr. Course Lect., Vol 35. St. Louis, C.V. Mosby Company, 1986.
8. Chandler, H.P. and Penneberg, B.L.: Bone Stock Deficiency in Total Hip Replacement—Classification and Management. Thorofare, NJ, Slack, Inc., 1989.
9. Charnley, J.: Low Friction Arthroplasty of the Hip: Theory and Practice. New York, Springer-Verlag, 1979.
10. Chiari, K.: Medial displacement osteotomy of the pelvis. Clin. Orthop. 98:55, 1974.
11. Engh, C.A. and Bobyn, J.D.: Biological Fixation in Total Hip Arthroplasty. Thorofare, NJ, Slack, Inc., 1985.
12. Eppright, R.H.: Dial osteotomy of the acetabulum. J. Bone Joint Surg. 58A:283, 1976.
13. Evarts, C.M.: Endoprosthetic Replacement for Femoral Neck Fractures. Surgery of the Musculoskeletal System. New York, Churchill Livingstone, 1983.

14. Garvin, K.L., Salvati, E.A., and Brause, B.D.: Role of gentamycin-impregnated cemented in total joint arthroplasty. Orthop. Clin. North Am. 19:3, 1988.
15. Gingras, M.B., Clarke, J., and Evarts, C.M.: Prosthetic replacement in femoral neck fractures. Clin. Orthop. 152:147, 1990.
16. Greene, K.A., Wilde, A.H., and Stulberg, B.N.: Pre-operative nutritional status of total joint patients: Relationship to post-operative wound complications. American Academy of Orthopaedic Surgeons Annual Meeting, Las Vegas, NV, 1989.
17. Harris, W.H., Crothers, O., and Oh, I.: Total hip replacement and femoral head bone grafting for severe acetabular deficiency in adults. J. Bone Joint Surg. 59A:752, 1977.
18. Hirohata, K., Shiba, R., and Shimizu, T.: Follow-up results of Chiari pelvis osteotomy for patients with acetabular dysplasia. Hirohata Joint Surgery Up to Date. New York, Springer-Verlag, 1989.
19. Jensen, J.E., Jensen, T.G., Smith, T.K., et al.: Nutrition in orthopaedic surgery. J. Bone Joint Surg. 64A:1263, 1982.
20. Kaell, A.T., Bennett, R.S., and Hamburger, M.I.: Rheumatologic Management of the Arthritic Hip. Edited by Stillwell, W.T. The Art of Total Hip Arthroplasty. Orlando, Grune & Stratton, 1987.
21. Kavanagh, B.F. and Fitzgerald, Jr., R.H.: Multiple revisions for failed total hip arthroplasty not associated with infection. J. Bone Joint Surg. 69A:1144, 1987.
22. Kavanagh, B.F., Ilstrup, D.M., and Fitzgerald, Jr., R.H.: Revision total hip arthroplasty. J. Bone Joint Surg. 67A:517, 1985.
23. Liechti, R.: Hip Arthrodesis. Surgery of the Musculoskeletal System. New York, Churchill Livingstone, 1983.
24. Maquet, P.G.J.: Biomechanics of the Hip. Berlin, Springer-Verlag, 1985.
25. Merkow, R.C., Haly, D.P., and Salvati, E.A.: Total hip replacement for Paget's disease of the hip. J. Bone Joint Surg. 66A:752, 1984.
26. Nelson, C.L., Martin, K., Lawson, N., et al.: Total hip replacement without transfusion. Contemp. Orthop. 2:655, 1980.
27. OmniFlex Hip System. Osteonics, Inc., Allendale, NJ.
28. PCA Hip Systems. Howmedica, Rutherford, NJ.
29. Ranawat, C.S.: Total hip arthroplasty in protrusio acetabuli of rheumatoid arthritis. J. Bone Joint Surg. 62A:1059, 1980.
30. Russell, T.A.: Arthrodesis of lower extremity and hip. Campbell's Operative Orthopaedics. St. Louis, C.V. Mosby Company, 1987.
31. Salter, R.B., Hansson, G., and Thompson, G.H.: Innominate osteotomy in the management of congenital subluxation of the hip in young adults. Clin. Orthop. 182:53, 1984.
32. Salvati, E.A., Chekoofsky, K.M., Brause, B.D., and Wilson, Jr., P.D.: Reimplantation in infection: A twelve-year experience. Clin. Orthop. 170:62, 1982.
33. Sculco, T.P.: Orthopaedic Care of the Geriatric Patient. St. Louis, C.V. Mosby Company, 1985.
34. Sim, F.H. and Stauffer, R.N.: Management of hip fractures by total hip arthroplasty. Clin. Orthop. 152:191, 1980.
35. Stauffer, R.N. and Sim, F.H.: Total hip arthroplasty in Paget's disease of the hip. J. Bone Joint Surg. 58A:476, 1976.
36. Stillwell, W.T.: The Art of Total Hip Arthroplasty. Orlando, Grune & Stratton, 1987.
37. Strathy, G.M. and Fitzgerald, Jr., R.H.: Total hip arthroplasty in the ankylosed hip: A ten year follow-up. J. Bone Joint Surg. 70A:963, 1988.
38. Stulberg, S.D. and Harris, W.H.: Acetabular Dysplasia and the Development of Osteoarthritis of the Hip. The Hip. St. Louis, C.V. Mosby Company, 1974.
39. Wilson, Jr., P.D., Aglietti, P., and Salvati, E.A.: Subacute sepsis of the hip treated by antibiotics and cemented prosthesis. J. Bone Joint Surg. 56A:879, 1974.
40. Woolson, S.T., Dev, P., Fellingham, L., et al.: Three-dimensional imaging of bone from computerized tomography. Clin. Orthop. 220:239, 1986.

CHAPTER 16

Total Hip Arthroplasty: Preoperative Evaluation

WILLIAM PETTY

Careful evaluation of the candidate for total hip arthroplasty is essential for a successful procedure with a good long-term outcome. Extra care is needed in this patient population, because most surgical candidates are at an age when they are at risk for a number of common medical illnesses. Planning of the operative procedure is done as a team effort, supervised by the orthopaedic surgeon and including the anesthesiologist and any other specialists involved in the patient's care.

In addition to thorough assessment of the musculoskeletal system, evaluation includes a complete history and physical examination, neurologic assessment, studies of vascular status, appropriate blood and urine tests, chest radiograph, and electrocardiogram. It is as important to detect asymptomatic heart disease, lung disease, or other disease as it is to assess known disease processes (see Chapter 10, *Anesthesia for Joint Replacement Surgery*). Patients with certain conditions may require treatment before surgery is performed—examples are men with prostatic enlargements sufficient to cause urinary retention.

The patient's nutritional status must be evaluated because of its importance in wound healing and postoperative recovery. Assessment of the upper extremities must not be overlooked because of the need to use walking aids or other types of support. Patients' functional and psychologic well-being should also be considered. The surgeon should be aware of the emotional needs of individual patients.

HISTORY

A thorough history of the patient's problem is essential, even though the patient may be referred with a clear complaint of hip pain or a firm diagnosis of the hip problem. In most patients with hip joint disease, the pain occurs in the groin, often radiating down the anteromedial thigh. Pain may or may not reach the knee joint. Sometimes the pain occurs posteriorly. With posterior pain, sciatica or other disease related to the spine must be considered. The pain of hip joint disease may be constant. Usually it is worsened by weight-bearing, motion of the hip joint, or both.

Patients should be encouraged to describe their problem in their own words, without interruption, except when the interviewer needs clarification or when the narrative is getting away from the subject. The association between various activities and hip pain or disability is important in determining the diagnosis and extent of disability. For this reason, patients should be questioned about the degree of interference with occupation, avocations, and activities of daily living. Also, they should be asked about previous measures they have taken to relieve pain and continue functioning. The following are some important questions:

- Have you had to stop work, change jobs, or modify your work activities?
- Do you have trouble dressing, especially putting on stockings and tying your shoes?
- Do you have trouble rising from a chair or climbing stairs?
- Do you use a cane or other supportive aid for walking?
- Has your sexual function diminished?
- Have you had to take analgesics, narcotics, antiarthritic agents, or other medications to help you continue functioning?
- Have you consulted other physicians about this problem in the past? If so, what have they advised and what have you tried?

Questions about sexual activity are important because sexual dysfunction is not uncommon in patients with severe hip disease. In a patient with severe multijoint deformity, essential activities such as perineal care may be impaired. The patient's history of alcohol use may also be important in diagnosis. The orthopaedic surgeon should also ask about heavy alcohol intake because it influences operative and postoperative care. The other standard components of the history are previous surgical procedures and medical illnesses.

Preoperative interviews should include questions about the patient's expectations from total hip replacement. What the patient perceives as indications for surgery may not be valid. If for example, a patient is currently disabled only for vigorous activities such as running and jumping and wishes to resume them after the operation, surgery may not be warranted, as these are activities that should be avoided after total hip replacement.

PHYSICAL EXAMINATION

The physical examination really begins at the time of the surgeon's first glimpse of the patient. As the patient enters the office, the surgeon makes a practice of observing how he or she moves. When the patient is already in the examining room, the surgeon watches how that patient rises from a chair. Is it an easy or a difficult task? Must the patient hoist himself or

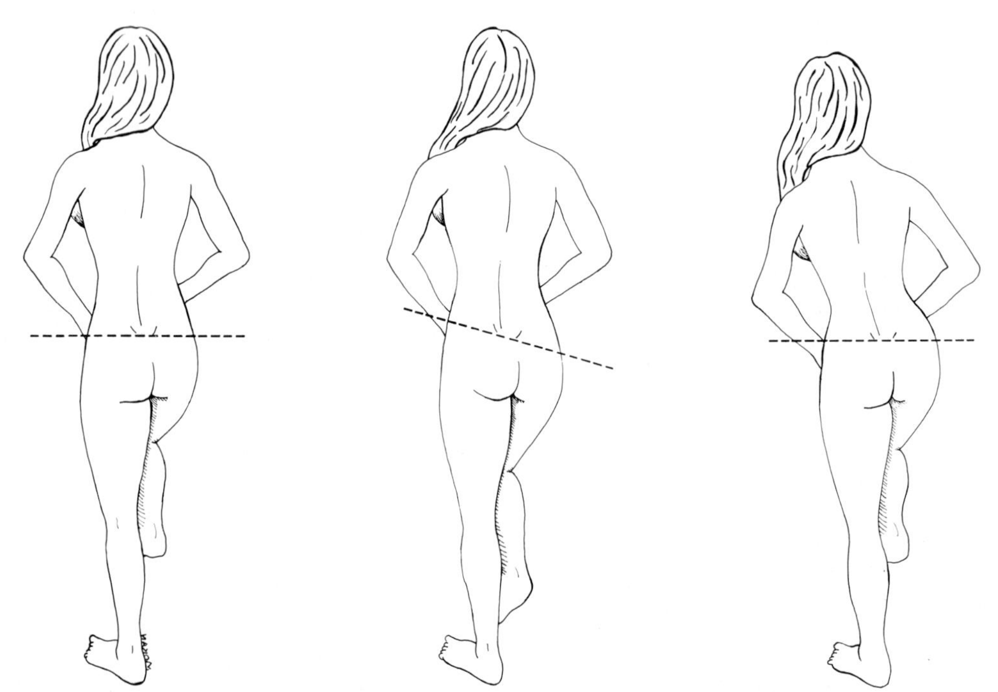

FIGURE 16–1. The Trendelenburg sign and Trendelenburg "lurch" (Duchenne sign). *Left,* Negative Trendelenburg sign and lurch. *Center,* Positive Trendelenburg sign. *Right,* Positive Trendelenburg lurch (Duchenne sign).

herself by the arms to get up? After rising from the chair, what posture does the patient assume? With appropriate respect for the patient's privacy, the surgeon can learn much about the disability by watching the patient remove their shoes, stockings, and outer clothing.

Observing the patient's upright posture can reveal important information about the disability. After rising from a chair, for example, a patient may show evidence of contracture or other deformity at the hip, knee, or other location. By asking the patient to stand first on one leg and then on the other, the surgeon may detect a dysfunctional abductor mechanism as revealed by a positive Trendelenburg sign. This sign is evidenced by dropping of the pelvis on the side opposite the involved hip. A patient often compensates for a dysfunction by leaning over the involved hip, shifting the body's center of gravity toward the involved side and reducing the abductor force required to remain standing (Trendelenburg lurch or Duchenne sign). The Trendelenburg lurch may or may not be associated with a positive Trendelenburg sign (Fig. 16–1).[3]

The patient's limb length can be assessed by having the patient stand with both legs straight while the examiner places one hand on each iliac crest and sights along them to detect any difference (Fig. 16–2). By having the patient stand with one foot on wooden blocks of various heights until the line of sight is parallel to the ground, the difference can be measured. A difference may not be due to unequal limb length but to hip deformity, usually flexion contracture, or to knee, ankle, or foot deformity.

By observing the patient walking, the surgeon can get clues to the abnormalities on the involved side. A patient should be asked to walk both with and without a cane or other walking aid, if possible. As the patient walks, the limp should be studied closely and its cause evaluated—is it pain, abductor dysfunction, or both?

When a limp is due primarily to pain, stride length and stance phase are shorter on the involved side. That knee is brought forward quickly, and pelvis rotation is exaggerated on that side. In an attempt to reduce discomfort, the patient decreases time and motion on the affected side.

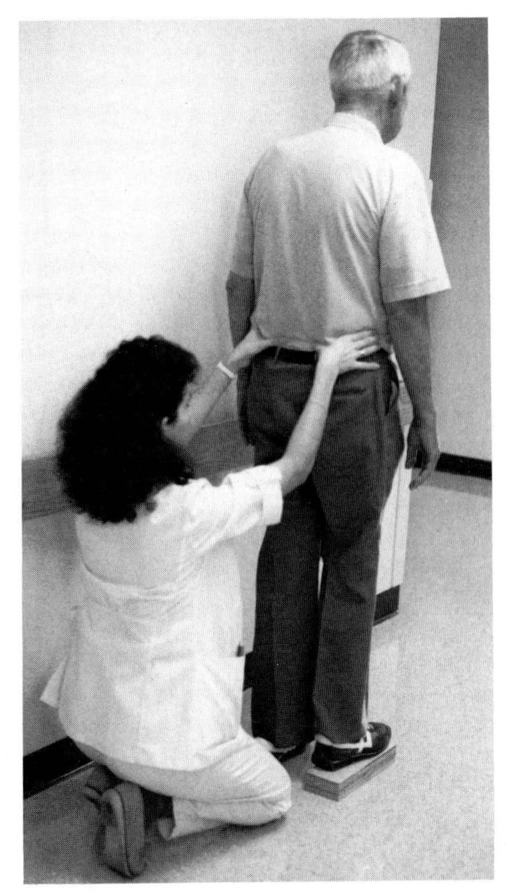

FIGURE 16–2. Estimation of limb length discrepancy in the standing position.

If abductor dysfunction is responsible, it may be caused by a single abnormality or several, including weak abductor muscles, short femoral head and neck segment, coxa vara, and arthritis pain (Fig. 16–3). The Trendelenburg limp resembles the Trendelenburg lurch (Duchenne sign), i.e., the body tilts over the involved hip to shift the body's center of gravity in that direction. Because this movement takes extra time, it may mask the shortened stance phase of the painful hip that also has abductor dysfunction.

When a patient with hip disease has the characteristics of both a painful hip and an abductor dysfunction, the presentation may be confusing to the examiner. However, with careful observation, the examiner can discern elements of both types of limp. It is important to note that the absence of a Trendelenburg sign or limp does not always mean that abductor function is

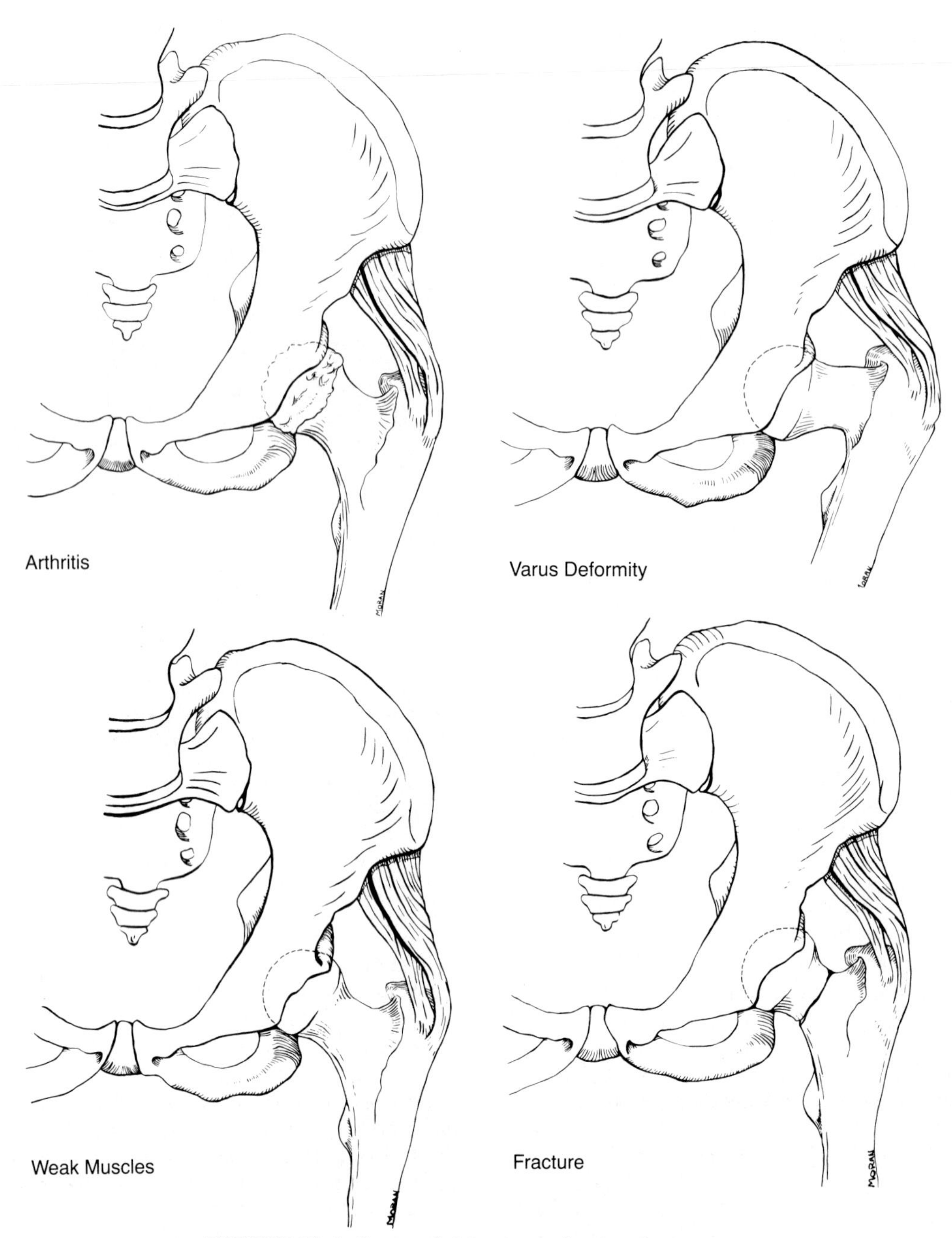

FIGURE 16–3. Causes of abductor mechanism dysfunction.

normal. The sign may be absent in cases of significant hip disease complicated by fibrous or bony ankylosis of the hip or spinal rigidity from spondylitis or extensive spinal fusion.

The position of the limbs should be observed with the patient supine on a firm examining table. Is contracture evidenced by lumbar lordosis or the position in which the patient holds the extremity (Fig. 16–4)? The patient should be asked to move the hip through various motions. If an abnormality is observed in any motion, the examiner may move the limb to determine any differences between passive and active motion. If the uninvolved hip is normal, the motion of the two hips can be compared. All areas of suspected pain should be palpated gently. A common cause of hip pain is greater trochanteric bursitis. It can be diagnosed by history and palpation.

One of the standard hip rating scales is completed as a part of the history and physical examination (see Chapter 21 for a discussion of hip ratings.)

OTHER STUDIES AND EXAMINATIONS

The plain radiograph remains the most valuable imaging study for the patient with hip disease. In certain instances, bone scans, plain or computerized tomography, and magnetic resonance imaging are helpful. Computerized tomography is especially useful in evaluating severe bony deformity, especially of the pelvis and acetabulum. A routine chest radiograph is made as part of the elderly patient's general examination.

Each patient scheduled for surgery undergoes a hemogram and urinalysis. Urine cultures are done if any suspicion has arisen about urinary tract infections. Some patients should also undergo laboratory tests for electrolyte values, liver function findings, and renal function findings (see Chapter 10, *Anesthesia for Joint Replacement Surgery)*.[4]

Because nutritional deficiency is common among elderly patients, nutritional status should be evaluated before surgery. Poor nutrition can compromise wound healing and can predispose the patient to infection of the wound site as well as to infection of the urinary tract, lungs, and so forth. In two studies of the nutritional status of patients scheduled for elective total hip arthroplasty, 27 percent and 29 percent were found to be malnourished[1, 2] Major wound complications were seven times more common in patients with nutritional deficiencies. For these reasons, patients with histories of weight loss greater than 10 lb, serum albumin levels of less than 3.4 gm/dl, or lymphocyte counts below 1500 cells/ml should undergo

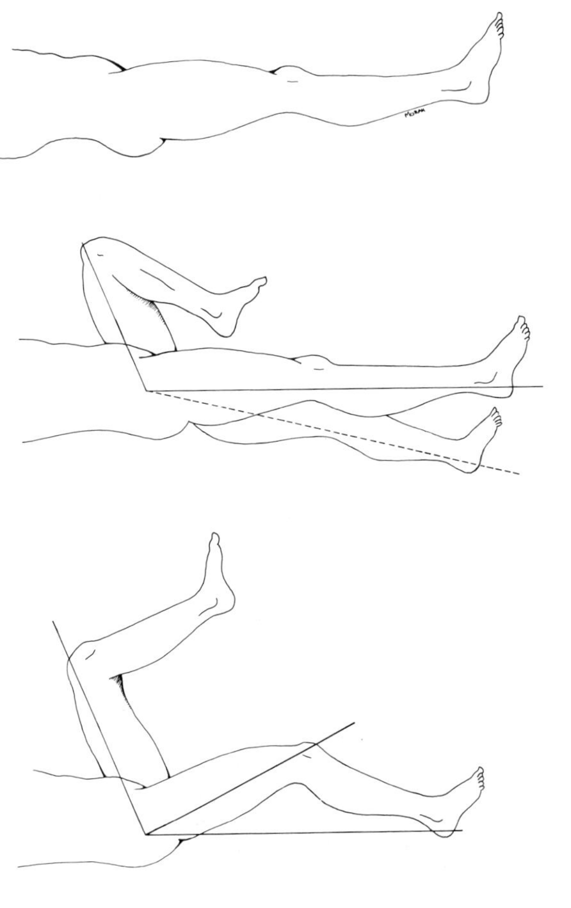

FIGURE 16–4. *Top,* Accentuated lordosis may be due to hip flexion contracture. *Center,* Negative Thomas test findings. With the opposite hip flexed to eliminate lumbar lordosis, the hip remains extended with the limb flat against the examining table. *Bottom,* Positive Thomas test findings. When the opposite hip is flexed to eliminate lumbar lordosis, the hip flexes. The angle between the thigh and table is the degree of hip flexion contracture.

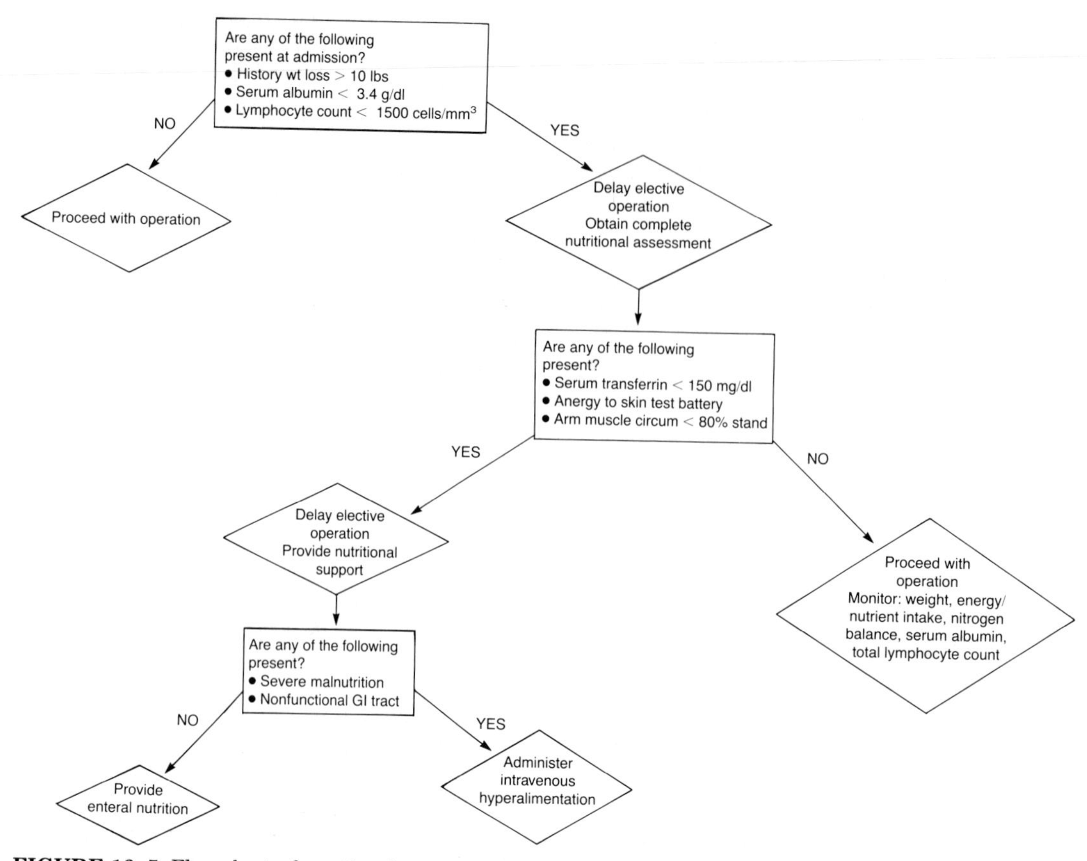

FIGURE 16–5. Flow chart of a rational screening approach to identify patients who are at risk for nutritional deficiencies, utilizing tests that are readily available. (Redrawn from Jensen, J. E., Jensen, T. G., Smith, T. K., et al.: J. Bone Joint Surg. 64A:1263–1272, 1982.)

further evaluation and correction of nutritional deficiency before surgery is scheduled (Fig. 16–5).[1,2]

PREOPERATIVE PREPARATION

The patient is oriented to the hospital environment, the plans for the operation, and the postoperative protocol. Brochures, videotapes, and illustrated books may all be helpful, but discussion with the physicians, nurses, and therapists, providing an opportunity for the patient to ask questions, is invaluable for setting the stage for a successful result and in allaying anxiety for the patient.

Orientation is especially important for the patient who will be admitted to the hospital the day of surgery. The patient showers or bathes with an antibacterial soap the night before and the morning of surgery. In the operating room, the surgeon assures proper positioning of the patient for the approach chosen. Preventive antibiotics are given in the operating room just before the operation.

References

1. Greene, K. A., Wilde, A. H., and Stulberg, B. N.: Preoperative nutritional status of total joint patients: Relationship to postoperative wound problems. Orthop. Trans. 13:622, 1989.
2. Jensen, J. E., Jensen, T. G., Smith, T. K., et al: Nutrition in orthopaedic surgery. J. Bone Joint Surg. 64A:1263–1272, 1982.
3. Johnston, R. C., Fitzgerald, Jr., R. H., Harris, W. H., et al: Clinical and radiographic evaluation of total hip replacement. J. Bone Joint Surg. 72A:161–168, 1990.
4. Sanders, D. P., McKinney, F. W., and Harris, W. H.: Clinical evaluation and cost effectiveness of preoperative laboratory assessment on patients undergoing total hip arthroplasty. Orthopedics 12:1449–1453, 1989.

CHAPTER 17

Total Hip Arthroplasty: Operative Technique

WILLIAM PETTY

Generally, a standard procedure for total hip arthroplasty, either with cemented or press-fit fixation, is performed for a patient with severe osteoarthritis, rheumatoid arthritis, or osteonecrosis (Table 17–1).[11] The first part of this chapter covers the operative technique for cemented and press-fit primary total hip arthroplasty. A small number of patients with other diagnoses require special modifications of these techniques. The second part of this chapter discusses the guidelines for the surgical procedures that involve special problems.

TOTAL HIP ARTHROPLASTY WITH BONE CEMENT

When a modern prosthesis is used and total hip arthroplasty with bone cement is performed with careful attention to detail, this operation is one of the most successful procedures performed today—in any field of surgery. The majority of patients with hip disease can expect excellent and durable results.

Femoral Neck Resection

The hip is exposed by the surgeon's chosen approach, and the hip joint dislocated (see Chapter 14, *Surgical Approaches for Total Hip Replacement*). The remaining capsular and synovial tissues are excised from the femoral neck. Precise osteotomy of the femoral neck is important in providing proper length reconstruction and in correctly seating the prosthetic collar, if the prosthesis has one.

One or more of four methods may be employed to determine the correct level of femoral neck resection: (1) use of an osteotomy guide, (2) measurement of the distance between the cephalad extent of the lesser trochanter and the resection level, (3) determination of the remaining cartilage and the amount of subchondral bone to be removed, and (4) placement of fixed markers in the ilium and greater trochanter or proximal femoral area.

Table 17–1. DIAGNOSES IN 2012 HIPS TREATED BY TOTAL HIP ARTHROPLASTY

Diagnosis	Percentage
Osteoarthritis	54.0
Failed prosthesis	12.6
Failed cup	5.9
Rheumatoid arthritis	5.8
Aseptic necrosis with osteoarthritis	5.1
Failed osteotomy	4.1
Traumatic arthritis	3.2
Congenital hip dysplasia	2.7
Slipped capital femoral epiphysis	0.9
Nonunion of fracture	0.9
Legg-Calvé-Perthes disease	0.4
Ancient sepsis	0.3
Miscellaneous	4.1

Modified from Coventry, M. B., Beckenbaugh, R. D., Nolan, D. R., and Ilstrup, D. M.: J. Bone Joint Surg. 56A:273–284, 1974.

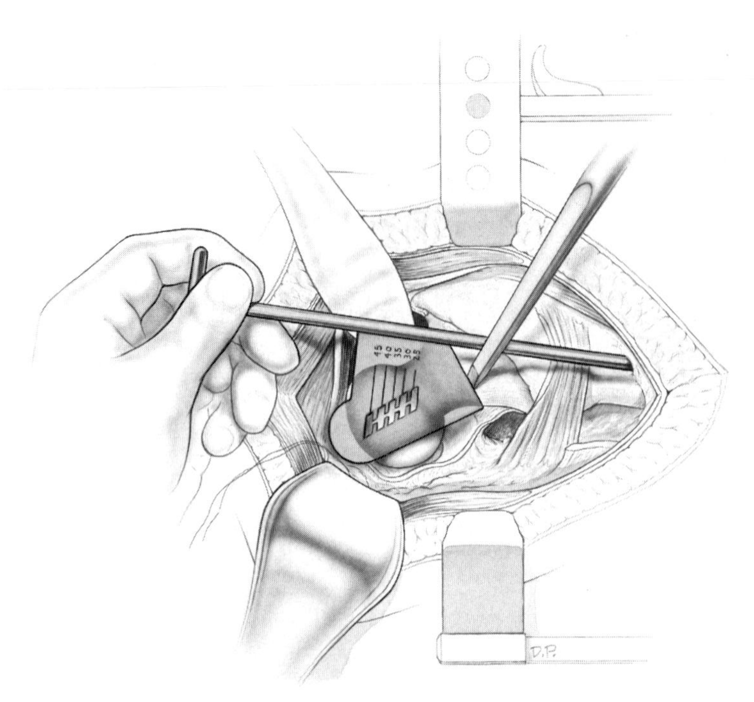

FIGURE 17–1. Neck resection level determined with an osteotomy guide.

Use of an Osteotomy Guide (Fig. 17–1). In this method, the surgeon marks the center of rotation of the femoral head, which is not the actual center of the head. A circular template with a hole in the center is helpful in selecting this point. In most hips, the center lies along a line extending from the tip of the greater trochanter and perpendicular to the longitudinal axis of the femoral shaft. Examination of radiographs will show any variance from this location, and appropriate adjustments may be made. The hole or slot of the osteotomy guide, representing the neck length that was selected preoperatively, is placed over the center of rotation, and the guide is aligned with the longitudinal axis of the femoral shaft. This procedure is done by palpating the femur through the muscles or by directing the guide toward the center of the knee joint or popliteal fossa. The resection level and angle are then marked.

Measurement of the Distance Between the Cephalad Extent of the Lesser Trochanter and the Resection Level (Fig. 17–2). During preoperative templating, the surgeon measures the distance between the cephalad extent of the lesser trochanter and the selected resection level. An osteotomy guide, a broach, or a trial prosthesis is used to aid in marking the appropriate resection angle.

Determination of the Remaining Cartilage and the Amount of Subchondral Bone to be Removed (Fig. 17–3). The amount of cartilage that must be removed, if any, and the amount of subchondral bone to be resected from the acetabulum are determined. Their combined height is subtracted from the height of the acetabular

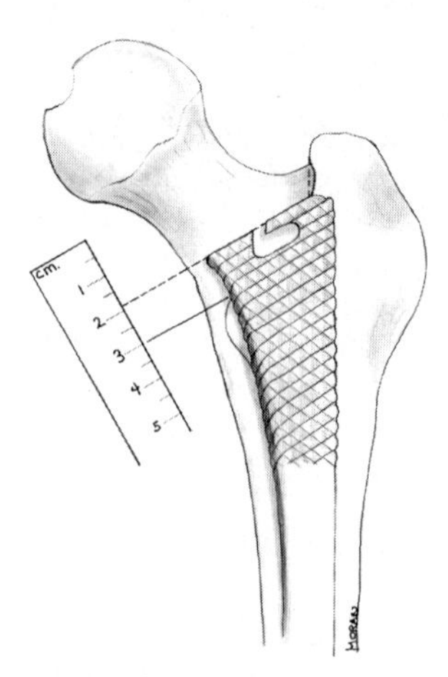

FIGURE 17–2. Determination of the neck resection level by measuring from cephalad extent of lesser trochanter to neck resection level as determined during preoperative templating.

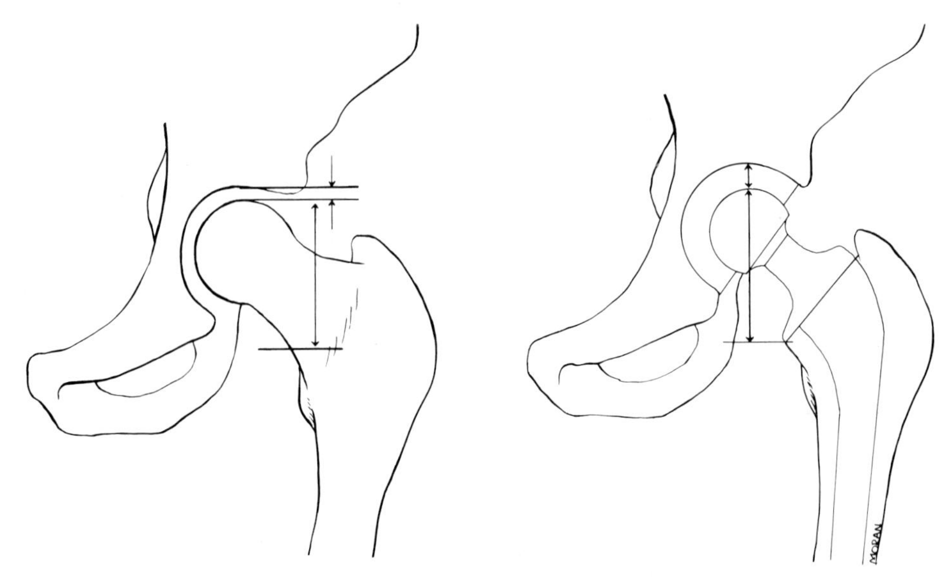

FIGURE 17–3. Determination of the neck resection level by measuring the remaining cartilage and bone to be removed and the prosthesis neck length (see text). (Modified from Woolson, S. T.: Orthopedics 13: 17–21, 1990.)

and head-neck portions of the femoral components to be implanted. The difference equals the height of the head-neck fragment to be removed. The distance is measured from the superior aspect of the femoral head to the medial border of the femoral neck where the osteotomy is made. If adjustments are necessary for length correction, the length of the prosthesis neck can be altered or the level of the neck osteotomy shifted upward or downward by the appropriate amount.[73]

Placement of Fixed Markers (Fig. 17–4). When the surgeon wishes to gauge length across the hip joint rather than just length of the proximal femur, fixed markers may be placed in the ilium and greater trochanter or proximal femoral area. These markers remain in place during surgery and are useful if a question arises about lengthening or shortening when the acetabulum is placed.[74] The distance between the two markers is measured with the leg in neutral abduction-adduction and preferably full extension. This distance, taking into account any length adjustments needed, is reproduced during trial reduction of the prosthetic components. For the method to be accurate, the leg must be placed in the same position for measurements before dislocation and after trial prosthesis placement. The level of resection is estimated and the angle set with the osteotomy guide, broach, or trial prosthesis.

After the osteotomy site is determined, the osteotomy is made with an oscillating saw (Fig. 17–5). To avoid cutting into the greater trochanter, it may be necessary to cut the superior portion of the femoral neck along the medial border of the greater trochanter.

Preparation of the Acetabulum

After the head-neck fragment has been removed, additional capsule is excised as needed to provide excellent exposure of the acetabulum. Cobra and similar retractors are ideal to achieve this exposure. Only smooth retractors are placed posteriorly to reduce the possibility of sciatic nerve injury. Superior exposure may be improved by utilizing an iliac retractor that is held in place with drill bits (Fig. 17–6).

Osteophyte formation may be extensive in patients with osteoarthritis and other disease processes. In some cases, the transverse acetabular ligament may be ossified. Osteophytes should be removed, with an

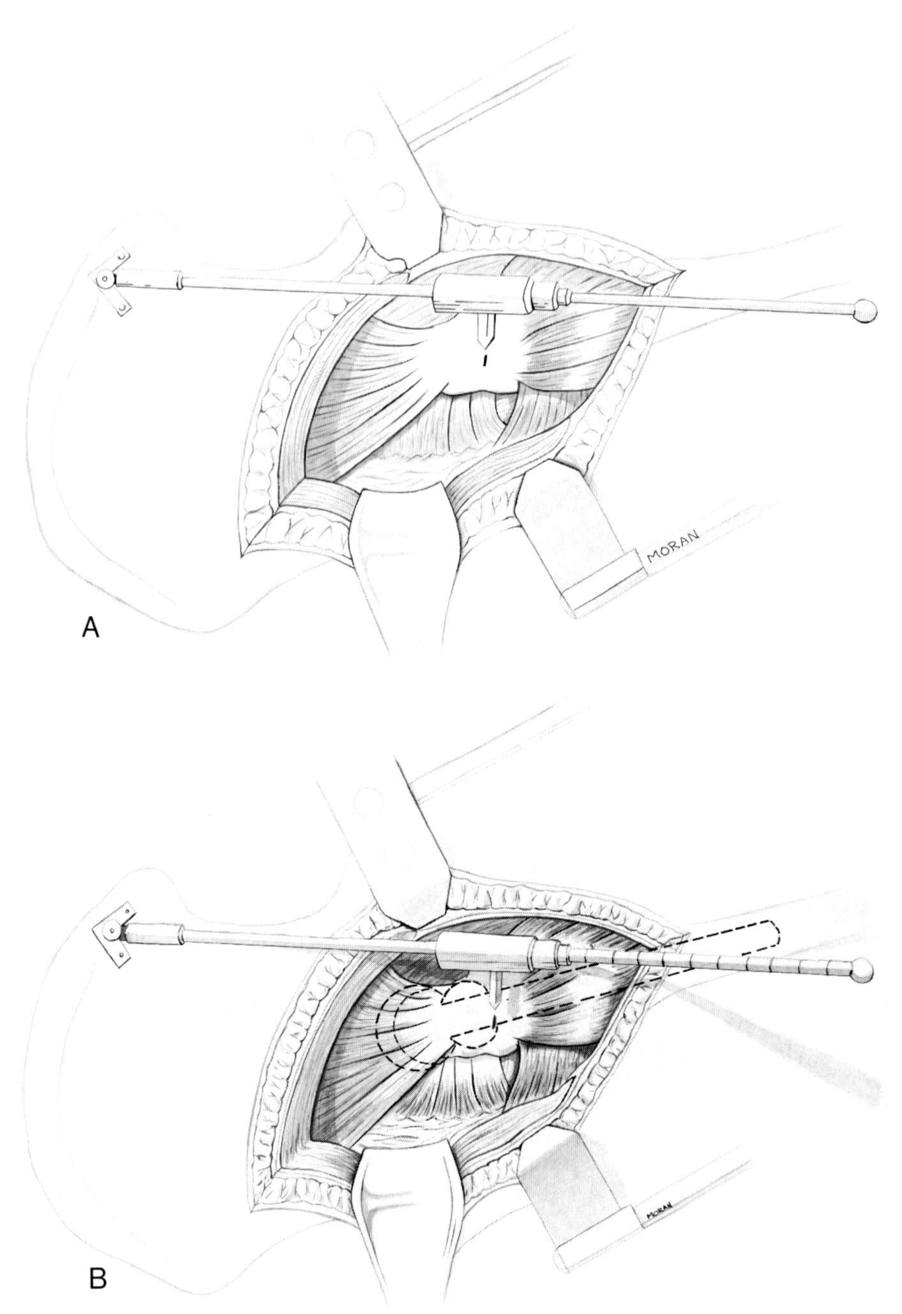

FIGURE 17–4. The use of markers fixed in bone to determine extremity length. *A*, Prior to hip dislocation. *B*, Evaluation during trial reduction.

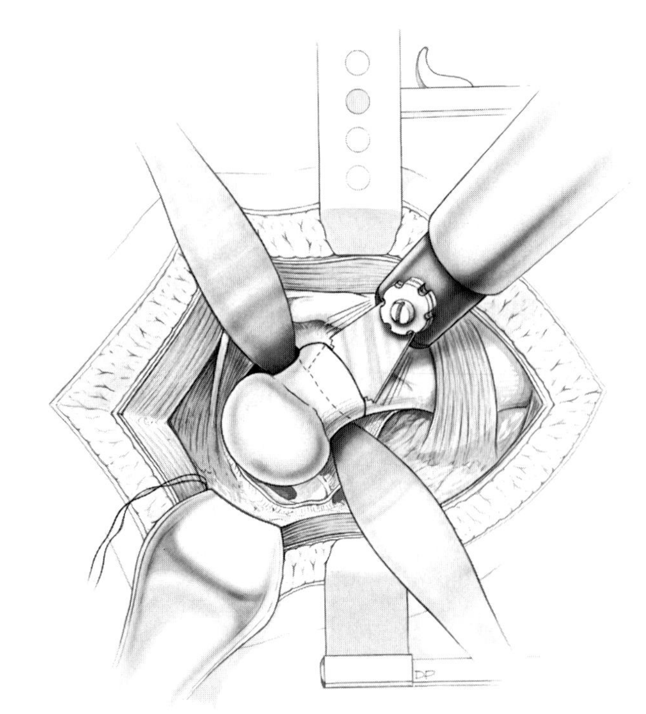

FIGURE 17–5. Femoral neck osteotomy.

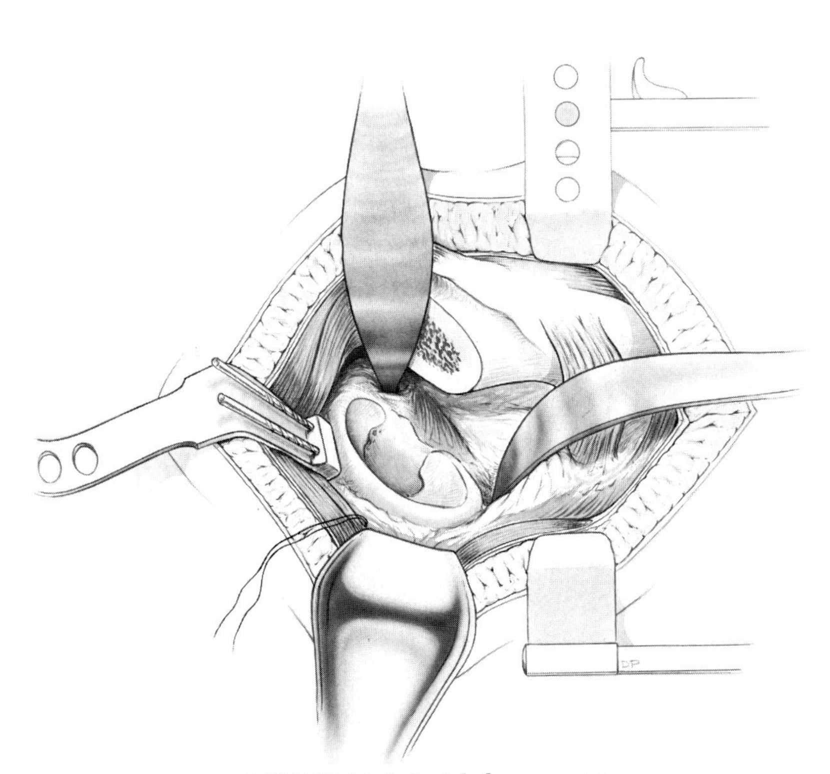

FIGURE 17–6. Acetabular exposure.

osteotome, a rongeur, or both, to provide accurate anatomic landmarks for prosthetic positioning and to avoid impingement on the prosthesis during insertion or during motion after implantation. Acetabular reamers may be helpful in removing medial osteophytes in the acetabular fossa. Initial reaming is done with an instrument several millimeters smaller than the prosthesis size selected during preoperative templating. To avoid superior placement of the acetabular component, initial reaming is directed more medially. Subsequent reaming is done in 30- to 40-degree abduction and 20-degree anteversion (forward flexion) (Fig. 17–7). The superior subchondral bone is preserved.[52, 57]

Integral bone cement spacers are provided with most modern acetabular prostheses.[50, 52, 69] The designated component size includes the spacers so that the reaming prepares for accurate prosthetic fit and cement. When reaming is complete, the trial prosthesis is placed and evaluated for fit. After satisfactory trial placement, the acetabulum is further prepared by removing any remaining soft tissue and clearing out cysts. Bone collected from the reamers may be employed to graft areas left by large cysts, if the bone is free of soft tissue. The resected femoral head and neck also provide an excellent source of cancellous bone for grafts. Small cyst cavities make ideal extra anchoring holes for cement. Several holes, 6 to 8 mm in diameter, are drilled into the iliac subchondral bone. If desired, they may also be made in the ischium and pubis (Fig. 17–8).[52, 57] Some surgeons prefer fewer but larger cement anchoring holes.[3]

The acetabular surface may be further roughened with additional very shallow holes. A way to enhance acetabular cement fixation is by vacuuming the cancellous bone. A hole the size of a suction tip is drilled in the ilium superior to the acetabulum, and the suction tip is placed in the hole. Just before cement is applied, the hole is suctioned to improve intrusion into the cancellous bone. This practice is especially useful when much bleeding occurs from the exposed bone. Some surgeons prefer hydrogen peroxide or dilute epinephrine to reduce bone bleeding at the time of cement application. Before cementation, the bone is thoroughly cleansed with pressure-pulsed lavage.

After the bone cement has been mixed

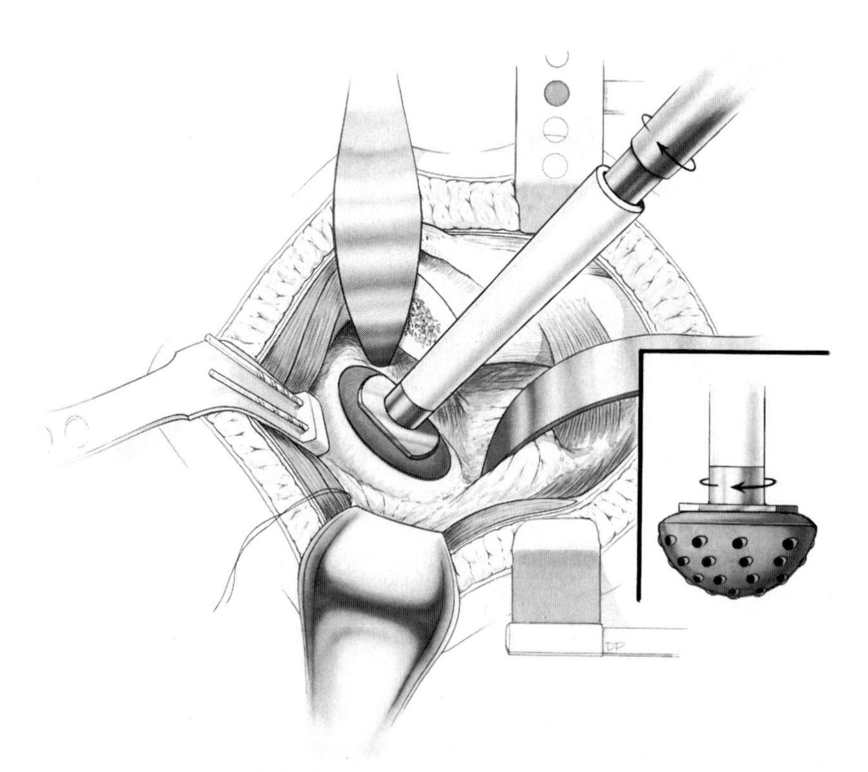

FIGURE 17–7. Acetabular reaming.

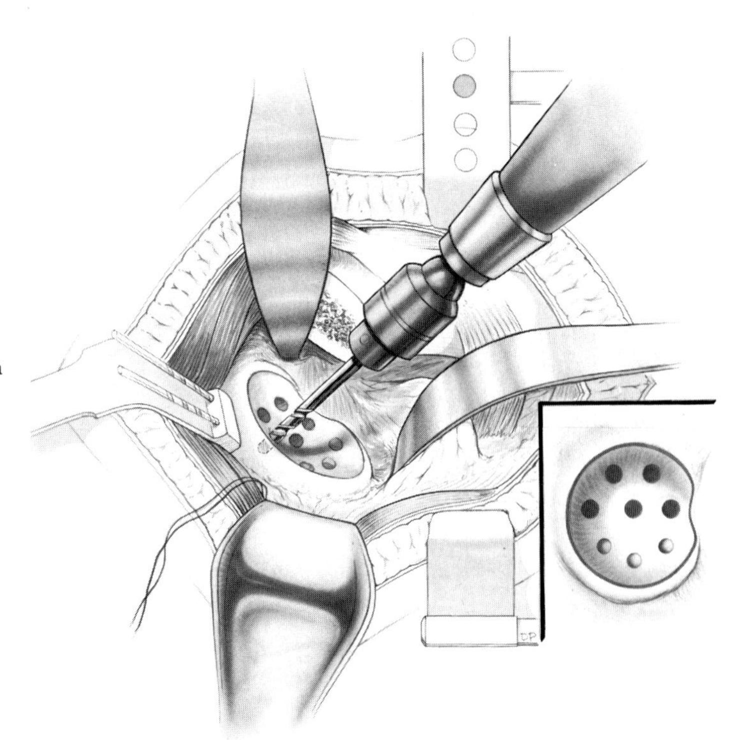

FIGURE 17–8. Cement fixation holes in the acetabulum.

under vacuum or centrifuge to reduce porosity (see Chapter 7, *Fixation Methods*), it is loaded in a syringe. Pressure from the syringe forces cement into the interstices of the bone in the anchoring holes and acetabulum. Pressure may be added with a mechanical device, the removed femoral head, or a smaller acetabular trial device placed over a rubber dam.[47, 49] Many modern acetabular components for cemented use have a peripheral extended lip or flange to add pressure to bone cement during insertion, which also helps maintain pressure throughout polymerization.[63]

The method employed to position the acetabular component varies with the surgeon's preference. When the patient is placed in the straight lateral, 30-degree posterior tilt, or straight supine position, positioner bars or pins may be utilized as guides. Local anatomic sites may also be used for orientation, e.g., the ilium, ischium, pubis, and acetabulum itself. The utilization of both methods is wise. Normally, the face of the polyethylene component is positioned in 30- to 40-degree abduction to keep the metal backing of the prosthetic component, if it has one, contained entirely within the acetabulum. The extended polyethylene roof of most modern acetabular components makes this possible. The prosthetic acetabulum is usually placed in 20- to 30-degree anteversion (Fig. 17–9). The component may be held in place with pressure from the positioner until the cement has polymerized. Alternatively, after the position has been established, the positioner can be replaced by a smooth-headed pusher that moves easily within the socket. This practice reduces the chances of moving the component while the cement polymerizes. If this is done, pressure should be held against the socket while the two instruments are being exchanged so that pressure on the cement is unrelieved until polymerization is complete. Although excess cement is best removed when it is still soft, remaining cement can be removed later with an osteotome. A sponge placed in the acetabulum protects it from bone fragments and other debris during femoral preparation.

Preparation of the Femur

The femur is fixed in an appropriate position, depending on the surgical approach, so it will not move during femoral preparation. The proximal femur is elevated with a retractor such as a hip skid. It is important to provide lateral access to

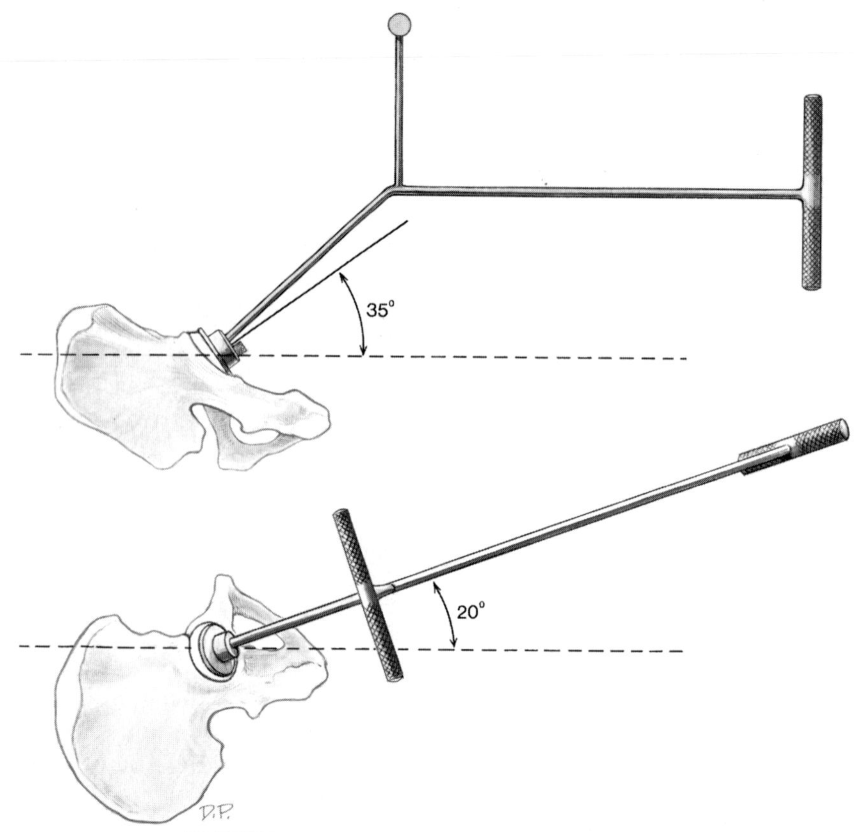

FIGURE 17–9. Acetabular component positioning.

the femoral canal, because modern femoral stems for cemented use have straight or nearly straight lateral borders. To provide straight entry into the femoral canal, any remaining lateral bone on the femoral neck and medial cortex of the greater trochanter is removed with a box osteotome (Fig. 17–10).

The canal is entered with a tapered reamer or similar instrument (Fig. 17–11). After entry, the endosteum is palpated with a long curved hemostat to be sure the femoral canal has not been perforated. This practice is especially important in osteoporotic bone with thin cortices. The discovery of inadvertent perforation is less difficult to deal with when it can be corrected intraoperatively, than when it is seen for the first time on a postoperative radiograph (see Fig. 19–8). When a system involves a flexible reamer, a guide wire is placed and reaming is usually performed in 1-mm increments, removing loose or soft bone and sizing the canal in the area of the isthmus (Fig. 17–12). The largest reamer that should be selected is that which gives cortical contact and "chatter." For systems with a device that centralizes the distal stem in the femoral canal, the largest flexible reamer used determines the size of the centralization device. Some systems have a hand or power reamer to prepare the mid stem and medial portion of the greater trochanter.

Broaching is usually started with the smaller broach or with a broach two sizes smaller than that templated during the preoperative planning (Fig. 17–13). As the broach is driven into the femur, it may rotate slightly into anteversion. If much resistance is met inserting the broach for the size chosen preoperatively, the surgeon should then choose the next smaller size femoral stem rather than risk femoral fracture.

For a prosthesis with a collar, an oscillating saw or a calcar planer is utilized to make final fit adjustments of the collar against the medial aspect of the femoral neck cortex when the broach is fully seated

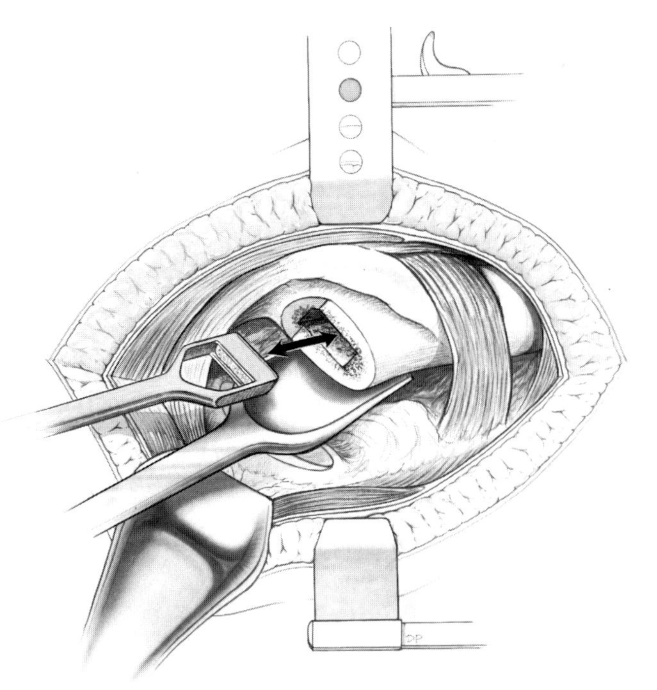

FIGURE 17–10. Lateralization of the entry point into the femoral canal with a box osteotome.

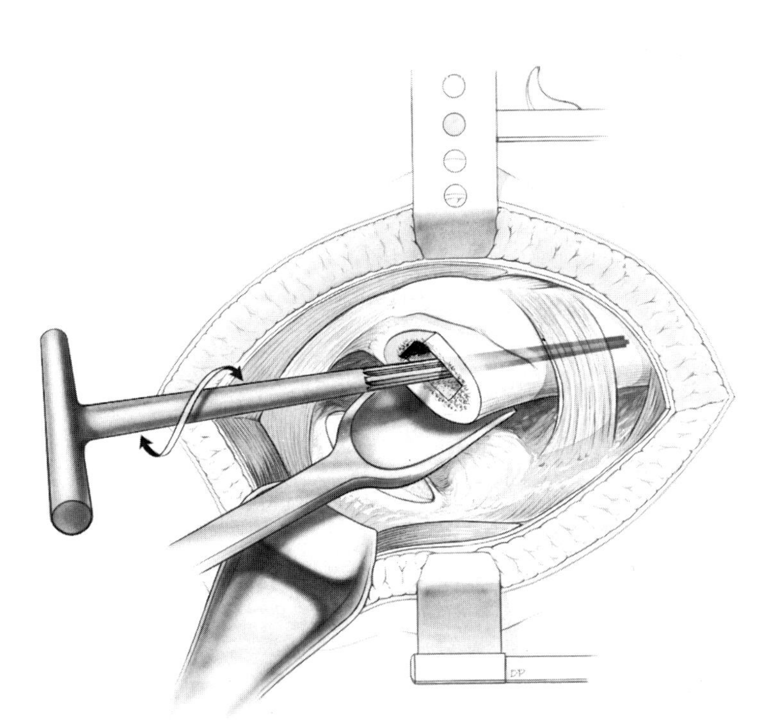

FIGURE 17–11. Entry into the femoral canal with a tapered reamer.

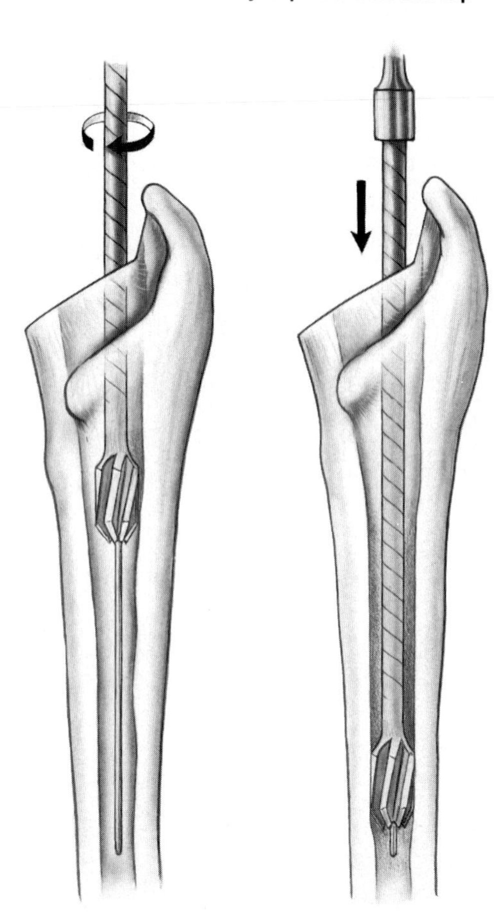

FIGURE 17–12. Flexible reaming of the intramedullary canal.

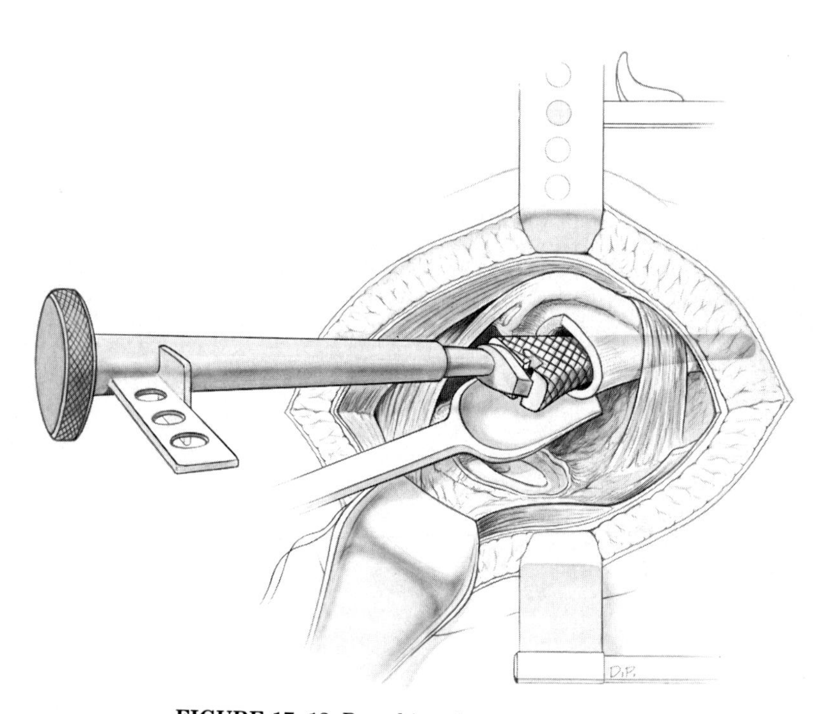

FIGURE 17–13. Broaching the proximal femur.

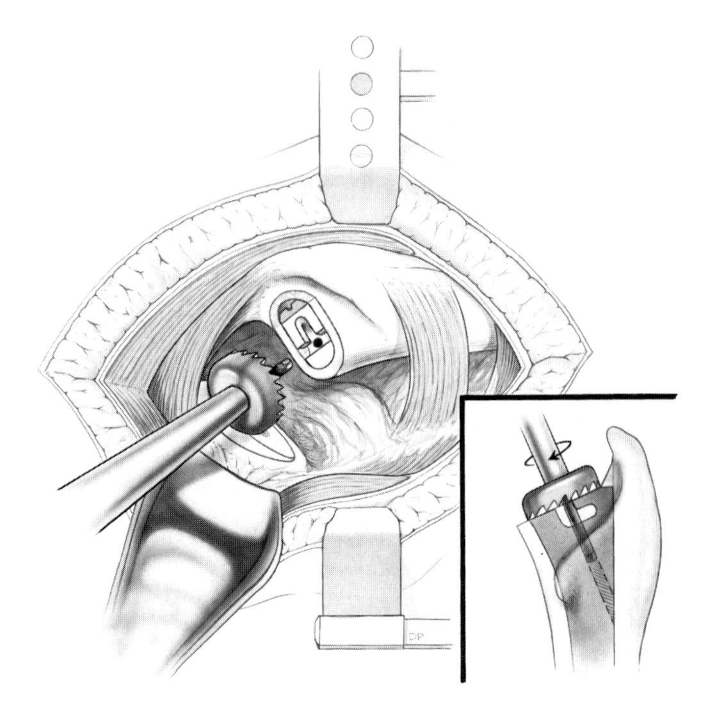

FIGURE 17–14. Preparation of the femoral neck for improved collar contact.

(Fig. 17–14). The trial head and neck or trial prosthesis is placed and the hip reduced (Fig. 17–15). The limb is held in a neutral position and its length assessed by evaluating the relationship of the level of the greater trochanter tip to the center of rotation of the femoral head. If markers have been placed in the ilium and proximal femur, measurements are taken to evaluate reconstruction length (see Fig. 17–4). Unless the acetabular component has been placed in a nonanatomic position, the center of rotation of the femoral head is at or near the level of the greater trochanteric tip, with the hip in neutral position, when the length is correct. When length adjust-

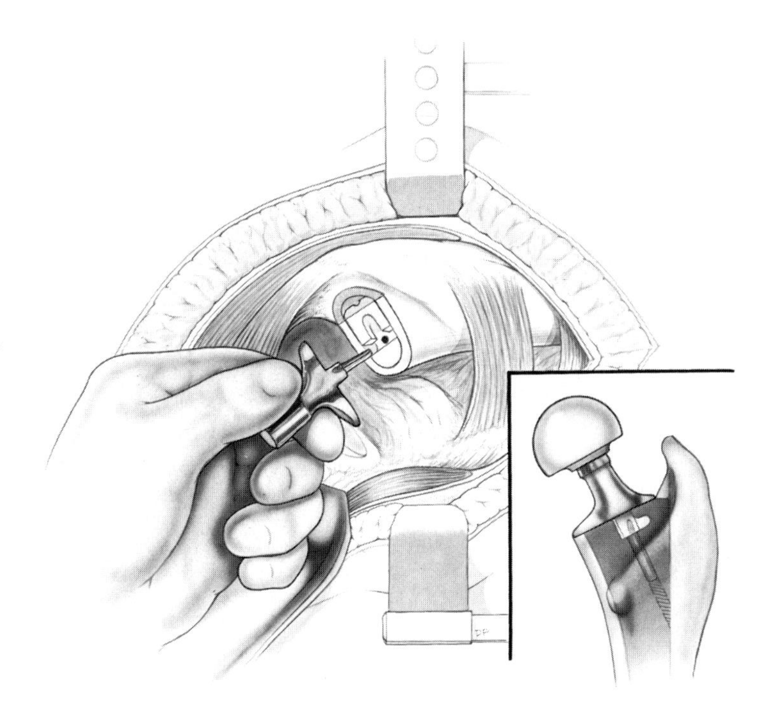

FIGURE 17–15. Placement of trial neck and head.

ments are needed, a trial head of different length is placed. For nonmodular systems, a trial prosthesis of different neck length is placed. Some surgeons use muscle tension as an indicator of accuracy of length reconstruction. However, this method is unreliable because muscle tension varies with the amount of preoperative soft tissue contracture, the amount of soft tissue release, and the anesthetic agents given during surgery.

Hip motion and stability of the reconstructed hip are evaluated in both extension and flexion. If remaining osteophytes cause impingement of the prosthetic components, they are removed. When length reconstruction, motion, and stability are satisfactory, the hip is dislocated and all trial components are removed.

To achieve an effective, durable surgical result, the femur must be prepared carefully to receive bone cement. First, the canal is cleaned with a brush and pressure-pulsed lavage to remove hematoma and debris from bone interstices (Fig. 17–16). This procedure improves cement intrusion, apposition of cement against bone, and strength of cement fixation.[2, 24, 34, 36, 42, 54] It also lowers the incidence of hemodynamic and blood gas changes during cement and prosthesis insertion.[8, 64] Second, the femoral canal is plugged to prevent the cement from travelling too distally and to allow for pressurization of the cement.[2, 5, 34]

Femoral Canal Plugs

The surgeon may choose one of three types of plugs for the femoral canal: cement plug (Fig. 17–17A), bone graft plug (Fig. 17–17B and C), or polymeric plug (Fig. 17–17D).

Cement plugs are placed by means of a syringe system (see Fig. 17–17A).[26, 46] The plug is allowed to polymerize before the bulk of the cement is placed for prosthesis fixation, preventing cement leakage around the plug and making it less likely to migrate. Plugs produced in this way have the greatest ability to withstand pressurization (Fig. 17–18).[5] However, the method has two disadvantages: (1) it adds to operating time and (2) some danger of pulling cement back up the canal during syringe removal exists, impeding placement of the prosthesis.

For a more physiologic plug, a bone graft plug may be cut from the femoral head or neck, avoiding the introduction of additional prosthetic material to the femur (see Fig. 17–17B). Standard cutting instruments may be employed; however, cutting and sizing are more likely to be precise by

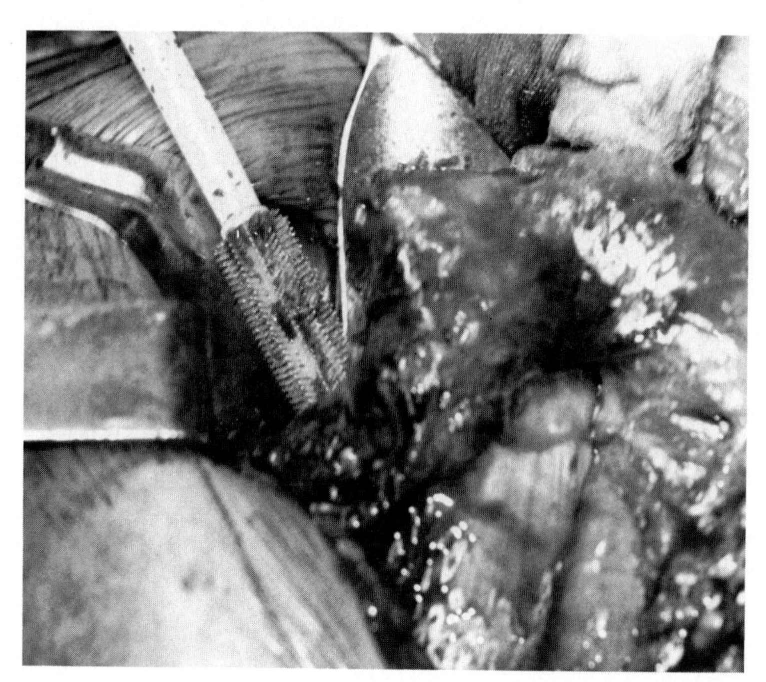

FIGURE 17–16. Intramedullary femoral brushing to remove hematoma and other debris to provide for improved cement intrusion.

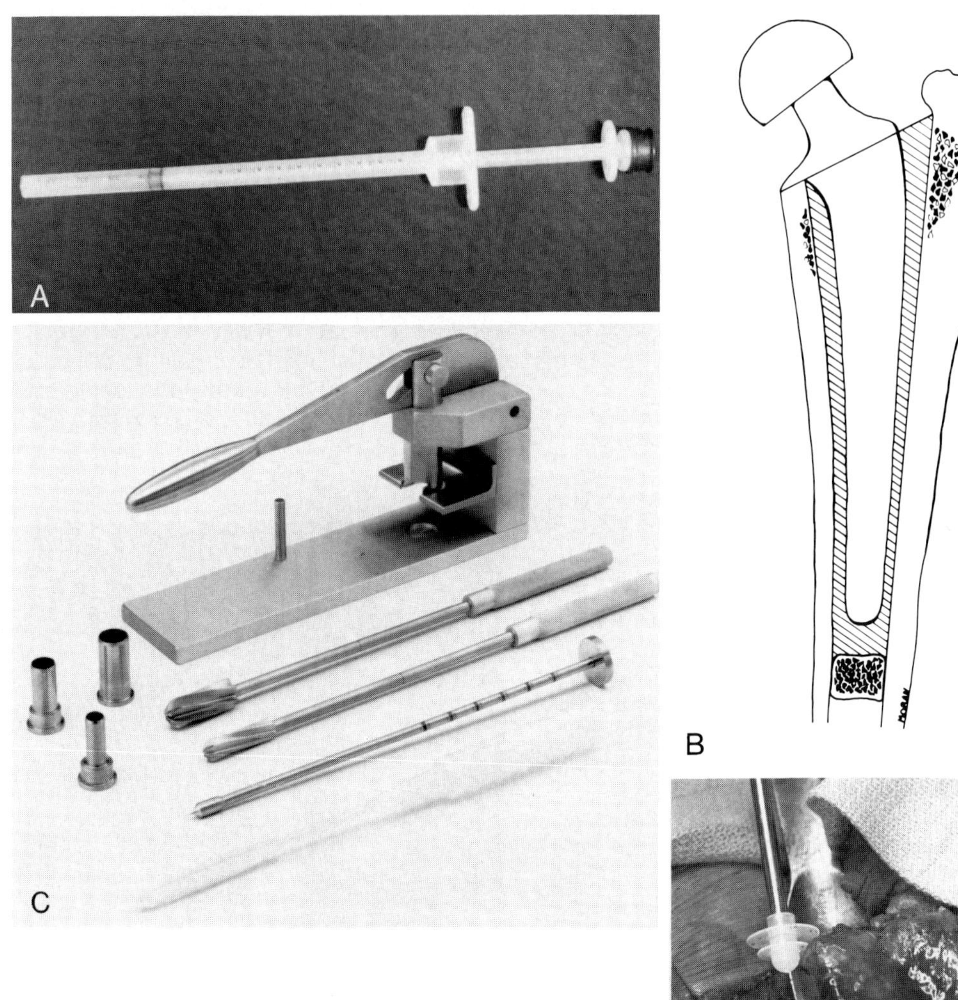

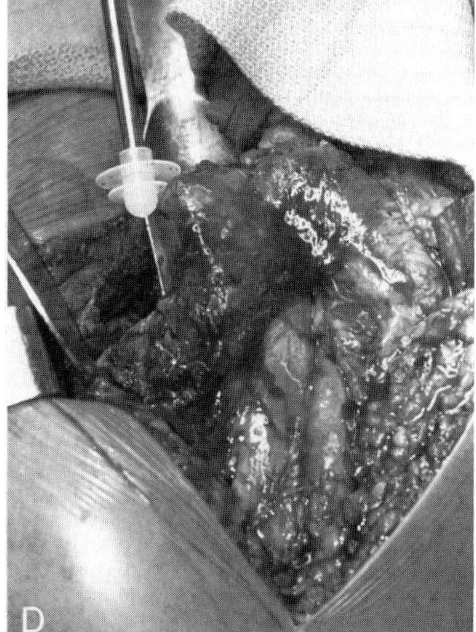

FIGURE 17–17. Restrictor plugs prevent cement from extending distally in the femoral canal and allow for improved cement pressurization. *A*, Syringe designed for placement of a cement plug. *B*, Bone graft plug placed distal to stem tip. *C*, Instrument system for making and inserting bone graft plug. (Courtesy of Zimmer, Inc.) *D*, Polymeric plug.

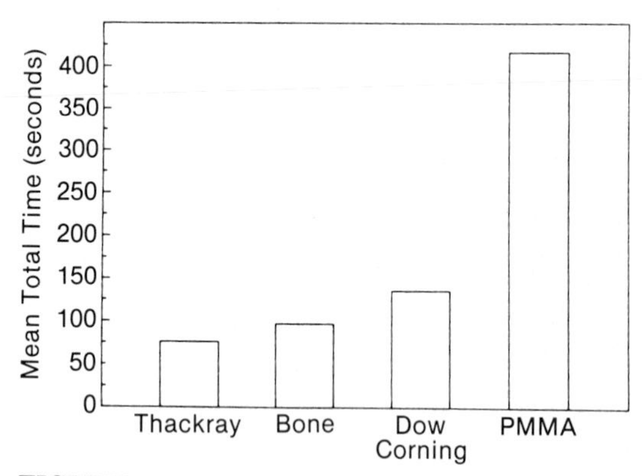

FIGURE 17–18. Relative ability of different types of bone restrictor plugs to withstand greater than 50 psi. (Redrawn from Beim, G.M., Lavernia, C., and Convery, F.R.: J. Arthrop. 4:139–141, 1989.)

employing an instrument system especially designed to prepare grafts (see Fig. 17–17C).[42, 75]

Many different designs of polymeric plugs are available commercially (see Fig. 17–17D). Their major advantages are convenience and rapidity of placement. As with other types of plugs, leakage is uncommon but can occur.

The plug is placed 1.5 to 2 cm distal to the tip of the femoral stem. Bone cement is mixed in a vacuum or centrifuge system. Because of the excellent canal fill attained with modern cementing techniques, at least two standard packs of cement are usually needed. Cement in a low-viscosity state improves intrusion into the bone. The syringe in which the cement is loaded must have a nozzle long enough to reach the cement-restricting plug in order to avoid debris entrapment and blood layering within the cement and to prevent inadequate cement pressurization (Fig. 17–19).[20, 35] After the canal is filled, the cement is pressurized with a mechanical device or with pressure from a finger over a rubber dam (Fig. 17–20). Short, high-level forces should be utilized to improve cement intrusion, whichever technique is selected.[38, 71]

When the surgeon has taken precautions to secure the patient's leg in the desired position, the prosthesis is inserted. Insertion is probably best controlled when the prosthesis is held in the surgeon's hand (Fig. 17–21). Although some systems provide prosthesis holders, they have the disadvantage of adding a longer lever arm and producing exaggeration of any unwanted movements of the prosthesis within the cement. The prosthesis should be inserted to within 1 cm of full seating, the excess cement cleared away, and the proper position ascertained. The prosthesis is then fully seated. Because the cement fills the femoral canal so effectively, the surgeon may sometimes need to complete seating of the prosthesis with a stem impactor and mallet. After excess cement is removed, the cement is allowed to polymerize without any movement of the prosthesis.[23, 25, 26, 36, 45–47]

With a modular head system, the surgeon may make a final check of length reconstruction with the trial heads. The taper on the femur stem is wiped clean, and the femoral head is impacted into place (Fig. 17–22). The acetabulum is cleaned and inspected, and the hip is reduced (Fig.

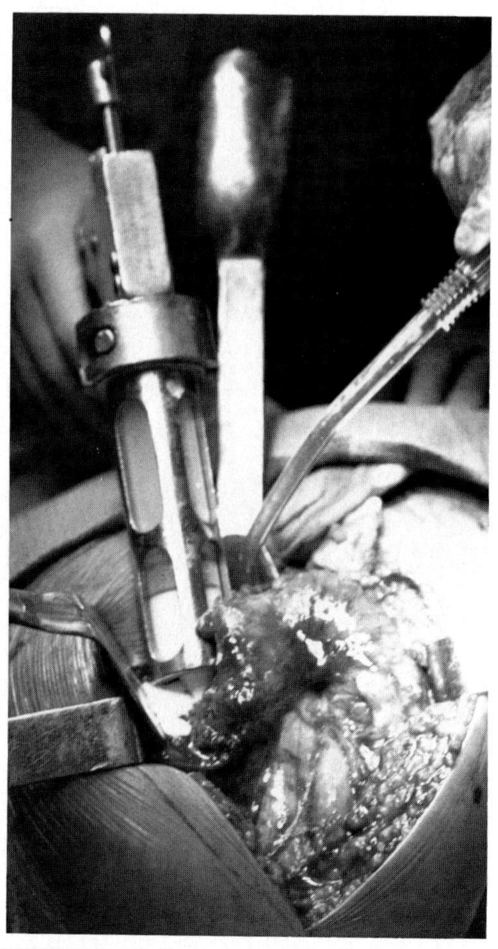

FIGURE 17–19. Cement placed in the femoral canal with a syringe.

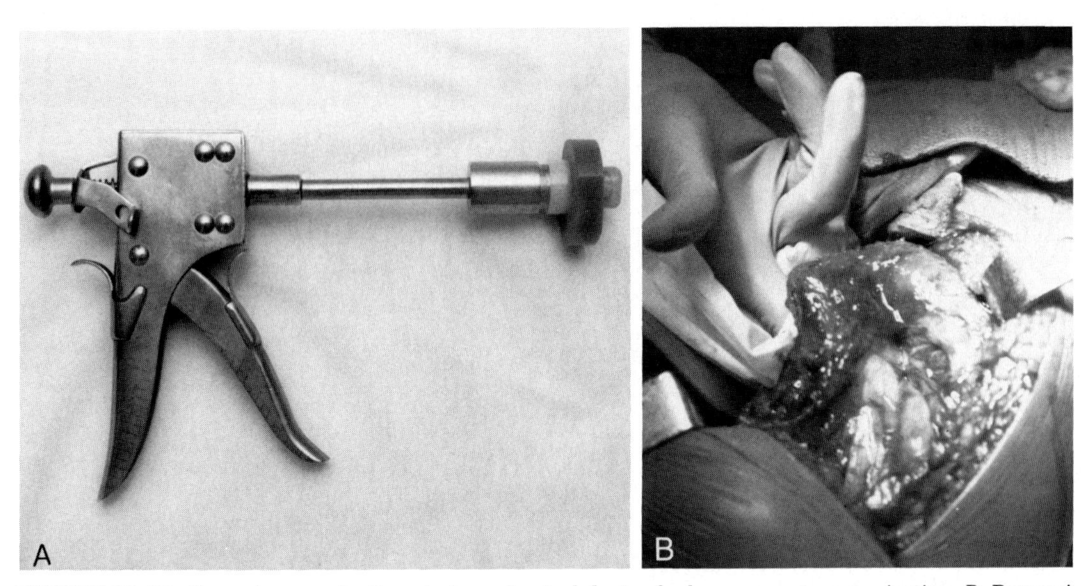

FIGURE 17–20. Cement pressurization. *A,* A mechanical device for bone cement pressurization. *B,* Pressurization of bone cement with a finger over a rubber dam.

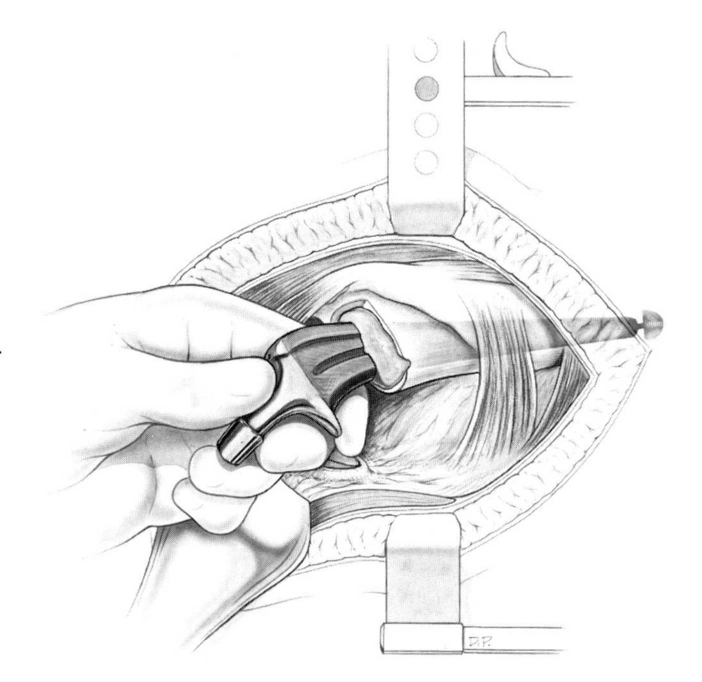

FIGURE 17–21. Femoral stem insertion.

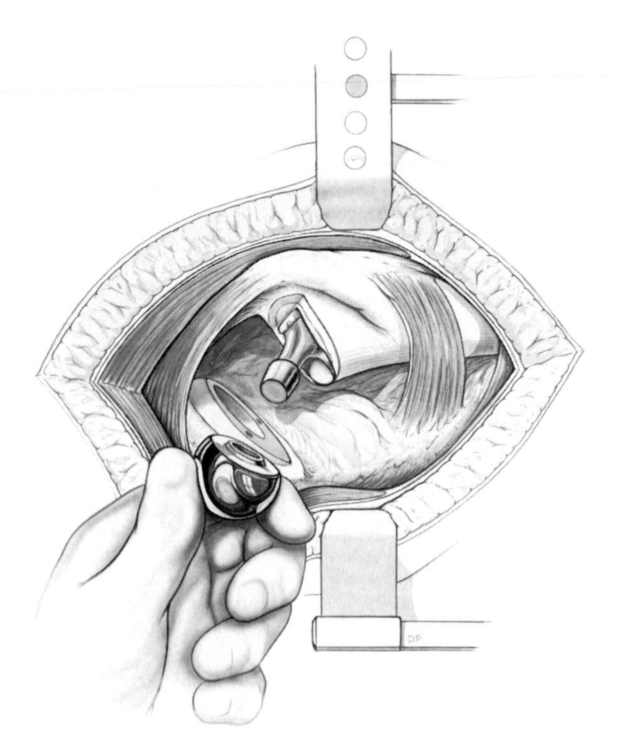

FIGURE 17–22. Femoral head placement.

17–23). A final check of length reconstruction, motion, and stability is made. Drains are placed, and the surgical wound is closed.

TOTAL HIP ARTHROPLASTY WITH PRESS-FIT FIXATION

Total hip arthroplasty with press-fit fixation actually preceded the procedure employing bone cement, primarily for hemiarthroplasty, but also for total hip replacement. However, major improvements have been made, including the development of porous-coated prostheses, a wide array of prostheses sizes, and instrument systems to help the surgeon size and place prostheses more accurately. The technique for press fitting a total hip prosthesis is similar for a prosthesis with or without a porous coat.

Preparation of the Acetabulum

The acetabulum is prepared and reamed as it is for cemented arthroplasty, although some acetabular prostheses for press-fit application have nonhemispheric shapes, requiring special reamers. Most systems have a trial prosthesis for verifying proper position, fit, and apposition to bone. Fit is accomplished in one of two ways: the prosthesis and reaming systems are designed for line-to-line fit of the prosthesis within the bone or the prosthesis is designed to be slightly oversized to provide an interference fit.

Some surgeons ream 1 to 2 mm smaller than the chosen prosthesis size to increase the interference fit. The surgeon must know when a prosthesis and its instrument system are designed for an interference fit and by how much, so that the system's interference fit plus that of the surgeon's are not excessive. Many surgeons do not "under-ream." They place the component with line-to-line fit. No clinical or laboratory studies have been published in which one of these fitting methods is superior to the other for press-fit acetabular prostheses.

If cysts are present in the acetabulum, all soft tissue is cleared away and bone grafts are prepared from the bone tissue collected during reaming, if it is free of soft tissue, or from the resected femoral head and neck. If the prosthesis has pegs or

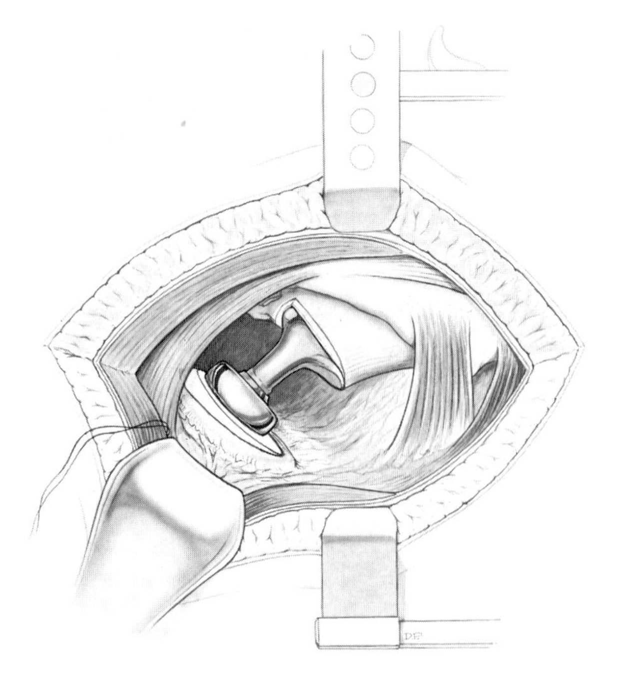

FIGURE 17–23. Final reduction.

spikes, a guide is usually provided to prepare the bone for them (Fig. 17–24). Pulsed-pressure irrigation is unnecessary during bone preparation for press-fit prostheses.

The prosthesis is placed employing the insertor, which usually has a guide to help position the component. If the surgeon selects a system with anteversion built into the neck of the femoral component, care must be taken to avoid excessive anteversion of the acetabular component, as it may compromise stability of the hip in external rotation. The prosthesis is impacted firmly

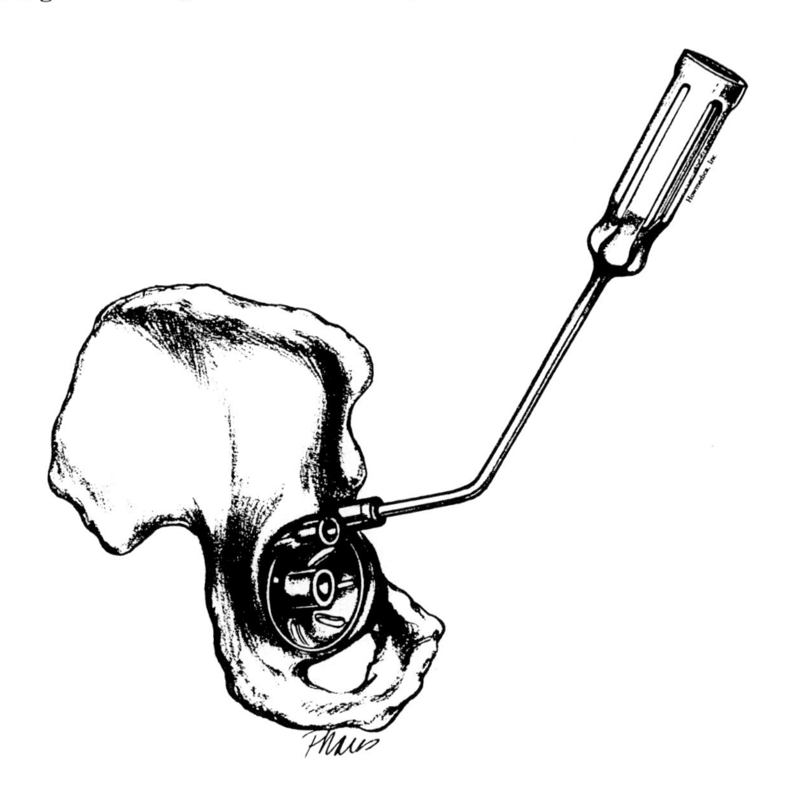

FIGURE 17–24. A drill guide designed for accurate placement of hole for socket peg. (Courtesy of Howmedica, Inc.)

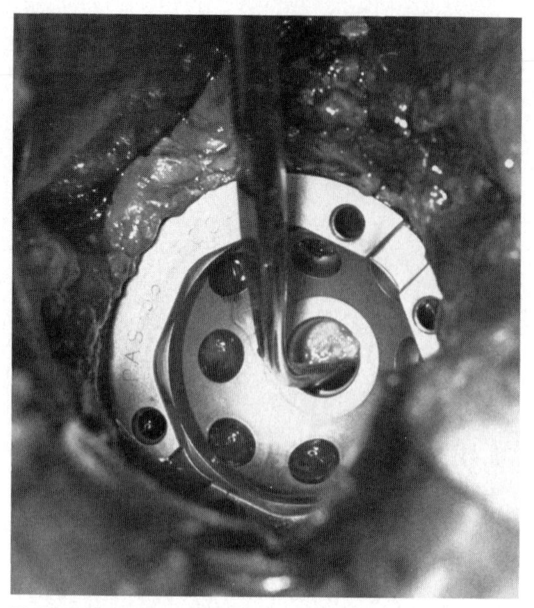

FIGURE 17–25. Screw holes and central hole allow evaluation of prosthesis-bone apposition.

into place, after which the central hole or screw holes, if present, are inspected to confirm close apposition of the component to the bone (Fig. 17–25). If the system is designed for screw fixation of the component, the holes are carefully drilled and the screws placed in the selected locations.

The quadrant system should be utilized as an added safety measure during acetabular screw placement (Fig. 17–26).[31, 70] That is, unless essential to provide stability, screws are placed neither in the anterior superior and inferior quadrants of the acetabulum nor in polar screw holes to avoid damaging the external iliac artery and vein and the obturator nerve, artery, and vein (Fig. 17–27). The quadrants are determined by an imaginary line running from the anterior superior iliac spine through the center of the acetabulum and bisected by a perpendicular line that creates the four quadrants (see Fig. 17–26).

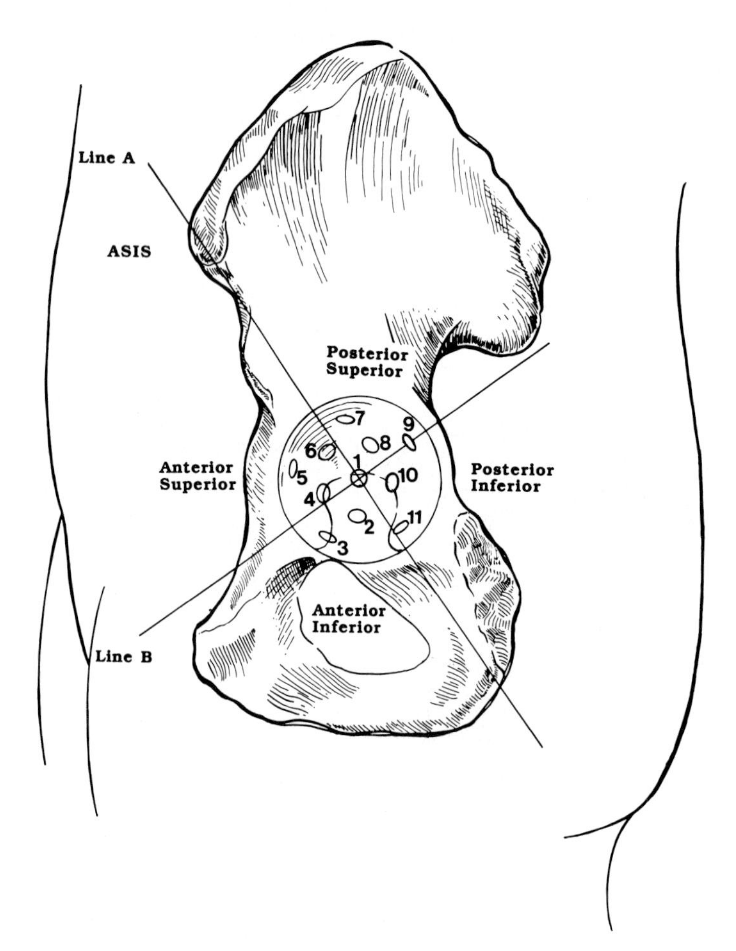

FIGURE 17–26. Quadrant system for determination of safer screw placement in acetabular prostheses. (Wasielewski, R.C., Cooperstein, L.A., Kruger, M.P., and Rubash, H.E.: J. Bone Joint Surg. 72A: 504, 1990. By permission.)

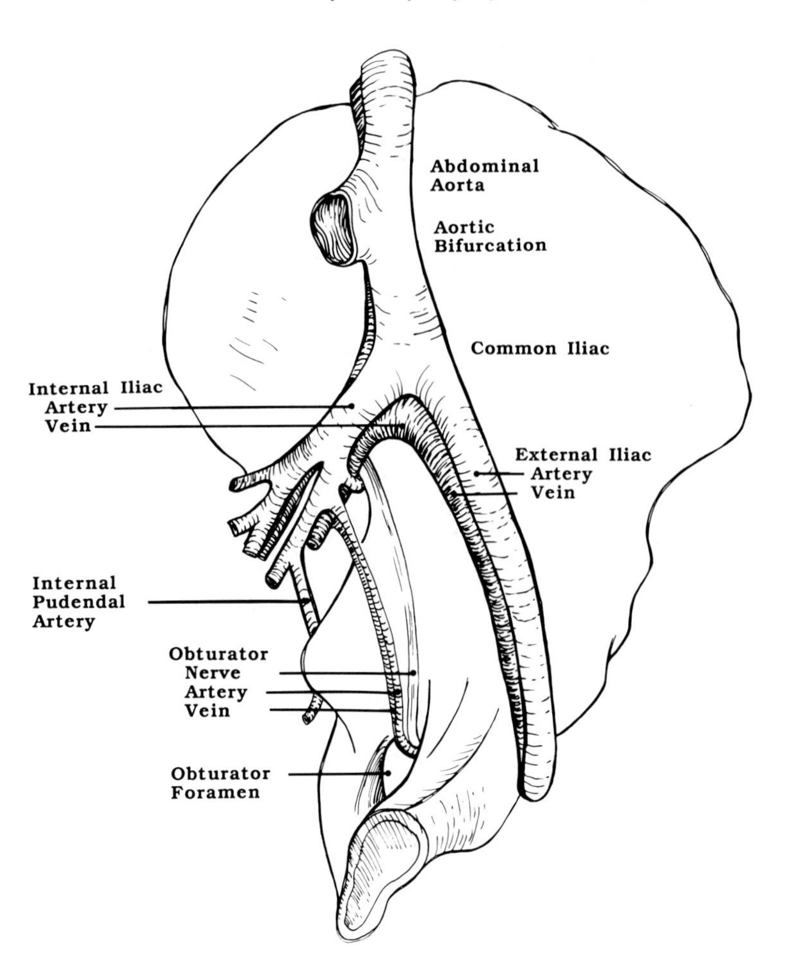

FIGURE 17–27. Structures at risk with acetabular screw placement. (Wasielewski, R.C., Cooperstein, L.A., Kruger, M.P., and Rubash, H.E.: J. Bone Joint Surg. 72A: 504, 1990. By permission.)

Placement of screws in the posterior superior or posterior inferior quadrants is relatively safe. Also, bone stock in these sites is better for screw placement. As an extra precaution, the sciatic notch area can be palpated during drilling and screw placement posteriorly. Because nerves and vessels may be injured in any quadrant, especially during plunging of the drill bit, care must be taken when any bone is drilled for placement of acetabular screws. Excessively long screws should be avoided.[31, 70] If a modular socket is selected, the final position of the polyethylene liner is determined and it is seated.

Preparation of the Femur

The femur is placed in a fixed position. The position depends on the surgeon's chosen approach. The proximal femur is raised with a hip skid or similar retractor. For most press-fit systems, femur preparation begins with removal of any remaining lateral portion of femoral neck and medial cortical portion of the greater trochanter. The proximal portion of the canal is entered with a box osteotome. Some systems require a flexible or rigid intramedullary reamer over a guide wire. If a rigid reamer is used, special care is needed to avoid partial or complete perforation of the femoral cortex. When the surgeon employs a system that requires reaming, the bone is reamed to the size needed for the patient's prosthesis, avoiding extensive bone removal.

Broaching is the next step. When possible, the first broach should be several sizes smaller than that templated during preoperative planning. In some systems, one always begins with the smallest broach; however, it is safer to do this with all systems. The surgeon should broach the canal slowly and carefully to fit the largest broach without fracturing the bone. If a small fracture appears around the proximal edge of the femur, broaching is stopped. If the crack does not widen and extends only a short distance, no special treatment may be needed other than careful insertion of the prosthesis. When the crack shows signs of widening or runs more than a short distance, a circumferential metallic band, cable, or wire should be applied.

When the broach has been fully seated, the trial neck and head or trial prosthesis and head are placed. The hip is then reduced; length reconstruction, motion, and stability are evaluated. After adjustments are made, the hip is dislocated and all trial components are removed. The femoral stem is impacted into place. Usually only moderate force is needed until the prosthetic component is almost seated. Greater force is then required for final seating. If necessary, another trial reduction is performed with the trial head. If the acetabular liner has not been impacted into place, this is done. The taper for the head is cleaned, and the selected femoral head impacted into place. After making sure the acetabulum is clear of all debris, the surgeon reduces the hip and performs a final check of length reconstruction, motion, and stability. Drains are placed, and the wound is closed.

TOTAL HIP ARTHROPLASTY FOR SPECIAL PROBLEMS

Congenital Dysplastic Hip

Adults with coxarthrosis associated with congenital dysplasia of the hip may present special technical problems when they undergo total hip arthroplasty. If the dysplasia is mild, selection of a small prosthesis may be sufficient (Fig. 17–28). However, in severe dysplasia, especially when the hip is completely dislocated, potential technical difficulties include the following:

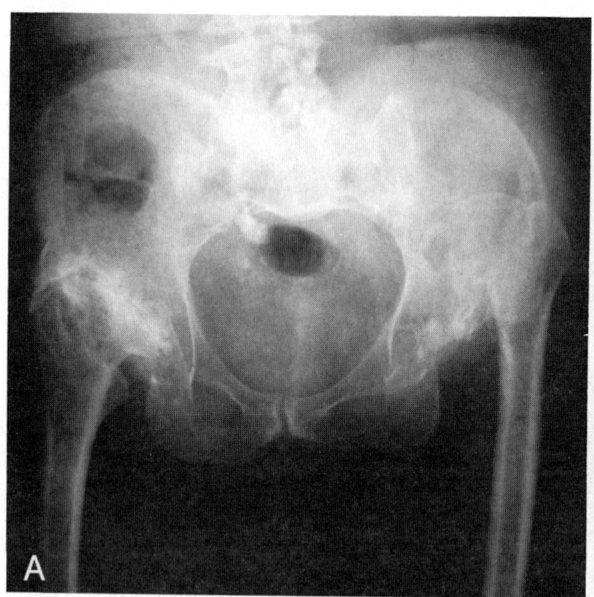

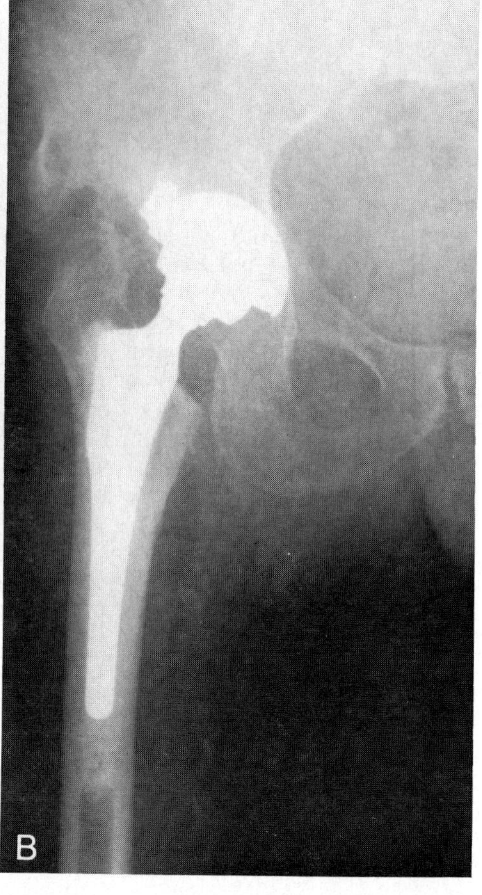

FIGURE 17–28. Treatment of patient with congenital dysplasia. *A*, Complete congenital dislocation on the left and subluxation and less severe dysplasia but severe degenerative arthritis on the right side. *B*, Treated on the right side by standard total hip arthroplasty using standard small components. Cementation of porous coated stem is not generally recommended.

1. A femoral head that articulates with a false acetabulum several centimeters superior to the level of the true acetabulum and limited bone stock in both the false and true acetabula (Fig. 17–28A)
2. Deficient proximal femur with a narrow intracortical canal requiring special small or custom prostheses
3. Marked anteversion of the proximal femur and acetabulum
4. Short soft tissues including muscle and neurovascular structures
5. Presence of previous hip reconstruction (e.g., acetabular osteotomy or arthroplasty, mold arthroplasty, femoral osteotomy).

Careful assessment of bone stock in the pelvis may be aided by computerized tomography.

An added challenge for the surgeon is that many patients with severe coxarthrosis associated with dysplasia are young (see Chapter 20, *Results of Primary Total Hip Arthroplasty*). Thorough preoperative planning is necessary for all patients with congenital dysplasia, and it must be done far enough in advance of the operation to be able to order prostheses of the appropriate sizes.

In the most severe cases, the transtrochanteric approach obtains adequate exposure. This approach allows placement of a bone graft to augment bone stock in the acetabulum, if needed, and shortening of the femur.[17, 40] Extensive additional release of soft tissue, including the iliopsoas and tendon of the gluteus maximus, is often necessary. The prosthetic acetabulum is usually placed in the true acetabulum because the bone stock is generally better there than high on the ilium (Fig. 17–29). Also, hip biomechanics are better with the acetabulum in its normal location. Russotti and Harris[59] report that high placement (an average of 43 mm above the interteardrop line) of the socket is an acceptable alternative in complex acetabular reconstruction, especially when bone stock in the high location is better than that at the true acetabulum. In a review by Shaughnessy and colleagues[62] no differences were reported in prosthesis survival between patients with high and low placement of the prosthetic socket.

After either the true or false acetabulum has been located, soft tissue is removed. Reaming is performed carefully with reamers of the appropriate size, and care is taken to avoid violation of the pelvic cortex. Some investigators recommend that a patient with severe dysplasia and a complete high-riding dislocation have a bone graft made from the femoral head placed superiorly and posteriorly to the acetabulum (Fig. 17–30).[13, 17, 29] Others have reported successful total hip replacements in patients with congenital dysplasia without bone grafts for bone stock augmentation; rather, superior defects are filled with bone cement.[40] With long-term follow-up, some surgeons have reported a high failure rate when bulk bone grafts are utilized in dysplastic acetabula (Fig. 17–31). In one study, 20 percent of patients who were followed at least 10 years required revision, and another 27 percent showed loose prostheses radiographically.[44]

Bulk grafting may be more successful when two thirds or more of the prosthetic socket is covered with host, rather than grafted, bone (Fig. 17–32). If the acetabular bone stock is augmented with bone graft, all soft tissue is removed from the femoral head and lateral ilium and the graft is fixed in place with screws. If the bone is so soft that screws do not hold, bolts with washers and nuts are employed. In a case in which the bone stock is deficient posteriorly, the femoral head graft is placed so that the femoral neck extends posteriorly.[17] Reaming is completed, and the socket component placed. Phillips and Rao[53] have had good intermediate term results in patients treated with a lateral acetabular autogenous femoral head graft and a bipolar acetabular prosthesis.

Substantial lengthening of the soft tissues is more dangerous in the patient with a limb that failed to grow fully during childhood than in a patient with a limb that shortened during adulthood. In order to place the femoral head into the prosthetic socket without dangerous stretching of nerves or vessels, it is necessary to shorten the proximal femur, often to below the level of the lesser trochanter. After this procedure is done, the remaining femur is quite straight and usually requires a small, straight prosthesis. Unfortunately, many femoral prostheses designed for press-fit application provide an unsatisfactory fit in this situation, especially those with curved stems. Another approach

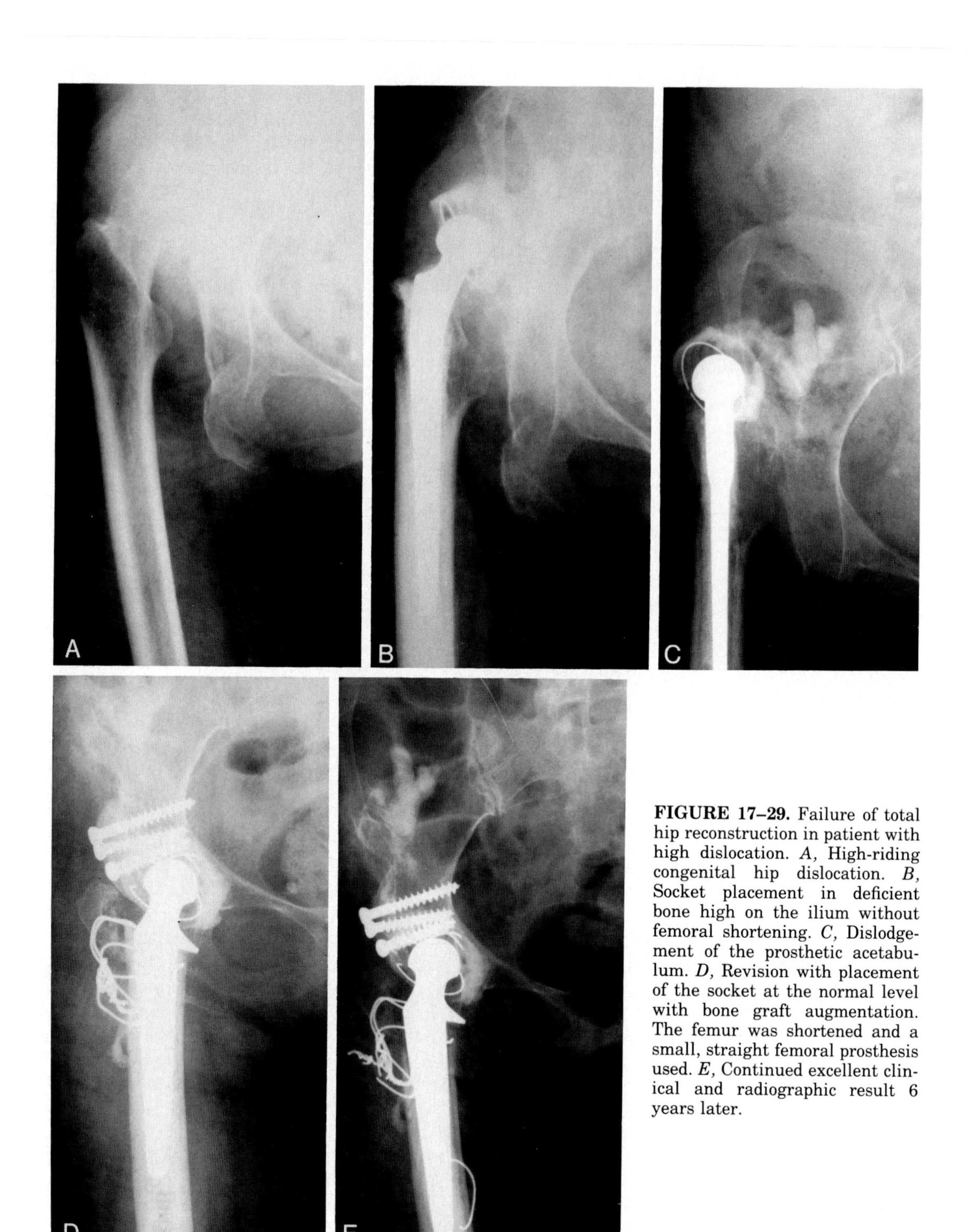

FIGURE 17–29. Failure of total hip reconstruction in patient with high dislocation. *A,* High-riding congenital hip dislocation. *B,* Socket placement in deficient bone high on the ilium without femoral shortening. *C,* Dislodgement of the prosthetic acetabulum. *D,* Revision with placement of the socket at the normal level with bone graft augmentation. The femur was shortened and a small, straight femoral prosthesis used. *E,* Continued excellent clinical and radiographic result 6 years later.

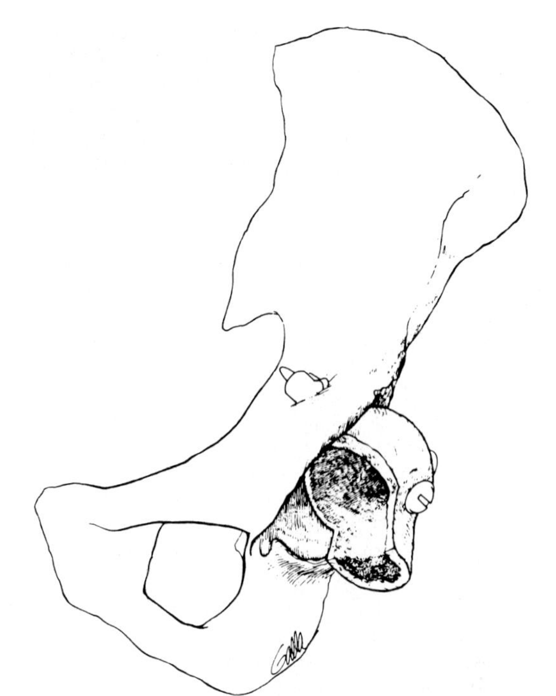

FIGURE 17–30. Placement of bone graft superiorly and posteriorly to augment deficient acetabular bone in dysplasia. (Gerber, S.D. and Harris, W.H.: J. Bone Joint Surg. 68A: 1241–1248, 1986. By permission.)

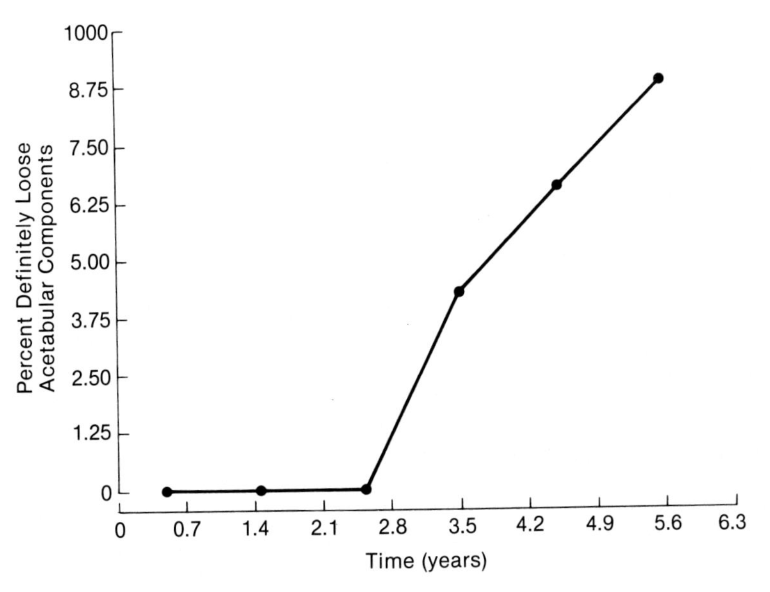

FIGURE 17–31. Increasing failure rate with time in dysplastic acetabula augmented with large bulk autografts for cemented total hip arthroplasty. (Gerber, S.D. and Harris, W.H.: J. Bone Joint Surg. 68A: 1241–1248, 1986. By permission.)

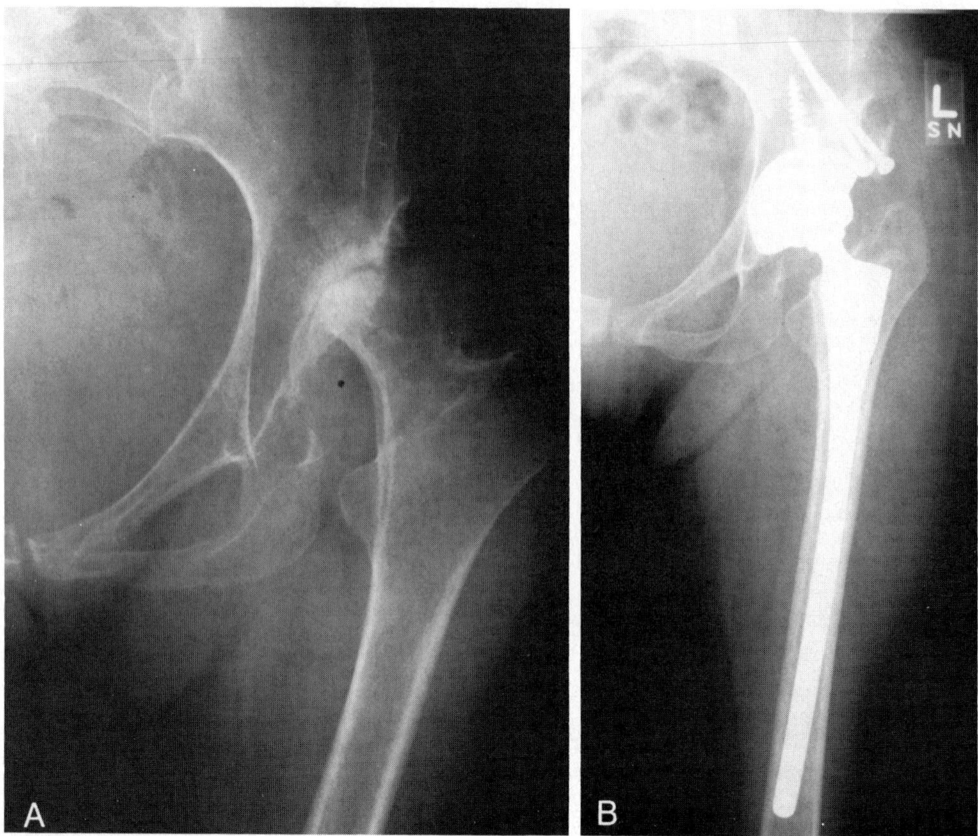

FIGURE 17–32. Total hip arthroplasty for a patient with congenital dysplasia. *A,* The bone is deficient superiorly. *B,* Bone graft was fixed in place to fill the superior defect; 80 percent of the prosthetic socket is covered with host, rather than grafted, bone.

to femoral shortening is a step cut osteotomy performed at the level of the lesser trochanter, allowing for better maintenance of the metaphyseal region of the proximal femur (Fig. 17–33).[51]

If the transtrochanteric approach has been utilized, the limb is abducted after placement of the prosthesis and the greater trochanter is reattached. If the abductor muscles are very tight with the limb in neutral position, balanced suspension may be required postoperatively, with the limb placed in abduction initially and gradually brought to the neutral position over a period of a few days to about 3 weeks. In a case in which structural bone has been grafted, the period of partial weight bearing may be extended. When apposition and fixation of the graft are good, this period need not be extended beyond 3 to 4 months because graft-to-host bone heals quickly in cancellous bone and the mechanism of cancellous bone remodeling normally does not weaken the bone.

Protrusio Acetabuli

In patients with protrusio acetabuli, the surgical technique must be modified because of excessive bone stresses on the medial wall of the protruded acetabulum with medial placement of the prosthetic acetabulum. This problem is avoided by placement of the prosthetic socket in a more lateral position.[12, 55] (See Chapter 23, *Revision Total Hip Arthroplasty,* for a description of a method for determining proper positioning of the acetabular component.[56]) Protrusio acetabuli occurs in about 20 percent of patients who require total hip arthroplasty for rheumatoid arthritis; it also occurs in association with Marfan's syndrome and Ehlers-Danlos syndrome and in an idiopathic form associated with coxarthrosis.[65, 72]

Since the early days of total hip arthroplasty, protrusio rings, protrusio sockets, and wire mesh have been recommended to reinforce the protruded medial acetabular

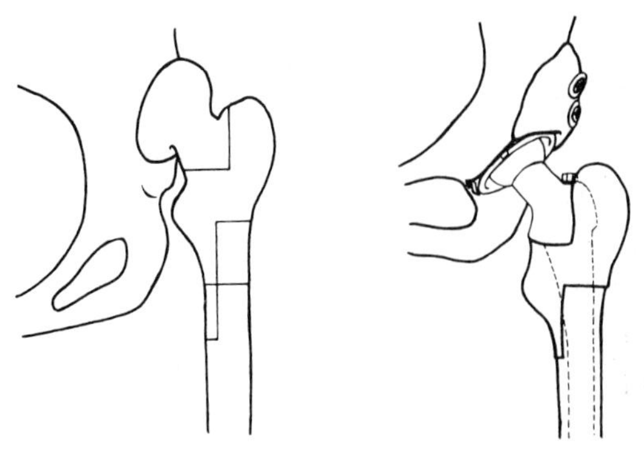

FIGURE 17–33. Shortening osteotomy of the femoral metaphysis to provide femoral shortening in total hip reconstruction for congenital dislocation. (Paavilainen, T., Hoikka, V., and Solonen, K.A.: J. Bone Joint Surg. 72B: 205–211, 1990. By permission.)

wall. A metal protrusio ring placed about the periphery of the acetabulum increases stresses in the lateral pelvic cortex but has little effect on stresses in the medial wall. A complete metal protrusio cup raises stresses on the periphery and reduces them on the medial wall. A metal-backed polyethylene cup reduces stress in the medial wall and reduces tensile stress in the bone cement. Metal reinforcement in just the medial portion of the socket has no significant effect on acetabular stress (Fig. 17–34).[12] Metallic acetabular reinforcement rings have been shown to prevent central migration of the acetabular component in protrusio acetabuli.[1] No special treatment for protrusio is needed under the following conditions: (1) protrusion less than 5 mm, (2) strong medial wall, and (3) minimal osteoporosis and no known collagen or other bone defects.

Bone grafting of the protruded medial wall is the preferred method of correcting protrusio acetabuli during total hip arthroplasty because it does the following: (1) lateralizes the acetabular component, (2) normalizes the center of rotation of the hip, and (3) offers potential biologic strengthening of the medial wall. Additional fixation devices are necessary only when the continuity through the acetabulum has been lost (see Chapter 23, *Revision Total Hip Arthroplasty*).[58] Bone graft placed between the medial wall of the acetabulum and the prosthetic socket provides the most physiologic means of lateralizing the socket to the normal position (Fig. 17–35). The graft may be cortical or cancellous or both and may come from the iliac crest or allograft. Autogenous femoral

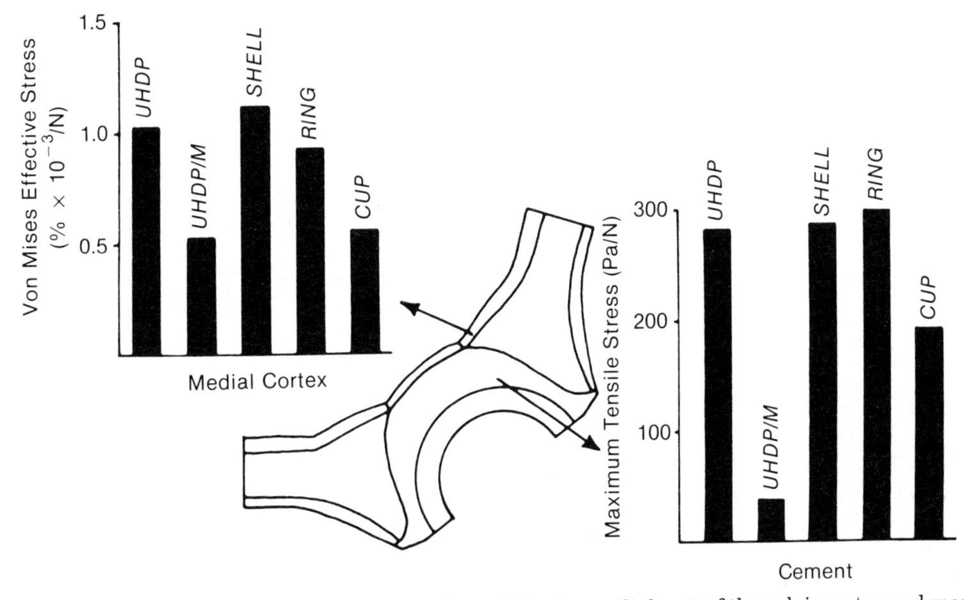

FIGURE 17–34. Von Mises effective stress occurring within the medial part of the pelvic cortex and maximum tension occurring within the cement in protruded acetabulum reconstructed with a normally placed acetabular component. (UHDP = polyethylene cup; UHDP/M = metal-backed polyethylene cup; SHELL = metal medial acetabular shell with polyethylene cup; RING = metal protrusio ring with polyethylene cup; and CUP = metal protrusio cup with polyethylene cup. (Crowninshield, R.D., Brand, R.A., and Pedersen, D.R.: J. Bone Joint Surg. 65A: 495–499, 1983. By permission.)

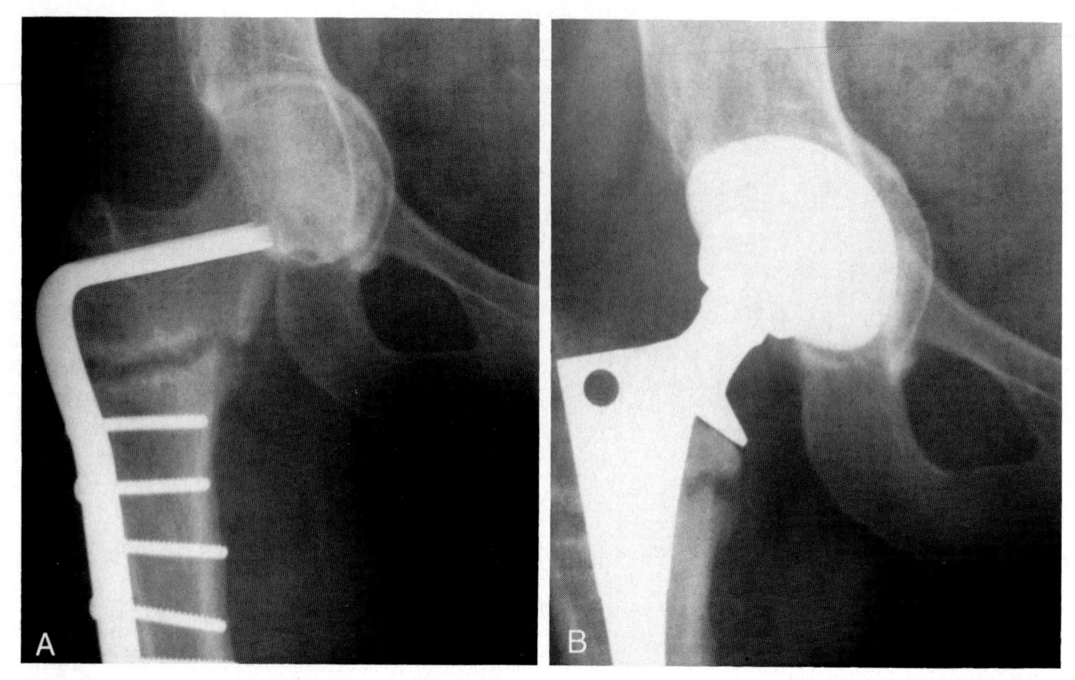

FIGURE 17–35. A patient with Marfan's syndrome with protrusio acetabuli. *A,* She was treated previously with a proximal femoral osteotomy. Healing of the osteotomy is delayed. She has continued severe groin pain. *B,* An acetabular bone graft was employed to provide socket lateralization. The patient had excellent pain relief and subsequent healing of the osteotomy.

head, from which all cartilage but not subchondral bone is removed, makes an ideal grafting material. The graft is placed with its articular surface directed into the acetabulum, and the graft may be held in place by installation of the acetabular component with or without bone cement.[14, 48] If the socket is cemented, the cement must be kept from intruding between the graft and the medial wall. When the protrusio is deep, the surgeon can fix the graft with screws, countersinking them into the subchondral bone and then reaming the graft *in situ.*[27, 30, 39, 66]

Ankylosing Spondylitis

When total hip arthroplasty is performed for a patient with ankylosing spondylitis, the procedure may differ only slightly from that performed for other diagnoses. Patients who have severe forms of the disease involving multiple joints, those who have marked rigid flexion of the spine and hips, and some of those who have had previous hip surgery present major technical problems from the standpoint of the anesthesia, positioning, and surgical procedure. The patient must be carefully and completely evaluated. Some have severely arthritic knees with associated flexion contracture; they may have a fixed equinus deformity. The surgeon's goal is to release contractures, providing a plantigrade foot and achieving equal limb length. When Achilles tendon lengthening and capsulotomies of the foot are necessary, they are done before hip replacement. If knee arthroplasty is required, it follows hip replacement. In patients with juvenile onset ankylosing spondylitis or those with severe adult onset ankylosis spondylitis, small or custom prostheses may be necessary.

Anesthesia may require special techniques, such as awake intubation and occasionally tracheostomy. Positioning of the patient on the operating table is often difficult and may require special supports. The transtrochanteric approach provides the best exposure for difficult operations. Because the hips are often solidly fused, the femoral neck may have to be osteotomized *in situ.* When the hips are fused with a large amount of bone, normal landmarks may be obscured. Placement of a guide wire followed by radiographic examination helps confirm the correct location for the osteotomy.

The acetabulum is first cleared with curette, gouge, rongeur, or all of these. The socket is then reamed. Either a cemented or an uncemented socket component may be placed. When the bone is very osteoporotic, cementing may be preferable. The femoral prosthesis is prepared in a standard manner, with great care taken to avoid cortical penetration or fracture due to osteoporosis and thin cortices. If full or nearly full extension cannot be achieved owing to tight soft tissues or if neurovascular structures might be damaged by attempts to correct the contracture, the femur may be shortened as is done with complete congenital dislocation of the hip. Preparation should include plans for using a longer neck size to provide greater separation between the pelvis and proximal femur. This technique allows for better motion and reduces the chances of refusion. Because of the poor bone quality, cemented placement of the femoral stem may be preferable to press-fit fixation, in some instances.

The patient is monitored closely after surgery for evidence of cardiac or respiratory compromise. Balanced suspension is helpful in protecting a tightly reattached greater trochanter and permitting more comfortable early motion. Preventive treatment is provided to avoid or reduce the formation of extensive heterotopic bone.[15] Not all investigators agree on the incidence of this complication. Some have reported no increase in significant heterotopic bone formation after total hip replacement in patients with ankylosing spondylitis and therefore doubt the need for preventive treatment.[18, 33]

Juvenile Rheumatoid Arthritis

Total hip replacement for children with juvenile rheumatoid arthritis requires careful preoperative planning. Mini-sized components or custom prostheses may have to be ordered for the procedure. Surgery often improves function dramatically in children and young adults with severe joint destruction or contracture. Frequently the primary indication for surgery is functional incapacitation rather than pain. If the patient is severely handicapped, skeletal immaturity may not contraindicate hip replacement. When both hip and knee replacement are indicated, hip replacement is usually performed first.

The transtrochanteric approach is best when the deformity is severe. Great care must be taken to provide adequate soft tissue release, which usually includes complete capsulotomy, release of the iliopsoas, and sometimes release of the gluteus maximus tendon. If this soft tissue release is not done, fracture of the small osteoporotic bone is more likely. Anteversion may be as much as 60 to 80 degrees; trochanteric osteotomy helps placement of the stem to correct this abnormal version.

In some patients, bone grafts are required owing to protrusio acetabula or deficient bone stock of the superior acetabulum (see Protrusio Acetabuli and Congenital Dysplastic Hip). When the patient has an open triradiate cartilage, the cartilage should be curetted and bone grafted. It may be necessary to shorten the femur (e.g., in cases of congenital dislocation of the hip) to avoid overstretching of neurovascular structures. As in other patients with severe deformity and contracture, these patients may benefit from balanced suspension of the extremity immediately after surgery.[4, 16, 21, 43, 60, 61]

Hip Arthrodesis

The patient with pain in the low back, opposite hip, or ipsilateral knee after previous arthrodesis or spontaneous fusion of a hip may be a candidate for hip replacement. The surgeon may choose the transtrochanteric, anterior, or posterior approach. If landmarks to determine the appropriate site of neck osteotomy are not apparent, a guide wire is placed and a radiograph made. The osteotomy is then performed, after which the acetabulum is cleared with curette, gouge, and rongeur. Hip replacement is performed in standard fashion. The tensor fascia may be attached to the proximal femur when abductor muscles are completely absent, but most reports indicate little or no abductor dysfunction without special techniques to substitute for apparently absent abductor muscles. Hip muscle strength may improve for 2 years or more after surgery. Unless the patient has had many previous operations resulting in substantial soft tissue and bone deformity, the quality of the result following total hip arthroplasty of an ankylosed hip will approach that of primary replacement for other diagnoses.[6, 9, 10, 22, 32, 37, 68]

Total Hip Replacement After Proximal Femoral Osteotomy or Previous Fracture

Some patients who have had a recurrence of symptoms after proximal femoral osteotomy may eventually require hip replacement after several years. Several procedural alternatives are possible for managing the proximal femoral deformity as follows:

1. If the deformity is minimal, standard stem placement may be possible, although a smaller prosthesis may be needed (Fig. 17–36). This technique may be more feasible with cemented stem placement.
2. A prosthesis designed for use after proximal femoral osteotomy may be employed.
3. A custom prosthesis may be selected.
4. The osteotomy may be corrected ("undone") at one stage and when healed, the hip arthroplasty done as a second stage.
5. The proximal femur may be reosteotomized at the time of total hip replacement and fixed with the prosthetic stem.

When osteotomy is not undone during total hip replacement, the danger of intraoperative femoral fracture is greater during femoral preparation. The chances of fracture are positively correlated with the amount of displacement of the osteotomy. In patients with cemented hip replacement, clinical and radiographic results after femoral osteotomy are as favorable as those in patients without previous osteotomy. Comparative follow-up data on press-fit hip replacement after osteotomy are currently unavailable.[7, 19, 28, 67]

Total hip replacement following malunion of fracture of the proximal femur should be planned in much the same manner as that following osteotomy, even though the bone may be more irregular. When configuration of the proximal femur appears to be especially complex due to fracture malunion or previous osteotomy, computerized tomography may aid in evaluation. Total hip replacement may be indicated in the treatment of nonunion of proximal femoral fractures. Total hip arthroplasty for a femoral neck fracture that has not healed is not usually complex. However, patients with unstable fractures in the trochanteric area may present with (1) distortion of the femoral canal, (2) substantial shortening of the femur, and (3) variable femoral bone stock deficiency. These features may cause increased potential for intraoperative technical problems. These problems are minimized by careful preoperative planning and assuring the availability of the appropriate prostheses.[41]

Whether a patient has had previous osteotomy or fracture, there is often an internal fixation device in place at the time total hip replacement becomes indicated. Some surgeons have recommended that these devices be removed at a separate operation. Healing of the bone is allowed. Total hip replacement proceeds at a later operation in order to avoid the problem of stress risers left in the bone when internal fixation devices are removed. At times, this practice may be necessary because of damage to the bone stock by an internal fixation device. Bone defects that would compromise total hip arthroplasty can be grafted and allowed to heal before proceeding with the arthroplasty. If defects left in the bone by removal of the internal fixation device are not extensive, it is usually feasible to remove the device and place the hip prosthesis at the same operation. When a cemented stem is used, the defects left by screws are plugged to avoid cement extrusion. Bone graft is the best material for filling the defects. For a press-fit stem this may not be as important, especially when the defect is traversed by the stem because the defects will heal in several weeks. If the defect is in the area of the stem tip with either a cemented or a press-fit stem, the surgeon might select a longer stem to avoid having the stem tip near a stress riser. If this step is not done, bone grafting of the defect becomes much more important and more caution is advised in the first 2 to 3 months of the postoperative period to reduce the possibility of fracture.

Resection Arthroplasty

When a patient who has undergone resection arthroplasty suffers persistent pain

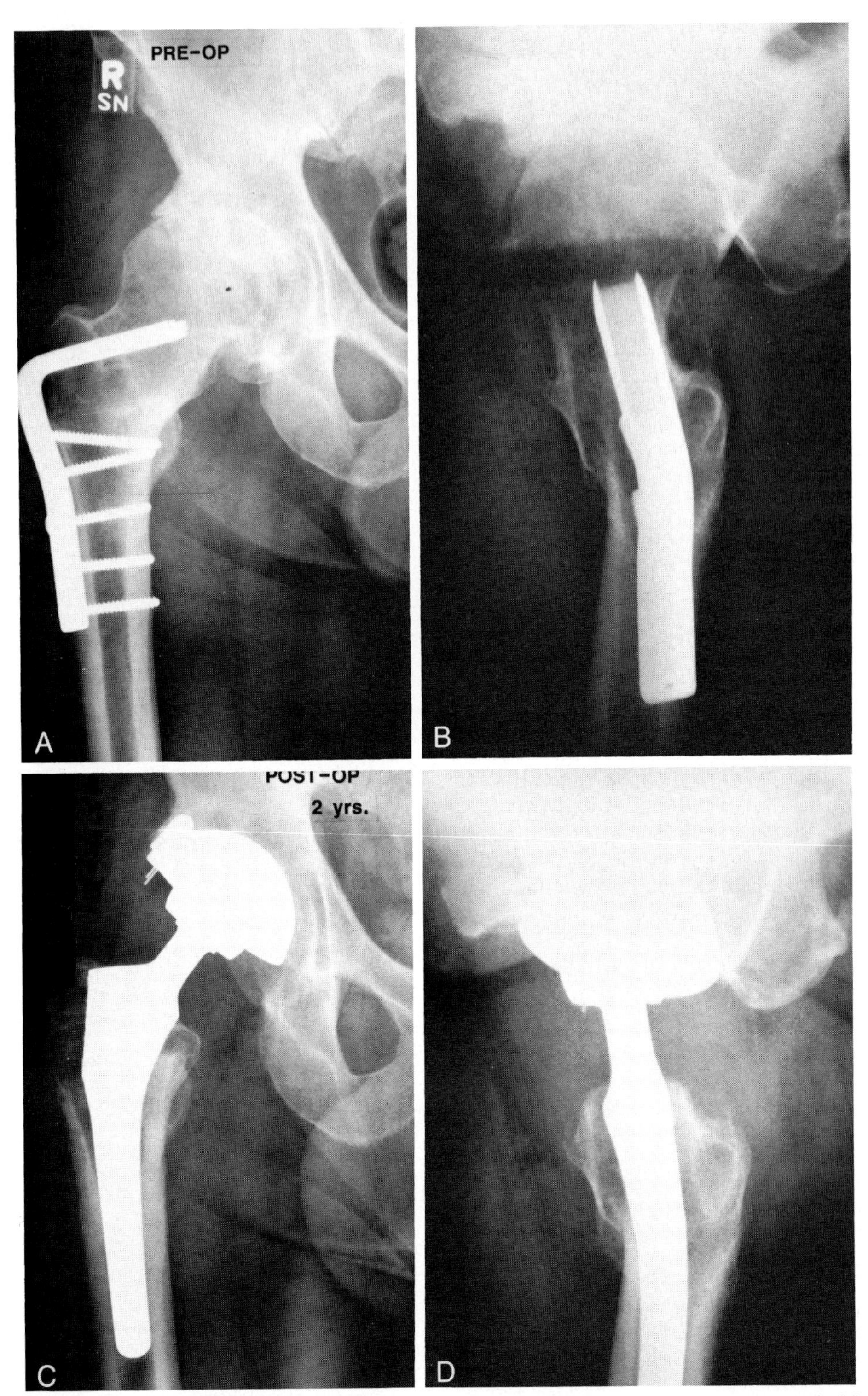

FIGURE 17–36. A hip with previous osteotomy treated by standard total hip replacement. *A*, Moderate deformity is seen preoperatively. *B*, Preoperative lateral radiograph. *C*, Postoperative anteroposterior radiograph. *D*, Postoperative lateral radiograph.

and functional incapacity, total hip arthroplasty may be indicated. If the resection arthroplasty was performed using the type of osteotomy described by Milch or Batchelor, it may be necessary to follow one of the procedures described in the previous section. However, the bone deformity after one of these procedures may be less severe than that after osteotomy for the treatment of osteoarthritis. Reattaching the trochanter in a normal anatomic position via the transtrochanteric approach may give all the correction needed in this situation. The thick, strong pseudocapsule that forms after resection arthroplasty must be excised to provide adequate exposure and allow for regaining extremity length. If the neck osteotomy done at the time of resection arthroplasty was lower than that normally done for total hip replacement, it may be necessary to utilize a longer neck prosthesis than usual.

Cup Arthroplasty

When a patient's hip that has had previous cup arthroplasty again becomes disabling, total hip arthroplasty may be indicated. Radiographs may show collapse of the cup on the femur. Usually there is adequate femoral bone stock remaining so that any deficiency can be managed by using a longer neck femoral component. Sometimes, on the socket side, the cup may erode the acetabular bone and protrude into the pelvis. This problem is managed as recommended in the section Protrusio Acetabuli.

References

1. Aebi, M., Ballmer, P., Richner, L., and Ganz, R.: The acetabular reinforcement ring in primary total hip replacement (145 cases). American Academy of Orthopaedic Surgeons Annual Meeting, Las Vegas, 1989.
2. Amstutz, H. C., Markolf, K. L., and McNeice, G. M.: Loosening of total hip components: Cause and prevention. The Hip. St. Louis, C. V. Mosby Company, 1976.
3. Amstutz, H. C., Yao, J., Dorey, F. J., and Nugent, J. P.: Survival analysis of T–28 hip arthroplasty with clinical implications. Orthop. Clin. North Am. 19(3):491–503, 1988.
4. Arden, G. P.: Surgical treatment of Still's disease (juvenile chronic arthritis). Ann. Acad. Med. Singapore 12(2):174–184, 1983.
5. Beim, G. M., Lavernia, C., and Convery, F. R.: Intramedullary plugs in cemented hip arthroplasty. J. Arthrop. 4:139–141, 1989.
6. Besser, M. I.: A muscle transfer to replace absent abductors in the conversion of a fused hip to a total hip arthroplasty. Clin. Orthop. 162:173–174, 1982.
7. Biedert, R. and Muller, W.: Repeat intertrochanteric osteotomy in the implantation of a cement-free straight total hip endoprosthesis following previous varization osteotomy. A case report. Z. Orthop. 125(6):648–651, 1987. (Published in German.)
8. Byrick, R. J., Bell, R. S., Kay, J. C., et al: High-volume, high-pressure pulsatile lavage during cemented arthroplasty. J. Bone Joint Surg. 71A:1331–1336, 1989.
9. Cameron, H. U. and Jung, Y. B.: Results of total hip arthroplasty without trochanteric osteotomy following hip fusion. Orthop. Rev. 16(9):646–650, 1987.
10. Courpied, J. P., Kerboul, M., Bellier, G., and Postel, M.: Total replacement of ankylosed hips. Rev. Chir. Orthop. 67(3):289–296, 1981. (Published in French. Author's transl.)
11. Coventry, M. B., Beckenbaugh, R. D., Nolan, D. R., and Ilstrup, D. M.: 2,012 Total hip arthroplasties: A study of postoperative course and early complications. J. Bone Joint Surg. 56A:273–284, 1974.
12. Crowninshield, R. D., Brand, R. A., and Pedersen, D. R.: A stress analysis of acetabular reconstruction in protrusio acetabuli. J. Bone Joint Surg. [Am]. 65(4):495–499, 1983.
13. Dooley, B. J., Clifford, M. J., and Hjorth, D. P.: Total hip replacement combined with bone grafting for acetabular dysplasia causing severe osteoarthritis of the hip joint. Aust. N. Z. J. Surg. 55(2):195–198, 1985.
14. Drabu, K. J. and Ring, P. A.: Uncemented acetabular cups in dysplastic and protrusio acetabuli. Clin. Orthop. 210:173–178, 1986.
15. Finsterbush, A., Amir, D., Vatashki, E., and Husseini, N.: Joint surgery in severe ankylosing spondylitis. Acta Orthop. Scand. 59(5):491–496, 1988.
16. Garcia-Morteo, O., Maldonado-Cocco, J. A., and Babini, J. C.: Ectopic ossification following total hip replacement in juvenile chronic arthritis. J. Bone Joint Surg. [Am.] 65(6):812–814, 1983.
17. Gerber, S. D. and Harris, W. H.: Femoral head autografting to augment acetabular deficiency in patients requiring total hip replacement. J. Bone Joint Surg. 68A:1241–1248, 1986.
18. Giordani, M., Penenberg, B. L., and Kaufman, R. L.: Heterotopic ossification following total hip arthroplasty in patients with ankylosing spondylitis. American Academy of Orthopaedic Surgeons Annual Meeting, Las Vegas, 1989.
19. Glassman, A. H., Engh, C. A., and Bobyn, J. D.: Proximal femoral osteotomy as an adjunct in cementless revision total hip arthroplasty. J. Arthroplasty 2:47–63, 1987.
20. Gruen, T. A., Markolf, K. L., and Amstutz, H. C.: Effects of lamination and blood entrapment on the strength of acrylic bone cement. Clin. Orthop. 119:25, 1976.
21. Gudmundsson, G. H., Harving, S., and Pilgaard, S.: The Charnley total hip arthroplasty in juvenile rheumatoid arthritis patients. Orthopedics 12(3):385–388, 1989.

22. Hardinge, K., Murphy, J. C., and Frenyo, S.: Conversion of hip fusion to Charnley low-friction arthroplasty. Clin. Orthop. 211:173–179, 1986.
23. Harris, W. H. and Davies, J. P.: Modern use of modern cement for total hip replacement. Orthop. Clin. North Am. 19(3):581–589, 1988.
24. Harris, W. H., McCarthy, J. C., and O'Neill, D. A.: Femoral component loosening using contemporary techniques of femoral cement fixation. J. Bone Joint Surg. 64A:1063–1067, 1982.
25. Harris, W. H., McCarthy, J. C., Jr., and O'Neill, D. A.: Loosening of the femoral component of total hip replacement after plugging the femoral canal. The Hip. St. Louis, C. V. Mosby Company, 1982.
26. Harris, W. H. and McGann, W. A.: Loosening of the femoral component after use of the medullary-plug cementing technique. Follow-up note with a minimum five-year follow-up. J. Bone Joint Surg. [Am.] 68(7):1064–1066, 1986.
27. Heywood, A. W.: Arthroplasty with a solid bone graft for protrusio acetabuli. J. Bone Joint Surg. [Br.] 62(3):332–336, 1980.
28. Holtgrewe, J. L. and Hungerford, D. S.: Primary and revision total hip replacement without cement and with associated femoral osteotomy. J. Bone Joint Surg. 71A:1487–1495, 1989.
29. Jensen, J. S., Retpen, J. B., and Arnoldi, C. C.: Arthroplasty for congenital hip dislocation. Techniques for acetabular reconstruction. Acta Orthop. Scand. 60(1):86–92, 1989.
30. Johnsson, R., Ekelund, L., Zygmunt, S., and Lidgren, L.: Total hip replacement with spongious bone graft for acetabular protrusion in patients with rheumatoid arthritis. Acta Orthop. Scand. 55(5):510–513, 1984.
31. Keating, E. M., Ritter, M. A., Faris, P. M., et al: Anatomic study of structures at risk with acetabular screw fixation of total hip replacement. Orthop. Trans. 13:497, 1989.
32. Kilgus, D. J., Amstutz, H. C., Wilgin, M. A., and Dorey, F. J.: Joint replacement for ankylosed hips. J. Bone Joint Surg. 72A:45–54, 1990.
33. Kilgus, D. J., Gorek, J., and Nambe, R. S.: Total hip replacement for ankylosing spondylitis with average six-year follow-up. Orthop. Trans. 13:498, 1989.
34. Krause, W. R., Krug, W., and Miller, J.: Strength of the cement-bone interface. Clin. Orthop. 163:290–299, 1982.
35. Krause, W. R., Krug, W., and Miller, J.: Strength of the cement-bone interface. Clin. Orthop. 163:291, 1982.
36. Lee, A. J. and Ling, R. S.: Improved cementing techniques. Instr. Course Lect. 30:407–413, 1981.
37. Lubahn, J. D., Evarts, C. M., and Feltner, J. B.: Conversion of ankylosed hips to total hip arthroplasty. Clin. Orthop. 153:146–152, 1980.
38. Markolf, K. L. and Amstutz, H. C.: Penetration and flow of acrylic bone cement. Clin. Orthop. 121:99, 1976.
39. Mayer, G. and Hartseil, K.: Hip replacement in acetabular protrusion. Acta. Orthop. Scand. 56(6):461–463, 1985.
40. McQueary, F. G. and Johnston, R. C.: Coxarthrosis after congenital dysplasia. Treatment by total hip arthroplasty without acetabular bonegrafting. J. Bone Joint Surg. [Am.] 70(8):1140–1144, 1988.
41. Mehlhoff, T., Landon, G. C., and Tullos, H. C.: Total hip arthroplasty following failed internal fixation of the proximal femur: a retrospective review of technical complications. Orthop. Trans. 12:742, 1988.
42. Miller, J., Burke, D. L., Stachiewicz, J. W., et al: Pathophysiology of loosening of femoral components in total hip arthroplasty. The Hip. St. Louis, C.V. Mosby Company, 1978.
43. Mogensen, B., Brattstrom, H., Ekelund, L., and Lidgren, L.: Total hip replacement in juvenile chronic arthritis. Acta Orthop. Scand. 54(3):422–430, 1983.
44. Mulroy, R. D., Jr.: Prohibitive failure rate of femoral head autografts in total hip replacement for acetabular deficiency by 12 Years. American Academy of Orthopaedic Surgeon's Annual Meeting, New Orleans, 1990.
45. Oh, I., Bourne, R. B., and Harris, W. H.: The femoral cement compactor. An improvement in cementing technique in total hip replacement. J. Bone Joint Surg. [Am.] 65(9):1335–1338, 1983.
46. Oh, I., Carlson, C. E., Tomford, W. W., and Harris, W. H.: Improved fixation of the femoral component after total hip replacement using a methacrylate intramedullary plug. J. Bone Joint Surg. [Am.] 60(5):608–613, 1978.
47. Oh, I. and Harris, W. H.: A cement fixation system for total hip arthroplasty. Clin. Orthop. 164:221–229, 1982.
48. Oh, I. and Harris, W. H.: Design concepts, indications, and surgical technique for use of the protrusio shell. Clin. Orthop. 162:175–184, 1982.
49. Oh, I., Merckx, D. B., and Harris, W. H.: Acetabular cement compactor. An experimental study of pressurization of cement in the acetabulum in total hip arthroplasty. Clin. Orthop. 177:289–293, 1983.
50. Oh, I., Sander, T. W., and Treharne, R. W.: Acetabular cup groove and pod design and its effect on cement fixation in total hip arthroplasty. Clin. Orthop. 189:308, 1984.
51. Paavilainen, T., Hoikka, V., and Solonen, K. A.: Cementless total hip replacement for severely dysplastic or dislocated hips. J. Bone Joint Surg. 72B:205–211, 1990.
52. Petty, R. W., Miller, G. J., and Piotrowski, G.: *In vitro* evaluation of the effect of acetabular prosthesis implantation on human cadaver pelves. Bull. Prosth. Res. 17:80–89, 1980.
53. Phillips, T. W. and Rao, D. R.: Bateman bipolar hips with autologous bone graft reinforcement for dysplastic acetabula. Clin. Orthop. 251:104–112, 1990.
54. Poss, R., Brick, G. W., Wright, R. J., et al: The effects of modern cementing techniques on the longevity of total hip arthroplasty. Orthop. Clin. North Am. 19(3):591–598, 1988.
55. Poss, R., Maloney, J. P., Ewald, F. C., et al: Six- to 11-year results of total hip arthroplasty in rheumatoid arthritis. Clin. Orthop. 182:109–116, 1984.
56. Ranawat, C. S., Dorr, L. D., and Inglis, A. E.: Total hip arthroplasty in protrusio acetabuli of rheumatoid arthritis. J. Bone Joint Surg. 62A:1059–1065, 1980.
57. Ranawat, C. S., Rawlins, B. A., and Harju, V. T.: Effect of modern cement technique on acetabular

fixation total hip arthroplasty. Orthop. Clin. North Am. 19:599–603, 1988.
58. Ranawat, C. S. and Zahn, M. G.: Role of bone grafting in correction of protrusio acetabuli by total hip arthroplasty. J. Arthroplasty 1(2):131–137, 1986.
59. Russotti, G. M. and Harris, W. H.: High placement of the acetabular cup: a long-term follow-up study. Orthop. Trans. 12:690, 1988.
60. Ruddlesdin, C., Ansell, B. M., Arden, G. P., and Swann, M.: Total hip replacement in children with juvenile chronic arthritis. J. Bone Joint Surg. [Br.] 68(2):218–222, 1986.
61. Scott, R. D., Sarokhan, A. J., and Dalziel, R.: Total hip and total knee arthroplasty in juvenile rheumatoid arthritis. Clin. Orthop. 182:90–98, 1984.
62. Shaughnessy, W. J., Kavanagh, B. F., and Fitzgerald, R. H., Jr.: Effects of acetabular component position on total hip arthroplasty: results in patients with congenital dislocation of the hip. American Academy of Orthopaedic Surgeon's Annual Meeting, New Orleans, 1990.
63. Shelley, P. and Wroblewski, B. M.: Socket design and cement pressurisation in the Charnley low-friction arthroplasty. J. Bone Joint Surg. [Br.] 70(3):358–363, 1988.
64. Sherman, R. M., Byrick, R. J., Kay, J. C., et al: The role of lavage in preventing hemodynamic and blood-gas changes during cemented arthroplasty. J. Bone Joint Surg. [Am.] 65(4):500–506, 1983.
65. Shore, A., Macauley, D., and Ansell, B. M.: Idiopathic protrusio acetabuli in juveniles. Rheumatol. Rehabil. 20(1):1–10, 1981.
66. Slooff, T. J., Huiskes, R., van Horn, J., and Lemmens, A. J.: Bone grafting in total hip replacement for acetabular protrusion. Acta Orthop. Scand. 55(6):593–596, 1984.
67. Soballe, K., Boll, K. L., Kofod, S., et al: Total hip replacement after medial-displacement osteotomy of the proximal part of the femur. J. Bone Joint Surg. [Am.] 71(5):692–697, 1989.
68. Strathy, G. M. and Fitzgerald, R. H., Jr.: Total hip arthroplasty in the ankylosed hip. A ten-year follow-up. J. Bone Joint Surg. [Am.] 70(7):963–966, 1988.
69. Vasu, R., Carter, D. R., and Harris, W. H.: Evaluation of bone cement failure criteria with applications to the acetabular region. J. Biomech. Eng. 105(4):332–337, 1983.
70. Wasielewski, R. C., Cooperstein, L. A., Kruger, M. P., and Rubash, H. E.: Acetabular anatomy and transacetabular screw fixation in total hip arthroplasty. J. Bone Joint Surg. 72A:501–508, 1990.
71. Weinstein, A. M., Bingham, D. M., Sauer, B. W., and Lunceford, E. M.: The effect of high pressure insertion and antibiotic inclusions upon the mechanical properties of polymethylmethacrylate. Clin. Orthop. 121:67–73, 1976.
72. Welch, R. B. and Charnley, J.: Low friction arthroplasty of the hip in rheumatoid arthritis and ankylosing spondylitis. Clin. Orthop. 72:22–32, 1970.
73. Woolson, S. T.: Leg length equalization during total hip replacement. Orthop 13:17–21, 1990.
74. Woolson, S. T. and Harris, W. H.: A method of intraoperative limb length measurement in total hip arthroplasty. Clin. Orthop. 185:207–210, 1985.
75. Wroblewski, B. M. and Van der Rijt, A.: Intramedullary cancellous bone block to improve femoral stem fixation in Charnley low-friction arthroplasty. J. Bone Joint Surg. [Br.] 66(5):639–644, 1984.

CHAPTER 18

Total Hip Arthroplasty: Postoperative Care and Rehabilitation

WILLIAM PETTY

Programs for postoperative hip rehabilitation vary widely at different surgery centers. Some programs are extensive; other are limited. In general, hip replacement requires a less intense program of rehabilitation than knee replacement. Most patients do well with basic instructions in how to use walking aids and explanations of precautions they must observe to avoid dangerous postures that might cause dislocation. A well-designed program that emphasizes the central role of the patient in carrying out rehabilitation results in more rapid and complete recovery. Both preoperative and postoperative patient education should be supported and encouraged by all members of the health care team. They should emphasize to the surgical candidates that the patients who follow guidelines closely achieve the best treatment outcomes for total hip replacements.

POSTOPERATIVE CARE

Management of the patient in the immediate postoperative period has many aspects. Preventive care is important—precautions must be taken against infection, thromboembolism, and heterotopic bone formation. If blood loss during surgery was significant, transfusions may be needed. These topics are discussed elsewhere in this text. Postoperative drains can usually be removed after 24 hours without increasing the risk of hematoma formation. When drains remain in place too long, contamination of the drain site by skin organisms is more likely. Also drain removal permits a more comfortable early movement of the hip.[19] Appropriate analgesic agents are provided for the patient. Patient-controlled analgesia offers the benefits of improved comfort and greater alertness.

After surgery, the limb is placed in balanced suspension or protected by an abduction pillow placed between the legs. Balanced suspension or limb slings maintain the appropriate position of abduction, allow for simple early motion of the operated hip, and elevate the operated extremity (Fig. 18–1A). An abduction pillow may be specifically designed for the purpose or a regular pillow may be placed properly (Fig. 18–1B). With either method of abduction, a small pillow or pad behind the knee provides enough knee flexion to make the patient more comfortable. If the patient has adduction deformity of the opposite hip, a smaller pillow should be placed or the pillow should be placed caudally. Otherwise, the operated extremity will be forced into more than 10 degrees of abduc-

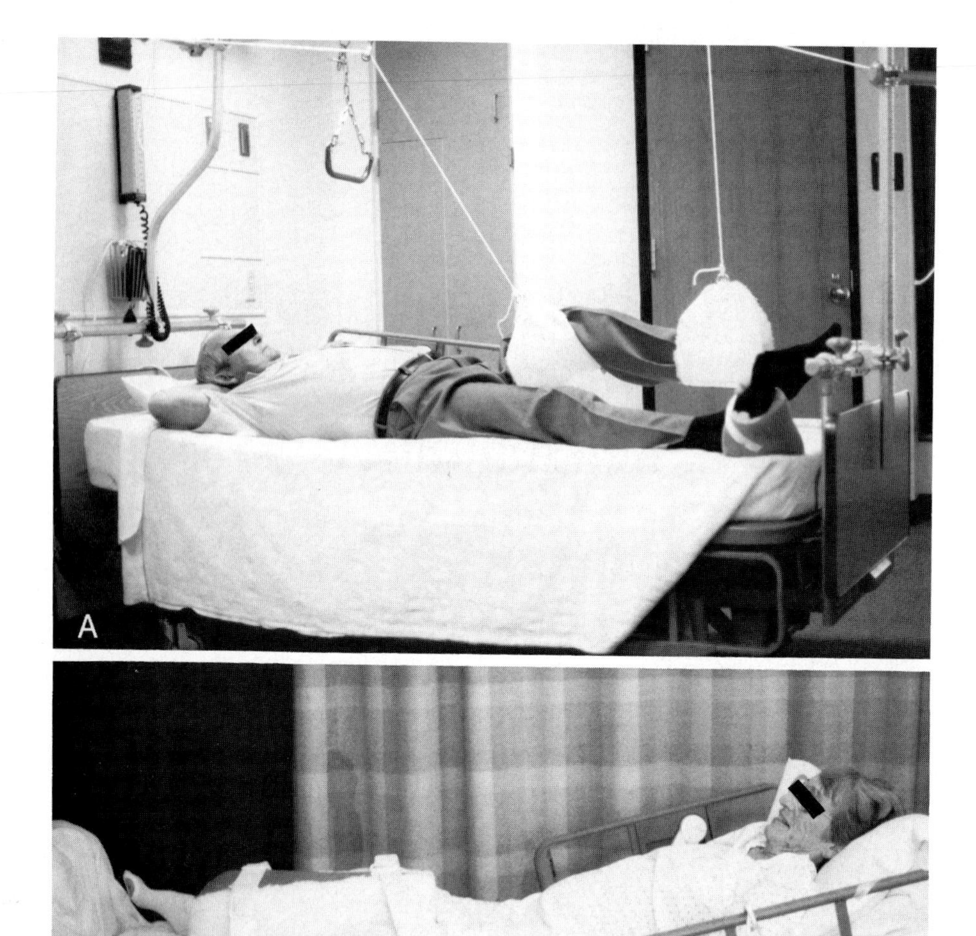

FIGURE 18–1. Methods for maintaining lower extremity position following total hip arthroplasty. *A,* Limb slings allow the patient to begin gentle movement of the hip soon after surgery. *B,* Abduction pillow with pad behind the knee.

tion, causing discomfort and shortening of the abductor muscles. Velcro straps on the abduction pillow must not be too tight and should not compress the peroneal nerve. If suspension is used, care is also needed to avoid pressure on the peroneal nerve area. Heel pads are placed on both feet but are removed from time to time to allow the patient to slide the heel and flex the knee as soon as the patient can. The extremity can be elevated by raising the foot of the bed.

REHABILITATION

Preoperative Assessment and Training

Rehabilitation actually begins preoperatively, as the patient provides the physical therapist with information about their home and work environment. The therapist responds by planning a postoperative rehabilitation program tailored to the patient's environment and needs. Education of the patient includes instructions about gait (walking), exercise and precautions for the newly operated hip.

The home environment of most patients is satisfactory for rehabilitation if they have someone to stay with them when they leave the hospital. Generally, patients can participate in basic activities of daily living without assistance. Although many patients who undergo hip replacements for unilateral hip disease achieve independence rapidly, they should not be expected to prepare meals or do housework right after returning home. For patients with extensive disability due to multiple musculoskeletal problems or those with severe medical illnesses, planning should begin early so that appropriate arrangements can be set in motion. The patient may need to go home with a family member or friend, to have household help, or to stay in an extended care facility temporarily.

By learning about the patient's home environment, the therapist can tailor a basic postoperative program to his or her specific needs. For example, patients with stairs to climb will require extra instruction and practice in stair climbing. The therapist should inquire about any safety hazards present in the patient's environment (e.g., loose rugs) so they can be removed before and not after an accident. Preoperative evaluation should include consideration of and planning for vocational and avocational activities during recovery.

The therapist's physical evaluation includes assessment of both the hip to be operated on and the opposite hip. Both lower extremities should be assessed for strength, range of motion, presence of contractures, and length. The therapist must also evaluate the patient's upper extremities for strength and look for any contractures or other deformities that might make using a walking aid difficult.

When patients know how to walk with a cane, crutch, or walker, their skill must be assessed. Frequently, patients use walking aids incorrectly and require more instruction than if they did not use them. Regardless of previous experience, patients approach early postoperative walking more confidently when they master walking aids preoperatively. The therapist provides instruction, shows the patient transfer techniques, outlines precautions, and describes the sequence of progression of the postoperative program.

Postoperative Rehabilitation

As soon as patients recover consciousness, nursing personnel remind them to begin the exercises practiced preoperatively: ankle dorsi- and plantar flexion, ankle circles, quadriceps and gluteal sets, alternating hip hiking, and bicycling of the knees (moving the knees up and down alternatively) (Table 18–1). On the second or third postoperative day, abduction and increased hip and knee flexion exercises are added. When the quadriceps muscles are strong enough, straight leg raising may be done. Patients who are unable to do this exercise at first should be reassured that this movement will come with continued quadriceps setting and time. Patients with significant preoperative hip flexion contractures should do the Thomas test while contracting the abdominal, gluteal, and quadriceps muscles to help fully extend the hip. Lying prone also helps. Patients with back pain from lying supine will find relief by flexing their hips and knees, pulling to a sitting position with the trapeze bar, and then arching the back and slowly lying back down.[2, 10]

Most patients are able to stand the day after surgery. Transfers, if practiced preoperatively, can usually be done without starting with a tilt table. A patient with a severe general disability may find a tilt table helpful in getting into an upright position safely (Fig. 18–2). However, some elderly patients are fearful of this device

Table 18–1. POSTOPERATIVE EXERCISES IN BED

Day 1	Ankle dorsi and plantar flexion Ankle circles Quadriceps and gluteal sets Alternating hip hiking Bicycling of the knees (moving the knees up and down alternately)
Day 2 or 3	Add abduction and increased hip and knee flexion When the quadriceps muscles are strong enough, straight leg raising may be done.

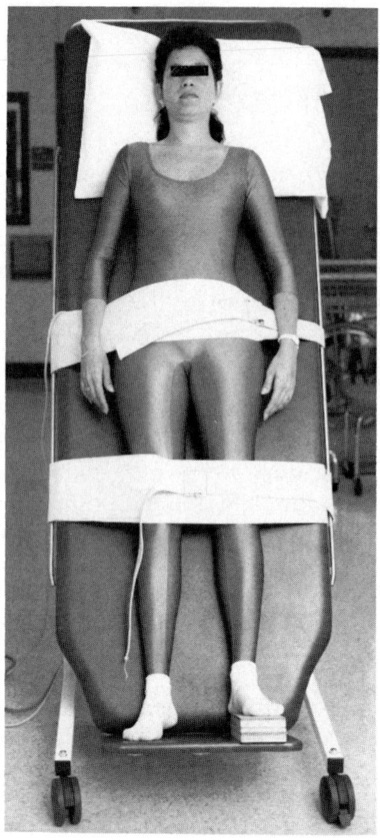

FIGURE 18–2. A tilt table may be helpful for some patients in gaining the upright posture following hip surgery.

Patients who can stand comfortably are assisted in taking a few steps the first or second time they stand, usually with walkers. Most feel somewhat uncomfortable moving about until drains, urinary catheters (if placed), and intravenous lines are removed.

For cemented arthroplasty, the prosthesis fixation is probably as strong at 24 hours as it will ever be, so from this standpoint, full weightbearing may begin immediately. Some surgeons express concern about bone necrosis adjacent to the implant and advocate guarded weightbearing. However, remodeling of this necrotic bone takes months, and no logical reason therefore exists to avoid weightbearing for a few weeks.[5, 8] No evidence has been found that early weightbearing jeopardizes long-term durability of the hip replacement. Weightbearing is gradually started, mainly for the patient's comfort and to allow the muscles the time needed to recover from the trauma of surgery and to regain the strength that was lost because of the protracted hip disease. For patients with poor balance and other disabilities, walking aids offer added protection.

The patient is instructed in standing exercises: toe raises with the knee fully extended on each side and partial weight placed on the operative side, quadriceps and gluteal setting, and stretching of the hips and knees into full extension. Gait training is begun—the goal is to help the patient achieve a normal gait pattern. Patients commonly walk with a shortened or half stride, on tiptoe on the operated side. They are taught to walk with equal stride length, placing the heel firmly with full knee extension during stance. Some patients must be reminded to keep their heads up and to look where they are going (Fig. 18–3). A full-length mirror often helps the patient develop a normal gait.

A patient who has undergone bilateral total hip arthroplasty under the same anesthetic or with a short interval between operations should use the four-point alternating gait (Fig. 18–4). This technique is

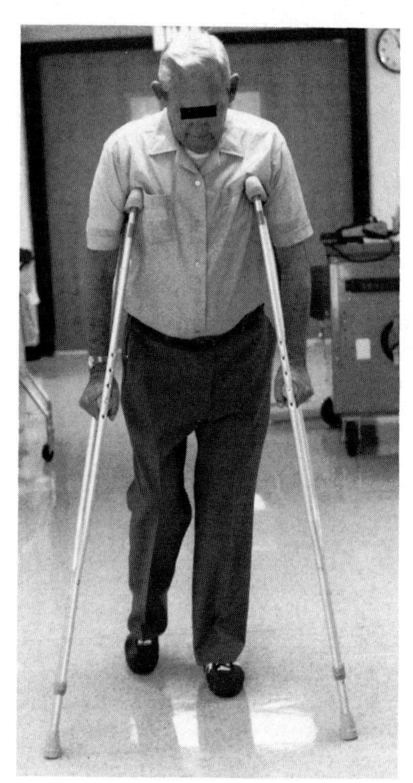

FIGURE 18–3. During the early phase of gait training following total hip replacement, a patient often needs reminding to keep the head up.

difficult to master and requires patience to teach. When patients have developed confidence in their walking, they can begin stair climbing, going up with the unaffected leg first, then the operated leg, and then the crutches. Going down, the crutches are first, then the operated leg, and then the unaffected leg. With this technique, the patient raises and lowers the body with the unaffected leg and crutches (Fig. 18–5). After bilateral operations, the stronger limb is considered as the unaffected limb.[2, 5]

Patients with good balance may prefer elbow crutches; these devices do not reduce weightbearing as much as regular crutches but are not as difficult to use unilaterally and allow easier transition to a cane (Fig. 18–6). Normally, this transition takes 2 to 4 weeks postoperatively in a patient who has no other disability. The speed of the transition depends on the patient's strength and balance. A therapist or physician should supervise the transition for at least one session to be sure the patient utilizes the cane properly and safely. When the patient no longer has a Trendelenburg limp without support, the cane may be put aside.

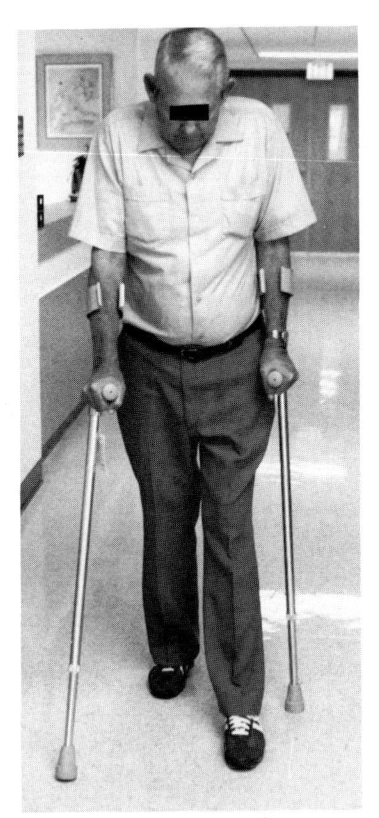

FIGURE 18–4. The four-point alternating gait is used after bilateral total hip arthroplasty. The crutch in the contralateral hand provides support for each hip in alternating fashion.

In a study comparing the effects of immediate versus delayed weightbearing in patients with porous-coated hip prostheses, no differences were found in hip rating, thigh pain, or radiographic appearance.[11] Still, most surgeons recommend gradual progression of weightbearing when total hip arthroplasty is performed with press-fit fixation, especially when porous-coated prostheses are employed. This conservative approach is based on data from animal studies demonstrating that early bone ingrowth requires 2 to 3 weeks and that strength of bone ingrowth fixation plateaus at about 12 weeks.[3, 9, 16, 18] Although tissue ingrowth in humans probably differs from that of experimental animals and may be more fibrous than osseous, restriction of motion between bone and prosthesis during early biologic attachment of the prosthesis is certainly logical. Variations in prosthetic design (e.g., straight or curved, collar or no collar) and differences in surgical technique may result in varying amounts of prosthetic motion within the bone. Because these effects are not well understood, a conservative policy regarding weightbearing may be safer at this time in a patient who has undergone total hip arthroplasty with a porous femoral stem. The argument for additional weightbearing protection in a patient with a porous-coated acetabular component mated with a cemented femoral stem is less sound because the socket component is well contained within the acetabulum and may be subjected to less potential motion between prosthesis and bone.

A reasonable approach in a patient who is having total hip replacement with a porous prosthesis, especially on the femoral side, appears to be partial weightbearing (one third of body weight) for 6 weeks followed by the use of a cane in the opposite hand for another 6 weeks. Patients may estimate the weight they are placing on the operated hip by stepping on a bathroom scale. Telemetric-force measurements across the hip after total hip or hemiarthroplasty have demonstrated that with straight leg raising or with a walker during the early postoperative period, forces

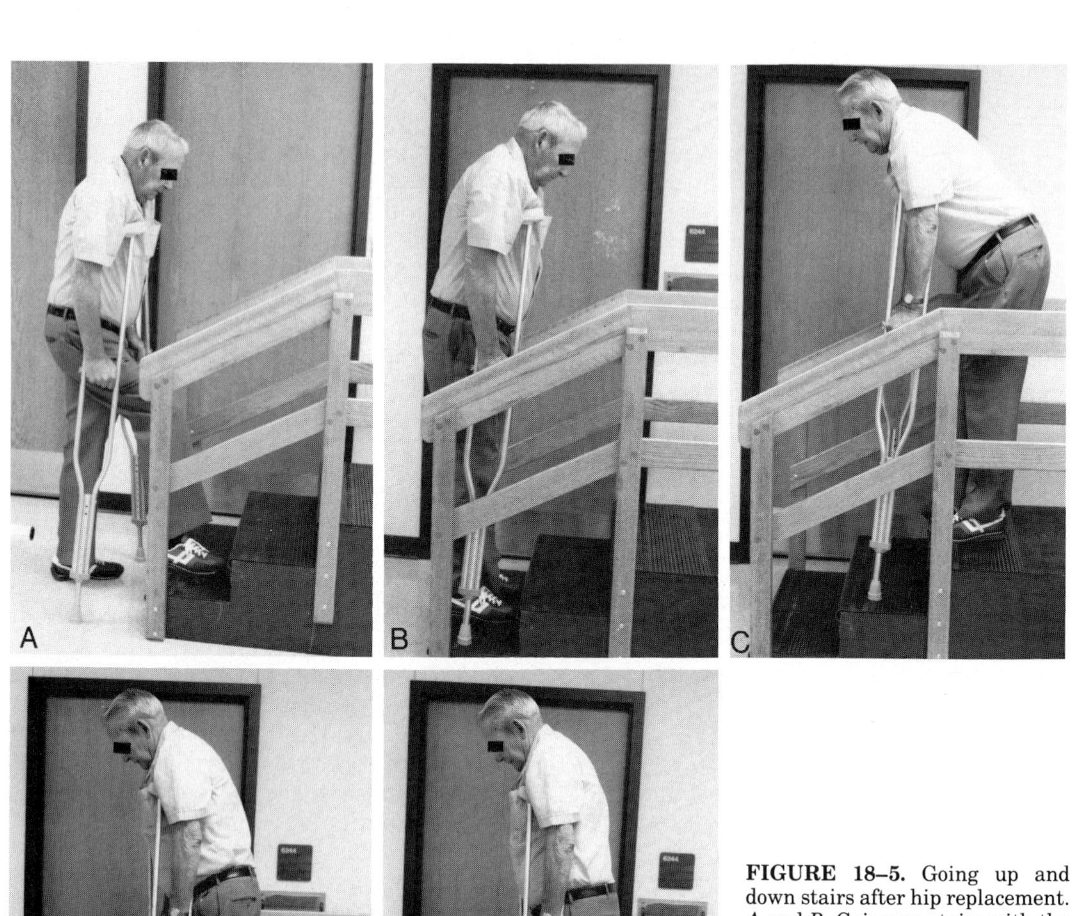

FIGURE 18–5. Going up and down stairs after hip replacement. *A* and *B*, Going up stairs with the unaffected leg first, then the operated leg, and finally the crutches. *C*, Going down stairs, the crutches come first (*C*), then the operated leg (*D*), and then the unaffected leg (*E*).

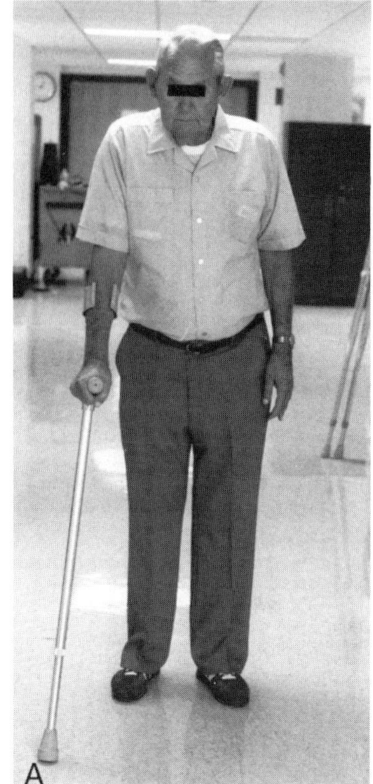

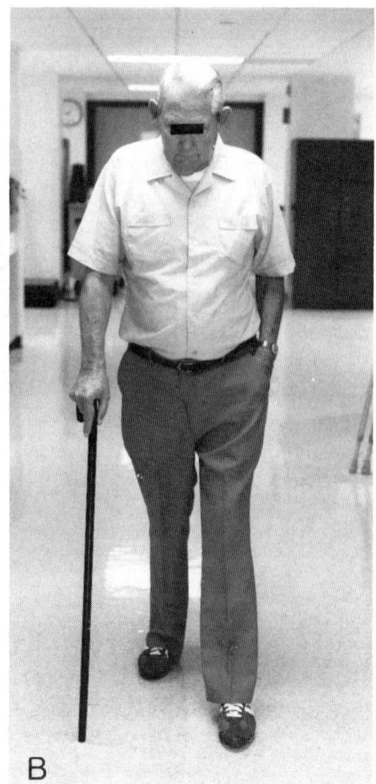

FIGURE 18–6. *A*, Elbow crutches are easier to use unilaterally than axillary crutches. *B*, The patient makes an easy transition from a single elbow crutch to cane.

are equal to body weight and increase with crutch and cane use. The highest forces are measured when patients rise from chairs. The greatest out-of-plane orientation of the resultant force occurs with rising from a chair, stair climbing, and straight leg raising (Table 18–2).[4, 7, 12]

The patient may sit in a chair within a few days of surgery, when the incision is comfortable. The patient's feet may rest on the floor for brief periods, but most of the time the feet should be supported on a stool with the knees extended to reduce dependent leg edema (Fig. 18–7). The sitting surface should be at least 50 cm from the floor and chairs should have arms to make getting up easier.[5, 17] The hospital and home bathrooms should be equipped with elevated toilet seats, preferably with arms. For several weeks after surgery, patients should avoid sitting for more than an hour without moving about and should exercise to avoid edema and a feeling of stiffness in the operated area.

Well-positioned prosthetic components

Table 18–2. MAXIMUM JOINT LOADS DURING VARIOUS ACTIVITIES

	Maximum Resultant Force (Percent Body Weight)			
Activity	***3 Days***	***6 Days***	***16 Days***	***31 Days***
Straight leg raising	—	1.0	1.5	1.8
Getting out of bed	0.8	1.0	1.2	1.4
Getting into bed	0.8	1.0	1.5	1.5
Double-limb stance	0.5*	0.7†	0.9	1.0
Ipsilateral single-limb stance	1.2*	1.3†	1.4†	2.1‡
Walking with aid	1.0*	1.5§	2.6§	2.4‖, 2.8¶

*Using a walker.

†Ipsilateral hand on crutch, contralateral hand in attendant's hand.

‡Contralateral hand in attendant's hand.

§Using crutches.

‖Between parallel bars.

¶With crutches, unsupported ipsilateral stance. (Davy, D. T., Kotzar, G. M., Brown, R. H., et al: J. Bone Joint Surg. 70A:45–50, 1988. By permission.)

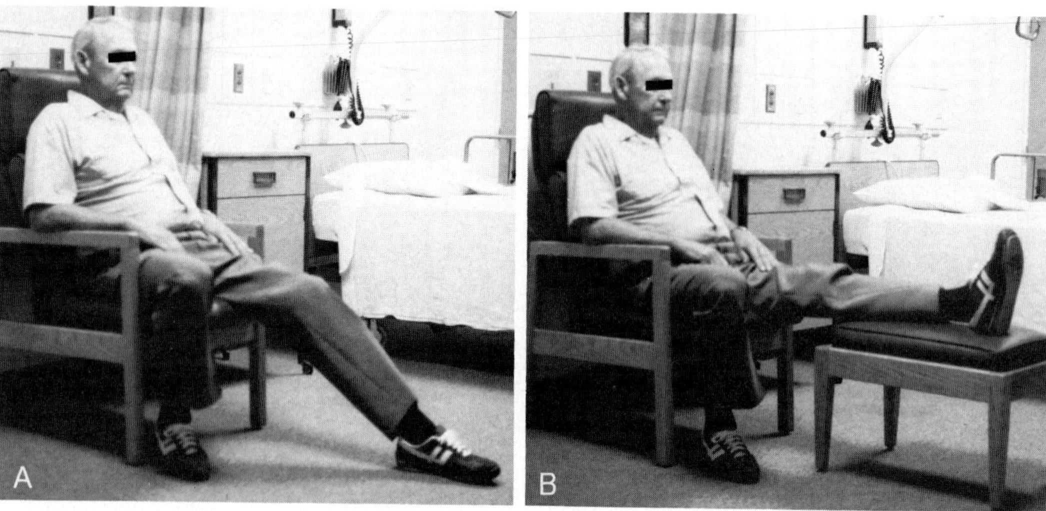

FIGURE 18–7. *A,* While sitting following hip arthroplasty, the feet may rest on the floor for brief periods (*A*), but most of the time the feet should be supported on a stool to reduce dependent leg edema (*B*).

provide the best protection against postoperative hip dislocations, but stability is not as good during the first few weeks after surgery as it is after a strong fibrous pseudocapsule has formed. Thus, patients should avoid certain motions during this period to reduce the risk of dislocation. The key is that abduction is safe and adduction is dangerous (Fig. 18–8). The risk of dislocation goes up when the patient adds excessive flexion and internal rotation to adduction, particularly the latter. The legs may be crossed with the ankle of the operated limb placed on the opposite knee. The legs should not be crossed with the operated thigh resting on the opposite thigh. Foot care and putting on stockings and shoes should be done in proper leg position. The patient should use a stool in the shower to avoid slipping or falling.

Rehabilitation After Hospitalization

The first postoperative follow-up evaluation should be scheduled with the surgeon in 6 to 12 weeks. Additional follow-up visits are usually scheduled at 6 and 12 months. The surgeon should give the patient telephone numbers to call if any problems or questions arise.

Patients who have undergone total hip replacements can expect to resume a normal lifestyle unless their preoperative vocational or avocational pursuits involved very high activity levels (e.g., running, jumping). Although no conclusive evidence is available to demonstrate that activities placing high impact loads on the prosthetic

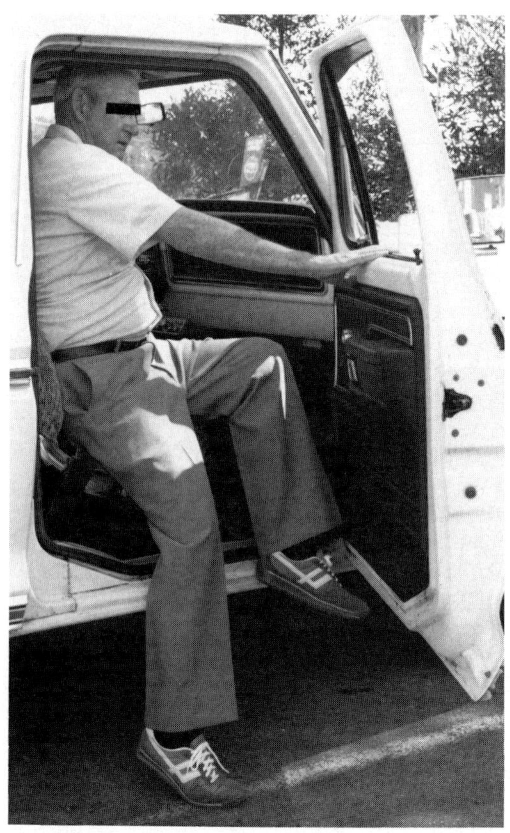

FIGURE 18–8. The patient is taught to get into a car or truck safely, avoiding adduction of the recently operated right hip.

hip lead to earlier failure, the fact is that patients who have had hip replacements and engage in high-stress sports have earlier failure of total hip arthroplasty, especially young men (see Chapter 20, *Results of Primary Total Hip Arthroplasty*). Therefore, it seems reasonable to warn patients with hip replacements to avoid such high-stress activities.

Many patients with sedentary occupations may return to work within 6 weeks after total hip replacements. Those who must lift and carry objects in their jobs may have to delay returning to employment for 3 to 4 months, perhaps longer. Age, sex, and whether the hip replacement was unilateral or bilateral have no effect on restoration of function, although bilateral operations may prolong convalescence. The worst prognostic factor for return to work in a patient with total hip replacement is a long preoperative sick leave.[13] This is an important reason for not delaying hip replacement in disabled patients. Many patients consider their recoveries complete by 3 months after surgery and most by 6 months. Muscle strength continues to improve for 6 months postoperatively. Flexion and abduction improve for 1 year; adduction and rotation improve over an even longer period. Preoperative range of motion is the most important determinant of postoperative range of motion. Patients who have had previous hip surgery usually achieve less ultimate motion than those who have not.[20]

Patients are generally able to stop using walking aids by 3 months after operation. Exceptions are patients with arthritis involving multiple joints, most commonly rheumatoid arthritis, who often need both walking aids and other devices to assist them in the activities of daily living.[10] Patients should be encouraged to walk outdoors in good weather. When pavements are icy or wet, exercise should be taken indoors. Gentle swimming and water exercises are excellent. Patients may resume sexual activity but should not be too vigorous for a few weeks. The position of hip abduction with flexion for a woman should be very safe. The man should be careful to avoid adduction, at least during the first few weeks postoperatively.

Patients are encouraged to progress toward living as normally as possible when they go home. Those who have only hip disease generally need no supervised physical therapy after leaving the hospital. Patients with multiple problems (e.g., inflammatory arthritis with widespread involvement) often need further therapy, either through a special rehabilitation facility with a therapist or through home visits by a therapist.

Nonambulatory Patients

Patients with severe functional disabilities, especially those who cannot walk preoperatively, have special requirements for rehabilitation both before and after total joint replacement surgery. If three or four major joints must be operated on, patients require great physical and psychologic stamina and the encouragement and support of the entire health care team. Total hip arthroplasty usually precedes total knee arthroplasty. If the destruction and deformity are such that two joints can be reconstructed during one hospitalization and the other joints can be done 2 to 3 months later, this should be arranged because it allows for both physical and psychologic recovery of the patient. When substantial flexion contracture or severe pain is present in both hips, the operations should be scheduled near the same time. Otherwise, the unoperated hip will impair ambulation and the patient will get an inferior result in the operated hip, often developing a recurrence of flexion contracture. The same is true for total knee replacement surgery. Some patients must have three or four joints reconstructed during the same hospitalization because of severe pain, or both.

The major cause of poor results in these patients is significant neurologic deficit or loss of motivation. Severe upper extremity involvement may make satisfactory rehabilitation more difficult but does not prevent it. These patients often have dramatic improvement, with most becoming walkers and developing increased independence.[1, 15]

References

1. Arafiles, R. P. and Gustilo, R. B.: Joint replacement in nonambulatory patients. J. Bone Joint Surg. [Am] 61(6):892–897, 1979.
2. Aufranc, O.: Constructive Surgery of the Hip. St. Louis, C. V. Mosby Company, 1962.

3. Bobyn, J. D., Pilliar, R. M., Cameron, H. U., and Weatherly, G. C.: Osteogenic phenomena across bone-implant spaces with porous surfaced intramedullary implants. Acta Orthop. Scand. 52:145–153, 1981.
4. Brand, R. A. and Crowninshield, R. D.: The effect of cane use on hip contact force. Clin. Orthop. 147:181–184, 1980.
5. Charnley, J.: Low Friction Arthroplasty of the Hip. Berlin, Springer-Verlag, 1979.
6. Davis, F. M., Laurenson, V. G., Gillespie, W. J., et al: Leg blood flow during total hip replacement under spinal or general anaesthesia. Anaesth. Intensive Care 17(2):136–143, 1989.
7. Davy, D. T., Kotzar, G. M., Brown, R. H., et al: Telemetric force measurements across the hip after total arthroplasty. J. Bone Joint Surg. [Am] 70(1):45–50, 1988.
8. Gebauer, D. and Blumel, G.: Extreme loading as cause of aseptic loosening of the total hip endoprosthesis socket and the resultant therapeutic consequences. Aktuel. Traumatol. 13(4):154–159, 1983. (Published in German.)
9. Harris, W. H. and Jasty, M.: Bone Ingrowth into Porous Coated Canine Acetabular Replacements: The Effect of Pore Size, Apposition, and Dislocation. The Hip. St. Louis, C. V. Mosby Company, 1985.
10. Haworth, R. J.: Use of aids during the first three months after total hip replacement. Br. J. Rheumatol. 22(1):29–35, 1983.
11. Hoblitzell, R. M., Simpson, J. M., Mikhail, W. E., et al: Effect of immediate versus delayed weightbearing on uncemented porous coated anatomic total hip arthroplasty. Orthop. Trans., 13:526, 1989.
12. Hodge, W. A., Fijan, R. S., Carlson, K. L., et al: Contact pressures in the human hip joint measured *in vivo*. Proc. Natl. Acad. Sci. USA 83(9):2879–2883, 1986.
13. Johnsson, R. and Persson, B. M.: Occupation after hip replacement for arthrosis. Acta Orthop. Scand. 57(3):197–200, 1986.
14. Keith, I.: Ethamsylate and blood loss in total hip replacement. Anaesthesia 34(7):666–670, 1979.
15. McElwain, J. P. and Sheehan, J. M.: Bilateral hip and knee replacement for rheumatoid arthritis. J. Bone Joint Surg. [Br] 67(2):261–265, 1985.
16. Pilliar, R. M.: Porous-surfaced metallic implants for orthopedic applications. J. Biomed. Mater. Res. 21(Suppl. A1):1–33, 1987.
17. Rodosky, M. W., Andriacchi, T. P., and Anderson, G. B. J.: The influence of chair height on lower limb mechanics during rising. J. Orthop. Res. 7:266–271, 1989.
18. Sandborn, P. M., Cook, S. D., Spires, W. P., and Kester, M. A.: Tissue response to porous-coated implants lacking initial bone apposition. J. Arthroplasty 3(4):337–346, 1988.
19. Willett, K. M., Simmons, C. D., and Bentley, G.: The effect of suction drains after total hip replacement. J. Bone Joint Surg. [Br] 70(4):607–610, 1988.
20. Woolson, S. T., Maloney, W. J., and Schurman, D. J.: Time-related improvement in the range of motion of the hip after total replacement. J. Bone Joint Surg. [Am] 67(8):1251–1254, 1985.

CHAPTER 19

Total Hip Arthroplasty: Complications

WILLIAM PETTY

Complications of total hip arthroplasty fit into several broad categories. Complications related to the technical aspects of the surgical procedure itself are one category. Nerves and, less often, blood vessels may be injured, and fractures of the bone or prosthesis may occur during or after total hip arthroplasty. Although limb length equality is a goal of total hip replacement, it may not be possible to achieve in some cases. This chapter begins with a description of the range of problems related to technical aspects of surgery and outlines measures that can reduce the likelihood of these complications.

Another complication of total hip replacement is heterotopic bone formation. Ossification of muscle and capsular tissues can be prevented and treated by methods discussed in *Heterotopic Ossification.*

Inappropriate positioning, soft tissue imbalance, and component malposition may lead to dislocation of the femoral head from the socket. Preoperative evaluation and careful surgical planning, as described in *Dislocation,* can lessen the incidence of this complication. Dislocation usually is managed by closed reduction.

Although infections are increasingly less common, they do sometimes occur after total hip replacements. Also, although the procedure is associated with a low mortality rate, some deaths are reported. The incidences of these complications are explored in *Infection* and *Mortality* at the end of the chapter.

COMPLICATIONS RELATED TO TECHNICAL ASPECTS OF SURGERY

Neural Injury

Injury to nerves may occur during or after total hip arthroplasty (Fig. 19–1). The nerve that is most commonly injured in association with total hip replacement is the sciatic, although the femoral nerve can also be involved. The obturator nerve may be injured but less commonly. The incidence of injury to the obturator nerve may be underreported, because the resulting functional disability is less than that with injury to the sciatic or femoral nerve.[53, 130]

The reported incidence of neural injury is 0.7 to 3.5 percent with primary surgery and up to 7.6 percent in revision total hip replacement.[7, 115, 130, 131] Nerve injury is more common in women, partly because of the excessive lengthening of completely dislocated congenital dysplastic hips. However, even when operations for dysplastic hips are excluded, nerve injury remains significantly more common in women than in men.[3, 53, 97, 130] Nerve injury is more likely in difficult reconstructions following pre-

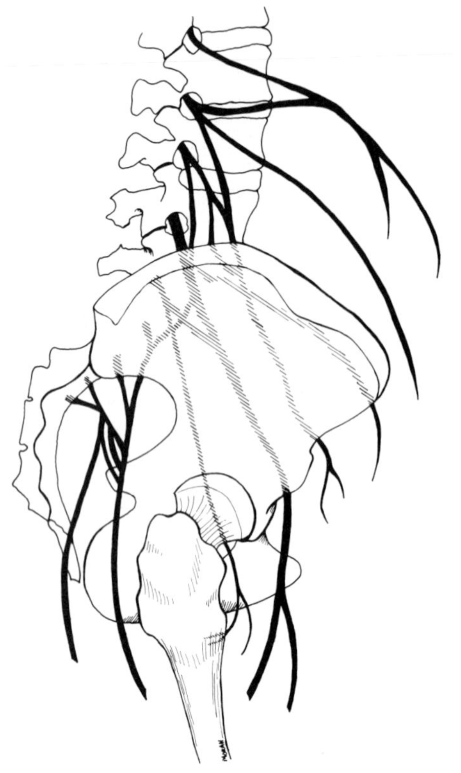

FIGURE 19–1. The relationship of the femoral, sciatic, and obturator nerves to the hip joint.

vious injuries or surgical procedures. The operating time and amount of blood lost are significantly greater in patients who develop neural injuries.[53]

Although neural injury may be clinically apparent, the more likely event is subclinical nerve injury that is detected by electromyographic study. In one series of hip replacements performed by an experienced surgeon through the transtrochanteric approach, 21 of 30 limbs had such evidence of nerve injury (six sciatic nerves, eight obturator nerves, one femoral nerve, five injuries to both the sciatic and obturator nerves, and one injury to both the sciatic and femoral nerves). No patient had symptoms of nerve injury, although slight muscle weakness was detected by careful examination in two patients.[130] This high incidence of subclinical nerve injury was not found in another similar study.[3] Subclinical nerve injuries may occur because of the flexion, adduction, and external rotation of the limb when the transtrochanteric approach is used. Clinically significant nerve palsies may occur with posterior, anterior, and transtrochanteric approaches.[3, 97]

In another study involving 50 patients, sciatic nerve function was assessed intraoperatively by somatosensory-evoked potential technique. Evidence of neural compromise was seen in 15 percent of primary cases and 36 percent of revision cases. Compromise was associated with acetabular retractors, reamer contact with the sciatic nerve, preparatory positioning of the femur, and reduction of an overlengthened femur.[118]

The causes of neural injury during operation include (1) stretching, (2) compression, (3) contusion, (4) thermal injury from bone cement, (5) laceration, and (6) vascular compromise. Postoperatively, nerves may be injured by dislocation of prosthetic components or compression by a hematoma, usually in association with anticoagulant therapy.[39] Stretching, the most common cause of nerve injury during total hip replacement, can be due to retraction or excessive lengthening of the limb. Direct compression of nerves usually occurs with placement of retractors (Fig. 19–2). Often the nerve is compressed between retractor and bone. An errant bolus of bone cement may injure a nerve by compression or by thermal injury. Compromise of the vascular supply is one mechanism of injury to nerves that are stretched or compressed. Both compression and stretch may occur in association with postoperative dislocation.

Prognosis is better for partial than for complete nerve injuries. Causalgia is a not uncommon complication of these neural injuries, persisting in some patients who have good return of muscle strength and sensation.

The following precautions can reduce the likelihood of nerve injuries:

1. Use careful retraction during the operation.
2. Expose and protect the sciatic nerve in difficult cases that involve previous injury or surgery but avoid overzealous retraction with a nerve tape.
3. Make certain the bone cement is contained. If the bone of the pelvis has been penetrated completely, place bone graft or other material to prevent the soft cement from exuding around a major nerve. The sciatic nerve may be injured

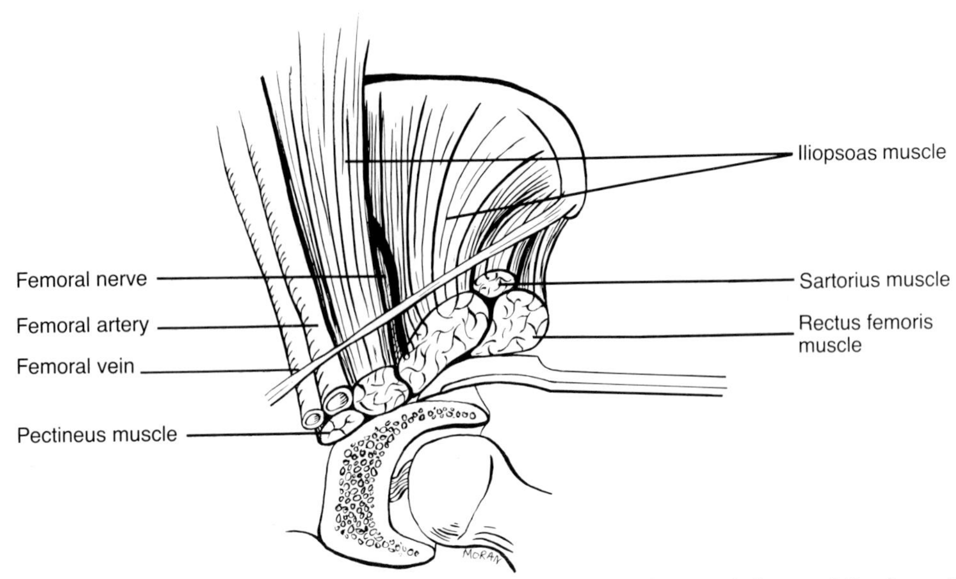

FIGURE 19–2. The relationship of the retractor placed anteriorly to the acetabulum and the femoral nerve and blood vessels.

by cement or the femoral stem when the femoral cortex is perforated. If femoral perforation occurs it must be repaired, and the stem and cement need to be contained within the canal.
4. Avoid overlengthening the limb.
5. Practice technically precise surgery, and to prevent direct injury, avoid blind cutting in the area of a nerve.
6. Maintain anticoagulant levels in the proper range.

The initial step in the treatment of clinically significant nerve injury is establishing an accurate diagnosis of the cause. When this step can be taken, treatment is directed toward removing the cause. As examples, a hematoma should be evacuated immediately and bone cement in the area of an injured nerve should be removed. If the limb has been lengthened and no other obvious cause of injury is found, the knee may be flexed to relieve stretch of the sciatic nerve. If knee flexion does not result in rapid improvement, or if injury is complete or severe, the best treatment may be closed dislocation of the hip to relieve traction on the nerve. A decision can then be made regarding revision of the reconstruction to lessen lengthening.

If the cause of the injury is not apparent, and especially if the paralysis is incomplete, the injury may be due to mild stretch or contusion from retraction during the operation. Recovery from a mild injury that consists of a transient conduction block may occur in days to weeks. But if the injury has been severe enough to cause axonal damage, recovery may not occur at all or may be incomplete after 1 or 2 years. Electromyographic studies are utilized to determine the prognosis and monitor the progress of those patients who do not recover in a short time.

Vascular Injury

Vascular injuries occur rarely in association with total hip replacement surgery. Series of at least several hundred hip replacements have been performed without vascular injury.[27] However, when vascular injuries do occur, as several small series and case reports reveal, the results may be devastating and include loss of the involved limb.[47, 88, 97]

Vascular injuries can be divided into those that are associated with acute intraoperative bleeding and those that become manifest sometime after surgery. Injuries may be caused by the following events during surgery:

1. Use of retractors, especially sharp, pointed ones that are placed blindly (see Fig. 19–2).

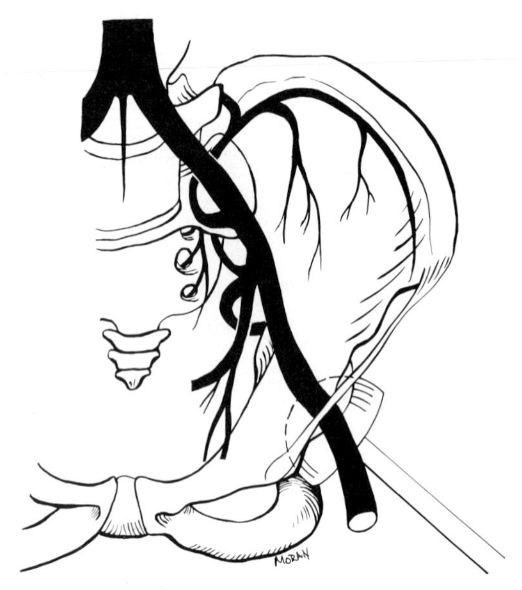

FIGURE 19–3. Proximity of the common iliac and femoral vessels to acetabulum.

2. Direct laceration with an osteotome, knife, or similar instrument.
3. Laceration by an osteophyte during joint manipulation.
4. Overreaming of the acetabulum, with direct injury by the reamer or, later, vessel erosion by the prosthesis (Fig. 19–3).
5. Vessel occlusion caused by the thermal effects of an errant cement bolus or, later, vessel erosion by direct contact with cement.
6. Use of drill bits to hold retractors.
7. Drilling for or placement of screws for uncemented acetabular components.
8. Tearing of the intima or vessel during manipulation of the extremity, which usually occurs in patients with scarring from previous surgery or injury or with severe atherosclerotic vessel disease.

Because vascular injury is more common in patients with previous surgery of the hip, it occurs more often during revision than during primary total hip arthroplasty. Similar to neural injury, vascular injury is more frequent in women than would be expected from the relative incidence of hip replacement operations in women and men. Vascular injury is more common with the anterior approach than with other approaches for total hip replacement, possibly because of retractor placement (see Fig. 19–2).

Prevention of vascular injuries requires careful surgical planning in difficult revision cases. Computerized tomography may be indicated to determine the relationship of neurovascular structures to prostheses, cements, or other implants that protrude into the pelvis.

The following precautions can help prevent vascular injuries:

1. When placing retractors adjacent to the acetabulum but inside the pelvis, position them against the bone.
2. Avoid the use of sharp or long, pointed retractors.
3. If either the acetabular wall or femur is perforated during reaming, repair the perforation prior to placement of the prosthesis.
4. Contain threads on acetabular components within bone to avoid soft tissue and vessel laceration.[103]
5. If an acetabular component is to be fixed with screws, drill meticulously, taking great care when the inner pelvic cortex is perforated. Screw fixation may be adequate without complete perforation of the inner pelvic cortex (see Chapter 17, *Total Hip Arthroplasty: Operative Technique*).
6. Observe precautions when drill bits or pins are used for self-retaining retractors.

Vascular injury may be recognized during surgery by the presence of a brisk uncontrollable bleeding or an unexplained drop in blood pressure. The injury must be accurately identified and repaired, which may require a separate incision, especially if the injured vessel is inside the pelvis. Occasionally, an injured vessel may be repaired directly but usually requires a graft. If the vessel is expendable, both ends should be ligated.

Symptoms of vascular compromise that may occur after hip replacement surgery include pain and coolness in the leg or foot. Arteriography is performed to diagnose and characterize the vascular defect. Four vascular complications may be considered as follows:

1. Thrombosis of a major vessel (Fig. 19–4)—the cause is the heat and pressure of bone cement or pressure of the prosthesis against the vessel.
2. False aneurysm—a small laceration in the wall of a large artery is followed by

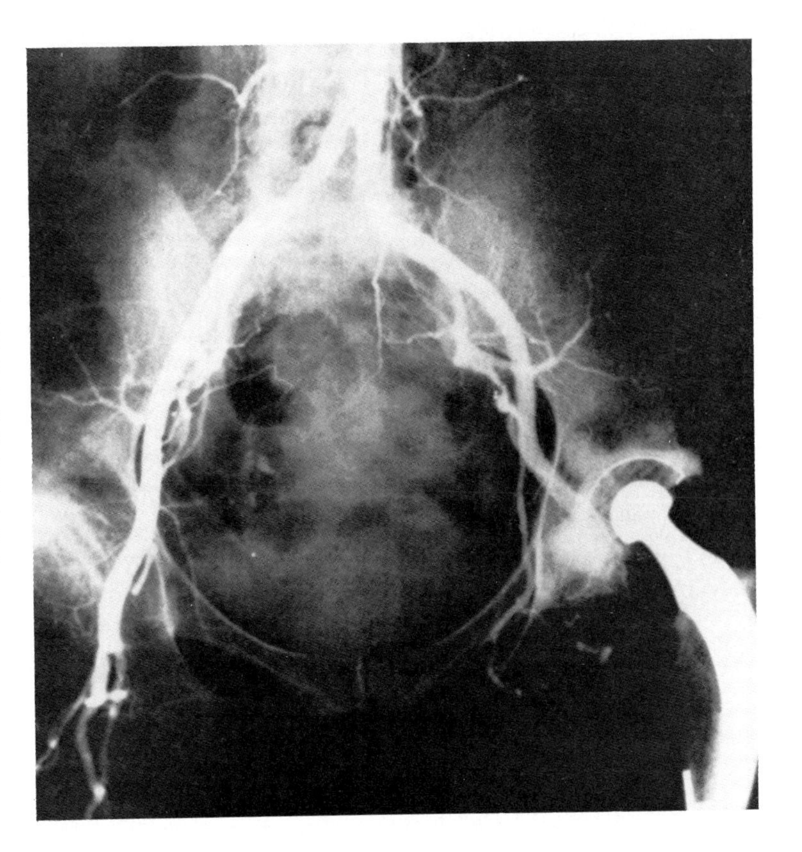

FIGURE 19–4. This patient had vascular compromise exhibited by a numb and cool foot and an absent femoral pulse 7 weeks after total hip arthroplasty. Arteriogram shows occlusion of the left common femoral artery. The patient was treated successfully by an endarterectomy and a vein patch. (Heyes, F.L.P. and Aukland, A. J. Bone Joint Surg. 67B: 533–535, 1985. By permission.)

the development of a laminated clot as blood continues to leak slowly into the surrounding tissues. A characteristic to-and-fro bruit is heard. Surgical treatment usually consists of ligation of the artery above and below the false aneurysm.

3. Arteriovenous fistula—after injury to an adjacent artery and vein, an arteriovenous fistula develops. The constant flow of blood from artery to vein causes a continuous machine-like murmur. The fistula can be treated in most cases by ligation of the vessels.

4. Interruption of critical collateral circulation. Vascular compromise in this case is probably a result of extensive manipulation and stretching of atherosclerotic vessels, which may cause intimal damage. Vascular supply usually can be improved with a bypass graft, but sometimes medical management or sympathectomy is the treatment of choice.[10, 47, 78, 85, 88, 97]

Fractures

Fractures associated with total hip replacements may occur in the prosthesis or in the bone. Fractures of prostheses are

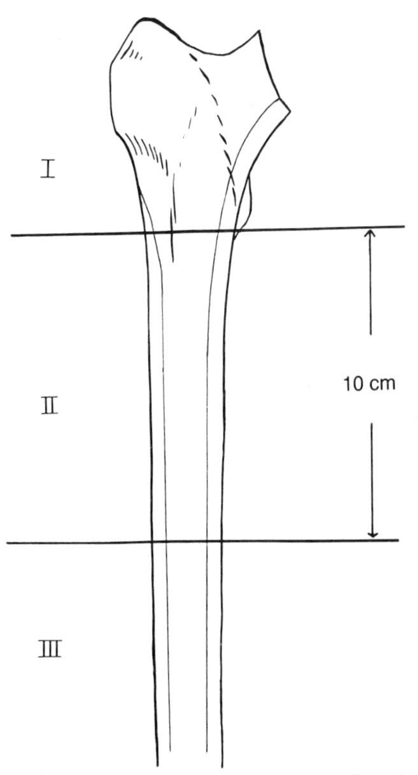

FIGURE 19–5. Fracture levels associated with total hip arthroplasty.

discussed in Chapter 23, *Revision Total Hip Arthroplasty*. Fractures of bone may occur preoperatively, intraoperatively, or postoperatively. Those occurring after surgery may or may not be associated with significant trauma. Fractures can be classified according to the following levels (Fig. 19–5) and types:[25]

Type I	Fracture that is proximal to the intertrochanteric line (level I) (Fig. 19–6A).
Type II	Vertical or spiral split that does not extend past the lower extent of the lesser trochanter (level I) (Fig. 19–6B).
Type III	Vertical or spiral split that extends past the lower extent of the lesser trochanter but not past the junction of the middle and distal third of the femoral stem (level II) (Fig. 19–6C).
Type IV	Fracture that traverses or lies in the area of the femoral stem tip (level III): Type IV A, spiral (Fig. 16–6D), and type IV B, transverse or short oblique (Fig. 19–6E).
Type V	Severely comminuted fracture between the lower extent of the lesser trochanter and the area of the stem tip (level III) (severely comminuted type III or IV) (Fig. 19–6F).
Type VI	Fracture that is distal to the area of the prosthesis (level III) (Fig. 19–6G).

Intraoperative Fractures

Intraoperative fractures have become more familiar to surgeons with the increased use of press-fit fixation for the femoral component of a total hip replacement.[32, 52, 56, 109, 128] In one series of reported intraoperative femoral fractures, the overall incidence in all press-fit cases was 6.3 percent, with a 7.2 percent incidence in revisions and 2.5 percent incidence in primary arthroplasties.[38] Intraoperative fractures also occur during cemented arthroplasty but less commonly. In one series, the incidence was estimated to be 0.4 percent.[54]

Because the stability of a press-fit prosthesis depends on close apposition between prosthesis and bone, the largest femoral stem that the bone will accept is chosen. Even with accurate preoperative templating, this practice sometimes leads to femoral fracture during broaching of the femoral canal. In systems in which the broach is slightly undersized relative to the prosthesis to provide a tight fit, fracture may occur during insertion of the prosthesis.

Fractures are most likely to occur in the following circumstances:

1. Presence of stress risers in some areas resulting from holes left by internal fixation devices or, in revision cases, from removal of bone cement or defects created by a loose prosthesis.
2. Presence of developmental or acquired bone deformity.
3. Soft tissue contractures that are not adequately released prior to dislocation or other manipulation.
4. Insertion of a broach or prosthesis that is too large for the femur.
5. Presence of weak bone due to osteoporosis or a less common condition, such as Gaucher disease.

Certain techniques can minimize the likelihood of fractures associated with stress risers as follows:

1. The stress riser is spanned completely by the prosthetic stem, and the stem extends a distance equal to two bone diameters beyond the stress riser.
2. The defect is bone grafted.
3. A circumferential wire is placed whenever any indication is given of fracture propagation from a stress riser.
4. Postoperative protection is provided by walking aids, casts, braces, or a combination of these devices.

Careful preoperative planning is especially important if the patient has substantial bone deformity, whether congenital, developmental, or acquired. It is helpful to draw the proposed reconstruction on the

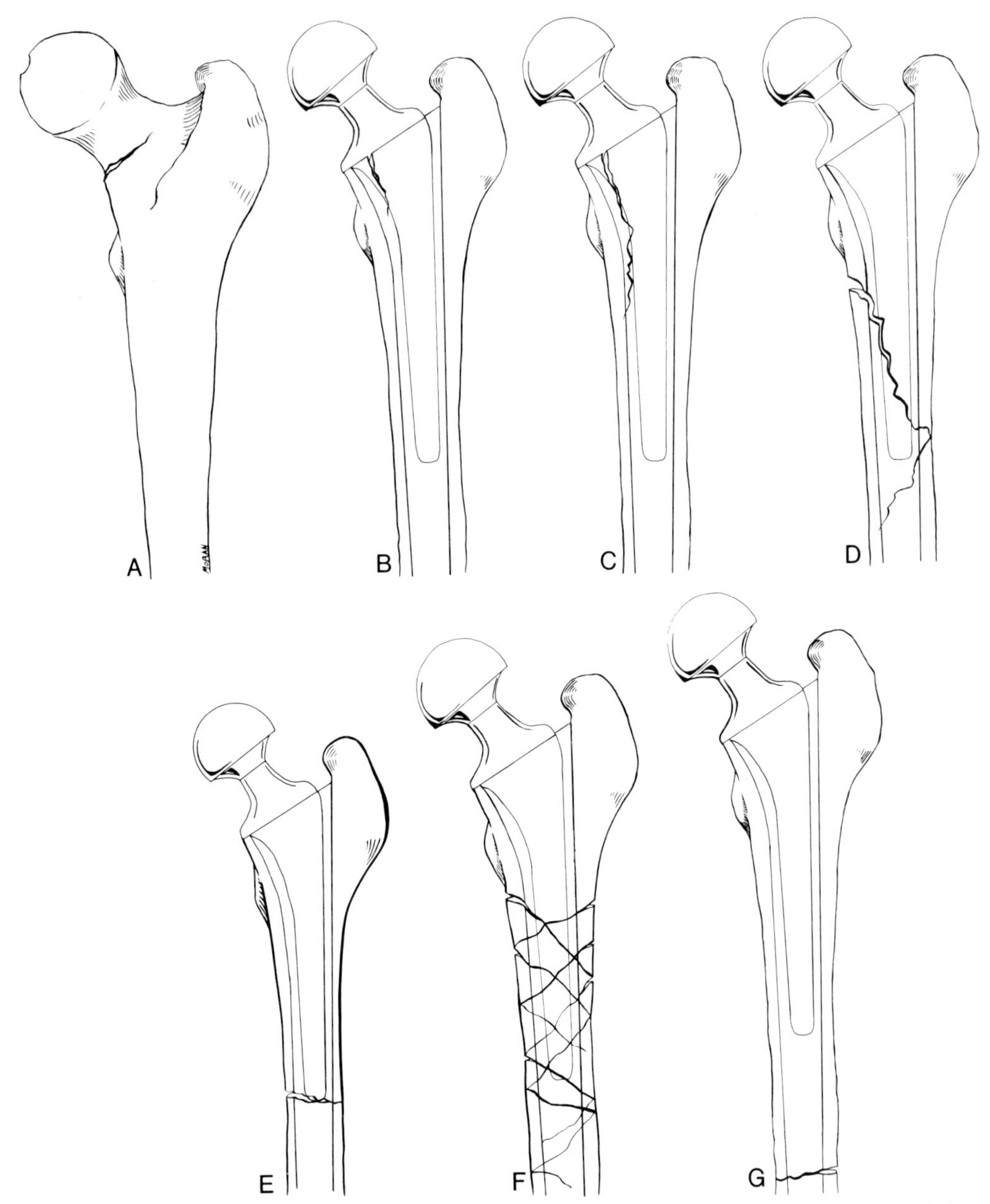

FIGURE 19–6. Classification of fracture types associated with total hip arthroplasty. *A,* Type I fracture proximal to the intertrochanteric line. *B,* Type II vertical or spiral split fracture does not extend past the lower extent of the lesser trochanter. *C,* Type III spiral or split fracture extends into level II. *D,* IV A spiral fracture involves the area of the stem tip. *E,* Type IV B transverse or short oblique fracture involves the area of the stem tip. *F,* Type V comminuted fracture. *G,* Type VI fracture below the prosthesis.

preoperative radiograph. Computerized tomography improves evaluation of the bone morphometry in difficult cases. The surgeon should plan for the most appropriate size and type of prosthesis. For example, it may be difficult to insert a curved prosthesis in the congenitally dislocated hip after the proximal femur has been resected to the level necessary for safe reduction.

Although soft tissue release must be adequate before dislocation is attempted in any hip, this maneuver is especially important when contractures are severe and bone is weak. The accuracy of preoperative templating may be enhanced by a measurement marker when the preoperative radiograph is taken, but sizing of the prosthesis by preoperative templating should always be considered no more than an estimate. The size of the broach and prosthesis that will fit the femur is not decided firmly until during the operation. In those systems that involve intramedullary reaming, overreaming by about 1 mm may be helpful when the fit is especially tight or a longer stem is being inserted (see Chapter 23, *Revision Total Hip Arthroplasty*).[36, 38, 54, 79, 110]

Intraoperative Fractures

Fractures proximal to the intertrochanteric line (type I) may occur when a dislocation is difficult or when an osteotome rather than a saw is employed for osteotomy of the femoral neck. The only change in the operative procedure that might be necessary is appropriate revision of the neck osteotomy and the selection of a prosthesis with a longer neck.

Vertical or spiral split fractures occur during broaching or prosthesis insertion. If they do not extend below the distal extent of the lesser trochanter (type II), they usually do not require special treatment, except perhaps for additional restriction on weightbearing during the first few weeks after surgery. However, if a type II fracture threatens greater trochanter detachment, a screw or wire placed across the fracture will protect the integrity of the greater trochanter until the fracture has healed. All fractures that appear to be limited to the area above the distal border of the lesser trochanter must be inspected carefully to be certain they do not extend further distally.

Type III fractures—those vertical or spiral fractures that extend beyond the lesser trochanter but not beyond the junction of the middle and distal third of the femoral stem—also usually occur during broach or stem insertion. The best treatment usually is placement of one to three circumferential wires to hold the fracture line together and to resist hoop stresses generated by the prosthesis.

Spiral fractures that traverse the stem tip (type IV A) are similar to type III fractures, but they often will not be sufficiently stable if treated only with circumferential wiring. These fractures often can be converted to type III fractures by placing a longer stem and then using circumferential wiring. If this maneuver is not possible, circumferential wiring and postoperative cast immobilization may be effective. Another alternative is an Ogden plate, which is designed for fixation with both screws in the bone distal to the prosthesis and heavy-duty Parham bands where the prosthesis fills the canal (Fig. 19–7).[83, 133]

Transverse or short oblique fractures (type IV B) probably are more common postoperatively than intraoperatively. They usually are associated with a stress riser near the stem tip. These fractures are often difficult to manage, because they may be very unstable. Type IV B fractures that occur intraoperatively are best treated by placement of a longer stem prosthesis, if this provides stability, or by an Ogden plate.

Severely comminuted fractures below the lesser trochanter (type V) are the most difficult to manage, especially when they also traverse the area of the stem tip. Management may be less difficult with placement of a longer stem that extends beyond the lower edge of the fracture. The multiple fracture fragments may be fixed with circumferential wires, screws, or both. In the area of the prosthesis, screws must be small, and they must be carefully placed to avoid the prosthesis. An Ogden plate may be helpful, especially when the fracture lines are concentrated below the stem. Onlay cortical allograft bone plates have been utilized successfully in the treatment of fractures occurring primarily below the stem.[92]

Type VI fractures—those occurring completely distal to the femoral stem—may be

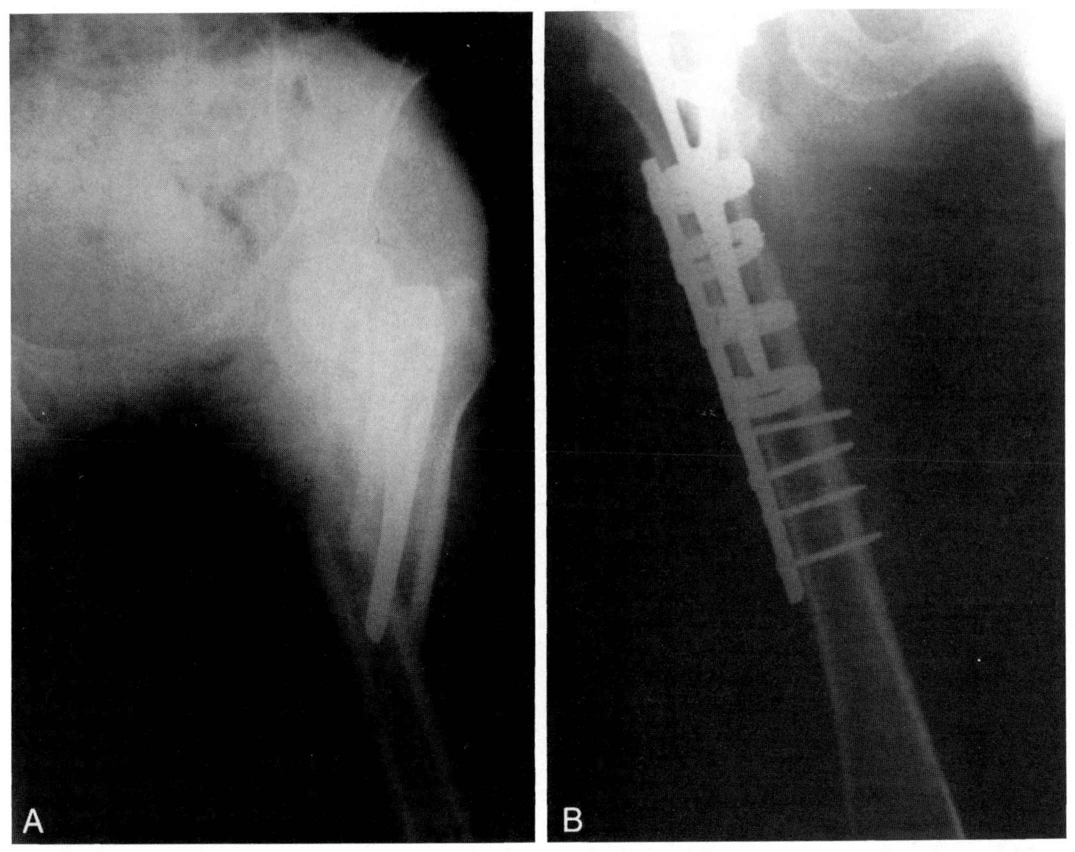

FIGURE 19–7. *A,* Fracture occurring in association with press-fit prosthesis. *B,* Stabilized with an Ogden plate.

amenable to standard fracture treatment, with or without open operation. A supracondylar fracture, for example, can be fixed with a blade plate or similar device, or it may be treated with traction, cast bracing, or both.[12] Obviously, standard intramedullary fixation cannot be done, although Ender and Kuntscher nailing has been applied successfully in the treatment of fractures at the distal tip of an uncemented endoprosthesis. The nails were passed adjacent to the prosthesis; therefore, this technique could not be employed when a prosthesis fills the canal almost completely, even if it is not cemented.[15, 93]

Cancellous bone grafting may allow for more rapid healing of complex fractures and may be advantageous for stress risers. Immobilization in the form of traction, a cast, or a brace may supplement the intraoperative fixation if the stability of a complex fracture, especially type IV or V, is in doubt.[36, 38, 50, 54, 76, 110]

The reported incidence of perforation of the femur with the stem during total hip arthroplasty is 0 to 4.4 percent. Despite isolated reports of satisfactory results when this complication is not discovered until after surgery, in general the results are poor (Fig. 19–8). These results are not unexpected, because a femoral stem protruding through a hole in the femoral shaft is in a mechanically unsound position, and the bone is weakened by the perforation.[124] Perforation of the femoral cortex must be discovered during the operation if this complication is to be managed properly. As a precaution, the endosteal surface of the femur should be palpated with a curved instrument after initial entry into the canal or after reaming and broaching to be certain that no perforation has occurred. This precaution is especially important in patients who have predisposing factors for this complication, such as previous hip surgery, hip dysplasia, and osteoporosis. If

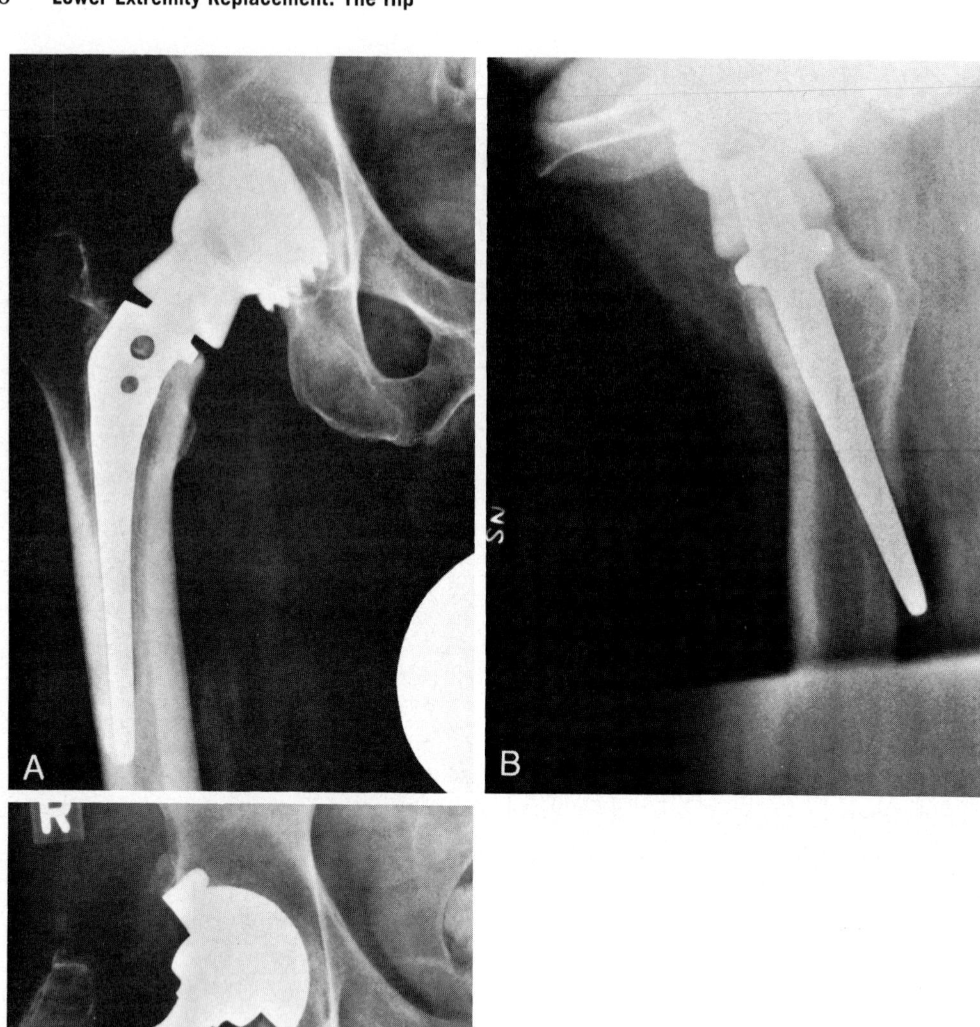

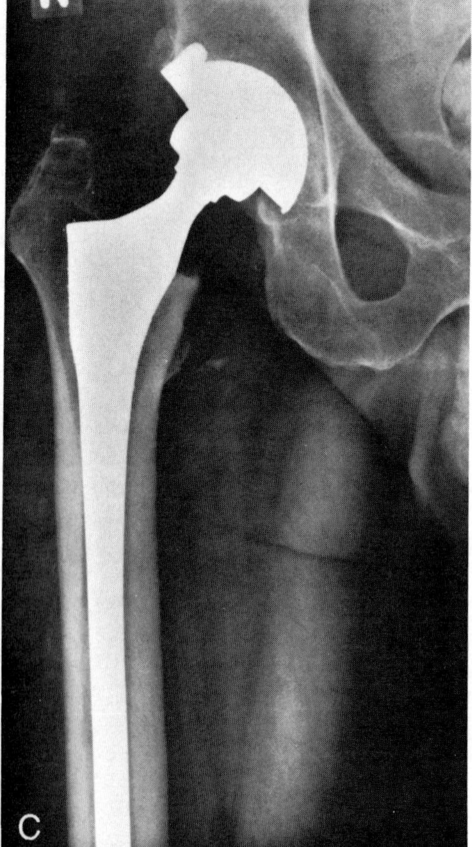

FIGURE 19–8. Inadvertent femoral perforation discovered several weeks postoperatively. *A,* Femoral perforation was not diagnosed on anteroposterior radiograph. *B,* Perforation is obvious on lateral radiograph taken several weeks later. *C,* The patient required revision because of associated loosening and pain.

perforation is discovered, the canal is entered and prepared properly. The defect should be occluded during installation of the cement, if used, and prosthesis. In most cases, the perforation is bone grafted.[124]

Postoperative Fractures

Type I fractures, i.e., those proximal to the intertrochanteric line, will not be seen after total hip replacement, of course. Type II fractures will not be seen as such, although it is theoretically possible for a type II fracture to become more severe if the extremity is exposed to excessive loads or significant trauma shortly after surgery. Other types of fractures can occur postoperatively.

The incidence of fractures after total hip replacement has been reported as 0.1 percent. These fractures occur within a few days of operation to many years after hip replacement.[12, 26, 62, 81, 110] Fractures occurring within days to weeks after surgery often represent unrecognized intraoperative fractures that were completed postoperatively or that developed from unprotected stress risers in the bone. Additional load on a femur that already is under high hoop stress due to a tight press-fit prosthesis might also lead to early fracture. Some late fractures after hip replacements are related to severe trauma, whereas others are related to loose prostheses and deficient bone quality.

When a fracture occurs postoperatively, the surgeon must choose between open and closed treatment. All postoperative fractures have a relatively high incidence of union when treated with a combination of traction and cast or brace. However, with types III, IV A, and V, later symptomatic loosening of the prosthesis may require revision. Early operation to repair the fracture and revise the prosthesis is a formidable procedure and usually is done in an elderly patient, but malunion and later loosening also require an extensive revision operation. If the surgeon elects to treat these fractures by closed means, the reduction should be as anatomic as possible so that later revision arthroplasty will not be more difficult. Type IV B fractures are not as likely to be associated with later loosening of the prosthesis, but both nonunion and malunion are more likely when treatment is by closed means. Fractures of the femur distal to the area of the prosthesis (type VI) can be treated by standard closed or open means without increased risk of later loosening of the prosthesis.[2, 12, 26, 50, 79, 81, 99] For postoperative fractures that are treated by open methods, the general principles previously discussed regarding intraoperative fractures apply. These methods are discussed further in Chapter 23, *Revision Total Hip Arthroplasty*.

Nondisplaced stress fractures may occur in areas of stress risers remaining after total hip arthroplasty. The pain is gradual rather than sudden in onset. Radionuclide bone scans or tomograms may be necessary to make the diagnosis. These fractures may heal with immobilization; if not, they may be bone grafted *in situ* (Fig. 19–9).[73]

Fatigue Fracture of the Pelvis

Fatigue fracture of the pelvis is an unusual complication following total hip arthroplasty, occurring in two of 5400 arthroplasties in one report. These fractures appear with a variable degree of groin pain, which may be severe enough to preclude weightbearing. Similar to other stress fractures, pelvic fatigue fractures may not be visible on initial radiographs. These fractures may be more likely in patients with rheumatoid arthritis or osteoporosis.

The location of pain in the groin may raise the concern of infection, but sedimentation rate and white blood cell count will be normal. Also, the aspirate findings will be negative for bacteria. Radionuclide scan is helpful in making the diagnosis.

Treatment consists of rest and supported weightbearing. The prognosis for healing and resolution of symptoms is good.[24, 29, 42, 63, 91, 111]

Limb Length Inequality

Both patient and surgeon would like total hip replacement to achieve equal limb length. This goal is not always possible because of preexisting shortening of the soft tissues, especially if the shortening developed during growth. Attempts to achieve lengthening in this situation may result in neurovascular injury (see *Neural Injury* and *Vascular Injury*). If the surgeon

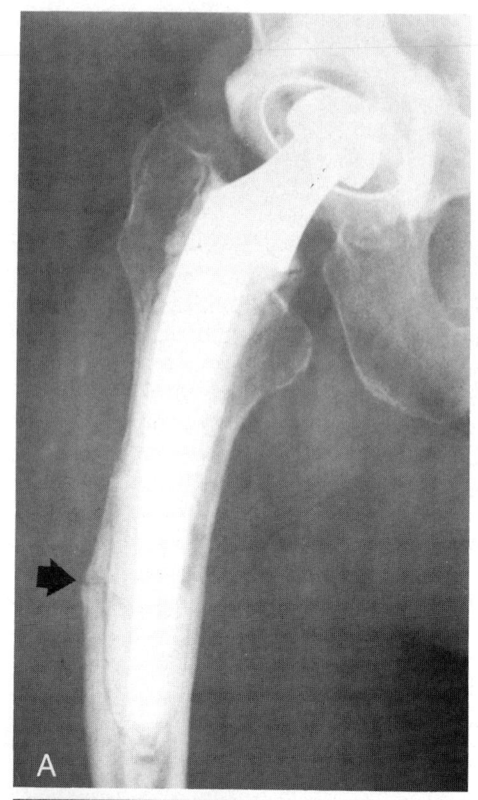

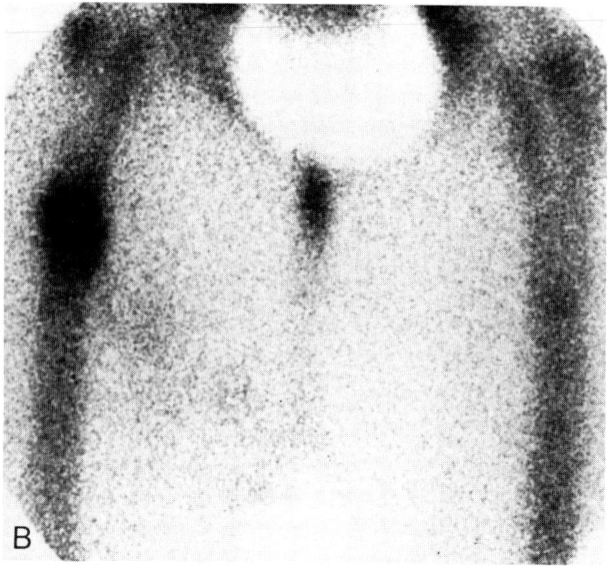

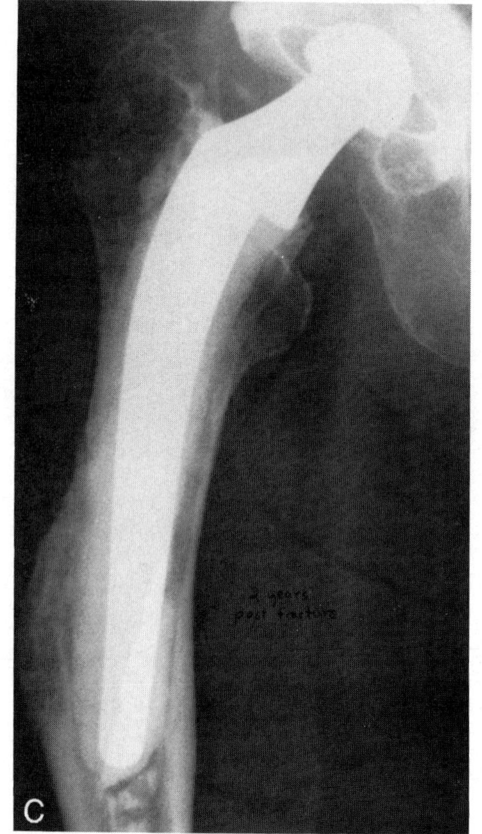

FIGURE 19–9. Fatigue fracture after total hip arthroplasty. *A,* Defect in the lateral cortex on the radiograph of a patient with thigh pain. *B,* Increased uptake on radionuclide bone scan. *C,* The appearance of healed fracture 2 years later. (Lotke, P.A., Wong, R.Y., and Ecker, M.L.: Clin. Orthop. 206:147–150, 1986. By permission.

explains why it will not be possible to achieve limb length equality, the patient is not likely to complain of limb length inequality.

However, patients are likely to be bothered by overlengthening of more than a few millimeters.[21] Whereas appropriate length should be restored to achieve stability, marked overlengthening can have catastrophic consequences due to neural or vascular injury. Even if such injuries are avoided, overlengthening by 2 cm or more can result in poor function due to flexion or abduction contracture, or both. These problems can be avoided by accurate length reconstruction measurements (see Chapter 17, *Total Hip Arthroplasty: Operative Technique*).

HETEROTOPIC OSSIFICATION

The etiology of heterotopic bone formation is unknown, although it probably involves a traumatic stimulus to the mesenchymal cells, resulting in their transformation to osteoblasts. Heterotopic ossification following total hip replacement seems related to myositis ossificans, or bone formation in muscle following trauma, but it differs from this condition in that after hip replacement not only muscle but also capsular tissues are involved.

The reported incidence of heterotopic bone formation after total hip arthroplasty ranges from 8 to 90 percent of cases. The incidence of functionally significant bone formation is much lower, ranging from 1 to 24 percent.[4, 16, 90, 94, 104, 112, 113] This complication may be seen more often in men than in women, in patients with hypertrophic osteoarthritis, and in patients with spinal hyperostosis and post-traumatic arthritis.[13, 33, 35, 45, 94, 112, 113] Heterotopic ossification may occur more commonly in patients with either juvenile or adult ankylosing spondylitis. Human leukocyte antigen B5 is found with increased frequency in patients with ectopic ossification.[41] The incidence of heterotopic bone formation is lower following total hip replacement for osteonecrosis than for other reasons.[101] Longer operative times are associated with increased heterotopic bone formation.[112] The incidence of this complication is higher with the anterior approach of Smith-Petersen and the lateral approach of McFarland and to a lesser extent with the transtrochanteric approach. A patient who develops heterotopic bone formation after previous hip surgery is almost certain to develop it with subsequent surgery on the same or the opposite hip.[94, 113, 121] The degree of ossification is likely to be more severe with recurrence in the same joint.[89, 94]

The amount of ossification is graded by Schmidt and colleagues as follows: *Grade 0*: No formation of heterotopic bone. *Grade I*: Formation of heterotopic bone occupying less than 50 percent of the distance between the femur and pelvis. *Grade II*: Formation of heterotopic bone occupying more than 50 percent of the distance between the femur and the pelvis but not bridging it (Fig. 19–10). *Grade III*: Formation of bridging heterotopic bone (Figs. 19–10 and 19–11).[107]

The classification of Schmidt[107] will be used in the following discussion. Another popular classification system is that described by Brooker and colleagues[16] (Table 19–1).

Some patients complain of pain, while the heterotopic bone is forming, as well as warmth about the hip. They occasionally have low-grade fevers. In a patient who has these symptoms 2 to 3 weeks after surgery, a radiograph may show the early wispy bone formation. A bone scan will reveal marked uptake. When these signs occur, it is too late for preventive measures to be effective. The best course is to allow the patient activity that is comfortable. Motion should not be forced; it will not be helpful, and it may increase the bone formation. Occasionally, patients with heterotopic bone formation will continue to have pain but most will not.

Patients who develop heterotopic bone extensively enough for it to be classified as grade II and especially grade III may have a significant decrease in range of motion. Limited motion in a poor position may aggravate problems in the lumbar spine, contralateral hip, or ipsilateral knee. Abduction strength is decreased in a patient with heterotopic bone but not enough to cause an abductor limp. Heterotopic bone formation has no adverse effect on strength of other muscle groups about the hip.[4]

Because ossification that falls into grade

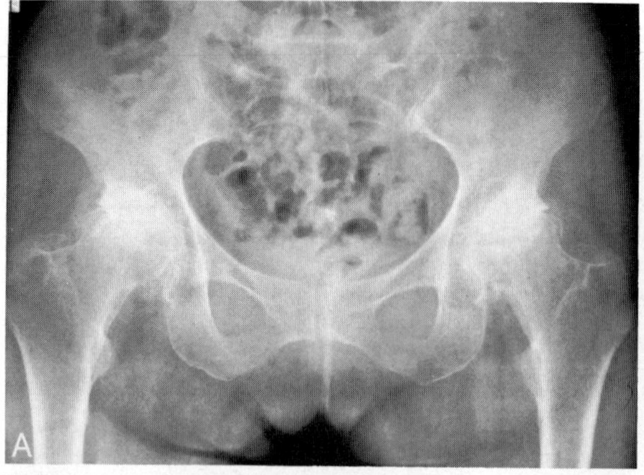

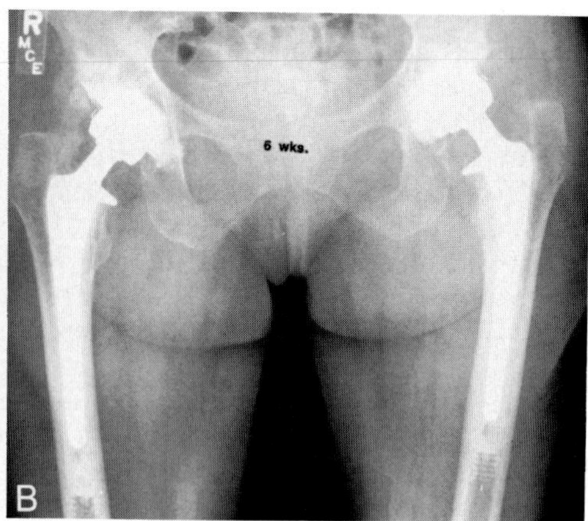

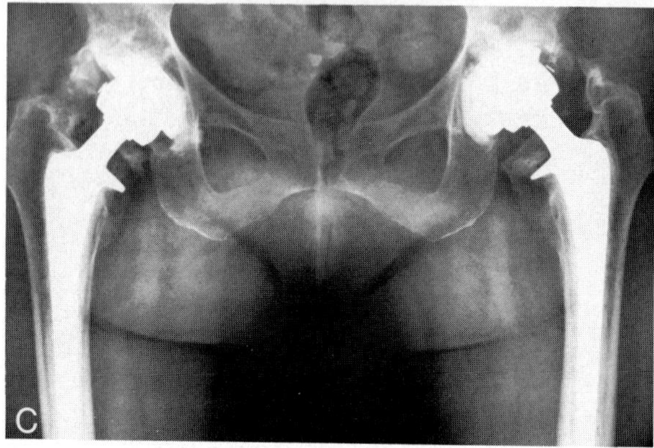

FIGURE 19–10. Development of heterotopic bone following total hip arthroplasty. *A,* Preoperative radiograph shows severe osteoarthritis bilaterally. *B,* At 8 weeks after total hip arthroplasty on the right and 6 weeks after surgery on the left early heterotopic bone is seen on both sides. The bone formation is more evident on the right. *C,* At 1 year postoperatively, grade II (Brooker grade III) heterotopic bone is seen on the left and grade III (Brooker grade IV) on the right. Although the patient has no pain, her function is poor.

I causes no decrease in range of motion or other functional problems, no treatment is indicated. Greater amounts of ossification may cause the total hip replacement to have a poorer outcome than either the surgeon or the patient expected. Patients with severe bilateral bone formations may be severely disabled. Therefore, measures to prevent heterotopic ossification may be indicated, at least in high-risk patients. The following may be candidates for preventive treatment:

1. Patients who have had previous hip surgery or trauma, especially those who had previous heterotopic bone formation to any degree.
2. Patients who underwent prolonged, difficult operations.
3. Patients who have hypertrophic osteoarthritis.
4. Patients who have ankylosing spondylitis.
5. Patients who had heterotopic bone formation after trauma or surgery in another site. Because it is impossible to predict accurately which patients will develop heterotopic bone sufficient to limit function, preventive treatment with indomethacin may be considered for those having total hip replacements.

Treatments that have been evaluated in the prevention of heterotopic bone formation following total hip replacement include diphosphonate, nonsteroidal anti-inflammatory agents, and radiation therapy.

Table 19–1. GRADING SYSTEM FOR POSTOPERATIVE HETEROTOPIC BONE FORMATION

Grade	Formation
Class I	Islands of bone within the soft tissues about the hip
Class II	Bone spurs from the pelvis or proximal end of the femur leaving at least 1 cm between opposing bone surfaces
Class III	Bone spurs from the pelvis or proximal end of the femur reducing the space between opposing bone surfaces to less than 1 cm
Class IV	Apparent bone ankylosis of the hip

Modified from Brooker, A. F., Bowerman, J. W., Robinson, R. A., and Riley, L. H., Jr.: J. Bone Joint Surg. 55A:1629–1632, 1973.

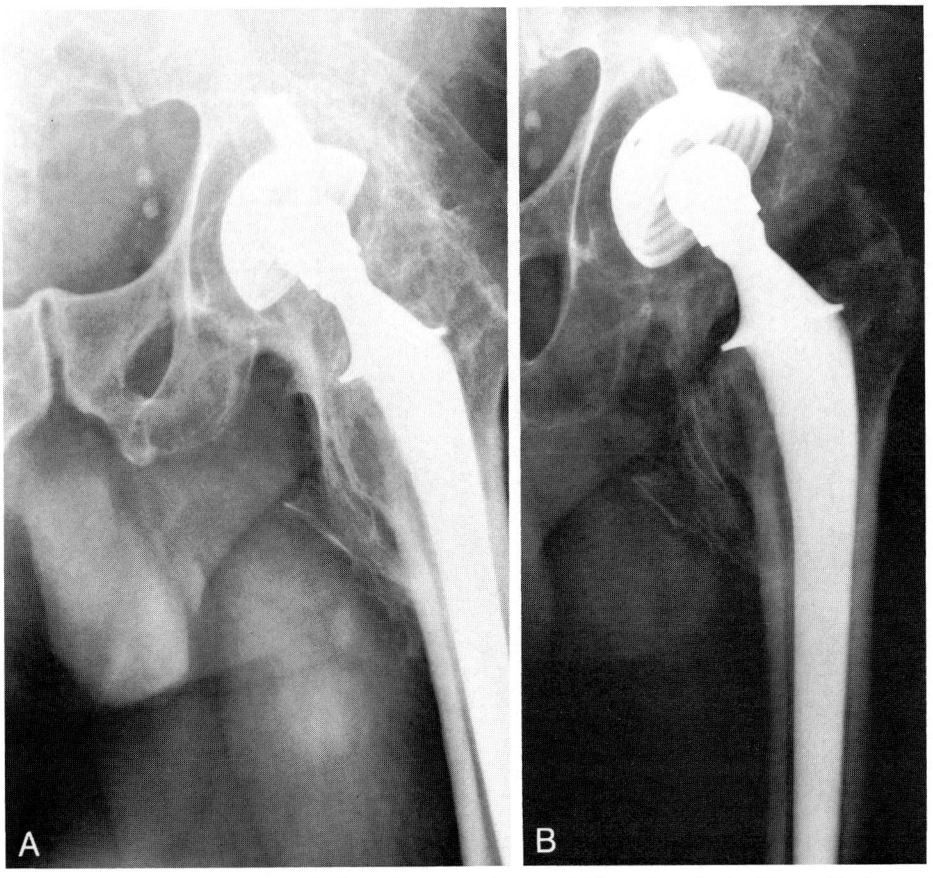

FIGURE 19–11. *A*, Massive heterotopic bone 2 years after total hip arthroplasty. The patient was treated with partial excision of bone and 1000 Gy. Flexion postoperatively was from 0 to 70 degrees.

Ethylhydroxydiphosphonate inhibits transformation of amorphous calcium phosphate into hydroxyapatite, thus inhibiting the mineralization of osteoid matrix. However, diphosphonate is not indicated in the prevention or treatment of heterotopic bone associated with total hip arthroplasty.[18, 37, 89, 125] Because diphosphonate has no effect on the formation of osteoid matrix, when the medication is discontinued the osteoid that formed during its administration will mineralize rapidly. Clinical evaluation has corroborated the lack of effectiveness of diphosphonate. The only effect seems to be a delay in the radiographic appearance of heterotopic bone. Long-term administration of diphosphonate results in osteomalacia and stress fractures.[18, 37, 89, 125]

Nonsteroidal anti-inflammatory agents that inhibit prostaglandin synthesis have, in addition to their anti-inflammatory effect, an inhibitory effect on local bone remodeling and repair of bone after trauma.[5, 120] Because of this effect, indomethacin and to a lesser extent ibuprofen have been given to retard the development of heterotopic bone.[6, 59, 66, 100, 102, 114] Indomethacin prevents or diminishes the recurrence of severe ossification after excision. Several investigators have reported no high-grade recurrence of excised heterotopic bone when indomethacin was taken.[59, 66, 100, 127] In a randomized, double-blind clinical trial, the incidence of ossification in patients having total hip replacements who received indomethacin was 13 percent (all grade I), whereas ossification developed in 73 percent of patients who received placebo (18 percent of cases grade III) (Table 19–2). The incidence of ossification in the soft tissues in the control group may have been high because no anti-inflammatory medications were permitted.[107] Knahr and colleagues[60] demon-

Table 19–2. COMPARISON OF THE RESULTS IN THE INDOMETHACIN TRIAL

Treatment	Total (No. of Patients)	Age (Yrs)		Diagnosis (No. of Patients)				Development of Osteophytes (No. of Patients)		Grade of Heterotopic Ossification (No. of Patients)				
		Mean	*Range*	*Osteo-arthritis*	*Avascular Necrosis*	*Revision Arthroplasty*	*Misc.*	*>10 mm*	*<10 mm*	*0*	*I*	*II*	*III*	*I–III*
Indomethacin	102	67	40–89	89	3	7	3	36	53	89	13	0	0	13
Placebo	99	68	28–87	86	5	5	3	33	53	27	24	30	18	72

Schmidt, A. S., Kjaersgaard-Andersen, P., Pedersen, N. W., et al: J. Bone Joint Surg. 70A:834–838, 1988. By permission.

strated a reduced incidence of heterotopic bone formation when anti-inflammatory medication was given to prevent thrombosis or for some other purpose. The dose of indomethacin usually has been 25 mg three times daily for 3, 6, or 12 weeks. Treatment for 6 weeks is effective and may result in fewer side effects than administration of the drug for a longer time.[107] Patients may have to discontinue indomethacin because of dyspepsia, although in one study this side effect was no more common with indomethacin than with placebo.[6]

Low-dose radiation therapy has been administered successfully to prevent heterotopic bone formation in high-risk patients who are having hip replacements and in those who have undergone excisions of massive amounts of heterotopic bone that developed after hip replacements. Ionizing radiation alters deoxyribonucleic acid in the cell nucleus. Its greatest effect therefore is on rapidly dividing cells, and this radiation may prevent the differentiation of mesenchymal cells into osteoblasts. In the early application of radiation therapy to prevent ectopic bone formation, a total of 2000 rads was administered. A total dose of 1000 rads (200 rads daily for 5 days) has since been found to be effective. Radiation therapy must begin within 4 days of surgery, preferably within 24 hours of the operation. In other studies, a single dose of 600 rads was given within 3 days of surgery to 17 patients at high risk for heterotopic bone formation, including 6 patients who had excision of previously formed heterotopic bone, and no patient developed heterotopic bone more severe than Brooker class I (scattered islands of bone).[8, 17, 28, 46, 123] A possible side effect of ionizing radiation is radiation-induced sarcoma, but this complication has not been found to develop with doses less than 3000 rads.[14, 57] Although radiation may slow tissue healing, wound healing problems have not been evident.[8, 28, 123]

Excision of heterotopic bone combined with adjunctive treatment may be indicated in those patients who have substantial loss of motion due to bone formation, especially when the loss of motion causes severe flexion or other contracture. Without this treatment, the total hip replacement may be a failure. Surgical excision of massive heterotopic bone is an extensive procedure. Blood loss may be substantial because of exposure of the large surface area of cancellous bone. The bone often has either partially or completely replaced the joint capsule and muscles surrounding the hip joint. Muscle replacement is especially common in the abductors, and care must be taken to preserve whatever muscle tissue remains. Excision alone will result in recurrence of bone in the soft tissues, often to a worse extent; therefore, adjunctive treatment with either radiation or indomethacin is indicated to prevent or diminish recurrence. A few patients have had successful excisions of heterotopic bone and prevention of recurrences by autologous free-fat interposition, but this method has not been studied thoroughly.[1, 98]

The measures to prevent heterotopic bone formation are administered systemically, in the case of prostaglandin-inhibiting medications, or are delivered to the proximal femur and acetabular region, in the case of radiation therapy. These treatments may interfere with tissue ingrowth into porous surfaces of press-fit prostheses. This issue has not been studied in depth, but it is not unanticipated that methods to retard the development of heterotopic bone will also retard bone ingrowth into porous implants. Bone formation in heterotopic bone, fracture healing, and ingrowth into prostheses is similar.[5, 120] One report indicated that ethylhydroxydiphosphonate markedly inhibits bone ingrowth into porous surfaces.[44] Radiation therapy retarded bone ingrowth temporarily, but ultimately ingrowth was unaffected. Indomethacin had no effect on bone ingrowth in one animal model,[44] but in another study in rabbits indomethacin was found to retard bone ingrowth into porous implants.[127] The deleterious effect was exhibited by failure of early ingrowth to increase and penetrate the deeper portions of the porous structure. The bone was more lamellar in structure compared with the bone in controls, which showed more cortical structure.[127] In a further investigation, indomethacin, ibuprofen, and aspirin in doses similar to those administered clinically were found to significantly retard bone ingrowth into porous chromium-cobalt implants in the rabbit, with higher doses causing more retardation of bone ingrowth than lower doses.[127]

DISLOCATION

Dislocation of the femoral head from the socket occurs in 0.4 to 8 percent of primary total hip arthroplasties.[11, 22, 27, 31, 64] The complication is more common after revision arthroplasty and in difficult primary cases, such as joint replacements for congenitally dislocated hips. In such circumstances, dislocations have occurred in up to 16 percent of cases.[132] Dislocation may be more common in patients who are mentally disoriented, who drink large quantities of alcohol, and who have diseases causing muscle incoordination, as well as those who underwent arthroplasty performed by a relatively inexperienced surgeon. Only rarely is dislocation after total hip replacement associated with significant trauma. Up to 40 percent of dislocations may recur.[30, 34, 65] Many reports have compared the dislocation rates with different surgical approaches, and although some favor one approach over others, overall the approach does not appear to be an important factor in determining the incidence of dislocation.

Dislocations may be classified according to cause as follows: *Type I*: Positional. *Type II*: Soft tissue imbalance. *Type III*: Component malposition. In type I dislocations, the components are positioned correctly and the soft tissues are well balanced, but the patient puts the hip into a position that is beyond the range that is possible with the prosthetic components. As a result, the femoral head disengages from the socket.

Evaluation

Soft tissues imbalance and component malposition can be determined by evaluation of radiographs of the pelvis and hip (Fig. 19–12).[34] Both preoperative and postoperative radiographs are evaluated. If the operated hip had considerable deformity before surgery and the opposite hip is more normal, evaluation of the opposite hip may be useful as well.

Soft Tissue Imbalance

Shortening in either the vertical or horizontal direction causes soft tissue imbalance, possibly resulting in dislocation. The following guidelines may help in the evaluation of the soft tissue balance on radiographs and in the planning of the hip reconstruction.

On the radiograph (see Fig. 19–12), the center of rotation of the femoral head is

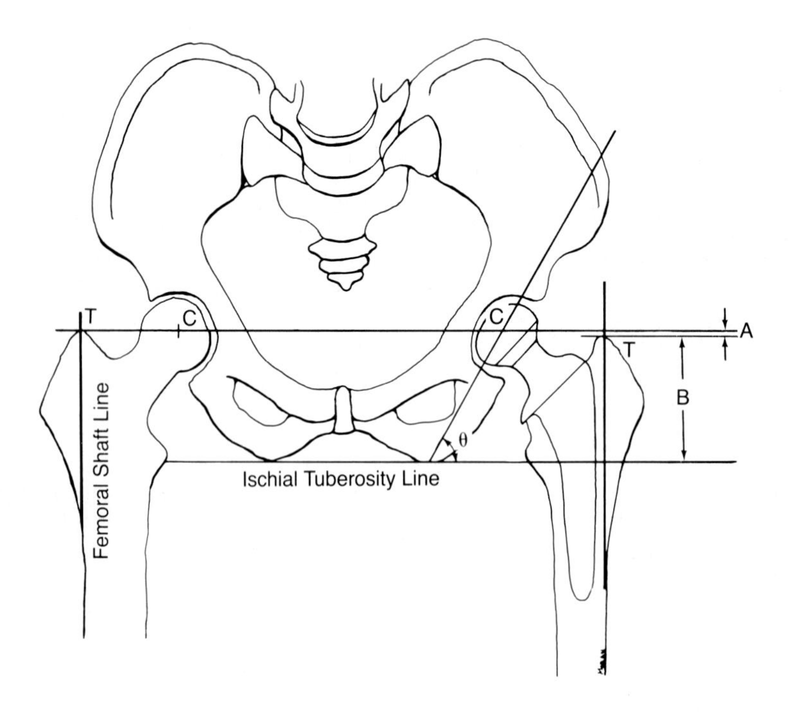

FIGURE 19–12. Diagram of the pelvis illustrating the reference lines and measurements made on radiographs for determining length reconstruction and soft tissue balance. (T = tip of greater trochanter; C = center of rotation.) (Redrawn from Fackler, C.D. and Poss, R.: Clin. Orthop. 151: 169–178, 1980.)

marked. The ischial tuberosity line touches the inferior aspect of each ischial tuberosity, and the femoral shaft line extends in both directions from the tip of the greater trochanter parallel to the long axis of the femoral shaft. A third line is extended in both directions from the tip of the greater trochanter perpendicular to the long axis of the femoral shaft, and a fourth line is drawn parallel to this line through the center of rotation of the femoral head. In most hips, these last two lines will be the same, because the center of rotation of the femoral head usually is at the level of the tip of the greater trochanter. The variation or congruence of these two lines in the operated hip—or the opposite (normal) hip if the deformity in the operated hip is too severe to provide useful evaluation—should be reproduced in the hip reconstruction. This practice provides appropriate length reconstruction, which can be confirmed by measuring the distance between the ischial tuberosity line and the horizontal line through the tip of the greater trochanter, the distance between the ischial tuberosity line and the tip of the lesser trochanter, or both distances.

The length of the line from the center of rotation of the head to the tip of the greater trochanter determines reconstruction of the abductor length in the horizontal direction. Avoiding soft tissue shortening of more than 5 mm in the horizontal direction may help prevent postoperative hip dislocation. Appropriate reconstruction of abductor length (within 5 mm of normal) can be achieved in most cases with a standard neck cut and appropriate vertical length reconstruction using a prosthesis with a fixed neck shaft angle and neck offset.[95] Some prosthesis systems provide a second neck offset for adjustment of horizontal abductor length.

For the few patients in whom the prosthesis angle and offset do not provide satisfactory horizontal abductor length reconstructions with a standard neck cut height, the neck cut height and prosthesis neck length can be varied. Vertical height—and, therefore, limb length reconstruction—is determined by a combination of neck lengths of the femoral bone and the prosthesis. With a fixed angle and offset prosthesis, the horizontal distance between the center of rotation of the femoral head and the greater trochanter can be increased by cutting more femoral neck and using a longer prosthetic neck. Conversely, this distance can be decreased by cutting less bone with the femoral neck osteotomy and using a shorter prosthetic neck. A shorter prosthetic neck length may increase the possibility of bony impingement, because it brings the remaining femoral bone closer to the pelvis. However, adjustments in bone or prosthesis neck length to provide proper horizontal length reconstruction nearly always require lengthening of the horizontal abductor length and therefore necessitate a longer prosthetic neck.

If acetabular reaming is directed too vertically, the prosthetic socket will be placed superior to the normal location, making both limb length and abductor length reconstruction difficult. This maneuver raises the dislocation rate because of the soft tissue imbalance and the increased likelihood of bony impingement. When the transtrochanteric approach is used, trochanteric detachment will result in soft tissue imbalance (see Chapter 14, *Surgical Approaches For Total Hip Replacement*).

Component Malposition

Evaluation of component malposition (type III dislocation) requires determination of the socket abduction angle and version of the socket and femoral component. To determine socket abduction, a line should be drawn through the longitudinal axis of the metal shell or the wire marker of an all-polyethylene socket. The angle between this line and the ischial tuberosity line is the socket abduction angle (angle *theta*). The safe zone for the abduction angle is 40 ± 10 degrees (Fig. 19–12).

The anteroposterior rotation of the prosthetic socket in relation to the anatomic position of the pelvis, or anteversion angle, is determined directly by measuring the angle between a line drawn through the axis of the metal shell or wire marker and the vertical on the cross-table lateral view of the acetabulum. Anteversion may also be estimated from the anteroposterior radiograph by the formula sin−1 D1/D2, where D1 is the minor length and D2 the major length of the ellipse formed by the edge of the metal socket or wire marker. The socket is anteverted if the lateral arc of the ellipse is more sharply defined than the medial arc. Several factors may interfere with the accuracy of this estimate; therefore, direct measurement of the cross-table lateral is preferable. The safe zone for anteroposterior rotation of the socket is 15 ± 10 degrees (Fig. 19–13).[30, 34]

Version of the femoral component is determined by fluoroscopy. The patient is placed prone with the knee flexed. The hip is rotated until the neck of the prosthesis is at its maximum length and thus is horizontal. The angle between the leg and the vertical determines the version. Internal rotation of the leg indicates anteversion, and external rotation indicates retroversion.[34] The femoral version angle may also be determined directly utilizing computerized tomography or calculations based on anteroposterior and lateral radiographs.[75] Excessive retroversion (> 0 degrees and excessive anteversion (> 20 degrees) are associated with increased rates of dislocation.[22, 27]

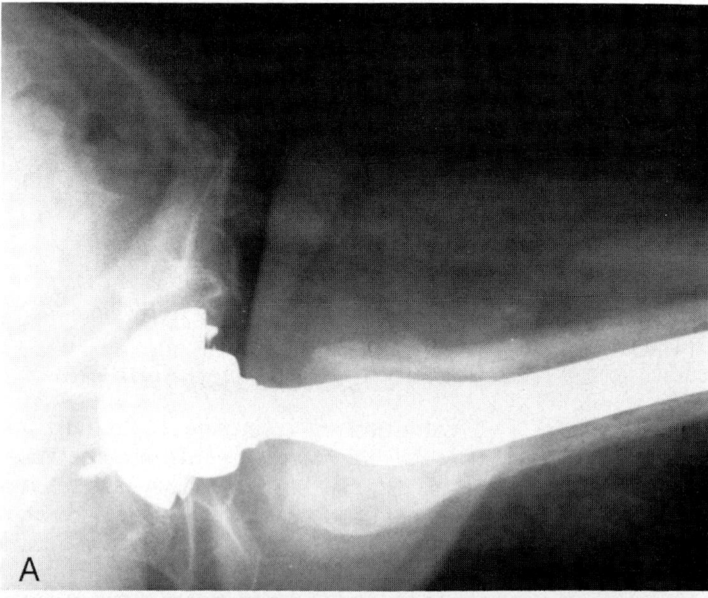

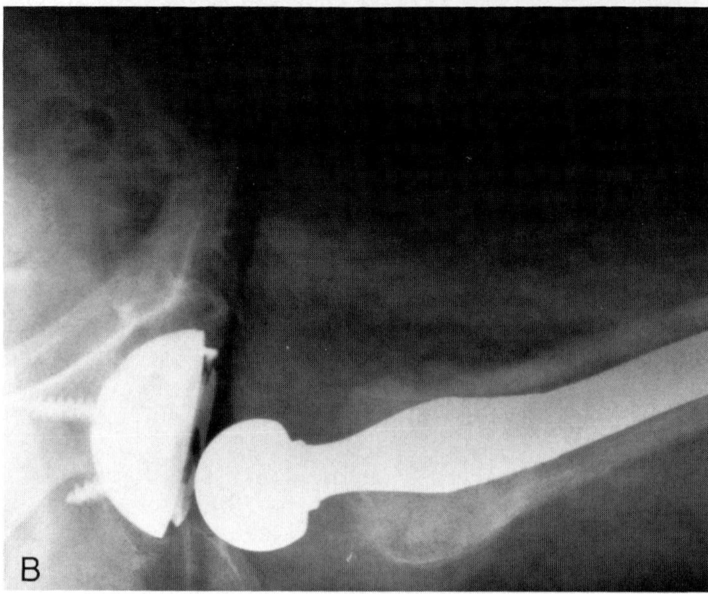

FIGURE 19–13. Malposition of acetabular component resulting in dislocation. *A,* On the lateral radiograph, the retroversion angle of the socket is 10 degrees or 15 degrees beyond the safe zone. *B,* The patient had recurrent posterior dislocations.

Management of Dislocation

The initial management of dislocation after total hip replacement is closed reduction. This is usually successful, except in the rare instance when soft tissue is interposed or the dislocation has remained untreated for several days, allowing muscle shortening.[34, 116] The reduction usually can be performed with analgesic, muscle-relaxing medication, or both, although more difficult cases, especially those with substantial muscle shortening due to delay in treatment, may require general anesthesia. Fluoroscopic control during reduction is helpful. The specific maneuver required for reduction depends on the location of the dislocated femoral head. Generally, the femoral head is brought to the level of the acetabulum by traction, and the head is then seated in the socket by rotation. When the head is posterior or superior, as is usually the case, adduction aids reduction. After reduction, stability is evaluated in various positions to determine those likely to lead to dislocation.

After closed reduction of a dislocated hip prosthesis, the patient should be carefully instructed again about avoiding positions that are dangerous to the stability of the hip (see chapter 18, *Total Hip Arthroplasty: Postoperative Care and Rehabilitation*). Instruction may be sufficient in many patients who have had positional dislocations. Immobilization, if indicated, can be achieved with a cast or brace, to avoid the disadvantages of bed rest, especially in elderly patients. Cast immobilization protects the hip from dangerous positions while the soft tissues heal. The preferred method is a pantaloon spica cast, which allows for walking and excellent mobility. If more complete restriction of rotation is indicated, a single full-limb hip spica cast with a knee hinge is effective. A brace can also protect the hip from dangerous positions while allowing motion within a specified range. If dislocation was posterior, flexion, adduction, and internal rotation are restricted. If dislocation was anterior, extension beyond 20 degrees of flexion is prevented and external rotation is restricted. Unlike a cast, a brace can be removed for bathing, but this may be a disadvantage if the patient is not totally compliant. Cast or brace protection usually is continued for 4 to 6 weeks. Meanwhile, a program to strengthen the muscles about the hip is instituted or continued.

In cases of severe malposition of components, operative revision may be considered, although it may be better to attempt continued closed treatment unless another dislocation occurs. Severe malpositions in which recurrent dislocations are likely include (1) an acetabular component outside the safe zone in both planes and (2) a femoral component in more than 20 degrees of retroversion. Adductor release is indicated in conjunction with closed reduction in patients with adductor contracture associated with acetabular abduction greater than 50 degrees. Revision and repair of a detached greater trochanter also may be indicated to correct muscle imbalance. During open reduction, the components can be inspected directly, and the surgeon should be prepared to proceed with correction of severe component malposition (see Chapter 23, *Revision Total Hip Arthroplasty*).

INFECTION

In the early history of total hip replacement, without antibiotics or environmental control, the infection rate was disturbingly high, up to 11 percent (Table 19–3).[86] When antibiotics began to be administered shortly before and for a brief time after surgery, the average infection rate for several series was reduced to 1.3 percent (Table 19–4).[86] In contemporary series, the infection rate was 0.7 percent with the use of "clean" rooms when antibiotics were not added and 0.6 percent when antibiotics were added (Tables 19–5 and 19–6).[86] The combination of an operating room with ultraviolet light and antibiotic administra-

Table 19–3. DEEP INFECTION IN REGULAR OPERATING ROOM AND WITHOUT ANTIBIOTICS

Investigators	No. of Cases/ Infections	Percent (%)
Charnley	190/13	6.8
Müller	683/27	4.0
Wilson et al	100/11	11.0
Patterson and Brown	368/30	8.2
Benson and Hughes	321/17	5.3
Murray	126/5	4.0
Ritter et al	96/6	6.5
Total	1880/109	5.8

Table 19–4. DEEP INFECTION IN REGULAR OPERATING ROOM AND WITH ANTIBIOTICS

Investigators	No. of Cases/ Infections	Percent (%)
Eftakhar et al	800/4	0.5
Fitzgerald	3215/42	1.3
Murray	622/7	1.1
Lowell and Kundsen	621/19	3.1
Leinbach and Barlow	275/4	1.5
Welch et al	150/0	0
Collis and Steinhaus	298/0	0
Irvine et al	167/4	2.4
Bentley and Simmonds	117/2	1.7
Salvati	526/8	1.5
Total	6791/90	1.3

tion resulted in an infection rate of 1.0 percent (Table 19–7).[86] The difference in infection rates with the regular operating room and no antibiotics versus all other groups was highly statistically significant ($p<0.001$). The incidence of infection in groups in which operations were performed in a "clean" room, whether or not antibiotics were given, was significantly less than the incidence in other groups ($p<0.01$).[86]

The efficacy of unidirectional airflow operating rooms in reducing infection rates for total hip replacement was confirmed by Lidwell and associates, and the efficacy of antibiotics has been validated in many studies.[67–69, 87] Infection rates have been especially low in large series of total hip replacements in which both unidirectional airflow and antibiotics were employed. In one series of 659 arthroplasties, the combined early and late infection incidence in procedures performed without structural bone grafts was 0.38 percent in primary operations. No infections were observed in 104 revisions. Infections were much more common when structural grafts were necessary, occurring in 6.8 percent of primary procedures and 3.0 percent of revision operations.[108] In another series of 1007 hip replacements, only 0.2 percent were associated with infections.[84] Another report revealed infections in 0.42 percent of primary arthroplasties and 0.47 percent of revision arthroplasties, for an overall incidence of 0.43 percent in 932 hip replacements.[48]

In most series, the incidence of infection has been lower in patients who had primary hip arthroplasties than in patients who had previous surgery, whether total hip arthroplasty or other procedures, such as internal fixation. In one series of 711 hip replacements, the incidence of infection with primary surgery was 1.6 percent, whereas that with secondary surgery was 3.5 percent.[87] Some investigators have reported a relatively high infection rate in patients with rheumatoid arthritis. In one large series of total hip replacement, the overall infection incidence was 0.89 percent, but 1.2 percent of patients with rheumatoid arthritis developed infections.[96] Other risk factors for infection include presence of remote infections at the time of operation, immunosuppression, operative or postoperative complications, and positive culture findings of bacteria from postoperative wound discharge.[122]

In the early development of total hip arthroplasty, previous infection in the hip, even if many years before, was considered a contraindication to this procedure.[20] Numerous reports now document that total hip arthroplasty can be performed successfully after previous sepsis, whether asso-

Table 19–6. DEEP INFECTIONS IN CLEAN ROOM OPERATING ROOM AND WITH ANTIBIOTICS

Investigators	No. of Cases/ Infections	Percent (%)
Nelson	243/0	0
Irvine et al	107/1	0.9
Welch et al	600/0	0
Leinbach and Barlow	425/3	0.7
Bentley and Simmonds	130/1	0.8
Salvati	1249/12	1.0
Total	2754/17	0.6

Table 19–5. DEEP INFECTIONS IN CLEAN ROOM OPERATING ROOM AND WITHOUT ANTIBIOTICS

Investigators	No. of Cases/ Infections	Percent (%)
Brady	300/3	1.0
Charnley	2152/12	0.6
Ritter et al	278/3	1.1
Total	2730/18	0.7

Table 19–7. DEEP INFECTIONS IN ULTRAVIOLET LIGHT OPERATING ROOM AND WITH ANTIBIOTICS

Investigators	No. of Cases/ Infections	Percent (%)
Lowell and Kundsen	665/5	0.8
Goldner et al	700/8	1.1
	1365/13	1.0

ciated with hip replacement, another implant, or some other factor. The prognosis is worse if sepsis is active at the time of hip replacement surgery and for certain bacteria, especially gram-negative organisms.[9, 19, 23, 51, 55, 61, 74, 82, 105, 129]

Staphylococci are the bacteria most commonly isolated from infected total hip replacements. In most series, *Staphylococcus epidermidis* is more common than *Staphylococcus aureus*. Gram-negative organisms occur much less commonly but may be more difficult to treat and eradicate, in part because of their antibiotic sensitivity profile. Anaerobes may be the causative infectious agents in total hip arthroplasty, and careful culture techniques for these organisms are essential (Tables 19–8 and 19–9).[19, 40, 80] Less commonly, infections may be associated with atypical mycobacteria and fungi.[43, 49] *Mycobacterium tuberculosis* may cause infection of total joint prosthesis, usually in a patient with previous infection of the hip associated with the same organism. Recurrence of infection is reduced by appropriate chemotherapy at the time of and after the hip replacement.[58, 106]

Most infections associated with total hip arthroplasty occur when bacteria gain access to the wound at the time of surgery. Infections resulting from hematogenous spread of organisms from remote sites have also been documented.[70, 72, 77, 117, 119, 126] These infections are usually associated with active infection elsewhere in the body. Bacteria from uninfected areas, such as those released during dental work or genitourinary manipulation, are much less common causes of infection in hip replacements.[117, 126] Lindquist and Slatis[72] reported three total hip replacements infected with microaerophilic *Streptococcus viridans* following dental procedures. Strazzeria and Anzel[119] reported a hip infection with *Actinomyces israelii,* an organism associated with dental caries and believed to exist almost exclusively in the mouth. This patient had not received antibiotics at the time of a tooth extraction.

These problems emphasize the importance of vigorous antibiotic treatment of any infection and a short course of antibiotic treatment for dental procedures, genitourinary and bowel manipulations, and similar procedures that are known to cause significant bacteremia in patients who have total joint prostheses. Antibiotic selection is based on the organisms commonly present in the area of manipulation. The medication should be given about 1 hour before the procedure, if taken orally, and closer to the time of the procedure if administered parenterally. An additional oral antibiotic dose 4 to 6 hours after the procedure may be wise.

Table 19–8. MICROORGANISMS ISOLATED FROM SPECIMENS TAKEN AT THE TIME OF RESECTION ARTHROPLASTY

Organism	No. of Isolates
Staphylococcus epidermidis	37
Staphylococcus aureus	19
Streptococcus viridans	10
Group-D *Streptococcus*	7
Escherichia coli	4
Proteus mirabilis	3
Pseudomonas aeruginosa	6
Enterobacter	4
Acinetobacter	1
Peptococcus	5
Bacillus sp.	3
Corynebacterium sp.	6
Bacteroides sp.	2
Beta-hemolytic *Streptococcus*	2
Propionibacterium acnes	1
No organism isolated	2

McDonald, D. J., Fitzgerald, R. H., Jr., and Ilstrup, D. M.: J. Bone Joint Surg. 71A(6):828–834, 1989. By permission.

Table 19–9. ORGANISMS CULTURED

Diagnosis	No. of Cases
Staphylococcus epidermidis	17*
Staphylococcus aureus	5*
Pseudomonas aeruginosa	2
Enterobacter	2
Microaerophilic *Streptococcus*	2
Escherichia coli	1
Propionibacterium acnes	1
Bacteroides fragilis	1*
Staphylococcus epidermidis and enterococcus	1

*Recurrence

Callaghan, J. J., Salvati, E. A., Brause, B. D., et al.: Reimplantation for Salvage of the Infected Hip: Rationale for the Use of Gentamicin-Impregnated Cement and Beads. The Hip. Edited by Robert H. Fitzgerald, Jr. St. Louis, C. V. Mosby Company, 1985. By permission.

MORTALITY

Some deaths are inevitable in association with any major surgical procedure, especially when the procedure is performed mostly in elderly individuals, many of whom have medical illnesses. Mortality rates in reported series of total hip replacements have varied from 0.4 to 3 percent. In a study in Sweden, the mortality rate for patients having total hip replacements for the diagnosis of coxarthrosis was little different than that expected in the general population. In women over age 70, mortality more than 1 year after surgery was less in those who had total hip replacement surgery than in the general population.[27, 71]

The most common fatal complication following total hip arthroplasty is pulmonary embolus (see Chapter 9, *Thromboembolic Disease*). Other common causes of death associated with total hip arthroplasties are coronary artery disease, cerebrovascular thrombosis, and cardiac arrest during the operation.

References

1. Abrahamsson, S. O., Ahlgren, S. A., Dahlstrom, J. A., et al.: Ectopic bone after hip replacement. Excision and free fat transplants in four cases. Acta Orthop. Scand. 55(6):589–592, 1984.
2. Adolphson, P., Jonsson, U., and Kalen, R.: Fractures of the ipsilateral femur after total hip arthroplasty. Arch. Orthop. Trauma Surg. 106(6):353–357, 1987.
3. Ahlgren, S. A., Elmqvist, D., and Ljung, P.: Nerve lesions after total hip replacement. Acta Orthop. Scand. 55(2):152–155, 1984.
4. Ahrengart, L. and Lindgren, U.: Functional significance of heterotopic bone formation after total hip arthroplasty. J. Arthroplasty 4(2):125–131, 1989.
5. Allen, H. L., Wase, A., and Bear, W. T.: Indomethacin and aspirin: Effect of non-steroidal anti-inflammatory agents on the rate of fracture repair in the rat. Acta Orthop. Scand. 51:595–600, 1980.
6. Almasbakk, K. and Roysland, P.: Does indomethacin (IMC) prevent postoperative ectopic ossification in total hip replacement? Acta Orthop. Scand. 48:556, 1977.
7. Amstutz, H. A., Ma, S. M., Jinnah, R. H., and Mai, L.: Revision of aseptic loose total hip arthroplasties. Clin. Orthop. 170:21–33, 1982.
8. Ayers, D. C., Evarts, C. M., and Parkinson, J. R.: The prevention of heterotopic ossification in high-risk patients by low-dose radiation therapy after total hip arthroplasty. J. Bone Joint Surg. 68A:1423–1429, 1986.
9. Balderston, R. A., Hiller, W. D., Iannotti, J. P., et al.: Treatment of the septic hip with total hip arthroplasty. Clin. Orthop. 221:231–237, 1987.
10. Bergqvist, D., Carlsson, A. S., and Ericsson, B. F.: Vascular complications after total hip arthroplasty. Acta Orthop. Scand. 54(2):157–163, 1983.
11. Bergstrom, B., Lindberg, L., Persson, B. M., and Onnerfalt, R.: Complication after total hip arthroplasty according to Charnley in a Swedish series of cases. Clin. Orthop. 95:91–94, 1973.
12. Bethea, J. S., 3d., DeAndrade, J. R., Fleming, L. L., et al.: Proximal femoral fractures following total hip arthroplasty. Clin. Orthop. 170:95–106, 1982.
13. Blasingame, J. P., Resnick, D., Coutts, R. D., and Danzig, L. A.: Extensive spinal osteophytosis as a risk factor for heterotopic bone formation after total hip arthroplasty. Clin. Orthop. 161:191–197, 1981.
14. Brady, L. W.: Radiation-induced sarcomas of bone. Skel. Radiol. 4:72–78, 1979.
15. Broad, C. P. and Hamami, M. N.: Kuntscher nailing of femoral fractures associated with Austin Moore's prosthesis. Injury 12(3):252–255, 1980.
16. Brooker, A. F., Bowerman, J. W., Robinson, R. A., and Riley, L. H., Jr.: Ectopic ossification following total hip arthroplasty. J. Bone Joint Surg. 55A:1629–1632, 1973.
17. Brunner, R., Morscher, E., and Hunig, R.: Para-articular ossification in total hip replacement: an indication for irradiation therapy. Arch. Orthop. Trauma Surg. 106(2):102–107, 1987.
18. Buovet, O. L. M., Nollen, A. J. G., Slooff, T. J. J. H., and Feith, R.: Effect of diphosphonate on para-articular ossification after total hip replacement. Acta Orthop. Scand. 45:926–934, 1974.
19. Callaghan, J. J., Salvati, E. A., Brause, B. D., et al.: Reimplantation for Salvage of the Infected Hip: Rationale for the Use of Gentamicin-Impregnated Cement and Beads. The Hip. Edited by Robert H. Fitzgerald, Jr. St. Louis, C. V. Mosby Company, 1985.
20. Charnley, J.: Acrylic Cement in Orthopaedic Surgery. Baltimore, Williams & Wilkins, 1970.
21. Charnley, J.: Low Friction Arthroplasty of the Hip. Berlin, Springer-Verlag, 1979.
22. Charnley, J. and Cupic, Z.: The nine and ten year results of the Charnley low friction arthroplasty of the hip. Clin. Orthop. 95:9–25, 1973.
23. Cherney, D. L. and Amstutz, H. C.: Total hip replacement in the previously septic hip. J. Bone Joint Surg. [Am] 65(9):1256–1265, 1983.
24. Chevrot, A., Lacombe, P., Zeny, J. C., et al.: Fatigue fractures of the obturator frame following hip arthroplasty. Rev. Rhum. Mal. Osteoartic. 53(2):129–132, 1986. (Published in french.)
25. Committee Exhibits of the AAOS: Classification and Management of Femoral Defects in Total Hip Replacement. Committee on the Hip. American Academy of Orthopaedic Surgeons Annual Meeting. New Orleans, 1990.
26. Cooke, P. H. and Newman, J. H.: Fractures of the femur in relation to cemented hip prostheses. J. Bone Joint Surg. [Br] 70(3):386–389, 1988.
27. Coventry, M. B., Beckenbaugh, R. D., Nolan, D. R., and Ilstrup, D. M.: 2,012 Total hip arthroplasties: A study of postoperative course and early complications. J. Bone Joint Surg. 56A:273–284, 1974.
28. Coventry, M. B. and Scanlon, P. W.: The use of radiation to discourage ectopic bone. A nine-

year study in surgery about the hip. J. Bone Joint Surg. [Am] 63A(2):201–208, 1981.
29. Cracchiolo, A.: Stress fractures of the pelvis as a cause of hip pain following total hip and knee arthroplasty. Arthritis Rheum. 24(5):740–742, 1981.
30. Dorr, L. D., Wolf, A. W., Chandler, R., and Conaty, J. P.: Classification and treatment of dislocations of total hip arthroplasty. Clin. Orthop. 173:151–158, 1983.
31. Eftakhar, N. S, and Stinchfield, F. E.: Experience with low friction arthroplasty. A statistical review of early results and complications. Clin. Orthop. 95:60–68, 1973.
32. Engh, C. A. and Massin, P.: Cementless total hip arthroplasty using the anatomic medullary locking stem. Clin. Orthop. 249:141–158, 1989.
33. Eyb, R. and Zweymuller, K.: Periarticular ossifications following implantation of cement-free total hip endoprostheses of the Zweymuller-Endler type. Z. Orthop. 123(6):975–980, 1985. (Published in German.)
34. Fackler, C. D. and Poss, R.: Dislocation in total hip arthroplasties. Clin. Orthop. 151:169–178, 1980.
35. Fahrer, H., Koch, P., Barandun, R., and Gerber, N. J.: Pelvic and skeletal hyperostosis (diffuse idiopathic skeletal hyperostosis, Forestier disease). Z. Rheumatol. 47(4):227–232, 1988. (Published in German.)
36. Federici, A., Carbone, M., and Sanguineti, F.: Intraoperative fractures of the femoral diaphysis in hip arthroprosthesis surgery. Ital. J. Orthop. Traumatol. 14(3):311–321, 1988.
37. Finerman, G. A. M. and Stover, S. L.: Heterotopic ossification following hip replacement or spinal cord injury. Two clinical studies with EHDP. Metabol. Bone Dis. 3:337–342, 1981.
38. Fitzgerald, R. H., Jr., Brindley, G. W., and Kavanagh, B. F.: The uncemented total hip arthroplasty. Intraoperative femoral fractures. Clin. Orthop. 235:61–66, 1988.
39. Fleming, R. E., Michelson, C. B., and Stinchfield, F. E.: Sciatic paralysis. A complication of bleeding following hip surgery. J. Bone Joint Surg. 61A:37, 1979.
40. Furno, P., Loubert, G., Lambin, Y., et al.: Acute primary infection due to slow-growing anaerobes after total hip arthroplasty. Nouv. Presse Med. 11(26):1991–1993, 1982. (Published in French. Author's transl.)
41. Garcia-Morteo, O., Maldonado-Cocco, J. A., and Babini, J. C.: Ectopic ossification following total hip replacement in juvenile chronic arthritis. J. Bone Joint Surg. [Am] 65(6):812–814, 1983.
42. Gaucher, A., Raul, P., Wiederkehr, P., et al.: Stress fractures of the pelvis. J. Radiol. 63(8–9):471–478, 1982. Published in French.)
43. Goodman, J. S., Seibert, D. G., Reahl, G. E., Jr., and Geckler, R. W.: Fungal infection of prosthetic joints: a report of two cases. J. Rheumatol. 10(3):494–495, 1983.
44. Haberman, E. T.: Panel on Radiation and Bone Ingrowth. Total Hip: Cement vs. Cementless. Boston, October 4, 1985.
45. Hartwig, C. H., Sell, S., and Kusswetter, W.: Periarticular ossification following cement-free and cement-fixed total endoprosthesis implantation in the hip joint. Z. Orthop. 127(3):296–301, 1989. (Published in German.)
46. Hedley, A. K., Mead, L. P., and Herndren, D. H.: The prevention of heterotopic bone formation following total hip arthroplasty using 600 rad in a single dose. J. Arthroplasty 4:319–325, 1989.
47. Heyes, F. L. and Aukland, A.: Occlusion of the common femoral artery complicating total hip arthroplasty. J. Bone Joint Surg. [Br] 67(4):533–535, 1985.
48. Hill, G. E. and Droller, D. G.: Acute and subacute deep infection after uncemented total hip replacement using antibacterial prophylaxis. Orthop. Rev. 18(5):617–623, 1989.
49. Horadam, V. W., Smilack, J. D., and Smith, E. C.: *Mycobacterium fortuitum* infection after total hip replacement. South. Med. J. 75(2):244–246, 1982.
50. Jahn, K. and Siegling, C. W.: Fractures of the femur following prosthetic replacement of the hip- and knee-joint. Zentralbl. Chir. 106(7):463–468, 1981. (Published in German. Author's transl.)
51. James, E. T., Hunter, G. A., and Cameron, H. U.: Total hip revision arthroplasty: Does sepsis influence the results? Clin. Orthop. 170:88–94, 1982.
52. Jantsch, S., Leixnering, M., Schwagerl, W., and Hackl, H.: Shaft fissures due to implantation of cementless total endoprostheses of the hip joint. An experimental study. Arch. Orthop. Trauma Surg. 107(4):236–241, 1988.
53. Johanson, N. A., Pellicci, P. M., Tsairis, P., and Salvati, E. A.: Nerve injury in total hip arthroplasty. Clin. Orthop. 179:214–222, 1983.
54. Johansson, J. E., McBroom, R., Barrington, T. W., and Hunter, G. A.: Fracture of the ipsilateral femur in patients with total hip replacement. J. Bone Joint Surg. 63A:1435–1442, 1981.
55. Jupiter, J. B., Karchmer, A. W., Lowell, J. D., and Harris, W. H.: Total hip arthroplasty in the treatment of adult hips with current or quiescent sepsis. J. Bone Joint Surg. [Am] 63A(2):194–200, 1981.
56. Kavanagh, B. F., Fitzgerald, R. H., and Ilstrup, D.: PCA uncemented THA. Orthop. Trans. 12:704, 1988.
57. Kim, J. H., Chu, F. C., Woodard, H. Q., et al.: Radiation-induced bone and soft tissue sarcoma. Radiology 129:501–508, 1978.
58. Kim, Y. Y., Ko, C. U., Ahn, J. Y., et al.: Charnley low friction arthroplasty in tuberculosis of the hip. An eight to 13-year follow-up. J. Bone Joint Surg. [Br] 70(5):756–760, 1988.
59. Kjaersgaard-Anderson, P. and Schmidt, S. A.: Indomethacin for prevention of ectopic ossification after hip arthroplasty. Acta Orthop. Scand. 57:12–14, 1986.
60. Knahr, K., Salzer, M., Eyb, R., and Blauensteiner, W.: Heterotopic ossification with total endoprostheses in various models of thrombosis prophylaxis. J. Arthroplasty 3:1–8, 1988.
61. Laforgia, R., Murphy, J. C., and Redfern, T. R.: Low friction arthroplasty for old quiescent infection of the hip. J. Bone Joint Surg. [Br] 70(3):373–376, 1988.
62. Larsen, E., Menck, H., and Rosenklint, A.: Frac-

tures after hemialloplastic hip replacement. J. Trauma 27(1):72–74, 1987.
63. Launder, W. J. and Hungerford, D. S.: Stress fracture of the pubis after total hip arthroplasty. Clin. Orthop. 159:183–185, 1981.
64. Lazansky, M. Z.: Complications revisited. The debit side of total hip replacement. Clin. Orthop. 95:96–103, 1973.
65. Lewinnek, G. E., Lewis, J. L., Tarr, R., et al.: Dislocations after total hip-replacement arthroplasties. J. Bone Joint Surg. 60A:217–220, 1978.
66. Lidgren, L. and Nordstrom, B.: Treatment of periarticular calcification after total hip arthroplasty. Arch. Orthop. Trauma Surg. 94(1):67–70, 1979.
67. Lidwell, O. M.: Airborne bacteria and surgical infection. Am. J. Med. 70(3): 693–697, 1981.
68. Lidwell, O. M.: Infection following orthopaedic surgery in conventional and unidirectional airflow operating theatres: The results of a prospective randomized study. Br. Med. J. 285:10, 1982.
69. Lidwell, O. M., Lowbury, E. J., Whyte, W., et al.: Infection and sepsis after operations for total hip or knee-joint replacement: influence of ultraclean air, prophylactic antibiotics and other factors. J. Hyg. (Lond). 93(3):505–529, 1984.
70. Limbird, T. J.: *Hemophilus influenzae* infection of a total hip arthroplasty. Clin. Orthop. 199:182–184, 1985.
71. Lindberg, H., Carlsson, A. S., Lanke, J., and Horstmenn, V.: The overall mortality rate in patients with total hip arthroplasty, with special reference to coxarthrosis. Clin. Orthop. 191:116–120, 1984.
72. Lindquist, C. and Slatis, P.: Dental bacteremia—a neglected cause of arthroplasty infections? Three hip cases. Acta Orthop. Scand. 56(6):506–508, 1985.
73. Lotke, P. A., Wong, R. Y., and Ecker, M. L.: Stress fracture as a cause of chronic pain following revision total hip arthroplasty. Report of two cases. Clin. Orthop. 206:147–150, 1986.
74. Lynch, M., Esser, M. P., Shelley, P., and Wroblewski, B. M.: Deep infection in Charnley low-friction arthroplasty. Comparison of plain and gentamicin-loaded cement. J. Bone Joint Surg. [Br] 69(3):355–360, 1987.
75. Magilligan, D. J.: Calculation of the angle of anteversion by means of horizontal lateral roentgenography. J. Bone Joint Surg. 38A:1231–1246, 1956.
76. Mallory, T. H., Kraus, T. J., and Vaughn, B. K.: Intraoperative femoral fractures associated with cementless total hip arthroplasty. Orthopedics 12(2):231–239, 1989.
77. Maniloff, G., Greenwald, R., Laskin, R., and Singer, C.: Delayed postbacteremic prosthetic joint infection. Clin. Orthop. 223:194–197, 1987.
78. Matos, M. H., Amstutz, H. C., and Machleder, H. I.: Ischemia of the lower extremity after total hip replacement. J. Bone Joint Surg. 61A:24–27, 1979.
79. Mayer, G., Seide, H. W., and Patzak, P.: Femur shaft fractures in artificial hip joint replacement. Zentralbl. Chir. 110(12):739–748, 1985. (Published in German.)
80. McDonald, D. J., Fitzgerald, R. H., Jr., and Ilstrup, D. M.: Two-stage reconstruction of a total hip arthroplasty because of infection. J. Bone Joint Surg. [Am] 71(6):828–834, 1989.
81. McElfresh, E. C. and Coventry, M. B.: Femoral and pelvic fractures after total hip arthroplasty. J. Bone Joint Surg. 56A:483–492, 1971.
82. Miley, G. B., Scheller, A. D., Jr., and Turner, R. H.: Medical and surgical treatment of the septic hip with one-stage revision arthroplasty. Clin. Orthop. 170:76–82, 1982.
83. Montijo, H., Ebert, F. R., and Lennox, D. A.: Treatment of proximal femur fractures associated with total hip arthroplasty. J. Arthroplasty 4(2):115–123, 1989.
84. Mulier, J. C., Vandepitte, J., Stuyck, J., et al.: Long-term study of the preoperative infection rate in 1007 total hip replacements using prophylactic cefamandole and other precautions. Arch. Orthop. Trauma Surg. 106(3):135–139, 1987.
85. Nachbur, B., Meyer, R. P., Verkkala, V., and Zurcher, R.: The mechanisms of severe arterial injury in surgery of the hip joint. Clin. Orthop. 141:122–133, 1979.
86. Nelson, J. P.: The Operating Environment and its Influence on Deep Wound Infection. The Hip. St. Louis, C. V. Mosby Company, 1977.
87. Nelson, J. P., Glassburn, A. R., Jr., Talbott, R. D., and McElhinney, J. P.: The effect of previous surgery, operating room environment, and preventive antibiotics on postoperative infection following total hip arthroplasty. Clin. Orthop. 147:167–169, 1980.
88. Nieder, E., Steinbrink, K., Engelbrecht, E., and Siegel, A.: Injury to pelvic vessels in total hip replacement surgery. Chirurgie. 50(12):780–785, 1979. (Published in German.)
89. Nollen, A. J. G.: Effect of ethylhydroxydiphosphonate on heterotopic ossification. Acta Orthop. Scand. 57:357–361, 1986.
90. Nollen, A. J. G. and Slooff, T. J. J. H.: Para-articular ossifications after total hip replacement. Acta Orthop. Scand. 44:230–241, 1973.
91. Oh, I. and Hardacre, J. A.: Fatigue fracture of the inferior pubic ramus following total hip replacement for congenital hip dislocation. Clin. Orthop. 147:154–156, 1980.
92. Panenberg, B. L., Chandler, H. P., and Young, S. K.: Femoral fractures below hip implants: A new and safe technique of fixation. Orthop. Trans. 13:1989.
93. Pankovich, A. M., Tarabishy, I., and Barmada, R.: Fractures below non-cemented femoral implants. Treatment with Ender nailing. J. Bone Joint Surg. [Am] 63A(6):1024–1025, 1981.
94. Pedersen, N. W., Kristensen, S. S., Schmidt, S. A., and Pedersen, P., Kjaersgaard-Andersen, P.: Factors associated with heterotopic bone formation following total hip replacement. Arch. Orthop. Trauma Surg. 108(2):92–95, 1989.
95. Petty, W.: Evaluation of abductor length reconstruction in total hip arthroplasty. (Unpublished data.) 1989.
96. Poss, R., Maloney, J. P., Ewald, F. C., et al.: Six- to 11-year results of total hip arthroplasty in rheumatoid arthritis. Clin. Orthop. 182:109–116, 1984.

97. Ratliff, A. H.: Vascular and Neurologic Complications Following Total Hip Replacement. The Hip. St. Louis, C. V. Mosby Company, 1981.
98. Riska, E. B. and Michelsson, J. E.: Treatment of para-articular ossification after total hip replacement by excision and use of free fat transplants. Acta Orthop. Scand. 50(6):751–754, 1979.
99. Ritschl, P. and Kotz, R.: Fractures of the proximal femur in patients with total hip endoprostheses. Arch. Orthop. Trauma Surg. 104(6):392–397, 1986.
100. Ritter, M. A. and Gloe, T. J.: The effect of indomethacin on para-articular ectopic ossification following total hip arthroplasty. Clin. Orthop. 167:113–117, 1982.
101. Ritter, M. A. and Meding, J. B.: A comparison of osteonecrosis and osteoarthritis patients following total hip arthroplasty. A long-term follow-up study. Clin. Orthop. 206:139–146, 1986.
102. Ritter, M. A. and Sieber, J. M.: Prophylactic indomethacin for the prevention of heterotopic bone formation following total hip arthroplasty. Clin. Orthop. 196:217–225, 1985.
103. Roberson, J. R.: Late hemarthrosis from a threaded acetabular component. J. Arthroplasty 3:61–65, 1988.
104. Rosendahl, S., Christoffersen, J. K., and Norgaard, M.: Para-articular ossification following hip replacement 70 arthroplasties ad modum Moore using McFarland's approach. Acta Orthop. Scand. 48:400–404, 1977.
105. Salvati, E. A., Chekofsky, K. M., Brause, B. D., and Wilson, P. D., Jr.: Reimplantation in infection: a 12-year experience. Clin. Orthop. 170:62–75, 1982.
106. Santavirta, S., Eskola, A., Konttinen, Y. T., et al.: Total hip replacement in old tuberculosis. A report of 14 cases. Acta Orthop. Scand. 59(4):391–395, 1988.
107. Schmidt, A. S., Kjaersgaard-Andersen, P., Pedersen, N. W., et al.: The use of indomethacin to prevent the formation of heterotopic bone after total hip replacement. J. Bone Joint Surg. 70A:834–838, 1988.
108. Schutzer, S. F. and Harris, W. H.: Deep-wound infection after total hip replacement under contemporary aseptic conditions. J. Bone Joint Surg. [Am] 70(5):724–727, 1988.
109. Schwartz, J. T., Mayer, J. G., and Engh, C. A.: Femoral fracture during non-cemented total hip arthroplasty. J. Bone Joint Surg. 71A:1135–1141, 1989.
110. Scott, R. D., Turner, R. H., Leitzes, S. M., and Aufranc, O. E.: Femoral fractures in conjunction with total hip replacement. J. Bone Joint Surg. 57A:494–501, 1975.
111. Sleeswijk, V.: Accidental femoral shaft fractures following hip arthroplasty of the same leg. Ned. Tijdschr. Geneeskd. 124(24):962–964, 1980. (Published in Dutch.)
112. Soballe, K., Christensen, F., and Kristensen, S. S.: Ectopic bone formation after total hip arthroplasty. Clin. Orthop. 228:57–62, 1988.
113. Sodemann, B., Persson, P. E., and Nilsson, O. S.: Periarticular heterotopic ossification after total hip arthroplasty for primary coxarthrosis. Clin. Orthop. 237:150–157, 1988.
114. Sodemann, B., Persson, P. E., and Nilsson, O. S.: Prevention of heterotopic ossification by nonsteroid anti-inflammatory drugs after total hip arthroplasty. Clin. Orthop. 237:158–163, 1988.
115. Solheim, L. F. and Hagen, R.: Femoral and sciatic neuropathies after total hip arthroplasty. Acta Orthop. Scand. 51:531, 1980.
116. Soudry, M., Juhn, A., and Mendes, D. G.: Interposed soft tissue obstructing the reduction of a dislocated Charnley hip arthroplasty. Orthopedics 8(3):389–390, 1985.
117. Stinchfield, F. E., Bigliani, L. U., Neu, H. C., et al.: Late hematogenous infection of total joint replacement. J. Bone Joint Surg. [Am] 62(8):1345–1350, 1980.
118. Stone, R. G., Weeks, L. E., Hajdu, M., and Stinchfield, F. E.: Evaluation of sciatic nerve compromise during total hip arthroplasty. Clin. Orthop. 201:26–31, 1985.
119. Strazzeri, J. C. and Anzel, S.: Infected total hip arthroplasty due to *Actinomyces israelii* after dental extraction. A case report. Clin. Orthop. 210:128–131, 1986.
120. Sudman, E. and Bang, G.: Indomethacin-induced inhibition of haversian remodeling in rabbits. Acta Orthop. Scand. 50:621–627, 1979.
121. Sundaram, N. A. and Murphy, J. C.: Heterotopic bone formation following total hip arthroplasty in ankylosing spondylitis. Clin. Orthop. 207:223–226, 1986.
122. Surin, V. V., Sundholm, K., and Backman, L.: Infection after total hip replacement. With special reference to a discharge from the wound. J. Bone Joint Surg. [Br] 65(4):412–418, 1983.
123. Sylvester, J. E., Greenberg, P., Selch, M. T., et al.: The use of postoperative irradiation for the prevention of heterotopic bone formation after total hip replacement. Int. J. Radiat. Oncol. Biol. Phys. 14(3):471–476, 1988.
124. Talab, Y. A., States, J. D., and Evarts, C. M.: Femoral shaft perforation. A complication of total hip reconstruction. Clin. Orthop. 141:158–166, 1979.
125. Thomas, B. J. and Amstutz, H. C.: Results of the administration of diphosphonate for the prevention of heterotopic ossification after total hip arthroplasty. J. Bone Joint Surg. 67A:400–403, 1985.
126. Thomas, B. J., Moreland, J. R., and Amstutz, H. C.: Infection after total joint arthroplasty from distal extremity sepsis. Clin. Orthop. 181:121–125, 1983.
127. Trancik, T., Mills, W., and Vinson, N.: The effect of indomethacin, aspirin, and ibuprofren on bone ingrowth into a porous-coated implant. Clin. Orthop. 249:113–121, 1989.
128. Vaughn, B. K. and Mallory, T. H.: Porous-coated anatomic total hip replacement—Clinical and roentgenographic results with minimum two-year follow-up. Orthop. Trans. 12:686, 1988.
129. Vidal, J., Salvan, J., Orst, G., and Marnay, T.: Total hip arthroplasty in the presence of sepsis. Rev. Chir. Orthop. 74(3):223–231, 1988. (Published in French.)
130. Weber, E. R., Daube, J. R., and Coventry, M. B.: Peripheral neuropathies associated with total hip arthroplasty. J. Bone Joint Surg. 58A:66–69, 1976.

131. Wilson, J. N. and Scales, J. T.: The Stanmore metal on metal total hip prosthesis using a three pin type cup. Clin. Orthop. 95:239–249, 1973.
132. Woolson, S. T. and Harris, W. H.: Complex total hip replacement for dysplastic or hypoplastic hips using miniature or microminiature components. J. Bone Joint Surg. [Am] 65(8):1099–1108, 1983.
133. Zenni, E. J., Jr., Pomeroy, D. L., and Caudle, R. J.: Ogden plate and other fixations for fractures complicating femoral endoprostheses. Clin. Orthop. 231:83–90, 1988.

CHAPTER 20

Results of Primary Total Hip Arthroplasty

WILLIAM PETTY

Total hip arthroplasty usually results in good or excellent outcomes, both clinically and radiographically. The success rates and types of failures reported in numerous studies are reviewed in this chapter.

Meaningful comparison of surgical results is possible only with consistent and objective measurements for assessment. Rating systems developed to quantify clinical results of total hip replacements are described in the opening of the chapter. Other evaluation methods, including assessment of radiographic findings and survivorship analyses, are also discussed.

Many studies have followed patients for over 10 years after cemented total hip arthroplasty. Shorter follow-up studies have been done for modern cementless hip replacements. Review of such studies is the focus of this chapter. Findings are separated according to clinical and radiographic results. To summarize these findings, the chapter concludes with an analysis of characteristics useful in predicting the likelihood of successful results.

METHODS OF EVALUATING RESULTS

Rating Methods

Various numeric scales have been created to provide objective, comparative information about short-term and long-term results of total hip arthroplasty. Despite the limitations of numeric rating scales, they do enable comparisons of different operations, alternative prostheses, operations performed for different diagnoses, results at various times after operations, and preoperative and postoperative status.

The rating scales for hip function described by D'Aubigne and Postel and modified by Charnley are used throughout the world. D'Aubigne and Postel developed the scale in 1954, and Charnley modified it to grade the results of the total hip arthroplasty procedure he described in 1972 (Tables 20–1 and 20–2).[13, 19] This grading system consists of a numeric scale from 1 (worst) to 6 (best) for three categories: pain, movement, and walking ability. According to Charnley, most patients for whom hip arthroplasty is indicated have Grade 3 or 4 pain; Grade 1 is rare, and Grade 5 is too mild to consider for operative treatment. Postoperatively, Grade 6 is considered excellent, and Grade 5 is good or satisfactory. In the Charnley modification, the numeric score for movement is determined by adding scores for total flexion-extension, abduction-adduction, and rotation. Arthroplasty often is indicated when the movement score is Grade 3. Such a hip may have reasonably well-maintained flexion but little abduction-adduction or rotation. A successful hip replacement will score

Table 20–1. METHOD OF GRADING FUNCTIONAL VALUE OF HIP—D'AUBIGNE AND POSTEL

Grade	Pain	Mobility	Ability to Walk
0	Pain is intense and permanent.	Ankylosis with bad position of hip.	None.
1	Pain is severe even at night.	No movement; pain or slight deformity.	Only with crutches.
2	Pain is severe when walking; prevents any activity.	Flexion under 40 degrees.	Only with canes.
3	Pain is tolerable with limited activity.	Flexion between 40 and 60 degrees.	With one cane, less than 1 hour; very difficult without cane.
4	Pain is mild when walking; disappears with rest.	Flexion between 60 and 80 degrees; patient can reach his foot.	A long time with a cane; short time without cane and with limp.
5	Pain is mild and inconstant; normal activity.	Flexion between 80 and 90 degrees; abduction of at least 15 degrees.	Without cane but with slight limp.
6	No pain.	Flexion of more than 90 degrees; abduction to 30 degrees.	Normal.

D'Aubigne, M. and Postel, M.: J. Bone Joint Surg. 36A:451–475, 1954. By permission.

Grade 5 or 6 on movement. The numeric score for walking indicates the functional capacity of a patient with disease of the hip.

In addition to the minor modifications Charnley made to the numeric scoring system of D'Aubigne and Postel, he added the alphabetic prefixes A, B, and C to indicate the general functional status of the patient:

A — The patient has one diseased hip and no other condition that interferes with walking.

B — Both hips are involved, but no other impediment to walking exists.

C — A generalized problem interferes with the ability to walk. This may be a problem of the musculoskeletal system, such as widespread rheumatoid arthritis or osteoarthritis in many joints, or a condition of another organ system, such as cardiovascular or respiratory disease or paraplegia.

Table 20–2. NUMERIC CLASSIFICATION OF THE CLINICAL STATE OF AFFECTED HIP JOINTS—CHARNLEY

Grade	Pain	Movement	Walking
1	Severe and spontaneous.	0–30 degrees	Few yards or bedridden. Two sticks or crutches.
2	Severe on attempting to walk.	60 degrees	Time and distance very limited without sticks.
3	Tolerable, permitting limited activity.	100 degrees	Limited with one stick. Difficult without a stick. Able to stand long periods.
4	Only after some activity.	160 degrees	Long distances with one stick. Limited without a stick.
5	Slight or intermittent. Pain on starting to walk but less with normal activity.	210 degrees	No stick but a limp.
6	No pain.	260 degrees	Normal.

Charnley, J.: J. Bone Joint Surg. 54B:61–76, 1972. By permission.

Charnley contended that only patients in category A and those in category B with bilateral hip replacements could be evaluated for walking ability with any validity. The replaced hip of a patient in category C might function well, yet the patient would receive a low score for walking because of an unrelated problem. This is a drawback of the functional portion of all rating scales.

Many surgeons, including those who use other numeric scales, have adopted the alphabetic rating scale for the purpose Charnley intended. This scale also can be employed to rate activity level in relation to the incidence of prosthesis failure. Charnley also advocated decimals and fractions in the D'Aubigne-Postel system to provide a more accurate picture of the results for groups of patients. The rating scales for hip function described by D'Aubigne and Postel and modified by Charnley have widespread use throughout the world.

The Hospital for Special Surgery Hip Rating System is another modification of the scale described by D'Aubigne and Postel. A numeric designation up to 10 is assigned for the categories of pain, function, and walking ability as well as an additional category: muscle power and motion (Table 20–3).[88] The University of California, Los Angeles, rating scale is almost identical to the Hospital for Special Surgery Hip Rating System, but it also includes an activity level rating (Table 20–4).[2]

In 1963, Larson[53] described what has become known as the Iowa Hip Rating, which is now popular in many areas of the United States (Table 20–5). This scale rates function, pain, gait, deformity, and range of motion. Muscle strength is recorded also, but no points are assigned for it. Function and pain represent 70 of the 100 points possible. The function score comprises 11 categories of daily living, weighted according to their importance for most people. The six pain categories range from no pain, for which the maximum 35 points is assigned, to continuous pain, which receives no points. The gait score is based on the need for walking aids and accounts for 10 of the 100 points. The deformity score is determined by the presence or absence of functionally important deformities and has a value of 10 points. Because 1 point is assigned to each 30 degrees of motion, the normal range of 300 degrees or more results in a motion score of 10.

In reporting the results of mold arthroplasty in 1969, Harris[38] used an evaluation system that has become known as the Harris Hip Rating (Table 20–6). As in the Iowa Hip Rating, pain and functional capacity are the two most important considerations, because they represent the indication for surgery in most patients. Pain accounts for 44 and function 47 of the maximum 100 points. The full 44 points are given if pain is totally absent, whereas no points are given if there is severe pain even at rest. Intermediate points are assigned for less extreme degrees of pain. The assessment of function consists of four categories: (1) activities of daily living, 14 points; (2) limp, 11 points; (3) walking aids, 11 points; and (4) maximum walking distance, 11 points. The complex method for evaluating the maximum of 5 points assigned to range of motion is simplified greatly if calculated by computer. Finally, 1 point is lost for each of the four functionally important deformities. This rating system and its modification have gained wide popularity in the United States.

The Mayo Clinic utilizes a modification of the Harris Hip Rating to report its extensive follow-up investigations of total hip arthroplasties. The Mayo Clinic's system assigns 45 points for pain, 45 for function, 8 for motion, and 2 for absence of deformity.[5]

Radiographic Evaluation

Radiographic comparison of the quality of the result of total hip arthroplasty in different series is difficult. Radiologic evaluation of loosening of the femoral component is usually based on a combination of the zonal method proposed by Gruen and colleagues[33] for the femoral component and the Charnley method for the acetabular component (Figs. 20–1 and 20–2).[20] Although most evaluations of loosening are based on the zonal method, the criteria for loosening vary. Some workers have adopted the criteria of Harris for defining loosening of the femoral component. Definite loosening is present when evidence exists of migration, which may take one of several forms: (1) a radiolucent line at the prosthesis-cement interface that was not visible on the postoperative radiograph; (2)

Table 20–3. HOSPITAL FOR SPECIAL SURGERY HIP RATING SYSTEM

Grade	Pain	Walking			Muscle Power (MP) and Motion*	Function
0	All the time. Unbearable. Strong medication frequently.	Bedridden.			Ankylosis with deformity.	Completely dependent and confined.
2	All the time but bearable. Strong medication occasionally. Salicylates frequently.	Wheelchair. Transfer activities with walker.			Ankylosis with good functional position.	Partially dependent.
4	None or little at rest. With activities. Salicylates frequently.	No support. One support. Bilateral support.	Housebound OR Less than one block Less than three blocks	Markedly restricted	MP—poor to fair. Arc of flexion less than 60 degrees. Restricted lateral and rotary movement.	Independent. Limited housework, shopping.
6	When starting, then better, or after a certain activity. Salicylates occasionally.	No support. One support. Bilateral support.	Less than one block Up to five blocks Unrestricted	Moderately restricted	MP—fair to good. Arc of flexion up to 90 degrees. Fair† lateral and rotary movement.	Most housework, unlimited shopping, desktype work.
8	Occasionally and slight.	No support. One support.	Limp No limp	Mildly restricted	MP—good or normal. Arc of flexion over 90 degrees. Good‡ lateral and rotary movement.	Very little restriction. Can work on feet.
10	No pain.	No support or appreciable limp.		Unrestricted	MP—normal. Motion—normal or almost normal.	Normal activities.

*Precedence in rating was given to active movement, but usually both active and passive movements were the same.
†Fair lateral movement: 10 degrees abduction, 10 degrees adduction. Fair rotary movement: internal rotation 10 degrees, external rotation 20 degrees.
‡Good lateral movement: 20 degrees abduction, 20 degrees adduction. Good rotatory movement: internal rotation 20 degrees, external rotation 40 degrees.
Wilson, P. D., Jr., Amstutz, H. C., Czerniecki, A., et al: J. Bone Joint Surg. 54A: 207–236, 1972. By permission.

Table 20–4. UCLA ACTIVITY LEVEL RATINGS

Grade	Activity Level
1	Wholly inactive: dependent on others; cannot leave residence.
2	Mostly inactive: very restricted to minimum activities of daily living.
3	Sometimes participates in mild activities such as walking, limited housework, and limited shopping.
4	Regularly participates in mild activities.
5	Sometimes participates in moderate activities such as swimming and can do unlimited housework or shopping.
6	Regularly participates in moderate activities.
7	Regularly participates in active events such as bicycling.
8	Regularly participates in very active events such as bowling or golf.
9	Sometimes participates in impact sports such as jogging, tennis, skiing, acrobatics, ballet, heavy labor, or backpacking.
10	Regularly participates in impact sports.

Modified from Amstutz, H., Thomas, B. J., Jinnah, R., et al: J. Bone Joint Surg. 66A:228–241, 1984.

Table 20–5. IOWA HIP RATING

Category	Points
A. Function (35 points)	
Does most of housework or job that requires moving about	5
Dresses unaided (includes tying shoes and putting on socks)	5
Walks enough to be independent	5
Sits without difficulty at table or toilet	4
Picks up objects from floor by squatting	3
Bathes without help	3
Negotiates stairs foot over foot	3
Carries objects comparable to suitcase	2
Gets into car or public conveyance unaided and rides comfortably	2
Drives a car	1
	____
B. Freedom from Pain (35 points) (Circle 1 only)	
No pain	35
Pain only with fatigue	30
Pain only with weightbearing	20
Pain at rest but not with weightbearing	15
Pain sitting or in bed	10
Continuous pain	0
	____
C. Gait (10 points) (Circle 1 only)	
No limp; no support	10
No limp using cane	8
Abductor limp	8
Short leg limp	8
Needs two canes	6
Needs two crutches	4
Cannot walk	0
	____
D. Absence of Deformity (10 points)	
No fixed flexion over 30°	3
No fixed adduction over 10°	3
No fixed rotation over 10°	2
Not over 1-inch shortening (ASIS-MM)	2
	____
E. Range of Motion (10 points)	
Flexion-extension (normal 140°)	____°
Abduction-adduction (normal 80°)	____°
External-internal rotation (normal 80°)	____°
Total degrees	____°
Points (1 pt/30°)	____
Muscle Strength (no points)	
Straight leg raising:	
Less than gravity ____ Gravity ____	
Gravity + resistance ____	
Abduction:	
Less than gravity ____ Gravity ____	
Gravity + resistance ____	
Extension:	
Less than gravity ____ Gravity ____	
Gravity + resistance ____	

Modified from Larson, C. B.: Clin. Orthop. 31:85–93, 1963.

Table 20–6. HIP EVALUATION SYSTEM—HARRIS

Category	Points
I. Pain (44 points possible)	
A. None or ignores it	44
B. Slight, occasional, no compromise in activities	40
C. Mild pain, no effect on average activities, rarely moderate pain with unusual activity, may take aspirin	30
D. Moderate pain, tolerable but makes concessions to pain. Some limitation of ordinary activity or work. May require occasional pain medicine stronger than aspirin	20
E. Marked pain, serious limitation of activities	10
F. Totally disabled, crippled, pain in bed, bedridden	0
II. Function (47 points possible)	
A. Gait (33 points possible)	
1. Limp	
a. None	11
b. Slight	8
c. Moderate	5
d. Severe	3
2. Support	
a. None	11
b. Cane for long walks	7
c. Cane most of the time	5
d. One crutch	3
e. Two canes	2
f. Two crutches	0
g. Not able to walk (specify reason)	0
B. Activities (14 points possible)	
1. Stairs	
a. Normally without using a railing	4
b. Normally using a railing	2
c. In any manner	1
d. Unable to do stairs	0
2. Shoes and socks	
a. With ease	4
b. With difficulty	2
c. Unable	0
3. Sitting	
a. Comfortably in ordinary chair 1 hr	5
b. On a high chair for ½ hour	3
c. Unable to sit comfortably in any chair	0
4. Enter public transportation	1
III. Deformity	
Absence of deformity points (4) are given if the patient demonstrates:	
A. Less than 30° fixed flexion contracture.	
B. Less than 10° fixed adduction.	
C. Less than 10° fixed internal rotation in extension.	
D. Limb length discrepancy less than 3.2 cm.	
IV. Range of Motion	
Index values are determined by multiplying the degrees of motion possible in each arch by the appropriate index.	
A. Flexion: 0–45° × 1.0; 45–90° × 0.6; 90–110° × 0.3	
B. Abduction: 0–15° × 0.8; 15–20° × 0.3; Over 20° × 0	
C. External rotation in extension: 0–15° × 0.4; Over 15° × 0	
D. Internal rotation in extension: any × 0	
E. Adduction: 0–15° × 0.2	
To determine the overall rating for range of motion, multiply the sum of the index values × 0.05. Record Trendelenburg test as positive, level, or neutral.	

Harris, W. H.: J. Bone Joint Surg. 51A: 737–755, 1969. By permission.

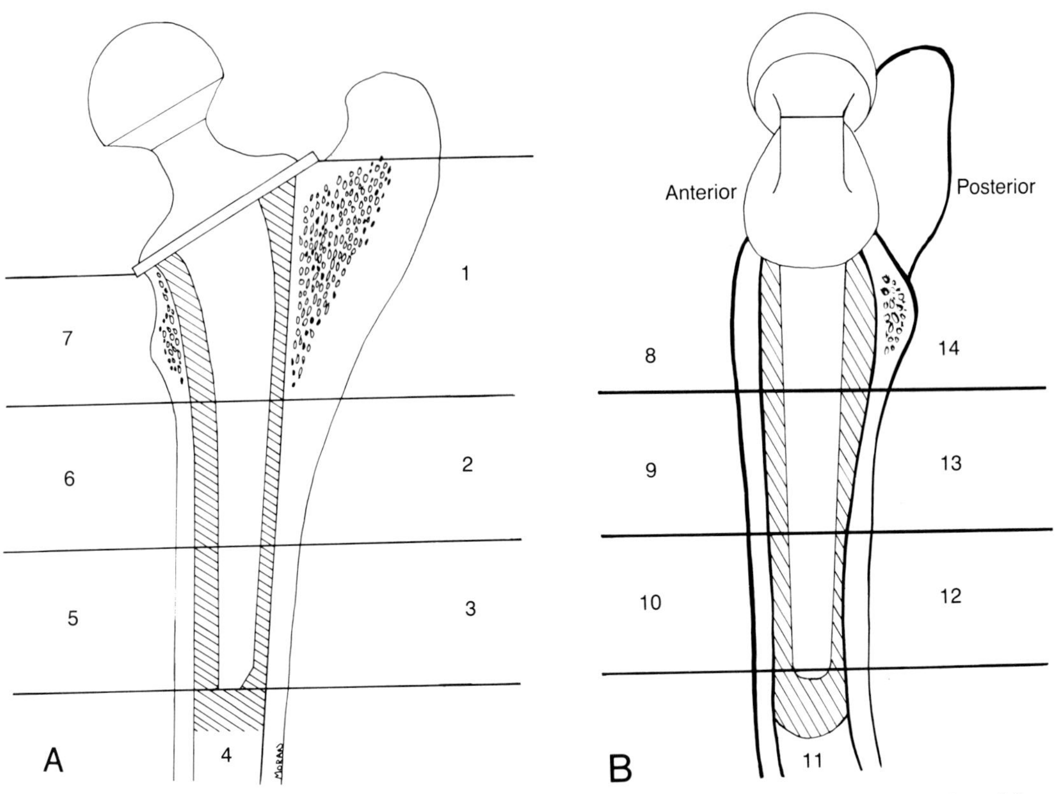

FIGURE 20–1. Zones for evaluation of loosening of the femoral component. *A*, Anteroposterior view of femur. *B*, Lateral view of femur.

a shift in the position of the prosthesis or cement; and (3) a fracture of either the stem or cement. Probable loosening is suspected when a continuous radiolucent line is present at the bone-cement interface and completely surrounds the cement mantle on either the anteroposterior or lateral radiograph. Possible loosening is characterized by a bone-cement lucency surrounding between 50 and 100 percent of the cement mantle on the anteroposterior or lateral radiograph that was not visible on the postoperative radiograph (Table 20–7).[40]

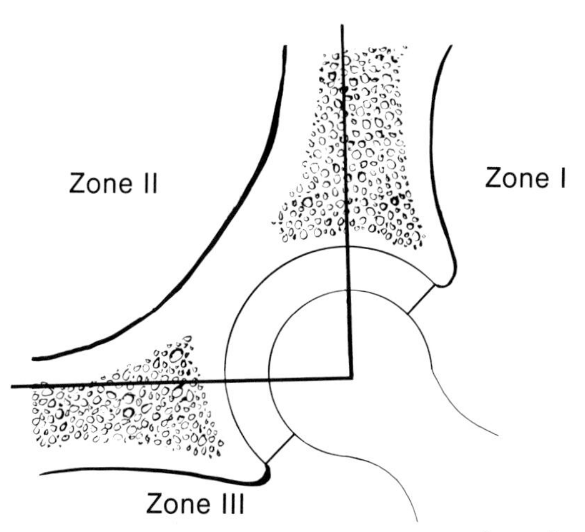

FIGURE 20–2. Division of circumference of acetabulum into zones I, II, and III.

Russotti and coworkers[77] adapted this method for acetabular loosening. Definite loosening of the socket is characterized by a shift in the prosthesis or a fracture of the component or cement. Evidence of probable loosening is a continuous radiolucent line at the bone-cement interface surrounding the entire cement mantle. The line is at least 2 mm wide in at least one of the acetabular zones described by DeLee and Charnley (Table 20–8).[20] Lines at the bone-cement interface that are progressive in either width or extent of the mantle sometimes are considered to represent possible loosening, although these lines may stabilize and not progress further.

Comparison of radiographs over time is important for all signs of loosening except obvious ones such as implant fractures. Consistency in positioning the hip, magnification, and energy and time of exposure

Table 20–7. TOTAL HIP STEM LOOSENING

Definite	Evidence of migration
Probable	Complete bone-cement interface lucency
Possible	Bone-cement interface radiolucency surrounding 50–100% of cement mantle

make the comparisons more valid. These parameters should be standardized as much as possible (see Chapter 11, *Imaging of Total Joint Replacement*).

The Hip Society, the Societe Internationale de Chirurgie Orthopedique et de Traumatologie Commission on Documentation and Evaluation, and the American Academy of Orthopaedic Surgeons Task Force on Outcome Studies agree on a common system of nomenclature that they have recommended for reporting both clinical and radiographic results of operations on the hip.[47] They encourage the use of standardized forms for recording data (Tables 20–9, 20–10, and 20–11). These data forms do not provide a numeric rating, but the investigator can derive various numeric ratings from the information recorded on the form (Table 20–12). Investigators may combine or expand the data as they choose.[47]

Survivorship Analysis

In evaluating any clinical or radiographic parameter over time, the number of patients available for evaluation will vary. Some patients will have died, and some patients' total hip replacements will have been revised. Patients may be lost to follow-up for various reasons. Percentages based on the number of patients evaluated at any one time do not provide an accurate estimate of failure or success because of these factors.

Many investigators have adopted the actuarial analysis method described by Kaplan and Meier[48] to provide a better estimate of survivorship or failure of total hip replacements. This method assumes that those patients lost to follow-up have the same general failure rates and other characteristics as those patients not lost to follow-up. If some patients with failed prostheses see other surgeons or if those patients with excellent results fail to return for follow-up examination, the survivorship estimates will be correspondingly biased. The estimates are less accurate when few patients (less than 20) are observed at a given time. The higher the percentage of patients who are still being evaluated, the more accurate the analyses.[21]

Table 20–8. ACETABULAR LOOSENING

Definite	Shift or fracture of prosthesis or cement.
Probable	Complete bone-cement radiolucency at least 2 mm wide in at least one zone.

LONG-TERM RESULTS OF CEMENTED TOTAL HIP ARTHROPLASTY

Clinical Results

The results of cemented total hip arthroplasty remain excellent for at least several years unless a significant complication occurs. When long-term follow-up has been possible, several investigators have reported worrisome radiographic findings, but clinical performance is usually good in these patients. Overall, the results of long-term studies of cemented hip replacement, even those performed with relatively unrefined operative techniques, have been remarkable for their high percentage of good and excellent clinical results and durability.

Charnley Hip Replacements

The longest follow-up for Charnley hip replacements has been reported by Wroblewski,[89] who described results 15 to 21 years after surgery in 93 patients. Their mean age was 53 years at the time of operation. At follow-up, 85 percent had no pain, and another 11 percent had only occasional discomfort. Although patient function was much improved after hip replacement, it tended to deteriorate over time, possibly because of infirmity associated with advancing age. In this series, 68 percent of the patients had nearly full motion and another 10 percent had normal motion.[89]

Older[64] reported long-term follow-up (10 to 12 years) of 153 Charnley hip replacements performed in 126 patients (survivors of an original 184 patients in whom 217 arthroplasties were performed). Of these, nine had revision arthroplasties: three for aseptic loosening (2 percent of the series), five for stem fracture (3 percent), and one for infection (less than 1 percent). At 10 to 12 years, 88 percent of the patients stated that their hip was "near perfect"; another 4 percent rated the hip as "satisfactory."

Brady and McCutchen[8] reported the results for 170 Charnley hip replacements in 145 patients followed for 10 to 13 years or until revision surgery. Revisions were required in 15 patients (9 percent). Six of the 15 revisions were performed for loosening (two of the socket, two of the femur, and two of both components). In the remaining nine patients, five revisions were performed for infections, three for broken stems, and one for dislocation.

Dall and associates[18] followed 98 patients with Charnley hip arthroplasties for a mean of 12 years. Of these, 14 patients needed revision: seven for stem fracture, four for socket loosening, two for dislocation, and one for stem loosening. The remaining 84 patients had mean ratings of 5.57 for pain, 5.35 for function, and 4.90 for motion on the Charnley scale.[18]

McCoy and colleagues[58] reported the results of Charnley hip arthroplasties in 100 patients after a mean of 15 years of follow-up—88 percent had either good (30 percent) or excellent results (58 percent). The results were lower than the 95 percent incidence of good or excellent results found at 10 years. The difference at 15 years was largely explained by three patients whose result was considered only fair, owing to general debilitation, and two others who required revision.[58]

Welch and associates[86] reported a series of 40 patients at 15 years after Charnley hip arthroplasty. They were survivors of an original series of 100 patients. Results were still excellent in 33 of the 40 and good in five. Only two patients had poor results at 15-year follow-up. The average clinical ratings on the D'Aubigne-Postel score were pain 5.7, walking 5.3, and motion 5.3.

Eftekhar and Tzitzikalakis[24] reported 5- to 15-year follow-up of 499 primary Charnley hip arthroplasties. The overall failure rate was 5 percent; 4 percent were due to mechanical causes and 0.7 percent to infection. Of the 11 mechanical failures requiring revision, five were due to stem fracture, two to stem loosening, three to socket loosening, and one to loosening of both components. Failure rates due to mechanical causes were not significantly different for primary and secondary arthroplasties. However, when failures due to infection were included, the total failure rate was almost twice as high for secondary surgery (7 versus 4 percent).

Wejkner and Stenport[84] reported the results of 325 Charnley hip replacements at 5-year and at 10- to 14-year follow-up (mean 11.7 years for the latter group). Both primary cases and revisions for failed arthroplasty or osteotomy were included. After 5 years, 86 percent of hips were rated good or excellent and 5 percent fair. In the remaining 20 cases (8 percent), the arthroplasty failed. The reasons were femoral loosening (nine cases), socket loosening (two cases), loosening of both components (one case), stem fracture (five cases), unexplained pain (two cases), and technical error (one case). At 5 years, the failure rate for secondary operations was 24 percent; for primary operations it was only 6 percent. By 10 years, another 13 arthroplasties had failed, representing an additional 5 percent of the group available for review. Patients who had lower ratings at 5 years were found to be at significantly higher risk of hip failure at 10- to 14-year follow-up. After 10 to 14 years, the average Charnley rating was 5.61 for pain, 5.81 for walking, and 5.29 for motion.

Kavanaugh and colleagues[50] reported the results of long-term follow-up in 139 surviving patients who had undergone 170 Charnley total hip replacements at least 15 years previously. The original series comprised 333 replacements in 300 patients. Of the 333 replacements performed, 37 (11 percent) required revision. The remaining 89 percent continued to function, with good or excellent results in 78 percent. The mean Harris Hip Rating was 92, and the Mayo Clinic combined clinical/radiographic score was 85. The Mayo Clinic score was lower because inclusion of the radiographic evaluation resulted in more good than excellent results. Overall

Text continued on page 328

Table 20–9. CLINICAL EVALUATION

Pain
  Degree
    ___ None—no pain
    ___ Mild—slight and occasional pain; patient has not altered patterns of activity or work.
    ___ Moderate—patient is active but has had to modify or give up some activities, or both, because of pain.
    ___ Severe—major pain and serious limitations
  Occurrence
    ___ None
    ___ With first steps, then dissipates (start-up pain)
    ___ Only after long (30-min) walks
    ___ With all walking
    ___ At all times
Work/level of activity
  Occupation (specify, including homemaker): ______________________
    Retired
      ___ No
      ___ Yes
    Nursing home
      ___ No
      ___ Yes (date entered: ____________)
  Level of activity
    ___ Bedridden or confined to a wheelchair
    ___ Sedentary—minimum capacity for walking or other activity
    ___ Semisedentary—white-collar job, bench work, light housekeeping
    ___ Light labor—heavy housecleaning, yard work, assembly line, light sports (e.g., walking $\leq$5 km)
    ___ Moderate manual labor—lifts $\leq$23 kg, moderate sports (e.g., walking or bicycling >5 km)
    ___ Heavy manual labor—frequently lifts 23–45 kg, vigorous sports (e.g., singles tennis or racquetball)

Time walked
  Without support
    ___ Unlimited (>60 min)
    ___ 31–60 min
    ___ 11–30 min
    ___ 2–10 min
    ___ <2 min or indoors only
    ___ Unable to walk
  With support
    ___ Unlimited (>60 min)
    ___ 31–60 min
    ___ 11–30 min
    ___ 2–10 min
    ___ <2 min or indoors only
    ___ Unable to walk
Satisfaction of patient
  Op. increased your function?
    ___ Yes
    ___ No
  Op. decreased your pain?
    ___ Yes
    ___ No
  Op. decreased your need for pain medication?
    ___ Yes
    ___ No
    ___ Not applicable
  Satisfied with results?
    ___ Yes
    ___ No
  Status of hip compared with your last visit?
    ___ Better
    ___ Same
    ___ Worse

Work capacity in last 3 mos.
- ___ 100%
- ___ 75%
- ___ 50%
- ___ 25%
- ___ 0

Putting on shoes and socks
- ___ No difficulty
- ___ Slight difficulty
- ___ Extreme difficulty
- ___ Unable

Ascending and descending stairs
- ___ Normal (foot over foot)
- ___ Foot over foot using banister or assistive device
- ___ 2 feet on each step
- ___ Any other method
- ___ Unable

Sitting to standing
- ___ Can arise from chair *without* upper-extremity support
- ___ Can arise *with* upper-extremity support
- ___ Cannot arise independently

Walking capacity

Usual support needed
- ___ None
- ___ 1 cane for long walks
- ___ 1 cane
- ___ 1 crutch
- ___ 2 canes
- ___ 2 crutches
- ___ Walker
- ___ Unable to walk

Physical examination

Limp *without* support
- ___ None—no limp
- ___ Slight—detected by trained observer
- ___ Moderate—detected by patient
- ___ Severe—markedly alters or slows gait

Range of motion of hip

Fixed flexion
- Left: ___°
- Right: ___°

Further flexion to
- Left: ___°
- Right ___°

Abduction/adduction
- Left: ___°/___°
- Right: ___°/___°

External/internal rotation (hip in 0° of flexion or maximum extension)
- Left: ___°/___°
- Right: ___°/___°

Trendelenburg sign

Positive
- ___ Left
- ___ Right

Negative
- ___ Left
- ___ Right

Unable to test
- ___ Left
- ___ Right

Trendelenburg lurch (abductor lurch or Duchenne sign)
- ___ Present
- ___ Absent

Limb lengths
- ___ Equal
- Short left: ___cm
- Short right: ___cm
- Method of measurement (radiograph, blocks, other): ________

Johnston, R. C., Fitzgerald, R. H., Harris, W. H., et al: J Bone Joint Surg. 72A:161–168, 1990. By permission.

Table 20–10. RADIOGRAPHIC EVALUATION: CEMENTED PROSTHESES

Acetabulum	Femur	
Migration of component (measurement must be related to teardrop) ___ No ___ Yes Superior: ___ mm Medial: ___ mm Location of center of rotation of hip relative to teardrop Superior: ___ mm Lateral: ___ mm Broken cement ___ No ___ Yes Zone (specify 1–3): ______ Cement-bone radiolucency (DeLee and Charnley) ___ No ___ Yes Maximum width Zone 1: ___ mm Zone 2: ___ mm Zone 3: ___ mm Continuous ___ No ___ Yes Maximum width: ___ mm Radiolucency around screws ___ No ___ Yes Not applicable Breakage of screws ___ No ___ Yes ___ Not applicable Wear of socket: ___ mm Position of component Inclination (abduction): ___° Version of cup Retroversion: ___° ___ Neutral Anteversion: ___°	Migration of stem Varus-valgus ___ No ___ Yes ___ Varus } qualitative only; ___ Valgus } choose one Subsidence (must be related to fixed landmarks on femur: prox. tip of greater trochanter and midpoint of lesser trochanter) ___ No ___ Yes (___ mm) ___ Within cement ___ With cement Broken cement ___ No ___ Yes Stem ___ Intact ___ Bent ___ Broken Radiolucency Prosthesis-cement (anteroposterior radiograph) ___ No ___ Yes Cement-bone Anteroposterior radiograph ___ No ___ Yes Maximum width Zone 1: ___ mm Zone 2: ___ mm Zone 3: ___ mm Zone 4: ___ mm Zone 5: ___ mm Zone 6: ___ mm Zone 7: ___ mm Lateral radiograph ___ No ___ Yes Maximum width Zone 8: ___ mm Zone 9: ___ mm Zone 10: ___ mm Zone 11: ___ mm Zone 12: ___ mm Zone 13: ___ mm Zone 14: ___ mm	Resorption of medial part of neck (calcar) ___ No ___ Yes Loss of height (exclusive of rounding): ___ mm Loss of thickness: ___ mm Resorption or hypertrophy of shaft ___ No Resorption (zones: ______) Hypertrophy (zones: ______) Change in density ___ No Patchy loss (zones: ______) Uniform loss (zones: ______) Increased trabecular bones (zones: ______) Endosteal cavitation ___ No ___ Yes Zones: ______ Length: ___ mm Width: ___ mm Ectopic ossification ___ Brooker I (none) ___ Brooker II (mild) ___ Brooker III (moderate) ___ Brooker IV (severe) Position of stem ___ Neutral ___ Valgus } qualitative only; ___ Varus } choose one Greater trochanter ___ Not osteotomized ___ Osteotomized ___ Healed ___ Not healed ___ Displaced ___ Non-displaced

Johnston, R. C., Fitzgerald, R. H., Jr., Harris, W. H., et al: J. Bone Joint Surg. 72A:161–168, 1990. By permission.

Table 20–11. RADIOGRAPHIC EVALUATION: UNCEMENTED PROSTHESES

Acetabulum

Migration of component (measurement must be related to teardrop)
- ___ No
- ___ Yes
  - Superior: ___ mm
  - Medial: ___ mm

Location of center of rotation of hip relative to teardrop
- Superior: ___ mm
- Lateral: ___ mm

Prosthesis-bone radiolucency (DeLee and Charnley)
- ___ No
- ___ Yes
  - Maximum width
    - Zone 1: ___ mm
    - Zone 2: ___ mm
    - Zone 3: ___ mm
  - Continuous
    - ___ No
    - ___ Yes
    - Maximum width: ___ mm

Radiolucency around screws
- ___ No
- ___ Yes
- ___ Not applicable

Breakage of screws
- ___ No
- ___ Yes
- ___ Not applicable

Porous coating
- ___ Intact
- ___ Dislodged
- ___ Progressive loss
- ___ Not applicable

Wear of socket: ___ mm

Position of component
- Inclination (abduction): ___°
- Version of cup
  - Retroversion: ___°
  - ___ Neutral
  - Anteversion: ___°

Femur

Migration of stem
- Varus-valgus
  - ___ No
  - ___ Yes
    - ___ Varus } qualitative only;
    - ___ Valgus } choose one
- Subsidence (must be related to fixed landmarks on femur: prox. tip of greater trochanter and midpoint of lesser trochanter)
  - ___ No
  - ___ Yes (___ mm)

Porous coating
- ___ Intact
- ___ Dislodged
- ___ Progressive loss
- ___ Not applicable

Stem
- ___ Intact
- ___ Bent
- ___ Broken

Prosthesis-bone radiolucency
- Anteroposterior radiograph
  - ___ No
  - ___ Yes
  - Maximum width
    - Zone 1: ___ mm
    - Zone 2: ___ mm
    - Zone 3: ___ mm
    - Zone 4: ___ mm
    - Zone 5: ___ mm
    - Zone 6: ___ mm
    - Zone 7: ___ mm
- Lateral radiograph
  - ___ No
  - ___ Yes
  - Maximum width
    - Zone 8: ___ mm
    - Zone 9: ___ mm
    - Zone 10: ___ mm
    - Zone 11: ___ mm
    - Zone 12: ___ mm
    - Zone 13: ___ mm
    - Zone 14: ___ mm

Resorption of medial part of neck (calcar)
- ___ No
- ___ Yes
  - Loss of height (exclusive of rounding): ___ mm
  - Loss of thickness: ___ mm

Resorption or hypertrophy of shaft
- ___ No
- Resorption (zones: ______)
- Hypertrophy (zones: ______)

Change in density
- ___ No
- Patchy loss (zones: ______)
- Uniform loss (zones: ______)
- Increased trabecular bone (zones: ______)

Endosteal cavitation
- ___ No
- ___ Yes
- Zones: ______
- Length: ___ mm
- Width: ___ mm

Ectopic ossification
- ___ Brooker I (none)
- ___ Brooker II (mild)
- ___ Brooker III (moderate)
- ___ Brooker IV (severe

Position of stem
- ___ Neutral
- ___ Valgus } qualitative only;
- ___ Varus } choose one

Greater trochanter
- ___ Not osteotomized
- ___ Osteotomized
  - ___ Healed
  - ___ Not healed
    - ___ Displaced
    - ___ Non-displaced

Johnston, R. C., Fitzgerald, R. H., Harris, W. H., et al: J. Bone Joint Surg. 72A:161–168, 1990. By permission.

Table 20–12. COMPARISON OF HIP SCORES FOR A PATIENT 10 YEARS AFTER TOTAL HIP REPLACEMENT

	Hip Score (Points)					
Rating System	***Pain***	***Function***	***Mobility***	***Motion***	***Radiographic Findings***	***Total***
D'Aubigne-Postel	6	6	—	5	—	6-6-5
Harris	44	47	4	3	—	98
Iowa	35	35	20	10	—	100
Mayo Clinic	40	20	20	—	18	98

Modified from Johnston, R. C., Fitzgerald, R. H., Jr., Harris, W. H., et al: J. Bone Joint Surg. 72A:161–168, 1990.

patient satisfaction was reported as excellent in this series. (See Table 20–13 for a summary of long-term clinical results of Charnley hip replacements.)

Other Cemented Hip Replacements

In a follow-up of 426 Exeter hip replacements, Fowler and associates[27] were able to evaluate 88 percent of patients 11 to 16 years after surgery. The remainder were lost to follow-up. The revision rate was 2 percent for loose stems, 4 percent for loose sockets, 3 percent for infection, and 5 percent for broken stems (total 14 percent). For the hips that required no revision, the mean Charnley ratings were 5.65 for pain, 4.57 for walking, and 5.06 for motion.

A report by Amstutz and colleagues[3] on hip replacements performed with the T-28 prosthesis prior to 1978 (n = 699) revealed a total revision rate of 10 percent. Of the total 69 revisions, 21 were required for femoral loosening; 14 of these involved stem fracture. A total of 14 hips were revised for acetabular loosening. The mean time between surgery and stem loosening was 7.5 years; that between surgery and acetabular loosening was 11 years. Mean clinical scores by the University of California, Los Angeles, rating system were 8.2 for pain, 7.1 for walking, 7.2 for function, and 4.9 for activity. The majority of patients in this series were over 60 years old and had declining activity due to advancing age. At 10 years postoperatively, the failure rate among survivors was 2 percent for the acetabular component and 6 percent for the stem. Excluding stem breakage, the failure rate for aseptic loosening of the stem was 2 percent. Contrary to the suggestions of other investigators,[80, 81] no indication of accelerated acetabular loosening with time was observed in this group.

Van Der Schaaf and coworkers[82] followed 83 patients who had undergone a total of 92 hip replacements with the Stanmore prosthesis at least 9 years previously. Over the 9-year period, five revisions were required, four for loosening and one for stem fracture. The survival rate of hip replacements at 9 years was 95 percent. All surviving hips had good or excellent clinical results.

The clinical results of 100 Müller curved stem hip replacements were less satisfactory. After 10 years, 25 arthroplasties had required revision. Of the remaining 53 hip replacements in surviving patients, 18 had Harris Hip Ratings of less than 80.[81] Similar poor results were reported by Pavlov,[66] who described a 15-year revision rate of 40 percent for hip replacements with the Müller prosthesis.

A study of the DF-80 prosthesis in 47 hip replacements in 40 patients was performed by Robinson and coworkers,[76] who noted early radiographic failure in ten cases (see *Radiographic Results*, discussed hereafter). The revision rate after an average follow-up of only 37 months was 4 percent. The markedly inferior clinical results in patients with Müller and DF-80 prostheses, all of whom had surgery performed by experienced surgeons, suggests that prosthesis design plays an important role in survivorship of total hip replacements (see Chapter 13, *Biomechanics and Design*).

Table 20–13. LONG-TERM CLINICAL RESULTS OF CHARNLEY TOTAL HIP ARTHROPLASTY

	Follow-up (Years)	Minimal or No Pain (%)	Revision Rate (%)
Wroblewski[89]	15–21	96	
Older[64]	10–12	92	6
Brady[8]	10–13		9
Dall[18]	12		14
McCoy[58]	10	95	
McCoy[58]	15	88	
Eftekhar[24]	5–15		5
Kavanaugh[50]	15+	78	11

Bilateral Replacement

Two groups of investigators have reported results in patients who had bilateral Charnley arthroplasties. In one study, patients had both procedures done at the same time. In the other, the average interval between arthroplasties was 9 months.

Agins and coworkers[1] reported 9- to 15-year follow-up of 178 arthroplasties performed bilaterally in one procedure from an initial series of 244. During the follow-up period, 22 revisions (12 percent) were required—five were for femoral loosening, two for socket loosening, four for loosening of both components, six for stem fracture, and five for infection. Two other patients had infections but were successfully treated by debridement. Clinical survivorship analysis, using revision for any reason as the end point, predicted 91 percent hip survival at 10 years and 76 percent hip survival at 15 years. With revision for mechanical failure as the end point, predicted survival was 97 percent at 10 years and 87 percent at 15 years.

Wejkner and Stenport,[85] reporting results for 58 patients who underwent hip arthroplasties at separate times, found an overall success rate (good and excellent results) of 92 percent at 5 years and 86 percent at 10 years. At 5 years, Charnley ratings were 5.84 for pain, 5.81 for walking, and 5.3 for motion. At 10 years, the ratings were 5.55 for pain, 5.95 for walking, and 5.32 for motion. All clinical failures were caused by fractured stems.

The arthroplasties described in the report of Agins and colleagues[1] involved five types of prostheses: Charnley, T-28, McKee-Farrar, Müller, and CAD. When the data for the various types were compared, Charnley stems performed significantly better than Müller stems, based on radiographic and revision criteria.[1]

Radiographic Results

Most investigators who have reported long-term radiographic results of cemented total hip replacements have observed interface demarcation and definite signs of prosthesis loosening, such as cement fracture and prosthesis migration. These radiographic signs have been reported in patients with clinical failure of their prostheses, as well as those with success.

In the long-term study of Charnley arthroplasties reported by Wroblewski,[89] 25 sockets (23 percent) were found to have migrated. Radiographs showed complete demarcation in 36 hips (32 percent) and demarcation less than 1 mm in the outer third (zone 1) in 20 hips (17 percent). Only 32 hips (28 percent) showed no change in bone-cement interface since surgery 15 to 21 years previously. The stem or stem-cement composite subsided in 29 percent of cases, and the cement fractured in 15 percent. Of the 17 fractures, 16 were at the tip only. The other occurred at the tip and midportion of the stem. Endosteal cavitation was found in 24 cases (21 percent)—17 at the calcar, six at the tip of the stem, and one at both sites. Loss of definition of the medial femoral neck (calcar resorption) was observed in 44 percent (Table 20–14). Polyethylene socket wear averaged 0.096 mm per year and was highly correlated with time but not with patient weight. Pointing to the relationship of socket wear to socket migration, Wroblewski suggested that the wear or penetration of the femoral head into the polyethylene socket results in progressive restriction of angular motion. Impingement of the neck of the stem on the edge of the socket causes shock loading of the prosthetic components, which may contribute to loosening (Fig. 20–3).

In Older's[64] 10- to 12-year follow-up of Charnley arthroplasties, 21 percent of the hips not requiring revision (i.e., 94 percent of the series) had medial femoral neck resorptions, but none was greater than 2 cm. Although fractured cement at the tip of the stem was observed 1 year after surgery in 21 percent of cases, no further deterioration was found. On the socket side, no demarcation was observed in 63 percent of arthroplasties; slight demarcation occurred in zone 1 in 22 percent, continuous demarcation of any width in 7 percent, and migration in 8 percent. Although Older[64] had predicted that the hips with migration might need revision, all were functioning well at long-term follow-up 10 to 12 years after surgery.

Brady and McCutchen[8] evaluated 130 hips radiographically after 10 years. In all, 29 hips had resorption of the medial calcar from 1 to 20 mm (average 5.1 mm); five hips had subsidence from 1 to 25 mm.

Table 20–14. LOSS OF HEIGHT OF THE MEDIAL FEMORAL CORTEX IN 115 CHARNLEY HIP REPLACEMENTS

Loss of Height (mm)	No.	%
0	68	58.6
>5	36	31.0
5–10	7	6.0
>10	4	3.4

Modified from Wroblewski, B. M.: Clin. Orthop. 211:30–35, 1986.

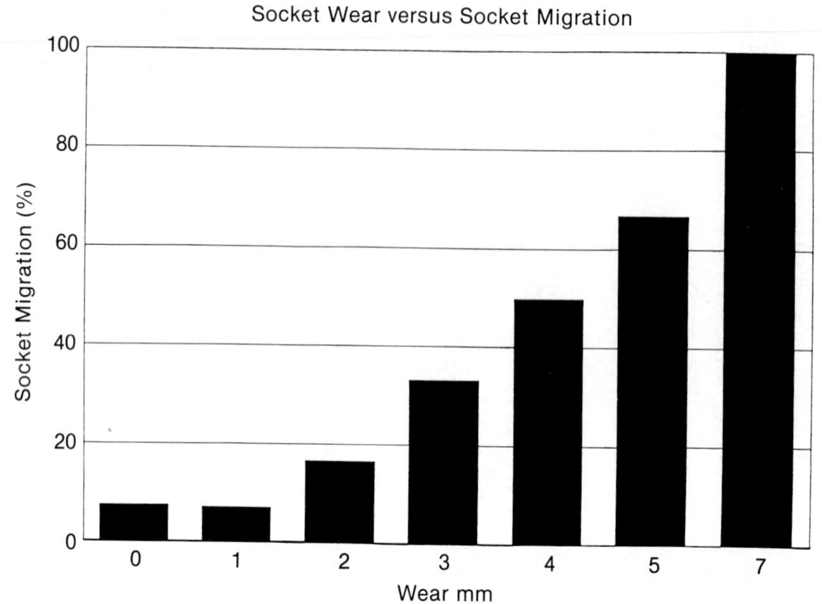

FIGURE 20–3. Socket wear versus socket migration.

Although eight hips showed continuous demarcation in all three acetabular zones, all patients were doing well clinically (Table 20–15).

Dall and coworkers[18] reviewed 84 hips radiographically and found that 36 (43 percent) had acetabular demarcation. In six of these cases (four of which had migrated), the findings were thought to be significant. Three stems had significant demarcation at the bone-cement interface and had subsided. In two of the three cases, endosteal cysts suggestive of granulomatous reaction were noted. Calcar resorption greater than 5 mm occurred in 12 hips (14 percent).

Table 20–15. CONTINUOUS ACETABULAR DEMARCATION

Patient	Degree of Lucency	Charnley Rating
1	3 mm, all three zones	6-6-5
2	1–3 mm, all three zones	3-3-2
3	1–4 mm, zones 1 and 2	6-5-5
4	1–3 mm, all three zones	6-5-5
5	1–3 mm, all three zones	6-6-5
6	1–3 mm, all three zones	6-6-5
7	1–3 mm, all three zones	5-6-6
8	1–5 mm, all three zones	6-6-5

Modified from Brady, L. P., and McCutchen, J. W.: Clin. Orthop. 211:51–54, 1986.

McCoy and colleagues[58] evaluated 30 hips radiographically 15 years after arthroplasty. On the femoral side, half (15 hips) had no interface demarcation or cement cracks. Demarcations were most common in zones 1, 4, and 7. Radiographs showed that two stems were grossly loose and had distal demarcations. Eight had cement cracks in the femur; four were found in zone 3 and four in zone 5. In the socket, ten radiographs (33 percent) showed no demarcation, 19 (63 percent) had demarcation in zone 1, ten (33 percent) in zone 2, and 14 (47 percent) in zone 3. Of these, three showed complete or nearly complete demarcation, and two had migrated. When radiographs made at 10 and 15 years were compared, only two hips showed deterioration. In one socket, demarcation in zones 1 and 2 had progressed from 1 to 2 mm, and one stem had 3 mm of subsidence.

In the review of Welch and associates,[86] radiographs indicated that two of 19 sockets were loose; 1 had migrated and the other showed complete demarcation. Two stems were loose, both having subsided, and two exhibited signs of probable loosening.

The overall failure rate of 5 percent in the 499 Charnley hip arthroplasties reported by Eftekhar and Tzitzikalakis[24] in-

Table 20–16. GRADING OF CLINICAL RESULTS IN RELATION TO RADIOGRAPHIC FINDINGS IN 140 HIPS AT THE 10-YEAR FOLLOW-UP EXAMINATION

Grade	Intact Stem and Socket *No. of Hips (%)*	Loose Stem *No. of Hips (%)*	Loose Socket *No. of Hips (%)*	Loose Stem and Socket *No. of Hips (%)*
Excellent	50(71)	31(56)	5(71)	1(13)
Good	15(21)	21(38)	2(29)	2(25)
Fair	5(7)	3(5)	—	5(63)
Total	70	55	7	8

Wejkner, B. and Stenport, J.: Clin. Orthop. 231:113–119, 1988. By permission.

cluded impending failures based on radiographic findings. These included five loose sockets and four loose stems. All loose stems occurred in secondary arthroplasties. In three cases, loose stems were replaced, and in one case conversion from arthrodesis was performed.

In their follow-up study, Wejkner and Stenport[84] employed three criteria to define femoral loosening: (1) radiolucency at least 1 mm wide and of any length between the metal and cement, (2) migration of the stem within the cement, and (3) migration of the stem-cement composite. A socket was considered loose if continuous lucency of 1 mm or more was observed in all three zones of the socket or if the socket had migrated. The number of loose components and the relationship of loosening to the clinical result are shown in Table 20–16. No statistically significant relationship was found between radiographic loosening and good and excellent results except when both components were considered loose. In that case, the quality of the clinical results fell precipitously. Within the group with loose stems, more hips were rated good than excellent compared with the groups without loose components or with loose sockets.

In the review of 333 Charnley hip replacements by Kavanaugh and colleagues,[50] probable loosening was defined as migration of the component, fracture of the cement, a radiolucent line between prosthesis and cement, or a complete radiolucent line wider than 1 mm in at least one zone. Radiographic evaluation revealed probable loosening of the acetabular component in 2 percent of cases at 1 year, 10 percent at 5 years, 12 percent at 10 years, and 14 percent at 15 years. For the same time intervals, probable loosening rates for the femoral components were in order 6, 15, 23, and 38 percent. Other investigators have suggested that loosening increases dramatically with time and that increased loosening of the acetabular component and decreased loosening of the femoral component are found over time. Previous reports from the Mayo Clinic have also suggested this.[80, 81] These suggestions were not borne out in the series reported by Kavanaugh and colleagues or that reported by Amstutz and associates.[3, 50] Kaplan-Meier survivorship analysis for various criteria, with failure defined as revision or clinical symptoms associated with probable radiographic loosening, is shown in Table 20–17.

Table 20–17. KAPLAN-MEIER PERCENT PROBABILITY ANALYSIS

Length of Follow-Up (Years)	Revision	Failure	Probable Loosening *Socket*	*Femur*
1	0.6	0.9	0.3	2.8
5	3.5	4.1	1.6	12.1
10	7.6	8.9	3.5	16.6
15	10.9	12.7	8.5	2.6

Kavanaugh, B. F., Dewitz, M. A., Ilstrup, D. M., et al.: J. Bone Joint Surg. 71A:1496–1503, 1989. By permission.

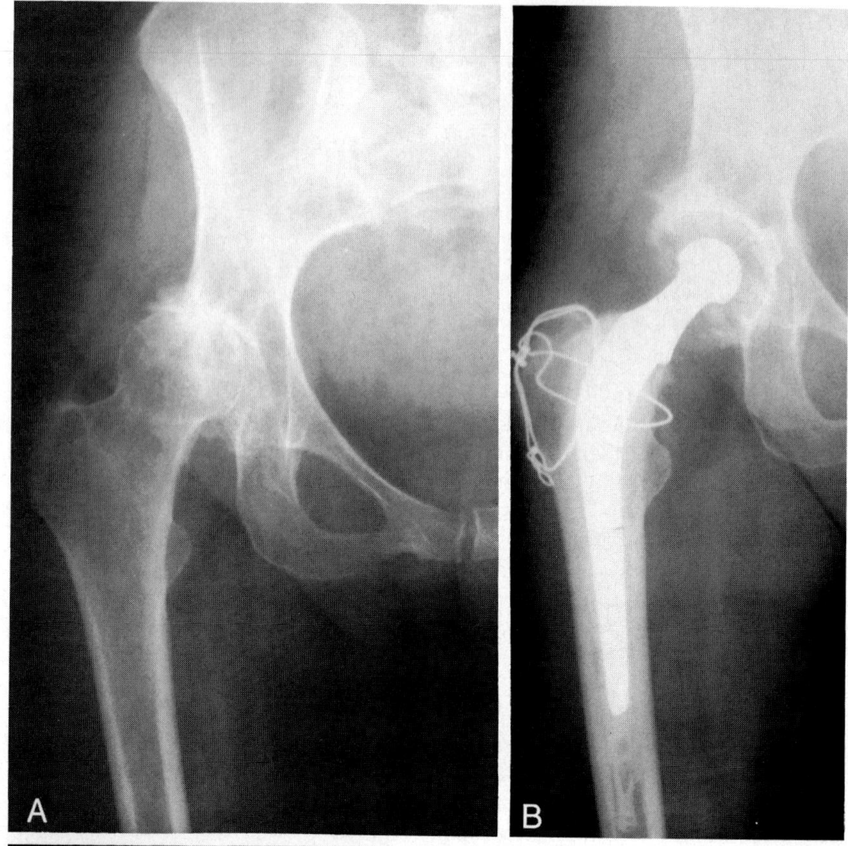

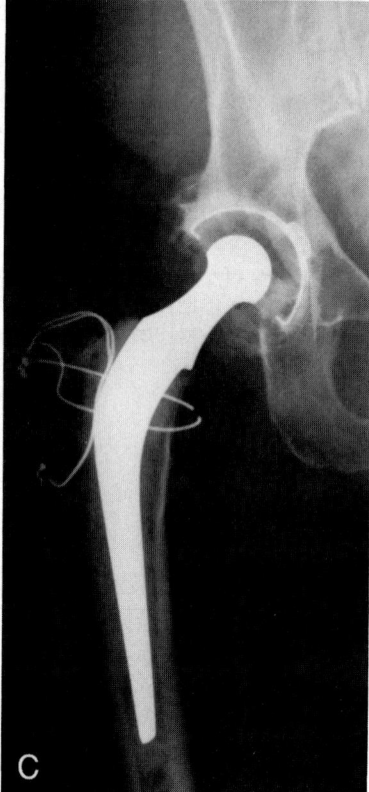

FIGURE 20–4. Charnley total hip arthroplasty successful for 15 years. *A*, Preoperative radiograph. *B*, Radiograph 6 months postoperatively. *C*, Radiograph 15 years postoperatively. No acetabular migration or demarcation has occurred. On the femoral side, osteopenia has increased. Iowa Hip Rating is 96.

Table 20–18. LONG-TERM RADIOGRAPHIC RESULTS OF CHARNLEY TOTAL HIP ARTHROPLASTY

		Socket		Femur			
	Follow-Up (Years)	*Migration* (%)	*Complete Demarcation* (%)	*Subsidence* (%)	*Stem Fracture* (%)	*Cement Fracture* (%)	*Calcar Resorption* (%)
Wroblewski[89]	15–21	23	32	29	*	15	44
Older[64]	10–12	8	7	2	3	21	21
Brady[8]	10	3	6	7	2	*	22
Dall[18]	12	4	6	4	7	27	14
McCoy[58]	15	7	3	7	*	*	*

*Information not given.

Stauffer[80] performed radiographic analysis on 231 of this same original group of 333 hips after 10 years and reported stem fractures in five hips (2 percent). Socket wear was not viewed as a significant problem. Calcar resorption of 1 to 9 mm was observed in 32 hips (14 percent) but was not related to loosening. Cement cracks occurred in 18 hips (8 percent), 16 of which progressed to gross loosening. Stauffer considered this an ominous sign. However, both Wroblewski[89] and Older[64] noted that cement cracks in the area of the stem tip of the Charnley prosthesis did not progress to failure during long-term follow-up (Fig. 20–4). (See Table 20–18 for a summary of the long-term radiographic results of Charnley hip replacements.)

In the 11- to 16-year follow-up of 426 Exeter hip replacements reported by Fowler and associates,[27] 21 percent had bone-cement radiolucency in zone 1 and 6 percent in zone 2. Calcar resorption of 1 to 7 mm was observed in 16 percent of cases, endosteal erosion in 8 percent, and diaphyseal hypertrophy in 29 percent. Cement cracks occurred in 20 percent of the hips, three fourths of them distally. Wear of polyethylene of 2 mm or less was found in 24 percent of the replacements. These radiographic findings did not correlate with inferior clinical results nor did migration of the stem distally from 1 to 10 mm, which occurred in 24 percent of cases (not a bad sign with this prosthesis design).

In the review of 699 T-28 hip arthroplasties by Amstutz and coworkers,[3] radiographs of two unrevised acetabular components showed migration and eight showed continuous demarcation. Hips with socket loosening tended to have more eccentric cement mantles, with the cement thicker in zone 3. This finding was associated with less bone coverage of the component. The use of large cement fixation holes (1.5 cm in diameter) was associated with better results than those with smaller holes, although other surgeons have documented excellent longevity of cemented acetabular fixation with small cement fixation holes (6 mm).[3, 24] Eight femoral components required revision, but another eight showed definite loosening, with subsidence of 7 to 8 mm. In addition, eight other femoral components showed 50 percent lucency, with at least a portion of the line wider than 1 mm. The progression of lucencies in this series is summarized in Table 20–19.[3]

In the series of 83 Stanmore cemented

Table 20–19. CEMENT-BONE LUCENCIES ON THE FEMORAL AND ACETABULAR SIDES (%)

Femoral Lucencies (>1 mm) in any Segment of Bone			Acetabular Lucencies (>1 mm)			Acetabular Lucencies (>2 mm)		
Zone	*5 Years*	*10 Years*	*Zone*	*5 Years*	*10 Years*	*Zone*	*5 Years*	*10 Years*
1	3.7	7.0	1	4.4	17.5	1	4.2	9.8
2	3.7	4.7	2	2.9	10.2	2	1.7	5.1
3	0.7	1.2	3	11.6	17.5	3	5.1	13.9
4	2.2	2.3						
5	2.2	4.7						
6	2.9	5.8						
7	0	3.5						

Amstutz, H. C., Yao, J., Dorey, F. J., et al: Orthop. Clin. North Am. 19:491–503, 1988. By permission.

hip replacements reviewed after a minimum of 9 years' follow-up, five revisions were performed. In patients not requiring revisions, one acetabular component (1.2 percent) migrated, and five femoral components (5 percent) subsided. None of these patients had significant clinical symptoms.[82]

Sarmiento and coworkers[78a] compared the results of total hip arthroplasties performed with the Charnley prosthesis, curved titanium alloy stems, and straight titanium alloy stems. The series were not comparable, however, because the Charnley procedures began 5 years before the titanium alloy series, and the female-to-male ratio was higher among patients receiving the straight titanium alloy stems. However, results were excellent with all three types of prostheses. Eleven-year survival rates of hip prostheses, based on radiographic criteria, were 92 percent for the Charnley prosthesis, 93 percent for the curved titanium stem, and 96 percent for the straight titanium stem. Titanium stems were associated with less calcar resorption and distal hypertrophy but a highly significant increase in bone-cement interface lucency compared with the Charnley prosthesis. Based on this criterion, prosthetic survival was 74 percent for the Charnley prosthesis, 37 percent for the curved titanium stem, and 34 percent for the straight titanium stem.

In the previously reported study of Müller hip replacements by Sutherland and coworkers,[81] in which the revision rate was 25 percent and Harris Hip Ratings were below 80 in 18 percent of cases, migration was observed in 23 percent of acetabular components and 28 percent of femoral components. In addition, a 4 percent incidence of osteolytic defects was reported in the femurs without migration. The overall loosening rate, combining revisions and radiographic findings, was 29 percent for the acetabulum and 40 percent for the femur. Loosening of the femoral component was positively correlated with heavier weight, male sex, varus position of the component, younger age, and wide femoral canal. As in Stauffer's study from the Mayo Clinic,[80] the femoral loosening rate decreased with time, whereas the acetabular loosening rate appeared to increase.

In his series of Charnley-Müller hip replacements, in which the revision rate was 40 percent, Pavlov[66] reported migration of 22 percent of acetabular components and 18 percent of femoral components after 15 years.

In the relatively short follow-up (average 37 months) of hip replacements with the DF-80 prosthesis, 23 percent of stems had subsided and 49 percent had extensive radiolucent bone-cement demarcation lines, indicating probable loosening of the femoral component (Fig. 20–5). Loosening was correlated with increased neck offset of the prosthesis, male sex, and tall stature. The investigators suggested that this early loosening was due to the design of the prosthesis and the use of material that created excessive proximal loading.[76]

Results with Modern Cementing Technique

Design concepts and surgical techniques for cemented total hip replacements have evolved throughout the 1970s and 1980s. "Modern" designs for cemented total hip prostheses include a relatively straight stem; a femoral cross-sectional geometry based on a broad medial border with a broader lateral border; a high-strength superalloy; and an avoidance of sharp borders or edges, which act as stress risers to the bone cement. On the acetabular side, modern design includes metal backing and cement spacers to provide a consistent, uniform cement mantle. In many designs, an extended acetabular roof and a lip enhance pressurization during socket insertion. Other important developments include improved delivery of cement to the bone as a result of thorough cleansing of blood clots and other debris from the interstices of bone, plugging of the femoral canal, retrograde delivery of cement into the canal, pressurization of the cement, and, more recently, reduction of cement voids by centrifugation or vacuum mixing. Femoral components with better material properties and the improvements in cement delivery were developed during the 1970s, and long-term assessments of these improvements are now available.

Poss and coworkers[66] compared the results of total hip arthroplasty utilizing the T-28 prosthesis with and without modern ce-

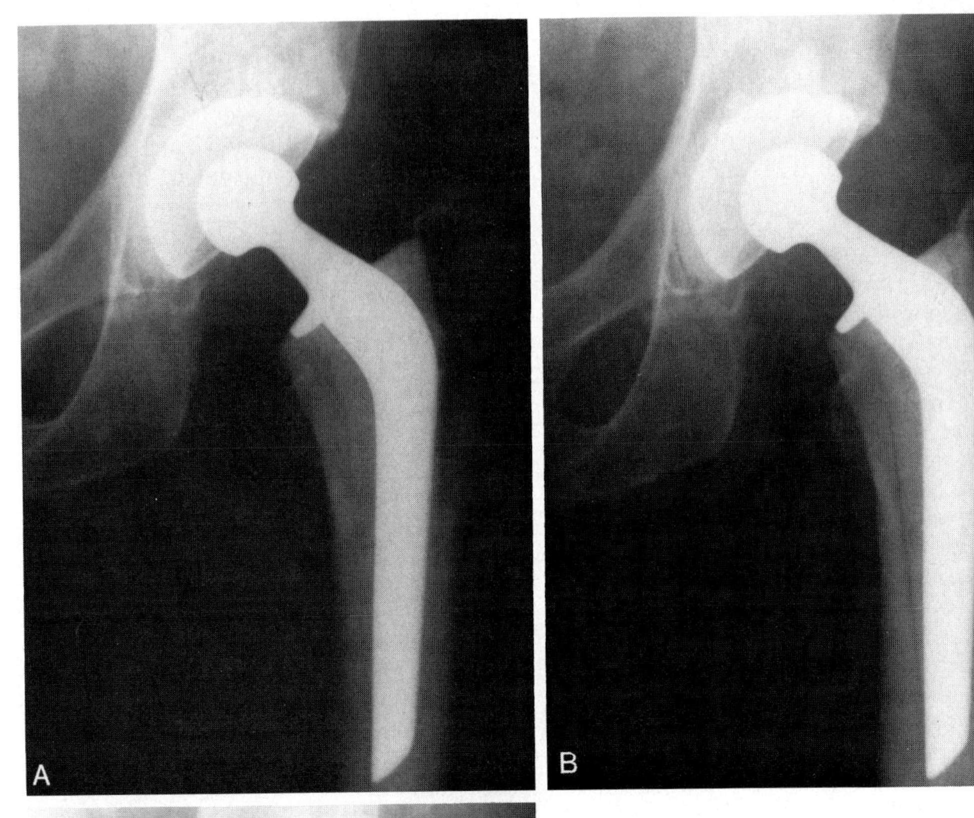

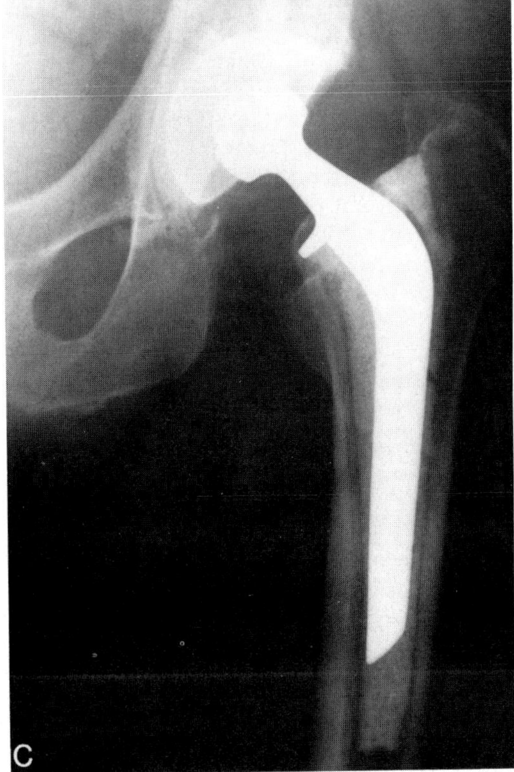

FIGURE 20–5. Postoperative radiographs of DF-80 prosthesis. *A*, Radiograph 1 week postoperatively. *B*, Radiograph 6 months postoperatively. *C*, Radiograph at 3 years showing loose cement stem composite with cement fracture. (Robinson, R.P., Lovell, T.P., Green, T.M., and Bailey, G.A.: J. Arthroplasty 4: 55–64, 1989. By permission.)

ment techniques.[69, 75] Mean follow-up was 4 years. Patients were matched for length of follow-up, diagnosis, height, weight, activity level, and use of assistive devices. "Modern techniques" included canal plugging, curettage of loose bone, and pressure-pulsed lavage of the bone surfaces. Based on the criteria of Harris and colleagues,[40] 21 percent of femoral components were definitely loose in the group with early cementing technique and less than 1.6 percent were possibly loose, whereas none were probably or definitely loose with "modern" cementing techniques. In the group that involved early cementing, when the initial postoperative radiographs showed inadequate cementation in one or two zones, the loosening rate was 6 percent; in three zones, 17 percent; and in four or more zones, 66 percent. Cement mantle adequacy seemed especially important in zone 4 (at the distal tip of the prosthesis); 66 percent of femoral components that loosened had inadequate cementation in zone 4. Cement homogeneity was also important, as 35 percent of the entire early group and 66 percent of those that loosened had poor cement homogeneity ($P<0.05$). More active patients younger than 45 years and weighing over 90 kg (200 lb) in Charnley Group A or B had higher rates of failure on 11- to 16-year follow-ups. All had early cementing techniques.[69, 75]

Ranawat and coworkers[71] compared the results of socket installation with early and modern techniques. The latter included the following: preservation of superior subchondral bone, multiple drill holes for cement penetration into the cancellous bone, cleansing of the bone with pressure-pulsed lavage, cement in the low viscosity state, and cement pressurization. No sockets were revised after 5 years, although socket migration occurred in 8 percent of hips from the early group. None of the arthroplasties in which modern techniques had been used exhibited migration. The radiolucency score was significantly inferior in the early cement group.

Harris and McGann[41] reported the results of total hip replacements performed using a canal plug, a retrograde cement delivery with a syringe, and a chromium-cobalt superalloy stem with a collar. Minimum follow-up was 5 years. One femoral component had been revised and one was definitely loose, for a total loosening rate of 1.7 percent. Two other components showed radiographic findings of probable loosening.

Russotti and associates[77] reviewed the clinical and radiographic results of 251 consecutive cemented total hip arthroplasties. Procedures were performed with pressure-pulsed lavage, a canal plug, retrograde cement delivery with a syringe, a chromium-cobalt high strength stem with a collar, and four different acetabular components, 87 percent of which were all polyethylene. After 5 to 7 years, 98 percent of hips showed excellent results, with an average Harris Hip Rating of 97 points. Three definitely loose femoral stems (1.2 percent), two probably loose, and one possibly loose, as well as one loose acetabular component, were reported. No revisions were performed (Table 20–20).

None of these reports involved the adoption of the innovations of the 1980s. These include cement pressurization, cement centrifugation or vacuum mixing, acetabular cement spacers, and cement fixation enhancement by precoating with bone cement or a macrotextured or microtextured surface on the prosthetic components. These additional measures may further improve the quality and longevity of cemented total hip replacements.

Table 20–20. RESULTS OF MODERN CEMENTING TECHNIQUES

		Socket			Femur		
	Follow-up (Years)	*Probable Loosening (%)*	*Definite Loosening (%)*	*Revision (%)*	*Probable Loosening (%)*	*Definite Loosening (%)*	*Revision (%)*
Harris[41]	5–8		0.8	0.8			
Poss[69, 75]	4	0	0	0	0	0	0
Ranawat[71]	5	0	0	0			
Russotti[77]	5–7	0	0.4	0	0.8	1.2	0

Results in Young Individuals

Large series of total hip replacements usually include patients younger than age 55, sometimes substantially younger. Some of these series report the results in different age groups. In addition, numerous investigations have specifically evaluated the results of total hip arthroplasties in younger individuals.

In patients under 45 years of age, White[87] found that 14 percent of hips required revision, whereas 80 percent of total hip replacements were excellent clinically 5 to 10 years after surgery. Radiographic appearance was not as good, with 34 percent of acetabular components and 25 percent of femoral components requiring revision or showing definite signs of loosening. Results were better in patients with osteoarthritis than in those with rheumatoid arthritis. The worst prognostic indicator was return to heavy manual labor, with arthroplasty failing in all six patients who did so.

In the long-term follow-up study of T-28 prostheses reported by Amstutz and coworkers,[3] patients aged 40 to 65 did as well as the entire group, but those younger than 40 at the time of operation had a markedly higher revision rate than the group as a whole. The failure rate was higher with individuals who continued to engage in high level activity or impact sports. Estimated failure rates for patients younger than 55 years were 9 and 21 percent at 5 and 10 years, respectively, compared with failure rates of 3.1 and 4.4 percent for those older than 55.

Chandler and coworkers[12] reported a 21 percent revision rate and an additional 36 percent impending failure rate after 5 years in patients younger than age 30. Results were better after an average follow-up of almost 10 years in the series of 49 Charnley total hip replacements reported by Halley and Wroblewski[36]; 80 percent of them were in patients with inflammatory arthritis. Although 14 percent of sockets failed, 28.6 percent had minimal demarcation in zone 1 only, and 53 percent showed no socket demarcation. Two femoral components failed, two subsided less than 2 mm, two had fractured cement at the tip, and two had cystic changes. All these changes stabilized, and the patients were doing well clinically. Polyethylene wear in younger patients was only slightly greater than that in older patients, averaging 1.7 mm at 10 years.[36]

Dorr and coworkers[23] reported a 19 percent revision rate and a total failure rate, including impending failure, of 45 percent. Nonetheless, 72 percent of hips were still satisfactory clinically after 5 years in patients aged 14 to 45 at the time of operation. Patients younger than 30 years and those with osteonecrosis had a worse prognosis, whereas those with collagen disease had a better prognosis. Sharp and Porter[79] reported that ten of 79 hip replacements in patients under age 40 required revision for loosening after an average follow-up of 6.6 years. Six other hips required surgery for trochanteric repair, and four others were judged loose radiographically. The failure rate was higher in patients with rheumatoid arthritis than in those with other diagnoses.[79]

Ranawat and coworkers[70] reported good or excellent clinical results in 90 percent of 103 cemented hip replacments 5 to 10 years after surgery in patients 40 to 60 years old. Nine femoral revisions were performed, eight for stem fracture and one for loosening. Two of the three acetabular revisions were done in association with femoral revision in sockets with complete demarcation. The other acetabular revision was for migration. Eight other sockets had migrated but had stabilized and were asymptomatic. The overall acetabular loosening rate was 9.7 percent, including those cases that required revision. The total loosening rate for the femoral component, including isolated lucencies in ten hips, was 29.9 percent. The definite loosening rate, including hips with subsidence and fractured stems, was 15.5 percent. When revision for any reason or radiographic evidence of migration of a component was the criterion for failure, the predicted survivorship of the hip replacement was 87.6 percent at 10 years.[17, 70]

Five to 11 years after surgery, Collis[15, 16] evaluated 45 cemented total hip replacements in patients under age 50. The average Iowa Hip Rating was 91.9 points, and the total revision rate was 8.9 percent. After a minimum follow-up of 10 years, the revision rate was 19.6. The majority of revisions were performed because of stem fracture, a problem that should be rare when superalloy prostheses are used. Collis attributed the success in his series in part to repeated admonition to avoid running, jumping, heavy labor, and lifting of more than 18 kg. This investigator found excessive body weight and heavy physical activity to be common among patients whose replacements failed.

In summary, total hip arthroplasty provides satisfactory results in patients older than 40 years if they are not overly active. It is anticipated that the improved results in cemented total hip arthroplasty will be reflected in these younger patients when longer-term results become available. Most total hip replacements in patients under the age of 60 years are now performed with cementless devices. It will be many years before we know if durability is better than or even equal to that seen with cemented hip replacments. Patients under age 40 and especially those under age 30 are less likely to have reasonably durable successful hip replacements; therefore, the procedure should be done rarely in this age group. However, total hip replacements may be indicated in very young patients with severe functional disability due to juvenile rheumatoid arthritis, because replacements may provide marked functional improvement. Even among these patients with relatively low activity levels, however, the complication rate is high.[34, 62]

RESULTS OF MODERN CEMENTLESS TOTAL HIP ARTHROPLASTY

Clinical Results

Although cementless total hip replacements have become very popular, composing perhaps half of all total hip replacements worldwide, data on early results with these prostheses are limited. Of course, no long-term information is available about the results of arthroplasty with modern cementless prostheses.

Porous Coated Cementless Prostheses

Cameron[10] evaluated Matchett Brown prostheses with a powder coating having an average pore size of 50 μm. Three years after hemiarthroplasties without acetabular reconstruction for fracture of the femoral neck or osteonecrosis of the femoral head, four hips required revision and 11 patients had slight or mild pain. The average Harris Hip Ratings were excellent in three, good in four, fair in six, and poor in seven.

Engh and coworkers[25, 26] reported the evaluation of total hip replacement with the Anatomic Medullary Locking stem in 307 patients after 2 years and 89 patients after 5 years. All stems were fully or two-thirds coated with a powder-made sintered porous surface. D'Aubigne-Postel average ratings were 5.8 for pain and 5.6 for walking. Pain, usually intermittent and mild, was present in 14 percent of patients, and limp was present in 21 percent. Patients judged to have good quality bone were less likely to have pain (11 percent) than those with poor quality bone (26 percent). Both pain and limp were less likely in reconstruction with a good stem fit in the femur. No evidence of significant deterioration in clinical results was apparent between the 2- and 5-year evaluations.

Hedley and coworkers[42] reported incidences of thigh pain in 4 percent and limp in 5 percent of 118 arthroplasties with Porous Coated Anatomic (PCA) prostheses. Revision had been necessary for one hip and was planned for a second. In the report of Callaghan and coworkers[9] on 50 PCA prostheses 2 years after surgery, the mean Harris Hip Rating was 92 points. Eighteen percent of the patients complained of mild thigh pain at 1 year and 16 percent at 2 years. Limp, present after 2 years in 28 percent of hips, was attributed in part to the direct lateral approach. After 2 years, 11 percent of patients still require a cane.

After a minimum 2-year follow-up, Kavanaugh and colleagues[50] reported that 97 percent of 102 hip replacements with PCA prostheses had good or excellent results. One hip had been revised, and another was scheduled for revision. In addition to those patients who required revisions, 22 percent complained of slight pain and 45 percent had a slight limp.

Vaughn and Mallory[83] reported a femoral revision rate of 14 percent for 50 PCA hip replacements with a minimum follow-up of 2 years. The average Harris Hip Rating was 84 points. Thigh pain was present in 37 percent, limp in 52 percent, and need for a cane in 25 percent. No clinical problems related to the acetabular component were apparent. Results were better in patients younger than 50 years as well as those in whom the femoral canal was filled well with the prosthesis.

In a 2-year follow-up involving 129 hips with HGP prostheses, moderate pain was present in 2 percent and moderate or severe limp in 4 percent. Intraoperative fractures or perforations occurred in 7 percent of cases. Three revisions (2.3 percent) of femoral components took place.[30, 68]

Gustilo and colleagues[35] found that patients had an average Harris Hip Rating of 92 points 5 to 7 years after hip replacement with a long stem femoral prosthesis with titanium fiber mesh pads placed proximally. The femoral component revision rate was 2.9 percent, the acetabulum revision rate was 8.9 percent, and the revision rate for bipolar components was 3.1 percent. Thigh pain was present in 5 percent of hips (Table 20–21).

In an attempt to solve the problem of stress shielding, Morrey[61] developed a short-stemmed prosthesis, which has been placed in 20 hips. With 1-year follow-up, he has performed one revision for loosening. Rehabilitation has been slower than that with conventional prostheses, but thigh pain has not been a problem.

Comparative Studies

Mikhail and coworkers[60] studied the results of Exeter cemented total hip replacement and PCA replacement after 2 to 4 years. Patients were satisfied with 100 percent of the cemented replacements and with 88 percent of the PCA replacements. Persistent thigh pain was present in 37 percent of the cementless PCA hip replacements. Bourne and colleagues[7] found slower rehabilitation with the PCA prostheses than with the cemented HD2 replacements, with 11 percent of the patients with the PCA prostheses complaining of thigh pain after 2 years. Petty[67] compared the results of 48 PCA hip replacements and 50 conventional cemented replacements after 2 years. In the group having uncemented arthroplasty, pain was present in 30 percent; pain was mild in 21 percent, and moderate in 9 percent. Limp persisted in 32 percent. In the group having cemented arthroplasty, 9 percent complained of mild pain and 4 percent limped. Although patients having cemented arthroplasty discarded walking aids earlier, the use of walking aids was similar in the two groups 1 year after surgery.

Ritter and Campbell[74] simultaneously implanted bilateral total hip prostheses in six patients. A conventional cemented stem was implanted on one side and a cementless porous polyethylene-coated titanium stem on the other. Cemented sockets were utilized on both sides. Patients preferred the cemented stems because they resulted in less pain and no limp.

Nonporous Surfaced Prostheses

Numerous prostheses are available for cementless use that do not provide for porous ingrowth. Instead, they have a rough surface for macrointerlock, a superficially rough surface, or a smooth surface.

O'Leary and coworkers[65] evaluated the results of 69 hip replacements with the Mittelmeier ceramic prosthesis, a design for macrointerlock. Although most patients were improved after an average fol-

Table 20–21. CLINICAL RESULTS OF MODERN POROUS COATED CEMENTLESS TOTAL HIP ARTHROPLASTY

	Follow-Up (Years)	Pain (%)	Limp (%)	Prosthesis	Revision (%)	
					Socket	*Femur*
Callaghan[9]	2	16	28	PCA	None reported	
Engh[25]	2–5	14	21	AML	None reported	
Galante[30]	2	2	4	HG	None reported	2
Gustilo[35]	5–7	5		Bias	None reported	3
Hedley[42]	2	4	5	PCA	None reported	2
Kavanaugh[50]	2	22	45	PCA	None reported	2
Vaughn[83]	2	37	52	PCA	None reported	14

low-up of 3 years, 25 percent of patients with surviving hips had mild pain and 84 percent of patients had limps. Revision was necessary in 19 hips (27 percent).

Jantsch and coworkers[45] reported that some patients complained of thigh pain for several months after hip replacement with the shaft system of Zweymüller, a stem with a rough, nonporous surface. They attributed these complaints, at least in part, to unrecognized fractures that occurred during surgery. In 5-year follow-up, Lord and Bancel[56] reported good or excellent results in 83 percent of hips with the Madreporic prosthesis.

The Ring uncemented plastic-on-metal prosthesis consists of a single-pegged, all-polyethylene offset conical cup available in four sizes and a straight-stemmed nonporous femoral component available in three sizes.[73] In a 2- to 7-year follow-up of 1402 total hip replacements with this prosthesis, Nunn[63] reported average Charnley ratings of 5.86 for pain, 5.96 for function, and 5.9 for motion. The revision rate was 1.5 percent. Clinical results were excellent in 93 percent of the entire group and in 87 percent of patients followed for at least 5 years. Using survivorship analysis, Nunn[63] predicted survival of 96.4 percent of hip replacements at 6 years.

Two groups of investigators have compared clinical results after implanting similar stems with and without proximal porous coatings. Levy and colleagues[55] reported comparable results with these two stem variations after 2 to 4 years. Hupfer and coworkers[43a] found that revision was necessary in 11 stems (32 percent) without porous coating and in only 1 stem (3 percent) with porous coating after an average follow-up of 4 years.

Polymer Prostheses

In an effort to reduce the stiffness of femoral stems, some surgeons have used polymer-coated prostheses. Griffin and Engh[32] reported that porous polysulfone-coated stems failed to provide consistent painless, stable fixation. By contrast, Andrew and coworkers[3a] reported satisfactory results in 92 percent of 400 hip replacements with the Isoelastic Prosthesis. This prosthesis system consists of a femoral component made from acetal-copolymer with a steel or titanium core and a pegged socket. The all-polyethylene design allows for supplemental screw fixation. The revision rate was 0.8 percent, and the average Harris Hip Rating was 87 points at an average follow-up of 28 months.

Jakim and colleagues[44] reported less favorable results using the Isoelastic Prosthesis. After an average follow-up of 42 months, 11 hips (32 percent) had been revised, and 16 (69 percent) of the remaining hips had poor Mayo Clinic scores. Only two hips (9 percent) were rated as good.

Radiographic Results

In a review of radiography an average of 21.8 months after surgery in 85 asymptomatic hips replaced with porous-surfaced prostheses, Kaplan and colleagues[49] found a variety of phenomena, listed here in decreasing order of frequency: (1) remodeling of the proximal medial edge of the cut femoral neck (rounding off) (98 percent); (2) linear lucency with a radiodense margin at the prosthesis-bone interface, which might increase in length or width over time (79 percent); (3) new bone formation at the prosthesis tip (36 percent); (4) heterotopic bone (24 percent); (5) cortical hypertrophy in the area of the stem tip (12 percent); (6) prosthesis subsidence or migration (7 percent); (7) evidence of intraoperative fracture (7 percent); and (8) periosteal reaction (4 percent). At the time of review, these findings could not be correlated with symptoms (Table 20–22). In Cameron's[10] study evaluating the results of porous-coated Matchett Brown prostheses, 50 percent of those that had not

Table 20–22. RADIOGRAPHIC FINDINGS OF POROUS SURFACED CEMENTLESS TOTAL HIP REPLACEMENT (%)

Finding	%
Rounding off of femoral neck	98
Linear lucency with radiodense margin at the prosthesis-bone interface, which may increase in length or width with time	79
New bone formation at the prosthesis tip	36
Heterotopic bone	24
Cortical hypertrophy in the area of the stem tip	12
Prosthesis subsidence or migration	7
Evidence of intraoperative fracture	7
Periosteal reaction	4

been revised developed a radiolucent line and a dense line of bone around the prosthesis by 1 year. These findings were not correlated with symptoms.

Engh and colleagues[25] determined that 259 implants with the Anatomic Medullary Locking stem (84 percent) had bone ingrowth. Fixation by bone ingrowth was defined as an implant without subsidence and without a radiopaque line. Stable fibrous ingrowth, defined as no progressive migration (although migration may have occurred) and a radiopaque line around the prosthesis associated with a radiolucency no wider than 1 mm, was seen in 42 implants (13 percent). These radiographic definitions of bone and fibrous ingrowth correlated with histology in 11 cases (Fig. 20–6). In a later survivorship analysis, Engh and Massin[26] estimated survival for stable fixation as 94 percent at 5 years and 88 percent at 8 years. No stems judged to have adequate fit in the femoral canal failed fixation, but 17 stems considered undersized migrated and 2 stems fractured.

In this group of fully and two-thirds porous-coated stems, bone remodeling was evaluated in 16 locations on the anteroposterior and lateral radiographs (Fig. 20–7). Stress shielding was classified on the basis of bone resorption or decrease in density: *First Degree*: Proximal medial edge rounding of cut femoral neck. *Second Degree*: Proximal medial edge rounding of femoral neck and loss of medial cortical density in level 1. *Third Degree*: More extensive loss of cortical density in level 1 and medial loss of cortical density in level 2. *Fourth Degree*: Loss of cortical density below levels 1 and 2. Of the 307 hips evaluated, 152 had no or first-degree stress shielding and 119 had second-degree, 23 had third-degree, and 13 had fourth-degree. Stress shielding was more extensive and severe in larger and thus stiffer stems and when the porous coating extended more distally on the stem. Although third- and fourth-degree resorption may be cause for concern for the future durability of the prosthesis, at the time of review resorption could not be correlated with symptoms.[25, 26]

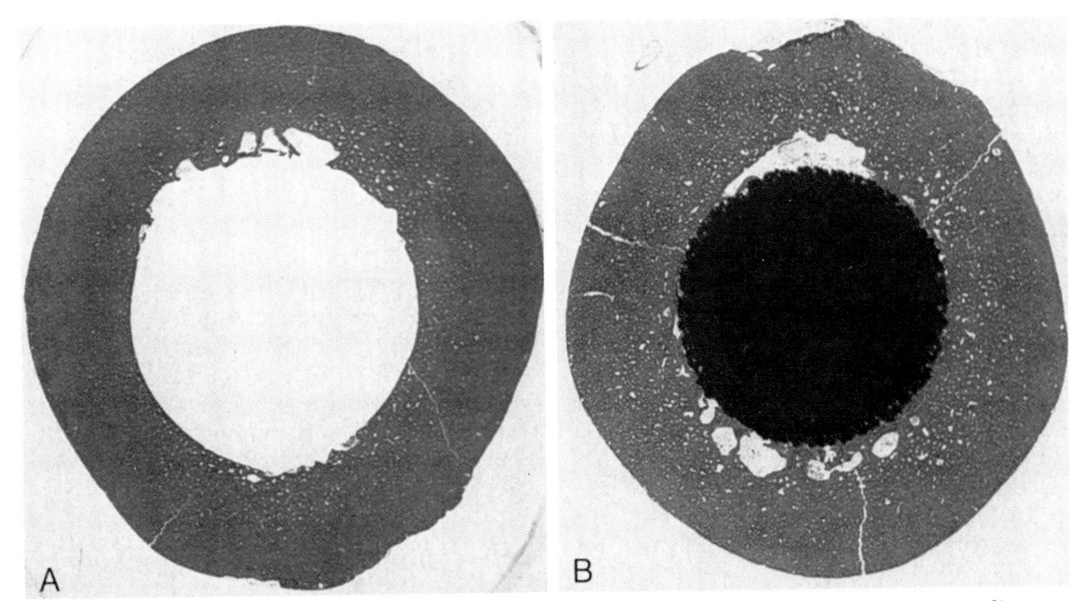

FIGURE 20–6. Post-mortem histologic sections retrieved 7 months after operation with a 16.5-mm diameter, cobalt chrome alloy stem on one side. The cortical thickness and density of both femora are similar. Bone ingrowth fixation is evident. More cortical osteopenia has occurred on the implanted side. *A*, Femoral cross-section without implant. *B*, Femoral cross-section with porous coated implant. (Engh, C.A., Bobyn, J.D., and Glassman, A.H.: J. Bone Joint Surg. 69B: 45–55, 1987. By permission.)

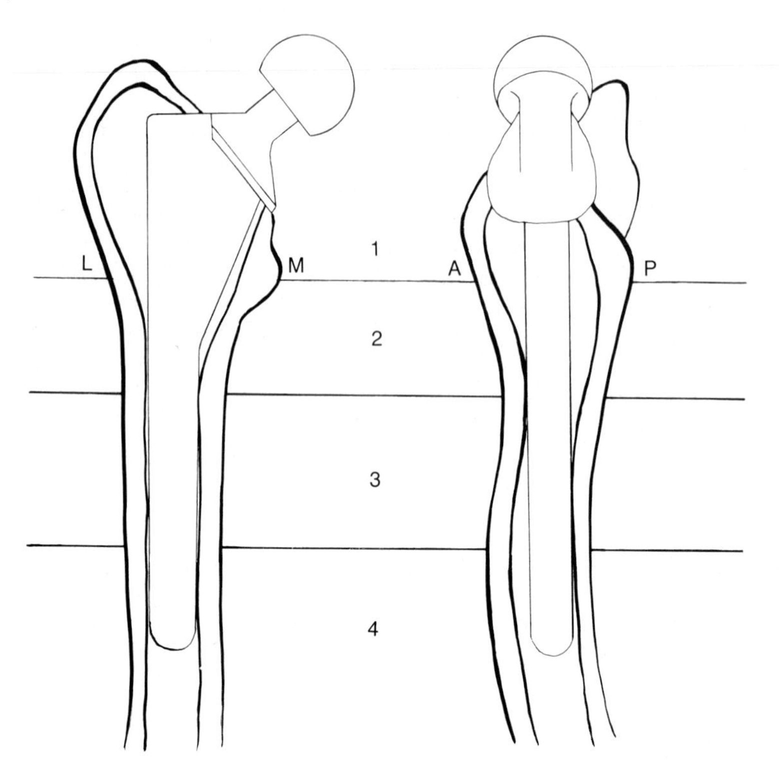

FIGURE 20–7. Schematic division of the femur into four levels for studying bone remodeling. At each level, the medial (M), lateral (L), anterior (A), and posterior (P) sites were examined for thickening or thinning and for radiographic evidence of increased or decreased bone density adjacent to the implant. (Engh, C.A., Bobyn, J.D., and Glassman, A.H.: J. Bone Joint Surg. 69B: 45–55, 1987. By permission.)

In a review of PCA hip replacements, Callaghan and coworkers[9] found a radiodense femoral line in 20 hips (41 percent) and a progressive acetabular line in 4 hips (8 percent). One femoral and one acetabular component migrated. Hedley and associates[42] found incomplete radiolucencies in 65 percent of the femoral and 52 percent of the acetabular components. Five femoral components subsided, and no sockets migrated.

Zweymüller and coworkers[90] reported excellent radiographic and histologic appearance with the rough but nonporous surfaced press-fit titanium shaft prosthesis in a few cases but provided no analysis of a series of cases. In Nunn's[63] review of a large number of Ring uncemented total hip replacements, radiographic analysis revealed a dense bony outline around the socket in most cases. Erosions around the peg were seen in 1.3 percent of hips. On the femoral side, subsidence occurred in 1 percent and demarcation in 7 percent.[63]

Bead shedding of powder-made sintered porous-surfaced prostheses and fiber mesh pad separation may occur from the acetabular and femoral components of hip prostheses (Fig. 20–8). These changes, probably associated with some degree of prosthesis looseness, may become increasingly common with time, at least with some prostheses. No correlation with increased symptoms has been reported. The potential long-term effects of abrasion or ion release under these conditions are not known.

Bone resorption that does not appear to be typical stress shielding has occurred with both titanium- and cobalt-based cementless prostheses. Because polymethyl methacrylate is not present in these reconstructions, bone resorption cannot be caused by bone cement particles. Polyethylene or metallic particles are potential causes of this phenomenon (see Chapter 12, *Histology and Pathology of Total Joint Replacement*).

Acetabular Components

Hybrid Total Hip Replacement

Although clinical and radiographic concerns are fairly prevalent with cementless femoral total hip prostheses, few problems

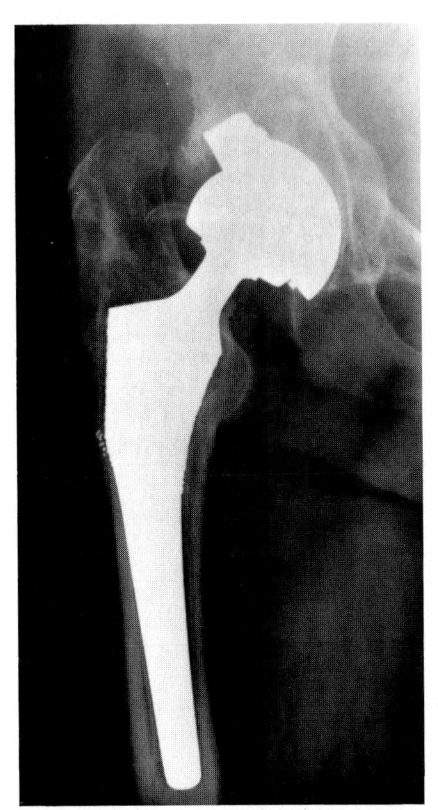

FIGURE 20–8. Bead shedding of powder-made, sintered, porous-surfaced prosthesis 5 years postoperatively.

have been found in early follow-up of porous-surfaced acetabular components. Follow-up of porous-surfaced acetabular components is much shorter than follow-up of cemented sockets, but the favorable early results, both clinically and radiographically, have made the hybrid technique popular (Fig. 20–9).

To separate possible symptoms of the acetabular component from those of the femoral component, Harris and Maloney[39] reviewed 126 primary total hip arthroplasties performed with cemented femoral components and a titanium fiber mesh–coated acetabular component with supplemental screw fixation. Minimum follow-up was 2 years (mean, 42 months). The mean Harris Hip Rating was 93 points; 96 percent of patients were rated good or excellent. Mild pain controlled by aspirin was reported by 6 percent, and no complaints of more severe pain were reported. Twenty percent of patients used a cane, 3 percent of them full time. No femoral components were definitely or probably loose. The one patient with an acetabular component that had migrated had no symptoms. There were no revisions.

Polyethylene Cementless Sockets

All-polyethylene cementless acetabular components have been implanted in a large number of patients, primarily in Europe. Bertin and colleagues[6] reported the results after an average follow-up of 2 years. Three different designs of pegged polyethylene sockets (those introduced by Morscher in 1977 and 1980 and by Ring in 1979) were used in 1878 total hip replacements. In this short follow-up, successful pain relief and walking ability were achieved in 97 percent of patients. Ten femoral components were revised, and two sockets were replaced at the revision because of slight motion. A uniform dense line adjacent to the prosthesis appeared consistently on radiographs.[6, 28] With a similar three-

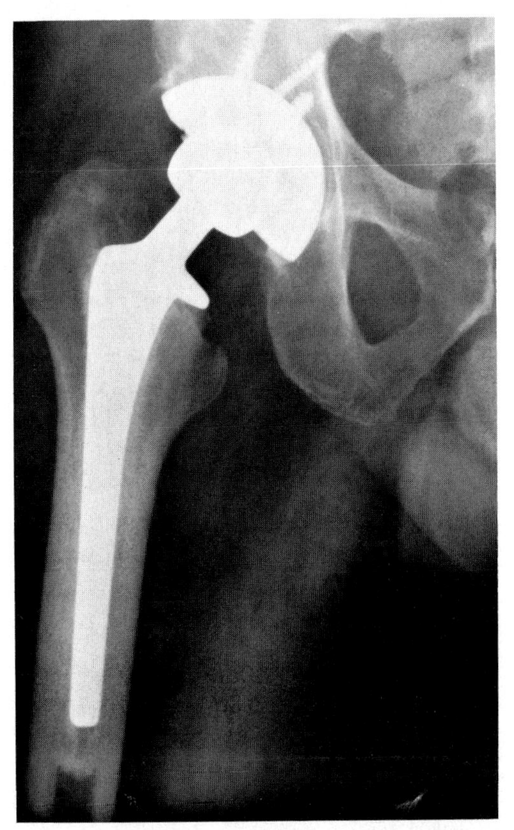

FIGURE 20–9. Hybrid total hip replacement with cemented femoral stem and porous coated acetabular component with supplemental screw fixation.

pegged polyethylene socket, Knahr and colleagues[52] reported 92 percent survival among 1316 hip replacements followed for a maximum of 5 years.

Threaded Socket

Threaded acetabular components are another means of cementless fixation in total hip replacement. *In vitro* experiments evaluating the effects of these devices on bone strain in cadaver acetabula and finite element studies have suggested that these sockets may not be clinically successful (see Chapter 13, *Biomechanics and Design*). Clinical investigation has confirmed an unacceptably high failure rate with threaded acetabular components if they do not have a microtextured porous coating to provide additional fixation.

Ayerza and coworkers[4] reported a revision rate of 9.6 percent for 64 conical, threaded ring, nonporous acetabular components 3 to 4 years after operation. Migration of 2 mm or more occurred in 27 hips (44 percent). Kennedy[51] implanted a threaded, truncated cone socket with no porous coating, porous coating at the dome only, or full coating. Only the fully coated design performed well at the 1-year follow-up. With the other two designs, all patients had "start-up " pain, and radiographic interface lucencies were common. By 1 year, 9 percent of sockets with no porous coating and 2 percent with partial coating had been revised. At revision, five of 22 hips were found to have metallosis.[51] In a comparison of five threaded socket designs, Mallory[57] discovered that only the component with a microtextured surface was satisfactory. Capello[11] found it necessary to revise 20 percent of threaded sockets followed 1 to 4 years. Of the remaining patients, 21 percent had mild pain, 7 percent moderate pain, and 3 percent severe pain.

PATIENT CHARACTERISTICS AFFECTING RESULTS

Total hip arthroplasty is one of the most successful operative treatments performed today. It provides marked pain relief and functional improvement for patients suffering from arthritis and other diseases of the hip.

Most total hip replacements are done for osteoarthritis in relatively elderly patients, and a large number for rheumatoid arthritis. Some reports suggest that the prognosis is better when total hip replacement is performed in patients with osteoarthritis, whereas others suggest more favorable prognosis with rheumatoid arthritis. Generally, patients with osteoarthritis have better bone quality. Patients with rheumatoid disease tend to be less active. Review of all available reports suggests no significant differences in durability of hip replacements for these two diagnoses, perhaps because the differences in bone quality and activity level balance each other.

Total hip replacement is more likely to result in failure under certain circumstances (Fig. 20–10).[59] Revision total hip arthroplasty has a higher failure rate than primary hip replacement.[72] Regular participation in vigorous sports, involving the high impact loads of running and jumping, or in other strenuous activities, involving

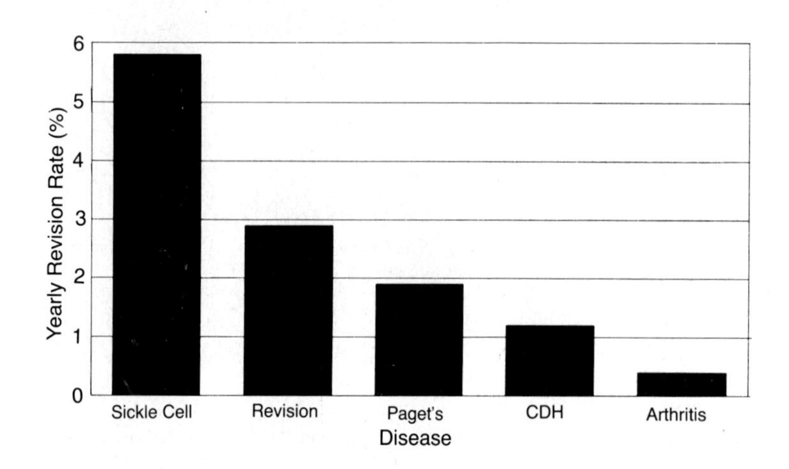

FIGURE 20–10. Annual revision rates for cemented total hip arthroplasties. (CDH = congenital dysplasia of the hip.) (Michelson, J.E. and Riley, L.H., Jr.: J. Arthroplasty 4:327–334, 1989. By permission.)

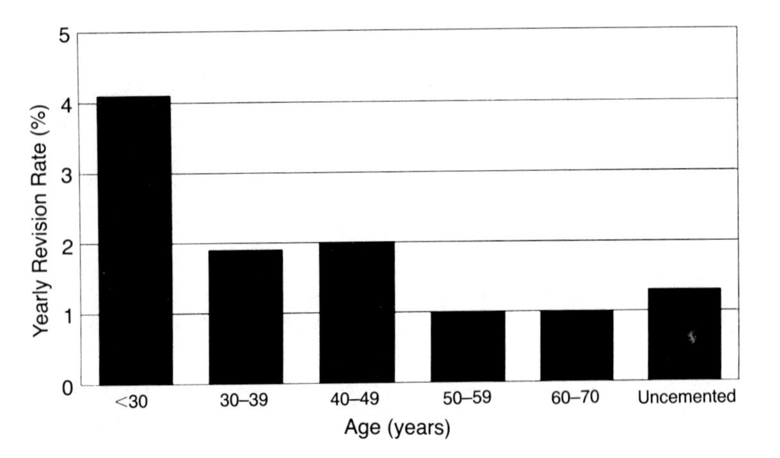

FIGURE 20–11. Annual revision rates for cemented total hip arthroplasties grouped by age and for uncemented arthroplasties. (Michelson, J.E. and Riley, L.H., Jr.: J. Arthroplasty 4: 327–334, 1989. By permission.)

heavy manual labor, reduces the durability of cemented and probably cementless hip replacements.[22]

Failure rates are higher for patients with congenital hip dysplasia; Paget disease; sickle cell disease; osteonecrosis; previous tuberculosis of the hip, especially if the disease has been quiescent for less than 10 years; and, perhaps, Gaucher disease.[14, 37, 54, 78] Patients who have had renal transplants generally have good results, but those on long-term dialysis often have poor results, with a very high complication rate.[29] No evidence exists that failure rates are higher in patients with systemic lupus erythematosus, although wound healing problems are more common. Failure does not appear more likely in cases of arthrodesis or ankylosis, in resection arthroplasty, or in association with obesity.

Total hip replacement is less successful in patients under age 50 at the time of operation, and the failure rate is especially high in patients under age 30 (Fig. 20–11).[59] The failure rate may be higher in males than females.[43]

The failure rate for cementless implants is slightly higher than that for cemented implants; however, this statement is based on analysis of data from the earliest cemented hip replacements, and the follow-up time is much shorter for cementless implants. Failure rates increase over time with cemented replacements, and it is not yet known whether the failure rate for cementless replacements will rise as follow-up times become more comparable with those for cemented replacements. The limited data available suggest that cementless femoral components perform better in young individuals and in patients with good quality bone than in older patients or in patients with poor quality bone. Cementless acetabular components have performed well over the relatively short follow-up period. Whether they will perform better or as well as cemented sockets over the long term cannot yet be determined. The relatively recent documented intermediate-term improvement in longevity of cemented total hip replacements and the expected long-term durability of cementless fixation offer promise that the excellent results of total hip arthroplasty will improve further.

References

1. Agins, H. J., Salvati, E. A., Ranawat, C. S., et al.: The nine- to fifteen-year follow-up of one-stage bilateral total hip arthroplasty. Orthop. Clin. North Am. 19:517–530, 1988.
2. Amstutz, H. C., Thomas, B. J., Jinnah, R., et al.: Treatment of primary osteoarthritis of the hip. A comparison of total joint and surface replacement arthroplasty. J. Bone Joint Surg. [Am.] 66(2):228–241, 1984.
3. Amstutz, H. C., Yao, J., Dorey, F. J., et al.: Survival analysis of T-28 hip arthroplasty with clinical implications. Orthop. Clin. North Am. 19(3):491–503, 1988.

3a. Andrew, T. A., Flanagan, J. P., Gerundini, M., and Bombelli, R.: The isoelastic, noncemented total hip arthroplasty. Clin. Orthop. 206:127, 1986.

4. Ayerza, M., Pierson, R., Sheinkop, M., et al.: A clinical review of a conocal screw-in acetabular design. Orthop. Trans. 12:662, 1988.
5. Beckenbaugh, R. D. and Ilstrup, D. M.: Total hip arthroplasty. A review of three hundred and thirty-three cases with long follow-up. J. Bone Joint Surg. 60A:306–313, 1978.
6. Bertin, K. C., Freeman, M. A., Morscher, E., et al.: Cementless acetabular replacement using a

pegged polyethylene prosthesis. Arch. Orthop. Trauma Surg. 104(4):251–261, 1985.
7. Bourne, R. B., Rorabeck, C. H., and Nott, L.: A prospective study of porous coated anatomic cementless and HD-2 cemented total hip replacements. American Academy of Orthopaedic Surgeons' Annual Meeting, Atlanta, 1988.
8. Brady, L. P. and McCutchen, J. W.: A ten-year follow-up study of 170 Charnley total hip arthroplasties. Clin. Orthop. 211:51–54, 1986.
9. Callaghan, J. J., Dysart, S. H., and Savory, C. G.: The uncemented porous-coated anatomic total hip prosthesis. Two-year results of a prospective consecutive series. J. Bone Joint Surg. [Am.] 70(3):337–346, 1988.
10. Cameron, H. U.: The results of early clinical trials with a microporous coated metal hip prosthesis. Clin. Orthop. 165:188–190, 1982.
11. Capello, W. N.: Early experiences with noncemented total hip replacements—screw-in rings. Orthop. Trans. 12:588, 1988.
12. Chandler, H. P., Reineck, F. T., Wixson, R. L., et al.: Total hip replacement in patients younger than thirty years old. A five-year follow-up study. J. Bone Joint Surg. [Am] 63A(9):1426–1434, 1981.
13. Charnley, J.: The long-term results of low-friction arthroplasty of the hip performed as a primary intervention. J. Bone Joint Surg. 54B:61–76, 1972.
14. Clarke, H. J., Jinnah, R. H., Brooker, A. F., et al.: Total hip replacement in sickle cell anemia. Orthop. Trans. 13:61, 1989.
15. Collis, D. K.: Cemented total hip replacement in patients who are less than fifty years old. J. Bone Joint Surg. [Am.] 66(3):353–359, 1984.
16. Collis, D. K.: Long-term results of an individual surgeon. Orthop. Clin. North Am. 19(3):541–550, 1988.
17. Cornell, C. N. and Ranawat, C. S.: Survivorship analysis of total hip replacements. Results in a series of active patients who were less than fifty-five years old. J. Bone Joint Surg. [Am.] 68(9):1430–1434, 1986.
18. Dall, D. M., Grobbelaar, C. J., Learmonth, I. D., et al.: Charnley low-friction arthroplasty of the hip. Long-term results in South Africa. Clin. Orthop. 211:85–90, 1986.
19. D'Aubigne, M. and Postel, M.: Functional results of hip arthroplasty with acrylic prosthesis. J. Bone Joint Surg. 36A:451–475, 1954.
20. DeLee, J. and Charnley, J.: Radiological demarcation of cemented sockets in total hip replacement. Clin. Orthop. 121:20, 1976.
21. Dorey, F. and Amstutz, H.: Survivorship analysis in the evaluation of joint replacement. J. Arthroplasty 1:63–69, 1986.
22. Dorey, F. J., Kilgus, D. J., and Amstutz, H. C.: The effect of patient activity, sports participation, and impact loading on the durability of cemented total hip replacement. American Academy of Orthopaedic Surgeons' Annual Meeting. Atlanta, 1988.
23. Dorr, L. D., Takei, G. K., and Conaty, J. P.: Total hip arthroplasties in patients less than forty-five years old. J. Bone Joint Surg. [Am.] 65(4):474–479, 1983.
24. Eftekhar, N. S. and Tzitzikalakis, G.: Failures and reoperations following low-friction arthroplasty of the hip. Clin. Orthop. 211:65–78, 1986.
25. Engh, C. A., Bobyn, J. D., and Glassmen, A. H.: Porous-coated hip replacement. J. Bone Joint Surg. 69B:45–55, 1987.
26. Engh, C. A. and Massin, P.: Cementless total hip arthroplasty using the anatomic medullary locking stem. Clin. Orthop. 249:141–158, 1989.
27. Fowler, J. L., Gie, G. A., Lee, A. J. C., et al.: Experience with the Exeter total hip replacement since 1970. Orthop. Clin. North Am. 19:477–489, 1988.
28. Freeman, M. A., Rasmussen, G. L., and Choy, W. S.: Replacement of the acetabulum with pegged press-fit components. The Hip. St. Louis, C. V. Mosby, pp. 261–268, 1985.
29. Fuchs, M. D., Hass, S., Goldstock, L., et al.: Hip replacement in patients with chronic renal failure. American Academy of Orthopaedic Surgeons' Annual Meeting, Las Vegas, 1989.
30. Galante, J. O.: Results of cementless HGP prosthesis. Orthop. Trans. 12:265, 1988.
31. Gore, D. R., Murray, M. P., Sepic, S. B., et al.: Anterolateral compared to posterior approach in total hip arthroplasty: differences in component positioning, hip strength, and hip motion. Clin. Orthop. 165:180–187, 1982.
32. Griffen, W. L. and Engh, C. A.: Porous polysulfone femoral components: short-term clinical and radiographic results in the elderly. American Academy of Orthopaedic Surgeons' Annual Meeting, Las Vegas, 1989.
33. Gruen, T. A., McNeice, G. M., and Amstutz, H. C.: "Modes of failure" of cemented stem-type femoral components. Clin Orthop. 141:17–27, 1979.
34. Gudmundsson, G. H., Harving, S., and Pilgaard, S.: The Charnley total hip arthroplasty in juvenile rheumatoid arthritis patients. Orthopedics 12(3):385–388, 1989.
35. Gustilo, R. B., Bechtold, J. E., Giachetto, J., et al.: Rationale, experience, and results of long-stem femoral prosthesis. Clin. Orthop. 249:159–168, 1989.
36. Halley, D. K. and Wroblewski, B. M.: Long-term results of low-friction arthroplasty in patients 30 years of age or younger. Clin. Orthop. 211:43–50, 1986.
37. Hanker, G. J. and Amstutz, H. C.: Osteonecrosis of the hip in the sickle-cell diseases. Treatment and complications. J. Bone Joint Surg. [Am.] 70(4):499–506, 1988.
38. Harris, W. H.: Traumatic arthritis of the hip after dislocation and acetabular fractures: treatment by mold arthroplasty. J. Bone Joint Surg. 51A:737–755, 1969.
39. Harris, W. H. and Maloney, W. J.: Hybrid total hip arthroplasty. Clin. Orthop. 249:21–29, 1989.
40. Harris, W. H., McCarthy, J. C., and O'Neill, D. A.: Femoral component loosening using contemporary techniques of femoral cement fixation. J. Bone Joint Surg. 64A:1063–1067, 1982.
41. Harris, W. H. and McGann, W. A.: Loosening of the femoral component after use of the medullary-plug cementing technique. J. Bone Joint Surg. 68A:1064–1066, 1986.
42. Hedley, A. K., Gruen, T. A., and Borden, L. S.: Two-year follow-up of the PCA noncemented total

hip replacement. The Hip. St. Louis, C. V. Mosby, pp. 225–250, 1987.
43. Herberts, P., Ahnfelt, L., Malchau, H., et al.: Multicenter clinical trials and their value in assessing total joint arthroplasty. Clin. Orthop. 249:48–55, 1989.
43a. Hupfer, T. A., Capello, W. N., and Hile, B. A.: A comparison of identical geometry nonporous and porous-coated stems. Orthop. Trans. 13:511, 1989.
44. Jakin, I., Barlin, C., and Sweet, M. B. E.: RM isoelastic total hip arthroplasty. J. Arthroplasty 3:191–199, 1988.
45. Jantsch, S., Leixnering, M., Schwagerl, W., et al.: Shaft fissures due to implantation of cementless total endoprostheses of the hip joint. An experimental study. Arch. Orthop. Trauma Surg. 107(4):236–241, 1988.
46. Jasty, M. and Harris, W. H.: Total hip reconstruction using frozen femoral head allografts in patients with acetabular bone loss. Orthop. Clin North Am. 18(2):291–299, 1987.
47. Johnston, R. C., Fitzgerald, R. H., Jr., Harris, W. H., et al.: Clinical and radiographic evaluation of total hip replacement. J. Bone Joint Surg. 72A:161–168, 1990.
48. Kaplan, E. L. and Meier, P.: Nonparametric estimations from incomplete observations. J. Am. Stat. Assoc. 53:457, 1958.
49. Kaplan, P. A., Montesi, S. A., Jardon, O. M., et al.: Bone-ingrowth hip prostheses in asymptomatic patients: radiographic features. Radiology 169(1):221–227, 1988.
50. Kavanaugh, B. F., Dewitz, M. A., Ilstrup, D. M., et al.: Charnley total hip arthroplasty with cement. J. Bone Joint Surg. 71A:1496–1503, 1989.
51. Kennedy, W. F.: Modes of failure of the threaded acetabular total hip replacement components. Orthop. Trans. 12:691, 1988.
52. Knahr, K., Bohler, M., Frank, P., et al.: 5 years' experiences with the Gersthof polyethylene peg-anchored acetabulum. Z. Orthop. 125(4):375–381, 1987. (Published in German.)
53. Larson, C. B.: Rating scale for hip disabilities. Clin. Orthop. 31:85–93, 1963.
54. Lau, M. M., Lichtman, D. M., Hamati, Y. I., et al.: Hip arthroplasties in Gaucher's disease. J. Bone Joint Surg. [Am.] 63A(4):591–601, 1981.
55. Levy, R. N., Capozzi, J. D., Levy, C. M., et al.: A prospective randomized comparison of press-fit and porous coated femoral stems of identical geometric designs: two to four year results. Orthop. Trans. 13:512, 1989.
56. Lord, G. and Bancel, P.: The Madreporic cementless total hip arthroplasty. Clin. Orthop. 176:67–76, 1983.
57. Mallory, T. M.: An experience with threaded acetabular components for cementless total hip replacement. Orthop. Trans. 12:589, 1988.
58. McCoy, T. H., Salvati, E. A., Ranawat, C. S., et al.: A fifteen-year follow-up study of one hundred Charnley low-friction arthroplasties. Orthop. Clin. North Am. 19(3):467–476, 1988.
59. Michelson, J. D. and Riley, L. H., Jr.: Considerations in the comparisons of cemented and cementless total hip prostheses. J. Arthroplasty 4:327–334, 1989.
60. Mikhail, W. E., Hoblitzell, R. M., Simpson, J. M., et al.: Comparison of cemented (Exeter) versus uncemented (porous coated anatomic) collarless femoral components: two to five year follow-up. American Academy of Orthopaedic Surgeons' Annual Meeting, Atlanta, 1988.
61. Morrey, B. F.: Short-stemmed uncemented femoral component for primary hip arthroplasty. Clin. Orthop. 249:169–175, 1989.
62. Neill, D. J., Granberry, W. M., Gooden, C., et al.: Long term results of total joint arthroplasty in patients twenty-one years of age and younger. Orthop. Trans. 13:511, 1989.
63. Nunn, D.: The Ring uncemented plastic-on-metal total hip replacement. J. Bone Joint Surg. 70B:40–44, 1988.
64. Older, J.: Low-friction arthroplasty of the hip: a 10–12-year follow-up study. Clin. Orthop. 211:36–42, 1986.
65. O'Leary, J. F., Mallory, T. H., Kraus, T. J., et al.: Mittelmeier ceramic total hip arthroplasty. J. Arthroplasty 3:87–96, 1988.
66. Pavlov, P. W.: A 15-year follow-up study of 512 consecutive Charnley-Müller total hip replacements. J. Arthroplasty 2:151–156, 1987.
67. Petty, W.: Comparison of cemented and uncemented primary total hip arthroplasty. Orthop. Trans. 12:589, 1988.
68. Pierson, R. H., Jacobs, J. J., Sheinkop, A. G., et al.: Primary total hip reconstruction with a cementless titanium fiber coated prosthesis. Orthop. Trans. 13:579, 1989.
69. Poss, R., Brick, G. W., Wright, R. J., et al.: The effects of modern cementing techniques on the longevity of total hip arthroplasty. Orthop. Clin. North Am. 19:591–598, 1988.
70. Ranawat, C. S., Atkinson, R. E., Salvati, E. A., et al.: Conventional total hip arthroplasty for degenerative joint disease in patients between the ages of forty and sixty years. J. Bone Joint Surg. [Am.] 66(5):745–752, 1984.
71. Ranawat, C. S., Rawlins, B. A., and Harju, V. T.: Effect of modern cement technique on acetabular fixation total hip arthroplasty. Orthop. Clin. North Am. 19:599–603, 1988.
72. Retpen, J. B., Varmarken, J., Sturup, J., et al.: Clinical results after revision and primary total hip arthroplasty. J. Arthroplasty 4:297–302, 1989.
73. Ring, P. A.: Ring UPM total hip arthroplasty. Clin. Orthop. 176:115–123, 1983.
74. Ritter, M. A. and Campbell, E. D.: Direct comparison between bilaterally implanted cemented and uncemented total hip replacements in six patients. Clin. Orthop. 207:77–82, 1986.
75. Roberts, D. W., Poss, R., and Kelley, K.: Radiographic comparison of cementing techniques in total hip arthroplasty. J. Arthroplasty 1:241, 1986.
76. Robinson, R. P., Lovell, T. P., Green, T. M., et al.: Early femoral component loosening in DF-80 total hip arthroplasty. J. Arthroplasty 4:55–64, 1989.
77. Russotti, G. M., Coventry, M. B., and Stauffer, R. M.: Cemented THA using contemporary techniques; a minimum five-year follow-up study. Clin. Orthop. 235:141–147, 1988.

78. Saito, S., Saito, M., Nishina, T., et al.: Long-term results of total hip arthroplasty. Clin. Orthop. 244:198–207, 1989.
78a. Sarmiento, A., Natarajan, V., Gruen, T. A., and McMahon, M.: Radiographic performance of two different total hip cemented arthroplasties. A survivorship analysis. Orthop. Clin. North Am. 19:505, 1988.
79. Sharp, D. J. and Porter, K. M.: The Charnley total hip arthroplasty in patients under age 40. Clin. Orthop. 201:51–56, 1985.
80. Stauffer, R. N.: Ten-year follow-up study of total hip replacement, with particular reference to roentgenographic loosening of the components. J. Bone Joint Surg. 64A:983–990, 1982.
81. Sutherland, C. J., Wilde, A. H., Borden, L. S., et al.: A ten-year follow-up of one hundred consecutive Müller curved-stem total hip-replacement arthroplasties. J. Bone Joint Surg. [Am.] 64A:970–982, 1982.
82. Van Der Schaff, R. K., Deutman, R., and Mulder, T. J.: Stanmore total hip replacement. J. Bone Joint Surg. 70B:45–48, 1988.
83. Vaughn, B. K. and Mallory, T. H.: Porous coated anatomic total hip replacement—clinical and roentgenographic results with minimum two-year follow-up. Orthop. Trans. 12:686, 1988.
84. Wejkner, B. and Stenport, J.: Charnley total hip arthroplasty. A ten- to 14-year follow-up study. Clin. Orthop. 231:113–119, 1988.
85. Wejkner, B. and Stenport, J.: Long-term results of bilateral Charnley total hip arthroplasty. J. Arthroplasty 3(4):305–308, 1988.
86. Welch, R. B., McGann, W. A., and Picetti, G. D.: Charnley low-friction arthroplasty. A fifteen- to seventeen-year follow-up study. Orthop. Clin. North Am. 19:551–555, 1988.
87. White, S. H.: The fate of cemented total hip arthroplasty in young patients. Clin. Orthop. 231:29–34, 1988.
88. Wilson, P. D., Jr., Amstutz, H. C., Czerniecki, A., et al.: Total hip replacement with fixation by acrylic cement. J. Bone Joint Surg. 54A:207–236, 1972.
89. Wroblewski, B. M.: 15–21 year results of the Charnley low-friction arthroplasty. Clin. Orthop. 211:30–35, 1986.
90. Zweymüller, K. A., Lintner, F. K., and Semlitsch, M. F.: Biologic fixation of a press-fit titanium hip joint endoprosthesis. Clin. Orthop. 235:195–206, 1988.

CHAPTER 21

Bipolar Hip Arthroplasty

WILLIAM PETTY

Bipolar hip prostheses are used most commonly for the treatment of displaced femoral neck fractures. In the treatment of other diseases of the hip, including arthritis and osteonecrosis, bipolar devices can be employed instead of the fixed acetabular components of conventional total hip replacements. Bipolar arthroplasty for revision of loose acetabular total hip replacement sockets is discussed in Chapter 23, *Revision Total Hip Arthroplasty*.

MOTION

Some patients who have fixed-head hemiarthroplasties of the hip develop articular erosion and perhaps protrusio acetabuli. Experimentally, cartilage responds to articulation against metal with early loss of proteoglycan, followed by surface damage to the cartilage and progressive degenerative changes.[6, 7] The basic design principle of the bipolar prosthesis is that the motion between the prosthetic head and inner-bearing insert reduces the motion, stress, and wear or erosion of the acetabulum (Fig. 21–1). Several studies have indicated little or no persistent motion between the two bearings of the prosthesis; thus, the bipolar prosthesis behaves in a manner similar to that of a unipolar prosthesis.[4, 19] Others have found some persistent movement of the interprosthetic bearing.[2, 10, 16] These differences may be due in part to the differences in prosthesis design.

In a comparison of movement in the Bateman prosthesis, a patient having replacement for fracture moved the hip joint primarily between the outer bearing and the acetabulum, whereas a patient having replacement for arthritis moved primarily at the interprosthetic bearing. This difference indicates that the condition of the articular cartilage influences the action of the prosthesis. Mess and Barmada[14] found that motion was about equal between the inner and outer bearings when unloaded. However, interprosthetic motion increased and outer bearing motion decreased with increased load.

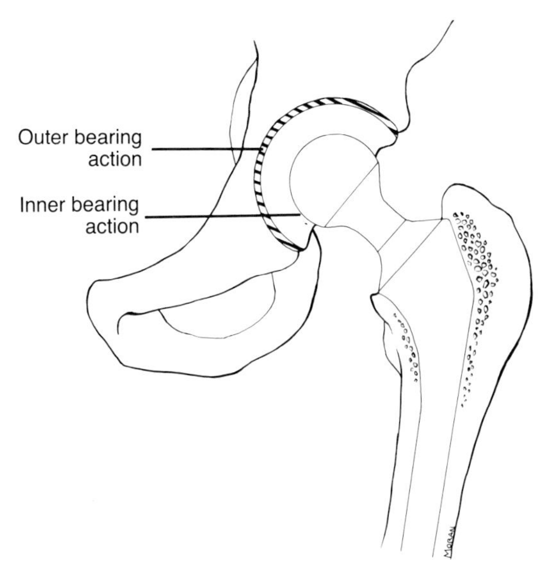

FIGURE 21–1. Two-bearing principle of the bipolar prosthesis.

CLINICAL RESULTS

Fracture

Lausten and colleagues,[11a] with a follow-up average of 51 months, reported good or excellent results in 75 percent of patients treated with bipolar prostheses for femoral neck fractures. Three hips (4 percent) had to be converted to total hip replacements, and three exhibited acetabular protrusions. Bochner and colleagues,[2] after a minimum follow-up of 2 years, reported that 93 percent of 90 patients were free of major pain and that 92 percent had satisfactory motion and muscle power. Functionally, 83 percent of patients returned completely to prefracture levels or used a cane that had not been necessary previously.

In a comparative study with fixed-head prostheses, Suman[16] found improved results in patients with femoral neck fractures treated with bipolar prostheses. Yamagata and associates[22] reported more acetabular erosions and higher reoperation rates following fixed-head hemiarthroplasties compared with bipolar replacements. Prosthesis survivorship estimate at 8 years was 86.3 percent for the bipolar prosthesis and 77.1 percent for the fixed-head prosthesis. Cement fixation led to a higher prosthesis survival rate with both types of head. Other investigators also have reported better results with bipolar prostheses compared with unipolar prostheses in the treatment of femoral neck fractures.[11, 12, 15]

Waddell[20] described improved results in bipolar arthroplasties for femoral neck fractures using more modern cementless femoral components. Of 110 arthroplasties, followed for 1 to 4 years, only one was removed because of infection. No revisions were necessary. Acetabular erosion was found in two cases. No acetabular protrusion was found.

Arthritis and Osteonecrosis

In a study of the Bateman prosthesis in the treatment of osteoarthritis, Bateman and colleagues[1] reported excellent results overall. Some deterioration in hip scores was observed with longer follow-up periods, which the investigators attributed to decreased function with advancing patient age rather than to prosthesis problems. McConville and associates[13] followed 70 patients for an average of 4.3 years after bipolar arthroplasties for osteoarthritis. Their patients had a mean Harris hip score of 78.8, with good or excellent results in 75.8 percent of the group. Six patients (8.6 percent) required revision. Wetherell and Hinves[21] evaluated 47 hips an average of 5 years after bipolar arthroplasties for osteoarthritis and found that 74 percent had no or slight pain. Estimated hip survival at 7 years was 86.2 percent. Although 22 percent of hips exhibited acetabular erosion greater than 2 mm, this finding did not correlate with symptoms. Results were best in patients older than 80 years.

Torisu and coworkers[17] evaluated the results of 25 bipolar arthroplasties with acetabular bone grafts 2 to 6 years after operation in patients with rheumatoid arthritis. The mean hip rating improved from 42.6 to 72.8. Of 25 hips, 24 were painless (96 percent). Acetabular migration ranged from 0 to 10 mm, with mean central migration of 2.7 mm and superior migration of 3.7 mm. In patients with either osteoarthritis or rheumatoid arthritis, Bowman and colleagues[3] found good or excellent results in 72.9 percent, fair results in 19.1 percent, and poor results in 8.5 percent of hips treated with bipolar arthroplasties.

Fischer and Capello[8] reported groin or buttock pain in 15 of 76 hips (19.7 percent) an average of 31 months after bipolar arthroplasty. Osteonecrosis was the underlying diagnosis in 64 cases and fracture in 12 hips. In 110 patients having arthroplasties primarily for the treatment of osteoarthritis and osteonecrosis, Gannon and colleagues[9] found a better range of motion but less reliable pain relief with bipolar arthroplasty compared with total hip arthroplasty (Figs. 21–2 and 21–3).

CONCLUSION

For the treatment of displaced femoral neck fractures, most series suggest better results with bipolar arthroplasties compared with fixed-head replacements. For the primary treatment of hip diseases, such as arthritis and osteonecrosis, motion is

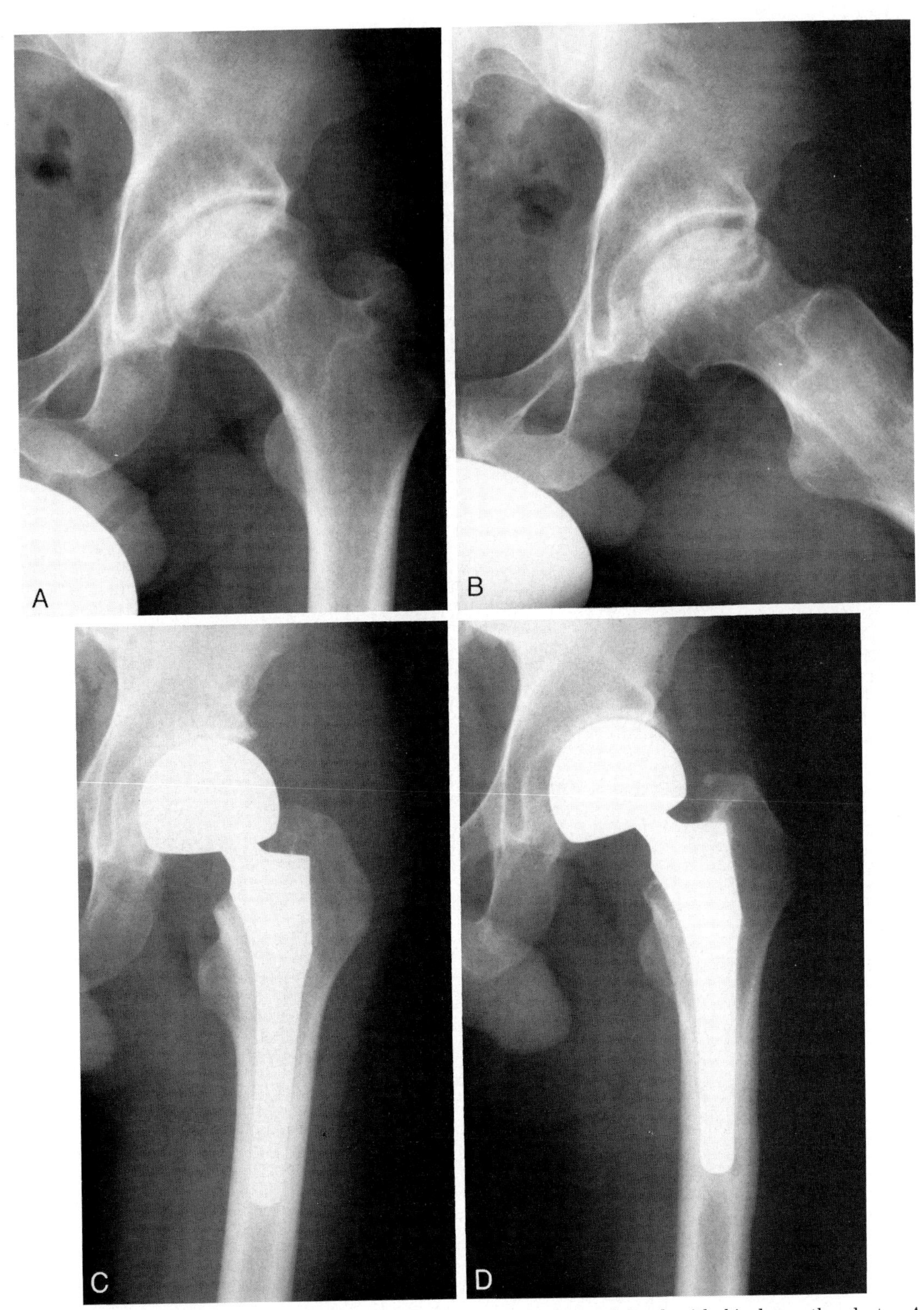

FIGURE 21–2. Treatment of disabling osteonecrosis of the femoral head with bipolar arthroplasty. *A*, Anteroposterior radiograph showing a large area of bone infarct. *B*, Osteochondral fracture and collapse are seen best on the lateral radiograph. *C*, Patient was treated with a bipolar cementless arthroplasty. *D*, The Harris hip rating is 96 five years later. Bone hypertrophy and a small area of bone lysis have occurred at the stem tip. No acetabular erosion has occurred.

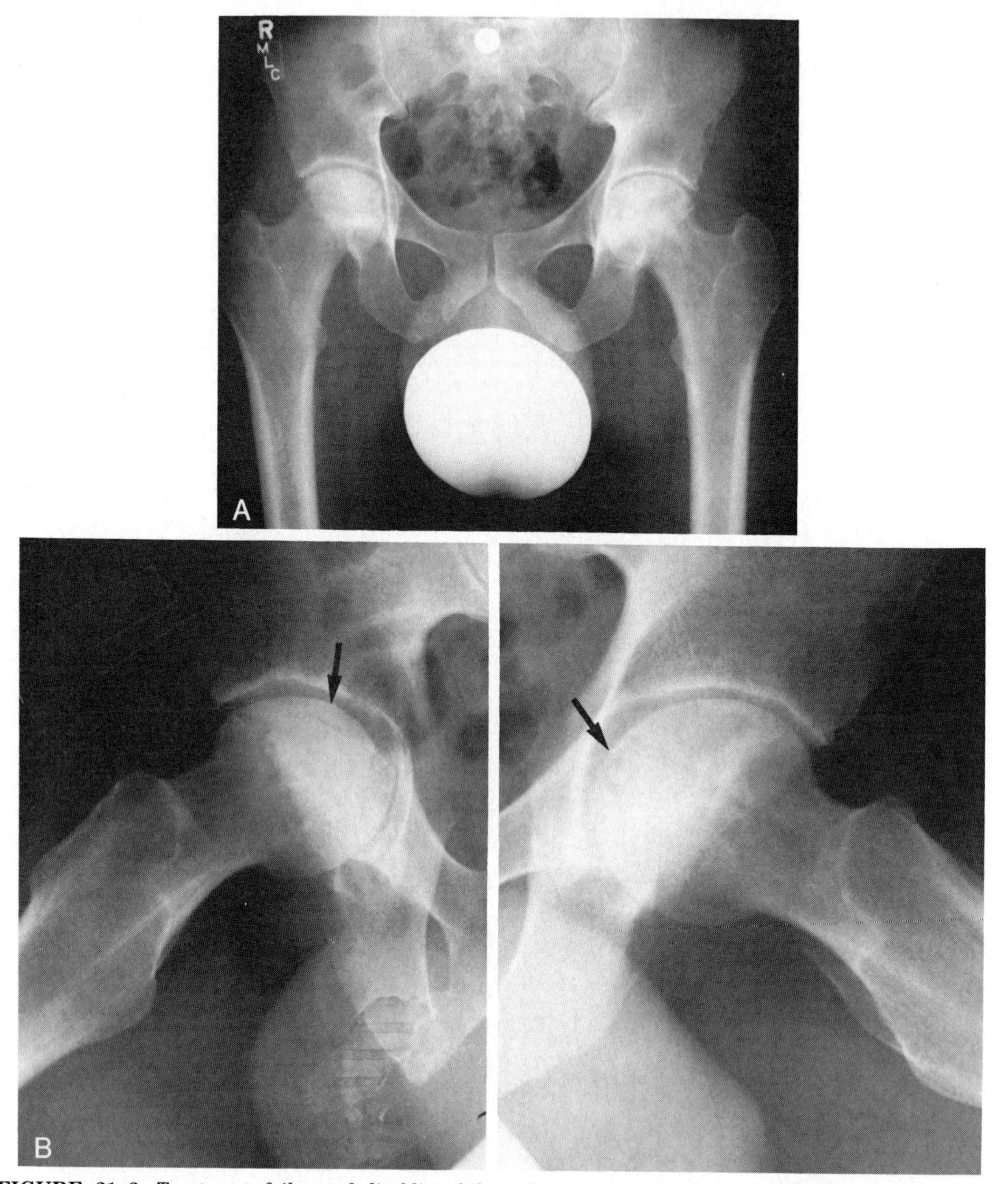

FIGURE 21–3. Treatment failure of disabling bilateral osteonecrosis of the femoral head with bipolar arthroplasty. *A*, Anteroposterior radiograph shows signs of osteonecrosis. *B*, Lateral radiograph shows osteochondral fracture.

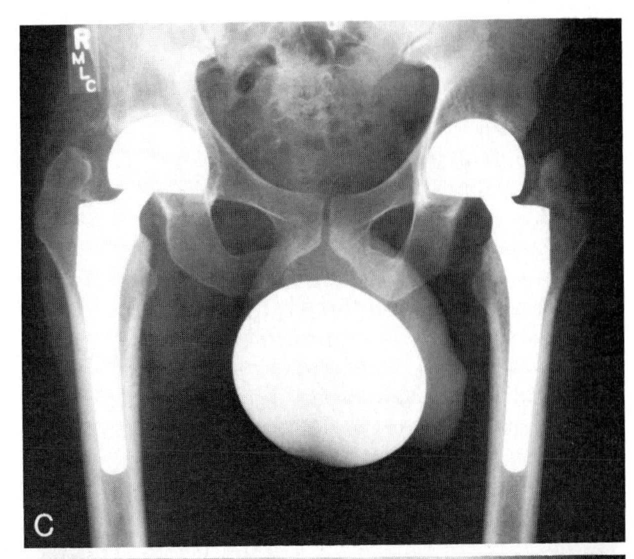

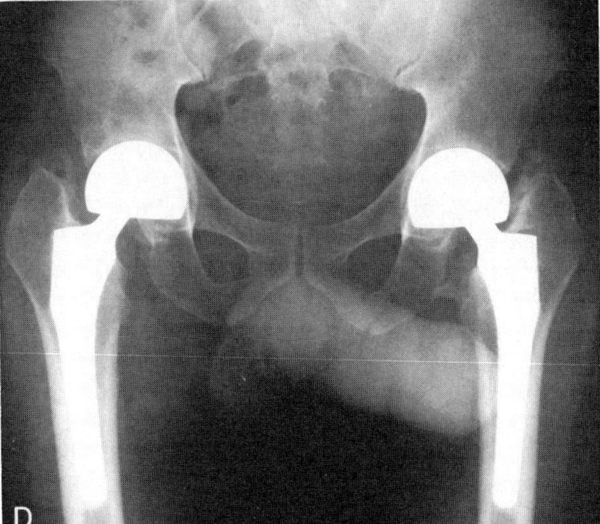

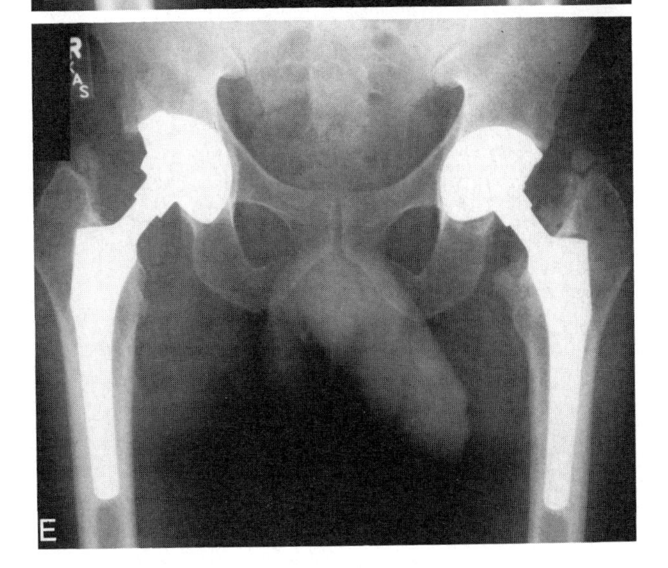

FIGURE 21–3 *Continued* *C*, Postoperative radiograph of bilateral, bipolar arthroplasties. *D*, The patient had disabling hip pain 2 years later. The radiograph showed acetabular erosion bilaterally. *E*, All hip symptoms resolved after conversion to fixed acetabular components.

more likely to occur at the interprosthetic bearing. Motion is usually excellent, but relief of pain is a less reliable outcome than with a fixed acetabular component for total hip arthroplasty.

General complications of bipolar arthroplasty procedures are similar to those with other hip arthroplasty procedures. Specific complications associated with the bipolar prostheses include failure of the polyethylene bearing inserts, which may be more likely with certain designs, and disassociation of the bipolar components, usually accompanying dislocation. When disassociation occurs, open reduction and reassembly or revision are necessary.[1, 11–13, 15, 18]

References

1. Bateman, J. E., Berenji, A. R., Bayne, O., and Greyson, N. D.: Long-term results of bipolar arthroplasty in osteoarthritis of the hip. Clin. Orthop. 251:54–66, 1990.
2. Bochner, R. M., Pellicci, P. M., and Lyden, J. P.: Bipolar hemiarthroplasty for fracture of the femoral neck. Clinical review with special emphasis on prosthetic motion. J. Bone Joint Surg. [Am] 70(7):1001–1010, 1988.
3. Bowman, A. J., Jr., Walker, M. W., Kilfoyle, R. M., et al.: Experience with the bipolar prosthesis in hip arthroplasty. A clinical study. Orthopedics 8(4):460–467, 1985.
4. Chen, S. C., Badrinath, K., Pell, L. H., and Mitchell, K.: The movements of the components of the Hastings bipolar prosthesis. A radiographic study in 65 patients. J. Bone Joint Surg. [Br] 71(2):186–188, 1989.
5. Chen, S. C., Sarkar, S., and Pell, L. H.: A radiological study of the movements of the two components of the Monk prosthesis (hard-top 'duopleet') in patients. Injury 12(3):243–249, 1980.
6. Cook, S. D., Thomas, K. A., and Kester, M. A.: Wear characteristics of the canine acetabulum against different femoral prostheses. J. Bone Joint Surg. [Br] 71(2):189–197, 1989.
7. Cruess, R. L., Kwok, D. C., Duc, P. N., et al.: The response of articular cartilage to weight-bearing against metal. A study of hemiarthroplasty of the hip in the dog. J. Bone Joint Surg. [Br] 66(4):592–597, 1984.
8. Fischer, D. A. and Capello, W. N.: Bipolar Hip Prostheses in Intact Acetabula. Annual Meeting of the American Academy of Orthopaedic Surgeons, Atlanta, Georgia, 1988.
9. Gannon, J. M., Kyle, R. F., Simonet, W. T., and Gustilo, R. B.: Comparison of results of bipolar and fixed acetabular components in total hip replacement using the BIAS femoral component. Orthop. Trans. 12:716, 1988.
10. Hodgkinson, J. P., Meadows, T. H., Davies, D. R., and Hargadon, E. J.: A radiological assessment of interprosthetic movement in the Charnley-Hastings hemiarthroplasty. Injury 19(1):18–20, 1988.
11. Labelle, L. W., Colwill, J. C., and Swanson, A. B.: Bateman bipolar hip arthroplasty for femoral neck fractures. Clin. Orthop. 251:20–25, 1990.
11a. Lausten, G. S., Vedel, P., and Nielsen, P-M.: Fractures of the femoral neck treated with a bipolar endoprosthesis. Clin. Orthop. 218:63, 1987.
12. Lestrange, N. R.: Bipolar arthroplasty for 496 hip fractures. Clin. Orthop. 251:7–19, 1990.
13. McConville, O. R., Bowman, A. J., Jr., Kilfoyle, R. M., et al.: Bipolar hemiarthroplasty in degenerative arthritis of the hip. Clin. Orthop. 251:67–74, 1990.
14. Mess, D. and Barmada, R.: Clinical and motion studies of the Bateman bipolar prosthesis in osteonecrosis of the hip. Clin. Orthop. 251:44–47, 1990.
15. Moshein, J., Alter, A. H., Elconnin, K. B., et al.: Transcervical fractures of the hip treated with the Bateman bipolar prosthesis. Clin. Orthop. 251:48–53, 1990.
16. Suman, R. K.: Prosthetic replacement of the femoral head for fractures of the neck of the femur: a comparative study. Injury 11(4):309–316, 1980.
17. Torisu, T., Utsunomiya, K., Masumi, S., and Maekawa, M.: Bipolar hip arthroplasty in rheumatoid arthritis. Clin. Orthop. 244:188–197, 1989.
18. Vazquez-Vela, G., Vazquez-Vela, E., and Dobarganes, F. G.: The Bateman bipolar prosthesis in osteoarthritis and rheumatoid arthritis. Clin. Orthop. 251:82–86, 1990.
19. Verberne, G. H.: A femoral head prosthesis with a built-in joint. A radiological study of the movements of the two components. J. Bone Joint Surg. [Br] 65(5):544–547, 1983.
20. Waddell, J. P.: The use of noncemented bipolar hip prosthesis in the management of subcapital fractures of the femur. Orthop. Trans. 11:496, 1987.
21. Wetherell, R. G. and Hinves, B. L.: The Hastings hip in osteoarthritis. A study of 47 cases with a 5-year follow-up period. J. Arthroplasty 4(2):143–149, 1989.
22. Yamagata, M., Chao, E. Y., Ilstrup, D. M., et al.: Fixed-head and bipolar hip endoprostheses. A retrospective clinical and roentgenographic study. J. Arthroplasty 2(4):327–341, 1987.

CHAPTER 22

Surface Replacement Arthroplasty

HARLAN C. AMSTUTZ

Conventional acrylic-fixed total hip joint replacement has been one of the most successful orthopaedic procedures devised, revolutionizing the treatment of elderly patients with arthritis by relieving pain and permitting return to relatively normal function.[30] With early operative techniques, many older patients had serviceable hips for their lifetimes. However, the hip replacements of younger patients, even when the procedures were technically correct, lacked sufficient durability as evidenced by stem fractures in the "presuperalloy" era and, especially, by loosening.[29, 63, 95, 101] Surface ("double-cup") arthroplasty was introduced to address the needs of these younger patients.

Surface replacement arthroplasty offers several advantages over conventional total hip replacement. Surface replacement preserves femoral bone stock, because little bone is removed from the femoral head to accommodate the metal shell. The natural anatomy and joint biomechanics are preserved. The intramedullary canal is not violated.

The increased diameter of the femoral shell is necessary because the size of the femoral head can be reduced only to neck size. This necessitates a thinner-walled polyethylene shell for the acetabular component than that utilized in conventional replacement. Even with reduction of the femoral head to the size of the neck with surface replacement, preparation of the acetabular bone at best resembles that employed for conventional replacements; thus, no more acetabular bone is preserved. However, the large diameter of the femoral shell enhances joint stability, and unit interface pressure is lower at the articular surface. When the surface replacement technique is mastered, the operating time (incision to closure) is shorter than that for conventional stemmed replacement, the blood loss is less, and the incidence or effect of sepsis may be reduced.[5]

The ability of modular sockets to achieve cementless bone ingrowth has been a significant advance in surface replacement design. Hybrids with cemented femoral or all-cementless applications are now practical. The prospects for long-term durability are better. Previously, even the most enthusiastic advocates of surface replacement admitted that long-term durability was jeopardized by the unavoidable use of thin-walled acetabular components and thin acrylic cement mantles.

EVOLUTION OF SURFACE REPLACEMENT

Resurfacing hip arthroplasty evolved from the original cup arthroplasty conceived by Smith-Petersen in the 1940s.[83] He believed that a favorable tissue reaction to a material placed between the reamed, diseased surfaces of a hip joint could provide a smooth functional articular surface. Although pain relief with improved function and durability was observed in some patients, success was unpredictable, and the technique was abandoned when total hip replacement appeared.

In the early 1950s, Charnley[31, 32] experimented with two thin cups (2 to 3 mm) of polytetrafluoroethylene (Teflon) pressed into position in the acetabulum and over the reshaped femoral head. An intense tissue reaction ensued. In 1953, Haboush[53] reported two cases of double-cup arthroplasties in which two metal cups fixed with acrylic cement were used. The follow-up period was short, however. In 1960, Townley[89, 90] employed a polyurethane acetabular cup combined with a metallic femoral cup that had a slender intramedullary stem. In 1977, he modified the design to include a polyethylene acetabular component. This femoral component, still in use, has a short, curved intramedullary stem, thus differing from a true surface replacement. In our analysis, this design has distinct disadvantages that are related to the inevitable stress concentration around the stem and peripheral stress shielding. A detailed analysis is needed of long-term outcome.

In 1968, Müller and Boltzy[74] reported a series of 18 double-cup arthroplasties in which uncemented metal components were used. The results were unsatisfactory, and the procedure was abandoned. In 1974, Gerard and coworkers[49, 50] implanted double cups of metal. Their theory was that this procedure would allow motion to occur between components and between component and bone. Polyethylene was utilized later, but the design was changed in 1975 because of an excessive wear reaction of the cup articulating against bone. A metal-backed polyethylene acetabular component was then tried, and the cylindric portion of the femoral component was lengthened. This press-fit system is still being utilized.[39]

In 1971, Paltrinieri and Trentani[77] began clinical trials of the first all-cemented system with a high-density polyethylene acetabular component and a metal femoral cup with a neck skirt. Furuya and colleagues[46, 47] began clinical trials in 1971 employing stainless-steel acetabular and high-density polyethylene femoral components. Between 1972 and 1974, Freeman and coworkers[45] inserted a similar prosthesis having a high-density polyethylene femoral component and a metal acetabulum. Because the convex femoral polyethylene component wore rapidly, the femoral and acetabular component materials were reversed in 1977. In addition, the trochanteric osteotomy was discarded in favor of partial abductor release. In these early designs, the femur was shaped into a cylinder.

In 1973, Eicher began clinical trials with the first spheric design, the "Indiana Conservative Hip." A high rate of failure was observed in an early series reported by Capello,[24] but the rate of failure was later reduced by improvements in technique and design and by a change in indications, which excluded all but osteoarthritis.[25]

Tanaka,[85] the first to describe eccentric sockets, reported on the results of 57 procedures performed between 1975 and 1977. However, he and Furuya were the first to abandon the procedure, perhaps because their Japanese patients were small in stature and had hip dysplasia, a difficult combination to manage when resurfacing in that era. In 1978, Wagner[97] initially used the anterior approach to preserve the posterior capsular vessels with spheric surface replacement. Later, he reduced the head to neck size, reporting the results in 426 patients who were followed from 6 months to 4 years. Subsequently, ceramic (aluminum oxide) was employed for the femoral component, with improved but as yet unpublished results.

ACRYLIC-FIXED THARIES SURFACE REPLACEMENT

In 1973, we designed a method of resurfacing that would allow resection of nonviable bone while preserving as much femoral head and neck as possible. We called the system THARIES: Total Hip Articular Replacement using Internal Eccentric Shells. With an internal chamfered cylindric contour, instrumentation was specifically developed to optimize precision during preparation of the femoral head (Fig. 22–1).[4, 35] We have followed the results of 585 resurfacing hip replacements for 6 to

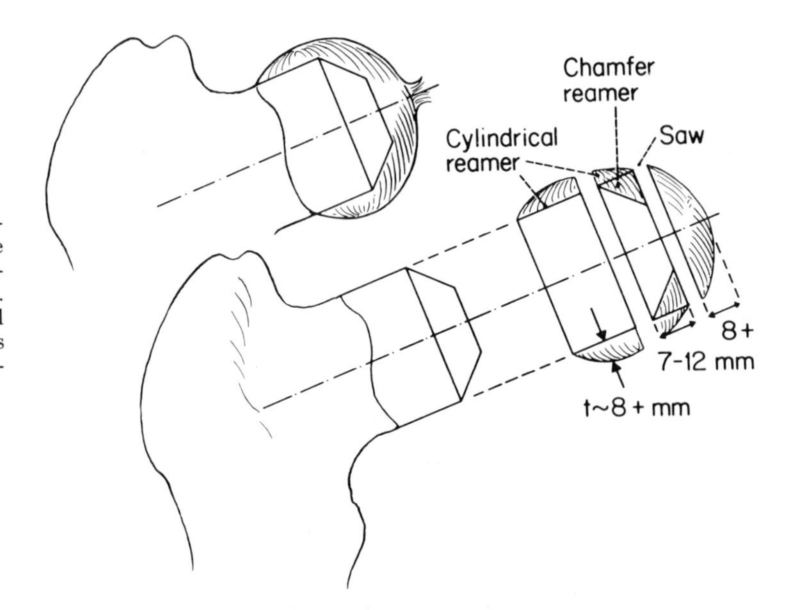

FIGURE 22–1. Removal of diseased (cystic and sclerotic) bone from the femoral head in preparation for femoral component. Note that the reamed cylindrical surface of the femoral head has approximately the same diameter as the neck.

16 years. Data are continually updated. The patients' primary diagnoses were osteoarthritis (44 percent), avascular necrosis (16 percent), rheumatoid arthritis/juvenile rheumatoid arthritis (15 percent), congenital hip dysplasia (9 percent), posttraumatic arthritis (4 percent), and other diagnoses (12 percent). All patients were young enough (mean age at time of surgery, 48 years; range 20 to 67 years) at the time of implant insertions that revisions would probably be needed in their natural lifetimes. The ratio of males to females was approximately equal (47/53). Many patients with 16-year follow-ups from all the diagnostic groups continued to function well. As of June 1990, 170 patients from the series had revision surgery performed at our institution for resurfacing failures. Another 49 patients were known to have undergone revision surgery elsewhere, for an overall failure rate of 37 percent.

A patient from this series is a 50-year-old insurance salesman, retired because of a lung disability and ankylosing spondylitis. He also has a history of two bowel resections for regional ileitis. His major disability preoperatively was degenerative arthritis secondary to osteonecrosis, resulting from chronic steroid administration for bowel disease. Before surgery, he had severe pain and limitation of walking, function, and range of motion. He underwent cemented T-28 and 6 weeks later, left THARIES replacement. Over the next 15 years, his activity level varied, often being limited by the systemic diseases (Fig. 22–2). At last follow-up evaluation, he had radiographic signs of loosening of the femoral stem component but no symptoms. Radiographically, the THARIES components were still stable.

Aseptic Loosening

The predominant cause of prosthetic failure was aseptic loosening of one or both components. This problem accounted for 86 percent of the failures. In two thirds of these patients, loosening started on the acetabular side. By the time of revision, one third of them also had femoral loosening due to osteolysis generated by debris and granuloma reaction. Most failures occurred at the cement-bone interface. The symptomatic loosening was often preceded by widening radiolucency leading to migration or component shift.

One of our patients, a 28-year-old mother and homemaker with congenital dysplasia and a previous shelf procedure at 4½ years of age, had increasing pain due to secondary osteoarthritis and a limb length discrepancy of 2 cm. The shelf was osteotomized and moved to the level of the normal acetabulum, and a THARIES replacement was performed. After surgery, this young woman was able to care for her small children. She later worked as a legal sec-

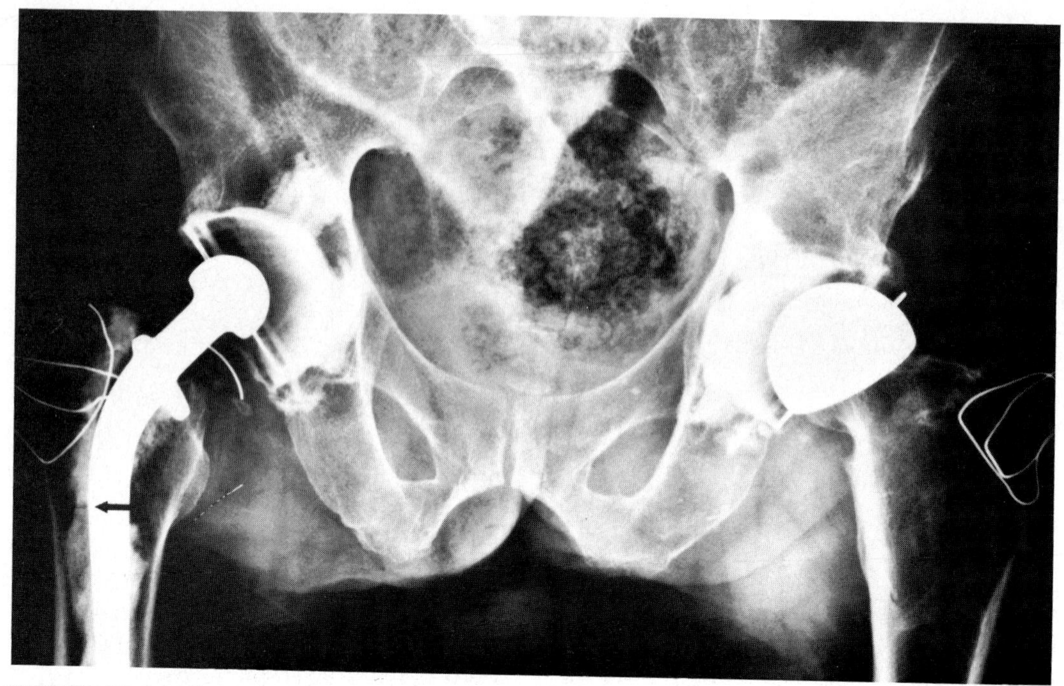

FIGURE 22–2. Follow-up 15 years after left total hip arthroplasty with internal eccentric shells (THARIES) and right T-28. Note less than 2 mm interface lucency about the acetabular component in zone I bilaterally. Some left femoral neck attenuation is present. The right femoral component is in a cantilever fatigue mode IV, with a lucent gap between the cement and femoral component in zone 1 and an acrylic crack in zone 2 shown at the arrow.

retary and was active bicycling and swimming for 9 years before acetabular failure required conversion to a conventional press-fit stem-type device (Fig. 22–3). At revision surgery, the femoral component was not loose, although some minor erosion of the neck had occurred adjacent to the component. The femoral head and neck portions were employed to graft the socket revision.

In some patients, serial radiography demonstrated progressive lucent changes at the acetabular interfaces consistent with those found in cement bone loosening after traditional procedures. Among the acetabular failures were 13 cases in which the sockets dislodged from the supporting cement mantle without significant loosening at the bone-cement interface. Previously considered rare, this complication was caused by polyethylene wear on the outer surface of the socket due to initial micromotion and then macromotion. Dislodgement was exacerbated by the shallow tapered grooves on the acetabular component used for fixation. The first failures occurred in dysplastic patients in whom the shallow acetabula precluded complete bony support of the polyethylene shells. We have since observed these failures in other diagnostic categories and in our long-term follow-ups of patients with conventional replacements. Fragmentation of thin zone 1 acrylic was common with localized osteolysis occurring in the cases of socket cement dissociation (Fig. 22–4).

Femoral loosening was identified radiographically by tilting and subsidence of the component. Subtle changes (< 1 mm) could be evaluated only with precise, reproducible grid radiographic techniques, which achieved good superposition of bony landmarks and superposition of trochanteric wires.[16] Scanning as described by Thomas and associates[86] and Capello and associates[26] was helpful in identifying early stages of femoral loosening because direct visualization of the bone-cement interface beneath the metal shell was impossible.

Pathologic studies demonstrated fragments of acrylic cement in association with variable quantities of metal and polyethylene debris within an exuberant mem-

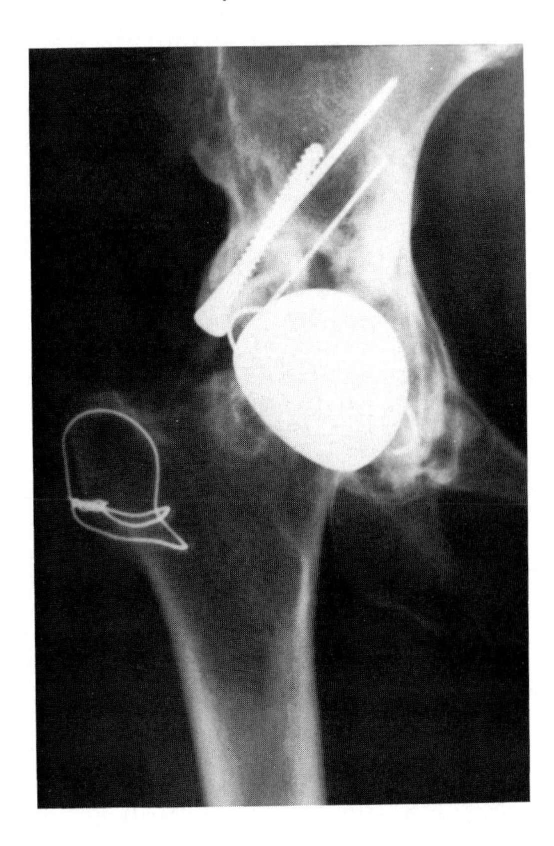

FIGURE 22–3. Follow-up 9 years after total hip arthroplasty with internal eccentric shells (THARIES) replacement and iliac grafting with loosening of the acetabular component. Note the 4 mm of lucency around the pubic acrylic peg and the 1.5 mm of lucency in the other bone cement areas. A mottled, cystic, and sclerotic area is seen at the lateral head-neck margin, but serial radiographs reveal no change in component position. The femoral component was not loose at revision.

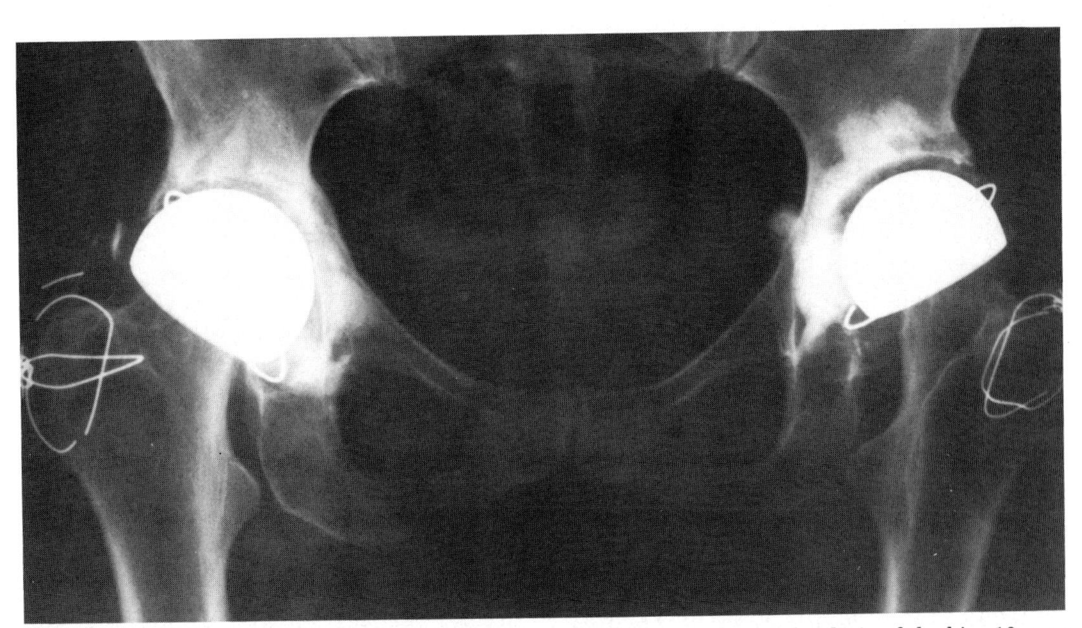

FIGURE 22–4. A 53-year-old woman developed pain in both hips secondary to dysplasia of the hips 10 years after a left total hip arthroplasty with internal eccentric shells (THARIES) and 8.5 years after a right THARIES. On the right side, the thin acrylic layer in zone 1 fragmented and caused localized osteolysis, further fragmentation of the acrylic, and abrasive wear of the acetabular side of the polyethylene, permitting an escaped liner from the acrylic bed that was otherwise intact. Since conversion to a press-fit prosthesis, the patient has resumed normal activities. The left THARIES continues to function 12 years after replacement, although early signs of socket loosening are seen radiographically.

brane with macrophages and giant cells. This effect resulted in osteolysis of bone. It has been postulated that the osteolysis may be induced by histiocytes participating in the elaboration of osteoclast-activating factor (interleukin-1) and prostaglandin E_2.[28, 38, 52, 67, 72, 100]

At revision surgery in patients with loose femoral components, the femoral necks were covered with thick yellowish membranes saturated with histiocytes. Small focal areas of necrosis were sometimes seen, but the bone remnants were generally well vascularized. In several cases of primary acetabular loosening, variable amounts of femoral neck thinning and cysts were observed. Ground sections of these specimens revealed structural compensation by hypertrophy of the remaining bone.

The demanding role that technique plays in this procedure is documented by our own experience. In 1978 and 1979, we changed our cement fixation technique. The large central cement fixation hole (10 mm diameter, 10 to 15 mm long) was discontinued, and multiple smaller drill holes were made in the prepared femoral bone. Unfortunately, loosening rates on the femoral side rose. However, surprising femoral durability was demonstrated in our earlier series, especially involving osteoarthritis.

Overall, the risk of failure in this and any other revision procedure is higher in young patients, highly active patients, patients whose diagnoses are associated with bone stock deficiency (avascular necrosis, congenital dysplasia of the hip, and revision of prior surface replacements), and patients whose revisions are performed by a surgeon with limited experience in the resurfacing hip procedure. In our series, osteoarthritic patients were at reduced risk of failure.

In patients without gross osteolysis secondary to acetabular loosening, few femoral neck fractures (n = 8) have occurred. The fracture line of these femora extended from the internal rim of the femoral cup across the dome to the opposite internal rim. The bone proximal to the fracture line was viable. Along the fracture surface, microfractures were occasionally observed with healing callus characteristic of fatigue fracture. The surrounding membranes contained normal tissue with no histiocytes and implant particulate debris or osteolysis. In patients with osteolysis-induced femoral neck erosion, eight fractures occurred because of substantial weakening of the supporting bone structure. There were three traumatic cervical fractures.

Neck Cysts of the Femoral Neck

Eight patients in our series had "enigmatic pain" severe enough to warrant reexploration, although examination findings were otherwise unremarkable clinically and radiographically. The time to reoperation ranged from 9 to 74 months. In all the specimens available for analysis, pathologic cystic lesions were identified within the femoral head, neck, or both. In three patients, the number and size of the cysts varied but were not extensive enough to cause loss of fixation among the femoral shell, the acrylic cement, and the supporting bone (Fig. 22–5). Unfortunately, the femoral head of the patient in Figure 22–5 was studied at a time when we examined only one or two sections histologically. The

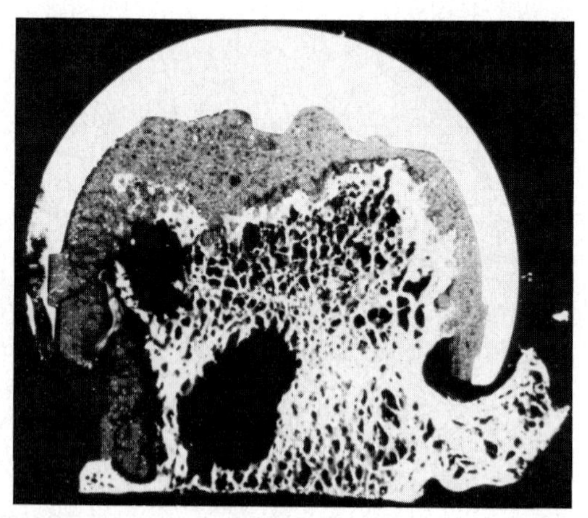

FIGURE 22–5. Microradiogram of the femoral head and neck of a patient 50 months after total hip arthroplasty with internal eccentric shells (THARIES) replacement at age 28 for post-traumatic osteochondritis dissecans. Neither component was loose but conversion to a stem-type device was performed because of the unexplained pain. Note the large cyst that contained a membrane with abundant mononuclear histiocytes and macrophages with synovial lining–like cells.

quality of the histologic preparation was less than optimal. The cyst contained variable numbers of histiocytes and giant cells associated with implant particulate debris, including small threads of polyethylene, metallic particles, and acrylic cement particles. Because most patients with cysts of the femoral necks or heads had no secondary arthritis at the time of the original operation and no protective secondary hyperemia in the bone, we initially thought that the cysts could have been related to avascular necrosis. However, microscopic examination of available surrounding tissue made this explanation unlikely.

Sepsis

Of the revisions, four percent (1.2 percent of the entire series) were performed for septic loosening. Two patients had previous histories of sepsis. In two others, sepsis was associated with the primary surgery. Only one patient had a late occurrence unrelated to the surgery. One patient with bilateral procedures had both sides fail because of sepsis.

Summary of Acrylic-Fixed THARIES Results

Except in cases of dysplasia and osteonecrosis and following surface replacement revision, our results with the THARIES system have been comparable with those of conventional hip replacements at similar follow-up periods when patients were matched for surgeon, age, sex, bone stock deficiency, and activity level. These results are in contrast to the disappointing results reported from other centers with much smaller groups of patients. However, most of the surgeons at these centers challenged the THARIES system by operating on young and often bone stock–deficient patients.[8, 17, 63, 87] We also found that the majority of our high-risk arthritis patients who had THARIES resurfacing that failed still benefited indirectly from the procedure. It bridged the time needed to bring them into the era of cementless prostheses before revision surgery was required. The revision employed grafting with a cementless socket. The procedure also allowed insertion of a virgin femoral prosthetic replacement, either cemented or cementless, into a nonviolated intramedullary canal. We learned the most important lesson—that the procedure produces remarkable femoral durability—only after analysis of our THARIES failures for the period 1987 to 1990. Most failures were due to socket loosening.

CEMENTLESS POROUS SURFACE REPLACEMENT

In the early 1980s, we introduced a new system involving a chamfered cylinder design for both the femur and acetabulum. The system had a porous surface for biologic ingrowth because we hoped to preserve the advantages of surface replacement. At the time, we were unaware of the femoral durability of the THARIES system.

Investigation into biologic ingrowth resurfacing at our institution began with animal experiments in the late 1970s and included many technique, design, and material changes. Many of our failures in dogs were related to technical errors.[13, 15] For example, neck fractures occurred as a result of inferior acetabular component impingement. These were eliminated by a design change incorporating an inferior relief into the socket. Dislocations resulted from failure to repair the external rotators and from improper component orientation. These dislocations were minimized by improved technique. Loosening occurred only with failure to achieve rigid fixation at the time of operation. Loosening did not occur when a precision interference fit was accomplished.

The most important lessons derived from resurfacing studies in dogs include (1) femoral head viability could be preserved; (2) bone ingrowth could be achieved on both the femoral and the acetabular sides, into either beads or mesh material but the degree was stress related; and (3) in the absence of complications, "anatomic" remodeling could take place. However, our enthusiasm for totally noncemented resurfacing was tempered by the development of metal-laden cysts and neck erosions in one third of the animals that carried implants for 18 to 24 months. The metallic debris originated primarily, we deduced, from inadequately sintered porous layers of titanium mesh and cobalt-chrome beads. Although these cysts did not compromise the 2-year functional results, failure was expected after a longer period.[62] We believed that clinical trials could commence when durable sintering could be accomplished. They were begun in 1983.

Component Design

The femoral and acetabular components incorporate a chamfered cylinder design based on the model developed in animal experiments.[15] We also introduced a hemispheric design with titanium beads to use with adjuvant screw fixation.[12] The chamfered cylinder was designed to preserve bone stock, maintain integrity of the pelvis, and achieve immediate component stability at the time of surgery without adjuvant fixation.[57] With the chamfered cylindric design, reaming is performed to achieve an exact fit for the chamfered and dome portions and, most importantly, an interference fit of 0.75 mm on the cylindric region. Thus, extremely close bony apposition is achieved with the cylindric area, providing an immediately stable component fixation.

Commercially pure titanium fiber mesh was sintered onto the internal and external surfaces of the femoral and acetabular Ti-6Al-4Va alloy shells, respectively. The mesh was 1.5 mm thick with a pore size of 300 to 500 μm and a porosity of 35 to 50 percent.[48] The system was designed so that less bone was removed in depth and circumferentially than in a comparable implantation in the acrylic-fixed THARIES system. Femoral preparation, similar to the latest technique in the THARIES design, allowed for removal of pathologic bone, preservation of enough bone for fixation, and maximization of the component surface area in contact with the bone (see Fig. 22–1).[10, 19] Removable snap-in socket inserts made of ultrahigh molecular weight polyethylene facilitated interchangeability of different femoral component sizes (Fig. 22–6).

Results

Each of the hemispheric and chamfered cylinder socket designs has undergone several changes in 7 years of clinical experience. The current design has a modular socket and femoral component of cobalt-chrome alloy. Technique changes were instituted to facilitate socket implantation in a more horizontal position and to permit direct apposition of the ingrowth surfaces to the prepared socket bed. Although these simplified the technique, the procedure is still exacting. Both of the socket designs, hemispheric and chamfered cylinder, have been successful with respect to durability of fixation (Fig. 22–7). No migration has been observed and neither has failure of bone ingrowth with the earliest chamfered cylinder designs or with the later hemispheric designs. The earliest hemispheric design incorporated hubs to accommodate regular screws, but the complexity of the insertion and the design of the hubs always increased the vertical inclination angle. However, two of three removed components of the earliest design, of nine implanted, were fixed by bone ingrowth. The ingrowth was all fibrous in one postmenopausal patient (Fig. 22–8). All these components were removed because of femoral failure; the sockets were removed because of their extreme vertical orientation. The

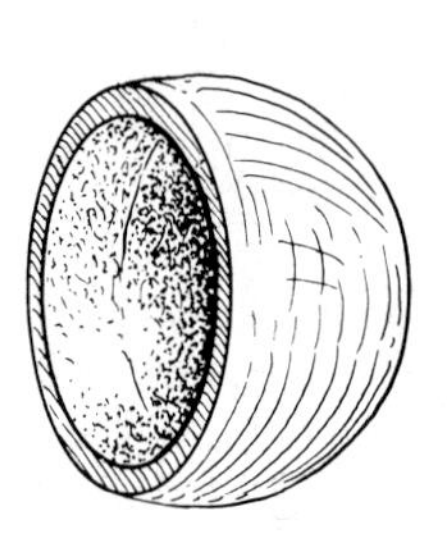
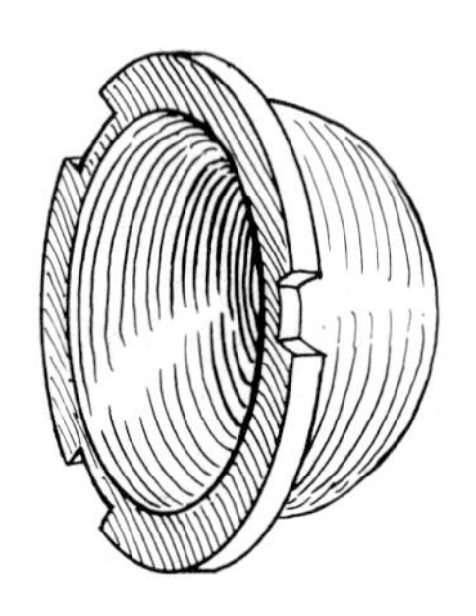
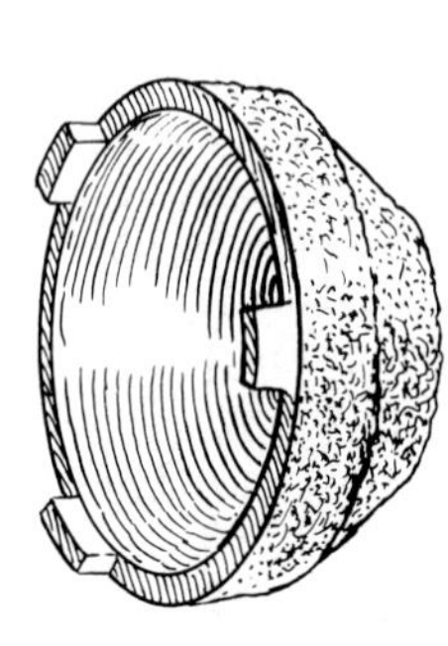

FIGURE 22–6. Current porous surface replacement components. The femoral component is cobalt-chromium alloy with a chamfered cylinder shape and an average pore size of 200 μm. The modular acetabular component has a shell of Ti-6Al-4V alloy and a commercially pure titanium porous surface. The polyethylene liner is modular and snaps into the acetabular shell.

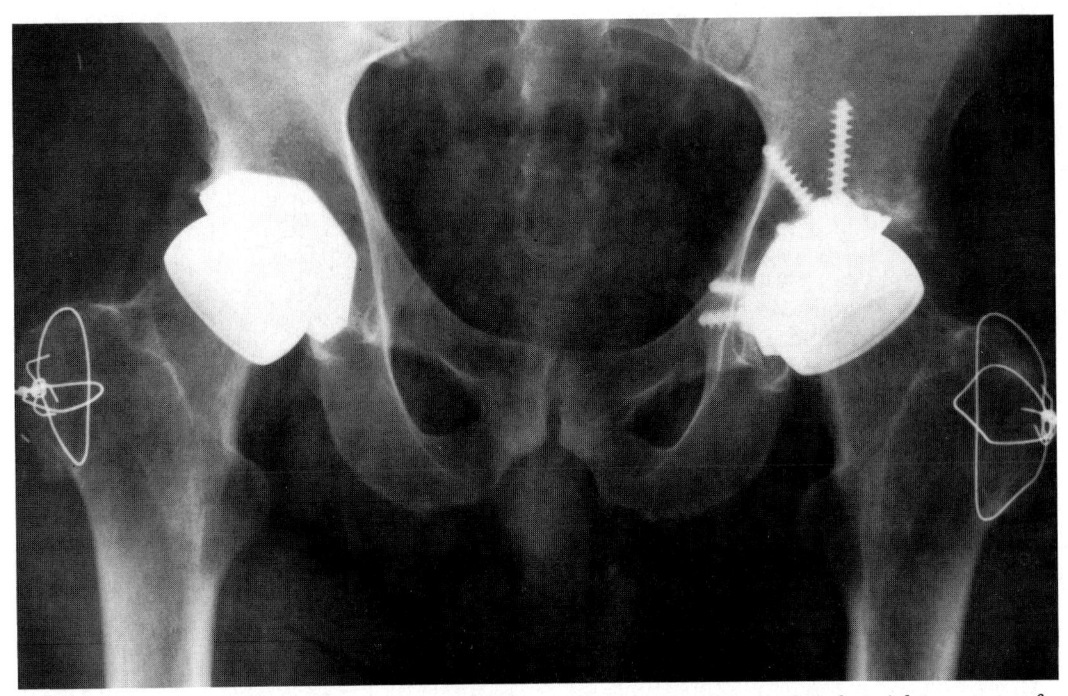

FIGURE 22–7. Follow-up radiograph of a 46-year-old man 6 years and 3 months after right porous surface replacement and 5 years and 6 months after left porous surface replacement, chamfered cylinder design–type, for severe degenerative osteoarthritis. He was pain free and functioning at a high level.

FIGURE 22–8. Follow-up radiograph of a 53-year-old woman with osteoarthritis of the left hip secondary to epiphyseal growth disturbance following hip surgery of unknown type at the age of 5 because of severe coxa valga. Radiograph was made 6 years after surface replacement with porous hemispheric acetabular component, autogenous femoral head dome graft to pelvis, and cemented femoral component (hybrid). At this follow-up examination, the patient had minimal discomfort and walked with a mild limp. She functioned at an 8 level with an activity level of 6 and had a functional range of motion. Note the thin radiolucency in zone 2 at the socket bone interface with a surrounding sclerotic line.

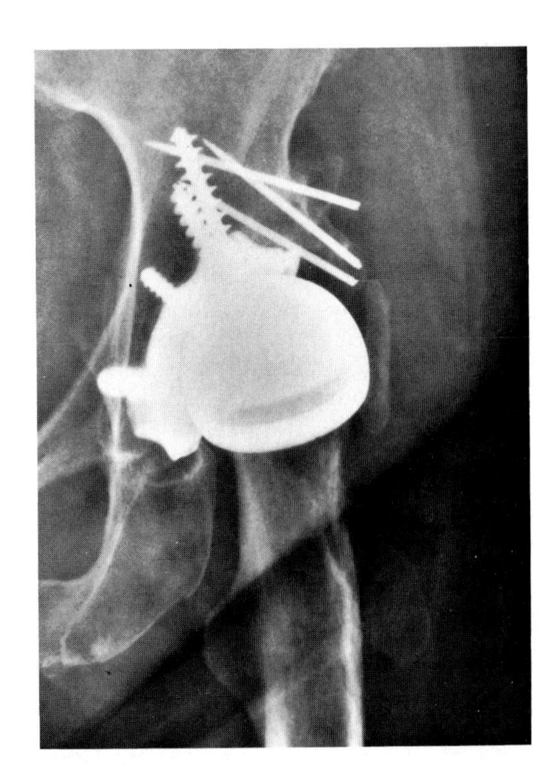

remaining components (six) appear on radiographs to be well fixed by bone.

The chamfered cylinder socket has been especially useful because it conserves bone. Roughly 3 mm is saved on the diameter as compared with the hemispheric design for a similar all-around thickness of polyethylene. Currently the term chamfered cylinder describes the exterior shape, the interior having been changed to a hemispheric design to facilitate manufacture of the modular liner and its implantation. The number of chamfered cylinder sockets implanted is now over 300. The chamfered cylinder has advantages that include removal of sufficient pathologic bone, minimal removal of normal bone, large ingrowth surface area, inherent stability with an interference fit, and lack of need for adjuvant fixation. Modular liner exchange capability has been demonstrated through revisions necessitated because of femoral failure.[14]

Although the expected durability has not been achieved in all patients, the improved socket design has eliminated failure due to socket loosening that plagued the era of cemented systems. Unfortunately, when the porous modular sockets were designed in 1982 and 1983, we had not yet recognized the potential for cemented femoral durability. Instead, we replaced the all acrylic–fixed system with an all-cementless system. Our first femoral component was chamfered cylinder Ti-6Al-4V with commercially pure titanium mesh. Despite the fact that no acrylic was used, the replacements have been plagued by femoral failures. Our hip survivorship values at 5 years are now slightly worse than our initial all acrylic–fixed THARIES experience. Essentially, we found ways to avoid the early acetabular failures of the era of the THARIES cemented system only to encounter an equal number of femoral-sided failures in the era of the porous systems. Had we selected a hybrid system initially, cementing the femoral component of cobalt-chrome, our failure rates might have been extremely low or nonexistent to date. Our lone long-term hybrid at 6 years, despite complex reconstruction, remains an excellent result (Fig. 22–9). Hybrids during the past 2 years have increased. These hybrids have been as successful as anticipated after our critical long-term analysis of femoral durability with cement fixation. However, the follow-up period is too short to confirm that this change will markedly improve long-term results.

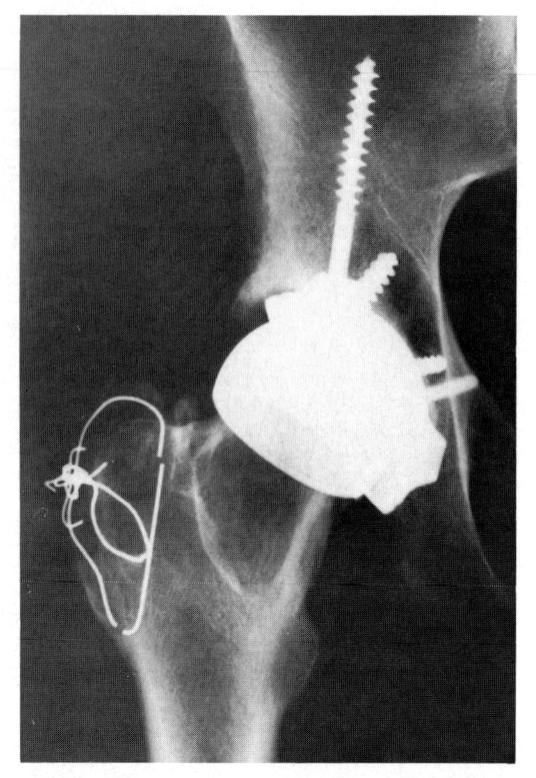

FIGURE 22–9. Five-year follow-up radiograph of a 53-year-old woman after porous surface replacement with early hemispheric design. She was extremely active (backpacking and skiing), but radiolucency progressively developed in the femoral neck with surrounding sclerotic halo. Note the wear (> 1 mm) with migration of the femoral component. The socket had a lucency with a surrounding sclerotic line suspicious of primary fibrous ingrowth confirmed at the time of revision surgery. "Metallosis" and neck cavitation were noted. The membrane lining contained macrophages and osteoclasts. Conversion was performed to a press-fit prosthesis.

We have had an excellent opportunity to study the quality of the bearing surface and assess its relation to failure because of surgical retrieval of 22 femoral components, 21 at revision and one in a patient who died of causes unrelated to the implant. The removals at revision were necessitated by mesh debonding in the hip of one patient, neck fractures in four (two in patients with juvenile rheumatoid arthritis), fractures or loosenings (no tissue ingrowth at revision) in two postmenopausal patients, and cyst formation in the femoral neck in 16 patients. Because 20 of 21 failures appeared to be caused by osteolysis induced by polyethylene debris in concert with titanium debris, we concluded that the titantium bearing is unsatisfactory and has directly or indirectly led to failure in all cases (Fig. 22–8). In reviewing our results with those of conventional replacements utilizing titanium bearings for nonmodular revision stems between 1980 and 1985, we found the same type of increasing wear and pending need for revision in highly active patients. Furthermore, we have retrieved titanium bearings from other replacement systems that have failed with the same identified wear mechanism. We believe that the soft titanium surface produced an excessive amount of particulate debris, primarily polyethylene, and this induced a macrophagic response causing severe osteolysis with resulting fracture or loosening. Under scanning electron microscopy, the femoral component surfaces have gouges 0.1 to 1.5 μm deep, with the magnitude related to the length of time of implantation and the patient's activity level. When we recognized that this was a serious problem, we changed to cobalt-chromium alloy for the femoral component. In addition, our procedures now include the increased use of hybrid acrylic-fixed devices.

The opportunity to observe sections of femoral specimens serially has enabled us to analyze bone ingrowth, which was demonstrated in all but two of the components. Bone ingrowth was observed in all of the men and in all of the premenopausal women who underwent the procedure. The depth and extent varied—bone ingrowth was more prominent in the chamfered portion and less prominent in the cylindric portion, particularly at the cup and in the dome. Bone ingrowth was present even in a specimen obtained 4 months postoperatively, at the time of one patient's death from causes unrelated to the replacement. The percentage of ingrowth in our surface replacement model has been much better than that reported in other retrieval analyses of systems with stemmed components and other socket designs. This difference is probably due to the rigid initial fixation and intimate contact we achieved at surgery. However, unlike the favorable bone ingrowth observed in relation to tilted socket components, which on occasion had gaps postoperatively that subsequently filled in with bone, this did not occur on the femoral side. Where the bone was in contact with the ingrowth surface, bone ingrowth occurred; where they were not in contact, stress shielding and loss of trabecular bone occurred.

Because many of the initial components were tilted, owing to the technical difficulties of implanting with an interference fit, we developed improved techniques to optimize results, including new lucent see-through contour contact gauges that improved our ability to assess the precison of the chamfered cylinder–prepared surface. We improved the precision of the dome cut perpendicular to the neck by close observation. The bone preparation and subsequent implantation orientation were also enhanced. Further, we found that even when the bone was prepared correctly, the component often tilted during the impaction process. We needed better instrumentation to seat the component correctly. The seating gauge was created to accomplish the objective of full contact of the components, as judged by the anteroposterior and frog lateral radiographs. Although we have not had to remove any specimens yet, and therefore have not had the opportunity to evaluate the uniformity of bone ingrowth, we expect the results to be better. The implantation technique still remains complex.

In order to make the procedure simpler for the surgeon, the interior configuration for the femoral component has been changed in order to self-center the component utilizing a tapered cone design. We have not had enough experience with the new technique to judge whether our objectives will be met, but we are encouraged by the results with the modular socket, which eliminates the main cause of failure in the acrylic-fixed surface systems.

INDICATIONS AND CONTRAINDICATIONS FOR SURFACE REPLACEMENT

We believe that surface replacement should be considered for the patient who might require a revision and a second replacement. Young or active patients are included as well as older patients who want to participate in activities thought to shorten the durability of replacements and who are willing to accept the risk that a revision may be required eventually. Several especially good indications exist for this surgery that should be considered for any age. One is deformity of the proximal femur that would make a stemmed replacement impossible or extremely difficult technically or that would prejudice the result. Another is high risk of sepsis because of a previous sepsis in the hip region or because of a high susceptibility due to disease, to drug therapy with steroids or other immunosuppressive drugs, or to both. If sepsis does occur at some later time, the magnitude of revision surgery is reduced. One other indication that should be considered is neuromuscular disease, because the large diameter ball of the surface replacement makes the replacement more stable and minimizes the risk of dislocation.

Generally, candidates for this procedure are in the age range of 40 to 60 years. Men who are candidates may be older, but postmenopausal women should be no older than 55 years. Slightly older patients are acceptable if a combination of characteristics is present such as heavy build, potentially high activity level (athletics, heavy labor), and other physiologic factors known to contribute to loosening or other complications of conventional replacement. We also consider the procedure for some patients younger than 40 who have no suitable alternatives. These patients include those with osteoarthritis secondary to slipped capital-femoral epiphysis, congenital hip dysplasia, dwarfism, coxa vara, Legg-Calvé-Perthes, or post-trauma with significant symptoms and functional losses. This patient group also includes those with osteonecrosis, who often have bilateral disease as young or middle-aged adults; those with multiple joint arthropathy; those with juvenile rheumatoid arthritis; and those with other arthritides who have increased risk of postoperative sepsis due to administration of steroids or other immunosuppressive drugs and general debility. Patients with primary osteoarthritis are candidates and their results are clearly the best.

The few absolute contraindications are active sepsis and open epiphyseal plates. Relative contraindications are loss of bone stock and severe limb length discrepancy. The alternatives of osteotomy and arthrodesis should be carefully considered for young, active patients; stem-type replacements should be considered for older patients.

TECHNIQUE FOR SURFACE REPLACEMENT

We recommend the lateral transtrochanteric approach using the lateral decubitus position. A trochanteric osteotomy is performed extracapsularly leaving the gluteus minimus attached initially to the capsule and trochanteric base. We still perform total capsulectomy but are evaluating circumferential acetabular capsular release. We are attempting to preserve extraperiosteal neck vessels, especially in the femoral neck in patients with only moderate arthritis, who may not have the hyperemia that is associated with advanced osteoarthritis. With a centering guide, we insert a 1/8-in Steinmann pin down the central neck axis. A guide for cylindric reaming down to neck size is thus provided. The pin is removed, and the dome is resected with the saw cut-off guide. Preparation of the femoral head is completed with either a chamfered cylinder or tapered cone facing reamer. The final reaming is performed with a pin reinserted down the center of the femoral head neck axis, which serves as a guide to prevent eccentric reaming. If cysts remain in the femoral head, the membrane linings are meticulously removed with a curette and high-speed burr.

For acetabular preparation, Hohmann retractors are placed around the acetabulum inferiorly and posteriorly. The femoral head, with the leg on the operating table, is displaced anteriorly. A special retractor is inserted to provide wide access to the acetabulum. The acetabulum is assessed for bone stock, and one of two socket configurations is chosen. The first is a hemispheric traditional socket, although the surgeon must be aware that it requires about 3 mm more of anteroposterior as well as mediolateral space for the same polyethylene thickness that a chamfered cylinder socket requires. However, the type of socket is the surgeon's choice. A hemispheric bed is prepared in the traditional manner with expanding reamers until the size of the bed corresponds to the size of the femoral component. The socket is prepared with a line-to-line contact. Sometimes a reamer of slightly smaller outside diameter is used for the socket if there is any tendency to ream eccentrically.

To prepare the acetabulum for the other choice, chamfered cylinder socket design with interference fit, the acetabular reamer guide must be fixed to the pelvis with care. The socket must be properly oriented in 15 degrees anteversion and 40 to 45 degrees acetabular lateral opening. If the slope of the acetabular walls is excessive, it is better to remove some of the anterior and posterior wall together with osteophytes in order to make the guide attachment less difficult, with an opening of 45 degrees or less. Threaded Steinmann pins are placed into the pelvis to provide rigid fixation with double-lock nuts (Fig. 22–10). Orientation provides 10 to 15 degrees of anteversion. Single-stage reaming is performed employing an appropriate-sized chamfered cylinder reamer. The direction is carefully checked to ensure proper orientation of the socket. Reaming is interrupted periodically to assess depth and quality of bone. A translucent contour contact gauge is inserted to check the extent of bone removal and to assess the contact areas. In an extremely dysplastic acetabulum, it is occasionally desirable to penetrate medially and inferiorly. This technique has created no problems when peripheral stability of the component after impaction has been adequate. The interference fit is 0.50 mm. Acetabular cyst lining membranes are removed with curettes and a high-speed burr. The cysts can be packed with bone removed from the femoral head or bone paste. Additional bone graft should not be applied because it only impedes ingrowth of bone.

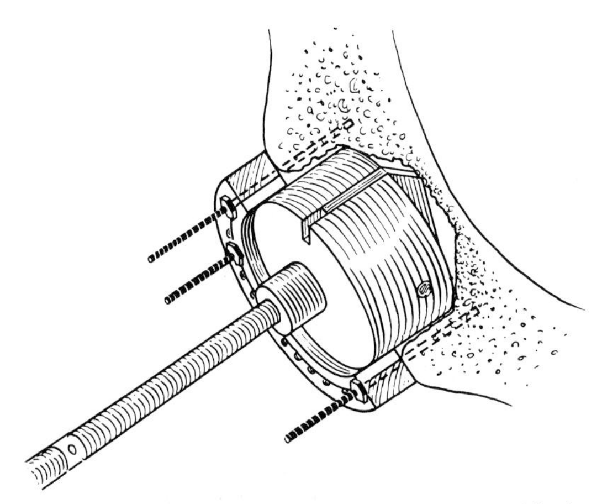

FIGURE 22–10. The acetabular reamer guide is temporarily fixed to the pelvis with three ⅛-in Steinmann pins and double-lock nuts for acetabular reaming.

When the hemispheric socket is inserted, circumferential screw fixation is preferred because it provides multiple contact areas. These include fixation into the ischium and pubis as well as the superior ilium. The liners are then inserted and carefully impacted.

If the femoral bone is of uniformly good quality, we recommend an ingrowth femoral component attached with an interference fit. When cystic cavities or residual defects are present, hybrid application employing a cemented femoral component is recommended. In either case, a seating guide is inserted around the neck inferior to the contour contact gauge. The guide is pressed into contact with bone to help determine when the component is fully seated. In the case of hybrid application, a central fixation hole ($\approx$ 1 cm diameter) is placed into the head 1 to 1.5 cm deep. Additional sclerotic areas of bone are drilled with a ⅛-in drill into softer cancellous bone distally. A sterilized rubber band is placed around the neck temporarily at the level at which the component will be fully seated. A balloon is filled with regular bone cement in a relatively low-viscosity state. The balloon filled with the acrylic is placed over the femoral head, contained around the neck with a circumferential wire, and the cement is pressurized into the cancellous bone. To make certain that the acrylic thickness is uniform all around, 2-mm spacers are placed on the dome of the femoral head. Acrylic cement is carefully trimmed around the neck circumferentially.

The greater trochanter is reattached with two wires placed approximately 5 and 10 mm under the trochanteric base. We employ a two-wire interlocking technique. If the patient is to receive radiotherapy and the trochanter may not be adequately shielded, we recommend placing two vertical wires and a single horizontal wire in a three-wire interlocking technique. Before wound closure, the wound is thoroughly irrigated and drained with two tubes inserted into the deep layers.

Postoperatively, all patients are placed in balanced suspension and treated with prophylactic antibiotics and warfarin. The patient begins walking on crutches at 3 days. Patients who have an all-cementless system are kept nonweightbearing for 2 months. Over the next 2 months, they gradually begin weightbearing. We believe that the cemented femoral component in a hybrid application with cementless socket requires approximately 2 months' protection before the patient should progress to a single support.

Fortunately, the current procedure for failed surfacing is less extensive than the primary procedure. Revision requires only a socket liner exchange and can be performed without trochanteric osteotomy. Less blood is lost and operative time is shorter than with primary replacements.

References

1. Akeson, W. H., Miyashita, C., Taylor, T. K. F., et al.: Experimental arthroplasty of the canine hip: Extracellular matrix composition in cup arthroplasty. J. Bone Joint Surg. 51A:149, 1969.
2. Amstutz, H. C. and Dorey, F.: The Development and Nine-Year Results of THARIES Resurfacing Arthroplasty. The Young Patient with Degenerative Hip Disease. Edited by J. Sevastik and I. Goldie. Uppsala, Almqvist & Wiksell, 1985.
3. Amstutz, H. C. and Graff-Radford, A.: THARIES Approach to Surface Replacement of the Hip. AAOS Instructional Course Lectures. St. Louis, C. V. Mosby Company, 30:688–737, 1981.
4. Amstutz, H. C., Clarke, I. C., Christie, J., and Graff-Radford, A.: Total hip articular replacement by internal eccentric shells. Clin. Orthop. 128:261, 1977.
5. Amstutz, H. C., Dorey, F., and O'Carroll, P. F.: THARIES resurfacing arthroplasty—evolution and long-term results. Clin. Orthop. 213:29–114, 1986.
6. Amstutz, H. C., Graff-Radford, A., Gruen, T. A., and Clarke, I. C.: THARIES surface replacement: A review of the first 100 cases. Clin. Orthop. 134:87, 1978.
7. Amstutz, H. C., Graff-Radford, A., Mai, L. L., and Thomas, B. J.: Surface replacement of the hip with the THARIES system: Two-to five-year results. J. Bone Joint Surg. 63A(8):1609–1677, 1981.
8. Amstutz, H. C., Kabo, J. M., Kim, W. C., and Yao, J.: Risk Factors for Femoral Head Resurfacing—Experimental Canine and Clinical Experience. Non-cemented Arthroplasty. Edited by R. H. Fitzgerald. New York, Raven Press, 1988.
9. Amstutz, H. C., Kabo, J. M., O'Carroll, P. F., and Kim, W. C.: Experimental and Preliminary Clinical Results of Porous Hip Resurfacing. The Young Patient with Degenerative Hip Disease. Edited by J. Sevastik and I. Goldie. Uppsala, Almqvist & Wiksell, 1985.
10. Amstutz, H. C., Kabo, M., Hermens, K., et al.: Porous surface replacement of the hip with chamfer cylinder design. Clin. Orthop. 222:140–160, 1987.
11. Amstutz, H. C., Kilgus, D. J., Thomas, B. J., and Webber, M. M.: Evaluation of Bone Ingrowth by Technetium Diphosphonate and Sulfur Colloid Scanning in Porous Hip Resurfacing. The Hip. St. Louis, C. V. Mosby Company, 1986.
12. Amstutz, H. C., Kabo, M., Hermens, K., et al.: Porous surface replacement of the hip with chamfer cylinder design. Clin. Orthop. 222:140–160, 1987.
13. Amstutz, H. C., Kim, W. C., O'Carroll, P. F., and Kabo, J. M.: Canine porous resurfacing hip arthroplasty—Long-term results. Clin. Orthop. 207:270–289, 1986.
14. Amstutz, H., Kilgus, D., Kabo, M., and Dorey, F.: Porous surface replacement of the hip with chamfered cylinder component. Arch. Orthop. Trauma Surg. 107:73–85, 1988.
15. Amstutz, H. C., O'Carroll, P. F., and Kim, W. C.: Comparative Experience with Canine and Human Titanium Fiber and Beaded Acetabular Components. The Hip. St. Louis, C. V. Mosby Company, 1985.
16. Amstutz, H. C., Ouzounian, T., Grauer, D., et al.: A simple technique for consistent visualization of the hip: The grid radiograph. J. Bone Joint Surg. 68A:1052–1056, 1986.
17. Amstutz, H. C., Thomas, B. J., Jinnah, R., et al.: Treatment of primary osteoarthritis of the hip. A comparison of total joint and surface replacement arthroplasty. J. Bone Joint Surg. 66A(2):228, 1984.
18. Amstutz, H. C.: Arthroplasty of the hip: The search for durable component fixation. Clin. Orthop. 200:343–361, 1985.
19. Amstutz, H. C.: The THARIES hip resurfacing technique. Orthop. Clin. North Am. 13:813, 1982.
20. Amstutz, H. C.: Surface Replacement of the Hip. The Hip. St. Louis, C. V. Mosby Company, 1980.
21. Aufranc, O. E.: Constructive hip surgery with vitallium mold. J. Bone Joint Surg. 39A:237, 1957.
22. Bierbaum, B. E. and Sweet, R.: Complications of resurfacing arthroplasty. Orthop. Clin. North Am. 13:761, 1982.
23. Capello, W. N. and Carter, D. R.: Finite-element Analysis of a Metal-backed Acetabular Component. The Hip. St. Louis, C. V. Mosby Company, 1983.
24. Capello, W. N., Ireland, P. H., Trammel, T. R., and Eicher, P.: Conservative total hip arthroplasty: A procedure to conserve bone stock. Clin. Orthop. 134:59–74, 1978.
25. Capello, W. N., Misamore, G. W., and Trancik, T. M.: Conservative total hip arthroplasty. Orthop. Clin. North Am. 13:833, 1982.
26. Capello, W. N., Wilson, N., and Wellman, H.: Bone Imaging—a Means of Evaluating Hip Sur-

face Replacement. The Hip. St. Louis, C. V. Mosby Company, 1980.
27. Capello, W. N.: Personal communication, 1986.
28. Chambers, T. J.: The cellular basis of bone resorption. Clin. Orthop. 151:283–293, 1980.
29. Chandler, H. P., Reineck, R. L., Wixon, R. L., and McCarthy, J. C.: Total hip replacements in patients younger than thirty years old. J. Bone Joint Surg. 63A:1426, 1981.
30. Charnley, J.: Low Friction Arthroplasty of The Hip: Theory and Practice. New York, Springer-Verlag, 1979.
31. Charnley, J.: Tissue reactions to polytetrafluoroethylene. Lancet 2:1379, 1963.
32. Charnley, J. C.: Arthroplasty of the hip: A new operation. Lancet 1:1129, 1961.
33. Clarke, I. C., Amstutz, H. C., Christie, J., and Graff-Radford, A.: The John Charnley Award Paper: THARIES Surface Replacement Arthroplasty for the Arthritic Hip: Rebirth of an Earlier Concept? The Hip. St. Louis, C. V. Mosby Company, 1977.
34. Clarke, I. C. and Amstutz, H. C.: Human Hip Joint Geometry and Hemiarthroplasty Selection. The Hip. St. Louis, C. V. Mosby Company, 1975.
35. Clarke, I. C., and Amstutz, H. C.: Design Concepts and Results of Surface Replacement Procedures for the Hip Joint. Disability. Proceedings of a Seminar on Rehabilitation of the Disabled, August 1978, Glasglow, Scotland. Edited by R. M. Kenedi, J. P. Paul, and J. Hughes. Great Britain, Macmillan Company, 1979.
36. Clarke, I. C.: Biomechanics. Multifactorial design choices—An essential compromise? Orthop. Clin. North Am. 13:681–707, 1982.
37. Cook, S. D., Georgette, F. S., Skinner, H. B., et al.: The fatigue properties of porous-coated and carbon-coated Ti-6Al-4Va implants. Transactions of the 29th Annual Meeting of Orthopaedic Research Society 8:332, 1983.
38. Cserhati, M. D., Oliveria, L. G., Jacob, H. A. C., and Schreiber, A.: Histomorphological investigations of coxa femoral ends following double-cup arthroplasty according to Freeman. Arch. Orthop. Trauma Surg. 94:233–240, 1979.
39. Delaunay, C.: Personal communication, 1986.
40. DeLee, J. G. and Charnley, J.: Radiological demarcation of cemented sockets in total hip replacement. Clin. Orthop. 121:20, 1976.
41. Dorey, F. and Amstutz, H. C.: Survivorship analysis in the evaluation of joint replacement. J. Arthroplasty 1(1):63–69, 1986.
42. Freeman, M. A. R. and Bradley, G. W.: ICLH double cup arthroplasty. Orthop. Clin. North Am. 13:799, 1982.
43. Freeman, M. A. R. and Bradley, G. W.: ICLH surface replacement of the hip. J. Bone Joint Surg. 65B(4):405–411, 1983.
44. Freeman, M. A. R., Cameron, H. U., and Brown, G. C.: Cemented double cup arthroplasty of the hip: A five-year experience with the ICLH prosthesis. Clin. Orthop. 134:45–52, 1978.
45. Freeman, M. A. R., Swanson, S. A. V., Day, W. H., and Thomas, R. J.: Conservative total replacement of the hip. J. Bone Joint Surg. 57B:114, 1975.
46. Furuya, K., Tsuchiya, M., and Kawachi, S.: Socket-cup arthroplasty. Clin. Orthop. 134:41–44, 1978.
47. Furuya, K.: Results of socket-cup arthroplasty. J. Jpn. Orthop. Assoc. 50:721, 1976.
48. Galante, J. O., Rostoker, W., Leuck, R., and Ray, R.: Sintered fiber metal composites as a basis for attachment of implants to bone. J. Bone Joint Surg. 53A:101, 1971.
49. Gerard, Y., Segal, P., and Bedoucha, J. S.: Hip arthroplasty by matching cups. Rev. Chir. Orthop. 60:281, 1974.
50. Gerard, Y.: Hip arthroplasty by matching cups. Clin. Orthop. 134:25, 1978.
51. Goldie, I. F., Bunketorp, O., Gunterberg, B., et al.: Resurfacing arthroplasty of the hip. Biomechanical, morphological, and clinical aspects based on the results of a preliminary clinical study. Arch. Orthop. Trauma Surg. 95:149–157, 1979.
52. Goldring, S. R., Schiller, A. L., Roelke, M., et al.: The synovial-like membrane at the bone-cement interface in loose total hip replacements and its proposed role in bone lysis. J. Bone Joint Surg. 65:575–584, 1983.
53. Haboush, E. J.: A new operation for arthroplasty of the hip based on biomechanics, photoelasticity, fast-setting dental acrylic and other considerations. Bull. Hosp. Joint Dis. 13:242, 1953.
54. Harris, W. H. and White, R. E.: Socket fixation using a metal-backed acetabular component for total hip replacement. J. Bone Joint Surg. 64A:745–748, 1982.
55. Head, W. C.: The Wagner surface replacement arthroplasty. Orthop. Clin. North Am. 13:789, 1982.
56. Head, W. C.: Wagner surface replacement arthroplasty of the hip. J. Bone Joint Surg. 63A:420–427, 1981.
57. Hedley, A. K., Kabo, J. M., Kim, W. C., et al.: Bone ingrowth fixation of new design acetabular components. A canine model. Clin. Orthop. 176:120, 1983.
58. Huiskes, R., Strens, P. G. E., Van Heck, J., and Slooff, T.: Interface stresses in the resurfaced hip. Finite element analysis of load transmission in the femoral head. Acta Orthop. Scand. 56:474, 1985.
59. Jolley, M. N., Salvati, E. A., and Brown, G. C.: Early results and complications of surface replacement of the hip. J. Bone Joint Surg. 64A(3):366–377, 1982.
60. Joyce, J. J.: Personal communication, 1982.
61. Kaplan, E. L. and Meier, P.: Nonparametric estimation from incomplete observations. J. Am. Stat. Assoc. 53:457, 1981.
62. Kim, W. C., Amstutz, H. C., O'Carroll, P. F., et al.: Porous Ingrowth in Canine Resurfacing Hip Arthroplasty: Analysis of Results with Up to Two-Year Follow-up. John Charnley Award Paper. The Hip. St. Louis, C. V. Mosby Company, 1984.
63. Kim, W. C., Grogan, T. J., Amstutz, H. C., and Dorey, F.: Survivorship comparison of THARIES and conventional hip arthroplasty in patients younger than 40 years. Clin. Orthop. 214:269–277, 1987.
64. Kim, W. C., Nottingham, P., Luben, R. A., et al.: Detection of osteoclast-activating factor in membranes removed at revision total hip arthroplasties. Trans. Orthop. Res. Soc. 9:276, 1985.
65. Lee, E. T.: Statistical Methods for Survival Data

Analysis. Belmont, California, Wadsworth, 1980.
66. Levack, B., Freeman, M. A. R., and Alencari, P. G. G.: Double Cup Replacement and Results up to 1984. The Young Patient with Degenerative Hip Disease. Edited by J. Sevastik and I. Goldie. Uppsala, Almqvist & Wiksell, 1985.
67. Luben, R. A., Mundy, G. R., Trummel, C. L., and Raisz, L. G.: Partial purification of osteoclast activating factor from physohaemagglutinin stimulated human leukocytes. J. Clin. Invest. 53:1473, 1974.
68. Ma, S. M., Kabo, J. M., and Amstutz, H. C.: Frictional torque in surface and conventional hip replacement. J. Bone Joint Surg. 65A(3):366–370, 1983.
69. Mallory, T. H., Ballas, S., and VanAtta, G.: Total articular replacement arthroplasty. A clinical review. Clin. Orthop. 185:131–136, 1984.
70. Markolf, K. and Amstutz, H. C.: Mechanical strength of the femur following resurfacing and conventional total hip replacement procedures. Clin. Orthop. 147:170–180, 1980.
71. McKellop, H., Clarke, I. C., Markolf, K., and Amstutz, H.: Friction and wear properties of polymer, metal, and ceramic prosthetic joint material evaluated on a multi-channel screening device. J. Biomed. Mater. Res. 5:619–653, 1981.
72. Mirra, J. M., Amstutz, H. C., Matos, M., and Gold, R.: The pathology of the joint tissues and its clinical relevance in prosthesis failure. Clin. Orthop. 117:221–240, 1976.
73. Moreland, J. R., Gruen, T. A., Mai, L. L., and Amstutz, H. C.: Aseptic Loosening of Total Hip Replacement: Incidence and Significance. The Hip. St. Louis, C. V. Mosby Company, 1980.
74. Müller, M. E. and Boltzy, X.: Artificial hip joints made from PROTOSOL. Bull. Assoc. Study Problems Internal Fixation, pp. 1–5, 1968.
75. Nasser, S., Campbell, P., Kilgus, J., et al.: Cementless total joint arthroplasty prostheses with titanium alloy articular surfaces: A human implant retrieval analysis. Clin. Orthop. 261:170–184, 1990.
76. Ouzounian, T. and Amstutz, H. C.: Evaluation of musculoskeletal sepsis utilizing indium-111 WBC imaging. Clin. Orthop. 221:304–311, 1987.
77. Paltrinieri, M. and Trentani, C.: A modification of the hip arthroprosthesis. Chir. Organi Mov. 60(11):85–95, 1971.
78. Pedersen, D. R., Crowninshield, R. D., Brand, R., and Johnston, R. C.: An axiosymmetric model of acetabular components in total hip arthroplasty. J. Biomech. 15:305–315, 1982.
79. Salvati, E., Wright, T., Burstein, A., and Jacobs, B.: Fracture of polyethylene acetabular cups. Report of two cases. J. Bone Joint Surg. 61A:1239–1242, 1979.
80. Salvati, E. A., Wilson, P. D., Jolley, M. N., et al.: A ten-year follow-up study of our first one-hundred consecutive total hip replacements. J. Bone Joint Surg. 63A:753, 1981.
81. Santore, R. F.: Cup Arthroplasty. Presentation. International Symposium on the Young Patient with Degenerative Hip Disease. Stockholm, 1984.
82. Shybut, G. T., Askew, M. J., Hori, R. Y., and Stulberg, D. S.: Theoretical and Experimental Studies of Femoral Stresses Following Surface Replacement Hip Arthroplasty. The Hip. St. Louis, C. V. Mosby Company, 192–224, 1980.
83. Smith-Petersen, M. N.: Evolution of the mould arthroplasty of the hip joint. J. Bone Joint Surg. 30B:59, 1948.
84. Strens, P. H. G. E.: An Analysis of Implant Failure in the Wagner Resurfacing Arthroplasty. Druk: Grafish Service Centrum Nijmegen b.v., pp. 1–224, 1986.
85. Tanaka, S.: Surface replacement of the hip joint. Clin. Orthop. 134:75, 1978.
86. Thomas, B. J., Amstutz, H. C., Mai, L. L., and Webber, M. M.: Identification of hip surface arthroplasty failures with TcSc/TcmDP radionuclide imaging. Clin. Orthop. 167:106–112, 1982.
87. Tooke, S. M., Moreland, J., and Amstutz, H. C.: Results of conventional and resurfacing replacements in congenital dysplastic hips: Two to 7.5 year results. Clin. Orthop. (In preparation.)
88. Tooke, S. M., Amstutz, H. C., and Hedley, A. K.: Results of transtrochanteric rotational osteotomy for femoral head osteonecrosis. Clin. Orthop. 224:150–157, 1987.
89. Townley, C. O.: Conservative total articular replacement arthroplasty (the TARA procedure) with the fixed femoral cup. Orthop. Trans. 5:463, 1981.
90. Townley, C. O.: Intramedullary cup-stem arthroplasty of the hip joint. A 16 mm film. Chicago, AAOS Audio-Visual Film Library, 1964.
91. Trentani, C. and Montagnani, A.: Follow-up of 150 Cases for More Than Ten Years according to Paltrinieri-Trentani. The Young Patient with Degenerative Hip Disease. Edited by J. Sevastik and I. Goldie. Uppsala, Almqvist & Wiksell, 1985.
92. Trentani, C. and Vaccarino, F.: Complications in surface replacement arthroplasty of the hip: Experience with the Paltrinieri-Trentani prosthesis. Int. Orthop. 4:247–252, 1981.
93. Trentani, C. and Vaccarino, F.: The Paltrinieri-Trentani hip joint resurface arthroplasty. Clin. Orthop. 134:36, 1978.
94. Trentani, C. and Vaccarino, F. P.: The Paltrinieri-Trentani hip joint resurface arthroplasty. Orthop. Clin. North Am. 13:857, 1982.
95. Turner, R. H. and Scheller, A. D.: Revision Total Hip Arthroplasty. New York, Grune & Stratton, 1982.
96. VanSycle, P. and Walker, P.: Parametric analysis of design criteria for acetabular components of surface replacement hip devices. Trans. 26th Ann. Meet. Orthop. Res. Soc. 5:292, 1980.
97. Wagner, H.: Surface replacement arthroplasty of the hip. Clin. Orthop. 134:102–130, 1978.
98. Wagner, H.: Symposium on Surface Replacement of the Hip. American Academy of Orthopaedic Surgeons Annual Meeting, Atlanta, February 10, 1980.
99. Wagner, H.: Personal communication, 1986.
100. Willert, H. G., Ludwig, J., and Semlitsch, M.: Reaction of bone to methacrylate after hip arthroplasty. A long-term gross, light microscopic, and scanning electron microscopic study. J. Bone Joint Surg. 56A:1382, 1974.
101. Wroblewski, B. M.: The mechanisms of fracture of the femoral prosthesis in total hip replacement. Int. Orthop. (SICOT) 3:137–139, 1979.

CHAPTER 23

Revision Total Hip Arthroplasty

WILLIAM PETTY

Although the results of primary total hip arthroplasties are, in general, excellent, some fail after a variable period of time. Approximately 10 percent of total hip arthroplasties in the United States are revisions of previous total hip replacements. Revision operations are nearly always more difficult than primary hip replacements for both the patient and the health care team. Patients often are considerably older than at the time of the primary arthroplasties and may have increased general medical and musculoskeletal disabilities. Previous operations on the hip often result in deficiencies of hip muscles and other soft tissue. Soft tissue scarring may be extensive, involving vital structures such as the sciatic nerve. At the time of revision, the hip may be infected, and the bone stock is usually deficient, sometimes severely. The failed components must be removed before reconstruction can be done. Whether the previous arthroplasty was cemented or cementless, removal of the failed components may be difficult and may result in additional damage to the bone stock. Incidences of intraoperative and postoperative complications are greater with revision procedures.

PREOPERATIVE EVALUATION

Pain in the region of the hip or thigh and other symptoms, such as dislocation, after total hip replacement are distressing to both patient and surgeon. These problems contrast sharply to the expected result—an essentially asymptomatic hip.

The preoperative evaluation for revision total hip replacement is similar to that for primary total hip arthroplasty (see Chapter 16, *Total Hip Arthroplasty: Preoperative Evaluation*) but may be more extensive because of a patient's increased medical and musculoskeletal disability.

History

The same questions are posed to the patient as those for possible primary hip replacement, but the clinician should solicit further information on all previous hip operations. Of specific interest is the postoperative course. Did the wound heal primarily? Was there prolonged drainage, fever, or pain, suggesting the possibility of infection? Was a definite diagnosis of infection made? How did the postoperative rehabilitation program progress? Were there any specific problems?

Some patients develop pain after a symptom-free interval of many years. Others never achieve a pain-free status after a primary hip replacement. An initial pain-free period suggests aseptic loosening or possibly a late hematogenous infection. Continued pain after primary hip replacement suggests the possibility of early component instability or infection beginning at the time of surgery. If the initial hip replacement followed another failed operation, unrecognized infection may have been present at the time of the primary hip replacement.

Pain associated with loose arthroplasty components may be constant. More likely, the pain will be associated with weightbearing, and it is often worse when the patient first stands and takes the first few steps. The patient with a loose femoral component may feel the need to manipulate or position the hip into a more comfortable position before beginning to walk. This feeling is less common with a loose acetabular component. Some patients with grossly loose prostheses actually can feel the prostheses move inside the bone upon rotation or other movement of the hip. The pain attributable to a loose socket is usually in the groin, whereas the pain attributable to a loose femoral component is typically in the upper or mid thigh. Deep-seated constant pain, affected little by hip motion or weightbearing, suggests the possibility of infection without loosening. Pain in patients with total hip replacements may radiate down the anterior thighs to the knees, but this occurrence is less common than with primary hip disease. Lateral hip pain may be due to trochanteric bursitis; posterior or diffuse pain may be due to a problem with the hip replacement or to other conditions, such as spinal disease.

The patient should be asked about fever, swelling, or warmth about the hip, which suggest infection. The patient may describe dislocation or apprehension of dislocation when the hip is in certain positions, suggesting subluxation (see Chapter 19, *Total Hip Arthroplasty: Complications.*)

Obtaining the patient's medical records, especially operative reports and previous antibiotic therapy records, is critical to history taking. The patient can provide substantial information for the history but may not be aware of many details and, of course, has no knowledge of the technical aspects of previous surgery. Operative notes provide helpful information about the prosthesis used for the hip replacement.

Physical Examination

Physical examination of the patient with failed total hip arthroplasty is similar to examination of the patient with possible primary hip replacement. Knowledge of previous incisions about the hip and status of soft tissues are important in planning revision surgery. Abductor function is analyzed carefully because a patient who has had previous hip surgery, especially multiple operations, often has avulsion of the greater trochanter or other deficiencies of important muscles.

The "push-pull" test may be helpful in evaluation for loose components, especially the femoral component (Fig. 23–1). The test is performed by either pushing or pulling on the extremity in a longitudinal direction, with the hip in full extension. The push or pull force is then suddenly reversed. Pain associated with the maneuver is suggestive of a loose prosthesis.

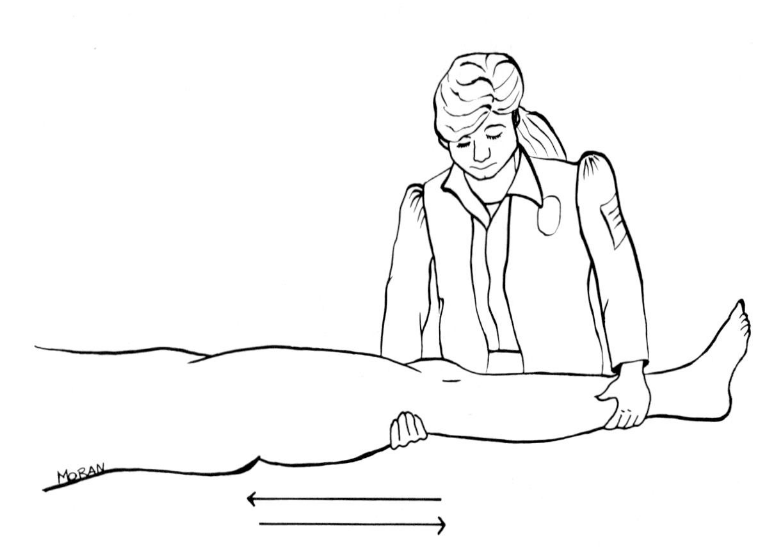

FIGURE 23–1. The "push-pull" test is used to evaluate loose total hip components, especially the femoral component. The test is performed by pushing or pulling on the extremity longitudinally and then reversing the force. Pain associated with the maneuver is suggestive of a loose prosthesis.

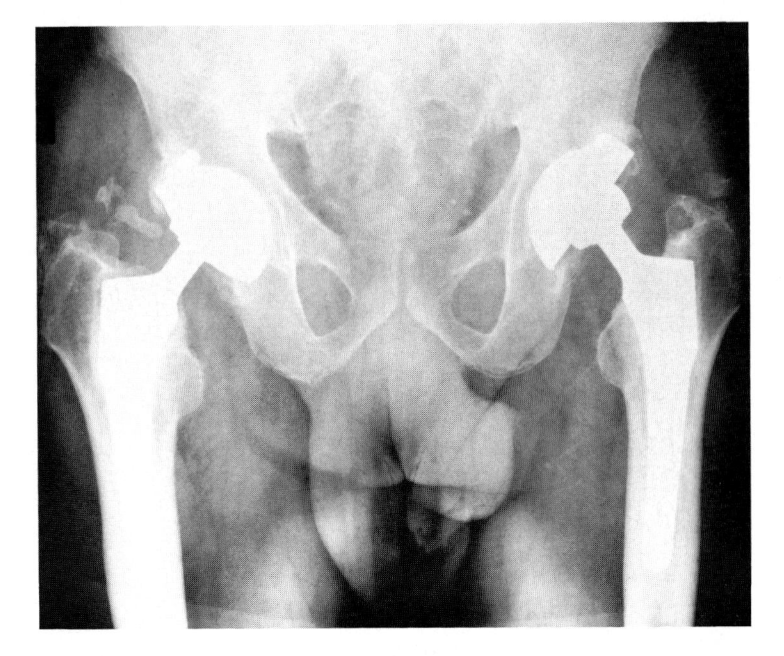

FIGURE 23–2. Orthopelvis view radiograph is centered on the symphysis pubis. This view provides visualization of the hip joint and most standard length femoral stems.

Radiographic and Laboratory Examinations

As with other hip diseases, the plain radiograph is the most valuable imaging study for evaluating the patient with problems following total hip replacement. The anteroposterior radiograph of the pelvis is centered on the symphysis pubis instead of on a point halfway between the symphysis pubis and the level of the superior iliac crest (Fig. 23–2). This ortho-pelvis radiograph provides excellent visualization of the hip joint and of most standard-length femoral stems. When longer stems are in place, additional views of the femur are necessary to see the entire prosthesis. The frog lateral position gives the best lateral visualization of the proximal portion of the femoral component (Fig. 23–3). The cross-table lateral view enables evaluation of the position of the acetabular component (anteversion or retroversion) and the status of the bone stock in the posterior column and neck of the ilium (Fig. 23–4).[63] In some instances, these standard views are supplemented with pelvic inlet and outlet or Judet oblique views to better evaluate the status of the socket and pelvic bone stock. Serial radiographs—starting with the one taken a few days after surgery—are invaluable in assessing septic or aseptic loosening. Additional imaging studies, including radionuclide scanning, tomography (either plain or computer-assisted), magnetic resonance, and angiography, may be helpful in the evaluation of failed total hip arthroplasty (see Chapter 11, *Imaging of Total Joint Replacement*).

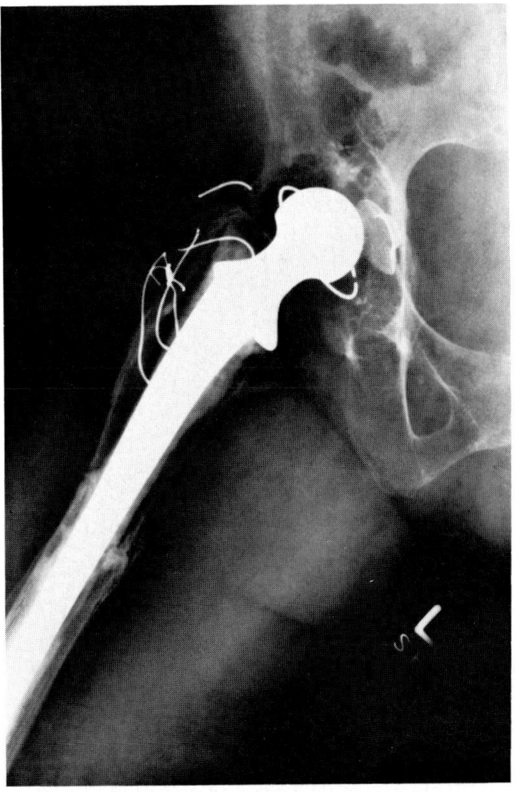

FIGURE 23–3. The "frog" lateral radiograph. A lateral view of the femoral component is provided.

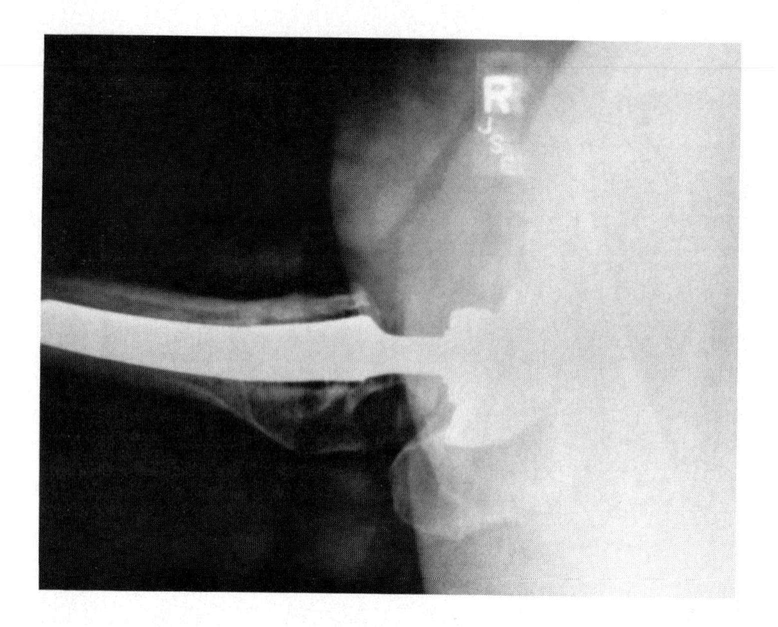

FIGURE 23–4. The cross-table lateral view. This view provides visualization of the acetabular component position and the status of the bone stock in the posterior column and superior neck of the ilium. It also provides a lateral view of the proximal femur.

Elevation of the erythrocyte sedimentation rate (ESR) is suggestive of infection or some other inflammatory condition, such as active rheumatoid arthritis. The ESR reaches a maximum (up to 64 mm/hr) 6 days after primary hip replacement and then decreases, remaining slightly elevated at 1 year (Fig. 23–5).[1] Normally, the ESR rises gradually with advancing age. As a rule of thumb, an ESR value up to half the patient's age is normal. Another finding suggestive of infection is elevation of C-reactive protein serum level. It reaches maximum levels (up to 134 mg/L)

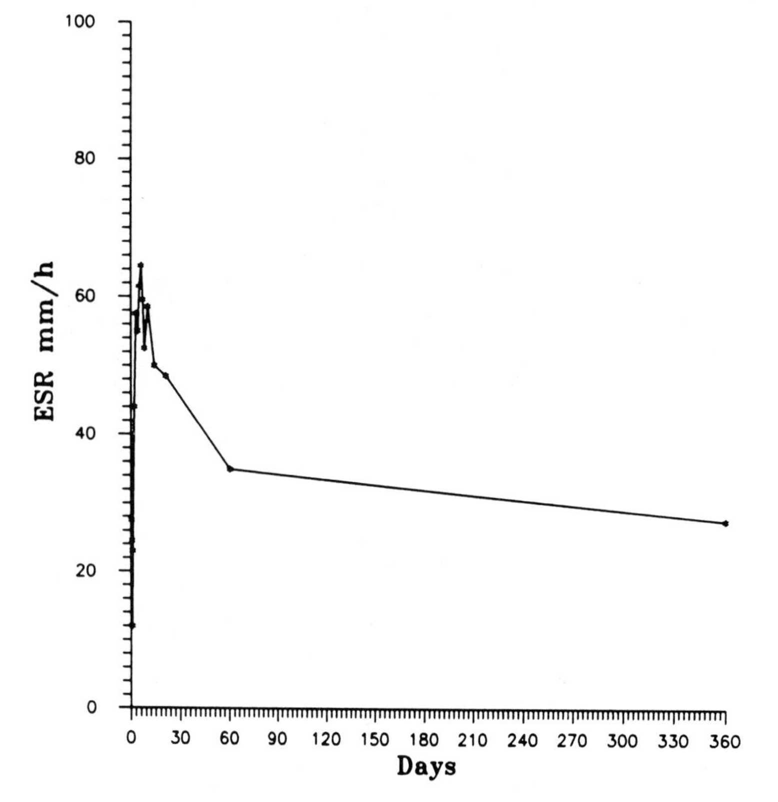

FIGURE 23–5. Erythrocyte sedimentation rate (ESR) after total hip arthroplasty.

on the second postoperative day and declines to normal levels by the third postoperative week (Fig. 23–6).[1] If either the ESR or C-reactive protein value is significantly elevated, careful evaluation for infection in the hip is essential.

Radionuclide imaging studies are helpful in evaluating infection associated with hip prostheses (see Chapter 11, *Imaging of Total Joint Replacement*). However, the most important investigation for suspected infection is cell count and culture of fluid aspirated from the joint. Staphylococci, which grow relatively well in culture, are the most common pathogenic bacteria in infected total joint replacements. Some bacteria causing infection in total joint replacements are anaerobic and difficult to culture. Therefore, fluids must be placed immediately in appropriate culture media, including broth, and maintained for at least several days so that the causative bacteria have an opportunity to grow.

Preoperative Planning

Successful rehabilitation of the patient with a failed total hip replacement begins with an accurate assessment based on the preoperative evaluation and continues with thorough planning of the proposed reconstruction. However, the situation encountered intraoperatively may vary, sometimes substantially, from that expected on the basis of the preoperative evaluation. The incidence of intraoperative complications is relatively high with this difficult surgery. Because of these factors, full preparation includes analysis of potential intraoperative complications and development of contingency plans for dealing with them. This planning often necessitates having available a wide array of instruments and prostheses. Templates for estimating the fit of the revision prosthesis are helpful, as they are in primary total hip replacements.

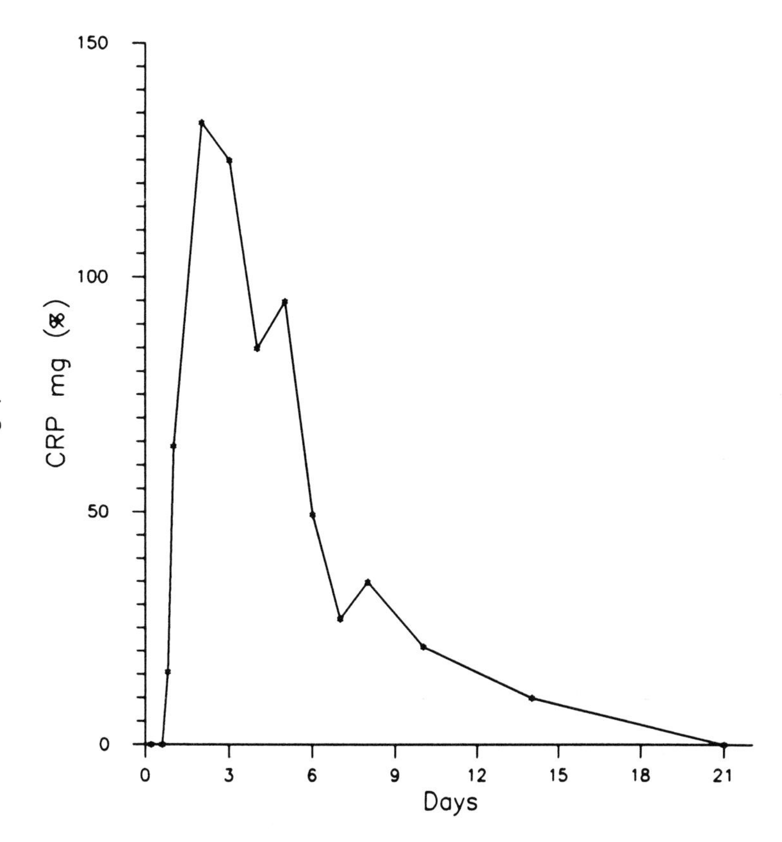

FIGURE 23–6. C-reactive protein (CRP) level after total hip arthroplasty.

INSTRUMENTS FOR REVISION ARTHROPLASTY

Many of the instruments for revision arthroplasty are the same as those for primary hip replacement. The difficulty in removing failed prostheses and the subsequent reconstruction make certain instruments especially valuable in these technically demanding operations.

Flexible osteotomes are often helpful in curved areas of the proximal femur, although not much driving force can be applied. Once the femoral component has been loosened adequately for removal, a stem extraction device often works best. Another option is to strike against the stem with a bone impactor and mallet. Long, narrow-handled osteotomes are essential for removing cement from the femoral canal (Fig. 23–7). These should have both straight and curved tips and both positive and negative cutting angles. The negative cutting angle provides some protection against penetration of the bone cortex (Fig. 23–8), whereas the positive angle allows precision in cutting between cement and bone (Fig. 23–9). A cement-

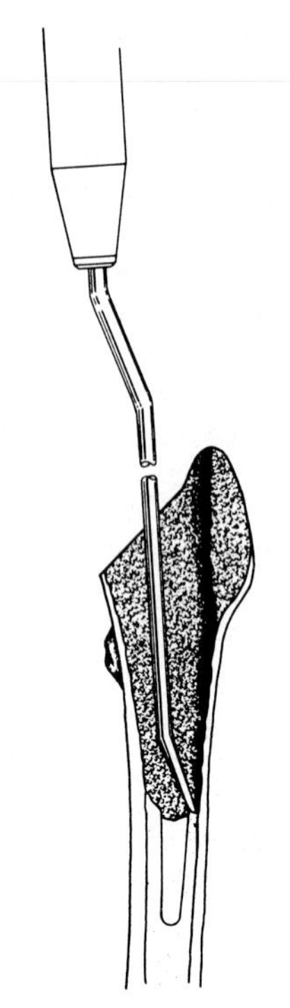

FIGURE 23–8. Long-handled osteotome with negative cutting angle. Protection is provided against penetration of bone cortex.

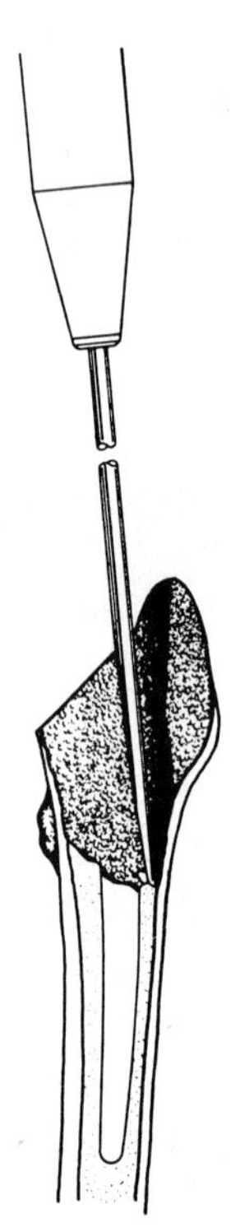

FIGURE 23–7. Long-handled straight osteotome for removing cement.

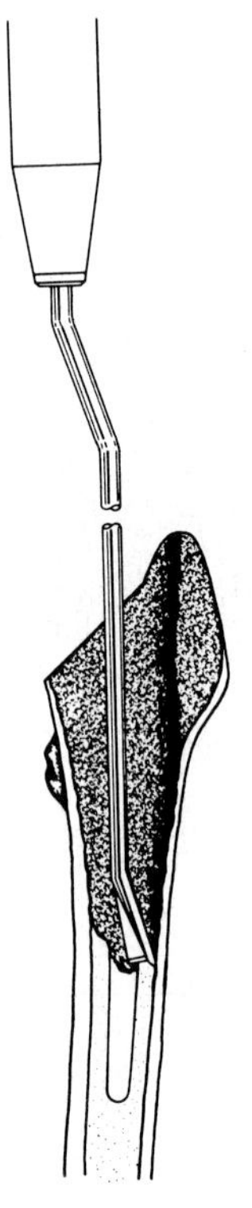

FIGURE 23–9. Long-handled osteotome with positive cutting angle allows precision cutting between cement and bone.

splitting chisel helps in breaking the cement into smaller pieces for extraction (Fig. 23–10). A gouge made to fit the curvature of the acetabular component is essential for removing a fixed socket without substantially damaging the bone (Fig. 23–11). Long, narrow, yet strong pituitary rongeurs facilitate removal of cement fragments from the femoral canal (Fig. 23–12). A long-handled curette or "crochet hook" is helpful in removing cement fragments and membranes from the intramedullary canal (Fig. 23–13).

High-speed air-driven drills are highly efficient for cutting away cement, but they also cut through bone rapidly (Fig. 23–14). These instruments are valuable in removing failed prostheses—provided the clinician has had adequate training and practice in the laboratory before using them in surgery. High-speed drills are especially useful for removing the distal fragment of a broken femoral stem. Special instruments can be combined with the drill to tap a hole into the fixed distal fragment, to secure a removal bar in the fragment, and to remove the fragment with a mallet (Fig. 23–15). High-speed drills are also helpful in preparing bone graft for acetabular or femoral reconstruction.

Adequate visualization is essential for safe removal of failed prostheses. Good surgical exposure facilitates visualization, which can be enhanced by special lighting (head lamps, probe lights, and fiberoptic lights). Standard fiberoptic sources designed for arthroscopy provide a brilliant light within the femoral canal. Image-intensified fluoroscopy is important if cement is to be removed from deep within the femoral canal without extensive exposure of the femur (Fig. 23–16).

SOCKET FAILURE

Preoperative Analysis and Planning

Socket (Hip Center) Location

As in primary total hip arthroplasty, in revision arthroplasty the normal hip center should be restored when possible to enable the return of limb length, to achieve proper muscle balance, and to avoid abnormally high forces across the reconstructed hip joint.

If the opposite hip is normal, the proper position of the center of rotation of the acetabular component is determined from it. If the contralateral hip is abnormal, the method described by Ranawat and associates[58] provides an accurate estimate of the proper position of the center of rotation of the hip (Fig. 23–17). In this method, two horizontal lines are drawn on a standard anteroposterior radiograph of the pelvis: one line at the level of the iliac crests and the other at the level of the ischial tuberosities. The distance between these two lines is the height of the pelvis. The two lines are connected by a perpendicular line passing through a point 5 mm lateral to the intersection of the Shenton and Köhler lines (point A). Point B is located above point A at a distance equal to one-fifth the height of the pelvis. A perpendicular to line AB and equal to it in length is constructed in the lateral direction ending at point C. An isosceles triangle is formed by joining points A and C. This triangle represents the appropriate position of the reconstructed acetabulum.

Classification of Acetabular Deficiencies

The planning for surgery for failed acetabular components is enhanced by classification of acetabular deficiencies (Table 23–1).[18] In the classification system devel-

Table 23–1. CLASSIFICATION OF ACETABULAR DEFICIENCIES*

Type I	Segmental deficiencies
	A. Peripheral
	1. Superior
	2. Anterior
	3. Posterior
	B. Central (medial wall absent)
Type II	Cavitary deficiencies
	A. Peripheral
	1. Superior
	2. Anterior
	3. Posterior
	B. Central (medial wall intact)
Type III	Combined deficiencies
Type IV	Pelvic discontinuity
Type V	Arthrodesis

*From the American Academy of Orthopaedic Surgeons Committee on the Hip.

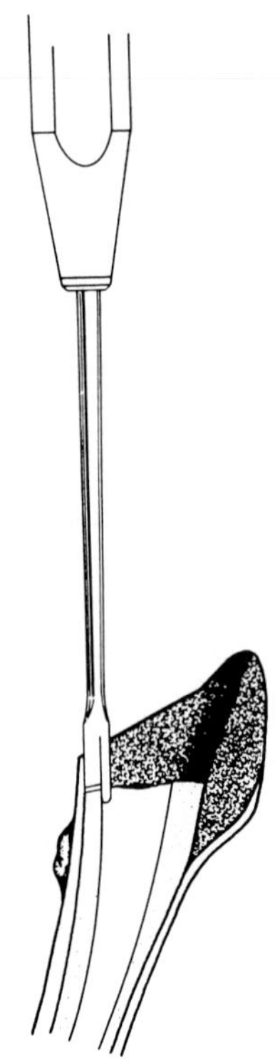

FIGURE 23–10. Cement-splitting chisel is helpful in breaking the cement.

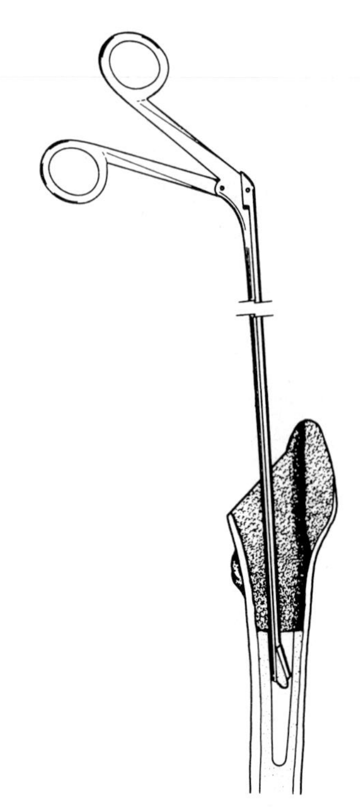

FIGURE 23–12. Long narrow yet strong pituitary rongeurs. These instruments facilitate removal of cement fragments from the femoral canal.

oped by the American Academy of Orthopaedic Surgeons Committee on the Hip, deficiencies are divided into five types. Type I, a segmental deficiency, represents a complete loss of bone in some portion of the supporting hemisphere; this loss may be in the medial wall (Fig. 23–18). Type II, a cavitary deficiency, involves a loss of bone with the supporting rim, including the medial wall, remaining intact (Fig. 23–19). Both segmental and cavitary deficien-

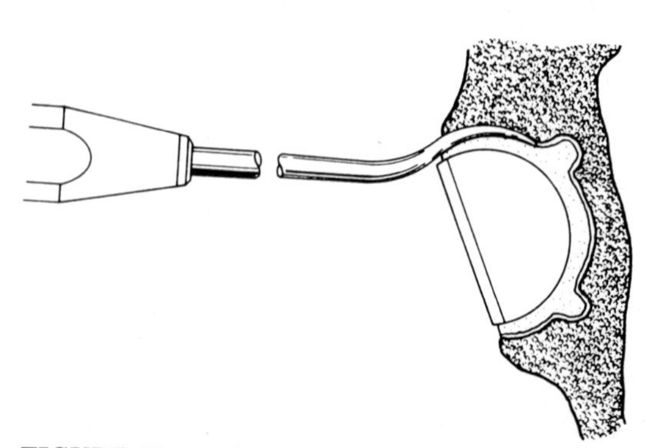

FIGURE 23–11. Gouge curved to fit the acetabular component. This tool is essential for removing a fixed socket without substantially damaging the bone.

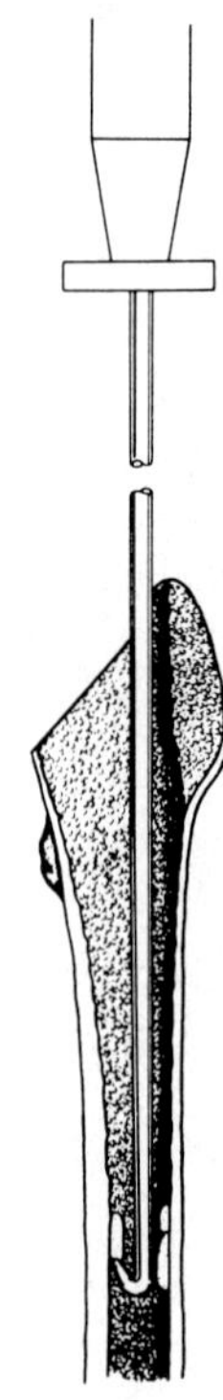

FIGURE 23–13. Long-handled curette or "crochet hook" for removing cement fragments and membranes from the intramedullary canal.

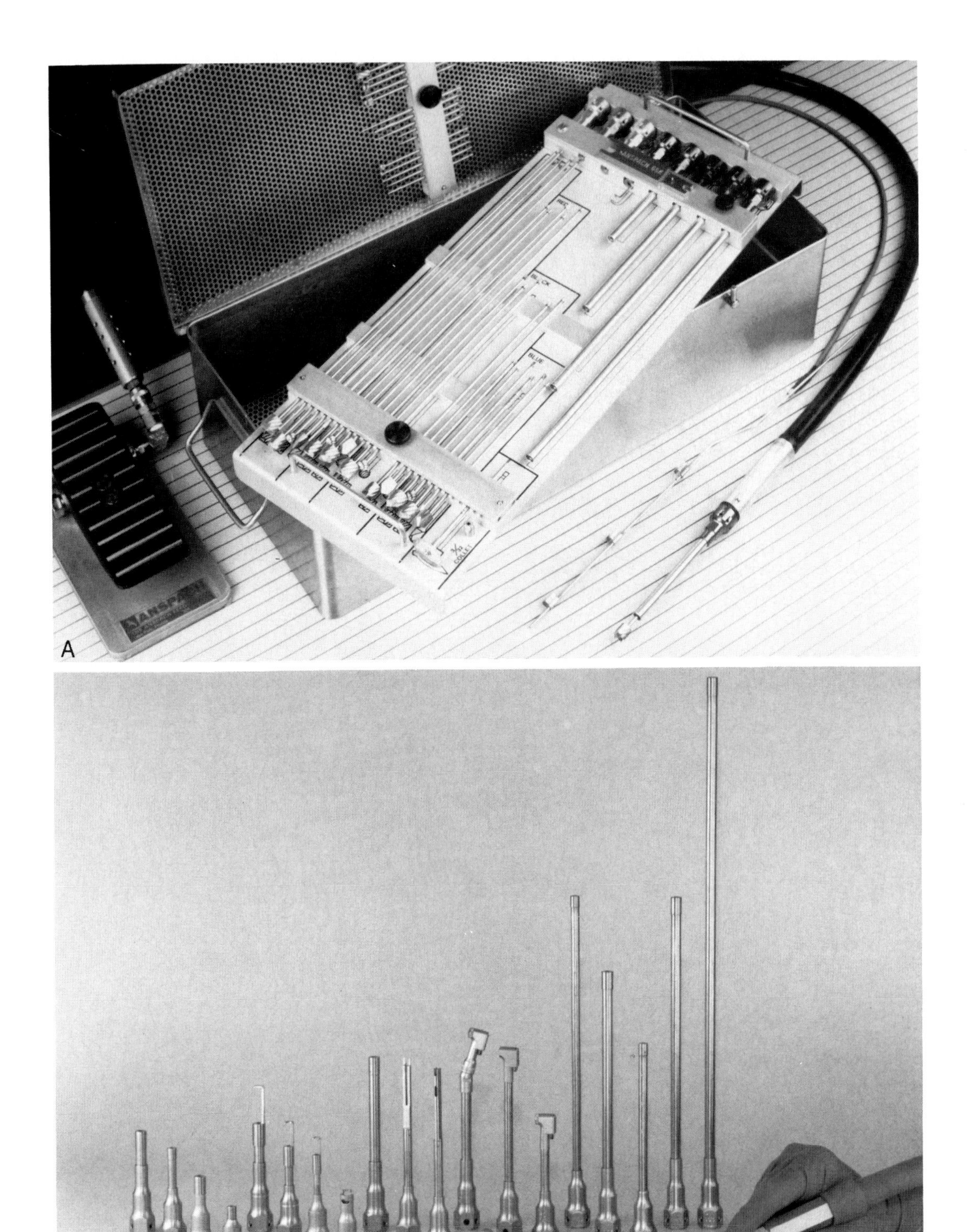

FIGURE 23–14. High-speed air-driven drills are highly efficient for cutting away bone cement. *A*, Anspach 65-K high-speed drill. *B*, Midas Rex high-speed drill.

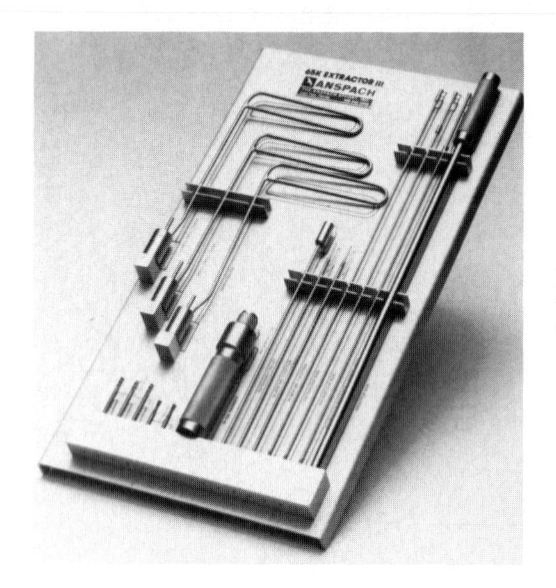

FIGURE 23–15. Special instruments used in combination with high-speed drills to remove the distal fragment of a broken femoral stem.

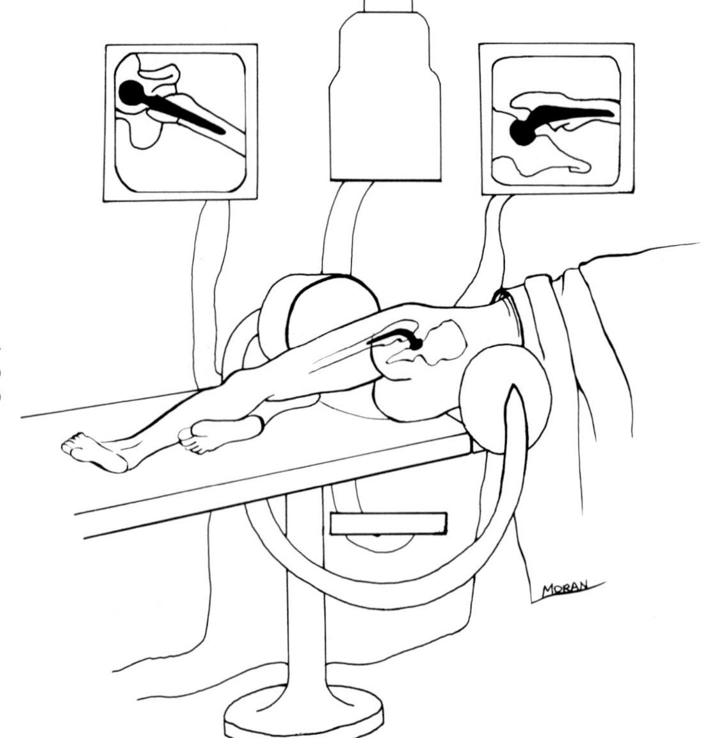

FIGURE 23–16. Image intensification. This technique may be used to guide cement removal from deep within the femoral canal.

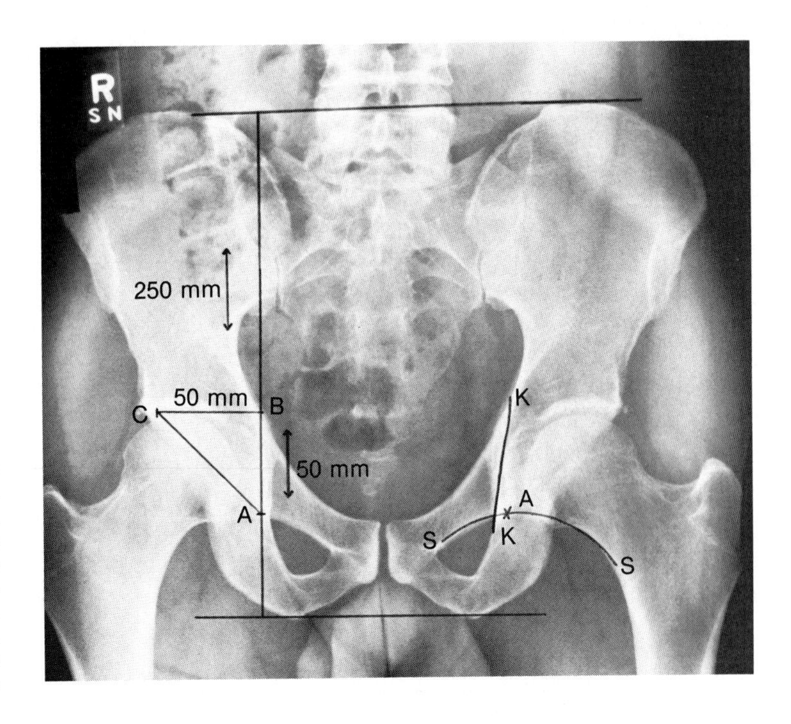

FIGURE 23–17. Method for estimating the correct location of the acetabulum. On the anteroposterior radiograph of the pelvis, horizontal lines are drawn at the level of the iliac crest and ischial tuberosities. The distance between these two lines is equal to the height of the pelvis. The two lines are connected by a perpendicular line passing through a point 5 mm lateral to the intersection of the Shenton and Köhler lines (point A). Point B is located above point A, at a distance equal to one fifth the height of the pelvis. A perpendicular line to line AB and equal in length is constructed in the lateral direction to point C. An isosceles triangle is completed by joining points A and C. This triangle represents the appropriate position of the reconstructed acetabulum. (Ranawat, C. S., Dorr, L. D., and Inglis, A. E.: J. Bone Joint Surg. 62A: 1059–1065, 1980. By permission.)

cies can be either peripheral or central, and peripheral deficiencies may be superior, posterior, or anterior (Figs. 23–20, 23–21, and 23–22). Type III, combined deficiencies, is designated by individual components. For example, a combined deficiency may consist of posterior and superior peripheral defects. Protrusio acetabuli includes a central cavitary deficiency and may or may not have a central segmental defect (Fig. 23–23). Type IV, pelvic discontinuity (Fig. 23–24), and type V,

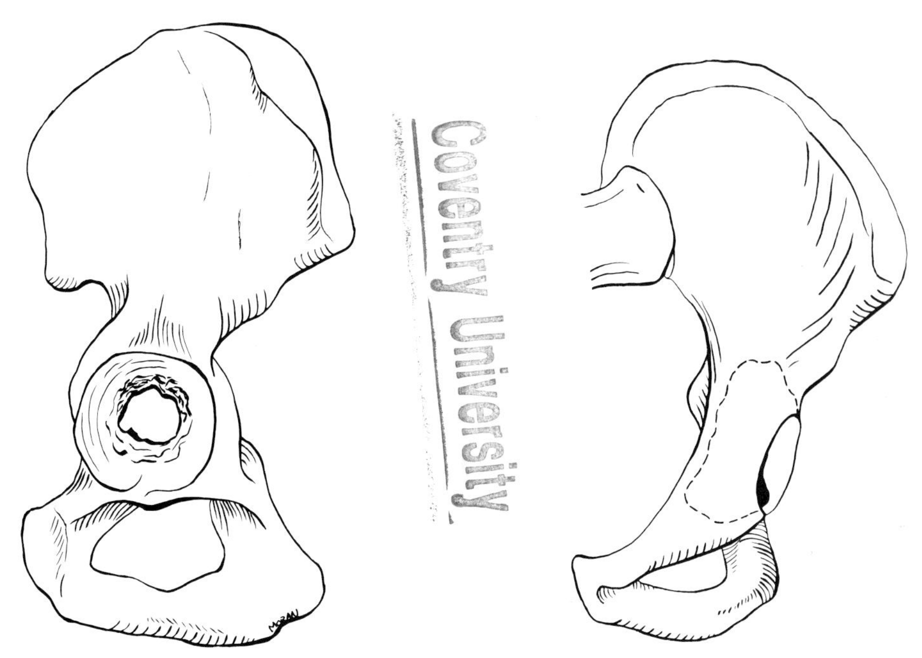

FIGURE 23–18. Lateral view showing a central segmental deficiency.

FIGURE 23–19. Anteroposterior view showing superior and inferior cavitary deficiency.

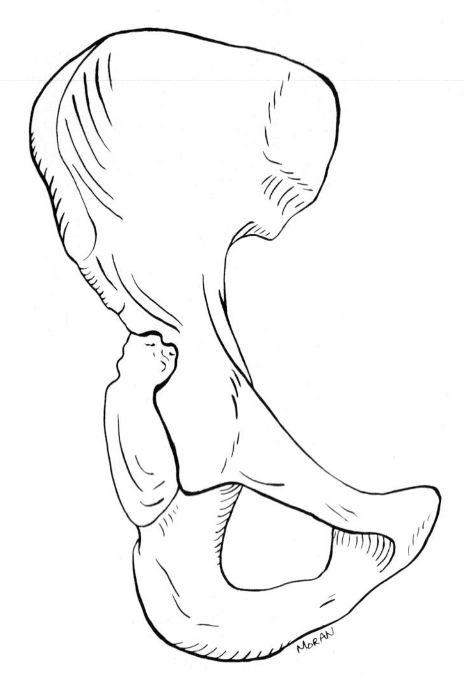

FIGURE 23–20. Anteroposterior view showing superior segmental defect.

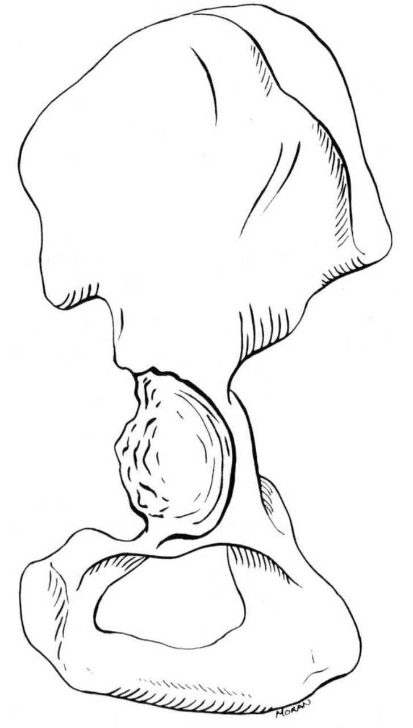

FIGURE 23–21. Lateral view showing posterior segmental defect.

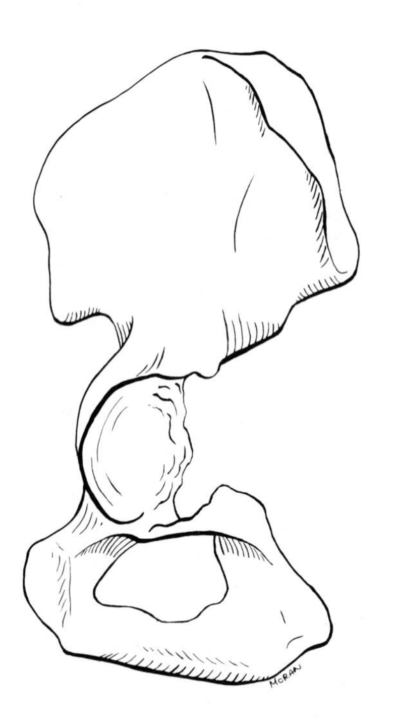

FIGURE 23–22. Lateral view showing anterior segmental defect.

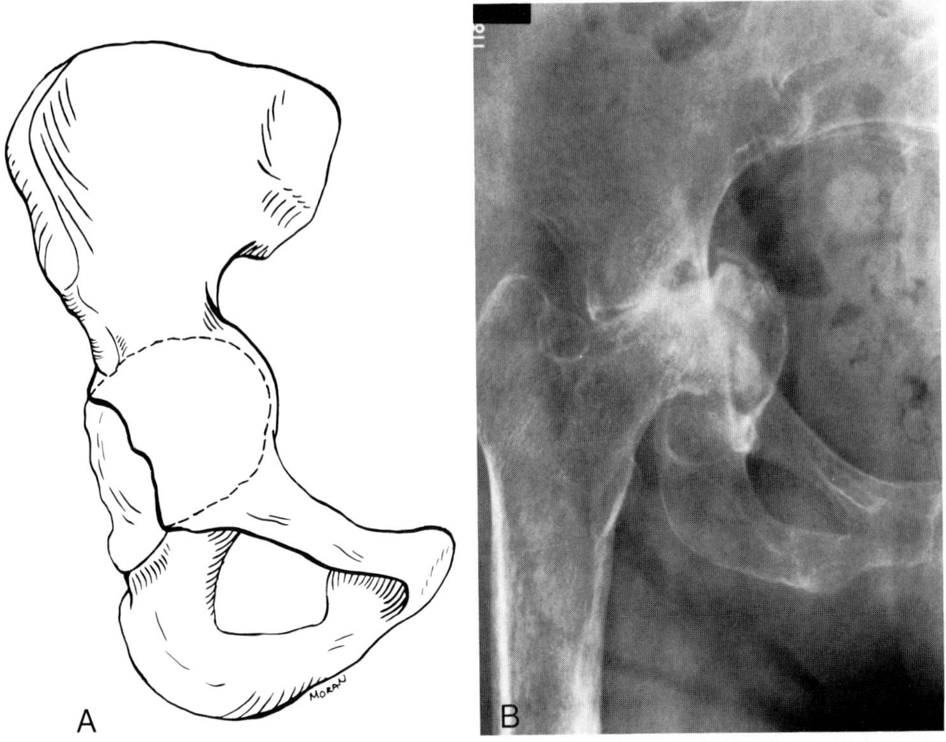

FIGURE 23–23. Protrusio acetabuli. *A*, Protrusio acetabuli consisting of central cavitary deficiency. *B*, Radiograph of a patient's hip affected by rheumatoid arthritis. Protrusio acetabuli consists of central cavitary and segmental deficiency.

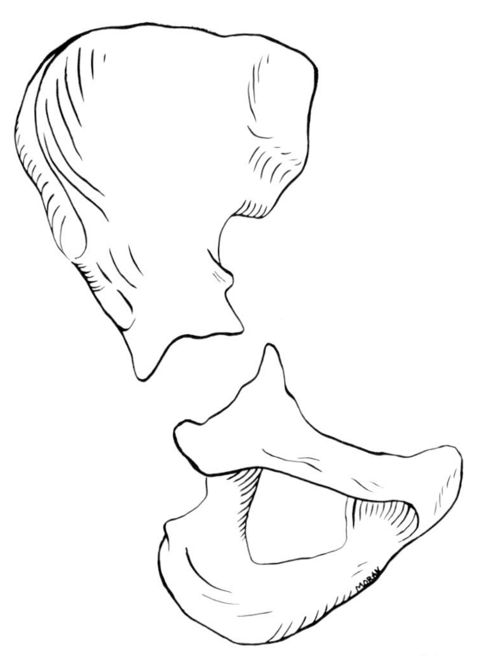

FIGURE 23–24. Pelvic discontinuity created by anterior, posterior, and central segmental deficiencies.

arthrodesis, complete the classification scheme.[18]

Material placed to fill a cavitary deficiency is contained by the intact rim, whereas material to fill a segmental deficiency must provide structural substitution for the missing bone. Cavitary deficiencies can be filled with a prosthesis in the form of a deep or protrusio socket, with bone cement, or with bone autograft or allograft (Fig. 23–25). Most surgeons prefer cementless acetabular components for revisions. However, if the cavitary defect is not too large and the bone quality after reaming is sufficient to provide mechanical interdigitation with cement, cement may be chosen. When failure has been associated with bone lysis, cement should be avoided for revision.[18, 49]

The key to successful reconstruction of segmental defects is provision of adequate structural support for the prosthetic acetabulum. It is important that the component be placed in the proper location and

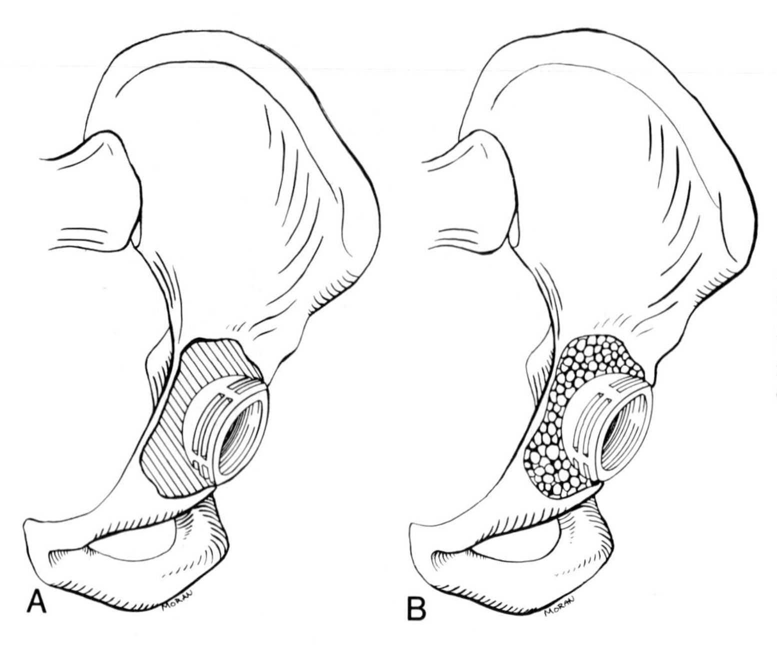

FIGURE 23–25. Reconstruction of cavitary deficiencies. *A*, Defect filled with bone cement. *B*, Defect filled with particulate bone graft. A protrusio socket may sometimes be helpful in dealing with cavitary defects.

that bone stock can be rebuilt biologically. Custom pelvic prostheses that have no biologic potential are usually reserved for special situations, such as after extensive bone resection for a malignant pelvic tumor (see Chapter 43, *Joint Reconstruction After Tumor Resection*). Most segmental defects can be reconstructed with either autogenous or allogeneic bone graft (see Chapter 5, *Allografts*). Autogenous graft has several advantages: complete tissue compatibility and potential for transfer of some viable bone cells to the grafted location. If the segmental defect is not too large, an adequate structural bone graft may be obtained from the iliac crest. When the defect is too large for replacement with an iliac graft or when the ilium has been depleted of adequate bone by previous graft harvesting, an allograft may be a source of structural bone graft material. Allografts have been utilized extensively for acetabular reconstructions both in difficult primary hip replacements like those for congenital dysplasia and in revision hip replacements (Figs. 23–26 and 23–27).

Many investigators have reported the results of structural autografts and allografts in the treatment of congenital dysplasia. The findings have been variable, with excellent results reported in short-term and medium-term follow-ups, but higher rates of failure have been reported in follow-ups of up to 10 years (see Chapter 17, *Total Hip Arthroplasty: Operative Technique*).[21, 26, 31, 38, 50, 52] Long-term results have been more favorable when two thirds or more of the acetabular prosthesis was covered with host rather than graft bone. All reports of allografts for treatment of segmental deficiencies in acetabular revision are based on short-term follow-ups, but these early reports suggest that structural autografts or allografts are helpful in providing immediate stability. In the short term, both cemented and cementless acetabular reconstructions augmented with structural bone grafts have high rates of success.[7, 17, 23, 31, 32, 44, 49, 65] Resorption of both allografts and autografts may occur, being more common and severe with allografts. Therefore, autografts should be employed when feasible, and as much host bone as possible should be preserved to provide structural support of the prosthesis.[17]

Cemented and Cementless Revisions

Although some investigators have reported good results in patients having cemented revisions of acetabular prostheses, most indicate a high incidence of failure, at least by radiographic criteria (see Chapter 24, *Results of Revision Total Hip Arthroplasty*).[65] This finding is not surprising because adequate fixation with cement re-

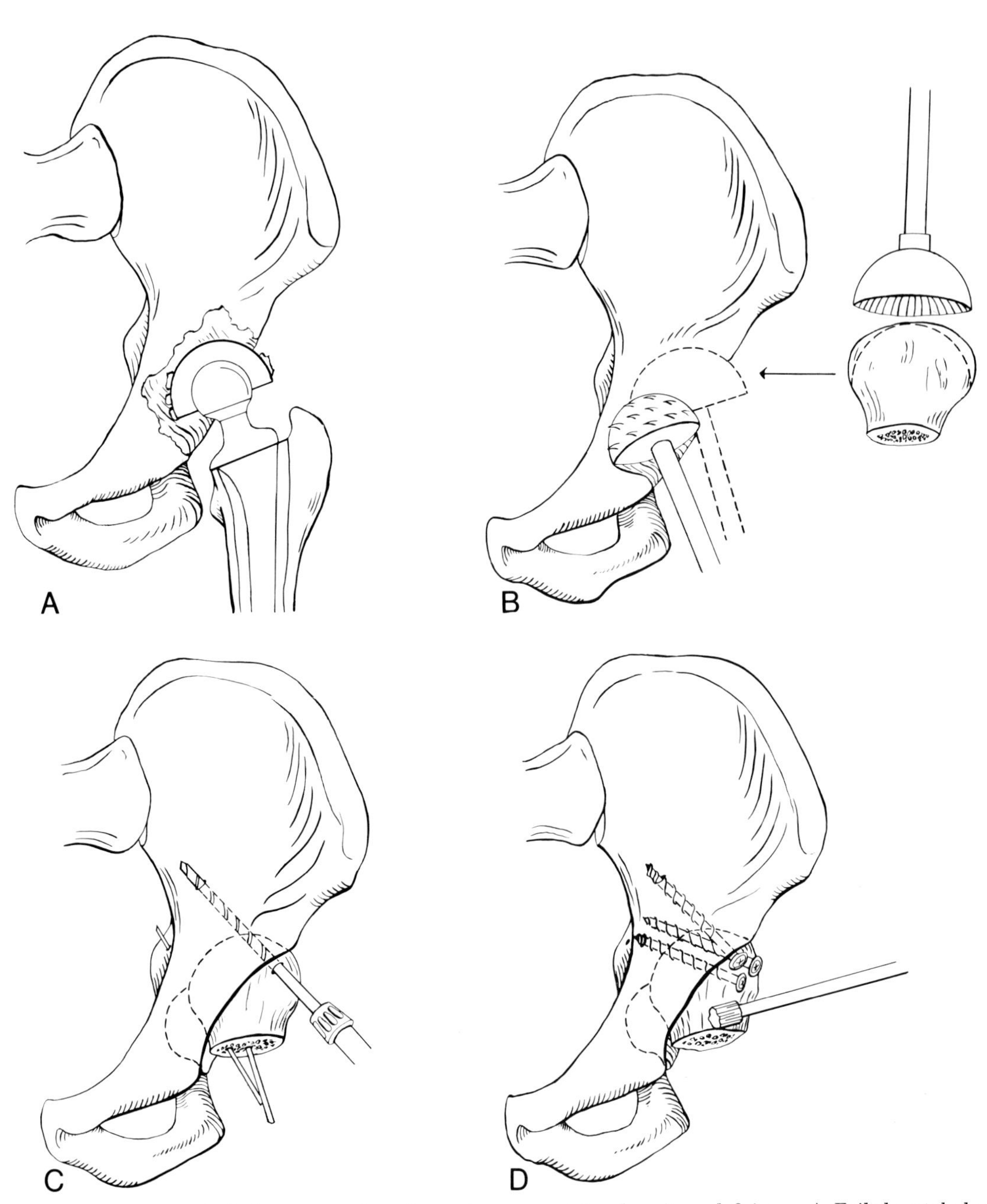

FIGURE 23–26. Method of reconstruction of superior segmental and cavitary deficiency. *A*, Failed acetabular component with superior segmental and cavitary deficiency. *B*, Locating the true acetabulum followed by limited reaming. The superior deficiency surface is cleaned and smoothed to accept bone grafts. This procedure may be done gently with an acetabular reamer. The femoral head is best prepared with female cup arthroplasty reamers. *C*, The femoral head graft held in place temporarily with smooth pins. Drilling is done for cancellous screws. *D*, The graft fixed in place with several screws. Screws are kept in the superior portion of the graft so they will not interfere with reaming. Initial reaming of the graft is performed with a high-speed burr.

Illustration continued on following page

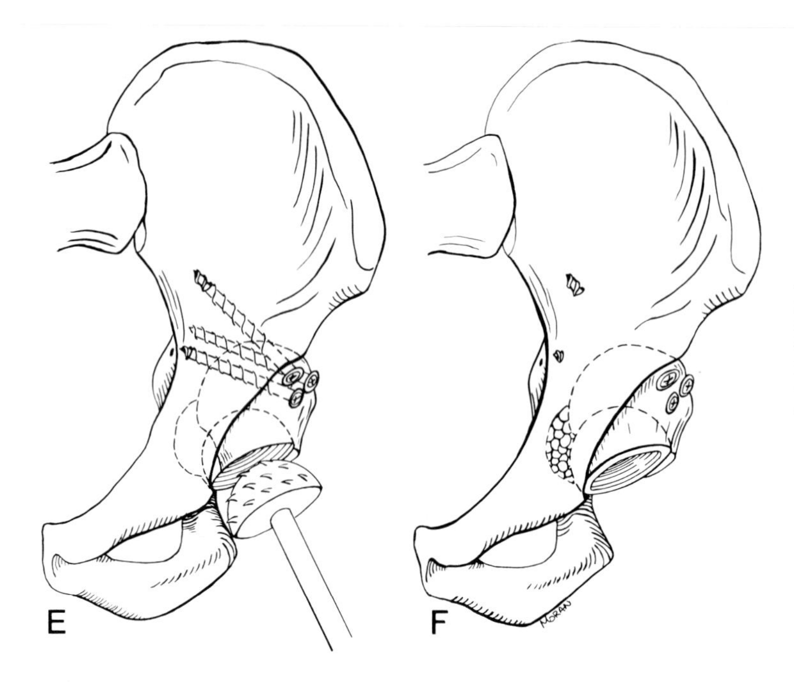

FIGURE 23–26 *Continued E,* Reaming completed at the level of the true acetabulum. *F,* Filling of remaining cavitary defect with particulate graft and insertion of the acetabular prosthesis.

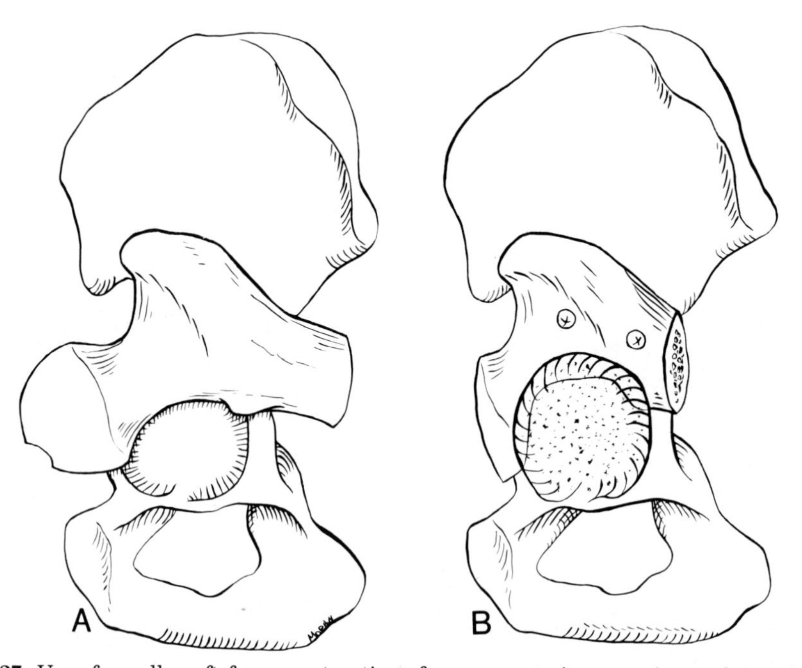

FIGURE 23–27. Use of an allograft for reconstruction of severe posterior, superior, and anterior segmental and cavitary deficiency. *A,* Curvature of the medial aspect of the femoral neck provides allograft material for reconstruction. *B,* Fixation of the allograft in place and reaming of the acetabulum. If the entire trochanteric portion of the allograft is not needed, it may be excised before or after fixation to the pelvis.

quires high-quality mechanical interdigitation with bone. In patients who require revision, the bone is often hard and little if any exposed cancellous bone is left. Because of these reasons, many surgeons prefer cementless acetabular components for revisions.

Numerous reports have been made of satisfactory results at short-term follow-up of revisions with cementless sockets.[17, 32, 44, 49] In the United States, cementless prostheses are usually porous coated. In Europe, they often are designed for macrointerlock or press-fit fixation. As in primary hip replacements, threaded sockets have not been as successful in revision procedures unless they have porous coatings.[23] Cementless sockets that provide for supplemental screw fixations enable enhanced fixations when stable press-fit fixations are difficult.

Some investigators have logically argued against a porous-coated press-fit prosthesis when most of the contact is with bone graft. They prefer a cemented prosthesis in this situation (Fig. 23–28). Some surgeons prefer to have press-fit sockets against grafts even though ingrowth into porous surfaces is likely to be of poor quality, if it occurs at all (Fig. 23–29). Fixation against graft, whether cemented or not, probably works well because the prosthesis is contained within a stable host bone-graft reconstruction.[17]

Operative Technique

Exposure

The operative approach for revision hip replacement is usually more extensive than for primary hip replacement. Some surgeons recommend an anterior approach if the primary acetabular defect is anterior and a posterior approach if the defect is posterior. The triradiate exposure allows for extensive visualization of the acetabulum and pelvis.[42] Whatever exposure is selected, the surgeon should avoid making sharp curves that compromise extension of the incision, should that become necessary during the operation (see Chapter 14, *Surgical Approaches for Total Hip Replacement*).[33]

Extensive scarring and obscuring of the normal tissue planes not only makes exposure and subsequent closure difficult but also makes damage to major nerves or arteries more likely. Two methods, alone or in combination, may reduce the likelihood of nerve damage. The most common means of protecting the sciatic or other nerve in these difficult operations is to expose the nerve throughout its course, adjacent to the hip joint. The sciatic nerve always is exposed first in an area of normal tissue distal to the scarring. The nerve then is exposed to its entry into the sciatic notch. The femoral nerve is less commonly endangered, but if it is, exposure is best begun proximally. The second method for reducing the danger of nerve damage is somatosensory evoked potential evaluation of the nerves during the operation. In a series of 25 operations monitored with this technique, Nercessian and colleagues[54] found 12 instances of neurologic compromise, associated with retraction in seven cases and with positioning in five. Once the compromise was relieved, the potentials recovered. No postoperative deficits were observed in this group, compared with two postoperative neurologic deficits (5.7 percent) after 35 operations without monitoring.

Major blood vessels may be involved in scar or may be located directly adjacent to a failed acetabular prosthesis. Intrapelvic protrusion of the acetabular prosthesis may expose vessels to damage during revision.[41] If migration of a failed socket places it in a position that might be close to a major vessel, angiography or other imaging studies should be done preoperatively (Fig. 23–30). The prosthesis usually can be moved away from the vessel by carefully stripping the scar tissue away from the prosthesis. The risk is higher when a major vein is involved, because of fragility of the vein's wall. At times, intrapelvic exposure may be necessary to free the prosthesis from vessels.

Removal of the Failed Prosthesis

When the acetabulum and surrounding bone have been adequately exposed, the next step is to remove the acetabular prosthesis. As much bone stock as possible

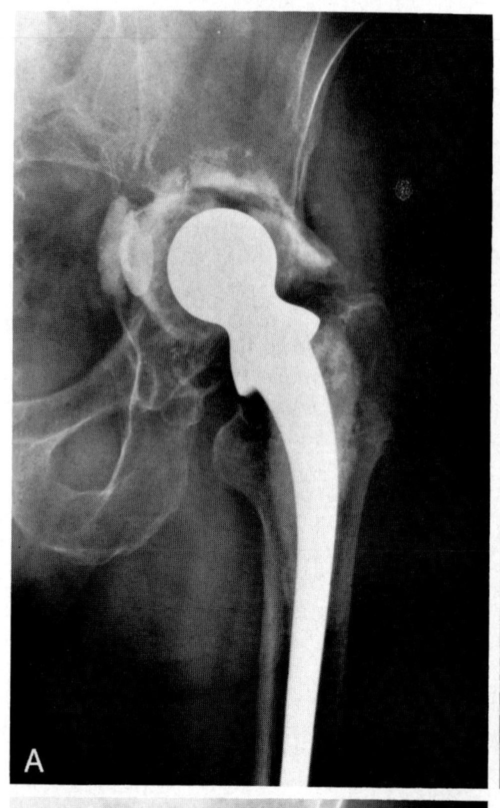

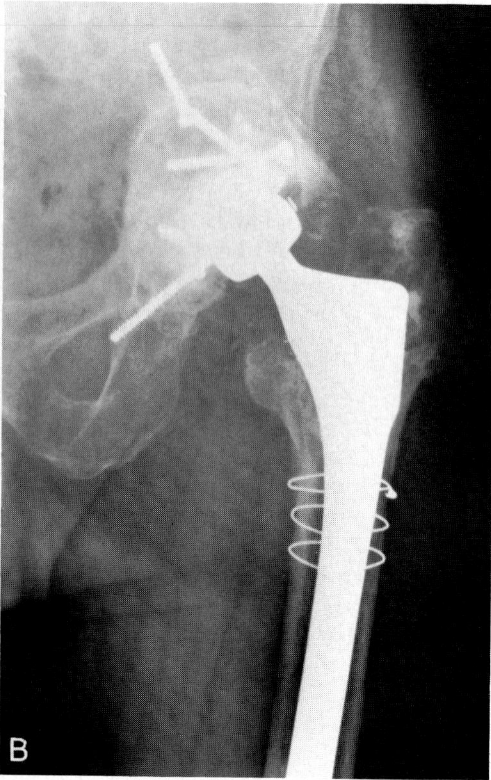

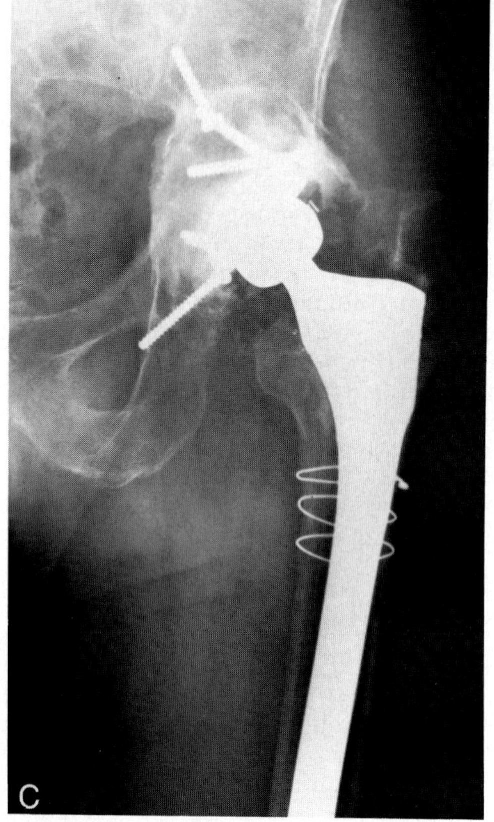

FIGURE 23–28. Acetabular deficiency reconstructed with allograft and cemented acetabular component. *A,* Loose acetabular component with segmental and cavitary deficiency. *B,* Acetabulum reconstructed with structural allograft fixed with screws and cemented acetabular component. *C,* Two years postoperatively, excellent incorporation of the graft has occurred. The patient has no pain and walks with a single cane.

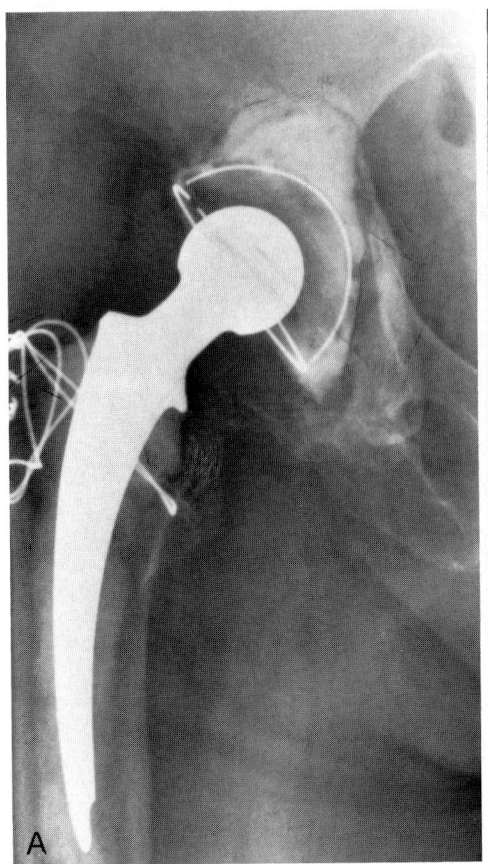

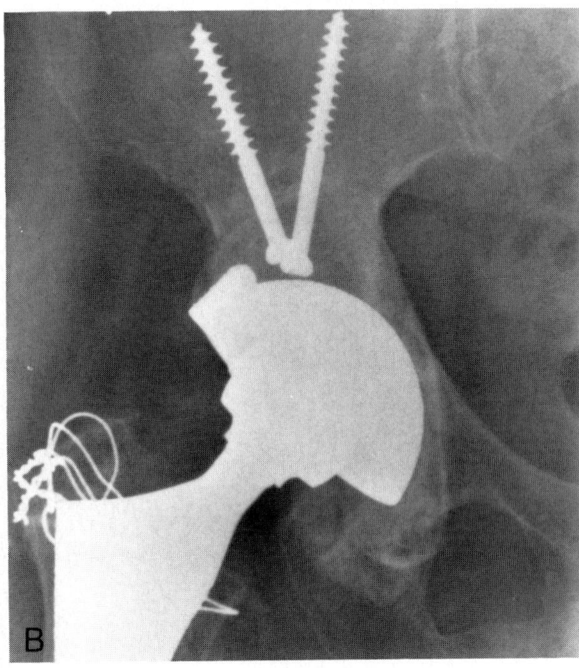

FIGURE 23–29. Acetabular deficiency reconstructed with allograft and porous-coated cementless acetabular component. *A,* Loose cemented acetabular component with superior cavitary deficiency. *B,* Acetabulum reconstructed with structural allograft fixed with two screws and porous-coated cementless acetabular component.

FIGURE 23–30. Preoperative angiogram in a patient with failed total hip arthroplasty with severe protrusio acetabuli prosthetica. The relationship of the migrated prosthesis to the intrapelvic vasculature is demonstrated.

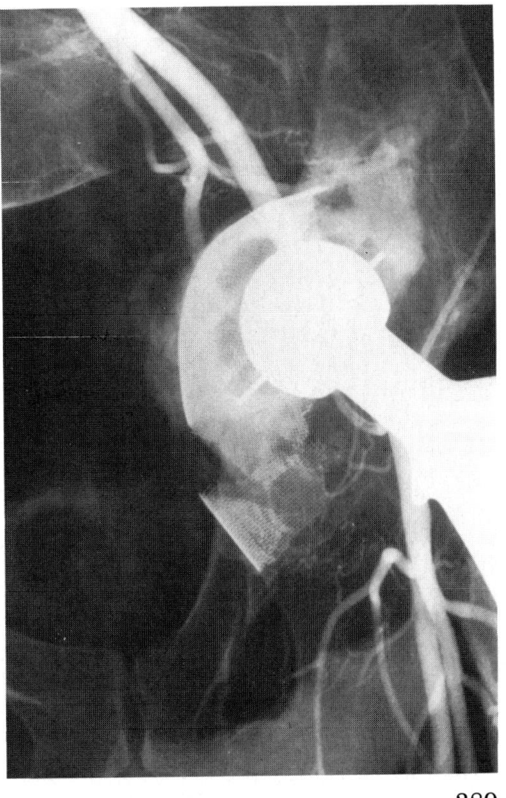

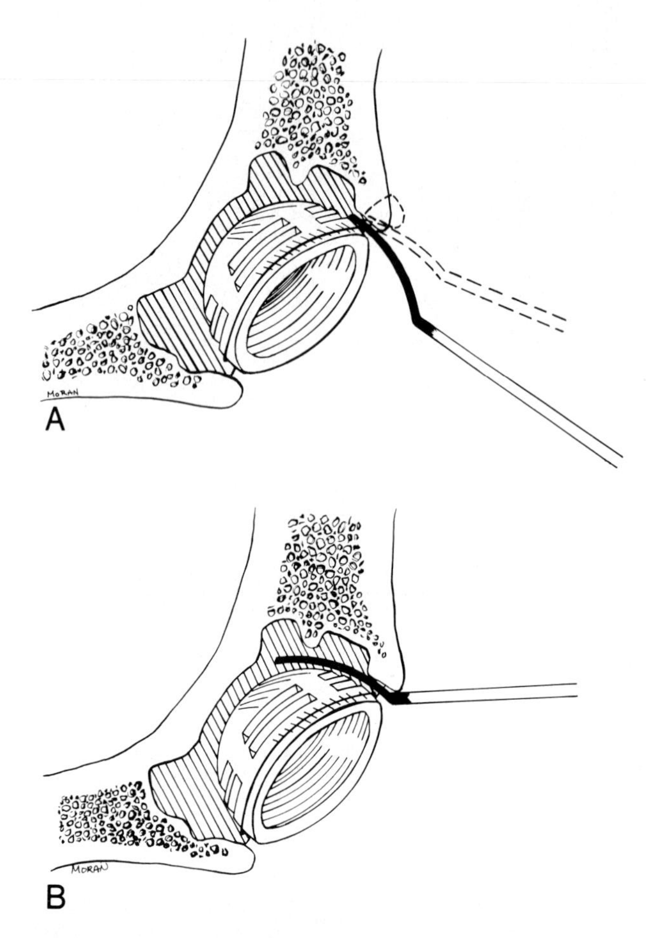

FIGURE 23–31. Cutting the prosthesis bone interface with an osteotome. *A*, Cutting with the curved osteotome or gouge is begun just outside the periphery of the socket. *B*, The curved osteotome or gouge is allowed to follow the curvature of the sphere. As much of the interface is cut as possible.

should be maintained. If acetabular failure involves gross loosening, removal of the prosthesis is often not difficult. When it is necessary to remove a well-fixed prosthesis, as for revision due to malposition, removal may be difficult.

Curved gouges help loosen the prosthesis with minimal bone damage. The gouge is directed just external to the outer hemisphere of the socket, following the curvature of the sphere (Fig. 23–31). The interface is cut in multiple locations by allowing the gouge to follow the curvature of the socket until it is loose. Wedging the gouge or other instrument against the bone to pry the prosthesis out before it is loose will damage the acetabular bone stock at the rim. An alternative method to remove the prosthesis, when the socket is well fixed and the bone stock poor, is to cut the socket into two or more pieces with a high-speed power burr and to remove each piece individually (Fig. 23–32). This maneuver is relatively uncomplicated with an all-polyethylene socket, but it is difficult and time consuming and generates abundant particles with a metal-backed socket. If the socket is modular and has been fixed with

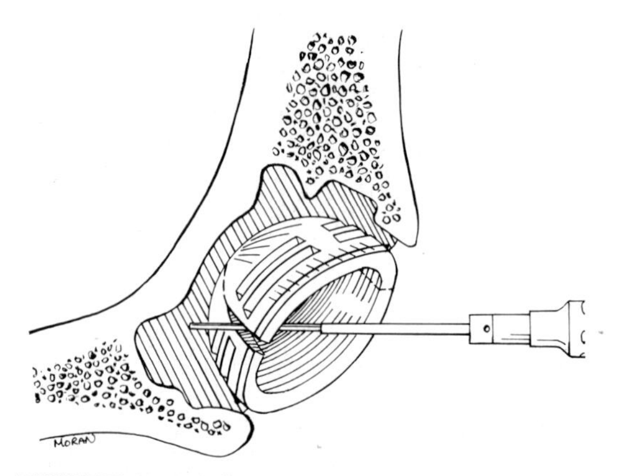

FIGURE 23–32. Cutting of the prosthesis into segments for removal. When the acetabular prosthesis is well fixed and the bone is weak, the bone may be preserved better by this procedure.

screws, the polyethylene liner is removed and the screws extracted before the interface is cut with a gouge. The interface of a porous socket must be thoroughly cut before removal is attempted to avoid removal of valuable bone. Even though bone ingrowth of a porous socket may be minimal, the prosthesis may be well fixed because of fibrous ingrowth.

On the one hand, threaded sockets may be so loose that they can be removed easily. On the other hand, one of the most difficult sockets to remove is a threaded one with a porous coating. The socket may be fixed very rigidly, with the threads obstructing passage of a gouge. Removal of a socket with these features usually will result in damage to the bone.

Cement may remain after a socket is removed, usually in holes drilled during the primary operation to enhance fixation. This cement often can be taken out by cutting around it with a small osteotome. If this maneuver is not effective, a high-speed burr may be.

After the prosthesis and cement are removed, the entire membrane is removed with a curette. This material is evaluated using histologic methods and bacterial culture methods.

Repairing Defects

The surgeon next inspects the acetabulum for deficiencies and plans the reconstruction. For defects that are minimal or cavitary, the acetabulum is reamed, but it is not reamed beyond its normal extent. Care is taken to avoid overreaming the anterior and posterior walls and sacrificing valuable bone. The surgeon should not attempt to freshen all bone surfaces with the reamer. Depths of cavitary defects and other irregularities are gently freshened with curettes. Although exposure of vascularized bone in the entire bed may be theoretically preferable, whether the revision socket is to be cemented or not, this exposure is often not feasible. If attempted, valuable bone may be sacrificed unnecessarily.

Cavitary defects should be bone grafted if a cementless socket is selected. For a cemented socket, cavitary defects may be either grafted or filled with cement (see Fig. 23–25). Grafting may be with either solid or particulate material. Solid autogenous graft probably performs better than solid allograft but either may be employed successfully. Most series suggest that particulate autograft and allograft incorporate equally well. Depending on the shape of the acetabulum, a deep or protrusio socket may be selected. Segmental defects are repaired with structural grafts. If sufficient bone is available from the iliac crest, it is harvested and shaped to replace the absent bone. If sufficient autogenous bone is not available, the graft is fashioned from allograft. The femoral head is the most common source for this allograft (see Fig. 23–26). Other sources include the trochanteric portion of the proximal femur, which is often an excellent source for large segmental defects because of its curvature (see Fig. 23–27); distal femur; and proximal tibia. The host and graft bone surfaces that will be in contact are freshened, but the structural integrity of both host and graft bone is maintained to allow for fixation. Screw fixation may be adequate for small grafts, but interfragmental screws combined with plate fixation are superior for repair of large defects.[23] After grafting, the acetabulum is reamed to assure appropriate fit of the prosthesis. Reaming of the graft may be initiated with a high-speed burr. Once a near-hemispheric shape is created, the preparation is completed with socket reamers (Fig. 23–26D and E).

Loss of pelvic continuity occurs when anterior, central, and posterior segmental defects are all present. All bony connection between the upper and lower hemipelvis is lost at the level of the acetabulum (see Fig. 23–24). These massive defects can be reconstructed by several methods, all of which are technically difficult. The likelihood of long-term success is unknown. These methods include (1) a repair of the segmental defects with massive structural grafts, using techniques similar to those for individual segmental defects (Fig. 23–33); (2) a half or whole allograft joint transplant; and (3) a custom prosthetic replacement similar to that used for reconstruction after massive resection for tumor (internal hemipelvectomy). For descriptions of the second and third techniques, see Chapter 43, *Joint Reconstruction After Tumor Resection.* Plates are especially helpful in achieving stable reconstruction

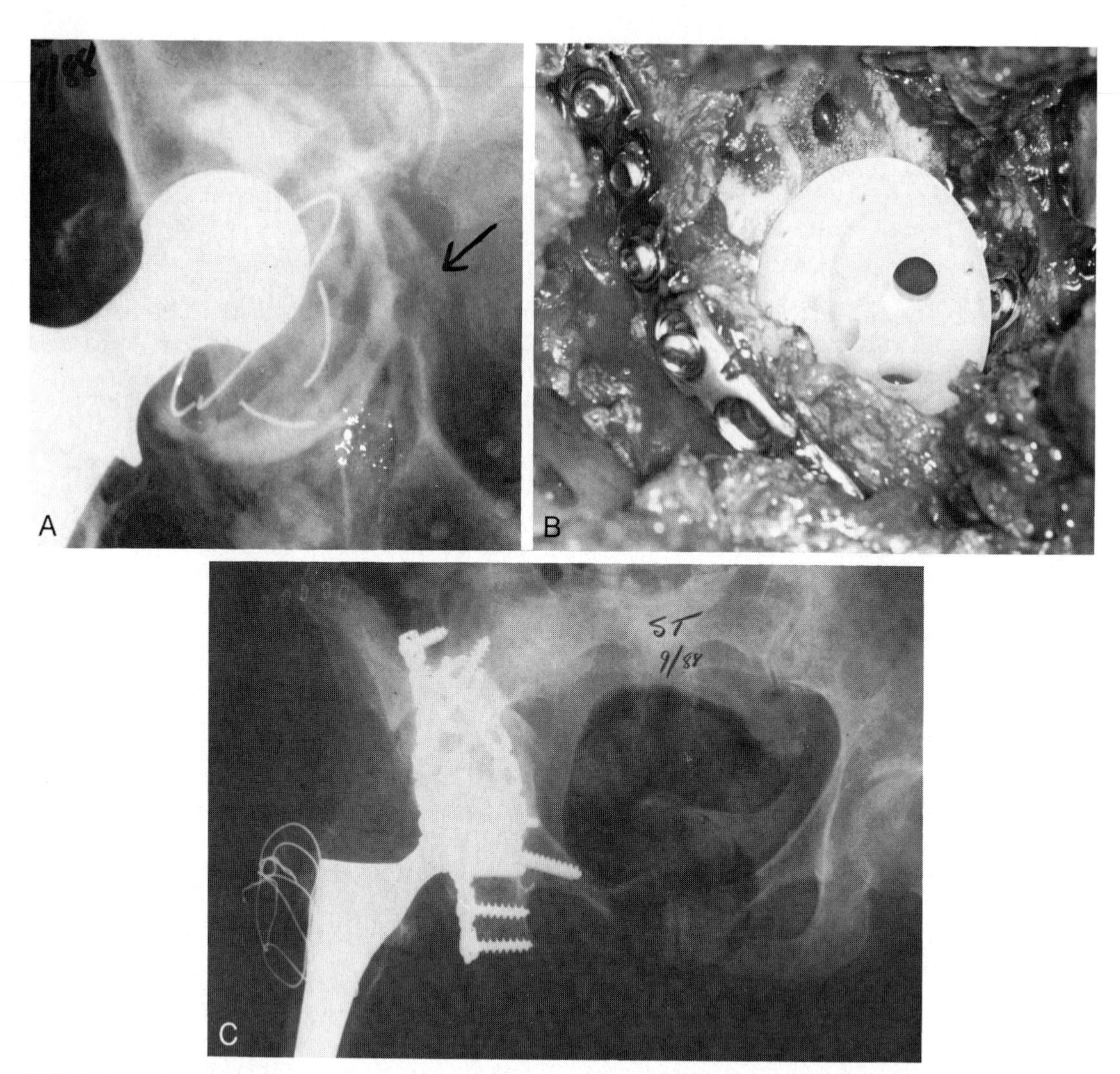

FIGURE 23–33. Pelvic discontinuity is reconstructed with large allograft. Reconstruction plates are used for fixation. *A,* Preoperative radiograph showing loose acetabular component with extensive and severe cavitary deficiency. The suggestion of a fracture may indicate pelvic discontinuity. *B,* Complete pelvic discontinuity found at surgery. Discontinuity was reconstructed with structural allograft and both anterior and posterior column reconstruction plates. *C,* Postoperative radiograph of reconstruction.

when pelvic discontinuity is present. Resection arthroplasty, although not likely to result in good function, may at times be preferable to these extensive reconstructions.[5, 55]

Socket Placement

If the socket is to be cemented, fixation holes are drilled where feasible. Removal of bone when drilling should be minimized. The acetabulum is further prepared with pulsed lavage, taking care to avoid disturbance of the graft. The prosthesis is then cemented into place. Interposition of cement between host and graft bone should be minimized.

When a cementless socket is utilized, whether or not it is porous coated, defects should be filled with graft. Particulate graft may be reverse reamed to pack it evenly into defects. Supplemental screw fixation may be especially advantageous in revision arthroplasty because a tight press-fit may be difficult to obtain. Screws are placed cautiously (see Chapter 17, *Total Hip Arthroplasty: Operative Technique*).

Bipolar Acetabular Prosthesis

The bipolar prosthesis, originally developed for the treatment of displaced femoral neck fractures, has been used for primary treatment of arthritis of the hip and osteonecrosis of the femoral head (see Chapter 10, *Bipolar Hip Arthroplasty*). The bipolar prosthesis has also been applied in the treatment of failed acetabular components of total hip arthroplasty. Preparation of the deficient acetabulum is similar to the technique for placement of a fixed acetabular component. After the acetabulum is cleared of debris and membrane and after the initial reaming is performed, segmental defects are repaired. Particulate bone graft is impacted into place in cavitary defects, the graft is reverse reamed to improve graft conformity, and the prosthesis is placed (Fig. 23–34). The prosthesis size is estimated by preoperative templating, but the final selection is determined intraoperatively. The key to successful reconstruction is a tight rim fit so that forces are mainly transmitted peripherally. The component should be well contained within the acetabulum to assure stability. An intraoperative radiograph is helpful for confirming proper size and fit (Fig. 23–35).[3, 11, 53, 59, 64, 67]

FEMORAL STEM FAILURE

Preoperative Analysis and Planning

Classification of Femoral Failure

As with the acetabular components of total hip arthroplasties that have failed, preoperative analysis and planning for the surgical treatment of femoral components that have failed are facilitated by classification. Several investigators have developed classification systems for reporting results of revisions for failed femoral components with their own techniques.[25, 46] It is difficult to assess the proposed operative planning and to compare results when a uniform classification is not employed. The American Academy of Orthopaedic Surgeons Committee on the Hip has developed a classification system for femoral failure similar to the format of the Committee's classification of acetabular failure (Table 23–2).[16] This classification system distinguishes six types of femoral defects: segmental (type I), cavitary (type II), combined segmental/cavitary (type III), malalignment (type IV), stenosis (type V), and discontinuity (type VI). Segmental de-

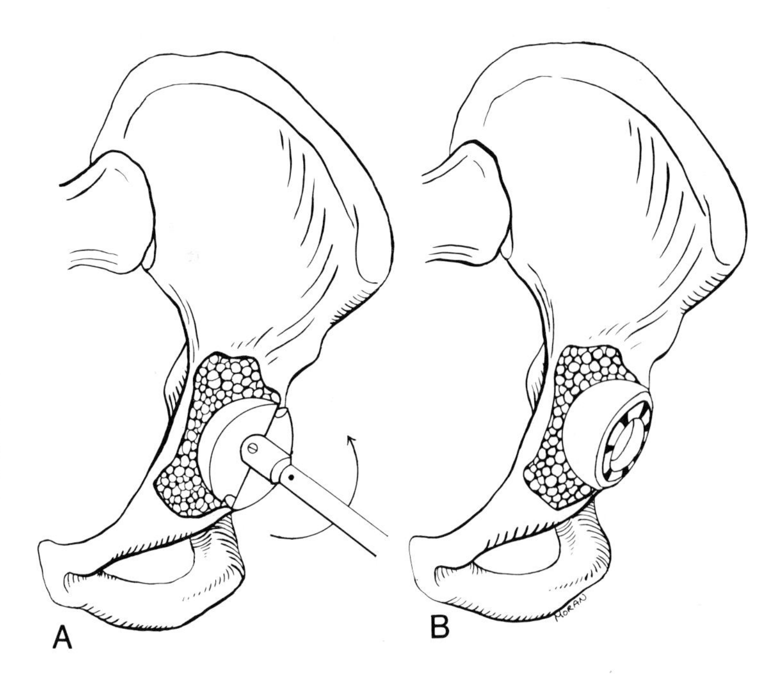

FIGURE 23–34. Reconstruction of the acetabulum using bipolar arthroplasty. *A*, Cavitary deficiency filled with particulate bone graft and reverse reamed. This procedure compresses the particulate bone graft and provides a hemispheric shape for the bipolar component. *B*, Well-contained bipolar component within the acetabulum. A tight rim fit assures that forces are primarily transmitted peripherally.

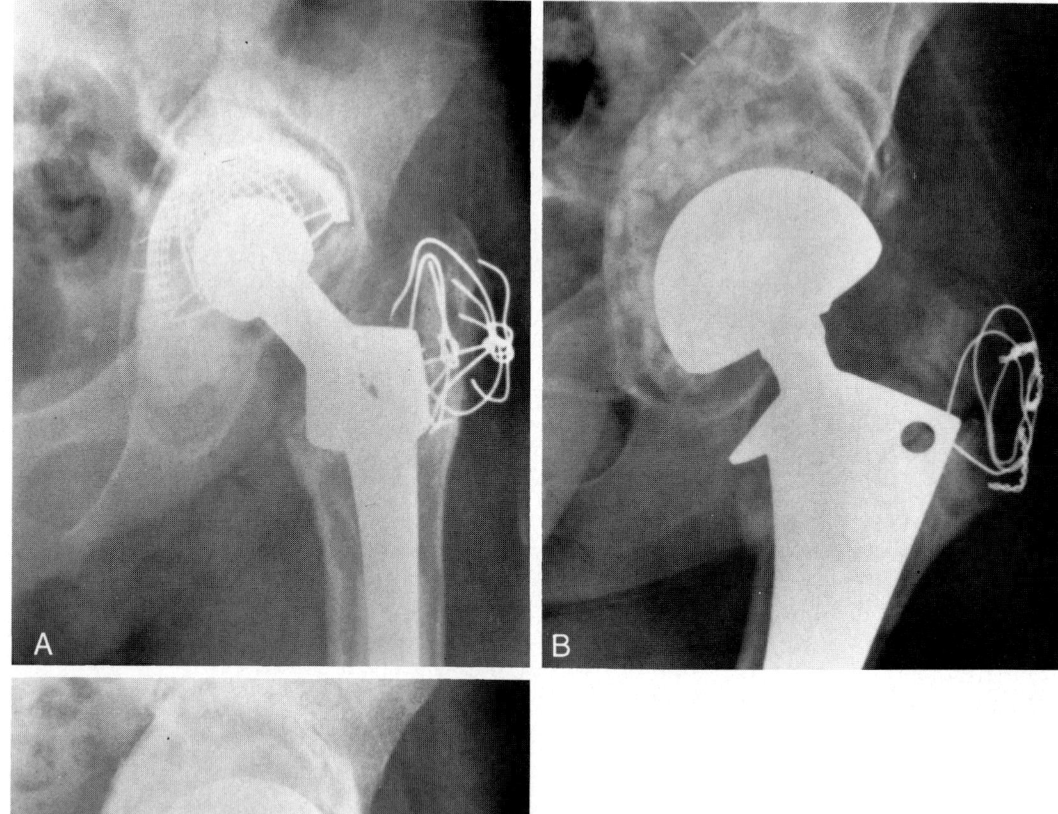

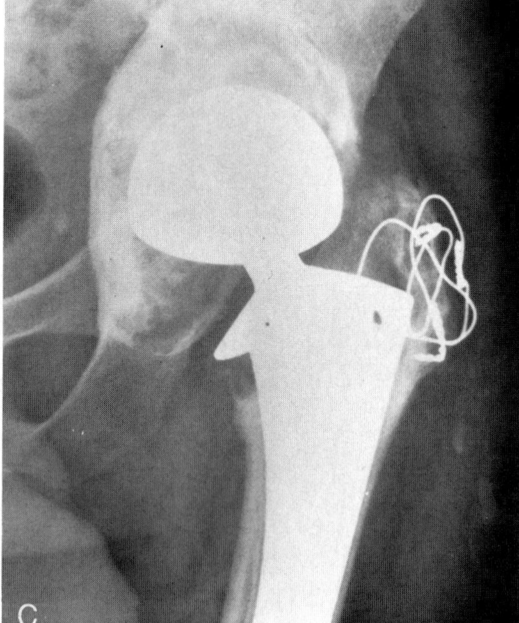

FIGURE 23–35. Radiograph showing acetabular reconstruction with bipolar prosthesis. *A,* Loose acetabular component with severe cavitary deficiency. *B,* Hip reconstructed with particulate bone graft and bipolar prosthesis. *C,* Some settling of bipolar prosthesis 1 year later but with good incorporation of bone graft.

Table 23–2. CLASSIFICATION OF FEMORAL DEFECTS*

Type I	Segmental deficiencies
	A. Proximal
	1. Partial
	2. Complete
	B. Intercalary
	C. Greater trochanter
Type II	Cavitary deficiencies
	A. Cancellous
	B. Cortical
	C. Ectasia
Type III	Combined deficiencies
Type IV	Malalignment
	A. Rotational
	B. Angular
Type V	Stenosis
Type VI	Discontinuity

*From the American Academy of Orthopaedic Surgeons Committee on the Hip.

fects involve deficiency of the cortical structure of the femur. Proximal segmental deficiency may be partial or complete (Fig. 23–36). Intercalary segmental deficiency is always partial (Fig. 23–37). A complete segmental intercalary defect is classified as discontinuity (Fig. 23–38). An absent or a deficient greater trochanter is a distinct form of segmental deficiency (Fig. 23–39). Cavitary deficiencies may involve cancellous or cortical bone or both, or the implant may have caused expansion of the bone (ectasia) (Fig. 23–40). Segmental and cavitary defects are often combined. Malalignment of the femur may be either rotational or angular, or the two deformities may be combined (Fig. 23–41). The final classification is stenosis (Fig. 23–42). The level of deficiency is also important (Fig. 23–43).

Cavitary deficiencies can be filled with cement, prosthesis, bone graft, or their combination. Most cavitary defects are filled with prosthesis or bone graft. The presence of large cancellous cavitary defects in the proximal femur may make it difficult to achieve stability of press-fit prostheses, but stability may be attained and the cavity filled with a combination of cortical and cancellous graft. Allograft or autograft cortical struts or fragments may be obtained from the ilium. Alternatively, stability is possible with three or more points of area contact in the middle and distal stem. Preferably, stability is provided by a combination of these two techniques (Fig. 23–44). When ectasia is present, accurate location of the intramedullary canal is essential to avoid cortical penetration and stem extrusion.

Combined segmental and cavitary deficiencies are managed by repair of the seg-

Text continued on page 400

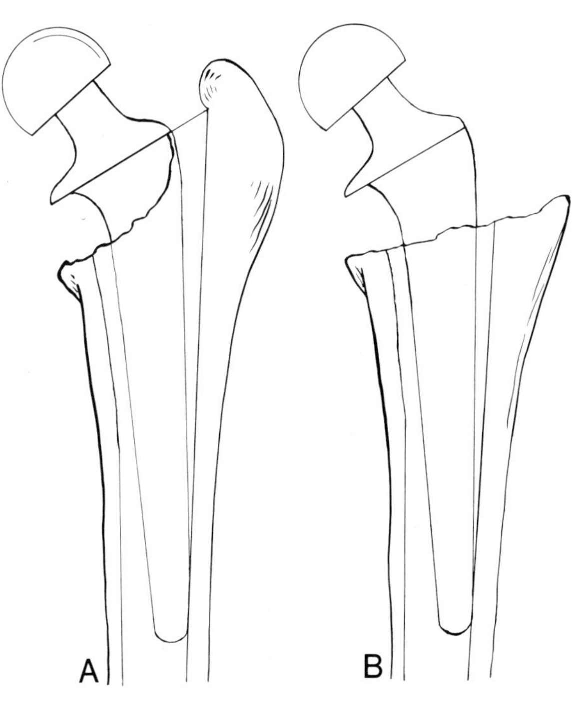

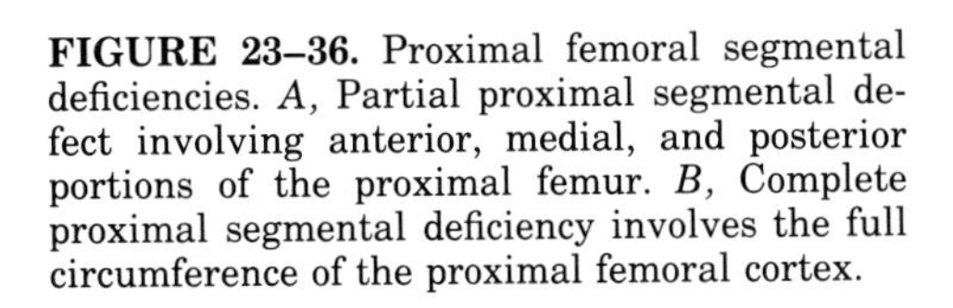
FIGURE 23–36. Proximal femoral segmental deficiencies. *A*, Partial proximal segmental defect involving anterior, medial, and posterior portions of the proximal femur. *B*, Complete proximal segmental deficiency involves the full circumference of the proximal femoral cortex.

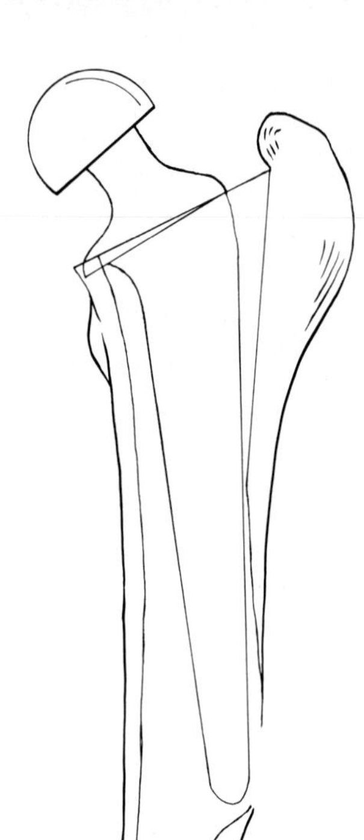

FIGURE 23–37. Intercalary segmental femoral deficiency at the tip of the prosthesis stem.

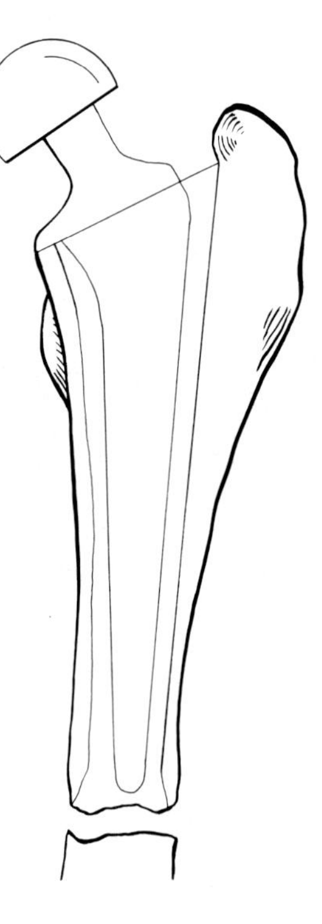

FIGURE 23–38. Femoral discontinuity consisting of a complete segmental intercalary defect.

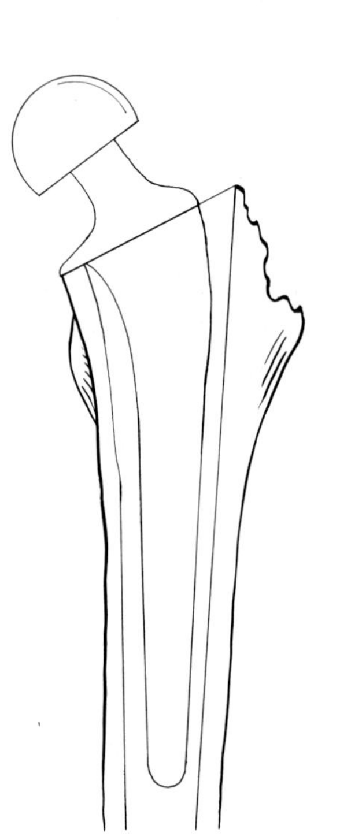

FIGURE 23–39. Segmental deficiency of greater trochanter.

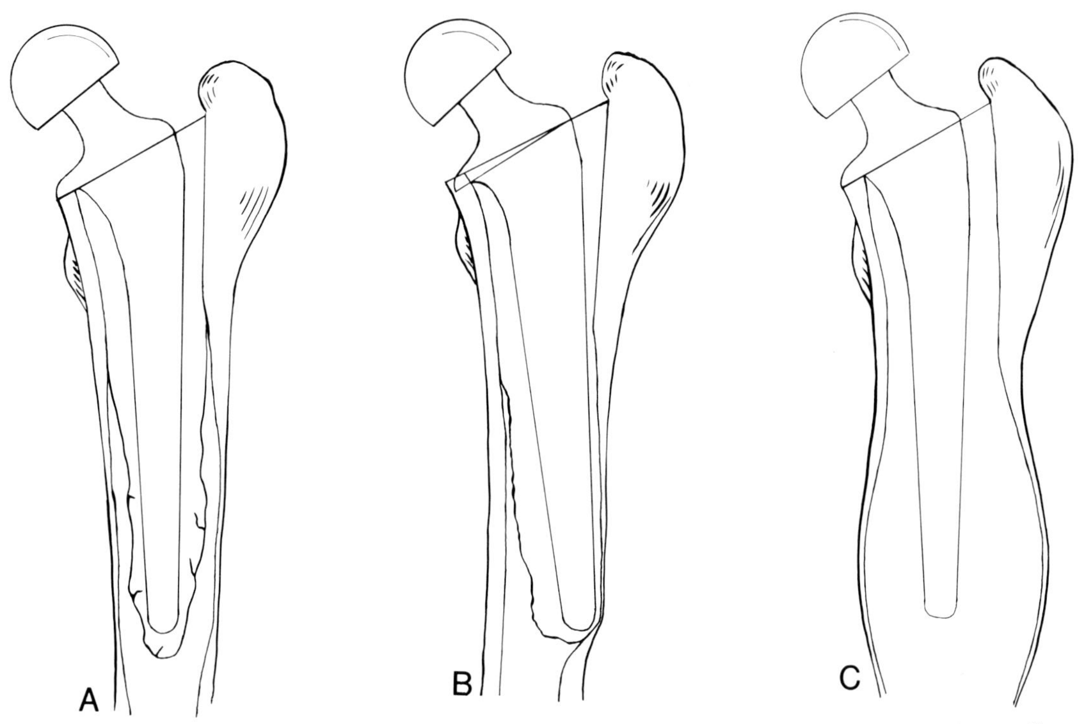

FIGURE 23–40. Cavitary femoral deficiencies. *A*, Symmetric cavitary deficiency involving primarily cancellous bone. *B*, Eccentric cavitary deficiency involving both cancellous and cortical bone. *C*, Ectasia involving cancellous and cortical bone with expansion of the cortex.

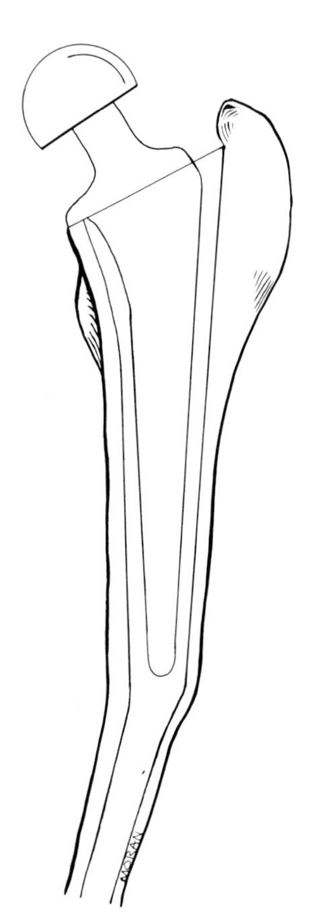

FIGURE 23–41. Angular malalignment.

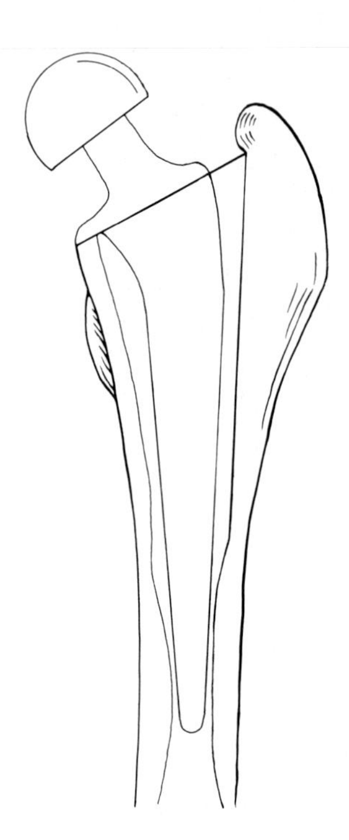

FIGURE 23–42. Femoral stenosis.

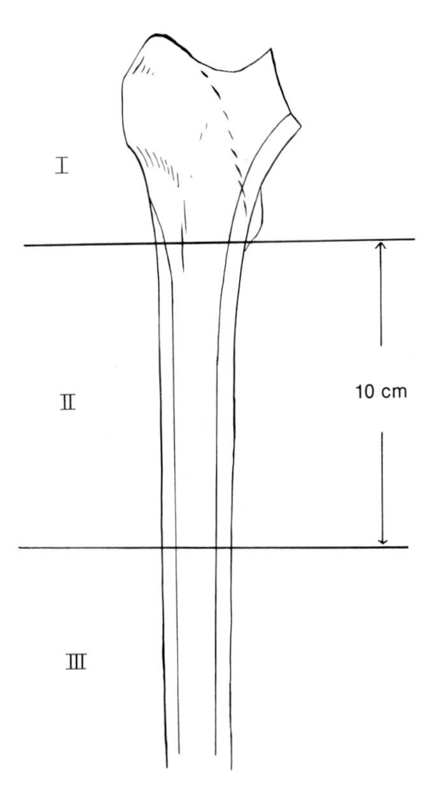

FIGURE 23–43. Level of femoral defect. Level I extends from the proximal extent of the femur to the caudad extent of the lesser trochanter. Level II extends 10 cm from the caudad extent of the lesser trochanter. Level III consists of the femur distal to level II.

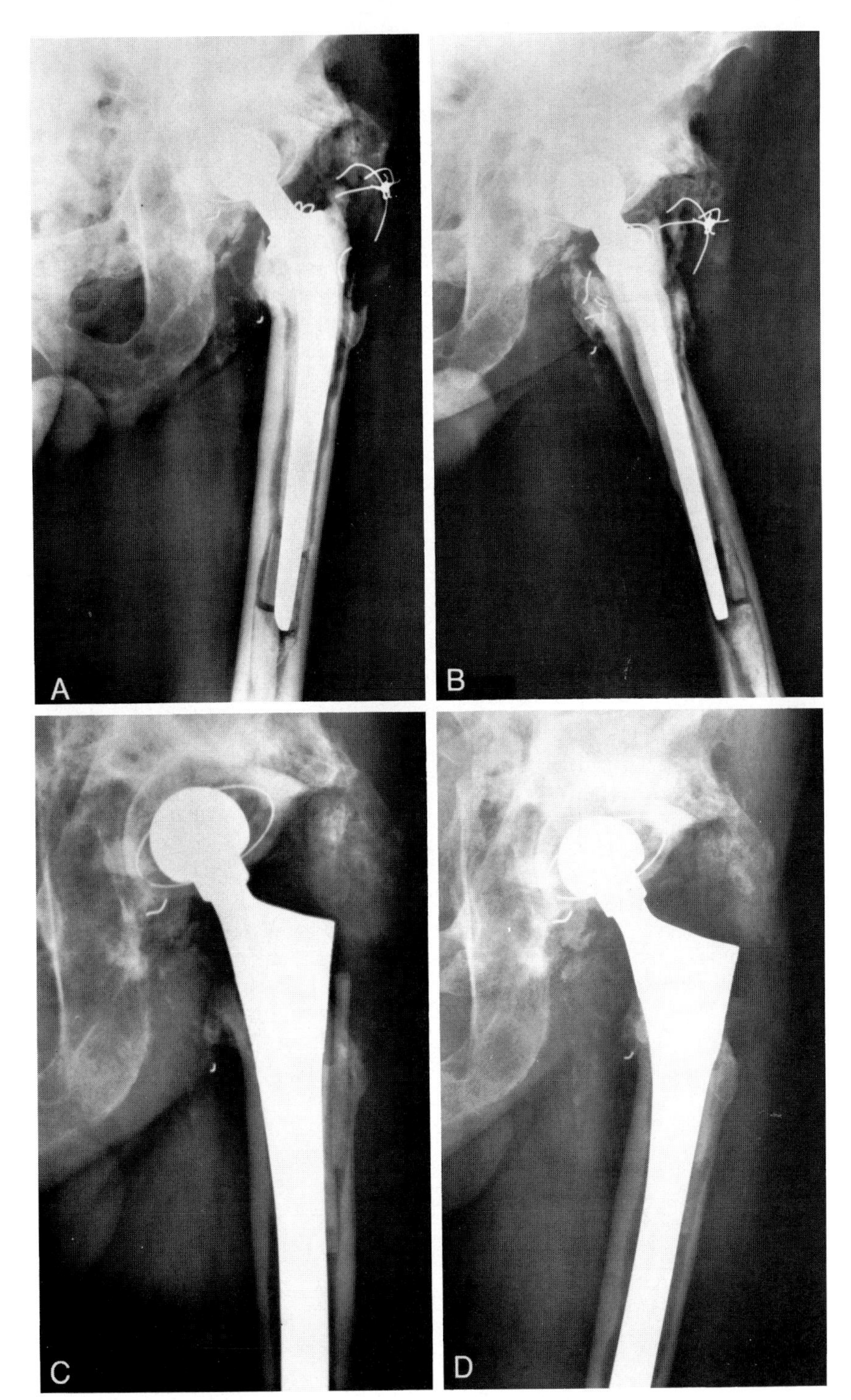

FIGURE 23–44. Cortical allograft struts are used in association with long-stem cementless femoral component to obtain stability. *A,* Preoperative anteroposterior radiograph demonstrating a loose femoral component with cement fracture, proximal segmental deficiency, and cavitary deficiency. *B,* Preoperative lateral radiograph showing, in addition to the findings in *A,* a probable intercalary segmental deficiency 4 cm above the stem tip. *C,* Postoperative radiograph showing reconstruction with a long-stem cementless femoral component. Proximal segmental deficiency was corrected with the proximal portion of the femoral stem and a long neck. The trochanter could not be repaired to the proximal femur; therefore, it was repaired to the fascia lata. Prosthesis stability could not be obtained with the prosthesis alone; therefore, multiple cortical allograft struts were placed in the proximal femur. Excellent stability was attained. *D,* Good incorporation of the cortical allograft struts 1 year postoperatively. Stability is maintained. The patient has occasional mild pain and walks well with one cane. No progression of cavitary deficiencies has occurred, but radiographically they appear to have filled in little.

mental defect first, followed by repair of the cavitary deficiency. Small partial proximal segmental defects may require no special treatment. Larger ones may be repaired with cortical graft. These partial defects, whether repaired or not, must not compromise stability of the prosthesis. Complete proximal segmental defects can be treated with structural grafts or replaced with prostheses. If the defect is short, a prosthesis with standard proximal design may be selected, although a longer neck may be indicated to restore length (Fig. 23–44D). Longer complete proximal segmental defects will require structural allografts or special proximal replacement prostheses (Figs. 23–45 and 23–46). The two best sources of grafts are proximal femur and proximal tibias (Figs. 23–45 and 23–47).

Intercalary defects are, by definition, partial. Small intercalary defects may have no effect on prosthesis stability, but they should be grafted with cancellous or cortical graft, or both, to improve bone stock and femoral strength. Whether larger defects affect stability or not, they are grafted with strong cortical graft, which is held in place with cerclage wire or cable (Fig. 23–48). These grafts are sometimes fixed with screws that are difficult to place so that they provide adequate fixation and yet remain clear of the femoral stem.

Partial absence of the greater trochanter, if the deficiency is small, may require no special treatment. A larger defect may be filled in with prosthesis. If the greater trochanter is absent or if the deficiency has resulted in abductor discontinuity, abductor function may be restored by reattachment. When this restoration is not possible, suturing the remaining abductor muscles to the iliotibial band during closure usually provides satisfactory abductor function. Methods for repairing a detached greater trochanter are detailed elsewhere in this text (see Chapter 14, *Surgical Approaches for Total Hip Replacement*).

Both angular and rotational deformities may be present in primary or revision arthroplasty, but angular deformity is usually present in the femurs that require revision arthroplasty. Such malalignment may result from malunion of fracture, most commonly at the stem tip or in the area of the stem (see Chapter 19, *Total Hip Arthroplasty: Complications*). A primary stem that fails in varus and results in plastic deformation of the femur into varus commonly requires revision (Fig. 23–49). Rarely, the femur and a long stem will deform together, making extraction of the stem especially difficult. The stem may be extracted by straightening the deformity manually. If the femur is not fractured, long stem extraction will require osteotomy at the site of deformity. Preoperative templating is vital for planning the osteotomy and selecting the prosthesis (Fig. 23–49B). The femur should be exposed extensively. Rigid mechanical fixation of the osteotomy is obtained with the stem of the revision prosthesis, when possible (Fig. 23–49C). Screws, wires, or small plates may be utilized as adjuncts and to provide rotational stability. Cortical bone graft struts held in place with cerclage wiring may be added for graft and supplemental fixation. A postoperative cast may supplement the internal fixation and provide rotational stability.[27,35] (See also Chapter 19, *Total Hip Arthroplasty: Complications.*)

Discontinuity of the femur results from a complete intercalary segmental defect. This type of deficiency is much less common than complete proximal segmental defects in failed total hip arthroplasty. It is more likely to result from trauma or tumor (Fig. 23–50A). Treatment of discontinuity resulting from fracture and with little segmental loss is similar to treatment of malalignment (Fig. 23–50). Larger intercalary defects may be filled with structural bone allograft, the femur being the best source of this graft.

Canal stenosis is usually associated with conditions such as congenital dysplasia of the hip and juvenile rheumatoid arthritis rather than with failed total hip arthroplasty. Obviously, patients who have had hip replacements because of these conditions may experience failure of primary arthroplasties and require revisions. Under these circumstances, the canal may be quite small. A small or even a custom prosthesis may be indicated for revision.

Cemented or Cementless Revision

Although the initial clinical results from cemented revision of total hip arthroplasty

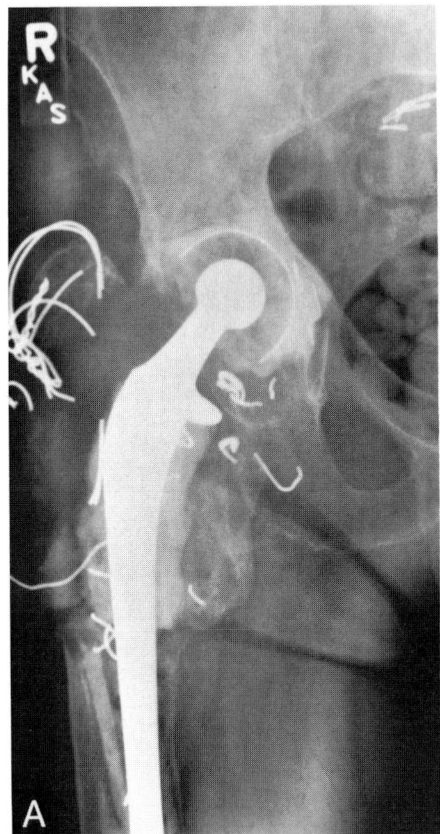

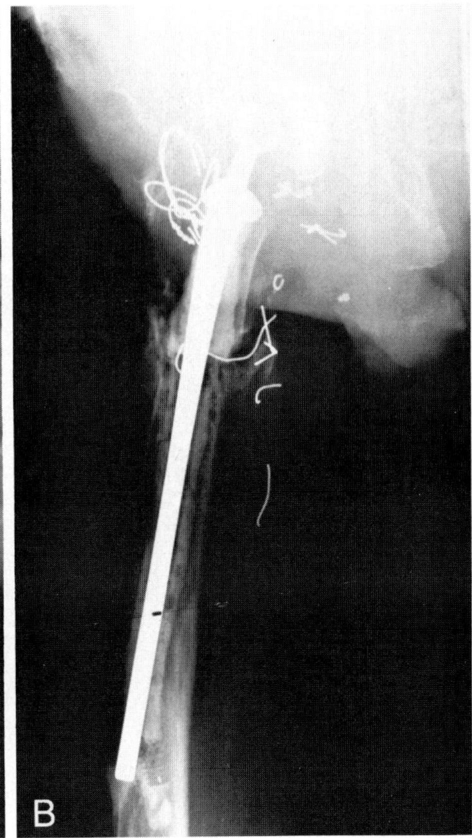

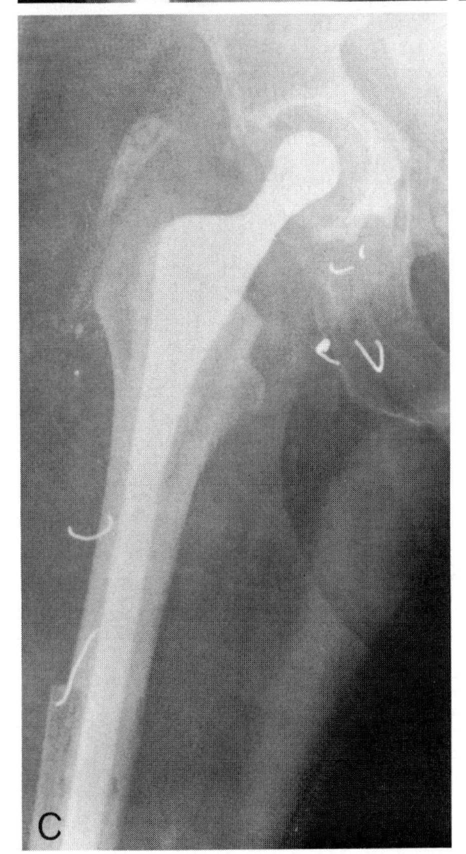

FIGURE 23–45. Cemented long femoral stem and proximal femoral allograft used to reconstruct proximal femoral segmental deficiency in a patient with Gaucher disease. *A* and *B*, Anteroposterior and lateral radiographs of failed femoral stem of previous revision arthroplasty show femoral discontinuity and absence of all but approximately 20 percent of the circumference of the proximal portion of the femur. *C*, Reconstruction of the femur with a proximal femoral allograft and a custom long-stem–cemented femoral component. The acetabular component showed no signs of loosening either radiographically or intraoperatively and therefore was left in place.

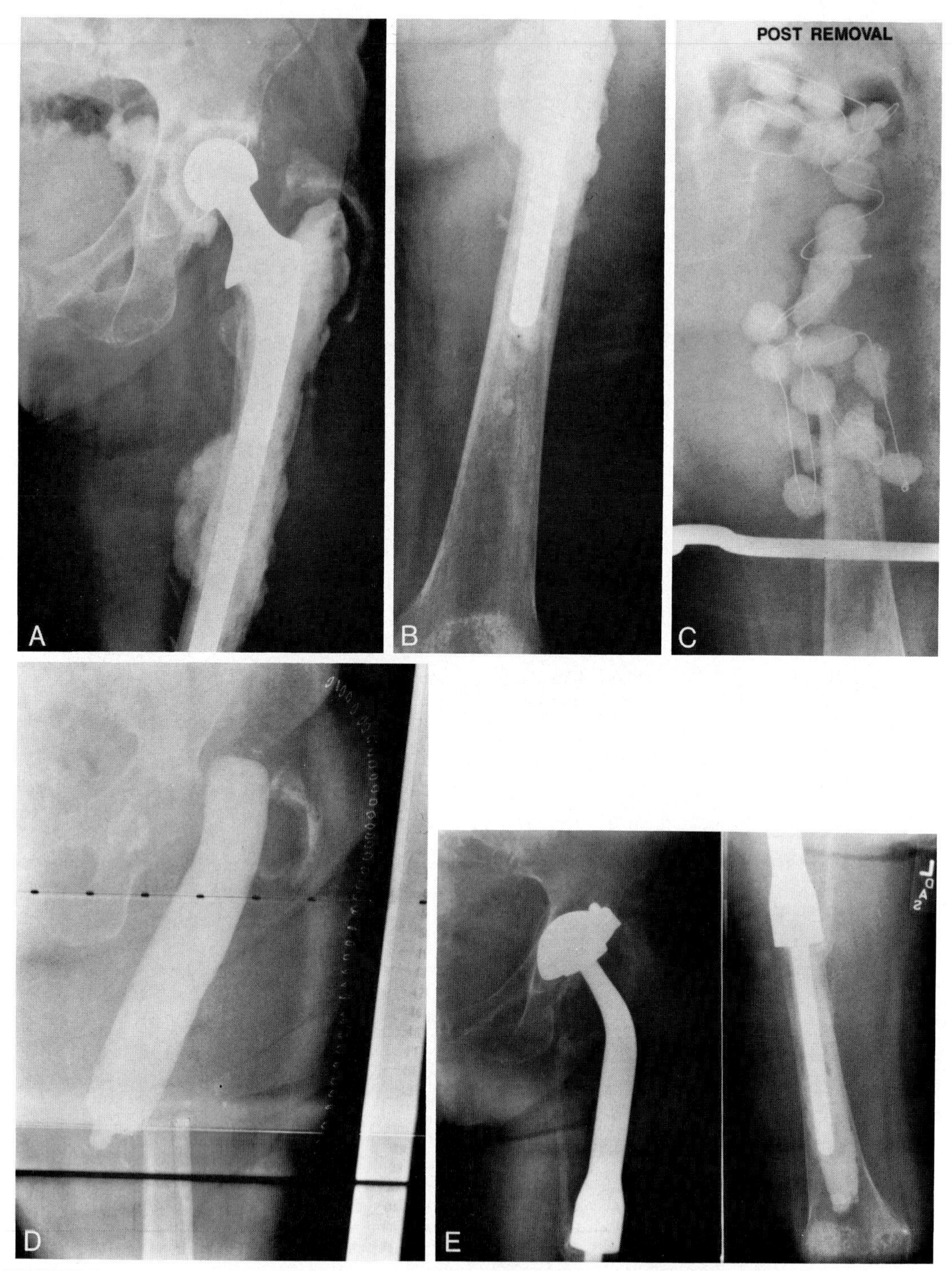

FIGURE 23–46. Patient with infected revision total hip arthroplasty. In previous revision most of the proximal half of the femur was replaced with cement. Revision was with cemented proximal femoral replacement prosthesis. *A* and *B*, Preoperative radiographs showing extensive bone loss with proximal femur replaced with bone cement. *C*, Resection of the prosthesis cement and remaining devascularized bone and placement of bone cement beads containing antibiotic. *D*, Maintenance of proximal femoral space after additional debridement by a bone cement–rod containing antibiotic. *E*, Radiograph of the hip 3 years postoperatively. The patient is free from infection and pain and walks with a single cane.

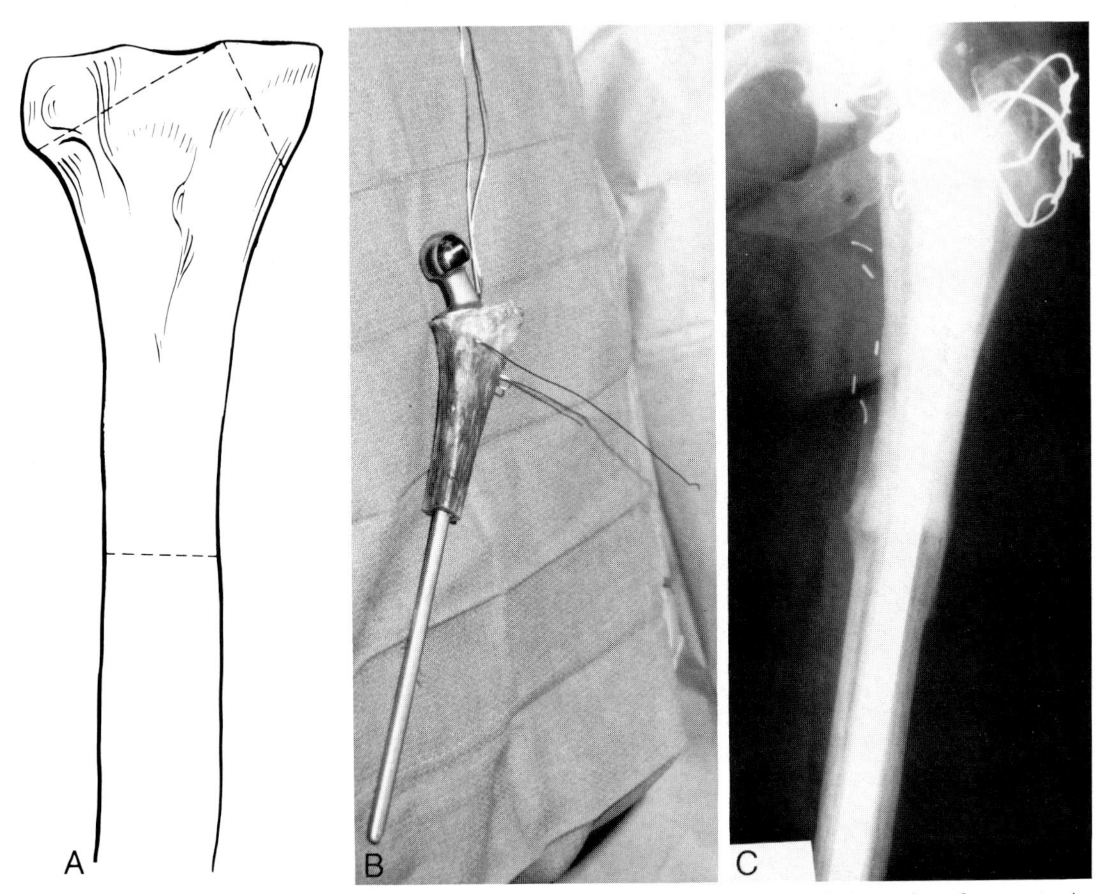

FIGURE 23–47. The proximal tibia, an excellent allograft source for proximal femoral replacement. *A*, Proximal cut to convert the proximal tibia to a proximal femoral replacement. *B*, Long-stem femoral prosthesis is placed in a proximal tibial allograft. Placement is done in preparation for proximal femoral reconstruction. *C*, Postoperative radiograph of proximal femoral reconstruction using long-stem femoral prosthesis and proximal tibial allograft.

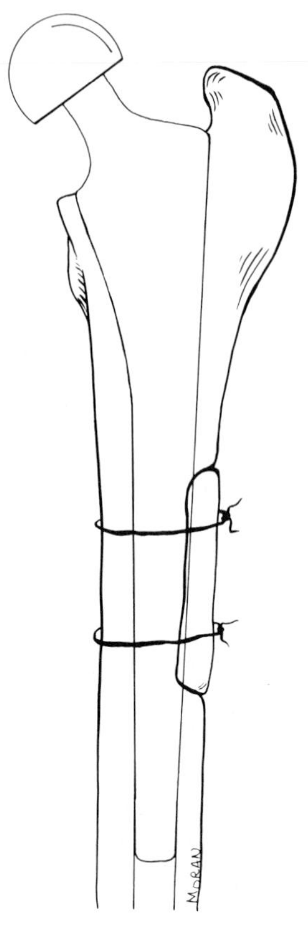

FIGURE 23–48. Intercalary deficiency repaired with cortical graft. Graft-host junctions are grafted with cancellous graft, preferably autograft.

failure are reasonably satisfactory, the incidence of failure rises substantially with longer follow-up periods. The radiographic appearance is worrisome, often even immediately after revision, but this is not surprising. Criteria for technically successful cementation seldom can be met in the revision situation, for the following reasons:

1. The endosteal bone surface usually is hard and smooth, with few if any remaining trabecular interstices for mechanical interdigitation with cement (Fig. 23–51). The result is marked decrease in shear strength of the bone-cement interface (Fig. 23–52).[20]
2. Because of the irregularity of the femoral canal, the cement mantle will be grossly nonuniform (Fig. 23–51).
3. It is difficult to occlude segmental defects sufficiently to provide pressurization of the cement.

In those femurs with massive bone loss, usually following multiple cemented revisions, massive filling of the irregular remaining bone is unlikely to provide a stable prosthesis. Bone grafts are often needed to fill both segmental and cavitary defects. It is difficult to prevent interposition of cement between large structural bone fragments. It is nearly impossible when multiple, small bone graft fragments are utilized.

For these reasons, some surgeons suggest that all revisions be done without cement. Others maintain that cemented revision may be preferable in some instances, particularly in elderly individuals, if the criteria for satisfactory cementation can be met. The rationale is that thigh pain can be avoided. Also, the long-term outlook with cementless prostheses is unknown. Most surgeons agree that cemented fixation is indicated in the unusual situation in which stability cannot be achieved with a cementless device. In revisions for failed prostheses associated with bone lysis, lysis sometimes recurs rapidly when cement is used. If evidence of bone lysis exists and stability cannot be achieved with a cementless stem and bone graft, one option is to leave the hip as a resection arthroplasty. Alternatively, the surgeon can bone graft the femur, allow time for this to heal, and operate later to place a cementless prosthesis. Cementation may be necessary when a long, proximal, complete segmental defect or discontinuity involving the entire isthmus area is reconstructed with a structural allograft or long proximal replacement prosthesis. Stable press-fit distal fixation is difficult to achieve in the widening femoral canal in this situation. Often, the distal bone is of good quality and allows for good cement fixation (see Figs. 23–45 and 23–46).

The major advantages of a cementless prosthesis in revision surgery are that it provides an opportunity to avoid further destruction of bone stock and, in many cases, to recover lost bone (see Fig. 23–44). Bone graft, whether autograft or allograft, is facilitated with a cementless femoral stem. Interference with healing because of cement between the grafts is avoided. Stability is the principal intraoperative goal with a cementless stem. Without stability, the reconstruction is almost certain to fail

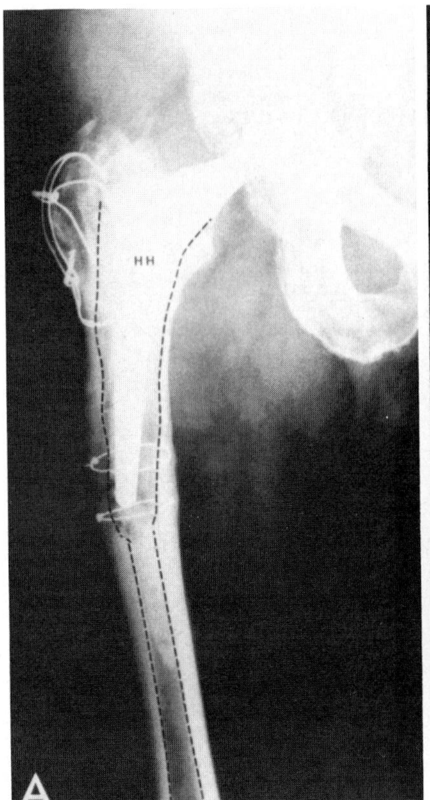

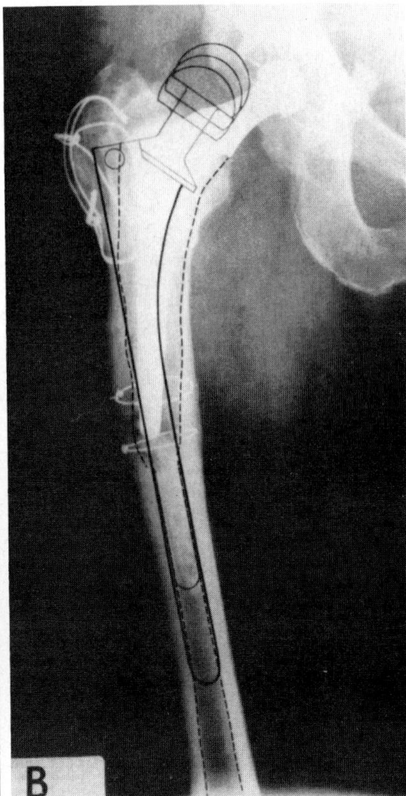

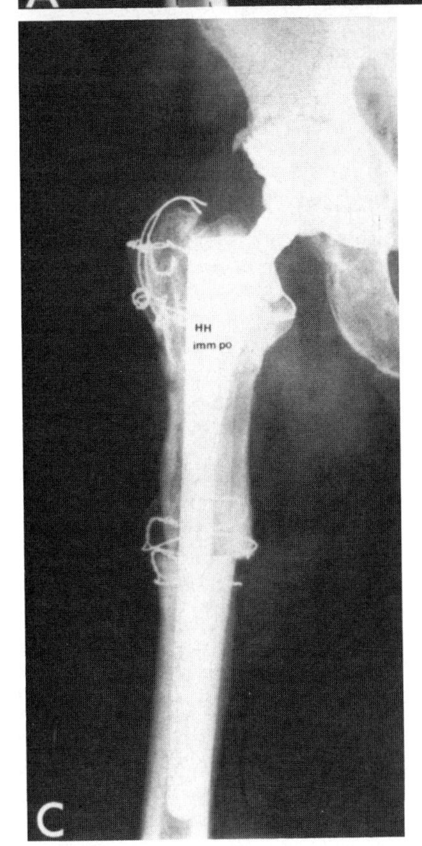

FIGURE 23–49. Reconstruction of failed total hip arthroplasty with varus malalignment. (Glassman, A. H., Engh, C. S., and Bobyn, J. D.: J. Arthroplasty 2:47–63, 1987. By permission.) *A,* Loose cemented femoral component, failed in varus, resulting in varus deformity of the femur at the stem tip. Dotted line outlines the deformity in the endosteal cavity of the distal femur and the proximal femur. *B,* Template of a long-stem prosthesis laid over the femur, demonstrating that an osteotomy will be required to place this femoral stem. *C,* Postoperative radiograph demonstrating correction of the deformity by osteotomy and fixation of the osteotomy with the femoral stem and wiring.

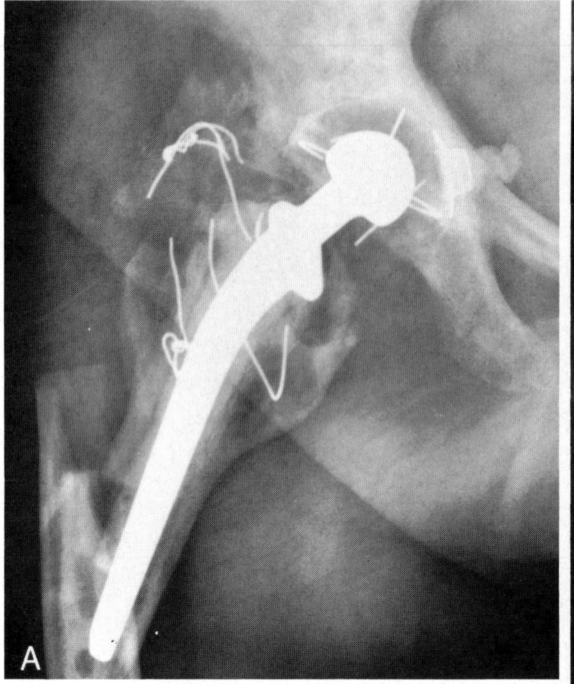

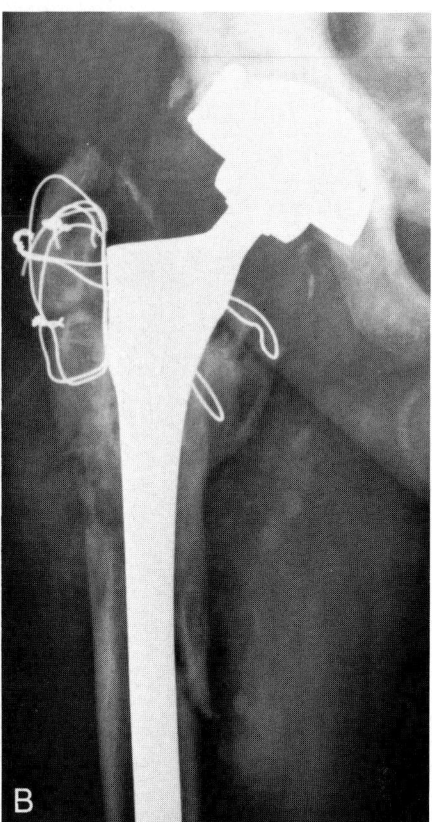

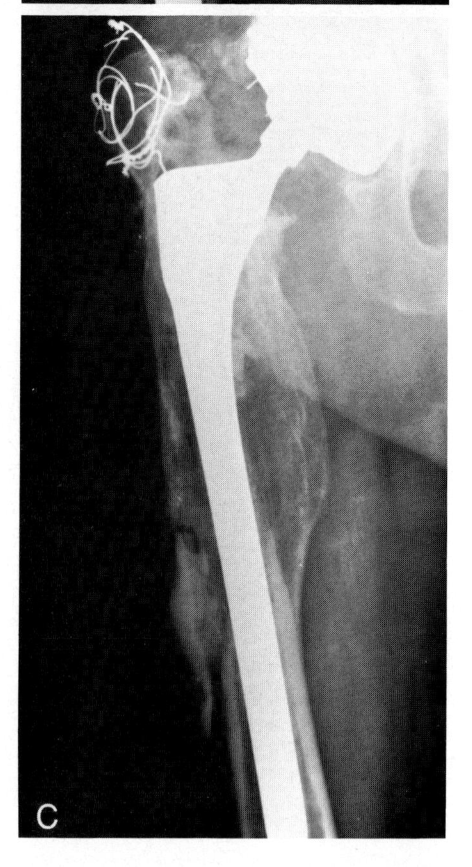

FIGURE 23–50. Femoral discontinuity resulting from fracture treated with long-stem cementless femoral component. *A,* Spiral fracture involving the area of the stem tip (Type IV-A fracture). (See Chapter 19, *Total Hip Arthroplasty: Complications.*) *B,* Reconstruction of the hip and fixation of the fracture with a long-stem femoral component. Stability was excellent without supplemental fixation. *C,* Fracture is well healed 1 year later. Patient walks with a cane and has no hip pain.

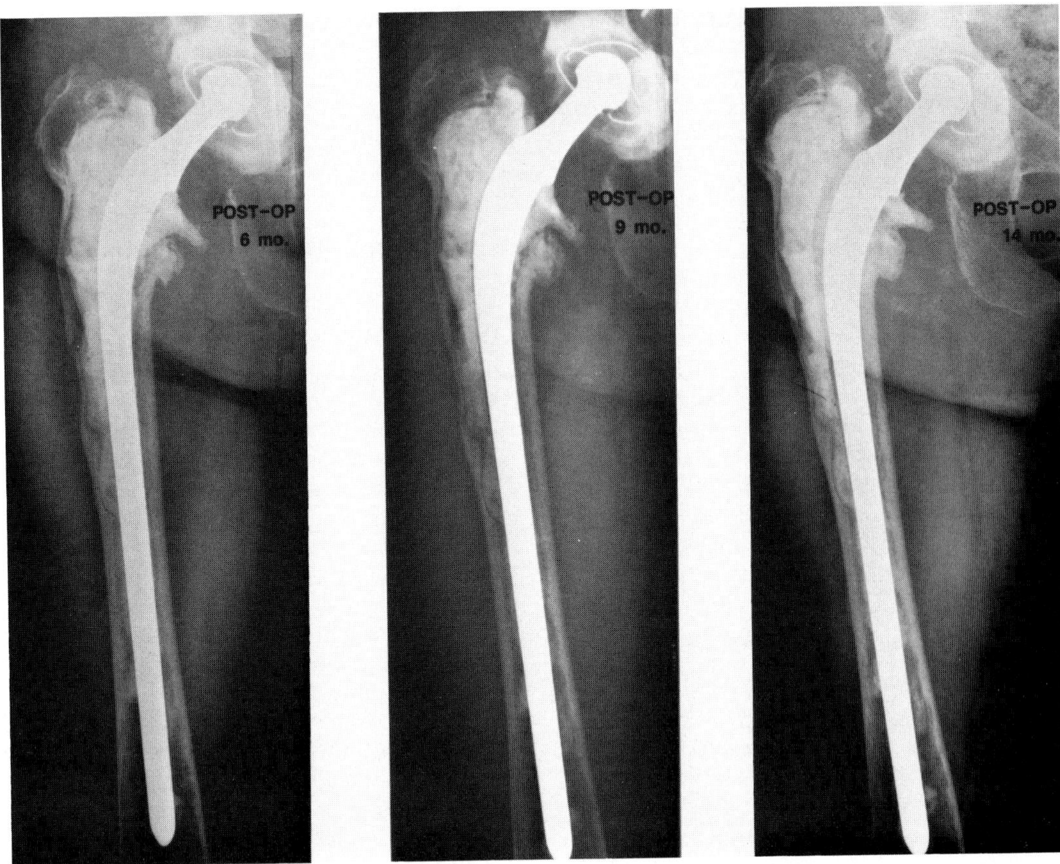

FIGURE 23–51. Cemented total hip arthroplasty revision. The patient's bone stock was poor for cemented revision. The patient rapidly developed recurrent femoral stem loosening.

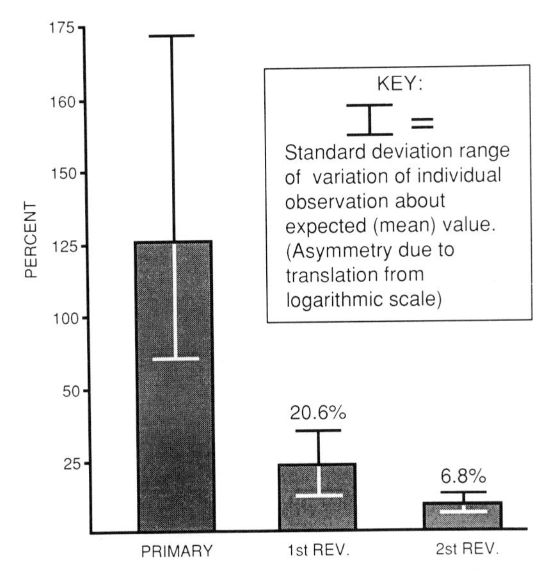

FIGURE 23–52. Reduction in shear strength at bone-cement interface after simulated revision joint replacement arthroplasty. (Dohmae, Y., Bechtold, J. E., Sherman, R. E., and Gustilo, R. B.: Orthop. Trans. 10:406–407, 1986. By permission.)

owing to subsidence, pain, motion of the prosthesis within the bone, and further bone destruction. In the bone with major deficiencies—whether segmental, cavitary, or combined—a long stem prosthesis may help achieve stability. Bone graft often effectively provides stability when it cannot be achieved with the prosthesis alone (see Fig. 23–44).[25, 29, 37, 46]

In most series of primary cementless femoral prostheses, the early results are inferior compared with those of cemented components owing to thigh pain, increased limp, increased use of walking aids, and slower rehabilitation (see Chapter 20, *Results of Primary Total Hip Arthroplasty*). The pain is usually mild, though, and ultimately recovery is satisfactory. Pain that appears to be associated with an abnormal concentration of stress in the area of the distal stem will probably resolve or at least improve with time, although this resolution may take 2 to 3 years. However, disabling thigh pain occasionally persists, and the only apparent cause is possible prosthesis instability. This may be an indication for revision. Surgeons do not agree on whether such a stem should be converted to another cementless one or to a cemented stem. A reasonable approach is to convert the cementless stem to a cemented stem in the patient over 60 or 65 years but to do a cementless revision in the younger patient. In converting to a cemented stem, great care must be taken in preparing the bone and providing a roughened surface for cement fixation, even though the endosteal surface is not likely to be as sclerotic as after failed cemented hip arthroplasty. When converting a failed primary cementless stem to another cementless stem, the surgeon must assure adequate sizing of the prosthesis to afford stability.

Prosthesis Selection

Decisions to be made in selection of the prosthesis include length of the stem; whether it is curved or straight; length of the porous coating, if any; and special requirements, such as the need for a proximal femoral replacement option (i.e., the Leinbach or similar design) or possibly for a custom prosthesis.

Excessive lengths may not be desirable. The stem should pass distally, by two femoral diameters, any segmental defects that are already present or that might be created during the operation. Whether the stem is curved or straight often is primarily a matter of the surgeon's preference. However, if preoperative evaluation reveals a prominent anterior bow and a long stem is indicated, a stem with an anterior curve may be selected.

Some investigators have suggested that porous coating should extend the entire length of the stem if substantial cavitation is present proximally, to provide diaphyseal fixation.[27] The long-term effect on stress remodeling of the femur is unknown, but experimental work as well as clinical follow-up in other situations suggest that such a reconstruction may lead to increased proximal bone resorption.[24, 34] A nonporous-coated stem and restriction of the coating to the proximal stem only rely more on bone apposition and fit for stability. When a proximal porous-coated stem is implanted in a femur with proximal cavitation, even with bone graft, any ingrowth is likely to be fibrous. A collar may provide an additional point of fixation for stability, but it should be considered supplemental to other modes of fixation.

Operative Technique

Specific surgical approaches are discussed in Chapter 14, *Surgical Approaches for Total Hip Replacement.* Because the femur usually has been weakened owing to cortical defects or cavitation, great care must be taken in dislocating the hip and exposing the femur to avoid fracturing it. Soft tissue release is extensive so that manual force can be minimal. The entire pseudocapsule around the proximal femur is excised or released. It is often necessary to release the iliopsoas and gluteus maximus tendons. Many surgeons prefer to expose the entire femur throughout the distance involved for removal of prosthesis and cement. This practice allows direct visualization of inadvertent femoral perforation, thereby minimizing bone damage, and provides exposure for controlled perforation or "windowing" the femur when indicated.[33] Extensive femoral exposure is the safer method when image-intensified fluoroscopy is not used, especially when cement must be cleared from deep within the femur. Trochanteric osteotomy offers more complete access to the proximal femur but compromises the stability provided by the greater trochanter to the press-fit stem. If the greater trochanter is left in place, visualization is improved by removing all soft tissue and any protruding bone from the medial aspect of the trochanter.

Removal of Cemented Femoral Stem

When the femoral stem is grossly loose, it sometimes can be removed easily by hand. Often, however, even when the stem can be moved within the canal, extraction is difficult. The stem is incarcerated because its geometry or the geometry of the attached cement will not allow it to pass through the proximal femoral envelope.

When the impeding material is the cement, it can be removed with osteotomes so that the stem can be extracted (Fig. 23–53). If the stem itself is impeding extraction, any soft tissue in the way is excised. Bone may be narrowing the envelope through which the prosthesis must pass usually because the stem has subsided into the bone. All bone that can be saved should be, but it is better to remove a small amount of bone to allow extraction of the stem than to fracture the proximal femur. Femoral components may be well fixed and difficult to remove even when they are loose enough to be painful or when conditions such as malposition, unacceptable limb length inequality (usually overlengthening), and certain types of prosthesis failure necessitate revision (Fig. 23–54).

Cement is cut with osteotomes and removed from around the proximal portion of the stem as far distally as can be done without damaging the bone (Fig. 23–55). As fracture occurs further distally in the cement, the stem can be removed by making mallet blows against a bone impactor applied to the collar or femoral head. A preferable method involves a specially designed extractor with a hammer (Fig. 23–56). Use of the specially designed extractors and mallet and the bone impactor is difficult on stems with modular heads, but with care an adequate grasping or striking surface can be located. If not, it may be necessary to cut a cortical window distal to the stem tip and to drive the stem out (Fig. 23–57). All windows cut from the cortex during revision surgery should be in the anterior cortex, where stress is less. The bone is saved for later replacement.

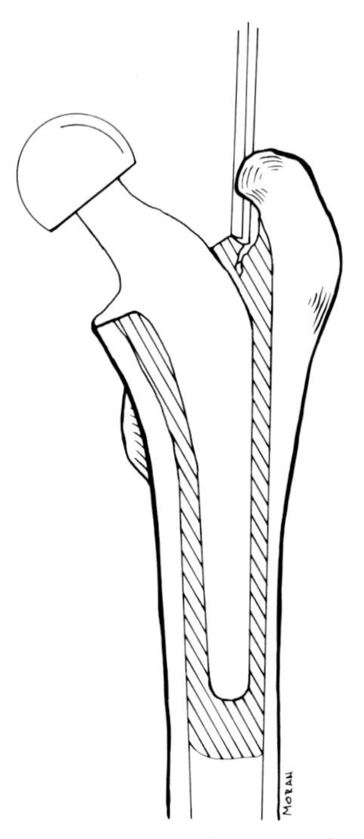

FIGURE 23–53. Incarceration of a loose femoral stem because of its geometry or that of the attached cement. If the proximal lateral cement is removed, the femoral stem will pass more easily through the proximal femoral envelope.

On occasion, the entire cement mass comes out with the stem or the cement mass can be grasped and extracted in one piece. One technique to remove the cement en masse is to place a threaded rod in the cavity that the stem occupied, inject fresh cement, allow it to polymerize around the rod, and then extract the rod and cement (Fig. 23–58).[13] However, even with grossly loose stems, some cement usually will be well fixed to bone. Some surgeons prefer to remove cement as far distally as possible with osteotomes, which is usually possible for 10 to 15 cm down the canal or up to the area where the stem tip was (Fig. 23–59). Remaining cement is then removed with a high-speed bur. When cement extends beyond the curvature of the femur, making straight access no longer possible, great care must be taken to avoid inadvertent bone damage (Fig. 23–60). Cement can be safely removed more distally through the proximal femur if the greater trochanter has been osteotomized or fluoroscopy is used (Figs. 23–61 and 23–16). Whatever technique is selected, a point may be reached where it is not safe to remove cement from the top. It is far preferable to make a controlled window in the femur to remove cement than to create inadvertent defects in the femur (Fig. 23–62). Several controlled windows spaced along the extent of the cement may make removal easier (Fig. 23–63).[46]

Several methods to enhance cement removal and minimize bone damage are under investigation. Under laboratory and early clinical investigation is laser vaporization of bone cement, which is based on the different response of bone and cement to light energy. The laser is directed through an instrument similar to the laparoscope.[62] Ultrasonic tools, based on tech-

Text continued on page 415

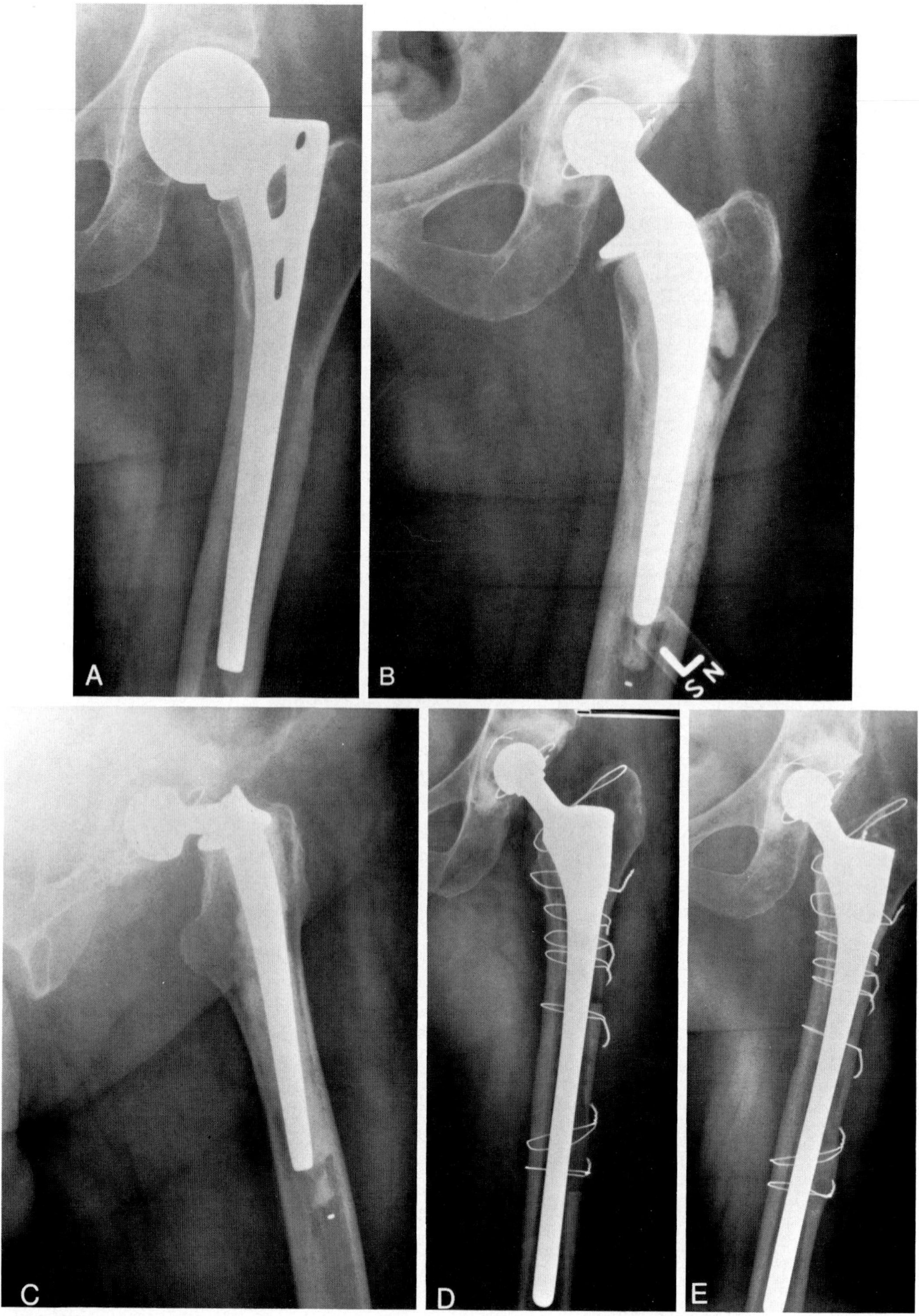

FIGURE 23–54. Well-fixed femoral stems. When stems must be taken out for reasons other than stem loosening, removal may be very difficult. *A,* Patient with a femoral neck fracture treated with an Austin Moore prosthesis. She had continuing pain probably due to a loose prosthesis. *B,* Conversion of the failed hemiarthroplasty to cemented total hip replacement. *C,* Fracture of the forged cobalt chromium alloy prosthesis through the femoral neck. Although the patient's result was excellent, 3 years postoperatively while working as a store clerk, she had sudden collapse of the extremity. Radiographs revealed this fracture. *D,* Revision of the femoral component to a long-stem cementless femoral component. The difficult cement removal resulted in a proximal femoral fracture. A controlled window was also used distally to remove the remaining cement. The proximal spiral fracture was treated with cerclage wiring. The cortical window removed to provide access for cement removal was replaced and wired in place with cerclage wiring. *E,* Radiograph of the hip 2 years later. The Iowa hip rating is 92.

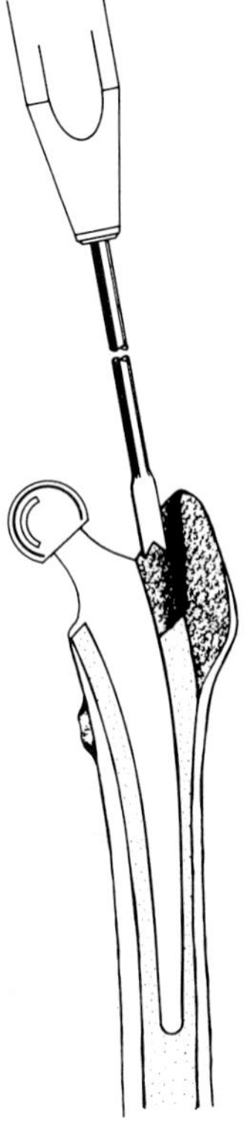

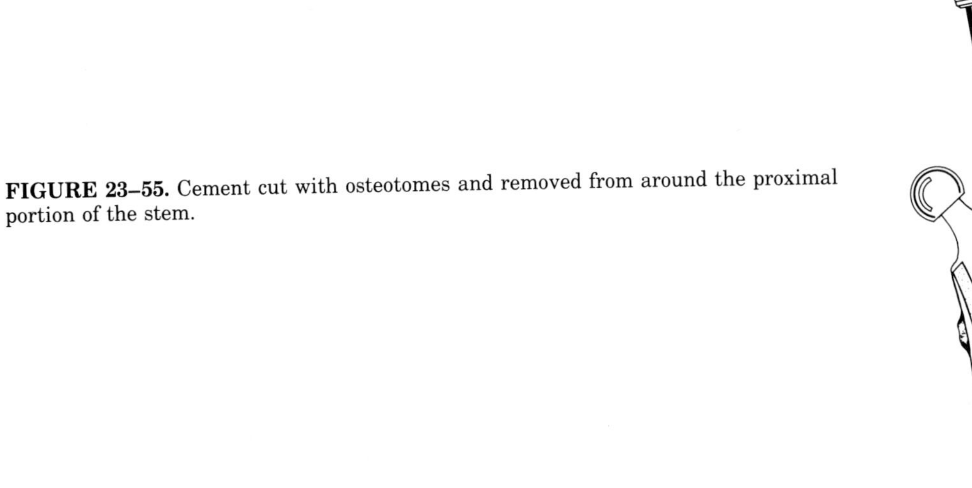

FIGURE 23–55. Cement cut with osteotomes and removed from around the proximal portion of the stem.

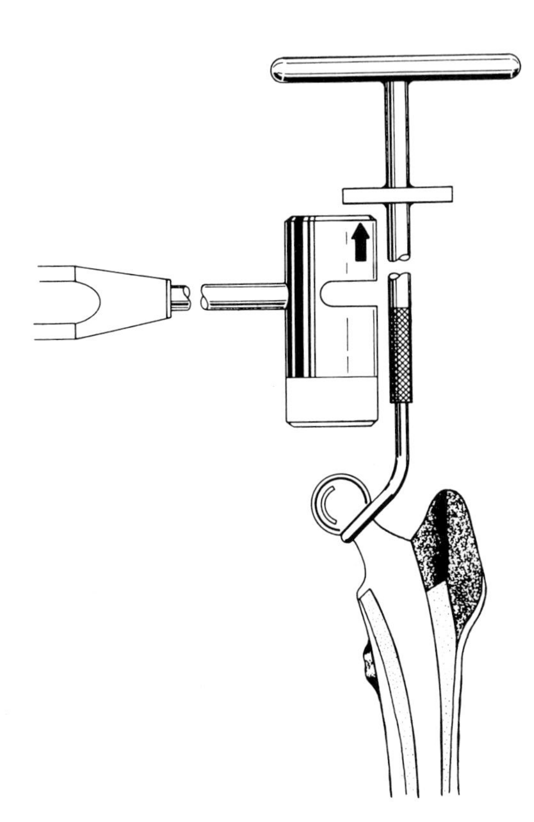

FIGURE 23–56. Removal of the failed stem with a stem extractor.

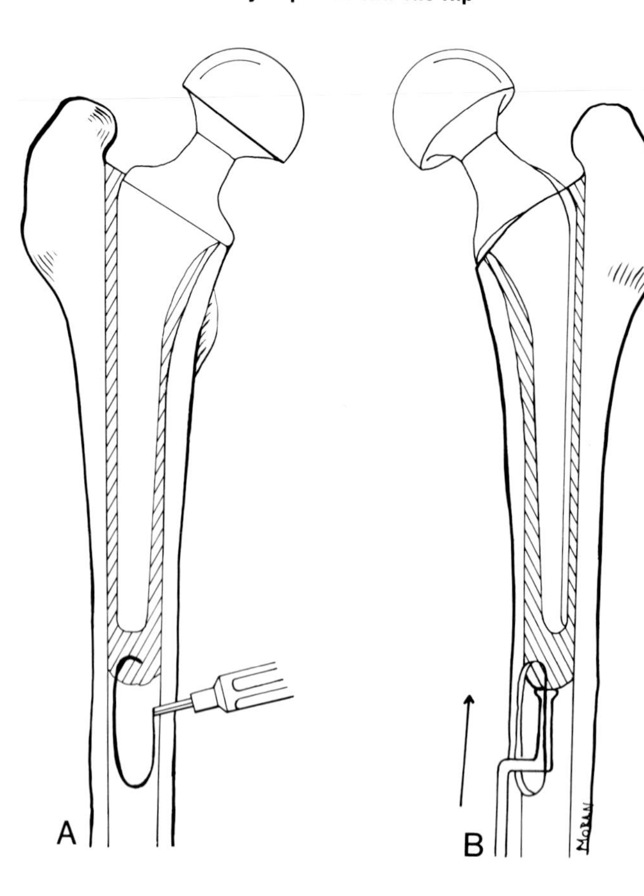

FIGURE 23–57. Cortical window cut distally to the stem tip, with the stem driven out. *A*, Making the cortical window. *B*, Driving the stem out from below.

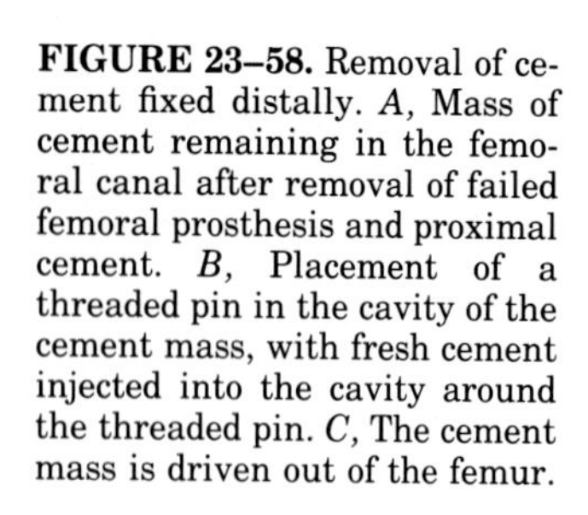

FIGURE 23–58. Removal of cement fixed distally. *A*, Mass of cement remaining in the femoral canal after removal of failed femoral prosthesis and proximal cement. *B*, Placement of a threaded pin in the cavity of the cement mass, with fresh cement injected into the cavity around the threaded pin. *C*, The cement mass is driven out of the femur.

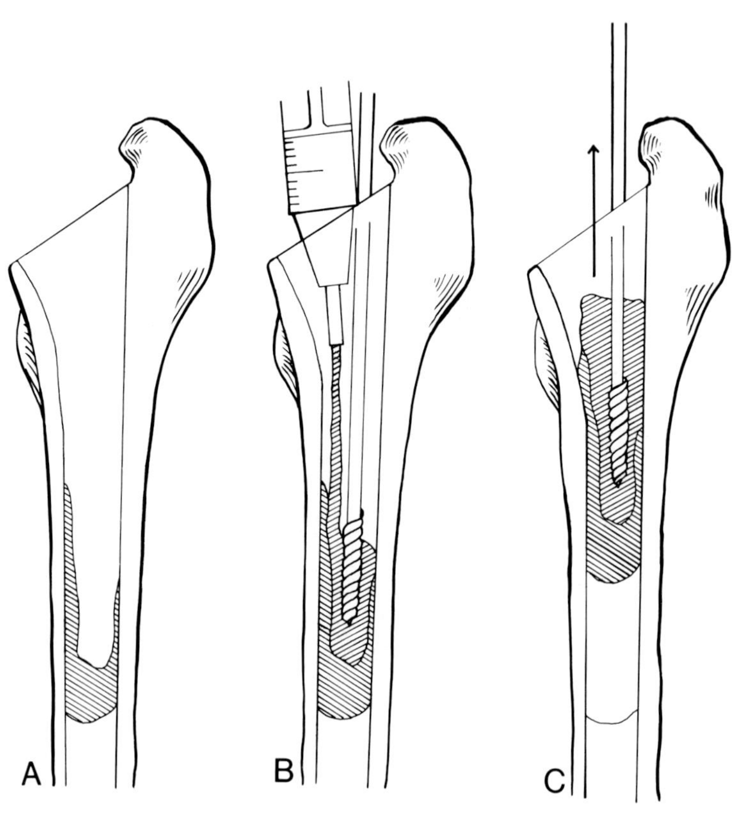

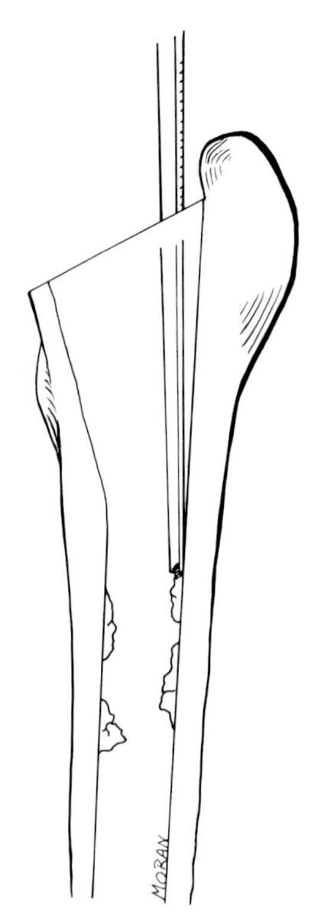

FIGURE 23–59. Removal of distal cement with osteotomes.

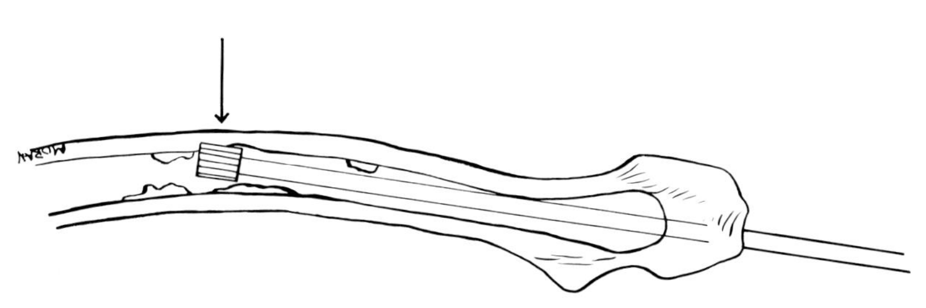

FIGURE 23–60. Cement extends beyond the curvature of the femur, and straight access is no longer possible. Great care must be taken to avoid inadvertent bone damage.

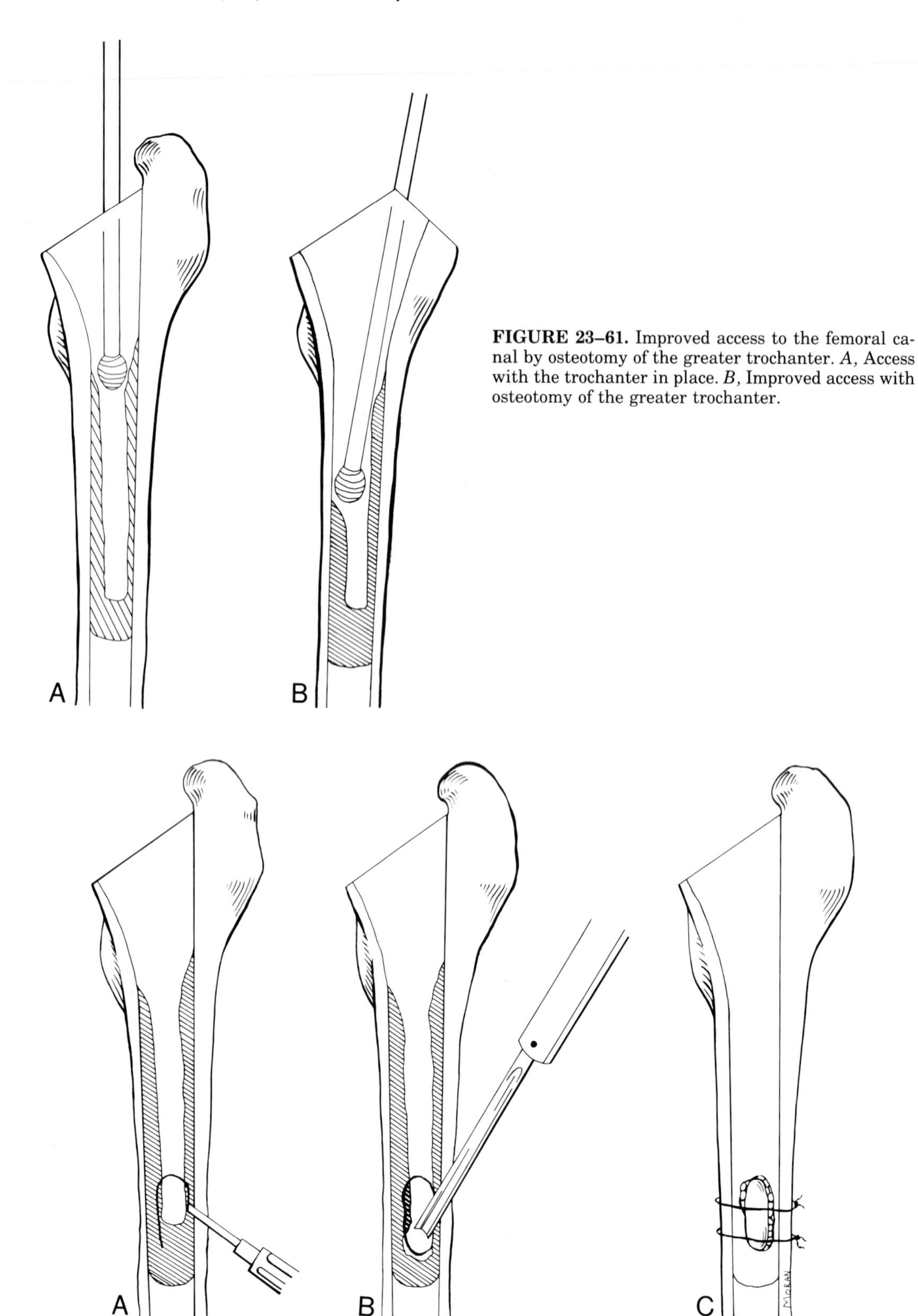

FIGURE 23–61. Improved access to the femoral canal by osteotomy of the greater trochanter. *A,* Access with the trochanter in place. *B,* Improved access with osteotomy of the greater trochanter.

FIGURE 23–62. Controlled window in the femur for cement removal. This procedure is far preferable to inadvertent penetration of the femur with an osteotome or high-speed burr. *A,* Cutting the window with a high-speed burr. *B,* Removing distal cement through the window. *C,* Salvage of the window. The cortical window removed is saved and repaired either after all cement is removed or after the new femoral stem is placed.

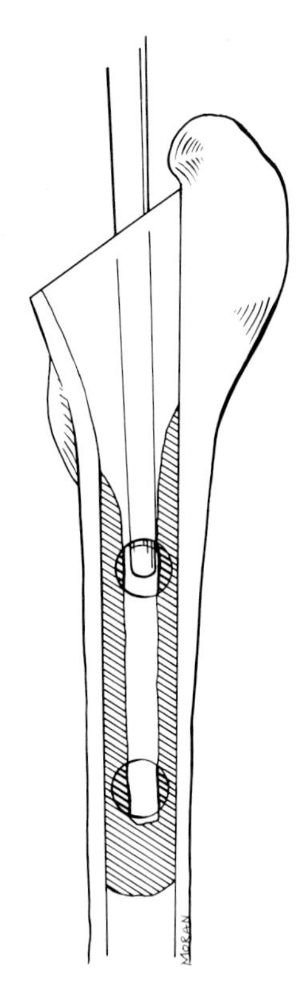

FIGURE 23–63. Several controlled windows made to visualize cement removal.

niques in dentistry, have been studied in the laboratory and to a limited extent in the clinical setting. The sonic energy has been applied directly to cement, softening it, and to a prosthesis, facilitating removal.[40] Extracorporeal shock wave lithotripsy has been studied in the laboratory to determine its potential for breaking up the bone-cement interface, but no clinical reports have been made of its use.[47]

Removal of Porous-Coated Stems

Porous-coated stems that must be removed for reasons other than loosening may be very rigidly fixed. Even painfully loose stems may be relatively well fixed with fibrous tissue, if not with bone ingrowth. Those stems that have porous coating extending far distally may be extremely difficult to remove. On occasion, plans to extract such a prosthesis have been abandoned.

The area of ingrowth, whether fibrous or bone, is first cut as far distally as possible by flexible osteotomes or a small power burr (Fig. 23–64). Although a power burr necessarily sacrifices some bone, this loss is better than fracturing the proximal femur because the bond was not broken adequately on attempted removal. If porous coating is only proximal, the femoral component can be extracted after the interface has been adequately cut. If the porous coating extends well distally or if the prosthesis has a roughened surface distally, especially titanium alloy stems, the interface between prosthesis and bone must be cut throughout most or all of the stem length before the stem can be removed.[69]

Even a small area of well-ingrown porous coating may prevent removal. A distal window for driving out the stem may not help. The safest method is to create an anterior cortical window about 1 cm wide throughout the entire length of the stem, saving the removed cortical bone for later repair (Fig. 23–65A). The interface around the rest of the stem's circumference is cut with flexible osteotomes (Fig. 23–65B). The stem can then be removed without difficulty (Fig. 23–65C). During reconstruction, the window is replaced and fixed in place with cerclage wiring (Fig. 23–65D). Cancellous bone graft may be added around the edges to speed healing.

Removal of Broken Stems

Sudden, catastrophic failure of femoral stems was seen more commonly when they were constructed of weaker metals and when optimal stem geometry was less well understood. This problem should occur less commonly as superalloy metals are utilized in optimally designed components. Catastrophic stem failure also occurred when femoral stems were placed in varus and when the stem was inadvertently scored with a drill, saw blade, or circumferential wire.

Generally, fracture of a femoral stem is a result of cantilever bending of a component that is well fixed distally and unstable proximally. The management of this problem requires broad exposure of the proximal femur, which can be achieved with a trochanteric osteotomy or a direct lateral

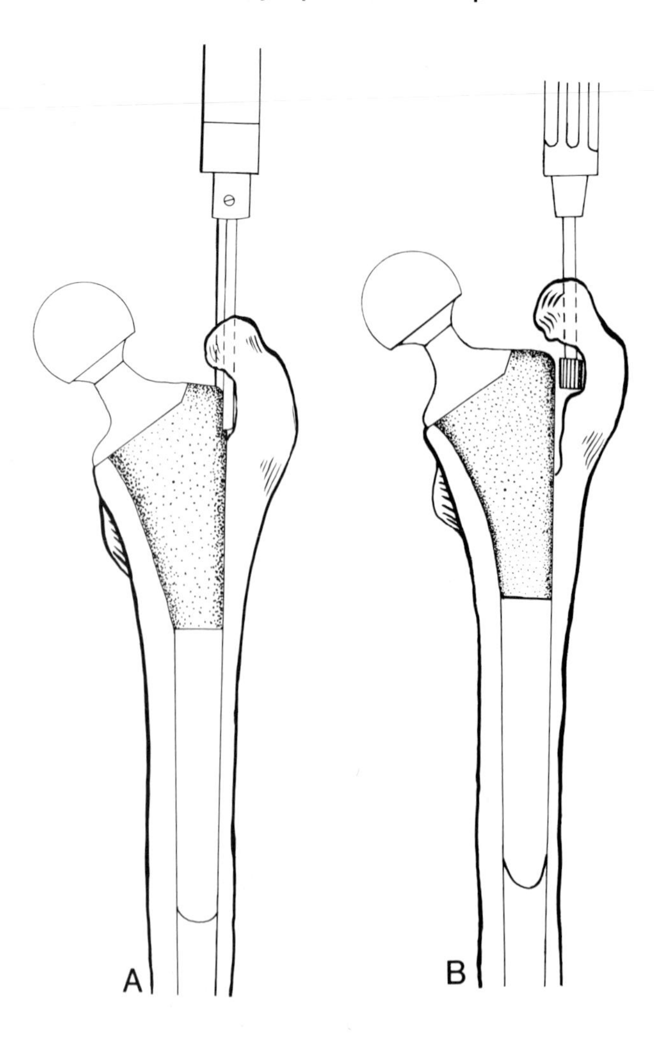

FIGURE 23–64. Cutting the bone-prosthesis interface of a porous-coated prosthesis. *A*, Cutting the interface with a flexible osteotome. *B*, Cutting the interface with a small high-speed burr.

approach. The removal of the proximal portion of the fractured component presents little problem. After a complete pseudocapsulectomy is performed to achieve wide proximal exposure, remnants of cement that lie proximal to the fractured stem surface are removed piecemeal with chisels and osteotomes.

Once the fractured surface is exposed adequately, one of three methods may be employed to remove the stem. In the first method, a high-speed low-torque burr system, such as the Midas Rex or the Anspach 65K, circumferentially exposes the upper centimeter of the broken stem tip. A hole is made in the upper portion of the stem with a femoral stem extraction drill bit. Undercutting is achieved with a second specialized high-speed burr. An extraction tool is engaged in the precut hole, and the stem is extracted. The second method involves chiseling the proximal cement until needle-nose pliers or similarly strong instruments can be applied to the stem for retrograde extraction. In the third method, a controlled femoral cortical window is created distal to the tip of the prosthesis, and the prosthesis is driven retrograde with a special curved metal tamp. Once the cemented stem has been extracted, the surgeon utilizes the high-speed burr or chisels to complete removal of the cement mantle.

Removal of a fractured femoral component that has a secure, porous-coated distal segment may sometimes be accomplished from the top by an extraction method described for broken cemented stems. How-

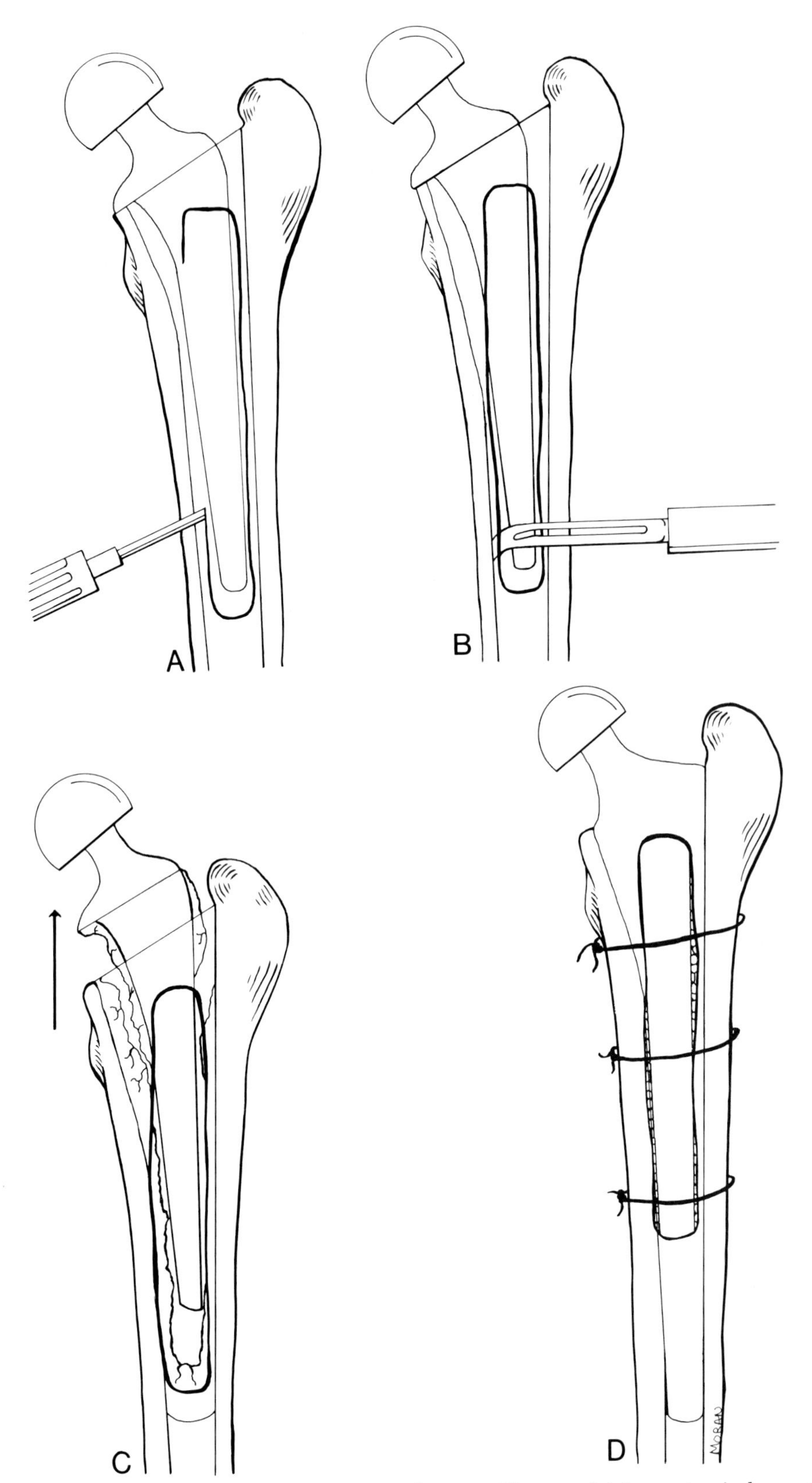

FIGURE 23–65. Removal of a well-fixed femoral stem that was either completely or extensively porous coated. *A*, Removal of the cortical window from the anterior femur throughout the length of the stem. *B*, Cutting of the interface with a flexible osteotome. *C*, Removal of the stem. *D*, Replacement of the cortical window removed earlier. The window is fixed with cerclage wiring. Cancellous bone graft is added around the edges of the window to enhance healing.

ever, if the stem is well fixed, a cortical window usually must be created and the interface cut with flexible osteotomes.

Femoral Reconstruction

After the femoral stem and cement are removed, all soft tissue membrane is removed with a curette or crochet hook (see Fig. 23–13). This material is sent for histologic and bacteriologic evaluations.

The femur and its deficiencies are carefully evaluated. If bone grafting of segmental deficiencies is necessary, autogenous graft is harvested or allograft obtained. The high-speed burr is an excellent tool for preparing the graft for a precise fit to host bone. Grafts for large trochanteric and partial segmental proximal or intercalary defects are fixed in place with cerclage wiring, screws, or small plates (Fig. 23–66). Care is taken to avoid intrusion of screws into the femoral canal (Fig. 23–67). For small defects, the graft may be added after femoral reaming and broaching.

The femur is prepared with reaming and broaching. When a long stem is necessary, intramedullary reaming with either flexible or rigid reamers is essential to assure proper sizing of the femur for the chosen prosthesis. When a standard length stem is sufficient, reaming may or may not be necessary, depending on the prosthesis system. Broaching is performed carefully, because the thin cortex can be fractured easily. After broaching is complete, the inside of the femur is evaluated for remaining cavitary defects, which will be grafted with particulate allograft or autograft (Fig. 23–68). Proximal cavitary defects that do not affect stability are grafted as the prosthesis is being inserted. If the graft is placed earlier, it is likely to be forced distally as the prosthesis is inserted. The broach or trial prosthesis is fully seated; a trial head is placed; and the hip is reduced to evaluate length reconstruction, motion, and stability. These are done with care to avoid excess stress on the weakened bone.

A complete segmental defect can be re-

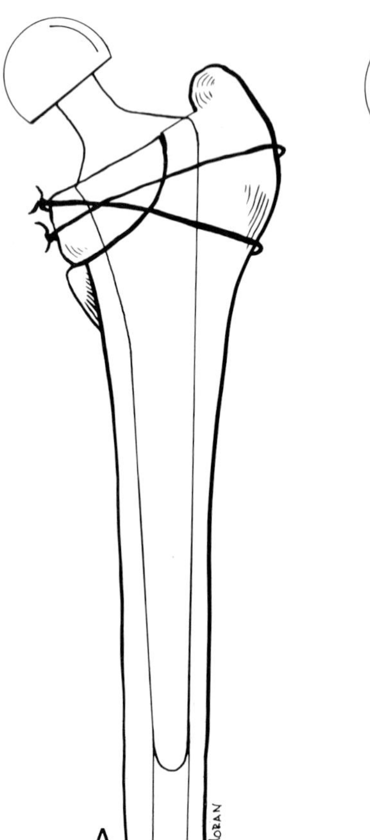

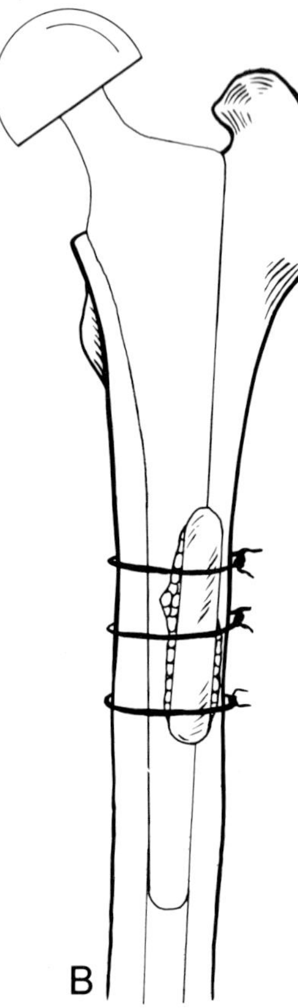

FIGURE 23–66. Grafting of segmental femoral defects. *A,* A large partial proximal segmental defect replaced with an appropriately shaped bone graft. The bone graft is held in place with cerclage wires. *B,* A large intercalary defect also repaired with bone graft and held in place with cerclage wires.

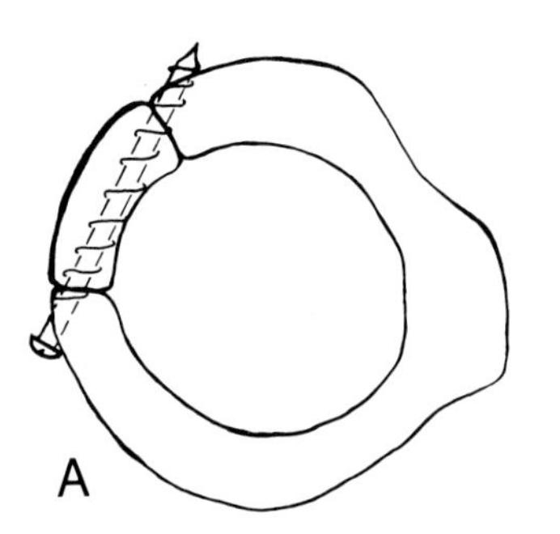

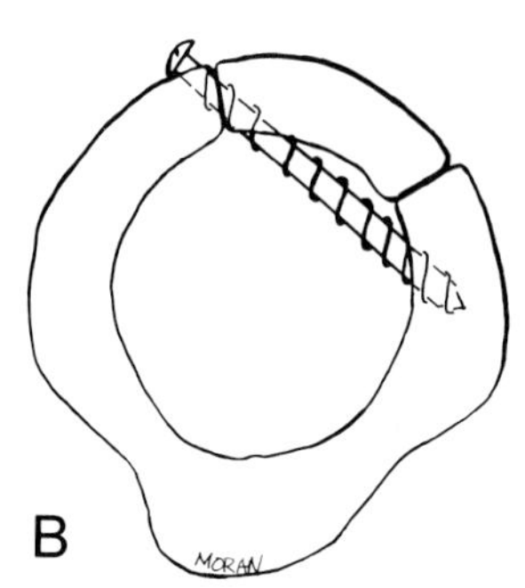

FIGURE 23–67. Use of screws for fixation of femoral bone graft. *A*, Screws utilized for fixation of fracture or bone graft. Screws must avoid intrusion on the medullary canal. *B*, Obstruction of the passage of the prosthetic stem by a screw that invades the medullary canal.

constructed in several ways. With a proximal replacement prosthesis, the fit is checked and a trial reduction is done. Alternatively, proximal allograft and cemented prosthesis are assembled for trial reduction, with special attention given to length reconstruction and rotational alignment. If the reconstruction is being done with a cementless prosthesis, the reduction is performed with a trial prosthesis. A trial prosthesis usually is not available when a custom prosthesis is being employed, and length and rotational alignment must be carefully analyzed for final reconstruction. Once the trial evaluation of a cementless stem is satisfactory, the graft, stem, and host bone fragment are assembled. Any supplemental internal fixation is added, and any additional proximal particulate graft is placed (Fig. 23–69).

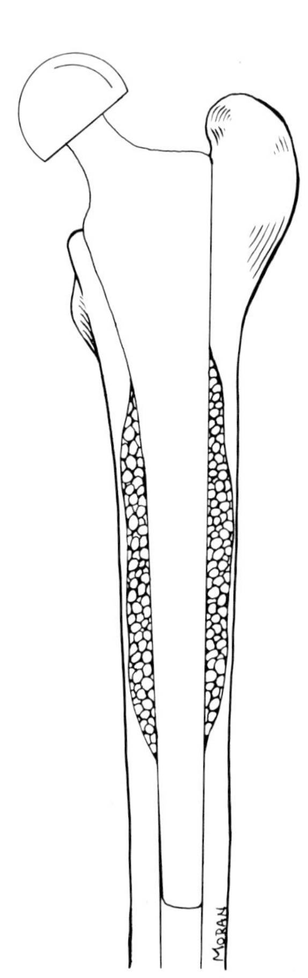

FIGURE 23–68. Large cavitary femoral defects grafted with particulate graft.

For cemented reconstruction, a distal canal restrictor is placed. Because the femoral canal widens distally, the most effective plug is made of cement. The surgeon has two alternatives for assembly with cement:

1. Mix cement for two or three syringes, fill the distal host bone canal and the allograft, and assemble all the parts.
2. First cement the prosthesis to the allograft, providing proper rotation and length placement within the graft (see Fig. 23–47). With a second cementation, cement the graft-prosthesis composite into the host bone. It is less difficult to assure good cementation with the two separate processes. With either method, care is taken to avoid cement between the graft and host bone. After placement of any necessary structural graft and the femoral prosthesis, cancellous graft may be added to graft-host junctions.

The greater trochanter is repaired (see Chapter 14, *Surgical Approaches for Total Hip Replacement*). The trochanter may be osteoporotic and may require wire mesh to prevent pull-through. The junction between the trochanter and proximal femur is usually of poor quality and should be grafted with cancellous bone. If the greater trochanter is absent or impossible to attach to the femur, the remaining abductors are

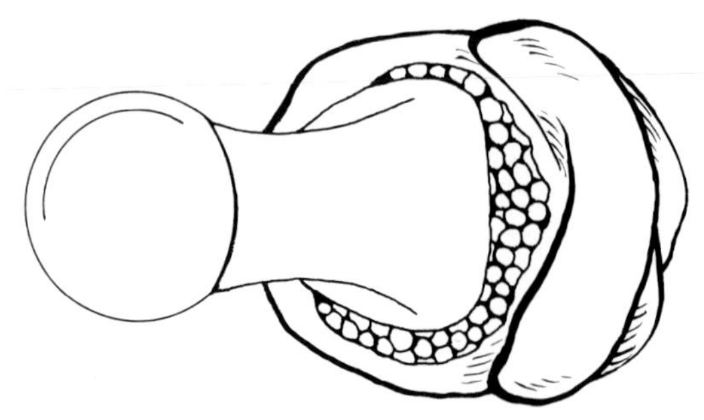

FIGURE 23–69. Grafting of cavitary deficiency of proximal femur after or during placement of cementless prosthesis.

repaired to the fascia lata with heavy suture.

Drainage tubes are placed. Careful closure of the tissue planes is important to improve soft tissue stability.

MANAGEMENT OF INFECTED TOTAL HIP ARTHROPLASTY

Except for death and major vascular injury, infection is the most feared complication associated with joint replacement surgery. Infection is uncommon, but it is nonetheless of major concern because of the enormous monetary and personal costs required to resolve the complication (see Chapter 8, *Prevention of Postoperative Infections*).

Diagnosis

Infection is suspected whenever pain occurs in the hip that has had total arthroplasty. Constant pain that is relatively unaffected by weightbearing and motion suggests infection without loosening. Infection is considered in the differential diagnosis of any loose prosthesis. The operative and postoperative course of the primary operation, any intercurrent infections, and recent procedures that are known to cause bacteremia are important components of the history. The physical examination includes determination of the patient's temperature and evaluation of the wound for warmth, redness, swelling, and drainage. Wound drainage is a near-certain indication of infection. If there is drainage, the area surrounding the sinus is cleansed, and cultures of the fluid are taken.

Important laboratory studies include determination of ESR, C-reactive protein level, and white blood cell count and differential.[1] Imaging studies may include radiography, sinography (if there is a sinus), and radionuclide scanning (see Chapter 11, *Imaging of Total Joint Replacement*).

Joint aspiration for culture is essential. After aspiration, dye may be injected and a radiograph taken to confirm the location of the aspiration. Cultures are performed for all potential infecting organisms, including anaerobes (Table 23–3).[48] If the culture report documents minimal growth of bacteria known to reside on the skin, such as *Staphylococcus epidermidis,* the aspiration is repeated. If the same organism is cultured again, infection is likely. When infection is strongly suspected but culture findings of aspirate are negative, cultures should be repeated. Persistent negative culture findings despite strong evidence of infection, such as those on scanning, may call for further investigation. Culture of tissues and scrapings from the prosthesis taken at surgery may reveal the causative organism.

Table 23–3. MICROORGANISMS ISOLATED FROM SPECIMENS TAKEN AT THE TIME OF RESECTION ARTHROPLASTY

Organism	Number of Isolates
Staphylococcus epidermidis	37
Staphylococcus aureus	19
Streptococcus viridans	10
Group-D *Streptococcus*	7
Escherichia coli	4
Proteus mirabilis	3
Pseudomonas aeruginosa	6
Enterobacter	4
Acinetobacter	1
Peptococcus	5
Bacillus sp.	3
Corynebacterium sp.	6
Bacteroides sp.	2
Beta-hemolytic *Streptococcus*	2
Propionibacterium acnes	1
No organism isolated	2
Total	112

McDonald, D. J., Fitzgerald, R. H., Jr., and Ilstrup, D. M.: J. Bone Joint Surg. 71A:828–834, 1989. By permission.

Wound Care

Tissue planes may be distorted in hips with infected prostheses. Every effort is made to define or recreate appropriate planes during exposure and closure.

The chemical nature and coating are major determinants of bacterial adherence to suture material. Synthetic monofilament and braided absorbable sutures are most resistant to infection and therefore are best for closure of wounds that have been infected.[15, 60] Wire sutures or staples are also appropriate for closure of the skin. Natural suture materials are less resistant to infection than are synthetic suture materials.

The popularity of closed irrigation-suction drainage systems has diminished because of the potential for secondary bacterial contamination and consequent infection. The alternative is a closed-suction drainage system as is chosen for other extensive wounds. Both irrigation-suction drainage and closed-suction drainage should be limited to no more than 2 to 3 days to reduce the possibility of secondary contamination.

Treatment

Treatment of infection in association with total hip arthroplasty may include (1) early debridement with retention of the prostheses, (2) suppression of infection with antibiotic therapy, (3) one-stage revision, (4) two-stage revision, and (5) resection arthroplasty.

Early Debridement with Retention of Prostheses

Early debridement and antibiotic therapy may be indicated in a patient who develops acute infection within 3 to 6 weeks following total hip replacement. With a cementless prosthesis, when infection occurs even within a few days, the best course is to remove all prosthetic components, treat the infection, and replace the prostheses later. A cemented prosthesis is much more difficult to remove shortly after surgery. Because the infection may be restricted to soft tissues and because the bacteria may not have become embedded yet in a protective glycocalyx on the implant surface, immediate extensive debridement may be successful.[2, 30]

When possible, these wounds should be closed primarily. If the appearance of the wound suggests that a second debridement may be necessary, the wound surfaces are lined with gauze and a few sutures are placed to prevent skin retraction. The patient returns to the operating room in 2 to 3 days, the wound is inspected and debrided further, and the wound is then closed. An alternative is to close the wound over antibiotic beads and have the patient return to the operating room after several days, reopening the wound at that time for further debridement. A wound that contains a prosthesis should be exposed only in the operating room under full sterile precautions, and it should be closed as early as possible.

Thorough surgical debridement is supplemented by antibiotic therapy. If this treatment fails, the prostheses will have to be removed to clear the infection.[2]

Suppression of Infection with Antibiotics

Antibiotic therapy alone is not curative for infection associated with total hip arthroplasty. It is indicated only in patients who are old and frail or who have definite medical contraindications to the extensive surgery involved in one-stage and two-stage revisions. Occasionally, a patient will refuse to have an infected prosthesis removed, usually because the hip is functioning well. Components must be well fixed to pursue this course. The patient should be tolerant to oral antibiotics to which the bacteria are sensitive and should not have systemic sepsis. Close follow-up is mandatory.[2, 28]

With antibiotic treatment alone, Goulet and colleagues[28] found that nine of 19 hips (47 percent) did not deteriorate clinically or radiographically with an average follow-up of 4.1 years. The other ten hips deteriorated, and seven prostheses had to be removed. Six of the seven patients had successful second-stage revision arthroplasties.[28]

One-Stage Revision

In addition to the planning and operative considerations discussed for revision total hip arthroplasty, special considerations are related to the infection.

One-stage revision has been popularized primarily by surgeons in Europe and has been performed elsewhere too. Conditions for which a one-stage revision arthroplasty may be considered are given in Table 23–4, and contraindications are listed in Table 23–5.[51] Callaghan and colleagues[10] have agreed that primary exchange should be limited to the patient who has an infection caused by organisms very sensitive to antibiotics and who has no wound purulence. Buchholz and associates,[9] in their extensive experience with primary exchange using cement-containing antibiotics, reported an overall success after one exchange of 77 percent. However, the success rate was reduced to 50 percent when virulent organisms (gram-negative bacilli or group D streptococci) were isolated.

The operative technique requires extensive debridement of the prosthesis, all cement, all necrotic bone, and all soft tissue. When the debridement is complete, there must be no visible evidence that infection was ever present. The infection recurrence rate is reduced with cemented revision when antibiotic is added to the cement.[9, 10, 45, 57, 66] (For techniques of adding antibiotics to cement, see Chapter 7, *Fixation Methods*.)

Two-Stage Revision

Two-stage revision of infected total hip arthroplasty is the preferred method for treating this problem in the United States. The popularity of this treatment results from its relatively high success rate.

Table 23–4. CONDITIONS FOR WHICH A ONE-STAGE REVISION ARTHROPLASTY MAY BE CONSIDERED

Organisms that are sensitive to at least three, preferably six, antibiotics
Gram-positive organisms
Absence of superinfection and multiple organisms
Healthy well-vascularized tissues
Absence of draining sinuses
Radiographic evidence of healthy femoral cortical bone
Reasonably good bone to support fixation both in the acetabulum and femur

Modified from Miley, G. B., Scheller, A. D., Jr., and Turner, R. H.: Clin. Orthop. 170: 76–82, 1982. By permission.

Table 23–5. INDICATIONS FOR GIRDLESTONE RESECTION

Virulent resistant organisms
Gram-negative organisms
Two or more concomitant strains of organisms
Unhealthy and edematous soft tissues
Draining sinus or sinuses
Radiographic evidence of well-established osteomyelitis with bone erosion
Severe loss of bone substance

Modified from Miley, G. B., Scheller, A. D., Jr., and Turner, R. H.: Clin. Orthop. 170: 76–82, 1982. By permission.

The initial operation includes extensive debridement of all implant material and infected or necrotic tissue. Leaving cement in the bone raises the rate of recurrence fourfold after the second-stage revision.[36, 48] Timing of the second stage has varied from a few days to more than a year after the first stage. The tendency is for a longer interval when the infection was caused by virulent organisms. McDonald and coworkers[48] found a significantly higher recurrence of infection when the interval was less than 1 year.

Preoperative planning and operation for the second-stage revision are similar to those for a revision arthroplasty that has not been infected. Preoperative evaluation for infection, including determination of ESR or C-reactive protein level, radionuclide scanning, and culture of hip aspiration, is especially important. At surgery, material for histology and culture are taken from several areas of the wound before any antibiotics are given. Tissue that arouses suspicion may be sent for frozen section examination. Microabscesses indicate continued infection. The finding of more than a few polymorphonuclear leukocytes suggests that infection may still be present.

Resection Arthroplasty

Resection (Girdlestone) arthroplasty is effective in clearing the infection and sometimes results in adequate pain relief. However, function often is poor, especially compared with a successful total hip replacement.[6, 8, 39, 48, 56] Surgical debridement must be thorough. All cement should be removed to avoid the higher incidence of infection after revision total hip replacement, should that be necessary in the future.[6, 8, 48, 56] All viable bone is preserved to provide stock for stability or for possible revision total hip replacement.

One element of postoperative care is obtaining traction sufficient to reduce muscle spasm and maintain comfort in balanced suspension. Traction may be applied through the skin or a proximal tibial pin. Pin traction is preferable, if more than very light weight is required or if traction will be needed for more than a few days. Some surgeons maintain traction for 2 to 6 weeks before the patient is allowed out of bed. I have shortened the patient's time in traction and have noted no difference in results. With this shorter regimen, the patient is maintained in bed in traction for several days during which both active and passive exercises are begun. After 3 to 5 days, whenever the patient is comfortable, walking is started without weightbearing on the involved limb. A day or two later, sitting is allowed. The patient returns to traction when in bed. Most patients are discharged from the hospital within 2 weeks. Light skin traction, suspended over the end of the bed at home, may be continued for a little longer, if desired. The patient uses a walker or crutches and bears minimal or no weight on the involved limb for the first 6 weeks. He or she is then advanced to partial weightbearing with walker or crutches, as tolerated. Many patients are strong enough to advance to a cane after 3 months, although some may take longer or never feel comfortable without a walker or crutches.

Antibiotics

Antibiotic therapy, although usually not adequate alone, is a critical element in the treatment of infected total hip arthroplasty. Consultation with an infectious disease specialist can help the surgeon select the appropriate antibiotic, determine the duration of therapy, and evaluate the response to treatment.

Antibiotics are selected on the basis of specific sensitivity to organisms cultured from tissue samples, preferably samples taken at the time of surgery. Antibiotics should not be given until these cultures are obtained. Tube dilution methods are employed to determine bacterial sensitivity. After antibiotic therapy is started, serum antibiotic levels and serum bactericidal levels help determine the effectiveness of the antibiotic against the organism causing the infection. If more than one organism is cultured from infected tissue, more than one antibiotic may be necessary. Some have proposed the administration of two or even three antibiotics against single-organism infections, because of the possible synergistic effect. However, whenever multiple antibiotics are given, the potential for complications rises. Occasionally, a combination of antibiotics may have an antagonistic effect, which can be determined by serum antimicrobial assay.[61]

Systemic Administration of Antibiotics

Patients with infected total hip arthroplasties usually require intravenous administration of the antimicrobial agents.[10, 48] In the study of two-stage revisions reported by McDonald and colleagues,[48] the treatment failure rate was significantly higher in patients with infections caused by virulent bacteria if they had systemic antibiotic therapy for less than 4 weeks.

If the patient's condition otherwise permits discharge from the hospital, parenteral antibiotic therapy can be continued at home. Hickman and Broviac catheters have been utilized successfully for long-term administration of antimicrobial agents, both in the hospital and at home. The major advantages of these catheters include their long-term durability and the reduced incidence of thrombosis, breakage, and septic complications. The disadvantage is that placement of the catheter requires an operation. Implantable administration ports have been introduced lately for long-term administration of parenteral medication. Their placement also requires an operation. Studies of treatment of infected total hip arthroplasties primarily have involved the application of intravenous therapy. Until adequate analysis of the effectiveness of orally administered agents is available, such agents should be substituted only cautiously. After a course of parenteral therapy, some surgeons and infectious disease specialists continue the patient's therapy with oral agents for up to 3 to 6 months. The importance of this therapy to successful treatment of infected total joint arthroplasty has not been determined.

Local Delivery of Antimicrobial Agents

Systemic administration of antibiotics will deliver bactericidal levels of the agent to the wound, but higher levels may be achieved locally while keeping systemic levels low. This may be especially advantageous with antibiotics with a high potential for toxicity. Antibiotics may be delivered locally to wounds by (1) an irrigation system; (2) an implantable port or infusion pump; and (3) their placement in a material, such as bone cement, that is left in the wound. Depot administration of antibiotics released from other materials, including absorbable polymers, is under investigation.

Because prolonged closed-suction irrigation is generally to be avoided, this is not a suitable method for local delivery of antibiotics. When this technique was utilized extensively, local levels of antibiotic higher than those achieved with systemic administration could not be maintained without increasing the systemic levels to the toxic range, because of systemic absorption from the wound. The effectiveness of the second option, implantable ports or infusion pumps for local administration of antibiotics, has not yet been established.

Experimental studies in animals indicate that the antibiotic-bone cement combination is highly effective in preventing infections of implants in wounds contaminated with bacteria.[57]

At the time of writing, antibiotic-cement combinations have not been approved by the United States Food and Drug Administration (FDA) in either bulk or bead form. Commercially prepared products are available only under the investigational device exemption FDA-approved protocols. Bone cement, both in bulk form and in beads, has been studied extensively for depot administration of antibiotics (see Chapter 7, *Fixation Methods*, and Chapter 8, *Prevention of Postoperative Infections*). All bone cements release most of the antibiotics studied, but Palacos-gentamicin has been shown to have better elution properties than other combinations. Aminoglycosides are preferred for depot administration in bone cement because of their broad-spectrum and bactericidal activity, low potential for allergic reactions (none have been reported), thermal stability, and solubility in water. Aminoglycosides have been applied extensively. Although usually given for treatment of infections caused by gram-negative bacteria, aminoglycosides are highly effective against staphylococci and moderately effective against streptococci.[10]

Cement-antibiotic combinations in bulk form have been shown to lower the infection rate after cemented revision, but their effectiveness after primary total hip arthroplasty is not as certain.[45] When they are administered in routine primary arthroplasties, infections that do occur may be associated with highly antibiotic resistant bacteria.[36] Extensive European studies of cement containing an antibiotic, usually an aminoglyside, for revision of infected total hip arthroplasty (often one-stage revision), have yielded a success rate ranging from 60 to 90 percent cure of infection.[9, 12]

Chains of beads for antibiotic delivery in the wound are placed extensively throughout the wound, including inside the femoral canal. The wound must be closed and suction drainage discontinued as early as feasible to maintain a high concentration of the antibiotic in the wound. Most of the antibiotic is released in the first several days. If the beads are left in the wound for longer than 2 to 3 weeks, they may be difficult to remove because extensive scar tissue forms around them.[10]

Other materials, including some that are absorbable, are under investigation for local delivery of antibiotics. If these materials are found to be safe and effective, they will prove to have a major advantage: they could deliver high local concentrations plus controlled release of the antibiotic without requiring an operation for removal.

REHABILITATION AFTER REVISION TOTAL HIP ARTHROPLASTY

The goals for rehabilitation after revision total hip arthroplasty are similar to those for primary total hip arthroplasty, and in some instances the rehabilitation program can be similar (see Chapter 18, *Total Hip Arthroplasty: Postoperative Care and Rehabilitation*). However, because surgical exposure is often more extensive, and reconstruction may be required for weakened skeletal structures and deficient soft tissue components, the rehabilitation program may require modification. The modified rehabilitation program is designed to protect (1) the hip against dislocation, (2) the structural integrity of the skeletal-prosthesis reconstruction until bone has healed, and (3) the soft tissue repair. The rehabilitation program also improves muscle strength.

Hip Joint Stability

Dislocation occurs more commonly after revision total hip arthroplasty than after primary total hip arthroplasty.[4, 14, 22, 43, 68] Contributing factors include the more extensive exposure required and the soft tissue deficiencies. If components are well placed, component malposition should not contribute to the increased incidence of dislocation (see Chapter 19, *Total Hip Arthroplasty: Complications*).

When the greater trochanter was not united preoperatively and when the trochanteric approach is selected for revision arthroplasty, trochanteric repair is especially important. In some instances, the trochanter is absent or impossible to repair, and the abductor muscles are therefore repaired to the fascia lata. Under either circumstance, the repair must be protected postoperatively. Limb suspension in abduction, with gradual reduction of the abduction over several days, will allow for gradual stretching of tight abductor muscles. After this initial stretching, a pantaloon hip spica cast or brace provides additional protection for soft tissue repair and against dislocation until a fibrous pseudocapsule has formed around the hip joint (Fig. 23–70). If a high degree of protection is needed, especially against rotation, immobilization is extended to include the foot. A knee hinge may be added to allow motion. The cast or brace may be applied with the hip in up to 10 degrees of abduction. If excessive abduction is held by a cast for several weeks, a contracture may result. The cast or brace may be applied immediately postoperatively, but usually this is delayed for several days

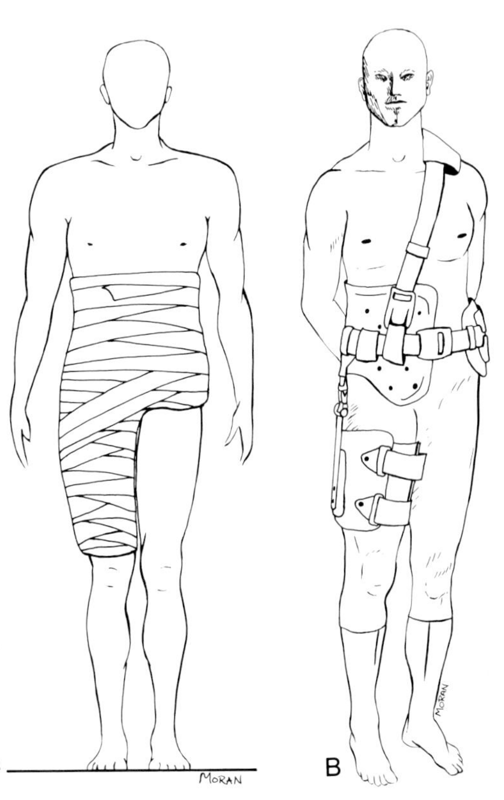

FIGURE 23–70. Immobilization to protect against dislocation after revision of total hip arthroplasty. *A*, Pantaloon cast. *B*, Brace.

until the wound has healed. While protecting the hip from dangerous positions, a brace may allow motion within a specified range.

Davey and Harris[19] reported the effective use of reverse skeletal traction applied through a proximal tibial pin for 3 weeks, followed by an abduction brace for an additional 6 weeks. The two patients had severe instability after complex revision total hip arthroplasties (Fig. 23–71).[19]

Bone Healing

Internal stability of bone defect repairs in revision total hip arthroplasty is usually sufficient, and external immobilization is not necessary. However, if any concern exists about the adequacy of internal fixation or the patient's compliance in following instructions, casts or braces may be used to protect repaired fractures or graft-host junctions until early healing has occurred.

Most revision hip replacements require more protection from weightbearing than do primary hip replacements. If no significant segmental or cavitary defects required bone grafting and if the soft tissues are in good condition, it is probably safe to progress to weightbearing as for primary total hip arthroplasty (see Chapter 18, *Total Hip Arthroplasty: Postoperative Care and Rehabilitation*). Patients with fractures or repair of significant segmental defects should bear only limited weight until the fracture lines or graft-host junctions show healing on radiographs. Patients with significant cavitary defects in the acetabulum, whether repaired with a fixed or bipolar component, will require protected weightbearing until the cancellous graft has consolidated, which may not be for a year. Otherwise, the incidence and degree of component migration are increased. After bone healing, the hip may be protected for several more months with the use of a cane. The cane may be required indefinitely after especially complex reconstructions.

Muscle Rehabilitation

Muscles about the hip and throughout the extremity may become very weak in patients who undergo revision total hip arthroplasties due to (1) previous surgery, (2) limited use of the hip prior to revision, (3) complex surgical procedures, and (4) immobilization of the extremity postoperatively. These patients often have generalized weakness as well.

Isometric exercises of muscles about the hip usually can be started immediately after surgery. Active assisted and active exercises are usually delayed until soft tissues have healed and external immobilization is removed. Exercises for the remainder of the operated limb are pursued as vigorously as possible with external immobilization. The contralateral lower limb and both upper extremities are exercised regularly. By the time external immobilization is ended, active exercises of the operated hip usually can be done. The muscle-strengthening program is contin-

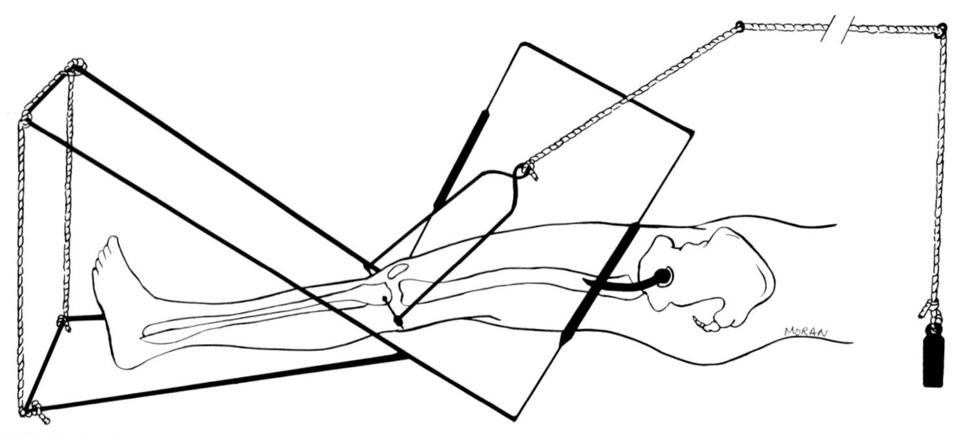

FIGURE 23–71. Reverse skeletal traction for severe instability after complex revision of total hip arthroplasty.

ued until sufficient results are obtained, which may take many months after revision hip replacements.

If external immobilization is not necessary postoperatively, precautions to prevent dislocation should be taken after revision arthroplasty. Patients ought to be reminded of these precautions when external immobilization is discontinued.

SUMMARY

Revision total hip arthroplasty often presents one of the most difficult challenges of musculoskeletal surgery. Successful surgical reconstruction requires careful analysis of the problem to distinguish between septic and aseptic conditions. Revision of a well-fixed femoral stem, whether cemented or porous, and extensive bone deficiency pose especially difficult problems. Preoperative planning of the reconstruction includes selection of the prosthesis and bone graft, if necessary, but the planning may have to be modified if bone deficiencies are found to be worse than expected during the operation.

Postoperative care following revision hip replacement is more extensive. The results of revision total hip arthroplasty should not be expected to be as good as the results of primary total hip arthroplasty. But with careful analysis and planning, skillful and biomechanically sound surgical reconstruction, and conscientious postoperative care, most patients with failed total hip replacements can achieve marked improvement from revision total hip arthroplasty.

References

1. Aalto, K., Osterman, K., Peltola, H., and Rasanen, J.: Changes in erythrocyte sedimentation rate and C-reactive protein after total hip arthroplasty. Clin. Orthop. 184:118–120, 1984.
2. Andrews, H. J., Arden, G. P., Hart, G. M., and Owne, J. W.: Deep infection after total hip replacement. J. Bone Joint Surg. 63B:53–57, 1981.
3. Bateman, J.: Salvage of failed hip arthroplasties using a multiple bearing implant. Orthop. Trans. 5:357, 1981.
4. Bergstrom, B., Lindberg, L., Persson, B. M., and Onnerfalt, R.: Complication after total hip arthroplasty according to Charnley in a Swedish series of cases. Clin. Orthop. 95:91–94, 1973.
5. Bittar, E. S. and Petty, W.: Girdlestone arthroplasty for infected total hip arthroplasty. Clin. Orthop. 170:83–87, 1982.
6. Bittar, E. S. and Petty, W.: Girdlestone arthroplasty for infected total hip arthroplasty. Clin. Orthop. 170:83–87, 1982.
7. Borja, F. J. and Mnaymneh, W.: Bone allografts in salvage of difficult hip arthroplasties. Clin. Orthop. 197:123–130, 1985.
8. Bosquet, M. M. J., Duncan, C. P., Mulier, J. C., and Patterson, F. P.: Girdlestone excision arthroplasty of the hip. A review of 49 patients. Orthop. Trans. 6:336, 1982.
9. Buchholz, H. W., Elson, R. A., Englebrecht, E., et al: Management of deep infection of total hip replacement. J. Bone Joint Surg. 63B:342–353, 1981.
10. Callaghan, J. J., Salvati, E. A., Brause, B. D., et al: Reimplantation for salvage of the infected hip: Rationale for the use of gentamicin-impregnated cement and beads. The Hip. St. Louis, C. V. Mosby Company, 1985.
11. Cameron, H. C. and Jung, Y. B.: Acetabular revision with a bipolar prosthesis. Clin. Orthop. 251:100–103, 1990.
12. Carlsson, A. S., Josephsson, G., and Lindberg, L.: Revision with gentamicin-impregnated cement for deep infection of total hip arthroplasties. J. Bone Joint Surg. 60A:1059–1064, 1978.
13. Cement Extraction System: Orthopedics Today 10(4):11, April 1990.
14. Charnley, J. and Cupic, Z.: The nine and ten year results of the Charnley low friction arthroplasty of the hip. Clin. Orthop. 95:9–25, 1973.
15. Chu, C. C. and Williams, D. F.: Effects of chemical configuration and chemical structure of suture materials on bacterial adhesion: A possible link to wound infection. Am. J. Surg. 147:197–204, 1984.
16. Committee Exhibits: Classification and Management of Femoral Defects in Total Hip Replacement. Committee on the Hip. American Academy of Orthopaedic Surgeons Annual Meeting, New Orleans, 1990.
17. Convery, F. R., Minteer-Convery, M., Devine, S. D., and Meyers, M. H.: Acetabular augmentation in primary and revision total hip arthroplasty with cementless prostheses. Clin. Orthop. 252:167–175, 1990.
18. D'Antonio, J. A., Capello, W. N., Borden, L. S., et al: Classification and management of acetabular abnormalities in total hip arthroplasty. Clin. Orthop. 243:126–137, 1989.
19. Davey, J. R. and Harris, W. H.: Reverse skeletal traction for instability following revision total hip arthroplasty. A report of two cases. Clin. Orthop. 234:110–114, 1988.
20. Dohmae, Y., Bechtold, J. E., Sherman, R. E., and Gustilo, R. B.: Bone/cement interface shear strength in revision joint replacement surgery. Orthop. Trans. 10:406–407, 1986.
21. Dooley, B. J., Clifford, M. J., and Hjorth, D. P.: Total hip replacement combined with bone grafting for acetabular dysplasia causing severe osteoarthritis of the hip joint. Aust. N.Z. J. Surg. 55(2):195–198, 1985.
22. Eftakhar, N. S. and Stinchfield, F. E.: Experience

with low friction arthroplasty. A statistical review of early results and complications. Clin. Orthop. 95:60–68, 1973.
23. Emerson, R. H., Jr., Head, W. C., Berklacich, F. M., and Malinin, T. I.: Noncemented acetabular revision arthroplasty using allograft bone. Clin. Orthop. 249:43, 1989.
24. Engh, C. A., Bobyn, J. D., and Glassmen, A. H.: Porous-coated hip replacement. J. Bone Joint Surg. 69B:45–55, 1987.
25. Engh, C. A., Glassman, A. H., Griffin, W. L., and Mayer, J. G.: Results of cementless revision for failed cemented total hip arthroplasty. Clin. Orthop. 235:91–110, 1986.
26. Gerber, S. D. and Harris, W. H.: Femoral head autografting to augment acetabular deficiency in patients requiring total hip replacement. J. Bone Joint Surg. 68A:1241–1248, 1986.
27. Glassman, A. H., Engh, C. A., and Bobyn, J. D.: Proximal femoral osteotomy as an adjunct in cementless revision total hip arthroplasty. J. Arthroplasty 2:47–62, 1987.
28. Goulet, J. A., Pellicci, P. M., Brause, B. D., and Salvati, E. M.: Prolonged suppression of infection in total hip arthroplasty. J. Arthroplasty 3(2):109–116, 1988.
29. Gustilo, R. B. and Pasternak, H. S.: Revision total hip arthroplasty with titanium ingrowth prosthesis and bone grafting for failed cemented femoral component loosening. Clin. Orthop. 235:111–119, 1986.
30. Harle, A.: Infection management in total hip replacement. Arch. Orthop. Trauma Surg. 108(2):63–71, 1989.
31. Harris, W. H.: Allografting in total hip arthroplasty in adults with severe acetabular deficiency including a surgical technique for bolting the graft to the ilium. Clin. Orthop. 162:150–164, 1982.
32. Harris, W. H., Krushell, R. J., and Galante, J. O.: Results of cementless revisions of total hip arthroplasties using the Harris-Galante prosthesis. Clin. Orthop. 235:126, 1988.
33. Head, W. C., Mallory, T. H., Berklacich, F. M., et al: Extensile exposure of the hip for revision arthroplasty. J. Arthroplasty 2(4):265–273, 1987.
34. Hedley, A. K., Clarke, I. C., Kozinn, S. C., et al: Porous ingrowth fixation of the femoral component in a canine surface replacement of the hip. Clin. Orthop. 163:300–311, 1982.
35. Holtgrewe, J. L. and Hungerford, D. S.: Primary and revision total hip replacement without cement and with associated femoral osteotomy. J. Bone Joint Surg. 71A:1487–1495, 1989.
36. Hope, P. G., Kristinsson, K. G., Norman, P., and Elson, R. A.: Deep infection of cemented total hip arthroplasties caused by coagulase-negative staphylococci. J. Bone Joint Surg. [Br] 71(5):851–855, 1989.
37. Hungerford, D. S. and Jones, L. C.: The rationale of cementless revision of cemented arthroplasty failures. Clin. Orthop. 235:12–24, 1986.
38. Jensen, J. S., Retpen, J. B., and Arnoldi, C. C.: Arthroplasty for congenital hip dislocation. Techniques for acetabular reconstruction. Acta. Orthop. Scand. 60(1):86–92, 1989.
39. Kantor, G. S., Osterkamp, J. A., Dorr, L. D., et al: Resection arthroplasty following infected total hip replacement arthroplasty. J. Arthroplasty 1:83–89, 1986.
40. Klapper, R. C. and Caillouette, J. T.: The use of ultrasonic tools in revision arthroplasty procedures. Contemp. Orthop. 20:273–279, 1990.
41. Korovesis, P., Siablis, D., Salonikidis, P., and Sdougos, G.: Abdominal-hip joint fistula. Complicated revision of total hip arthroplasty for false aneurysm of external iliac artery. A case report. Clin. Orthop. 231:71–75, 1988.
42. Krackow, K. A., Steinman, H., Cohn, B. T., and Jones, L. C.: Clinical experience with a triradiate exposure of the hip for difficult total hip arthroplasty. J. Arthroplasty 3(3):267–278, 1988.
43. Lazansky, M. Z.: Complications revisited. The debit side of total hip replacement. Clin. Orthop. 95:96–103, 1973.
44. Lord, G., Marotte, J., Guillamon, J., and Blanchard, J.: Cementless revision of failed aseptic cemented and cementless total hip arthroplasties. Clin. Orthop. 235:74, 1988.
45. Lynch, M., Esser, M. P., Shelley, P., and Wroblewski, B. M.: Deep infection in Charnley low-friction arthroplasty. Comparison of plain and gentamicin-loaded cement. J. Bone Joint Surg. [Br] 69(3):355–360, 1987.
46. Mallory, T. H.: Preparation of the proximal femur in cementless total hip revision. Clin. Orthop. 235:47, 1986.
47. Mat, T. C., Krause, W. R., Presler, A. J., et al: Use of high-energy shock waves for bone cement removal. J. Arthroplasty 5:19–27, 1990.
48. McDonald, D. J., Fitzgerald, R. H., Jr., and Ilstrup, D. M.: Two-stage reconstruction of a total hip arthroplasty because of infection. J. Bone Joint Surg. [Am] 71(6):828–834, 1989.
49. McGann, W. A., Welch, R. B., and Picetti, G. D., III: Acetabular preparation in cementless revision total hip arthroplasty. Clin. Orthop. 235:35–46, 1988.
50. McQueary, F. G. and Johnston, R. C.: Coxarthrosis after congenital dysplasia. Treatment by total hip arthroplasty without acetabular bonegrafting. J. Bone Joint Surg. [Am] 70(8):1140–1144, 1988.
51. Miley, G. B., Scheller, A. D., Jr., and Turner, R. H.: Medical and surgical treatment of the septic hip with one-stage revision arthroplasty. Clin. Orthop. 170:76–82, 1982.
52. Mulroy, R. D., Jr.: Prohibitive Failure Rate of Femoral Head Autografts in Total Hip Replacement for Acetabular Deficiency by 12 Years. American Academy of Orthopaedic Surgeons' Annual Meeting, New Orleans, 1990.
53. Murray, W. R.: Acetabular salvage in revision total hip arthroplasty. Clin. Orthop. 251:92–99, 1990.
54. Nercessian, O. A., Gonzalez, E. G., and Stinchfield, F. E.: The use of somatosensory evoked potential during revision or reoperation for total hip arthroplasty. Clin. Orthop. 243:138–142, 1989.
55. Petty, W. and Goldsmith, S.: Resection arthroplasty following infected total hip arthroplasty. J. Bone Joint Surg. 62A:889–896, 1980.
56. Petty, W. and Goldsmith, S.: Resection arthroplasty following infected total hip arthroplasty. J. Bone Joint Surg. 62A:889–896, 1980.
57. Petty, W., Spanier, S., and Shuster, J. J.: Prevention of infection after total joint replacement. Experiments with a canine model. J. Bone Joint Surg. [Am] 70(4):536–539, 1988.

58. Ranawat, C. S., Dorr, L. D., and Inglis, A. E.: Total hip arthroplasty in protrusio acetabuli of rheumatoid arthritis. J. Bone Joint Surg. 62A:1059–1065, 1980.
59. Roberson, J. R. and Cohen, D.: Bipolar components for severe periacetabular bone loss around the failed total hip arthroplasty. Clin. Orthop. 251:113–118, 1990.
60. Sharp, W. V., Belden, T. A., King, P. H., and Teague, P. C.: Suture resistance to infection. Surgery 91:61–63, 1982.
61. Shaw, J. A.: Triple antibiotics for the treatment of infected joint replacements. Case report and commentary. J. Arthroplasty 2(3):215–217, 1987.
62. Sherk, H. H., Kollmer, C., and Meller, M.: A laser osteoscope for PMMA removal in hip revision arthroplasty. Scientific Exhibit, American Academy of Orthopaedic Surgeons' Annual Meeting, Las Vegas, 1989.
63. Sutherland, C. J.: Radiographic evaluation of acetabular bone stock in failed total hip arthroplasty. J. Arthroplasty 3:73–79, 1988.
64. Torisu, T., Utsunamiya, K., Maekawa, M., and Ueda, Y.: Use of bipolar hip arthroplasty in states of acetabular deficiency. Clin. Orthop. 251:119–125, 1990.
65. Trancik, T. M., Stulberg, B. N., Wilde, A. H., and Feiglin, D. H.: Allograft reconstruction of the acetabulum during revision total hip arthroplasty. J. Bone Joint Surg. 68A:527–537, 1986.
66. Trippel, S. B.: Antibiotic-impregnated cement in total joint arthroplasty. J. Bone Joint Surg. [Am] 68(8):1297–1302, 1986.
67. Wilson, M. G. and Scott, R. D.: Reconstruction of the deficient acetabulum using the bipolar socket. Clin. Orthop. 251:126–133, 1990.
68. Woolson, S. T. and Harris, W. H.: Complex total hip replacement for dysplastic or hypoplastic hips using miniature or microminiature components. J. Bone Joint Surg. [Am] 65(8):1099–1108, 1983.
69. Zweymuller, K. A., Lintner, F. K., and Semlitsch, M. F.: Biologic fixation of a press-fit titanium hip joint endoprosthesis. Clin. Orthop. 235:195–206, 1988.

CHAPTER 24

Results of Revision Total Hip Arthroplasty

PETER F. GEAREN

The results of revision hip arthroplasty compare unfavorably to the results of conventional primary hip replacement, no matter what the method of revision. The clinical and radiographic results of revision total hip arthroplasty are influenced by many variables, which make comparison among series difficult. However, for clarity of reporting, these series can be analyzed as follows: revisions that were done either for aseptic failure and loosening of a previous implant or for infection; revisions that were either cemented or cementless; and revisions that required major structural grafts.

CEMENTED REVISION TOTAL HIP ARTHROPLASTY

Revision for Aseptic Loosening

Pellicci and coworkers[34] reviewed the results of 110 revisions in 107 patients with aseptic failure. The original arthroplasties failed because of femoral component loosening (in 44 hips), acetabular component loosening (in 17 hips), loosening of both components (in 23 hips), fracture of the femoral component (in 14 hips), recurrent dislocation secondary to malposition (in 7 hips), acetabular protrusion (in 3 hips), and fracture of the femoral shaft (in 2 hips). Technical deficiency with the primary arthroplasty could explain the failure in a majority of the cases. At the time of the initial review in 1982, 60 percent of cases (66 hips) were categorized as having good or excellent results after revision. Clinically, patients had mild, nondisabling pain or no pain at all. Radiographically, they had stable implants with no evidence of significant radiolucency. The outcome of revision in 25 hips (23 percent) was rated as fair. Mechanical failure was the principal cause of poor results in 15 of the 19 cases (17 percent). Two patients had recurrent dislocation and instability. Significant radiolucent lines were seen in over one fourth of the cases. Other significant complications included mechanical failure (14 percent), trochanteric problems (13 percent), and deep infection (3.6 percent). The reviewers concluded that the quality of revision arthroplasty potentially is as good as the quality of the primary procedure, but the significant complication rate, particularly the high incidence of radiolucent lines, might lead to unpredictable long-term results.

In 1985, these same reviewers published a report on the same group of patients after an average follow-up of over 8 years. The mechanical failure rate had risen from 14 to 29 percent. Clinical failure between the first and second studies was frequently in cases with progressive radiolucent lines.

A group of 146 revisions was reviewed

by Callahan and associates.[8] Most patients in this study had significant complications associated with revision operation, including perforation of the femoral cortex (13 percent), dislocation (8 percent), trochanteric complications (6.2 percent), and deep infection (3.4 percent). Average follow-up was 3.6 years. At that time, 34 percent of the patients had fair or poor results. Migration of one component occurred in 27 percent of cases, and progressive radiolucencies without evidence of migration occurred in 29 percent.

Amstutz and coworkers[1] reported the results of 66 revisions for aseptic loosening of conventional hip arthroplasties. The average time to revision was 4 years. The patients in this study were generally younger than most patients having primary hip arthroplasties. Improvement in hip scores an average of 2 years after revision was less than that after primary arthroplasty. Nearly 10 percent of the patients had already required a second revision at the time of the review. The quality of both the acetabular and femoral fixation was clearly inferior to that obtained with primary surgery. Progressive radiolucent lines were apparent in 20 percent of the cases and were considered radiographically significant, although no clinical loosening was present. Significant complications were noted in 56 percent of the cases.

In 1982, Broughton and Rushton[7] reviewed all revisions at Addenbrooke's Hospital in Cambridge. Of the 27 patients who had revisions for aseptic loosening, ten (37 percent) had poor results or had undergone Girdlestone arthroplasties at the time of the review. The results of the second revision generally were even worse, probably reflecting the increased technical difficulties with these additional operations.

Similarly, in a 1985 review by Kavanagh and colleagues,[24] the significant complication rate was high among the 166 hips that had been revised and followed over 2 years. Of the acetabular components, 20 percent and, of the femoral components, 44 percent showed radiographic evidence of probable loosening. The hip replacements that had been revised because of acetabular loosening had an even higher rate of radiographic and symptomatic loosening of the new acetabulum, presumably because of the poor bone stock available for reimplantation.

Stromberg and colleagues[42] reviewed the entire Swedish revision experience for the period 1979–1982 in patients younger than 55 years. This prospective, multicenter study included 65 patients having revision for aseptic loosening. By the study's conclusion, 13 patients (20 percent) had undergone revisions a second time for aseptic failure. Among the remaining patients the results were good or excellent in 29 percent, fair in 17 percent, and poor in 54 percent. Stromberg concluded that revision hip replacement utilizing cement in young and middle-aged patients with a cemented primary hip replacement leads to a high rate of aseptic failure.

Long-Stem Components

Turner and coworkers[46] reported their use of a cemented, long-stem femoral component in 165 hips. The patients were followed at least 5 years. Intraoperative complications occurred in 23 percent of the cases, with a 16-percent incidence of femoral perforation and a 5-percent incidence of femoral fracture. Functionally, results were rated excellent in 34 percent, good in 36 percent, fair in 17 percent, and poor in 13 percent. These investigations concluded that, compared with cemented conventional-length stems, cemented long-stem femoral components lowered the incidence of mechanical failure of revision cemented hip arthroplasty.

Multiple Cemented Revision Surgery

The Mayo Clinic experience with multiple revision surgery was summarized in 1987 by Kavanagh and Fitzgerald.[23] They documented a high failure rate for cemented re-revisions: 24 percent of the hips failed by 3.5 years. Significant postoperative complications occurred in 40 percent of the patients.

Revisions with Modern Cement Techniques

Rubash and Harris[38] reported the results of femoral component revisions employing modern cementing techniques in 43 hips revised for symptomatic aseptic failure, either loose or broken. The primary or original diagnosis was osteoarthritis in just over half the patients and congenitally dislocated hip in one third. The average age at the time of revision was 57 years. After follow-up of 6 years, the average postoperative Harris hip score was 87. Of the revisions, 10 percent were loose or possibly loose. Despite the significant intraoperative and postoperative complication rate, the investigators believed their results represented an improvement over other reports in the literature with respect to femoral loosening subsequent to cemented revision.

In 1990, Marti and associates[26] reported their results with cemented revision of failed total hip arthroplasty after follow-up of 5 to 14 years. The revision operations were done with meticulous technique and included bone grafting for both femoral and acetabular defects when necessary. They used antibiotic in the bone cement. Two infections (3 percent) required further surgery. Four revisions (7 percent) were needed for aseptic loosening. The revisions for aseptic loosening were at 6 months, 5 years, 6 years, and 9 years. Five femoral components subsided, and three sockets migrated. The average Harris hip score was 82 at follow-up. The score was 80 points or more for 38 hips (63 percent), 70 to 79 for 18 (30 percent), and less than 70 for 4 (7 percent). Predicted survival of the hip revisions in this series was 84 percent after 14 years.

Revision for Failed Surface Replacement Arthroplasty

Capello and colleagues[10] reported the results of revision for 24 failed resurfacing arthroplasties. For 15 patients who had conversions to conventional total hip arthroplasties, the average Iowa hip score following the procedure was 87. One patient required reoperation to remove an infected prosthesis. Another patient was awaiting revision for femoral component loosening. Salvage of a failed resurfacing hip arthroplasty was technically less difficult than a conventional revision procedure.

Based on their experience with 17 failed resurfacing arthroplasties, Thomas and Amstutz[43] reported that the clinical results of conversion from surface replacement to conventional hip arthroplasty were comparable to those of conventional revision surgery, but the outcome was less satisfactory than with primary hip arthroplasty. Significantly fewer technical problems were encountered as evidenced by the low rate of complications.

These reports are consistent with others in the literature, including those of Bradley and Freeman[6] and Steel and associates.[41]

CEMENTLESS REVISION TOTAL HIP ARTHROPLASTY

In Hungerford and Jones's[21] series of 87 hip revision arthroplasties, 90 percent of patients scored an average of 87 on the Harris hip scale after follow-up of 1 to 5 years. Two patients required a second revision. Three patients had persistent pain, and these arthroplasties were considered failures. The complications included three cases of dislocations, five of intraoperative femoral fractures, and four of subsidence.

Lord and colleagues[25] reported their experience with 284 revisions with cementless implants performed over 13 years. All cases involved aseptic loosening—71 required revisions for failed cementless femoral stems. At 5 years, 70 percent of the patients had good or excellent clinical results. The radiographic results in this series were not well detailed.

Another series with short follow-up was that reported by Hedley and coworkers,[20] who used Porous Coated Anatomic components. A total of 55 patients who had 61 revision procedures of one or both of the prosthetic components were evaluated both clinically and radiographically. The clinical results were good or excellent in 90 percent of the cases, fair in 5 percent, and poor in 5 percent. Symptomatic loosening and subsidence were the causes of the three failures. Minimal subsidence of one or both components, which stabilized with time, did not seem to affect the clinical result.

Engh and associates[14] reported the results of 160 cementless revision arthroplasties, which were followed for a mean of 4.4 years. Radiographic evaluation suggested four categories of component stability: (1) demonstrable bone ingrowth, (2) stable fibrous encapsulation, (3) questionable stability with signs of impending instability, and (4) definite implant instability with migration. Demonstrable bone ingrowth, which was graded as optimal, was observed in 84.3 percent of the femoral revisions. Almost 12 percent resulted in stable fibrous encapsulation, and 4 percent were definite failures. When press-fit stability was achieved at the time of surgery, subsequent failure was rare. Observations on acetabular components were less favorable, with 22 percent of the components classified as unstable. A large percentage of these were threaded acetabular rings, in conjunction with structural allografts.

Driessnach, Wiedel, and Law[12] also reviewed a series of uncemented revision procedures. Of 79 hips, two required revision again within the first year after surgery—one because of recurrent dislocation and the other because of femoral subsidence. The remaining patients were followed for an average of 21 months, and the average Harris score for 73 hips was 82. Results were 42.5 percent excellent, 19.2 percent good, 23.3 percent fair, and 15 percent poor. Scores tended to be lower in hips with significant bone loss and more previous arthroplasties. The reoperation rate was 11 percent, and the total failure rate was 26 percent. The combination of femoral component subsidence and instability was the most common indication for reoperation. In this series, structural bone allografts were utilized in 22 acetabula and 13 femora. These investigators noted that results were strongly influenced by the availability of autogenous structural bone and implant stability at the time of surgery.

Borden and colleagues[3] reported their experience with 249 cementless total hip revisions, with a minimum two-year follow-up period. Both components were revised in 180 cases, the acetabulum alone in 42 cases, and the femoral component alone in 27 cases. Of these patients, 90 percent achieved satisfactory grades on the Harris hip score. The most frequent complication was femoral component subsidence, which occurred in 6 percent. Dislocations occurred in 3 percent and deep infections in 1.5 percent.

Gustillo and Pasternak[16] reviewed the results of femoral component revision of 55 hips with the BIAS femoral component after follow-up for an average of 2.8 years. The average preoperative Harris hip score was 45.5, and the postoperative score was 82.5. Significant intraoperative and postoperative complications included dislocation in 4 percent, infection in 4 percent, and recurrent loosening in 6 percent. These workers concluded that uncemented femoral revision with this prosthesis and the addition of bone graft compared favorably with cemented femoral revisions.

Harris and colleagues[18] reported the results in 60 patients treated with the Harris-Galante prosthesis after nonseptic failure of cemented total hip arthroplasties. Minimum follow-up was 12 months. Despite the need for acetabular bone grafting in 86 percent of cases and femoral bone grafting in 57 percent, the average postoperative Harris hip score was 84. Excellent or good results were achieved in 71 percent of the patients. None of the components required revision. No socket migration occurred, and only one case of femoral component subsidence occurred.

REVISION TOTAL HIP ARTHROPLASTY FOR SEPTIC FAILURE

Four surgical options are available for the management of infected total hip replacement: (1) resection arthroplasty; (2) debridement and preservation of the existing components; (3) debridement and removal of components, followed by immediate reimplantation of new components; and (4) resection arthroplasty followed by delayed reimplantation. The advantages and disadvantages of resection arthroplasty are well known. Excision arthroplasty often provides a significant reduction in pain but poor and often disabling functional results. Patients are easily fatigued because of weakness of the lower extremity and the increased energy required by the use of external support.[5, 22, 28, 35]

One-Stage Exchange Arthroplasty for Septic Total Hip Replacement

Buchholz,[7a] a pioneer of one-stage exchange, has recommended this procedure as the treatment of choice for most deep infections involving a total hip replacement. The procedure requires excision of soft tissue and removal of the implant and cement. A new prosthesis is implanted immediately, using bone cement that contains antibiotics. Antibiotics are administered intravenously as well. Buchholz reported a 77 percent success rate in 583 patients and a 90 percent success rate when subsequent exchange procedures were performed after failure of the original revision.

Wroblewski[48] recorded a 75-percent success rate with one-stage revision without antibiotics in the cement. He later reported that the addition of gentamicin to the cement in revision surgery for deep infection increased the success rate from 75 to 91 percent.

In 1982, Miley, Scheller, and Turner[30] reviewed the results of one-stage reimplantations of 101 infected total hip arthroplasties. An antibiotic cement was used. After a minimum follow-up of 32 months, the infection had resolved in 87 hips.

Harris[17] reported the results of one-stage exchange arthroplasty in 18 patients followed for an average of 42 months. Treatment included antibiotic cement, intravenous antibiotics for 6 weeks, and oral antibiotics for several additional months. The success rate, as measured by the absence of sepsis and excellent functional results, was 78 percent.

Nasser, Lee, and Amstutz[32] reported the results of direct exchange arthroplasty for 30 septic total hip replacements after an average follow-up of 4 years. These direct exchanges were performed in patients who had antibiotic-sensitive organisms and viable soft tissues. Meticulous debridement was carried out to remove all infected implant, including all cement. Appropriate antibiotics, based on preoperative culture results, were placed in the cement in 28 of the 30 cases. On follow-up, all patients demonstrated good pain relief and improvement in function. No evidence of recurrent sepsis was observed. Two reoperations were necessary, both for aseptic loosening. These investigators concluded that direct exchange is an effective method for treatment of sepsis due to gram-positive organisms.

Balderston and colleagues[2] reported a success rate of 83 percent for revision of infected total hip arthroplasties. Statistically significant negative prognosticators included the number of previous operations, elevated sedimentation rates, and gross infections at the time of surgery. Every conversion to total hip arthroplasty due to infection associated with other hip implants, such as sliding hip screws and other fracture fixation devices, was successful.

Two-Stage Revision for Septic Total Hip Replacement

In the United States, two-stage revision is a more popular treatment for infected total hip arthroplasty than one-stage revision. Reported success rates vary from 60 to 95 percent.

None of the 82 two-stage revisions for infection reported by McDonald and colleagues[27] in 1989 incorporated antibiotics in the cement. Infection recurred in 13 percent of the cases, with an average follow-up of 5.5 years. Three of the seven patients in whom some cement had been left experienced a recurrence of infection. The incidence of recurrent infection was significantly higher when reimplantation was performed less than a year after the resection arthroplasty. Seven recurrent infections occurred among the 26 patients who had surgery within a year, whereas only four occurred among the 56 patients who had reimplantations more than a year after resection arthroplasty. The conclusion of this study was that a two-stage reconstruction is an effective, safe technique, even when the infection is caused by virulent organisms such as gram-negative bacilli, group D streptococci, or enterococci.

Gustilo and Tsukayama[15] treated 18 patients with removal of the infected implant and thorough surgical debridement, followed by insertion of antibiotic-bone cement beads. Parenteral antibiotics were administered, and cementless revision with autogenous bone graft was performed 6 weeks later. During follow-up, which averaged 19 months, infection recurred in two hips. These preliminary results suggested that a cementless revision is a reasonable alternative to a cemented revision.

Pinto and coworkers[36] evaluated the results of two-stage revision with cementless components in 17 patients managed with resection arthroplasty followed by 4 weeks of parenteral antibiotics. The interval between the first and second stage was 3 months for gram-positive infections and 12 months for gram-negative infections. The average Harris hip score was 86 after an average follow-up of 32.1 months. No recurrent infections occurred, and none of the patients required further surgery.

Both One-Stage and Two-Stage Revisions

Salvati and colleagues[39] evaluated antibiotic-impregnated cement in both one-stage and two-stage reimplantations. A total of 21 revision arthroplasties were performed in one stage, and eighteen were performed in two stages. The condition of 32 hips was assessed after 4 years, at which time 22 hips had excellent results, 8 had good results, and 2 had fair results. Three recurrences of infection were reported. Progressive radiolucencies were seen about the acetabulum in 13 percent of the cases, and femoral radiolucencies were seen in 16 percent.

Carlsson and associates[11] described early results in 59 patients who underwent one-stage reimplantations and 18 who underwent two-stage revisions. The interval between the resection and reimplantation in the latter group varied from 2 to 4 months. After follow-up of 6 months to 3½ years, five hips that had been treated with one-stage reimplantation were infected and eight were doubtful. Three recurrent infections and one doubtful after the two-stage procedure were noted. The difference between the two groups was not statistically significant.

COMPLEX TOTAL HIP ARTHROPLASTY WITH BONE GRAFT

Failure of the acetabular component of a cemented total hip replacement frequently leads to osseous defects in the acetabular bone stock. These defects complicate the technical aspects of revision and may affect the long-term results of revision. Sufficient autogenous bone graft from the femoral head is usually available for reconstruction of acetabular defects in primary total hip arthroplasty but for revisions, allograft is often necessary.

Allograft for Acetabular Insufficiency

Borja and Mnaymneh[4] reported on the use of allograft bone for acetabular wall reconstruction in eight revision total hip replacements. At follow-up after an average of 19 months, the acetabular grafts appeared to be united.

Trancik and colleagues[45] reviewed the results in 21 patients who had acetabular reconstructions with allografts after an average follow-up of 3.5 years. Of these, 17 patients had an average postoperative Harris hip score of 89. A second revision was required in one case because the allograft collapsed. Two patients had asymptomatic, progressive radiolucencies at the bone-cement interface. A total of 14 grafts (67 percent) appeared to be incorporated. Three-dimensional computerized tomography isotope scans showed uniform uptake, demonstrating revascularization and new bone formation in all grafts. No infections occurred.

Oakeshott and colleagues[33] categorized the results of 112 frozen allografts in 72 acetabular reconstructions according to the anatomic location of the defects and evaluated the results from 6 to 72 months after surgery. Of the 31 grafts for protrusio defects, 30 appeared consolidated at follow-up. Superior and medial migration occurred with 11 grafts, including 8 of the 9 bipolar prostheses and 2 of the 14 cemented prostheses. A total of 20 grafts had not changed position after initial insertion (65 percent).

In 11 of 18 shelf allografts from frozen femoral heads, cementless prostheses were employed. Union was present in 12 of the 18 cases, and four others showed partial union. None of the cases had graft fracture or fragmentation, although one graft resorbed completely. No evidence existed of implant migration in 16 of the 18 cases. The two cases that migrated involved bipolar prostheses.

A total of 20 other acetabular allografts were reported, and 11 were femoral head grafts done for column deficiencies. Nine total acetabular grafts were applied for defects that were too large to be replaced by femoral heads alone. Of these allografts, 15, including eight of the nine total acetabular grafts, showed evidence of union. Two components loosened, and two showed evidence of failure, in one case due to infection.

The investigators concluded that (1) protrusio defects can be managed with structural medial allograft and a cementless prosthesis, rather than particulate graft and a bipolar prosthesis; (2) shelf allografts are reliable when done by an experienced surgeon; and (3) whole allograft reconstructions for major defects are reasonable alternatives under difficult circumstances.

Cementless Components

Samuelson and colleagues[40] reported on 37 patients with extensive acetabular bone loss who had revisions with cementless sockets and large structural allografts. The component was stabilized on the maximum available surface area of host bone. Peripheral rim defects were filled with a bone held in place with screws, and central cavitary defects were filled with particulate graft. After mean follow-up of 1.5 years, 34 patients (92 percent) had no pain. Two components migrated in patients who were asymptomatic.

At the time of revision, an allograft plug was inserted into a predrilled hole in the iliac crest in six patients. In 6 weeks, the plug was removed and examined histologically. These workers concluded that allograft bone incorporates as well as autograft bone or a composite mixture of these grafts in the first 6 weeks following transplantation.

Emerson and colleagues[13] reviewed 106 acetabular revisions that required structural grafts for socket deficiencies. Three different acetabular components were evaluated: a bipolar component, a truncated-cone threaded cup, and a porous-coated hemispheric prosthesis. Component migration and graft resorption occurred with both the bipolar and threaded designs. The press-fit acetabular design showed little migration and resulted in a better clinical score. No revisions were performed for failure. If rim or column defects were present, a reconstruction plate with interfragmental screws formed a more successful construct than lag screws alone.

Both Allografts and Autografts for Acetabular Reconstruction

Young, Dorr, and Gruen[49] reported on the results of allograft and autograft reconstructions for deficient acetabula in 40 hips. At an average follow-up of 44 months, five of the 40 hips were classified as failures. Results were better when noncemented rather than cemented components were used and when greater than two thirds of the acetabular component was covered with host bone. When multiple grafts rather than a single allograft were selected, the results were inferior.

Acetabular Revision with Bipolar Prosthesis and Bone Graft

Murray[31] reported the results of 106 revision total hip arthroplasties done with bipolar acetabular components. After debridement of the acetabular component, cement, and fibrous membrane, defects were filled with bone graft. If necessary, allograft was employed to provide structural integrity to the peripheral rim of the acetabulum. After an average of 3 years, there were 43 good or excellent, 20 fair, and nine poor results. Of the 29 failures (30 percent), 14 required revision to a fixed cementless socket. Ten infections occurred. Murray concluded that the results of revision hip replacement with bipolar components were not as successful as results with fixed cementless acetabular components but were superior to the functional deficiencies produced by Girdlestone arthroplasty.

Cameron and Jung[9] suggested the need for an intact acetabular rim to prevent significant migration of the bipolar head. When massive bulk allograft was required to reconstitute the peripheral rim of the acetabulum, good or excellent results were achieved in 55 percent of cases.

Roberson and Cohen[37] found that 25 of 27 patients treated with bipolar prostheses in the management of failed total hip replacements had satisfactory results after a minimum of 2 years. The average postoperative Harris hip score was 81. Two patients had evidence of migration of the component. In one patient who required reoperation for dislocation, the bipolar component was inadequately sized to achieve peripheral bone support.

Torisu and coworkers[44] followed 37 patients for a minimum of 5 years after revision with bipolar components. The average hip score was 42.2 preoperatively and 82.7 postoperatively. Minimal migration of the prosthesis was recognized early in all 37 patients, but at 5 years 27 of the 37 hips had not migrated further.

Wilson and Scott[47] reported on 47 revisions with bipolar prostheses followed a minimum of 2 years. Acceptable levels of pain relief and improvement in function were achieved in all. The mean postoperative Harris hip score was 86, compared with a mean score of 48 preoperatively.

It is apparent from these series that when a stable press-fit can be achieved with a nonarticulating acetabular component, it is likely to yield a better functional result than a bipolar prosthesis. A bipolar implant is likely to migrate if the peripheral rim of the socket is not intact. If press-fit stability cannot be achieved with a fixed socket, a bipolar implant is a reasonable alternative. In some cases this may be the first procedure in a two-stage acetabular revision.

Proximal Femoral Allograft-Prosthesis Composite

When managing five patients who had severe structural bone deficiencies secondary to failed total hip replacements, McGann and associates[29] found generally good clinical results if no significant problems developed within the first 2 years. Complications included nonunion of the allograft to the host bone, fracture in association with stress risers in the allograft, infection, and dissolution of the graft. They stated that this form of treatment is an acceptable salvage procedure for patients with severe bone loss.

Oakeshott and associates[33] used allograft in the reconstruction of femoral defects, replacing the calcar of 26 patients with either segmental femoral calcar or segmental tibial diaphysis. In 12 patients, a portion of the proximal femur was replaced with proximal femoral metadiaphysis, segmental tibial metadiaphysis, or both. In the five cases in which the lateral femoral cortexes were deficient, segmental femoral struts were used. The best results of calcar allografts were achieved with metadiaphyseal grafts longer than 2 cm. Of the large-fragment femoral allografts, 58 percent had united at follow-up 6 to 72 months after surgery. One patient had a symptomatic nonunion. All of the lateral femoral cortical strut allografts had some form of union. These results suggest that osteolytic or significantly weakened lateral structural bone can be replaced with femoral allograft.

Head and associates[19] reported the results in 22 patients who had proximal femoral allografts for management of severe femoral bone loss. The average length of the allograft was 15 cm. Three methods of fixation were used. In ten patients, the prosthesis was cemented to the allograft and the host distal femur. In three cases, the prosthesis was cemented only to the host distal femur. Cement was not utilized on either the allograft or the host bone in nine cases. With evaluation an average of 2 years after surgery, functional improvement was found in 73 percent of the patients. Nine patients (41 percent) required additional surgical procedures to manage complications. The average postoperative Harris hip score was 65.

SUMMARY

The early results of cemented revision total hip arthroplasty were clinically satisfactory with short-term follow-up, but radiographic results were poor relative to primary hip replacement. Longer follow-up revealed an increased incidence of failure. Later reports of better cementing techniques, improved therapy for infection, and especially the use of cementless components that enable better rebuilding of deficient bone stock indicate an improvement in results for revision total hip arthroplasty. However, these results remain inferior to the results of primary total hip arthroplasty.

References

1. Amstutz, H. C., Ma, S. M., Jinnah, R. H., and Mai, L.: Revision of aseptic loose total hip arthroplasties. Clin. Orthop. 170:21–23, 1982.
2. Balderston, R. A., Hiller, W. D., Ianotti, J. P., et al: Treatment of the septic hip with total hip arthroplasty. Clin. Orthop. 221:231–237, 1987.
3. Borden, L. S., Hungerford, D. S., Hedley, A., et al: Cementless revision of failed cemented total hip replacement. Orthop. Trans. 12(3):590, 1988.
4. Borja, F. J. and Mnaymneh, W.: Bone allografts in salvage of difficult hip arthroplasties. Clin. Orthop. 197:123–130, 1985.
5. Bourne, R. B., Hunter, G. A., Rorabeck, C. H., and Macnab, J. J.: A six-year follow-up of infected total hip replacements managed by Girdlestone's arthroplasty. J. Bone Joint Surg. [Br] 66(3):340–343, 1984.
6. Bradley, G. W. and Freeman, M. A.: Revision of failed hip resurfacing. Clin. Orthop. 178:236–240, 1983.
7. Broughton, N. S. and Rushton, N.: Revision hip arthroplasty. A retrospective survey. Acta Orthop. Scand. 53(6):923–928, 1982.

7a. Buchholz, H. W., Elson, R. A., Englebrecht, E., et al: Management of deep infection of total hip replacement. J. Bone Joint Surg. 63B:342–353, 1981.

8. Callahan, J. J., Salvati, E. A., Pellicci, P. M., et al: Results of revision for mechanical failure after cemented total hip replacement, 1979 to 1982. A two- to five-year follow-up. J. Bone Joint Surg. [Am] 67(7):1074–1085, 1985.
9. Cameron, H. U. and Jung, Y. B.: Acetabular revision with a bipolar prosthesis. Clin. Orthop. 251:100–103, 1990.
10. Capello, W. N., Trancik, T. M., Misamore, G., and Eaton, R.: Analysis of revision surgery of resurfacing hip arthroplasty. Clin. Orthop. 170:50–55, 1982.
11. Carlsson, A. S., Josefsson, G., and Lindberg, L.: Revision with gentamicin-impregnated cement for deep infections in total hip arthroplasties. J. Bone Joint Surg. 60A:1059–1064, 1978.
12. Driessnack, R. P., Wiedel, J. R., and Law, J.: Revision total hip arthroplasty using uncemented prosthesis. Orthop. Trans. 13(1):76–77, 1989.
13. Emerson, R. H., Head, W. C., Berklacich, F. M., and Malinin, T. I.: Noncemented acetabular revision arthroplasty using allograft bone. Clin. Orthop. 249:30–42, 1989.
14. Engh, C. A., Glassman, A. H., Griffin, W. L., and Mayer, J. G.: Results of cementless revision for failed cemented total hip arthroplasty. Clin. Orthop. 235:91–110, 1988.
15. Gustilo, R. B. and Tsukayama, D.: Treatment of infected cemented total hip arthroplasty with tobramycin beads and delayed revision with the cementless prosthesis and bone grafting. Orthop. Trans. 12(3):739, 1988.
16. Gustilo, R. B. and Pasternak, H. S.: Revision total hip arthroplasty with titanium ingrowth prosthesis and bone grafting for failed cemented femoral component loosening. Clin. Orthop. 235:111–119, 1988.
17. Harris, W. H.: One-staged Exchange Arthroplasty for Septic Total Hip Replacement. Instructional Course Lectures. Edited by L. Anderson, St. Louis, C. V. Mosby, 1986.
18. Harris, W. H., Krushell, R. J., and Galante, J. O.: Results of cementless revisions of total hip arthroplasties using the Harris-Galante prosthesis. Clin. Orthop. 235:126, 1988.
19. Head, W. C., Berklacich, F. M., Malinin, T. I., and Emerson, R. H.: Proximal femoral allografts in revision total hip arthroplasty. Clin. Orthop. 225:22–36, 1987.
20. Hedley, A. K., Gruen, T. A., and Ruoff, D. P.: Revision of failed total hip arthroplasties with uncemented porous-coated anatomic components. Clin. Orthop. 235:75–90, 1988.
21. Hungerford, D. S. and Jones, L. C.: The rationale of cementless revision of cemented arthroplasty failures. Clin. Orthop. 235:12–24, 1988.
22. Hunter, G. and Dandy, D.: The natural history of the patient with an infected total hip replacement. J. Bone Joint Surg. [Br] 59(3):293–297, 1977.
23. Kavanagh, B. F. and Fitzgerald, R. H., Jr.: Multiple revisions for failed total hip arthroplasty not associated with infection. J. Bone Joint Surg. [Am] 69(8):1144–1149, 1987.
24. Kavanagh, B. F., Ilstrup, D. M., and Fitzgerald, R. H., Jr.: Revision total hip arthroplasty. J. Bone Joint Surg. [Am] 67(4):517–526, 1985.
25. Lord, G., Marotte, J., Guillamon, J., and Blanchard, J.: Cementless revision of failed aseptic cemented and cementless total hip arthroplasties. Clin. Orthop. 235:74, 1988.
26. Marti, R. K., Schuller, H. M., Besselaar, P. P., and Vanfrank Haasnoot, E. L.: Results of revision of hip arthroplasty with cement. J. Bone Joint Surg. 72A:346–354, 1990.
27. McDonald, D. J., Fitzgerald, R. H., Jr., and Ilstrup, D. M.: Two-stage reconstruction of a total hip arthroplasty because of infection. J. Bone Joint Surg. [Am] 71(6):828–834, 1989.
28. McElwaine, J. P. and Colville, J.: Excision arthroplasty for infected total hip replacements. J. Bone Joint Surg. [Br] 66(2):168–171, 1984.
29. McGann, W., Mankin, H. J., and Harris, W. H.: Massive allografting for severe failed total hip replacement. J. Bone Joint Surg. [Am] 68:4–12, 1986.
30. Miley, G. B., Scheller, A. D., Jr., and Turner, R. H.: Medical and surgical treatment of the septic hip with one-stage revision arthroplasty. Clin. Orthop. 170:76–82, 1982.

31. Murray, W. R.: Acetabular salvage in revision total hip arthroplasty. Clin. Orthop. 251:92–99, 1990.
32. Nasser, S., Lee, Y. F., and Amstutz, H. C.: Direct exchange arthroplasty in 30 septic total hip replacements without recurrent infection. Orthop. Trans. 13(3):519, 1989.
33. Oakeshott, R. D., Morgan, D. A., Zukor, D. J., et al: Revision total hip arthroplasty with osseous allograft reconstruction. A clinical and roentgenographic analysis. Clin. Orthop. 225:37–61, 1987.
34. Pellicci, P. M., Wilson, P. D., Jr., Sledge, C. B., et al: Revision total hip arthroplasty. Clin. Orthop. 170:34–41, 1982.
35. Petty, W. and Goldsmith, S.: Resection arthroplasty following infected total hip arthroplasty. J. Bone Joint Surg. 62A:889–896, 1980.
36. Pinto, M. R., Racette, J. W., and Fitzgerald, R. H.: Staged hip reconstruction following infected cemented total hip arthroplasty. Orthop. Trans. 13(3):612, 1989.
37. Roberson, J. R. and Cohen, D.: Bipolar components for severe periacetabular bone loss around the failed total hip arthroplasty. Clin. Orthop. 251:113–118, 1990.
38. Rubash, H. E. and Harris, W. H.: Revision of nonseptic, loose, cemented femoral components using modern cementing techniques. J. Arthroplasty 3(3):241–248, 1988.
39. Salvati, E. A., Callaghan, J. J., and Brause, B. D.: Prosthetic Reimplantation for Salvage of the Infected Hip. Instructional Course Lectures. Edited by L. Anderson. St. Louis, C. V. Mosby, 1986.
40. Samuelson, K. M., Freeman, M. A., Levack, B., et al: Homograft bone in revision acetabular arthroplasty. A clinical and radiographic study. J. Bone Joint Surg. [Br] 70(3):367–372, 1988.
41. Steele, R. A., Dempster, D., and Smith, M. A.: Total hip replacement of failed surface arthroplasty. Acta Orthop. Scand. 56(2):133–134, 1985.
42. Stromberg, C. N., Herberts, P., and Ahnfelt, L.: Revision total hip arthroplasty in patients younger than 55 years old. Clinical and radiologic results after 4 years. J. Arthroplasty 3(1):47–59, 1988.
43. Thomas, B. J. and Amstutz, H. C.: Revision surgery for failed surface arthroplasty of the hip. Clin. Orthop. 170:42–49, 1982.
44. Torisu, T., Utsunomiya, K., Maekawa, M., and Ueda, Y.: Use of bipolar hip arthroplasty in states of acetabular deficiency. Clin. Orthop. 252:119–125, 1990.
45. Trancik, T. M., Stulberg, B. N., Wilde, A. H., and Feiglin, D. H.: Allograft reconstruction of the acetabulum during revision total hip arthroplasty. J. Bone Joint Surg. 68A:527–537, 1986.
46. Turner, R. H., Mattingly, D. A., and Scheller, A.: Femoral revision total hip arthroplasty using a long-stem femoral component. Clinical and radiographic analysis. J. Arthroplasty 2(3):247–258, 1987.
47. Wilson, M. G. and Scott, R. D.: Reconstruction of the deficient acetabulum using the bipolar socket. Clin. Orthop. 251:126–133, 1990.
48. Wroblewski, B. M.: Revision of infected hip arthroplasty. J. Bone Joint Surg. 65B:224, 1983.
49. Young, S. K., Dorr, L. D., and Gruen, T.: Efficacy of allograft and autograft structural bone grafts in total hip arthroplasty. Orthop. Trans. 13(1):75, 1989.

CHAPTER 25

Prostheses for Total Hip Arthroplasty

WILLIAM PETTY

A wide array of hip prostheses are available to orthopaedic surgeons, with different designs offered by many different manufacturers. Prostheses are categorized by type of fixation: bone cement, porous-coated, and press-fit with or without macrointerlock. In addition, various custom prostheses are available. Most are used for special circumstances (e.g., after tumor resections, for difficult revision cases), but some surgeons select them routinely for primary total hip replacements. The surgeon's selection of a prosthesis for a specific patient depends on many factors, including the surgeon's knowledge, experience, and preference and the patient's condition. Fortunately, long-term evaluations by many investigators of patients with total hip replacements over the past two decades has generated much knowledge about the requirements for a high likelihood of success. Although our knowledge base is most extensive regarding cemented total hip arthroplasty, the most widely used fixation method, we are now gaining information rapidly regarding cementless methods of fixation.

This chapter contains information about the characteristics of various prosthesis systems. Descriptions of the prostheses and the figures included in this chapter were supplied by the manufacturers of the various prostheses. An attempt was made to include prostheses based on their popularity, either past or present, or on specific unique design features. Unfortunately, descriptions of some prostheses are excluded because the manufacturer did not supply the needed information.

TOTAL HIP PROSTHESES DESIGNED FOR BONE CEMENT FIXATION

Computer-Assisted Design (CAD) Hip Endoprosthesis

Developed in 1974 and manufactured by Howmedica, Inc., the CAD Hip endoprosthesis was a series of hip prostheses that reflected the most advanced design engineering techniques of the time (Fig. 25–1). It was the first device to utilize computer-assisted design techniques. By providing structural characteristics such as I-beam stem cross-section and rounded margins, designers recognized the need for stem strength and reduction of stress concentrations in the surrounding cement mantle. The CAD Hip was also the first hip prosthesis to offer a variety of stem sizes and types to accommodate varying patient anatomies. This prosthesis was made from cast cobalt-chromium alloy.

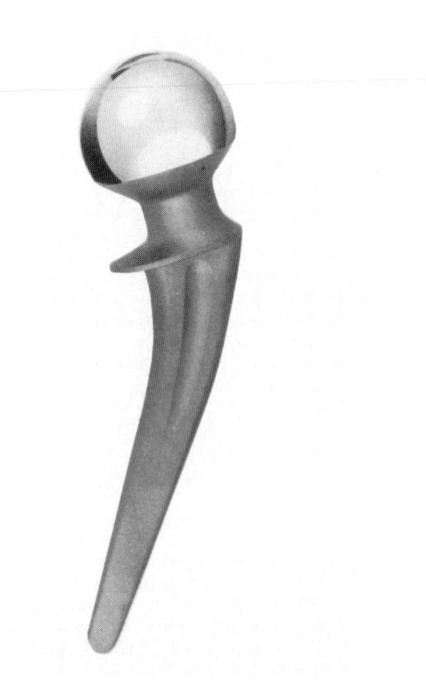

FIGURE 25–1. The computer-assisted design (CAD) hip endoprosthesis. (Courtesy of Howmedica, Inc.)

Charnley Hip Stem and Elite Modular Hip System

Nearly 30 years ago, Charnley set new standards for total hip replacement by introducing the combination of a 22-mm diameter stainless steel femoral head articulating with a thick-walled ultrahigh molecular weight polyethylene socket. He described this as the "low-friction (torque) arthroplasty." Both femoral and acetabular components were grouted into the bone using polymethyl methacrylate cement. This original design has been modified by a succession of refinements stimulated by long-term clinical data and significant improvements in materials (Fig. 25–2). The Elite Modular Hip System, manufactured by Chas. F. Thackray, Ltd., incorporates the most recent advances in the evolution of the Charnley prosthesis.

The Elite Modular Hip System offers a wide range of femoral stems, modular heads, and cup options (Fig. 25–3). The

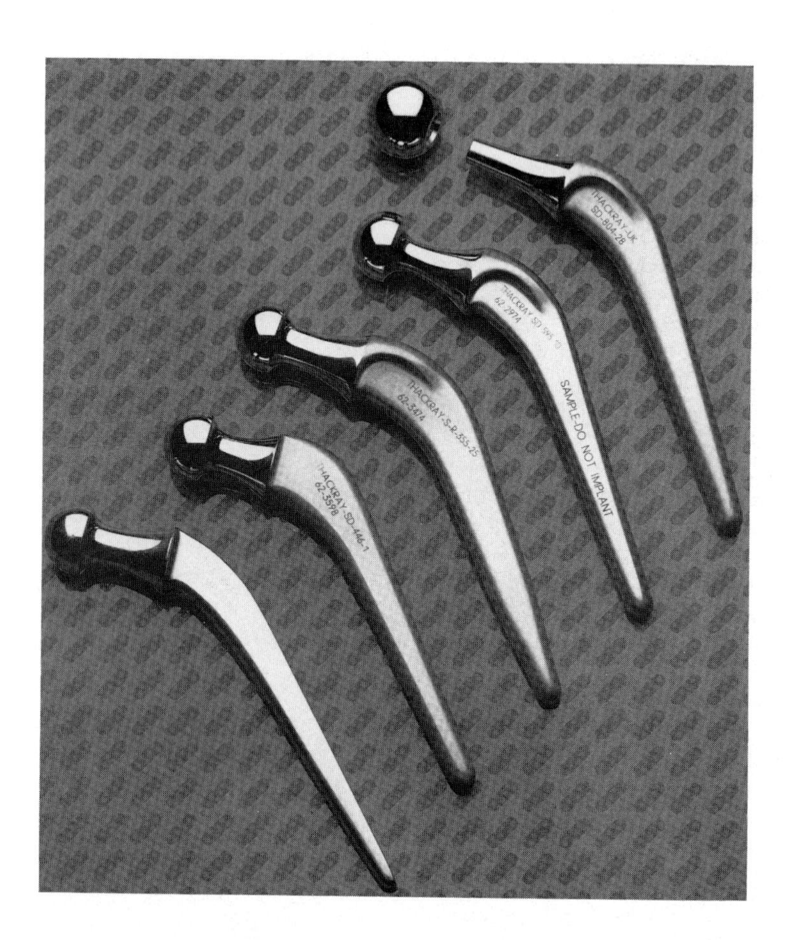

FIGURE 25–2. Refinements of the Charnley hip stem. (Courtesy of Thackray Reconstructive Systems.)

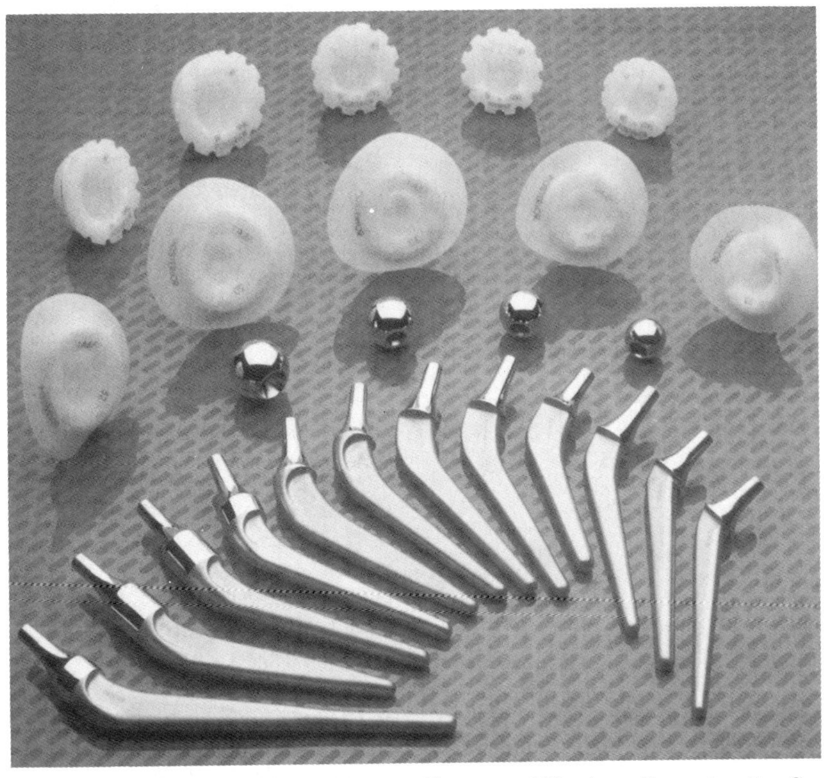

FIGURE 25–3. The Elite Modular Hip System. (Courtesy of Thackray Reconstructive Systems.)

femoral stems and heads are manufactured of Ortron 90, a stainless steel superalloy. The strength of Ortron 90 has permitted the reduced diameter neck in the design of the Elite, increasing the range of angular movement by 18 degrees, delaying the moment of impingement, lessening the possibility of dislocation, and thus extending theoretic cup life. The Elite Cobra cement-pressurizing flange on the proximal aspect of the femoral stem improves cement pressurization and provides increased resistance to subsidence. The shape and placement of the flange causes loads to be transmitted via cement to the endosteal surface of the proximal femur. Clinical evidence has shown that the flange provides increased resistance to subsidence when compared with a conventional "non-flanged" design.

The Elite Modular Hip System offers an integrated range of acetabular components including the pressurizing Ogee cup. This system provides a choice of cup sizes, materials, and methods of fixation. Each element is fully compatible with the Elite Modular Hip System. The Ogee flange is trimmed intraoperatively for customized fit within the rim of the acetabulum to facilitate cement pressurization. Studies have shown that a continuous flange is necessary to achieve adequate cement injection pressure.

Exactech Cemented Total Hip System

The Exactech Cemented Total Hip System, based on accumulated laboratory research and clinical experience over three decades, is an optimum hip prosthesis for cemented application (Fig. 25–4). The proximal stem design of maximum cross-section results in minimum cement stress, while still maintaining an even mantle of cement surrounding the stem. A stem centralizer also helps achieve cement mantle uniformity. Smooth, rounded surfaces, a broad medial collar, a broader lateral dimension, and a rounded shoulder are further elements of the stem geometry de-

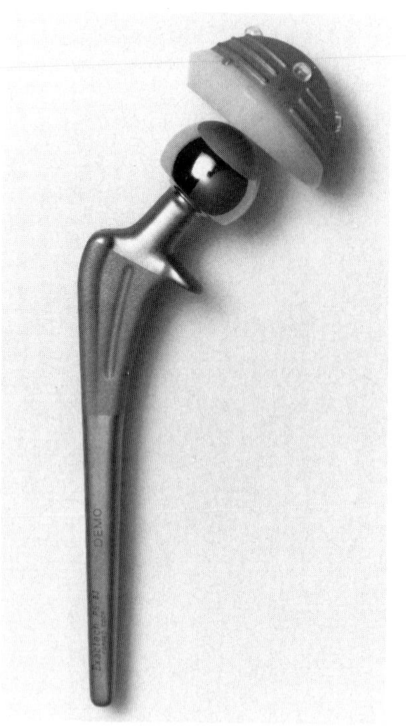

FIGURE 25–4. Exactech Cemented Total Hip System. (Courtesy of Exactech, Inc.)

signed to yield minimum cement stress in both tension and compression. Sizing of the cobalt-chrome femoral component features greater length in the larger stem sizes. This feature is intended to reduce the high bone cement stresses occurring across the prosthesis-femur composite in larger patients. An elliptic femoral neck design reduces socket impact and dislocation potential and improves range of motion. The proximal surface is microtextured to enhance cement fixation.

The stem mates with 26-mm, 28-mm, or 32-mm femoral heads by a taper locking mechanism. The femoral heads are produced in four neck lengths. The longer neck lengths are designed with a shorter sleeve to reduce the possibility of socket impact and dislocation caused by sleeve impingement.

The low-profile acetabular component has a cobalt-chrome metal shell bonded to an ultrahigh molecular weight polyethylene insert with integral polymethyl methacrylate spacers that provide for an even 3-mm mantle of cement. Cement fixation is enhanced by smooth ridges and a microtextured outer shell surface. The 10-degrees extended superior roof of the polyethylene allows improved stability while maintaining the metal shell completely within the acetabulum. *In vitro* studies reveal that this design produces nearly normal strain patterns in the pelvis after acetabular reconstruction.

Harris Precoat Plus Prosthesis

The Harris Precoat Plus Prosthesis manufactured by Zimmer, Inc., has a stem

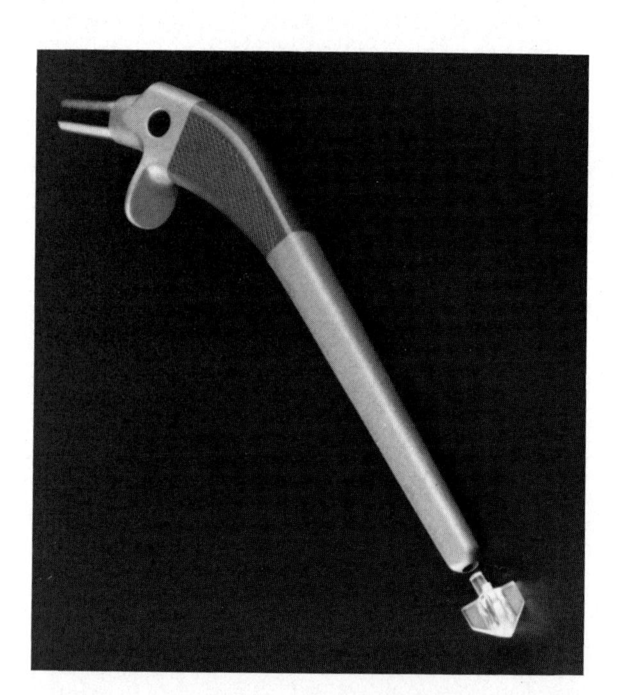

FIGURE 25–5. Harris Precoat Plus Prosthesis. (Courtesy of Zimmer, Inc.)

made from forged cobalt chromium. This prosthesis has polymethyl methacrylate precoating on the proximal stem for enhancement of cement fixation (Fig. 25–5). Other features include the following: a broad medial border to reduce peak stresses in cement by promoting a more uniform load distribution; a Morse-type taper for fitting femoral heads of multiple neck lengths; a calcar collar that extends medially, yet allows for anteroposterior access to disrupt the cement mantle interface if revision is required; graduated stem lengths to 300 mm for both primary and revision procedures; an elimination of sharp corners to prevent stress risers; and an optional distal centralizer to center the stem within the canal, promoting a uniform cement mantle. The socket is made of ultrahigh molecular weight polyethylene with a titanium alloy metal backing with cement spacers.

HD-2 Hip

The HD-2 Hip, manufactured by Howmedica, Inc., was the first major total hip prosthesis to be fabricated from a "superalloy," i.e., forged chrome-cobalt (Fig. 25–6). This prosthesis incorporated the positive aspects of the CAD Hip and added design enhancements, including a variety of head sizes, neck lengths, stem sizes, and a broad medial collar. The cross-section and teardrop configuration on the anterior and posterior aspects of the stem improved the relationship between the stem and the cement mantle. This system also introduced the concept of metal-backed acetabular cups with the Harris cup, featuring the first replaceable polyethylene liners.

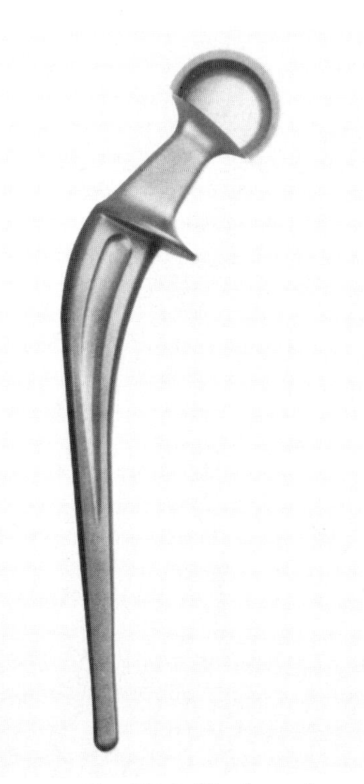

FIGURE 25–6. The HD-2 Hip femoral component. (Courtesy of Howmedica, Inc.)

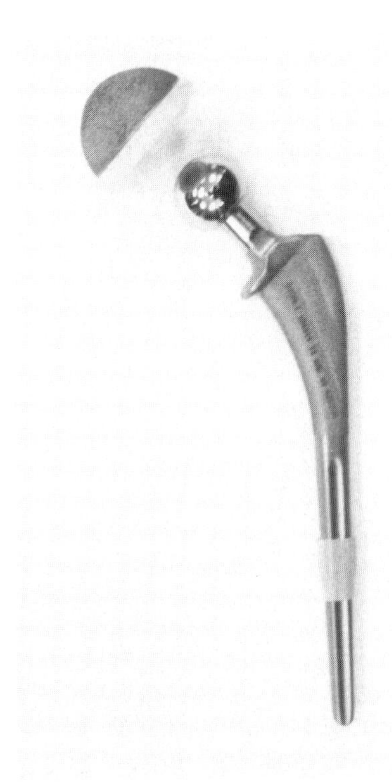

FIGURE 25–7. Mallory-Head Hip. (Courtesy of Biomet, Inc.)

Mallory-Head Hip

The Mallory-Head Hip is manufactured by Biomet, Inc. (Fig. 25–7). The design of the femoral component utilized in cemented procedures emphasizes proximal fixation, which is accomplished with a textured surface on the proximal portion of the prosthesis. A series of ribs along the proximal anterior and posterior surfaces are designed to contain the cement in the proximal femur. A small medial collar rests across the crest of the medial cortex. Extensions of the collar are created ante-

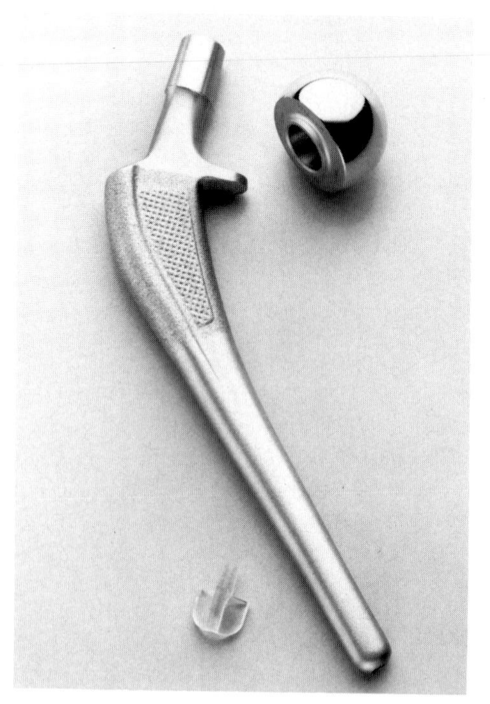

FIGURE 25–8. Precision Hip. (Courtesy of Howmedica, Inc.)

riorly and posteriorly with a cement mantle. The stem is modular in size to address anatomic variants. A precured polymethyl methacrylate sleeve placed independently at the distal one-third junction is provided to seat the component in axial alignment, leaving space for an adequate cement mantle (2 to 4 mm).

Precision Hip

The Precision Hip, manufactured by Howmedica, Inc., is a cemented total hip that seeks to optimize prosthesis/cement mantle/bone geometry to achieve a reproducible, long-lasting cemented arthroplasty (Fig. 25–8). Made from forged cobalt-chromium alloy, the Precision Hip has a proximal macrotexture plus a proximal surface-blasted finish. This feature enhances cement-prosthesis bonding. The system employs a distal cement spacer to centralize the stem within the cement mantle and distal canal. The Precision Hip has the only stem that uses a proximal cement spacer to help achieve proper prosthetic positioning. Instrumentation is an integral part of the Precision Hip system. A three-staged technique for preparation of the canal provides the basis for a precise cement mantle, which allows the proper mantle size for the particular prosthesis size.

Spectron EF

The Spectron EF Hip is manufactured by Richards, Inc. (Fig. 25–9). The femoral component consists of a forged cobalt-chromium alloy stem and modular femoral heads of different diameters and neck lengths. The proximal one third of the stem surface under the collar is roughened by "grit blasting," which strengthens fixation between the stem/cement interface. This feature, combined with the prominent wedge shape in the frontal and sagittal planes, helps convert interfacial shear stresses into compression of the cement mantle that will favorably load the proximal femur.

The Morse taper neck permits a wide selection of neck lengths and femoral head diameters for versatility and interchangeability. The circulotrapezoidal neck helps to increase the ratio of head-to-neck diameters, thus permitting a wide range of

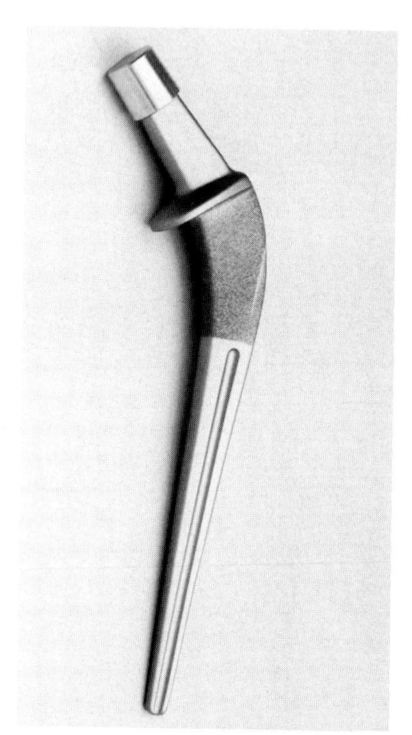

FIGURE 25–9. Spectron EF Hip. (Courtesy of Richards, Inc.)

hip motion. The anteroposterior and medial collar and the laterally flared cement locking wings on the Spectron EF femoral component help raise the intrusion pressure of the cement in the trabecular bone of the canal during insertion. The stem is tapered to increase cement intrusion pression and to even the stress transfer. The stem is wider on the lateral side to promote intrusion of the cement into the proximal medial bone. Six primary stems, two congenital dysplasia hip stems, as well as neck replacements, and long straight and proximal third stems are available in the Spectron EF system.

POROUS-COATED PROSTHESES

Anatomic Medullary Locking (AML) Total Hip System

Development of the original Anatomic Medullary Locking (AML) femoral component, manufactured by DePuy, Inc., was prompted by attempts to solve the problem of implant loosening due to cement failure. This was one of the major complications of total hip arthroplasty during the 1970s (Fig. 25–10). Given the long-term success of the Austin Moore, a stem with a similar design and excellent clinical record, designers theorized that enhanced fixation could be achieved with the addition of a three-dimensional porous coating that encouraged bone ingrowth. The main concept of the surgical procedure is to customize the internal anatomy of the femur to match the shape of the implant. Improvements in the instrumentation used during surgery have facilitated this "matching of the femur," leading to dramatic improvements in the mechanical failure rates associated with the AML Total Hip System.

For the hip joint, it is imperative to minimize micromotion if initial stable fixation is to be achieved. Also, rotational stability requires a design that resists out-of-plane loads, preventing rotation and thus motion at the bone-implant interface. The key implant features of the AML Total Hip System that help prevent micromotion and promote rotational stability are its porous coating and its instrumentation. The Porocoat porous coating is a sintered, three-dimensional matrix of small cobalt-chromium alloy beads, producing a rough, irregular, graded porous surface that is raised above the implant substrate. Instrumentation includes canal reamers and broaches that prepare a customized, slightly undersized endosteal envelope, enabling the Porocoat surface of the implant to achieve an interference fit. This extremely tight fit is possible because of the forgiving nature of the Porocoat porous coating, which produces less hoop stress than a smooth stem.

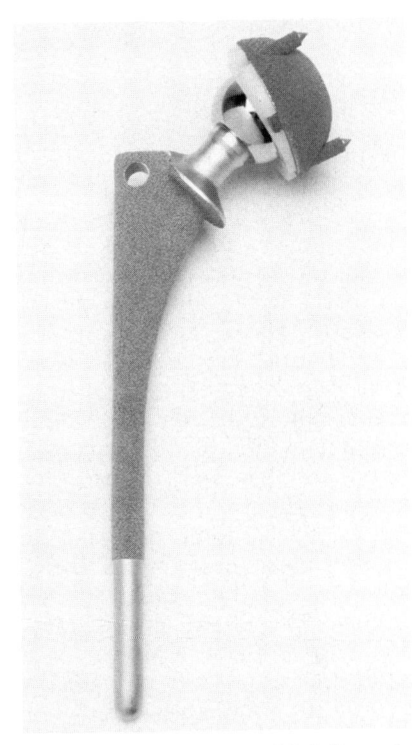

FIGURE 25–10. Anatomic Medullary Locking (AML) Total Hip System. (Courtesy of DePuy, Inc.)

To replicate the physiologic loading patterns of natural hip joints, the offset of total hip arthroplasty components should duplicate anatomic dimensions without altering limb length equality. The enhanced offset of the AML helps ensure this effect and reduces joint reaction forces.

Perhaps the key issue presented to the designers of the AML was reproducibility. They addressed it by incorporating anthropometric sizing into the system. Two metaphyseal geometries, seven rod diameters, three coating lengths, three stem lengths, collared and collarless designs, and modular heads in three diameters allow maximum flexibility in selecting an implant to accommodate the large variation in patient anatomy.

Anatomic Hip Prosthesis

The Anatomic Hip Prosthesis, manufactured by Zimmer, Inc., was designed to reestablish and restore the joint center of rotation, both in the anteroposterior and medial-lateral planes to help reproduce normal kinematics (Fig. 25–11). The contour of the stem matches the natural contour of the femoral canal. Additional key features include manufacture with Ti-6Al-4Va, proximal fiber mesh coating to provide enhanced fixation, and an extraction hole that facilitates removal of the stem if revision becomes necessary. The Morse-type taper accepts four different sizes of femoral heads: 22, 26, 28, and 32 mm. The proximal body promotes a precise fit at the prosthetic interface and provides rotational stability. An anteverted femoral neck and anterior head-neck offsets reestablish natural joint kinematics. The stem is available in nine sizes.

APR Hip System

The APR Hip System is manufactured by Intermedics, Inc. The APR II (Ti-6Al-4Va) stem is anatomically bent for better centralization within the femoral canal and is available in either a standard or large proximal body (Fig. 25–12). The wider proximal body allows the component to be customized in the anteroposterior plane. By choosing the proper medial/lateral size and adjusting the anteroposterior wedge, a better proximal fit is possible. Distal fit is achieved by employing full-length distal sleeves in +2-mm and +4-mm distal diameters. By locking on a sleeve, the distal diameter of the porous implant can be increased to provide better distal fill and overall component stability. A porous-coated medial collar is employed to load and maintain the calcar region. Proximal only porous coating (cancellous structured titanium) for proximal only fixation is located on the anterior, posterior, and medial aspects of the stem. The morphology of the porous coating allows for a pore size of approximately 500 μm (average) and 55 percent volume porosity. A single set of instruments is used to prepare the femur for the porous implant or the nonporous device. The nonporous stem (machined Ti-6Al-4Va alloy or forged Co-Cr alloy) incorporates distal and proximal polymethyl methacrylate centralizers for better placement within the cement mantle.

The same coating is utilized on the APR acetabular shell as on the femoral stem. The cup is hemispheric and offers a unique screw hole pattern for the best access to the superior ilial bone. Cancellous bone screws (6.5 mm) can be applied to anchor the shell in place. A variety of inserts can be snapped into the shell.

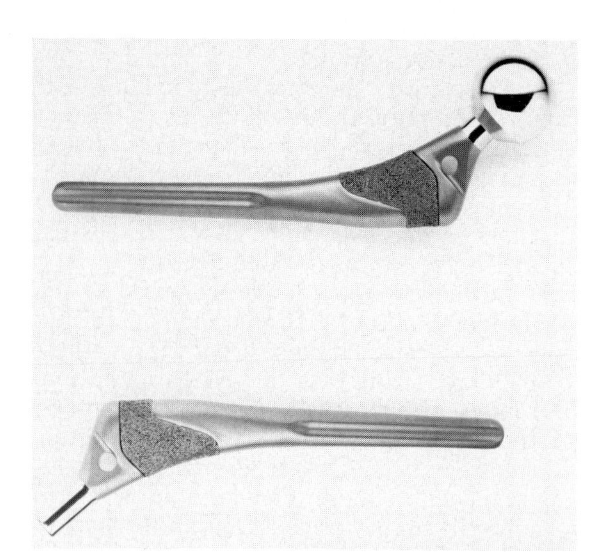

FIGURE 25–11. Anatomic Hip Prosthesis. (Courtesy of Zimmer, Inc.)

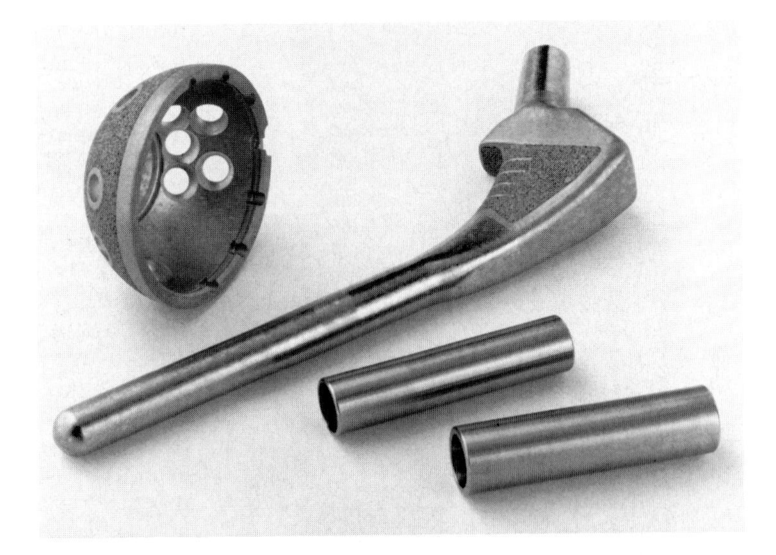

FIGURE 25–12. The APR Hip System. (Courtesy of Intermedics, Inc.)

BIAS Total Hip Prosthesis

The BIAS total hip prosthesis, manufactured by Zimmer, Inc., has a longer, intramedullary rod-like stem to provide initial stability while resisting bending forces. This prosthesis allows the bone itself to transmit compressive loads (Fig. 25–13). Available in 1-mm incremental sizes, the natural contour of the femur can be proportionally determined for optimal prosthesis-to-patient fit. An anatomic, wedge-shaped proximal prosthesis duplicates the natural femur, both in the straight lateral and curved medial aspects. The femoral neck is anteverted 12 degrees. A medial collar provides optimal load transfer to the weightbearing medial cortex of the proximal femur. The collar itself allows for anterior and posterior access if stem removal is necessary.

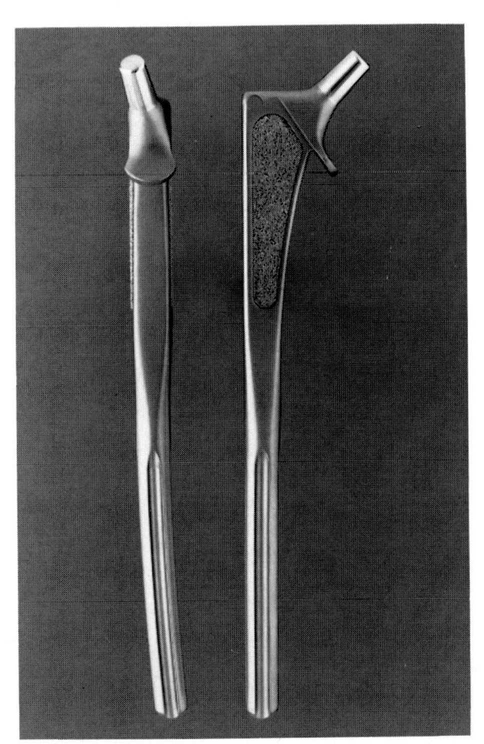

FIGURE 25–13. The BIAS total hip prosthesis. (Courtesy of Zimmer, Inc.)

Harris/Galante Porous-Coated Hip System

The Harris/Galante Porous-Coated Hip System, manufactured by Zimmer, Inc., uses thread-like, commercially pure titanium fiber-metal pads for biologic fixation. They are located proximally on the stem (Fig. 25–14) and on the outer surface of the acetabulum. The combination of advanced materials (commercially pure titanium pads and Ti-6Al-4Va alloy) provides exceptional biocompatibility and corrosion resistance. Additional features include a calcar-collar that extends medially, yet allows for anterior and posterior access if revision is necessary. An extraction hole permits rotation control during insertion and improves revision capability. The acetabular component has titanium fiber mesh on its outer surface and holes of 6.5-mm for titanium alloy screws. The polyethylene liner is available in various internal diameters.

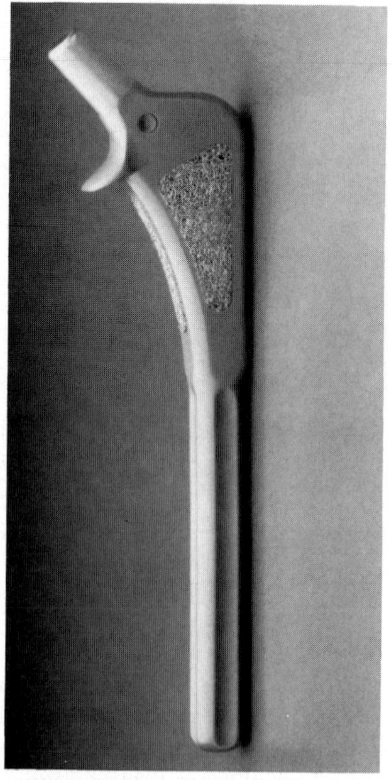

FIGURE 25–14. The Harris/Galante Porous-Coated Hip System. (Courtesy of Zimmer, Inc.)

Mallory-Head Hip

The Mallory-Head Hip is manufactured by Biomet, Inc. (Fig. 25–15). The acetabular component in the cementless system is essentially a hemisphere, with four fins about the periphery. The fins provide purchase within the anterior and posterior columns of the acetabulum and should seat within the dense bone around the periphery of the acetabulum. In osteopenic bone and in revision situations, supplemental screw fixation is advised when all the fins are not seated. A plastic insert can be placed within the metal shell to allow rotation, providing a high-wall ledge for increased stability in the preferred position.

The cementless femoral component is designed with fins in the proximal portion to anchor the prosthesis within the triangular portion of the upper femur. The femoral prosthesis is designed for proximal fixation only. Distal fixation of this component is contraindicated. The stem has straight anterior and posterior dimensions. The upper third of the stem has a plasma-spray porous surface, the middle third has a textured surface, and the distal third has a smooth surface.

MCS Porous-Coated Hip System

The MCS femoral stem, manufactured by Exactech, Inc., is designed to provide modulus compatibility and multiplane stability within the femur (Fig. 25–16). The cross-sectional geometry of the stem is trapezoidal, providing excellent proximal fill of the metaphyseal portion of the femur for better stress transfer to bone. The trapezoidal cross-section also provides maximum resistance to rotational forces. One of the design goals of the MCS femoral stem was to decrease or eliminate the thigh pain due to abnormal stress transfer to bone. The MCS femoral stem's design provides increased proximal stress transfer and minimizes stress transfer in the distal portion of the stem in several ways. The stem has been designed to increase contact surface area, especially with the strong bone at the periphery of the intramedullary canal. The stem tapers away from the bone gradually in its most distal portion

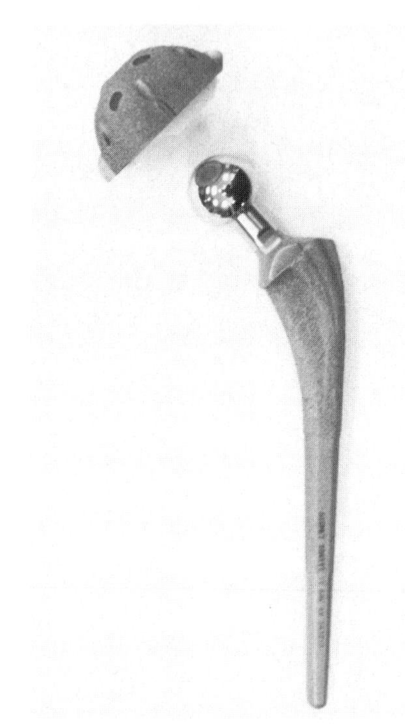

FIGURE 25–15. Mallory-Head Hip. (Courtesy of Biomet, Inc.)

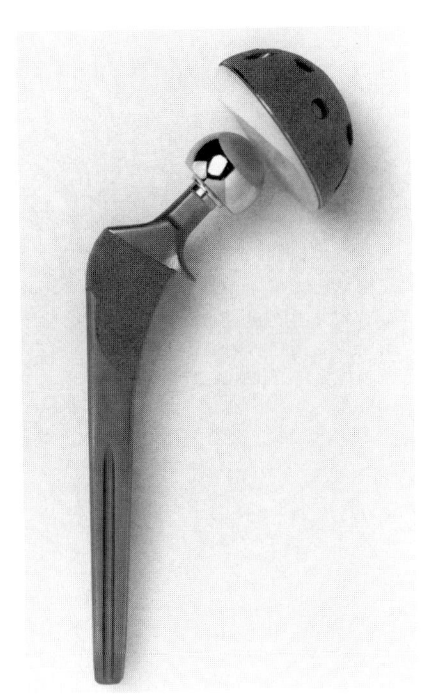

FIGURE 25–16. The MCS Total Hip Prosthesis. (Courtesy of Exactech, Inc.)

to avoid a sudden change in stress level in the bone at the stem tip. Fabricating the stem from forged Ti-6Al-4Va alloy with commercially pure titanium beads provides a twofold increase in flexibility when compared with stems of cobalt-chromium alloy. In addition, the larger sizes of the stem have grooves on all sides to reduce the amount of material used and the area moment of inertia, thereby reducing stem stiffness. The material is reduced further as the stem size increases to provide a more uniform flexibility throughout the range of sizes. The stem has a broad-based collar to provide improved immediate stability and more normal longitudinal stress to the proximal femur. Similar to the Exactech cemented stem, the MCS femoral neck is elliptic to provide greater range of motion with less possibility of neck impact against the acetabular component.

The MCS acetabular component consists of a titanium alloy shell and an ultrahigh molecular weight polyethylene liner. The shell has both central and peripheral screw holes to access the best pelvic bone stock. Peripheral holes accept 4.5-mm titanium screws, and central holes accept 6.5-mm titanium screws. Both screw configurations are designed to countersink the screws within the metal shell. The symmetric design of the shell allows optimum stress transfer of loads from prosthesis to bone. The internal configuration of the shell provides for versatility in placement of the 15-degree sloped roof of the polyethylene liner. The locking mechanism between the shell and liner permits simple assembly and disassembly, yet maintains excellent locking integrity.

Omnifit Femoral System

The Omnifit and Omniflex systems are manufactured by Osteonics Corp. The Omnifit Femoral System is designed to address the problems of femoral canal fill and fixation with bone cement (Fig. 25–17A). Sized proportionally, the Omnifit stems facilitate filling of the prepared canal with the largest stem cross-section possible for improved load distribution over a broad area. An anatomic neck/stem angle of 135 degrees, proportional neck length ranges, and Morse taper heads provide the ability to restore an anatomic head position for proper limb length and biomechanical function. Omnifit systems offer the advantage of choice of head sizes (22, 26, 28, and 32 mm) and neck lengths. The Omniflex system has a narrower stem with distal spacers. Stems are available with and without titanium bead proximal porous coating.

The titanium bead porous-coated Omnifit cup is a two-piece component that is assembled at the time of surgery after selection of the appropriate size (Fig. 25–17B). The commercially pure titanium metal shells are supplied in 2-mm increments and mate with ultrahigh molecular weight polyethylene cup inserts with bearing-head diameters of 22, 26, 28, and 32 mm. The plastic cup inserts lock securely in the metal shell but may be removed without disrupting the fixation of the metal shell, if it ever becomes necessary. Once locked into the metal shell, however, the cup insert must be destroyed to be removed. When the metal shell is implanted at an anatomic angle of inclination, the cup insert can be positioned so that the plastic cup face angle is aligned at 45 degrees of the inclination or indexed in various positions to attain joint stability or prosthetic head coverage. The dual ge-

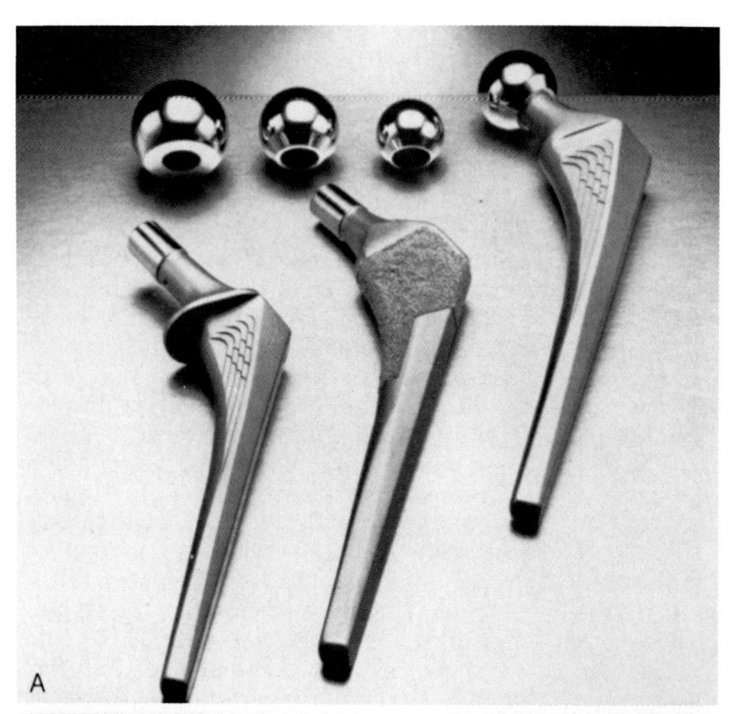

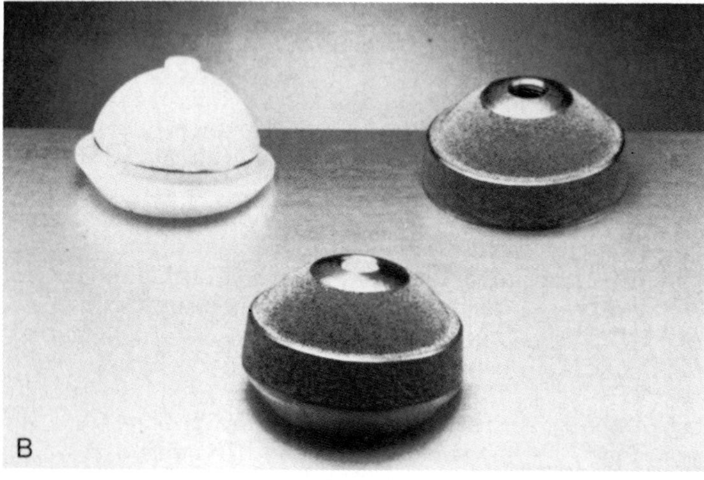

FIGURE 25–17. *A,* Omnifit Femoral System. *B,* Omnifit cup. (Courtesy of Osteonics Corp.)

ometry (conic and spheric) of the cup and corresponding instrumentation allows for an interference fit of the cup in the prepared acetabulum. The reamer prepares the acetabulum to be slightly smaller than the truncated cone of the implant. By impacting the cup into the prepared acetabulum, a stable press fit of the implant within the reamed conic cavity is achieved. The tight press fit offers significant stability of the implanted component against tilting and rotation, which is considered essential for biologic ingrowth.

Opti-Fix Hip System

The Opti-Fix Hip System, manufactured by Richards, Inc., is made of high-strength processed Ti-6Al-4Va alloy with a commercially pure titanium porous coating (Fig. 25–18). Opti-Fix has the biocompatibility and strength of titanium, and a special postsintering process increases the fatigue strength of the sintered titanium alloy substrate. The shape of the Opti-Fix Hip closely matches anatomic contours for a fit with greater surface contact in the medial femoral area. Here, the implant is subjected to compressive loading during bending. Opti-Fix femoral implants are available in 12 stem sizes with multiple neck lengths in either collared or collarless components.

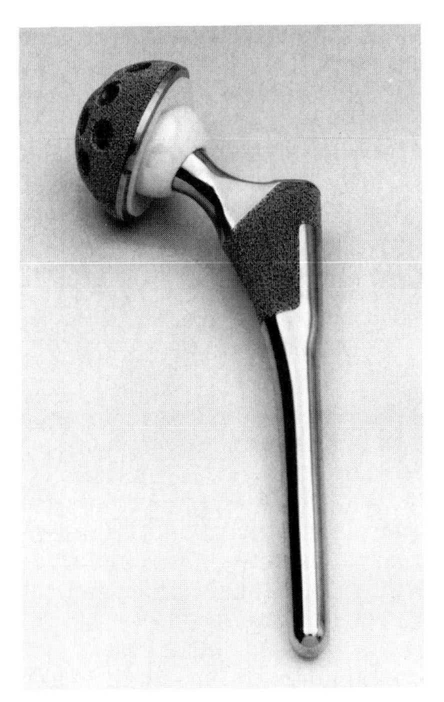

FIGURE 25–18. Opti-Fix Hip System. (Courtesy of Richards, Inc.)

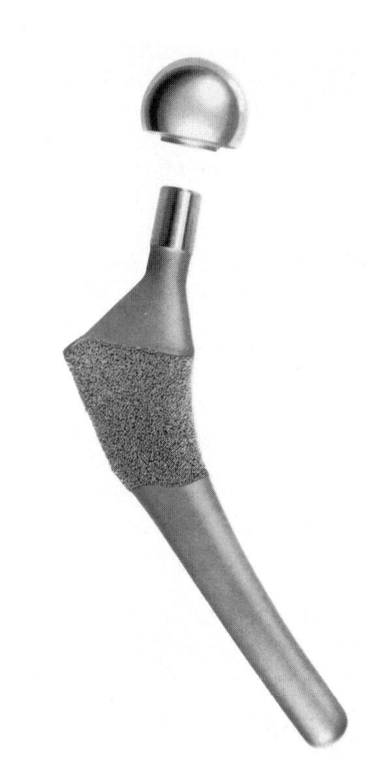

FIGURE 25–19. The PCA porous-coated hip. (Courtesy of Howmedica, Inc.)

The Opti-Fix acetabular component also consists of titanium alloy with commercially pure titanium beads. The hemispheric design closely matches natural anatomy. Multiple screw holes allow for intraoperative flexibility and accurate screw placement. The acetabular liner can be removed and placed in one of 24 positions. It is offered with a 0 degrees or 20 degrees overhang. The Opti-Fix acetabular component is available in 2-mm increments, from 44 to 70 mm.

PCA Porous-Coated Hip

The PCA porous-coated hip, manufactured by Howmedica, Inc., is made from forged cobalt-chromium (small sizes) and cast cobalt-chromium alloy (Fig. 25–19). The PCA stem is porous coated proximally with a posterior bow and an anteverted neck. It provides neck length variations through the provision of modular head components. The stem geometry was based on an anthropometric study and the sizing is not proportional. The shape of the stem is designed to maximize the distribution of the stresses in the metaphyseal region and to resist torsional and out-of-plane loading. The porous surface of the PCA hip consists of sintered cobalt-chromium beads that produce an average pore size of 425 μ. This system has evolved over time to include intermediate- and long-stem hips that share the features of the original PCA hip. These longer stems are also bulkier proximally to better fill large metaphyses and to address proximal bone losses in revision cases. Within the PCA system, several acetabular cup options are available, including shells with and without screw fixation capability.

Precision Osteolock Hip

Osteolock is a titanium, press-fit member of the Precision hip system, manufactured by Howmedica, Inc. (Fig. 25–20). This hip has the same broach envelope as the Precision cemented system but replaces the cement mantle with metal. The Osteolock stem has large integration channels on the "corners" of the proximal stem that engage the bone to provide acute stability. This stem also features a series of distal sleeves that allow independent sizing of the proximal and distal canal. The stem geometry is designed to provide better fits in patients with more varus anatomies.

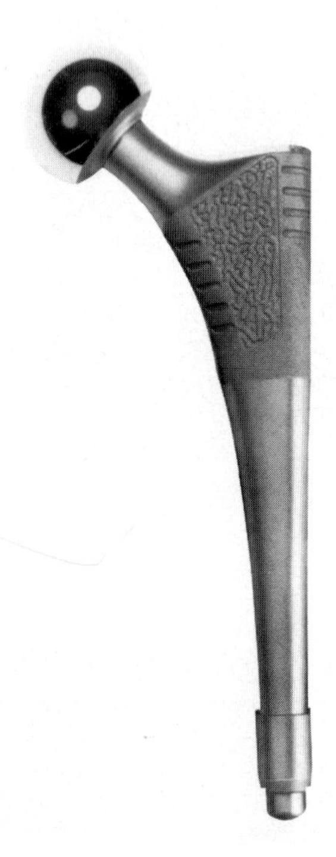

FIGURE 25–20. Precision Osteolock Hip. (Courtesy of Howmedica, Inc.)

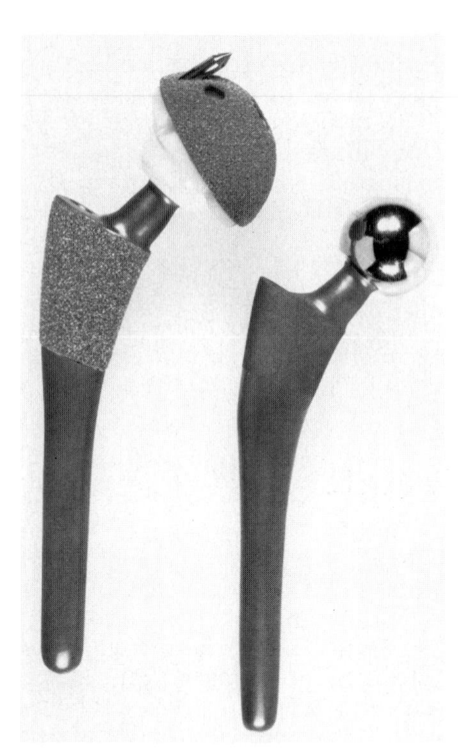

FIGURE 25–21. Profile Total Hip System. (Courtesy of DePuy, Inc.)

Profile Total Hip System

The Profile hip femoral prosthesis, manufactured by DePuy, Inc., was designed as a true anatomic device (Fig. 25–21). The initial design was based on the presumption that a stem shape closely resembling the internal anatomy of the femur, particularly in the proximal region, can achieve intimate contact and stability and can approximate the load transmission patterns of the normal femur. The fit achieved with such an anatomic design, with the emphasis on maximal fill and optimum fit in certain priority areas of contact, should result in increased load transfer to cortical bone and resist not only axial and bending loads, but the important torsional loads as well. These theories of stem design and load transfer are supported by previous clinical studies of various designs of press-fit stems.

The Profile's implant geometry was determined through anthropometric analyses of many femurs. Cadaveric specimens were sectioned and scanned by computer-assisted tomography in serial fashion to precisely determine the geometry of the endosteal cortex. The resulting surface formed the basic geometry of the component. Through a sophisticated stem design program with interactive computer graphics, the surface of the stem was smoothed to achieve a simple implant insertion. Priority contact areas, the proximal medial region and the distal lateral region, were identified as the areas where intimate cortical contact was most important.

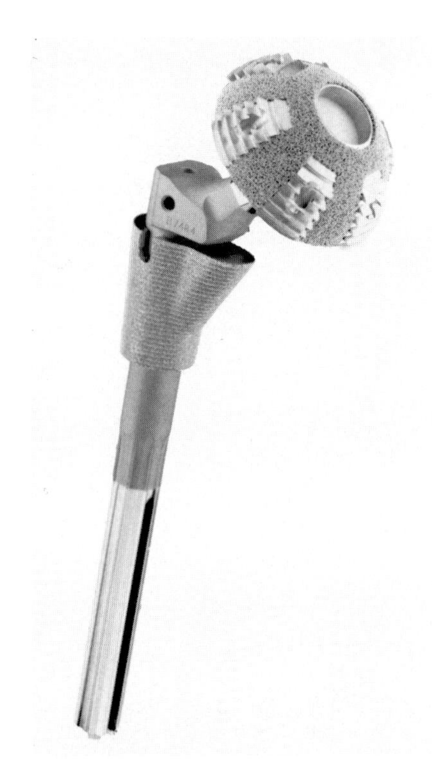

FIGURE 25–22. The S-ROM Total Hip System. (Courtesy of Joint Medical Products Corp.)

S-ROM Total Hip System

The modular femoral component of the S-ROM Total Hip System, manufactured by Joint Medical Products Corp., employs a titanium alloy proximal sleeve that locks onto a titanium alloy stem (Fig. 25–22). Up to ten proximal sleeves of varied size and geometry are available to fit each stem diameter. The rationale is to select a component to fit the femur distally and to combine it with the sleeve that best fits the femur proximally. Femoral preparation is accomplished precisely by use of reamers and milling cutters rather than broaches. The sleeve is implanted first to ensure maximum proximal stability. Because the stem is inserted through the sleeve and is locked to the sleeve by a Morse taper, the surgeon can select the exact neck version appropriate to each patient. The sleeve has a circumferential single layer of commercially pure titanium beads. Steps on the sleeve transmit compressive loads to the bone. Because no beads are applied to the stem, it retains its high fatigue strength. The distal portion of the stem is fluted to improve its rotational stability within the femur. A slot in the coronal plane of the distal stem reduces bending stiffness. Stems are available in varied lengths and a number of distal diameters, with various neck designs. Femoral heads are forged cobalt-chromium alloy.

The several hemispheric designs of S-ROM titanium acetabular component all incorporate S-ROM Poly-Dial acetabular insert bearings (ultrahigh molecular weight polyethylene), which allow the offset to be oriented with the hip reduced. The large selection of inserts includes both nonconstrained and constrained styles. The SuperCup acetabular cup provides immediate skeletal wall fixation and porous coating between the fixation devices and on the dome. The porous-coated Arthopor acetabular cup series includes cups with or without dome screws or with spikes. All S-ROM cups accommodate peripheral screws.

CHAPTER 26

Custom-Made Implants

DAVID STULBERG

Substantial anatomic variability of the proximal femur in humans has been demonstrated in a number of studies. Femurs also vary significantly in their dimensions. Often an unpredictable correlation occurs between the dimension of one portion of the proximal femur and another. This finding is particularly true of the anatomy of the femoral canal as it relates to that of the femoral neck region. Variations in normal femurs are exaggerated by the aging process, disease, and bone loss associated with failed hip implants.[9, 14, 28, 37–40, 42]

Most studies of proximal femoral anatomy have involved radiographic measurement of small numbers of anatomic specimens.[1, 8, 10, 18, 22, 31, 33, 44] Experience at our institution with computerized tomographic (CT) studies of the proximal femur indicates even greater anatomic variability than was previously reported. The conclusion seems inevitable that a large selection of implants is necessary to allow a reasonably accurate fit of implant to bone in the majority of patients. Studies suggest that a custom-made prosthesis offers an improved fit, especially when deformity is present.[15, 17, 30, 36, 37]

Custom-made prostheses in total hip arthroplasty may be cemented or uncemented. Uncemented implants appear to provide excellent pain relief and function when correctly inserted in properly selected patients.[16, 21, 25, 27, 29, 34, 35, 41, 46–48] Slower resolution of pain with walking and occasionally recurrent or persistent thigh pain have been associated with cementless femoral components.[3, 29]

RADIOGRAPHIC STUDIES

Radiographic results of clinical trials show that the remodeling changes following insertion of uncemented femoral components correlate with the design and fit of the prosthesis. When the femoral stem fits tightly within the femoral canal, resorption of the proximal femur is observed; resorption is more pronounced when fully porous-coated implants are utilized.[2, 4, 11–13] Implants that achieve initial rigid fixation by accurate proximal fit may be less likely to produce this stress shielding.[21, 43]

Precise fit of any component requires that its shape conform exactly to the space it will occupy. It must also be inserted accurately. Fit of both conventional press-fit and custom-made implants can be markedly affected by surgical technique. For this reason, careful preoperative planning and precision of intraoperative technique are essential.[19, 20, 23, 24, 26]

Although radiographic studies are essential to preoperative planning for the insertion of total hip implants, the information that one obtains can be misleading for a number of reasons.[5, 7, 45] The magnification of hip films may vary despite the efforts made to control this variable. My experience has revealed that the magnification of scaled radiographs can vary from 115 to 130 percent. This conclusion is based on experience with a protocol involving custom-made prostheses, in which scaled hip radiographs were made by technicians trained to achieve a magnification of 120 percent. The orthopaedic surgeon would not normally be aware of this phenomenon. Templates for determining the proper implant size are generally magnified 115 or 120 percent. Thus, the surgeon could easily make a sizing error of 10 to 15 percent if the source of information were templated radiographs.

Both the apparent width of the intramedullary canal into which the implant will be placed and the thickness of the femoral cortex vary with the penetration of the radiograph. We became aware of this issue when, as part of our custom-made prosthesis protocol, we compared the dimension of the intramedullary canal as measured on CT scan with that measured on radiographs.[5, 6] The differences between plain radiographs and CT scans with regard to the location and extent of cortical bone were particularly dramatic in patients who were relatively osteoporotic. We found that their plain radiographs frequently misrepresented the extent and location of cortical thinning. Consequently, accurate templating of such patients is difficult.

Patients with advanced degenerative arthritis of the hips often have contractures that make precise limb positioning difficult for anteroposterior and lateral radiographs. Yet, if the leg is not precisely positioned, the appearance of the femur will be markedly changed. On a plain radiograph, leg position affects the perceived width of the intramedullary canal, the shape of the femoral shaft, the length of the femoral neck, and the offset of the proximal femur. At best, preoperative planning based on radiographs can provide only an approximation of the proper size and shape of the femoral component that will fit most precisely. The final determination regarding the appropriate component must be made during the surgical procedure.

Another problem is that radiographs give the surgeon no opportunity to assess the cross-sectional anatomy of the proximal femur. Yet research emphasizes the importance of accurate cross-sectional fit in achieving rigid fixation and proper load transfer. With plain radiographs, accurate preoperative determination of the accuracy of cross-sectional fit and fill utilizing templates for the implant system selected by the surgeon is not possible. In addition, these films do not indicate the extent of anteversion of the femoral neck. Although this information can be obtained from comparative radiographs of the supracondylar femur, this is rarely done in practice. Information about anteversion of the proximal femur may be particularly important in a patient with arthritis resulting from a developmental or childhood hip abnormality.

ADVANTAGES OF CUSTOM-MADE IMPLANTS

Because the orthopaedic surgeon has imperfect tools with which to plan and execute the insertion of an uncemented femoral component, it is not surprising that the results are variable. Studies of patients operated upon by experienced surgeons who employed the same or similar uncemented implants have shown that the results are much more unpredictable than when these same surgeons employed cemented components. Custom-made components mitigate these difficulties. Clinical studies suggest that although conventionally made prostheses generally produce satisfactory results, outcomes might be improved if implant fit could be made more reliable and surgical technique for inserting the components more accurate.

DESIGN PRIORITIES

Although it is perhaps natural to envision custom-made prostheses as exact anatomic replicas of the bone into which they will be placed, such components could not be inserted into bone. The process of customization takes this into account and involves the defining of a specific set of design priorities. In the case of a custom-made femoral component, these priorities reflect outcomes planned by both the orthopaedic surgeon and the design engineer. When some of their goals conflict to some extent, design compromises are required. Together, the surgeon and engineer decide how tightly they wish the implant to fit at various points and how much, if any, cancellous or cortical bone should be removed from areas of the proximal femur. Because custom-made femoral components vary widely with regard to design priorities, extensive preoperative collaboration between the surgeon and design engineer is essential.

Implant design will depend to a considerable extent on the materials selected to make the custom component. Shapes that can be made with one material may be impossible with another. The strength of the material may limit the design options. If porous coating is selected, design preferences of the surgeon and engineer may have to be modified.

In general, custom-made femoral components are designed to achieve maximum fill of the proximal femur, achieving maximum contact of the prosthesis with the endosteal cortex. Precise proximal fit increases stability in the deformed femur and enhances proximal load transfer. In general, the stems of custom-made implants are designed to prevent implant subsidence by filling the proximal diaphysis. The design can incorporate the desired anteversion and horizontal offset.

A number of tools and techniques are employed to determine the design of the custom-made implant: scale radiographs, computer-assisted design technology, and intraoperative modeling. The manufacturer uses computer-integrated and computer-assisted manufacturing techniques. The information for each computer-assisted design is obtained from CT scans, plain radiographic films, or modeling. The CT scans are made of the proximal and supracondylar femur with a special protocol provided by the manufacturer. The tapes of these scans are sent to the manufacturer, along with scaled anteroposterior radiographs of the pelvis and scaled anteroposterior, "frog-lateral," and cross-table lateral radiographs of the involved hip. Edge detection computer analysis of the CT scan is performed, after which a three-dimensional computer reconstruction of the femur is made. Parameters that characterize the size and shape of the femur are obtained. Drawings of the femoral component are produced that reflect the design priorities determined for the patient. These drawings and radiographic templates of the implant are sent to the surgeon for evaluation and approval. The design is discussed with the engineer, and any needed modifications are made. Once approved, the drawing is signed and returned to the manufacturer. The signed drawing constitutes a prescription for the custom-made implant.

MANUFACTURING PROCESS

At the manufacturer, the component is constructed employing computer-integrated and computer-assisted manufacturing techniques. Manufacture of the implant usually requires 2 to 6 weeks after the design is approved.

The process for designing a custom-made prosthesis for revision of a previously failed cemented implant is slightly different from that for a primary procedure. Currently, CT scans are unable to accurately depict the bone anatomy surrounding a metallic implant. Thus, the cross-sectional anatomy of the femur—so important for obtaining a precisely fitting custom-made component—is not available when a revision prosthesis is designed. Scaled radiographs must be utilized in conjunction with CT scans to produce a revision implant.

To date, custom-made implants have been manufactured from titanium and cobalt alloys. Their surface treatment varies widely. In some, coatings are avoided completely. Other designs have sintered beads, pure titanium fiber mesh, or plasma-sprayed porous surfaces. Hydroxyapatite has also been applied to the surfaces of custom-made implants. Clinical studies are now in progress to evaluate implants cut from preformed titanium bar stock based on a mold of the proximal femur obtained at surgery. The actual manufacturing process requires only an hour or so

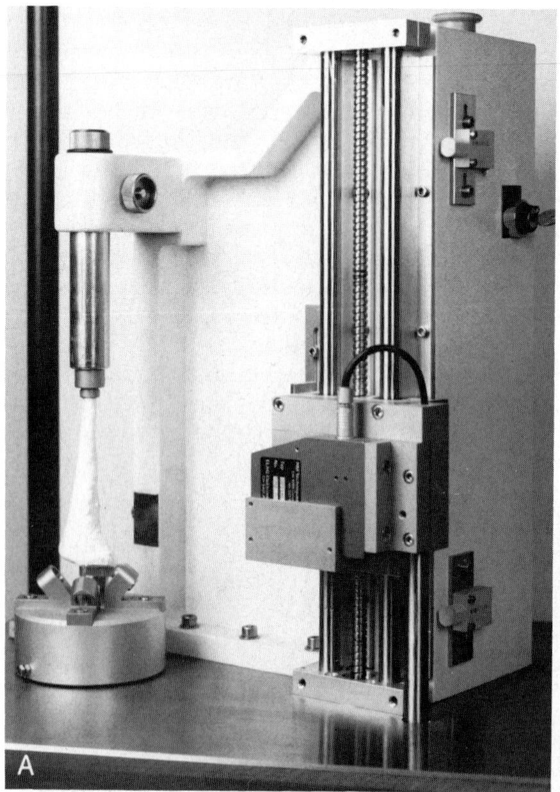

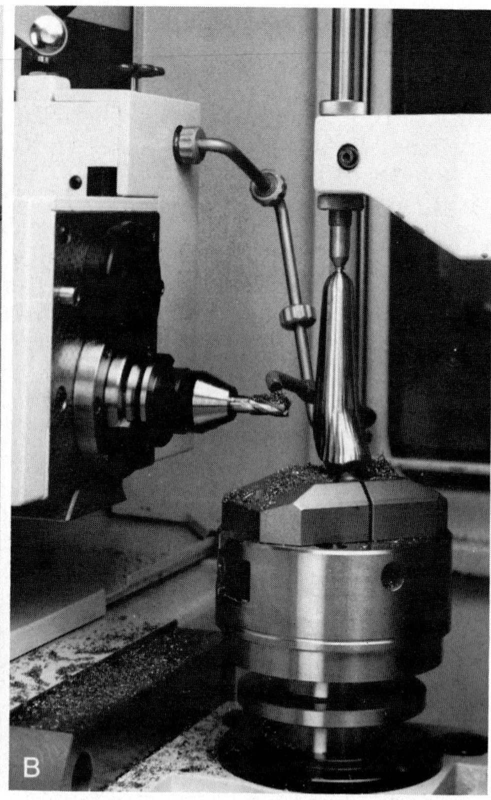

FIGURE 26–1. Intraoperative modeling and manufacture of custom implant. (Courtesy of Thackray Reconstructive Systems.) *A,* Computer-controlled scanning of silicone elastomer model made intraoperatively. *B,* Preformed prosthesis is modified in a computer-controlled milling machine.

and is carried out in an area adjacent to the operating room (Fig. 26–1).[32]

CLINICAL RESULTS

Follow-up studies of patients with custom-made implants have generally been under 2 years. The data suggest that custom-made prostheses for both primary and revision prostheses may produce rapid pain relief and return to function. However, intraoperative stability is essential (Fig. 26–2). If it is not achieved with implant or implant and bone graft, cementing may be necessary (Fig. 26–3). The most helpful current application of custom technology for total hip replacements appears to be in patients with significant hip deformities.

Clinical studies, as well as experimental and anatomic studies, indicate that implant fit within the proximal femur determines whether (1) optimal load transfer is achieved, (2) micromotion is controlled maximally, and (3) good early clinical results are obtained. Early clinical outcomes with custom implants are at least equivalent to those with conventionally made implants. The custom-made devices appear to fill the proximal femoral canal more completely and fit within the metaphyseal endosteal envelope more accurately than do conventionally made uncemented implants.

Theoretically, the anatomic conformity of uncemented custom-made components should be superior to that of ready-made components. In reality, fit is highly dependent on the accuracy and reproducibility of the surgeon's technique. The techniques required to implant these tight-fitting components differ substantially from those required to insert conventionally manufactured uncemented plants. The skills of inserting custom implants must be acquired. The achievement of ideal initial rigid fixation, long-term durability, and physiologic bone stress with femoral com-

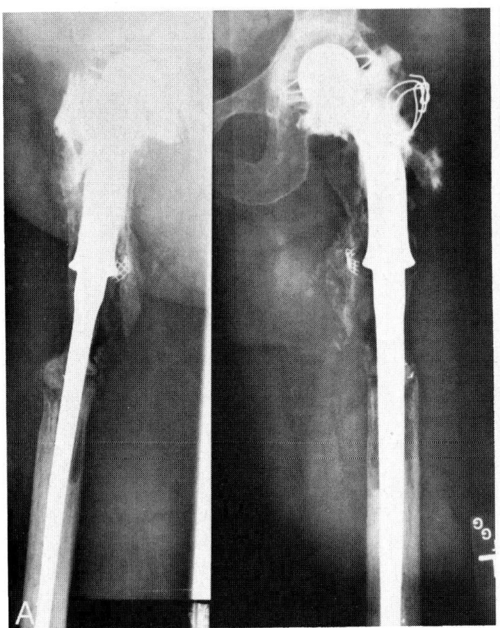
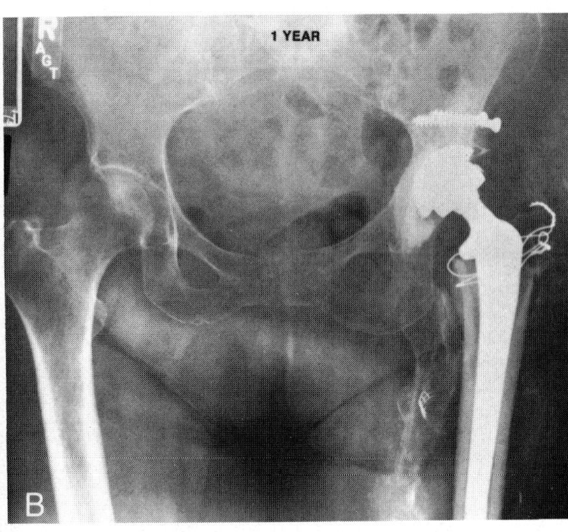

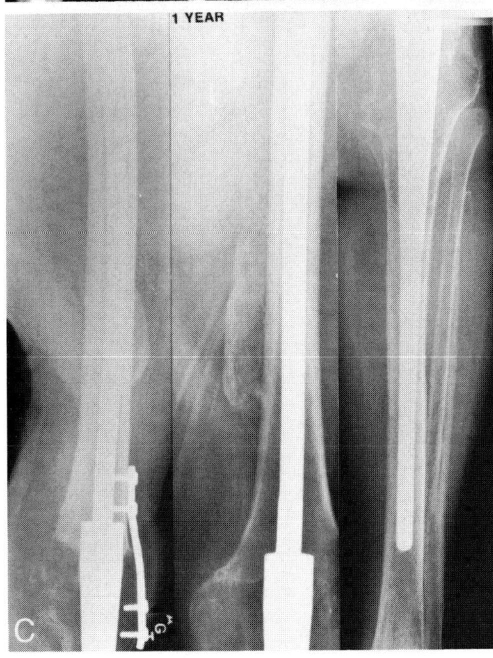

FIGURE 26–2. Custom uncemented total hip implant in complex revision arthroplasty in a patient with ipsilateral knee arthrodesis. *A*, Preoperative radiograph shows absent proximal femur replaced with prosthesis and cement. Intraoperatively, most of the remaining femoral cortex was extremely thin and the prosthesis was fractured in its midportion. *B* and *C*, Limb was placed in traction and reconstructed with custom, uncemented full limb–length femoral component and femoral allograft 4 weeks later. The long stem was joined at the level of the knee with a taper fitting. A small plate was added to assure rotational stability between the allograft and distal femur during healing. The patient achieved excellent healing of host bone to allograft. She has no pain and walks well with a cane 3 years postoperatively.

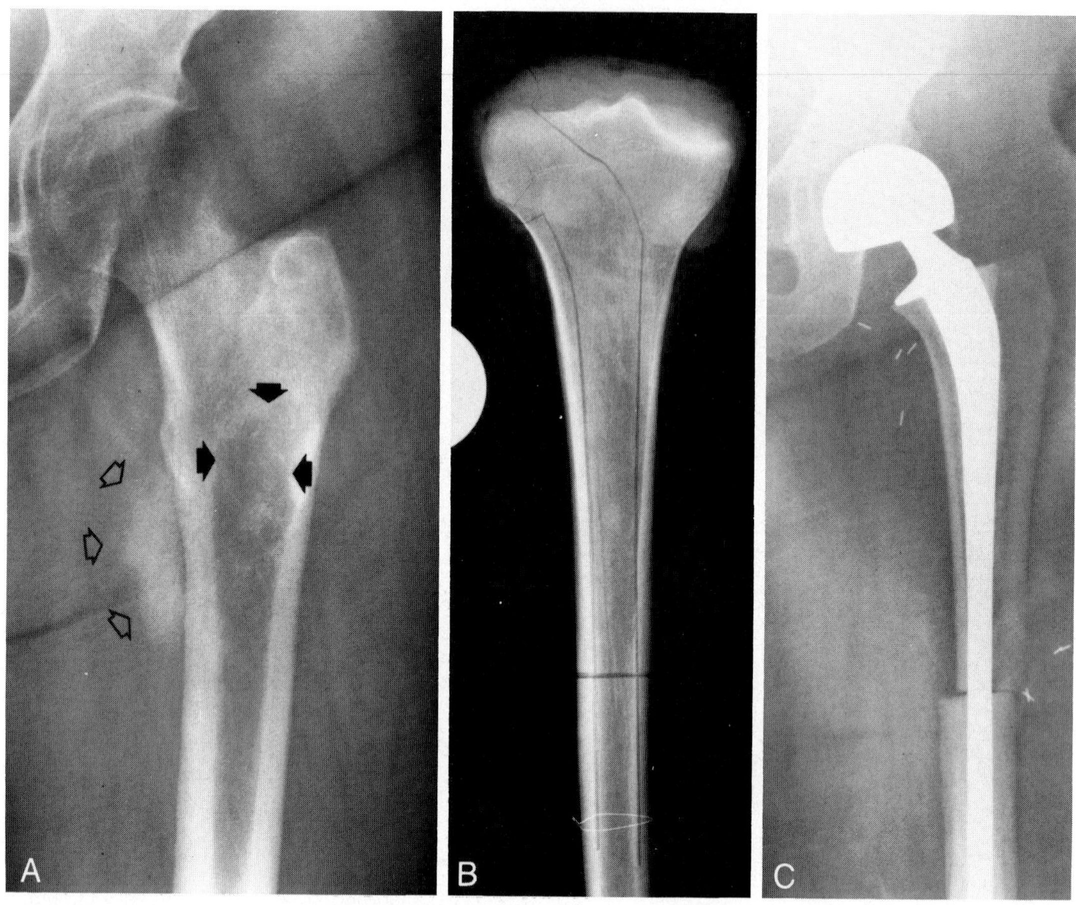

FIGURE 26–3. Patient with osteosarcoma of the proximal femur treated by custom cemented femoral component and tibial allograft. *A,* Osteosarcoma of the proximal femur with soft tissue extension. *B,* Templating of tibial allograft for custom femoral prosthesis. *C,* After tumor excision, the femur was reconstructed with custom cemented prosthesis and tibial allograft.

ponents also demands materials that will accommodate to the biologic environment in which they are placed. The methods and materials currently being employed to design and make custom implants represent the foundations upon which more elaborate and sophisticated custom technologies will evolve.

References

1. Averill, R. G., Pachtman, N., and Jaffe, W. L.: A Basic Dimensional Analysis of Normal Human Proximal Femora. Proceedings of the Eighth Annual Northeast Bioengineering Conference, Cambridge, Massachusetts, 1980.
2. Belec, L., Collier, J., Mayor, J., et al: The changes in stress distribution of femurs with bone ingrown porous-coated hip prostheses. Orthop. Trans. (in press)
3. Bourne, R. B., Rorabeck, C. H., and Nott, L.: A Prospective Study of Porous-Coated Anatomic Cementless and HD-2 Cemented Total Hip Replacements. Presented at the 55th Annual Meeting of the American Academy of Orthopaedic Surgeons, Atlanta, Georgia, February 4–9, 1988.
4. Brown, J. W. and Ring, P. A.: Osteolytic changes in the upper femoral shaft following porous-coated hip replacement. J. Bone Joint Surg. 67B:218, 1985.
5. Cherf, J., Stulberg, S. D., Wixson, R. L., and Pubols, S.: Characteristics of Fit in Uncemented Components. Presented at the Mid-America Orthopaedic Society Meeting, Bermuda, April 19–23, 1989.
6. Cherf, J., Stulberg, S. D., and Pubols, S. C.: Limitations of Plain Radiographs in Evolutionary Uncemented Femoral Components for Total Hip Arthroplasty. Presented at the Mid-America Orthopaedic Society Meeting, Alabama, March, 1990.
7. Clark, J. M., Freeman, M. A. R., and Witham, D.: The relationship of neck orientation to the shape of the proximal femur. J. Arthroplasty 2:99, 1987.
8. Dai, K. R., An, K. N., Hein, T., et al: Geometric and biomechanical analysis of the human femur. Orthop. Trans. 10:99, 1985.

9. Dorr, L. D., Faugere, M. C., Bognar, B., et al: Histologic Validation of a New X-ray Classification of Hip Changes in Patients with Osteoarthritis Requiring Total Hip Replacements. Presented at the 34th Annual Meeting of the Orthopaedic Research Society, Atlanta, Georgia, February 4–6, 1988.
10. El-Najjar, M. Y. and McWilliams, K. R.: Forensic Anthropology: The Structure, Morphology and Variations of Human Bone and Dentition. Springfield, Illinois, Charles C Thomas, 1978.
11. Engh, C. A.: Porous-coated hip replacement. The factors governing bone ingrowth, stress shielding, and clinical results. J. Bone Joint Surg. 69A:45–55, 1987.
12. Engh, C. A. and Bobyn, J. D.: Biological Fixation in Total Hip Arthroplasty. Thorofare, New Jersey, Slack, 1985.
13. Engh, C. A., Bobyn, J. D., and Glassman, A. H.: Porous-coated hip replacement. J. Bone Joint Surg. 69B:45, 1987.
14. Erickson, J. F.: Aging changes in the medullary cavity of the proximal femur in American blacks and whites. Am. J. Phys. Anthropol. 51:563, 1979.
15. Garg, A., Deland, J. T., and Walker, P. S.: Design of intramedullary femoral stems using computer graphics. Eng. Med. 14:89, 1985.
16. Giachetto, J. J., Pasternak, H. S., Gustilo, R. B., and Bzdyra, B.: Two- to 5-year Follow-up of Primary Total Hip Arthroplasty with the BIAS Femoral Ingrowth Prosthesis in Young Patients. Presented at the 55th Annual Meeting of the American Academy of Orthopaedic Surgeons, Atlanta, Georgia, February 4–9, 1988.
17. Granholm, J. W., Robertson, D. D., Nelson, P. C., and Walker, P. S.: Computer design of custom femoral prosthesis. IEEE Computer Graphics and Applications 7:26, 198.
18. Harper, M. C. and Carson, W. L.: Curvature of the femur and the proximal entry point for an intramedullary rod. Clin. Orthop. 220:155, 1987.
19. Harrigan, T. P., Jasty, M., and Harris, W. H.: The Effect of Surgical Precision on the Mechanics of Pressfit Femoral Components. Presented at the 34th Annual Meeting of the Orthopaedic Research Society. Atlanta, Georgia, February 4–6, 1988.
20. Harris, W. H.: Current Status of Noncemented Hip Implants. The Hip. Edited by R. C. Brand. St. Louis, C. V. Mosby, 1986.
21. Hedley, A. K.: Two-year Follow-up of the PCA Noncemented Total Hip Replacement. The Hip. Edited by R. C. Brand. St. Louis, C. V. Mosby, 1986.
22. Huang, H. K. and Suarez, F.: Evaluation of cross-sectional geometry and density distributions of humans and laboratory animals using computerized tomography. J. Biochem. 16:821, 1983.
23. Hungerford, D. S., Borden, L. S., Hedley, A. K., et al: Principles and Techniques of Cementless Total Hip Arthroplasty. The Art of Total Hip Arthroplasty. Edited by W. T. Stillwell. Orlando, Florida, Grune & Stratton, 1987.
24. Hungerford, D. S., Hedley, A., Habermann, E. T., et al: Total Hip Arthroplasty: A New Approach. Baltimore, University Park Press, 1984.
25. Itami, Y., Akamatsu, N., Tomita, Y., Nagai, J., and Nakajima, I.: A clinical study of the results of cementless total hip replacement. Arch. Orthop. Trauma Surg. 102:10, 1983.
26. Jasty, J., Harrigan, T. P., Henshaw, R. O., et al: Residual strains produced in the proximal femur during rasping and during the insertion of uncemented metal femoral components. Orthop. Trans. 12:399, 1987.
27. Levy, R. N., Capozzi, J. D., Levy, C. M., and Lewis, M. M.: A Prospective Randomized Comparison or Press-fit and Porous-coated Femoral Stems of Identical Geometric Designs: Two- to Four-year Results. Presented at the 56th Annual Meeting of the American Academy of Orthopaedic Surgeons, Las Vegas, Nevada, February 10–15, 1989.
28. Magee, F. P., Longo, J. A., and Hedley, A. K.: The effect of age on the interface strength between porous coated implants and bone. Orthop. Trans. 13:455, 1989.
29. Massin, P. and Engh, C. A.: Cementless total hip replacement using the anatomical medullary locking stem: Two- to Nine-year Result Using a Survivorship Analysis. Presented at the 56th Annual Meeting of the American Academy of Orthopaedic Surgeons, Las Vegas, Nevada, February 10–15, 1989.
30. McKellop, H., Ebramzadeh, E., Saramiento, A., and Neiderer, P.: Stem-bone Micromotion in Noncemented Hip Prostheses. Presented at the European Congress on Biomaterials, Bologna, Italy, September, 1980.
31. Morscher, E. W.: Cementless total hip arthroplasty. Clin. Orthop. 181:76, 1983.
32. Mulier, J. C., Mulier, M., Brady, L. P., et al: A new system to produce intraoperatively custom femoral prosthesis from measurements taken during the surgical procedure. Clin. Orthop. 249:97–113, 1989.
33. Noble, P. C., Alexander, J. W., Lindahl, L. J., et al: The anatomical basis of femoral component design. Clin. Orthop. 235:148, 1988.
34. Pierson, R. H., Ayerza, M., Sheinkol, M. B., et al: A Clinical and Radiographic Review of a Cementless Titanium Femoral Prosthesis. Presented at the 55th Annual Meeting of the Academy of Orthopaedic Surgeons, Atlanta, Georgia, February 4–9, 1988.
35. Ring, P. A.: Five- to fourteen-year interim results of uncemented total hip arthroplasty. Clin. Orthop. 137:87, 1978.
36. Robertson, D. D., Walker, P. S., Granholm, H. W., et al: Design of custom hip stem prosthesis using 3-D CT modelling. J. Comput. Assit. Tomogr. 11:804, 1987.
37. Robertson, D. D., Walker, P. S., Hirano, S. K., et al: Improving the fit of press-fit hip stems. Clin. Orthop. 228:134, 1988.
38. Ruff, C. B. and Hayes, W. C.: Subperiosteal expansion and cortical remodeling of the human femur and tibia with aging. Science 217:945, 1982.
39. Ruff, C. B. and Hayes, W. C.: Age changes in geometry and mineral content of the lower limb bones. Ann. Biomed. Eng. 12:573, 1984.
40. Ruff, C. B. and Torchia, M. E.: Diaphyseal Involution in Femora with Prosthetic Hip Implants. Presented at the 33rd Annual Meeting of the Orthopaedic Research Society, San Francisco, January 22, 1987.
41. Salzer, M., Knahr, K., and Frank, P.: Radiologic and Clinical Follow-ups of Uncemented Femoral

Endoprostheses with and without Collars. The Cementless Fixation of Hip Endoprostheses. Edited by E. Morscher. New York, Springer-Verlag, 1984.

42. Smith, R. W., Jr. and Walker, R. R.: Femoral expansion in aging women: Implications for osteoporosis and fractures. Science 145:156, 1964.
43. Stulberg, B. N., Bauer, T. W., Davis, A., and Higbie, H.: Bone Remodelling Capacity and the Clinical and Radiographic Performance of Cementless Total Hip Arthroplasty. Presented at the 34th Annual Meeting of the Orthopaedic Research Society, Atlanta, Georgia, February 4–6, 1988.
44. Trotter, M. and Peterson, R.: Transverse diameter of the femur on roentgenograms and on bones. Clin. Orthop. 52:233, 1967.
45. Wixson, R. L., Gilbert, J., Stulberg, S. D., et al: Personal communication.
46. Young-Hoo, K. and Nam-Hyun, K.: A Comparison of Porous-coated Anatomic and Anatomical Medullary Locking Cementless Total Hip Prosthesis. Presented at the 56th Annual Meeting of the American Academy of Orthopaedic Surgeons, Las Vegas, Nevada, February 10–15, 1989.
47. Zweymuller, K.: First Clinical Experience with an Uncemented Modular Femoral Prosthesis System with a Wrought Ti-6Al-4V Stem and an AL203 Ceramic Head. The Cementless Fixation of Hip Endoprostheses. Edited by E. Morscher. New York, Springer-Verlag, 1984.
48. Zweymuller, K.: A cementless titanium hip endoprosthesis system based on press-fit fixation: Basic research and clinical results. Instr. Course Lect. 35:203, 1986.

SECTION VII

LOWER EXTREMITY REPLACEMENT: THE KNEE

CHAPTER 27

Design of Total Knee Replacements

DONALD L. BARTEL
TIMOTHY M. WRIGHT

The primary design goal for a total knee replacement, as for any total joint replacement, is to restore joint function for the lifetime of the patient. To restore function, the prosthetic joint must be able to provide the motions between the bone segments that occur in a normal knee and must be able to transmit normal functional loads. The motions and the forces cannot be considered independently. If the motion of the joint is altered in any way, such as by loss of function of the posterior cruciate ligament (PCL), the forces transmitted by the joint and their distribution among the various structures of the knee are modified.[6] To assure long life—the second aspect of the primary design goal—the composite bone-implant structure must be able to withstand the loads that are applied to the bones in a normal knee joint. Otherwise, failure of the implants or the supporting cancellous bone or disruption of the interfaces between the implant and the bone could occur. Furthermore, the articulating surfaces must be designed to minimize surface damage, which generates debris. Accumulation of debris in the soft tissues surrounding the joint may contribute to late infection or implant loosening.

The design of total joint replacements must be based on the functional and structural characteristics of the normal joint. This chapter, therefore, begins with a discussion of the normal knee. Specific considerations and problems associated with the design of total knee replacements are then discussed.

THE NORMAL KNEE

Functional Considerations

The primary motion of the knee joint is flexion and extension in the sagittal plane. The motion of the femur with respect to the tibia in flexion is determined by the geometry of the condyles and the kinematic constraints of the cruciate ligaments.

When viewed from the side, each of the femoral condyles may be approximated by two radii, one for the anterior portion and the other for the posterior portion.[10, 32] The tibial plateaus are relatively flat. If it were not for the menisci, contact between the femoral condyles and the tibial plateaus would occur over a very small area, which would produce large contact stresses. The menisci distribute the functional loads more uniformly over a larger area and provide additional kinematic constraint.

As the knee is flexed, the contact areas between the condyles and the tibial plateaus move posteriorly. This motion of the femur with respect to the tibia (rollback) is controlled by the action of the PCL. This prevents soft tissue behind the knee from restricting the range of motion of the joint and increases the moment arm of the patellar tendon with respect to the point of contact.[6] As a result, the mechanical efficiency of the quadriceps mechanism is increased, an important advantage for functional activities such as ascending and descending stairs and rising from a chair.

For functions of daily living such as normal gait (walking) and ascending or descending stairs, the contact force between the femur and the tibia has been estimated to be about 4.5 times body weight.[36] The contact forces acting on the joint are large because the functional loads on the lower extremity produce large moments about the knee. The muscles that resist these applied moments have small moment arms with respect to the joint. Consequently, large muscle forces are required to maintain equilibrium, which in turn produces large contact forces between the femur and the tibia.

The relative motion of the femur with respect to the tibia in the mediolateral plane is very small during normal function. The primary motion that does occur is due to varus or valgus moments at the knee joint, which are produced by functional loads acting on the lower leg. The moment acting on the proximal tibia, which resists the functional moment, may be developed by redistribution of the contact force between the lateral and medial plateaus, which is possible because of the compliance of articular cartilage; by voluntary co-contraction of extensor and flexor muscles; or by stretching of the collateral ligaments.[6]

The primary motion of the patella with respect to the femur is in the sagittal plane. The motion of the patella is determined by two factors: (1) the geometry of the articulating surfaces of the patella and the patellar groove on the femur and (2) the forces applied to the patella by the quadriceps mechanism. The contact force between the patella and the femur is distributed between the lateral and medial facets of the patella.

The total resultant force on the distal femur is made up of a component due to patellofemoral contact and a component due to tibiofemoral contact. During normal gait, the contact points between the patella and the femur and between the tibia and the femur move, and the positions and magnitudes of the contact forces change. However, the positions and magnitudes of these forces vary in such a way that the direction of the total resultant force on the distal femur remains constant: the force is aligned approximately along the axis of the femur.

Structural Considerations

The primary loads acting on the proximal tibia are the distally directed loads of the femoral condyles on the tibial plateaus. In normal function, the loads applied to the proximal tibia by the cruciate and collateral ligaments are sufficiently small compared with the loads applied by the femoral condyles that they can be neglected.

The downward loads on the plateau of the proximal tibia are shared by the cancellous bone and the outer cortical shell. In axially loaded composite structures that have parallel load paths, the component that has the greatest structural stiffness carries the most load. The apparent density and the elastic modulus of the cancellous bone in the proximal tibia decrease distally. The outer shell nearest the joint line has properties similar to those of the cancellous bone.[28] The axial structural stiffness of the outer shell of the tibia increases from the proximal to the distal portion, whereas the structural stiffness of the cancellous bone decreases. Because the ratio of the loads carried by the cancellous bone and the outer shell is equal to the ratio of their structural stiffnesses, the axial load is carried entirely by the cancellous bone in the proximal aspect of the tibia. Axial loading is gradually transmitted from the subchondral cancellous bone to the cortical cone of the diaphysis as the stiffness of the cancellous bone decreases and the stiffness of the outer shell increases through the metaphysis.

The properties of cancellous bone also vary with position in the transverse planes of the proximal tibia. The bone of greatest density and elastic modulus is immediately beneath the areas of the plateau that are in contact with the femoral condyles. In other words, the most dense bone is located

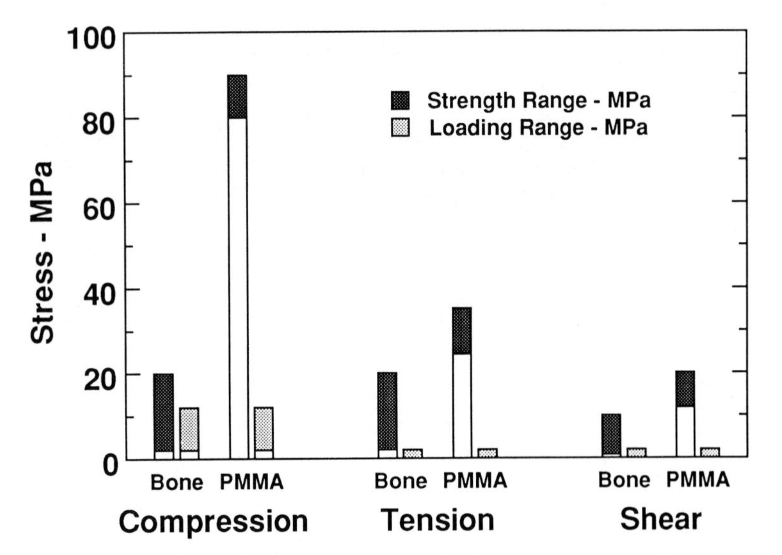

FIGURE 27–1. Strength and loading of cancellous bone and bone cement beneath the plateau of total knee prostheses.

in the lateral and medial aspects, and the least dense bone is in the central portion of the tibia.

Similar to the proximal tibia, the distal femur consists of cancellous bone and an outer cortical shell. The cancellous bone is most dense in the subchondral region immediately beneath the articular surfaces of the condyles. Both the distribution of density and the orientation of the bone in the distal femur show that the load is transferred from the dense subchondral bone to the cortical bone of the diaphysis over a relatively short metaphyseal region.

DESIGN CONSIDERATIONS

Load Transfer

Most contemporary total knee prostheses for primary repair of diseased or damaged joints are surface replacements. The components of these prostheses do not rely on intramedullary stems for fixation. Instead, they are designed to cap the cut surfaces of the remaining tibia, femur, and patella, thus transferring joint loads directly to the underlying cancellous bone. This effect is similar to the distribution of joint loads in the normal knee. Joint loads are borne by subchondral bone and thus are distributed over the cancellous bone of the distal femur and proximal tibia. The load is transferred through the cancellous bone to the cortical shell in the metaphyseal region.

A design goal in total knee arthroplasty is distribution of the joint loads to the underlying cancellous bone as uniformly as possible and over as large an area as possible. The subchondral bone, which serves this function in the normal knee, is often damaged or must be removed to fit the prosthetic components. The remaining cancellous bone usually is less stiff and less strong than normal subchondral bone and thus becomes the weak link in the bone-implant system.

Even when components are fixed to the bone with cement, failure may be most probable in the cancellous bone. The cement stresses under the tibial plateau are less than those that would cause failure of the cement. The stresses in the bone are of the same magnitude as the static strengths of cancellous bone (Fig. 27–1). The resistance to cyclic stresses that lead to fatigue failure of the bone is lower than the static strengths, suggesting that the bone is in even more jeopardy.

Metal Backing

Many contemporary prostheses have incorporated a metal layer to distribute the applied loads uniformly over a large area of cancellous bone. A metal backing is placed between the polyethylene portion of the tibial component and the cancellous bone. The effect of a metal layer can be seen in Figure 27–2, which compares maximum stresses occurring in the cancellous bone beneath a polyethylene tibial component with a polyethylene peg or with a metal backing and a metal peg.[3] The metal backing reduces the maximum compres-

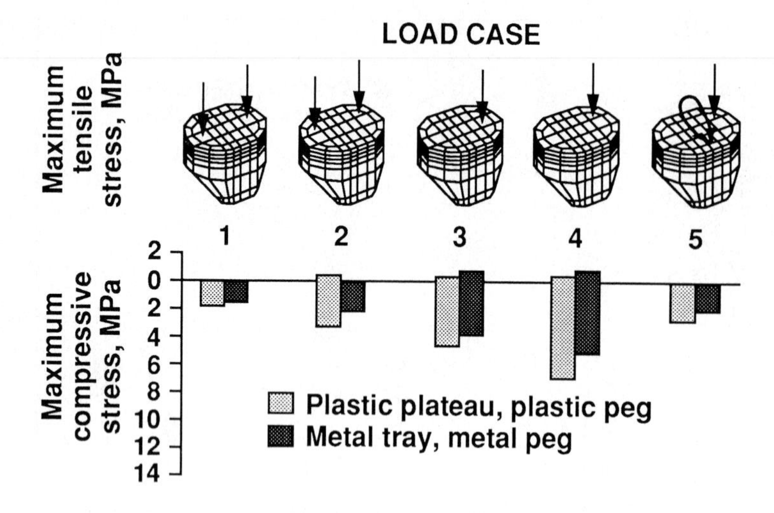

FIGURE 27–2. Maximum stresses in cancellous bone beneath the plateau of a total condylar knee prosthesis for various loading conditions.

sive stresses. The reduction in stresses is marginal when the loads are shared symmetrically between the plateaus. However, a substantial reduction occurs when the loads are applied asymmetrically (see Fig. 27–2). Asymmetric loads are often associated with failure of tibial component fixation secondary to bone failure. The decrease in compressive stress in the cancellous bone is due to the increase in stiffness of the component because of the metal backing, which allows for more uniform distribution of the loads. The presence of a metal peg does not explain the reduced compressive stress. The plateaus are directly coupled to the underlying dense cancellous bone, whereas the peg is coupled to the more porous, less stiff cancellous bone in the central region of the proximal tibia.

Although the addition of a metal backing decreases the maximum compressive stress in the underlying cancellous bone, it also increases the maximum tensile stress. This factor is most pronounced in cases in which the loads are applied asymmetrically (see Fig. 27–2). When an asymmetric load is applied to one plateau, the opposite plateau of the metal-backed component tends to lift off from the cancellous bone. To prevent this occurrence, tensile strength must be provided at this interface. Methods of providing tensile strength include dovetails or undercuts to allow both cement intrusion into the metal backing and screws through the backing into the cancellous bone. The addition of the metal backing also creates new design problems. For example, the polyethylene must be attached securely to the metal tray. A number of methods have been employed, including metal tabs and dovetails and direct molding of the polyethylene over the metal tray. The design must take into account the dimensional changes that occur in polyethylene components while implanted. Yet another disadvantage of the metal backing is that the polyethylene layer must be thinner to maintain the overall thickness of the tibial component. As the polyethylene thickness decreases, the stresses associated with wear and surface damage of the polyethylene increase.[2] Thus, the long-term performance of the component might be compromised. Lastly, the addition of a metal backing adds to cost.

Because of these drawbacks, some surgeons advocate the use of all-polyethylene tibial components for primary total knee arthroplasties with good ligamentous stability. With appropriate surgical technique, these joints can be reconstructed to assure primarily symmetric loading. Therefore, a metal backing would be less advantageous in terms of load transfer. With the development of new fabrication techniques, the mechanical properties of polyethylene may be altered,[21] which may allow for design of stiffer all-polyethylene components and extend the indications for these implants.

Plateau

Although one design goal for load transfer in the tibial component is to distribute the load over as large an area as possible, it is not necessary to extend the plateau so that it makes contact with the cortical shell at the outer edge of the tibia. This shell has mechanical properties similar to those of cancellous, rather than cortical, bone and can therefore carry little additional load.[28] Coverage of the entire plateau is important, however, because the intercondylar distance is related to the width of the tibial component in most contemporary designs. With a wider plateau, the intercondylar distance is increased, which reduces the loads imposed in the collateral ligaments and the joint contact forces when varus and valgus moments are applied across the knee joint.[6]

The discussion here has centered on the tibial component. The same considerations for load transfer apply to femoral and patellar components. Load transfer for these two types of implants has not been explored extensively, probably because fewer clinical problems are related to load transfer to these bones.

Kinematics

Motion during flexion and extension depends upon the geometry of the condyles of the femoral component and the plateau in the anteroposterior plane. Normal kinematics during flexion and extension can be achieved most simply by approximating the anteroposterior geometry of the condyles with two radii. The same two radii adequately represent the lateral and medial condyles.[36] As a result, it may not be essential to provide asymmetric designs with separate components for right and left knees.

In the mediolateral direction, the geometry between the contacting surfaces is represented most simply by a single radius for the femoral component and a single radius for the tibial component. The surfaces should conform in the mediolateral direction, but complete conformity of the radii would not allow sufficient joint laxity for axial rotation of the femoral component with respect to the tibia. This laxity enables soft tissue around the joint to share torsional loading, thus protecting the fixation interfaces.

Neither of the articulating surfaces should be flat in the mediolateral direction. If only the tibial surface is flat, the contact will be extremely nonconforming, and high stresses will be placed on and within the polyethylene. If both surfaces are flat, perfect conformity will occur only when both condyles are contacting the tibial component. Any angular displacement between the femoral and tibial components in the mediolateral plane results in contact at the outer margin of the femoral component, where the surfaces necessarily are highly nonconforming. High stresses on and within the polyethylene and an increased risk of surface damage result.

Rollback of the femoral component with respect to the tibia can be achieved in several ways.

1. The lowest point on the tibial surface can be placed posteriorly. As the knee joint is loaded in flexion, the femoral component tends toward the lowest point to achieve equilibrium.
2. Substitute posterior cruciate function can be provided by an upper constraint spine of the tibial component and a cam on the femoral component. Posterior stabilized designs of several contemporary prostheses are examples of this approach. As the knee is flexed, the substitute posterior cruciate function provides definite kinematic constraint.
3. Cruciate-sparing designs can be used. If the contacting surfaces of the artificial knee are not located properly with respect to the femur and the tibia, the PCL may overconstrain the joint and introduce additional forces on the tibial component. These effects could contribute to eventual loosening. Most cruciate-sparing designs have required nonconforming articulating surfaces for proper function. As discussed subsequently, the result may be higher stresses on and within the polyethylene components.

The anterior cruciate ligament also provides kinematic constraint by limiting posterior motion of the femur with respect to the tibia. This function does not seem as critical to clinical performance of the total knee replacement as does the function of the PCL. Nevertheless, some substitute anterior cruciate function can be provided by appropriate curvature of the posterior aspect of the tibial component in the anteroposterior plane.

Fixation

Fixation of total knee components with bone cement must be considered the current "gold standard." Cemented knee prostheses have long-term survival rates exceeding 90 percent.[30, 35] (See Chapter 33, *Results of Total Knee Arthroplasty.*) Loosening of cemented components, although still the most cited problem, is a rare complication in most large clinical series. Loosening occurs less frequently than in the femoral components in most series of total hip replacements followed for comparable periods of time. Despite excellent results, concern about the long-term survival of cemented prostheses continues. Some surgeons remain reluctant to use cemented prostheses in young active patients. Press-fit and porous-coated total knee replacements have been introduced with the aim of achieving stable biologic fixation.[13, 15]

Fixation between the cement and the implant is often enhanced with undercuts, small pegs, or blades on the implant, which provide tensile and shear resistance. Fixation between the cement and the cancellous bone, primarily a function of mechanical interlock, is enhanced by maximizing the area of cement between the component and the bone. Cement techniques that have evolved over the last two decades include extensive preparation of the bony bed and pressurization of the cement into the bone to ensure adequate penetration. The considerable work done to determine the optimal amount of cement penetration needed for good fixation suggests that little is to be gained in penetration beyond a few millimeters.[25] The cancellous bone remains the weak link in the composite structure formed by the bone, the cement-filled bone, and the cement.

Design goals for cementless fixation are much less clear. The relationship between the way loads are transferred in the initial period after implantation and the subsequent extent and distribution of tissue ingrowth is currently unknown, as are the remodeling rules that might relate the long-term stability of biologic fixation to implant design. Stable initial fixation must be achieved for adequate tissue ingrowth to occur.[9] Devices to provide this initial fixation include screws and pegs. Regardless of technique, a fibrous layer may form at the interface between the porous layer and the bone because of the repetitive motions that can occur at this interface.[37]

Implant designs that rely on ingrowth into a porous metal layer must by necessity have a metal backing. In addition to the disadvantages discussed previously regarding load transfer, the bond between the beads or fiber mesh that make up the porous layer and the underlying metal substrate presents a metallurgic problem. The strength of the substrate is adversely affected by the sintering heat treatment needed to secure the porous coating. Compromise must be achieved between the strengths of the bond and of the substrate itself. Inadequate attention to this problem can result in fracture of the porous layer from the substrate[23, 31] and fracture of the metal substrate itself.[27, 31]

Whether fabricated from polyethylene or metal, the pegs employed in many contemporary cementless designs can be thought of as supplemental fixation. When pegs are centrally located between the plateaus, they are coupled to more porous, less stiff cancellous bone. Little load sharing occurs between peg and bone. However, the pegs do provide additional resistance to shear and torsional loads between the implant and the bone. They can also supply redundant fixation if loosening occurs under the plateaus of the component.

Some press-fit knee prostheses incorporate polyethylene pegs with numerous protruding flanges.[14] The pegs are inserted into undersized drill holes beneath the plateaus so that the flanges deform. The intent of this design is that the small pegs will become mechanically interlocked with the trabeculae of the cancellous bone. Adaptive bone changes around the press-fit component, including bone ingrowth into the spaces between the polyethylene flanges, have been demonstrated with this type of fixation. Small pegs have also been incorporated into porous-coated prostheses to provide supplemental fixation.[15] However, preferential ingrowth of bone occurs into these pegs at the expense of adequate ingrowth into the rest of the undersurface of the plateau.[31]

Minimizing Surface Damage

The articulating surfaces of polyethylene components in total knee replacements

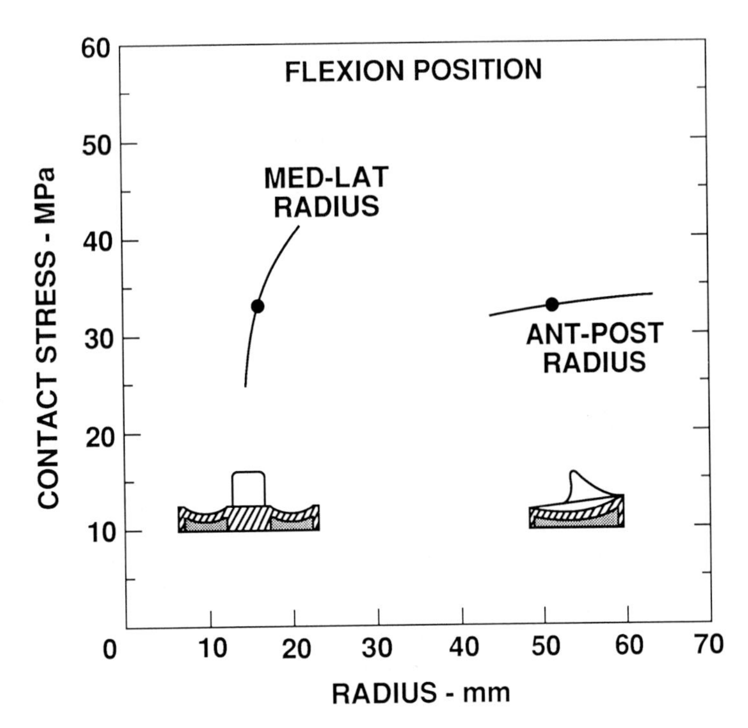

FIGURE 27–3. Compressive contact stress on the polyethylene layer of the tibial component as a function of the geometry of the contact surface.

eventually experience damage. Surface damage is caused by stresses due to contact between the metal and the polyethylene components and can occur in the absence of cement debris. Surface damage generates polyethylene debris that accumulates in the soft tissue and is associated with late loosening and late infection.[26] Nevertheless, a design goal in total knee arthroplasty is to minimize the stresses responsible for the generation of this debris through the choice of the geometry and the material properties of the polyethylene components.

The pits and delamination seen in tibial components are due to fatigue loading,[2] which causes cracks to propagate from surface or subsurface defects. The cyclic loading results from the movement of the contact area between the femoral and tibial components during functional loading of the knee. The stresses associated with crack propagation, the range of the maximum principal stress, and the maximum shear stresses are affected by the conformity of articulating surfaces, by the thickness of the component, and by the elastic modulus of the polyethylene.[2] Changes in these design variables also affect the contact stress in the same way they affect the stresses associated with crack propagation. Therefore, the goal of minimizing surface damage can be achieved by minimizing the contact stress between the components of the total knee replacement (see Chapter 3, *Polymers*).

Conformity of Articulating Surfaces

In principle, contact stress could be reduced by increasing the conformity between the femoral and tibial components in both the lateromedial and the anteroposterior directions. However, for total condylar type prostheses, the contact stress is relatively insensitive to changes in conformity in the anteroposterior direction, and changes in radii in the anteroposterior geometry can be rather limited if appropriate motion of the femur with respect to the tibia during flexion is to be maintained (Fig. 27–3). Consequently, with most contemporary designs, conformity between femoral and tibial components is achieved, if at all, only in the mediolateral direction.

The polyethylene-bearing surfaces of most contemporary knee replacements are fixed with respect to the tibia. Complete conformity would eliminate rotational laxity about the long axis of the tibia, which is necessary for soft tissue structures to

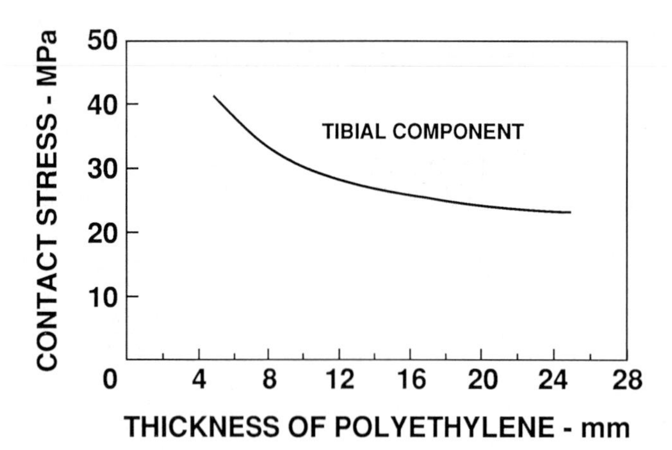

FIGURE 27–4. The maximum contact stress on the surface of a tibial component as a function of the thickness of the polyethylene layer.

carry part of the torsional loads applied to the knee. If the torsional load is taken entirely by the prosthesis, the fixation surfaces may be subjected to high stresses and loosening is more likely. Any design represents a trade-off between two objectives: minimizing contact stresses and minimizing fixation surface stresses.

Different combinations of the medial-lateral radius on the tibial component and the medial-lateral radius on the femoral component can be found that have the same contact stress or the same resistance to torsional loading. In the extreme, the contact surfaces can be flat. Flat surfaces would be completely conforming in the mediolateral direction and have little rotational constraint. As mentioned previously, such designs have a distinct disadvantage if a varus or valgus motion occurs between the femur and the tibia. In such a case, high contact stresses occur because of the high nonconforming contact between the edge of the femoral component and the tibial plateau.

An alternative design option to achieve greater conformity while maintaining rotational laxity is for the polyethylene to conform to the femoral component but move with respect to a metal tibial tray, which is fixed to the bone. Some designs (e.g., LCS and Oxford) include small polyethylene components that slide in tracks machined into the metal tibial tray. These polyethylene components are intended to function as artificial menisci. For such moving-bearing designs to be completely conforming, the femoral component must have a single anteroposterior radius. Wear has been observed in retrieved acetabular components even in completely conforming designs.

The use of a single radius to approximate the anteroposterior geometry of the femoral condyles changes the motion of the femur with respect to the tibia during flexion and extension. As a result, some compromise in the function of the collateral ligaments may occur. This disadvantage, as well as the greater complexity in surgical technique and prosthesis design and the possibility of polyethylene bearing dislodgement, must be weighed against the potential benefits of increased conformity with moving-bearing designs.

Thickness of Polyethylene Component

As the thickness of the polyethylene component increases, the contact stress decreases and becomes less sensitive to greater thicknesses (Fig. 27–4). At a thickness less than 10 mm, the contact stress is sensitive to further decreases in thickness. Very thin polyethylene components are associated with high contact stresses in nonconforming designs. Consequently, a minimum polyethylene thickness in the range of 8 to 10 mm should be maintained for tibial components if at all possible.

The thickness of the polyethylene may be limited with metal-backed components. Addition of the metal backing necessitates a decrease in the thickness of the polyethylene if the overall thickness of the component is to be maintained.

Elastic Modulus

Attempts to reduce surface damage by increasing the strength of the polyethylene have not been successful because they have resulted in stiffer materials. As the stiffness increases, the contact area decreases, and the stresses associated with surface damage also increase. Unless the increase in strength of the materials is greater than the increase in the stresses, such materials have no advantage.

The elastic modulus of the polyethylene also increases with length of implantation. The resulting change in modulus varies according to the depth beneath the articulating surface. This elevation in modulus results in higher stresses associated with surface damage. Because the greatest change in material properties occurs in the region with the greatest maximum shear stress, the increase in modulus probably is due to both loading and chemical degradation. The effects of stress and environment on the properties of polyethylene are topics of ongoing research.

Patellofemoral Joint

In the earliest knee replacement designs, the patellofemoral joint was not resurfaced. In most of these designs, unicondylar components replaced the medial and lateral tibiofemoral articulations and the patellar groove was not replaced. Even with those designs that substituted a metal flange for the patellar groove on the femur, such as the Guepar and Walldius designs, the patella was not resurfaced. Patellar pain was a continuing clinical problem with all of these early designs.[17]

Dome-Shaped Designs

To eliminate the alignment problems associated with separate unicondylar components and to improve fixation, total knee replacements evolved to include bicondylar components. Many of these designs address the patellar problem by including surface replacements for both the femoral groove and the posterior surface of the patella. The femoral groove is replaced by a concave groove on the extended flange of the metal femoral component. A dome-shaped implant fabricated from polyethylene substitutes for the patellar surface. The articulating geometries are simple: one spheric radius for the patellar component and one mediolateral radius for the femoral groove. Contact between the components conforms only near full extension. With flexion, the convex patellar surface articulates against the convex inner surfaces of the condyles on the femoral component.

With the dome-shaped design, precise rotational alignment is not necessary. Implantation of the patellar component involves simple bone cuts and does not require extensive instrumentation. Fixation of the patellar component is usually achieved with bone cement supplemented by a central peg or smaller peripheral pegs and a small extended flange around the circumference, providing resistance to torsional and shear loads.

The clinical results with dome-shaped patellar components have been excellent.[16] Nonetheless, retrieval studies have demonstrated considerable surface damage as well as gross deformation of the patellar components.[12] The components wear and deform. A more conforming shape results. Two concave areas of wear correspond to articulation against the femoral condyles, and a third area of wear across the dome corresponds to articulation against the bottom of the groove on the femoral flange. The greater conformity resulting from wear and deformation reduces the contact stresses and may contribute to the low incidence of complications reported with these types of components.

Metal-Backed Components

Despite the good clinical results with dome-shaped implants, other design changes have been introduced. Metal backing to improve load transfer in acetabular and tibial components led to development of patellar components with metal backing. The justification for metal-backed patellar components is less clear than that for other metal-backed components, because loosening of patellar components has never been a serious clinical problem.

Early results with metal-backed patellar components were poor. There were reports of many failures that were due to components wearing through the polyethylene layer, dissociation of the polyethylene layer from the metal backing, and fracture of the metal fixation pegs from the metal backing.[4, 22, 33, 34] Because of these failures, many surgeons have now abandoned metal backing for routine patellar replacement.

Anatomically Shaped Components

Another design change for patellofemoral replacement is the introduction of shapes for the articulating surfaces that are more anatomic. The two primary design goals are to maximize the contact area, thereby minimizing the contact pressures, and to create a more conforming articulation so that the patella will track better in the femoral groove, thereby decreasing the possibility of subluxation and dislocation.

The surgical techniques to achieve the appropriate alignment between anatomically shaped patellar and femoral components are demanding. Alignment is difficult to assess in the operating room, because it depends on the dynamic action of the quadriceps as it flexes the knee joint. A final disadvantage is the increased inventory, because right and left knee components are required in such a system.

Other Design Alterations

Less dramatic changes from the simple dome-shape have also been introduced. The spheric, convex polyethylene articulating surface has been altered to include a concave surface near the circumference. This contour, which mimics the profile of worn dome-shaped components, provides a more conforming surface to articulate against the femoral condyles in flexion. The spheric convex dome is maintained to articulate against the femoral groove near extension. An example of this design is the Press-Fit Condylar Knee prosthesis.

Another alteration to the dome-shaped patella is a deepened groove in the femoral component. An example is the Modified Total Condylar prosthesis. The rationale for deepening the groove is twofold: (1) to reduce the chance for subluxation or dislocation and (2) to maximize the contact between the patellar and femoral components.

Importance of Surgical Technique

Much of the success of patellofemoral replacements is dependent not on the design of the patellofemoral joint but on surgical technique. For example, the position of the joint line of the total knee replacement compared with the original joint line can significantly affect patellar pain and knee joint function.[11, 24] Similarly, the tracking of the patella in the femoral groove probably is more dependent on surgical placement of the components and on the soft tissue reconstruction than on the design of the patellofemoral groove.

Posterior Cruciate Ligament-Sparing Designs

Whether to sacrifice or to spare the PCL remains a controversial question. The main argument for preserving the ligament is based upon gait studies.[1, 20] In these studies, no significant differences between PCL-sparing and PCL-sacrificing designs were observed for level walking. However, patients with PCL-sparing designs performed better on stairs. Those in favor of sacrificing the cruciate ligaments argue that the surgical procedure is technically less difficult.[8] Absence of the cruciate ligaments facilitates correction of deformity and allows use of prostheses designed with more conforming articular surfaces.

A PCL-sparing design must allow for femoral rollback during flexion. Because of this requirement, most PCL-sparing designs have relatively flat tibial surfaces. Consequently, the tibiofemoral contact may be more nonconforming, which leads to relatively high contact stresses and a greater long-term risk of surface damage.

The design of a metal tray for a PCL-sparing device is more difficult, because a cutout is necessary to accommodate the ligament. Reports of fatigue failures of these trays have stated that the fracture initiates at a corner of the cutout.[27, 31]

Although it could be argued that the inclusion of substitute PCL function in a total knee replacement increases the loading on the tibial component and, therefore, increases the risk of loosening of the component, the stresses on the underlying cancellous bone are indeed no worse.[3] Radiographs show no increase in radiolucencies with designs with substitute PCL function compared with designs without substitute PCL function.

SPECIAL DESIGN PROBLEMS

Periarticular Fractures

A periarticular fracture about the joint in a total knee replacement presents a special design problem. Fracture fixation devices, such as plates, often can secure the fracture without disrupting the fixation and function of the implant components. But if the fracture has compromised reconstruction or if the fracture is located so close to the components that such fixation devices cannot be adequately secured to the bone, revision arthroplasty may be necessary.

In addition to the usual design considerations concerning load transfer, kinematics, fixation, articulating surfaces, and the patellofemoral joint, design goals for the revision knee components must include stable fixation of the fracture until healing occurs. In many cases, an intramedullary stem can be incorporated into the component (Fig. 27–5). The stem functions much like an intramedullary rod, sharing bending loads with the bone but allowing the fractured surfaces of the bone to transmit axial compressive loads. When flutes are designed to cut into the reamed endosteal surface of the cortex, torsional loads can be transmitted directly to the cortical bone. The fluted stem has little effect on the load transfer characteristics of the cancellous bone adjacent to the total knee replacement. Because the rod is press fit into the bone and is free to move within it under axial loads, most of the load applied to the condylar surfaces of the knee continues to be transferred through the underlying cancellous bone to the metaphyseal cortex. If the rod were strongly coupled to the cortex, such as by surrounding bone cement, it would transmit axial load directly to the cortex, but this effect is less desirable. In that case, the stem would substantially unload the cancellous bone in the region of the joint, which may lead to deleterious bone remodeling.

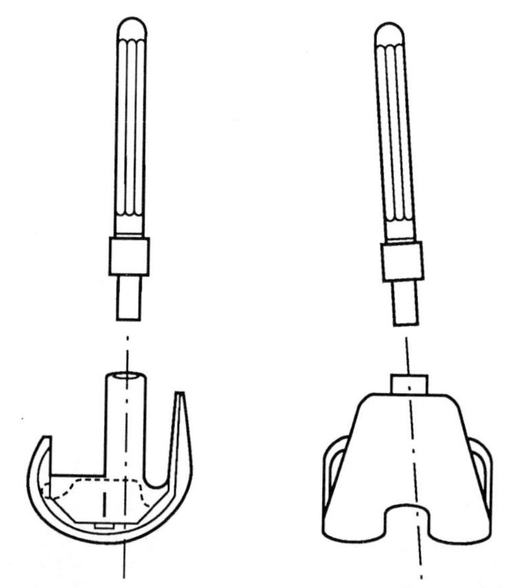

FIGURE 27–5. Femoral component of a revision prosthesis with a fluted rod for intramedullary fixation.

Many contemporary total knee systems have modular femoral and metal-backed tibial components. An intramedullary stem can be attached at the time of surgery. These systems enable treatment of periarticular fractures without design and fabrication of a custom implant.

Ligamentous Instability

The design goals for the total joint replacement of a knee with inadequate or absent collateral ligament constraints must extend to provision of adequate joint stability under the internal and external rotations and the varus and valgus movements encountered during daily activities. Many of the early hinged designs of total knee replacements routinely sacrificed the collateral ligaments. Ligament function was replaced with a linked component. One reason often cited for the poor clinical results achieved with these prostheses is the rigidity of the metal-to-metal hinge, which transferred much of the torsional load directly to the interfaces between the bone, cement, and prosthesis. This problem led to a high complication rate, including loosening and implant failures.[19]

More recently, a spine has been extended between the plateaus of the tibial component to fill more of the space between the condyles of the femoral component. By controlling the gaps between the spine and the condyles, the point at which contact occurs in rotation and in varus-valgus movements between the components can be controlled so that as much constraint as necessary is provided.[16, 18] Usually, the polyethylene spine is reinforced with an inner metal core extending from the metal backing of the tibial component. However, wear and deformation of the polyethylene will still occur, somewhat decreasing the constraint over time.

Bony Deficits

The design of total knee replacements must contend with the loss of bone stock caused by failure of a previous prosthesis or by disease. One of the most common modes of failure is the crushing of cancellous bone under the medial plateau, leading to loosening of the tibial component (Fig. 27–6A). The resulting bony deficit is a wedge-like defect, which must be reconstructed during revision surgery to provide a means of load transfer to the remaining cortex.

The defect may be filled with bone graft, bone cement, cement reinforced with a screw, or metal.[5] Reconstituting the bone is by far the optimal solution, provided that enough graft material is available and that it can be incorporated sufficiently to assume a load-bearing role. Cement can be molded *in situ* to completely fill the deficit, creating a mechanical bond to the remaining bone at the edges of the defect. However, because of the greater structural demands on the cement, eventual mechanical failure cannot be discounted. Metal implants are an effective alternative (Fig. 27–6B), although careful preparation of the remaining bony structures is required to match the geometry of the implant. The metal provides a stiff, strong load path between the joint line and the cortex.[3] Contemporary modular total knee replacement systems incorporate wedges and inserts that can be attached without difficulty to the tibial and femoral components at surgery.

Resections

A more perplexing design problem is the treatment of tumors about the knee. These

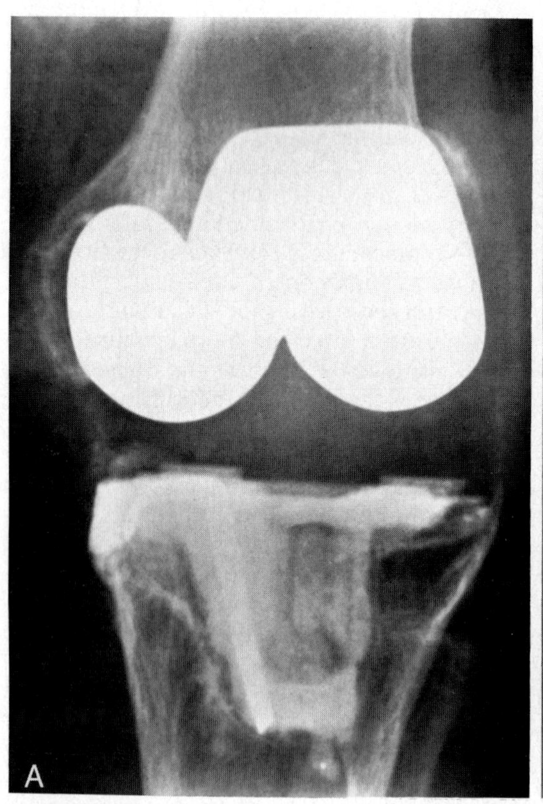

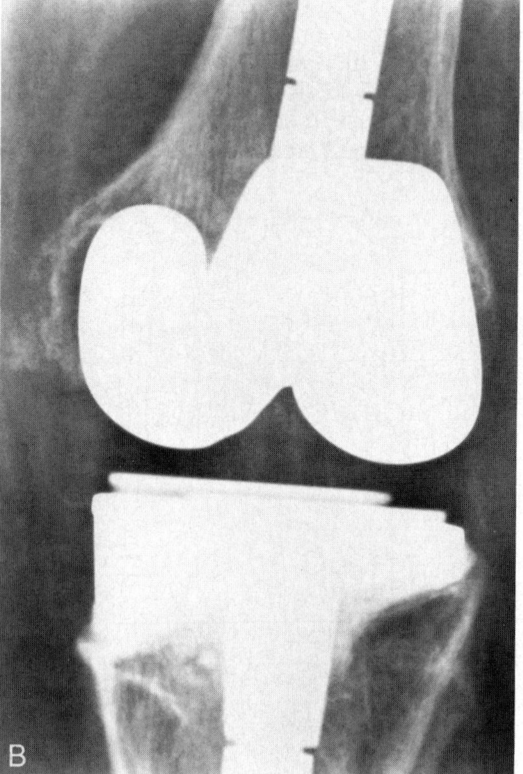

FIGURE 27–6. *A*, Radiograph of a failed knee replacement showing the crushing of the cancellous bone under the medial plateau. *B*, Radiograph of the revision prosthesis with a metal wedge to fill the bony defect.

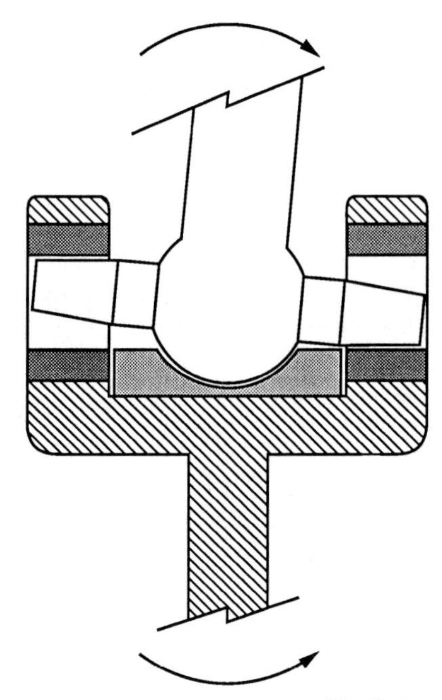

FIGURE 27–7. The bearing assembly that provides varus-valgus and rotational constraints in a segmental knee replacement. (Enneking, W. F. (ed.): Limb Salvage in Musculoskeletal Oncology. New York, Churchill Livingstone, 1987. By permission.)

require the resection of large amounts of bone and soft tissue. The soft tissue resection often includes the collateral ligaments and the main flexor and extensor muscles for the knee joint.

The design goals for a total knee replacement in this situation are quite different from ordinary design goals. The kinematics of the joint replacement must be consistent with the loss of both ligamentous constraint and muscle function. A metal-on-plastic hinged prosthesis can substitute for ligamentous constraint.[7, 29] Adequate rotational and varus-valgus laxity are assured by designing the hinge to allow a limited amount of internal-external rotation and varus-valgus motion, typically 5 degrees, before contact between the metal axle and the polyethylene bushings (Fig. 27–7). The ends of the axle are tapered to guarantee line contact over the entire width of the bushings, thus minimizing the contact stresses in the bushings.

The lack of a sufficient quadriceps mechanism can be managed by placing the center of rotation of the joint (i.e., the center of the axle linking the femoral and tibial components) posterior from the center of rotation in the normal extended knee. Because of the posterior placement, the line of action of the ground reaction force on the foot during heel strike will pass anterior to the center of rotation of the prosthesis. An extension moment will therefore be generated about the knee, and the knee will remain in extension as weight is transferred onto the limb.

The articulating surfaces, other than those of the polyethylene bushings, do not contribute to the kinematics of the prosthesis in such a design. Because these surfaces primarily transmit the large compressive joint load, they can be designed with one goal in mind: to maximize the contact area between the femoral and tibial components. The simplest geometry to accomplish this goal is a ball-and-socket joint (see Fig. 27–7).

Fixation of the component in a bone from which a tumor has been removed requires different considerations than fixation in a bone not involved with tumor. The component itself must act as a segmental replacement for the portion of bone removed because of disease. Therefore, fixation must be to the remaining diaphyseal cortex. The design considerations are similar to those of other total joint implants that rely on fixation to cortical bone, such as femoral components for total hip replacements. If the bone is sufficient for biologic attachment, fixation is most simply accomplished with an intramedullary stem that can be press fit into the medullary canal. If the quality of the bone is inadequate for press fit and porous ingrowth, an intramedullary stem can be cemented into the bone.

To transfer load to the cut end of the bone, to maximize the stress on the cut end, and to maximize the surface over which axial loads are borne, a cone-shaped taper may be incorporated into the beginning of the fixation stem, which is used for biologic fixation. The conic geometry ensures greater contact area between implant and bone compared with a straight shoulder. Special reamers are required to prepare the cut end of the bone to accept the cone. Fixation can be supplemented by extracortical bone ingrowth into a porous coating on the shaft of the component adjacent to the cone. Flutes are cut in the stem to provide torsional stability and to minimize axial load transfer along the straight portion of the stem (See Chapter 43, *Joint Reconstruction Following Tumor Resection*).

References

1. Andriacchi, T. P., Galante, J. O., and Fermier, R. W.: The influence of total knee-replacement design on walking and stair climbing. J. Bone Joint Surg. 64A:1328–1335, 1982.
2. Bartel, D. L., Bicknell, V. L., and Wright, T. M.: The effect of conformity, thickness, and material on stresses in ultra-high molecular weight components for total joint replacement. J. Bone Joint Surg. 68A:1041–1051, 1986.
3. Bartel, D. L., Burstein, A. H., Santavicca, E. A., and Insall, J. N.: Performance of the tibial component in total knee replacement: Conventional and revision designs. J. Bone Joint Surg. 64A:1026–1033, 1982.
4. Bayley, J. C., Scott, R. D., Ewald, F. C., and Holmes, G. B., Jr.: Metal-backed patellar component failure following total knee replacement. J. Bone Joint Surg. 70A:668–674, 1988.
5. Brooks, P. J., Walker, P. S., and Scott, R. D.: Tibial component fixation in deficient tibial bone stock. Clin. Orthop. 184:302–308, 1984.
6. Burstein, A. H.: Biomechanics of the Knee. Surgery of the Knee, pp. 21–39. Edited by J. N. Insall. New York, Churchill Livingstone, 1984.
7. Burstein, A. H., Otis, J. C., Lane, J. M., and Wright, T. M.: The B-L En Bloc Total Knee Prosthesis—Design and Performance. Proceedings of the Second Workshop on the Design and Application of Tumor Prostheses for Bone and Joint Reconstruction, pp. 200–202. Edited by R. Kotz. Vienna, Egermann Druckereigesellschaft, 1983.
8. Corces, A., Lotke, P. A., and Williams, J. L.: Strain Characteristics of the Posterior Cruciate Ligament in Total Knee Replacement. American Academy of Orthopaedic Surgeons 56th Annual Meeting, Las Vegas, Nevada, 1989.
9. Engh, C. A. and Bobyn, J. D.: Biological Fixation in Total Hip Arthroplasty. Thorofare, NJ, Slack, Inc., 1985.
10. Erkman, M. J. and Walker, P. S.: A study of knee geometry applied to the design of condylar prostheses. Med. Biol. Eng. 14, Jan., 1974.
11. Figgie, H. E., III, Goldberg, V. M., Heiple, K. G., et al: The influence of tibial-patellofemoral location on function of the knee in patients with posterior stabilized condylar knee prostheses. J. Bone Joint Surg. 68A:1035–1040, 1986.
12. Figgie, M. P., Wright, T. M., Santner, T., et al: Performance of dome-shaped patellar components in total knee arthroplasty. Trans. 35th Ortho. Res. Soc. 14:531, 1989.
13. Freeman, M. A. R., Blaha, J. D., and Bradley, G. W.: Cementless fixation of ICLH tibial component. Ortho. Clin. North Am. 13:141–154, 1982.
14. Freeman, M. A. R., McLeod, H. C., and Levai, J.-P.: Cementless fixation of prosthetic components in total arthroplasty of the knee and hip. Clin. Orthop. 176:88–94, 1983.
15. Hungerford, D. S. and Kenna, R. V.: Preliminary experience with a total knee prosthesis with porous coating used without cement. Clin. Orthop. 176:95–107, 1983.
16. Insall, J. N.: Total Knee Replacement. Surgery of the Knee, pp. 587–695. Edited by J. N. Insall. New York, Churchill Livingstone, 1984.
17. Insall, J. N., Ranawat, C. S., Aglietti, P., and Shine, J.: A comparison of four models of total knee replacement prostheses. J. Bone Joint Surg. 58A:754–765, 1976.
18. Insall, J. N., Tria, A. J., and Scott, W. N.: The total condylar knee prosthesis: The first five years. Clin. Orthop. 145:68–77, 1979.
19. Jones, E. C., Insall, J. N., Inglis, A. E., and Ranawat, C. S.: GUEPAR knee arthroplasty results and late complications. Clin. Orthop. 140:145–152, 1979.
20. Kelman, G. J., Biden, E. N., Wyatt, M. P., et al: Gait laboratory analysis of a posterior cruciate-sparing total knee arthroplasty in stair ascent and descent. Clin. Orthop. 248:21–26, 1989.
21. Li, S. and Howard, E. G.: Characterization and Description of an Enhanced Ultra High Molecular Weight Polyethylene for Orthopaedic Bearing Surfaces. Presented at 16th Meeting Society for Biomaterials, Charleston, SC, May, 1990.
22. Lombardi, A. V., Jr., Engh, G. A., Volz, R. G., et al: Fracture/dissociation of the polyethylene in metal-backed patellar components in total knee arthroplasty. J. Bone Joint Surg. 70A:675–679, 1988.
23. Manley, M. T., Kotzar, G., Stern, L. S., and Wilde, A.: Effects of repetitive loading on the integrity of porous coatings. Clin. Orthop. 217:293–302, 1987.
24. Martell, J. M., Andriacchi, T. P., Rosenberg, A. G., and Galante, J. O.: The relationship between changes in patellar height and function following total knee replacement. Trans. 36th Ortho. Res. Soc. 15:169, 1990.
25. Miller, J.: Fixation in Total Knee Arthroplasty. Surgery of the Knee, pp. 717–728. Edited by J. N. Insall. New York, Churchill Livingstone, 1984.
26. Mirra, J. M., Marder, R. A., and Amstutz, H. A.: The pathology of failed total joint arthroplasty. Clin. Orthop. 170:175–183, 1982.
27. Morrey, B. F. and Chao, E. Y. S.: Fracture of the porous-coated metal tray of a biologically fixed knee prosthesis: Report of a case. Clin. Orthop. 228:182–189, 1988.
28. Murray, R. P., Hayes, W. C., Edwards, W. T., and Harry, J. D.: Mechanical properties of the subchondral plate and the metaphyseal shell. Trans. 30th Ortho. Res. Soc. 9:197, 1984.
29. Otis, J. C. and Lane, J. M.: Nonmodular Segmental Knee Replacements: Design and Performance. Limb Salvage in Musculoskeletal Oncology, pp. 22–25. Edited by W. F. Enneking. New York, Churchill Livingstone, 1987.
30. Ranawat, C. S. and Boachie-Adjei, O.: Survivorship analysis and results of total condylar knee arthroplasty: Eight- to 11-year follow-up period. Clin. Orthop. 226:6–13, 1988.
31. Ranawat, C. S., Johanson, N. A., Rimnac, C. M., et al: Retrieval analysis of porous-coated components for total knee arthroplasty: A report of two cases. Clin. Orthop. 209:244–248, 1986.
32. Shinno, N.: Statico-dynamic analysis of move-

ment of the knee. Tokushima J. Exp. Med. 8:101–123, 1961.
33. Stulberg, S. D., Stulberg, B. N., Hamati, Y., and Tsao, A.: Failure mechanisms of metal-backed patellar components. Clin. Orthop. 236:88–105, 1988.
34. Sutherland, C. J.: Patellar component dissociation in total knee arthroplasty: A report of two cases. Clin. Orthop. 228:178–181, 1988.
35. Vince, K. G. and Insall, J. N.: Long-term results of cemented total knee arthroplasty. Ortho. Clin. North Am. 19:575–580, 1988.
36. Walker, P. S.: Human Joints and Their Artificial Replacements. Springfield, IL, Charles C Thomas, 1978.
37. Yang, A., Sumner, D. R., Choi, S., et al: Direct measurement of micromotion at the bone-implant interface: The tibial component in a canine model. Trans. 36th Ortho. Res. Soc. 15:233, 1990.

CHAPTER 28

Surgical Approaches for Total Knee Replacement

BERNARD STULBERG
TIMOTHY HUPFER

The long-term success of a total knee arthroplasty is closely related to proper realignment of the knee with appropriate soft tissue tension. Durable implant fixation requires the correct positioning of the implant on the bone, the correct size implants, and the balancing of ligamentous structures to restore good static reconstruction. In the primary knee arthroplasty, difficulties of exposure relate to limb deformity, joint contracture, osteophyte overgrowth, and prior procedures that may have altered the anatomy of the proximal tibia and distal femur. In revision arthroplasty, exposure can be further complicated by extensive scarring within the joint, soft tissue contracture, and malposition of the implants.

A number of factors influence the surgeon's choice of incision for total knee arthroplasty. Our discussion is limited to the most commonly used approaches for primary or revision arthroplasty. The choice is influenced primarily by the surgeon's plans for handling the extensor mechanism of the knee. As the approach to total knee replacement is always anterior, the challenge faced by the surgeon relates to displacement of the patella and attached quadriceps tendon and patellar ligament. The proximal tibia and distal femoral surfaces must be completely visualized without compromise of the patellar ligament insertion. If this visualization is impossible, the surgeon must decide whether the extensor mechanism should be released, and if so, by what method.

This first section of the chapter deals with the anterior approach and medial parapatellar entry through the extensor mechanism, as it is employed for primary and most revision and complex knee arthroplasties. The lateral approach is also discussed. This approach can be used for primary and unicompartment arthroplasties. The Coonse-Adams approach for dividing the quadriceps mechanism and the tibial tubercle osteotomy are discussed as exposures in complex circumstances. Although some variations of these are mentioned, the reader is referred to other publications for more extensive reviews of surgical exposures for the knee.[14, 16, 28]

In contrast to hip arthroplasty, in which the hip joint is deeply set and surrounded by many muscle groups, the knee joint is close to the skin and poorly covered by well-vascularized tissues. As a result, promotion of wound healing and avoidance of infection assume even greater importance. Operating room environment, laminar flow, perioperative skin handling, and surgeon and assistants' positioning must be considered.[10, 25] The surgeon also needs to be aware of any problems identified during the preoperative planning that will influence incision placement for the approach. Approaches that disrupt the quadriceps mechanism in some way often require modifications in postoperative rehabilitation. Prior injuries to the knee, including past surgeries, may have resulted in soft tissue loss, bony deformity, or implant placement of either internal fixation devices or prostheses that may hamper the surgeon's ability to approach the knee joint in standard ways. Plastic surgery may be needed in some situations.[6] Correction of deformity or exposure of the knee may displace soft tissues in such a way that closure is not possible without muscle transposition, particularly when trauma has caused soft tissue loss along the medial tibia or when severe varus deformity is evident.[6, 30] In addition to addressing soft tissue problems related to skin and subcutaneous tissues, the surgeon must consider problems due to muscle compromise, vascular insufficiency (either arterial or venous), nerve compromise, and tendon or ligamentous deficiency. Chapter 29, *Indications and Preoperative Planning for Total Knee Arthroplasty,* includes a more detailed discussion of these concerns.

This chapter also includes a discussion of the concepts of bone resection and ligament balancing. Although there are universally accepted surgical goals for primary and revision total knee arthroplasty, there are areas of controversy as well. In the following section we discuss "generic" concepts, pointing out areas in which the surgeon's philosophy, preference, and familiarity with an approach are most important.

SURGICAL APPROACHES

Many possibilities exist for placement of skin incisions. However, any incision must be placed so that it properly incorporates or avoids prior incisions. After the quadriceps tendon is exposed, the joint may be entered through a medial or lateral parapatellar incision. To facilitate exposure, a tibial tubercle osteotomy or proximal quadriceps turndown (Coonse-Adams) approach may be necessary.

Medial Parapatellar Approach

The three variations to the medial parapatellar arthrotomy are as follows: (1) a slightly medial incision in the quadriceps tendon (Fig. 28–1), (2) a more midline quadriceps tendon incision, and (3) an approach along the inferomedial border of the vastus medialis.[1] The medial parapatellar arthrotomy may be employed with a lateral skin incision. However, this maneuver requires an extensive subcutaneous dissection.

The incision starts in the quadriceps tendon and proceeds distally near to the patella, sweeping around the proximal medial margin. The incision must stay close enough to the patella so that tendinous tissue is present on the medial side. If the incision at the superomedial margin of the patella enters the vastus medialis muscle, the repair will be weakened. It is better to remain close to the patella and, if necessary, repair this tissue through drill holes than to preclude good tendon repair. The capsular incision proceeds distally along the medial border of the patellar tendon. The proximal medial tibia is subperiosteally exposed. At the anterolateral aspect of the tibia, the surgeon works deep to the patellar tendon where the major obstacle

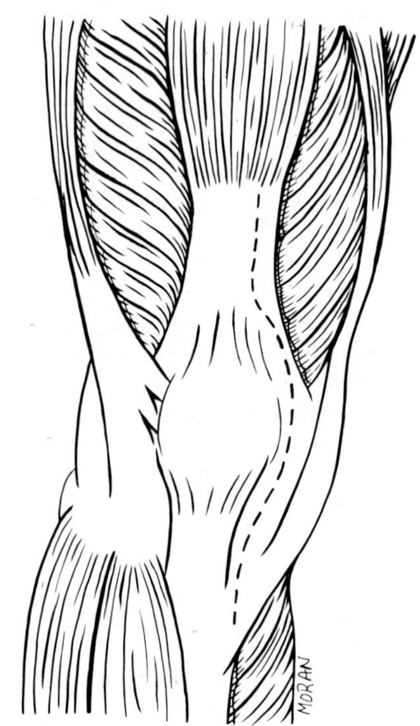

FIGURE 28–1. The standard approach for total knee arthroplasty involves a longitudinal incision in the medial portion of the quadriceps tendon and sweeps around the medial border of the patella and then along the medial border of the patellar tendon.

is retraction of the fat pad. No strong capsular attachment requires elevation laterally. Usually it is unnecessary to remove the fat pad or release a portion of the insertion of the patellar tendon. If the fat pad is large and redundant, the portion adjacent to the joint may be excised. The patella is retracted anterolaterally and the lateral gutter palpated for synovial scarring extending from the patella to the femoral condyle that can be released. If synovectomy is necessary, the synovium should be removed at this time and the underlying fat left intact. The patella is then everted and the knee flexed. Osteophytes are removed (Fig. 28–2). Soft tissue should be released enough to allow placement of the total knee alignment guides required for making the bone cuts. After the total knee components are inserted, closure of the quadriceps mechanism is performed, usually done over suction drainage. Sutures that are slowly resorbable or nonresorbable should be used.

The medial parapatellar approach offers adequate exposure of the knee for performing total knee replacement. However, the inferomedial geniculate artery may be sacrificed. Displacement of the patella laterally may be awkward, and lateral tibial exposure can be difficult in valgus knees or in knees with prior proximal tibial osteotomies. The infrapatellar branch of the saphenous nerve may require sacrifice. Although this may result in neuroma formation, denervation in the skin area is usually well tolerated.

Lateral Parapatellar Approach

In the lateral parapatellar approach, the incision begins proximally in the quadriceps tendon and extends to the superolateral pole of the patella (Fig. 28–3). Following around the patella, it is taken distally along the lateral border of the patellar tendon, sacrificing the superior and inferior lateral geniculate artery contributions to the patella. A longer incision in the quadriceps tendon may be necessary to mobilize the patella medially. After arthrotomy, the proximal medial and lateral tibia is exposed and osteophytes are removed. The knee is then flexed with the patella everted medially.

For valgus knees, this approach allows excellent exposure of the lateral tibial and femoral surfaces. If the skin incision necessitates a lateral approach, a lateral arthrotomy may minimize any subcutaneous dissection that is necessary. A major disadvantage with this exposure is the difficulty in mobilizing the patella medially. Also, most surgeons are relatively unfamiliar with this approach. Although patellar tracking may be improved through release of the lateral tissues, compromise of the blood supply with subsequent necrosis of the patella may accompany sacrifice of

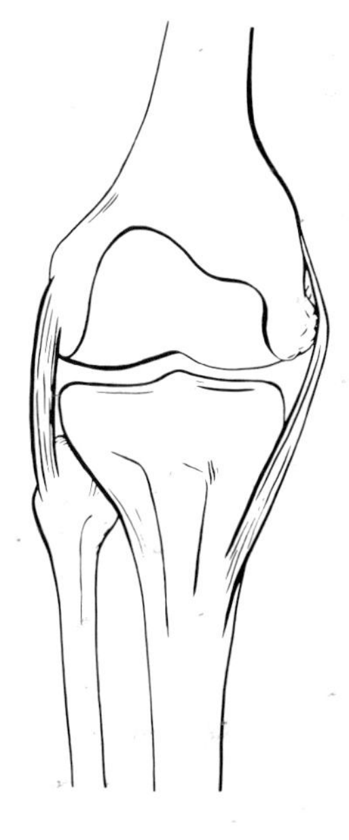

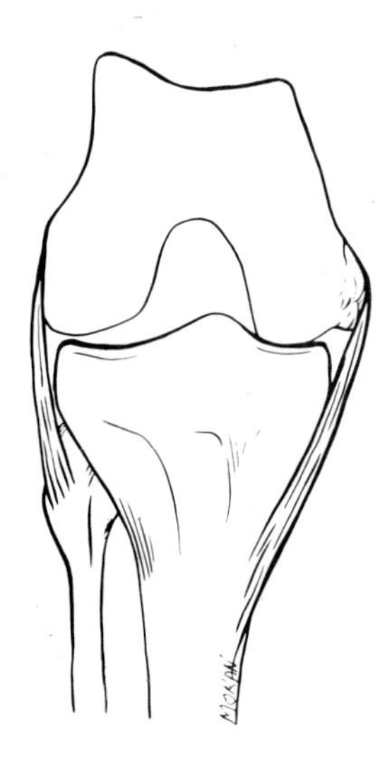

FIGURE 28–2. Osteophytes along the joint border may cause increased tension in the ligaments, resulting in difficulty providing ligamentous balance. These osteophytes must be removed.

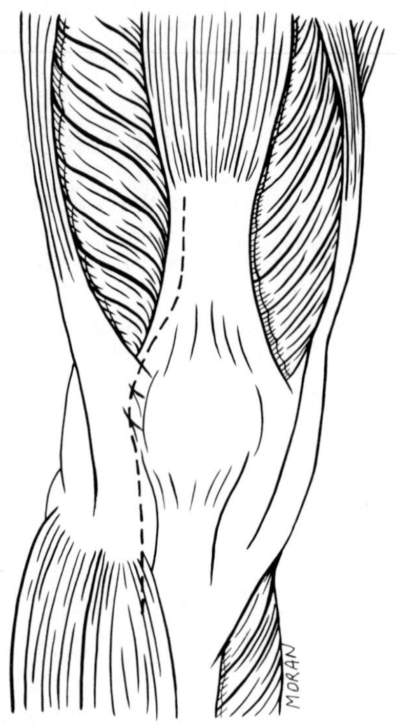

FIGURE 28–3. The lateral approach for total knee arthroplasty involves a longitudinal incision in the lateral portion of the quadriceps tendon and sweeps around the lateral border of the patella and then along the lateral border of the patellar tendon.

the contributions of the superior and inferior lateral geniculate arteries to the patellar.

Tibial Tubercle Osteotomy

After either medial or lateral parapatellar arthrotomy, a tibial tubercle osteotomy (Fig. 28–4) may be employed to displace the patella safely while distal femoral and proximal tibial bone resections are performed.[33] If the medial parapatellar approach is utilized, the fascia and muscle attachments laterally should be maintained. Osteotomy is performed after holes for repair are predrilled in the tubercle. An oscillating saw may be used, or multiple drill holes may be made and connected through the use of an osteotome.[16, 31] Fixation is performed with wires or screws placed in lag fashion. Postoperatively, the knee is placed in an immobilizer. The patient is allowed to do active and passive flexion but not active extension for up to 6 weeks.

This approach substantially improves visualization of the distal femoral and proximal tibial surfaces in markedly scarred knees. A disadvantage of the approach is that loss of fixation of the tibial tubercle can lead to a poor clinical result. In addition, rehabilitation is slowed and the overall functional gain from the knee arthroplasty may be compromised. A major concern with the tubercle osteotomy is maintenance of integrity of the patellar tendon attachment. One must obtain secure fixation to a fragment of suitable size to minimize loss of integrity.

Coonse-Adams Approach

The Coonse-Adams approach is also selected to facilitate exposure in knees with severe fibrosis (see Fig. 30–20).[5, 26] In this procedure, an oblique incision is made along the lateral border of the quadriceps and directed in a distolateral direction. The patella is "turned down," allowing direct *en face* visualization of the distal femur and proximal tibia. Closure is performed by direct suture apposition of the remaining tendon ends and may be adjusted to modify the arc of knee motion.

This approach facilitates exposure and does not require bone-to-bone healing in the postoperative period. It also allows adjustment of the tight quadriceps mechanism to increase flexion. However, the vascular supply to the quadriceps tendon is disrupted, sometimes leading to necrosis and subsequent wound complications. In addition, it weakens the quadriceps mechanism. Often, several months are needed to overcome this weakness.

SURGICAL GOALS

The long-term success of total knee arthroplasty depends on restoration of limb alignment and proper soft tissue tension at the time of the procedure. When these two goals are accomplished, the longevity of the arthroplasty becomes predictable, and prosthetic survival rates greater than 90 percent at 10 or more years can be expected.[22, 29] Functional improvement is less predictable, however, and relates to such variables as implant design, implant technique, soft tissue integrity about the

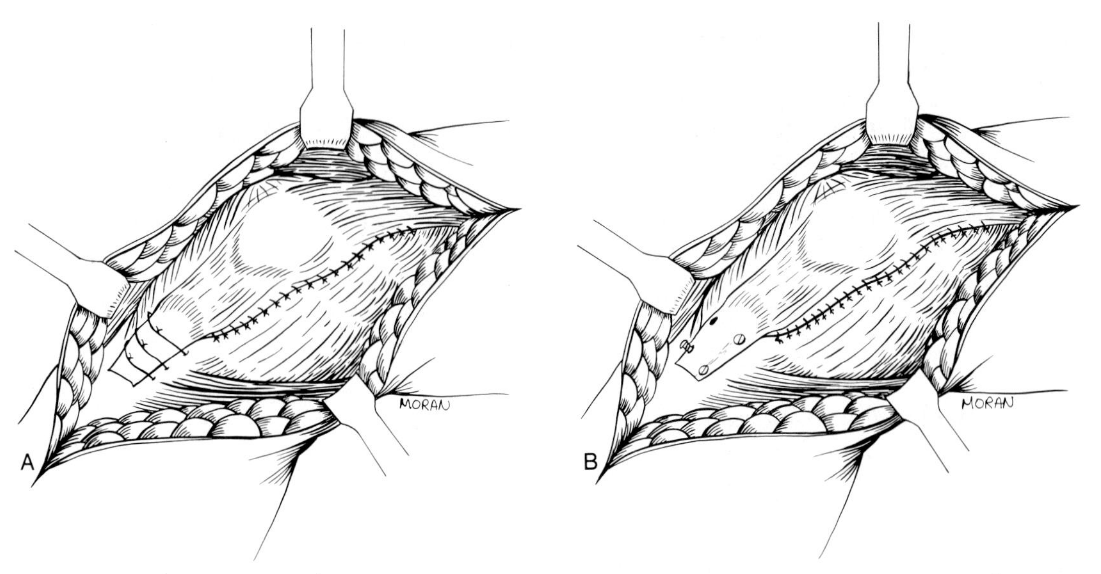

FIGURE 28–4. Fixation of the tibial tubercle after osteotomy. *A*, Fixation with wires. *B*, Fixation with screws.

knee, and patient motivation. The variables suggest that the longevity of the arthroplasty is almost entirely dependent upon technical factors of implantation. The six critical elements of technique are as follows:[15, 21] (1) proper instrumentation and understanding/familiarity with its use; (2) minimal bone resection, particularly of the proximal tibia; (3) resection of tibial and femoral surfaces at right angles (or within 3 degrees) to their respective mechanical axes;[13] (4) restoration of the joint line at anatomic levels to avoid tissue placement in abnormally stretched or shortened positions; (5) maintenance of soft tissue tension, equal in varus-valgus and anteroposterior stress in both flexion and extension (static stability); and (6) restoration of patellofemoral alignment to allow for proper extensor mechanism function. Each of these is discussed briefly.

Instrumentation

Instrumentation systems allow the surgeon to accomplish proper resection of bone and appropriate tension within the ligaments once the resection has been completed. These goals can be met in a number of ways, some of them influenced by implant style. Basically, however, there are bone resections that (1) align the implant, (2) space the implant to provide equal soft tissue tension in flexion and extension, and (3) shape the bones to allow proper sizing and seating of the implant. Resections of the distal femur and the proximal tibia in the anteroposterior plane are critical to restoration of limb alignment. Intramedullary and extramedullary guide systems allow the surgeon to identify landmarks that align these resections properly. Resections of the patellar surface must be in the correct alignment to facilitate restoration of proper patellofemoral tracking. Posterior femoral resection must accomplish two goals: (1) achieve correct rotational alignment of the femoral component and (2) achieve needed thickness to provide stability of the knee in flexion. In systems in which resection of the proximal tibia is done first and the tibial resection is used as a guide to posterior femoral resection, the amount of posterior femoral bone removed will vary. With this approach, the goal is to align the posterior resection parallel to the plane of the tibial resection. This resection should not be performed until soft tissue balancing has been accomplished. For systems in which distal femoral resection is done first, measured amounts of distal and posterior femoral bone are removed. Rotational alignment of the femoral component is achieved independently from tibial resection and is often performed before soft tissue balancing has been completed. For kinematic purposes, the surgeon's approach to resection and implantation will vary, depending on the implant design. For example, in some designs the posterior cruciate is retained and in others it is sacrificed. Anterior femur resections and chamfer resections and the depth of patellar resection are done to accommodate the size and internal architecture of the implants. Bone preservation is usually a goal of such resections, and instruments that determine the height and depth of resection are available and mated with appropriate cutting blocks and surfaces.

Instruments help the surgeon test proper tensioning in several ways. Some systems employ tensioning instruments ("tensors")[11, 15] with alignment rods that allow the surgeon to judge tensioning and restoration of limb alignment, usually before the distal femoral surface is resected. The level of resection varies in such an approach. When other systems are used, bone resections are made independently in relation to defined and identified axes. Either trial implants or spacers are then utilized to allow the surgeon to judge tension and alignment.[18–20, 32] In all approaches, good alignment requires knowledge of the location of the center of the femoral head (see Chapter 29, *Indications and Preoperative Planning for Total Knee Arthroplasty*).

Minimal Bone Resection

Kinematic advantages have been recognized to restoring the distal and posterior femoral surfaces to their anatomic positions (i.e., restoring the joint line). Many systems have distal femoral resection guides that set the amount of distal femoral resection based on a measured distance from the remaining distal surface, usually an amount equal to that replaced by the implant. The importance of minimal tibial bone resection to the maintenance of tibial fixation is well established.[2, 4] Depth gauges have substantially improved the surgeon's ability to minimize tibial resection. These devices attach to alignment guides and allow the surgeon to place a resection block for removal of minimal tibial bone. In addition, the amount of tibial bone that must be resected can be estimated and the best way to handle large bone defects can be determined (see Chapter 29, *Indications and Preoperative Planning for Total Knee Arthroplasty*). These systems should become a standard part of the surgeon's armamentarium.

The distal femoral joint line can be restored to its proper location by resection of a predetermined amount of distal femoral condyle in proper alignment, measured from the least involved femoral condyle (Fig. 28–5). Measured posterior resection is accomplished by instruments that place a distal femoral cutting block in the proper anteroposterior position on the resected distal femur and in the correct rotation. Correct anteroposterior placement of this block can be achieved with an intramedullary rod,[32] a guide with posterior runners that positions medial and lateral pinholes for a cutting block, or a guide that uses the anterior femur for placement of medial and lateral pinholes. These blocks must be placed in the correct rotation before fixation. However, this placement is difficult for the surgeon to judge and difficult for the designer to instrument. Some controversy exists regarding the best rotational position of the distal femoral block. The surgeon should be aware of the potential significance of such differences when posterior cruciate retaining and sacrificing designs are chosen.[15, 20]

Knee systems may differ in how they

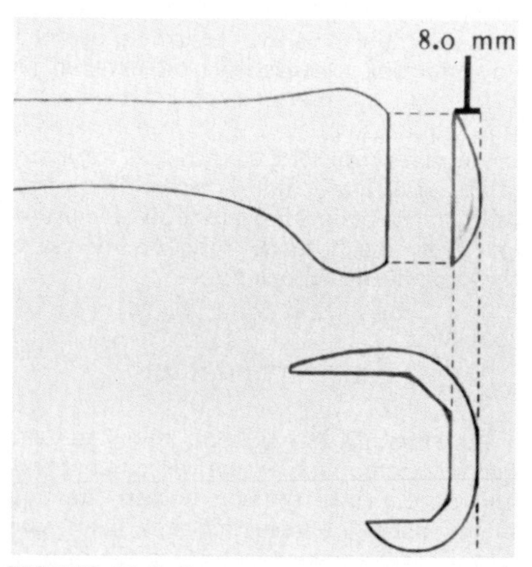

FIGURE 28–5. Resection at the distal femur by means of an oscillating saw. Amount of bone resected corresponds to thickness of distal portion of femoral implant when measured from least involved femoral condyle. (Courtesy of Johnson & Johnson.)

address femoral sizing. Some systems offer interchangeability in that all sizes of femoral components mate with all sizes of tibial components. Other systems are less flexible. The surgeon can compensate for this inflexibility by altering the amount of posterior femoral resection to accommodate the inner dimensions of the femoral implant, as is usually done in posterior cruciate sacrificing designs. Most systems provide methods for a surgeon to avoid anterior notching of the femur. Notching of the anterior femur results from improper placement of the femoral anteroposterior block in the anteroposterior plane, improper sizing of the anteroposterior resection (and thus of the femoral component), improper placement of the femoral block in the flexion-extension plane (excessive extension), or malrotation of the femoral cutting block.

Resection of Tibial and Femoral Surfaces

All instrument systems provide alignment guides to help the surgeon judge the mechanical axes of the femur and tibia. Philosophies of implantation differ, but agreement is universal regarding the importance of tibial-femoral alignment. Alignment can be judged by both intramedullary and extramedullary methods.

Extramedullary alignment of the femur is judged by identifying the center of the distal femur and the center of the femoral head. Radiographic positioning of a femoral head marker is the most accurate way to identify the center of the femoral head. Whether sterile or palpated through the surgical drapes, an externally placed hip marker provides the best estimate of the center of the hip joint. External guides place resection blocks at a right angle to this axis.

Intramedullary alignment involves placing a rod of sufficient length up the distal femoral canal until the rod is stabilized by the diaphyseal portion of the femoral canal. Care must be taken to ensure adequate opening of the hole at the level of the femoral attachment of the posterior cruciate ligament for three reasons: (1) to assure proper placement of the rod in the middle of the condyles;[32] (2) to avoid fat embolization;[8] and (3) to prevent inaccurate positioning of the rod in the lateral plane due to distal impingement (and thus extension of the femoral cut and component). This rod is then attached to the distal femoral resection guides at an angle sufficient to place the distal femoral resection perpendicular to the mechanical axis (Fig. 28–6). We prefer systems that offer attachments of extramedullary alignment devices as a check of this important resection (Fig. 28–7).

Systems providing extramedullary tibial guides rely on the surgeon's visual assessment for proper placement. The center of the tibial plateau and the center of the talus represent the mechanical axis in the mediolateral plane. The anteroposterior resection angle is determined by placing the guide parallel to the tibia in the lateral plane. This judgment is sometimes difficult to make for an obese patient. Rotational alignment is determined by placing the alignment jig parallel to the plane of the ankle joint. For some surgeons, this determination is less difficult to visualize as "having the foot face forward," with the ankle at neutral dorsiflexion-plantar flexion. Usually this maneuver means aligning the jig in the plane of the first and second web space. Alternatively, the surgeon can select either the malleolar axis parallel to the line from the medial to lateral malleolus or the medial third of the tibial tubercle. In most knees, these landmarks usually result in the same rotational position. In unusual cases involving alteration of alignment, however, the unsuspecting surgeon can be misled. Examples are hind foot malalignment (rheumatoid arthritis), prior proximal tibial procedures with alteration of anatomy (failed high tibial osteotomy), and prior tibial tubercle procedures.

Intramedullary alignment of the tibia is performed by making a minimal tibial resection at the level of the intercondylar eminence and placing an alignment rod through the center of the metaphysis to the diaphyseal portion of the tibia. A fixed cutting or planing surface is then attached.[32] Rotational adjustment is made when the surface is prepared for accepting the implant (placement of the peg, screw holes, or both). "Feeler" gauges can be added to these devices to judge the depth of tibial resection.

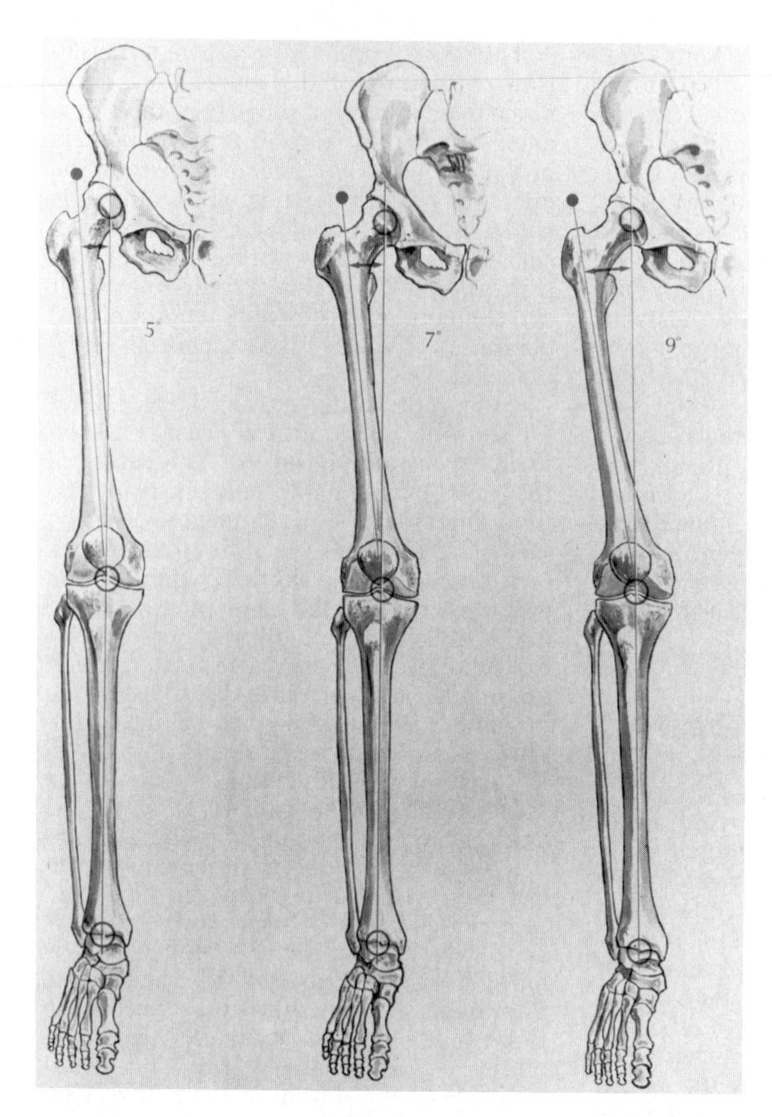

FIGURE 28–6. The angle between the mechanical and anatomic axis of the knee joint may vary by several degrees. When an intramedullary alignment system is used, the block is placed at an angle to the anatomic axis equal to the difference in the anatomic and mechanical axes. (Courtesy of Johnson & Johnson.)

The surgeon utilizes instruments to help judge alignment of knee components in three planes. Both femoral and tibial resections must restore correct mediolateral alignment (varus-valgus), anteroposterior alignment (flexion-extension), and rotational alignment. Instrumentation should be selected that helps the surgeon make these judgments accurately. We prefer intramedullary guides for femoral alignment, as their margin of error in flexion-extension and mediolateral alignment is small and rotational alignment is simpler to judge for most knees. We prefer extramedullary tibial alignment because visualization of mediolateral and rotational alignment is predictable, and anteroposterior resection can be addressed by sequential resection with appropriately angled resection blocks.

Restoration of Joint Line

Restoration of the joint line at near anatomic levels is important in achieving the correct tension of the ligaments. In addition, it may have substantial bearing on the performance of the patellofemoral joint.[12, 21] The distal femoral joint line is restored to its anatomic location by resection of the distal femur a measured amount from the most preserved condyle, at an angle perpendicular to the mechanical axis. This measured amount of resection is equal to the thickness of the distal portion of the femoral component to be used. This measurement is particularly important for knee designs that preserve the posterior cruciate ligament.

Joint line preservation is also important for the patellar surface, as motion can be

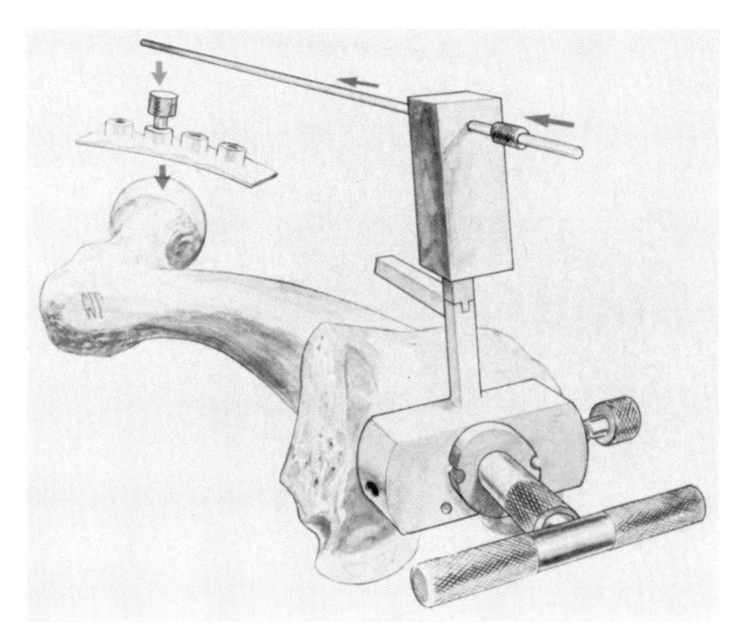

FIGURE 28–7. Assembly of the tower onto a femoral locating device in order to check the alignment established by the intramedullary device. (Courtesy of Johnson & Johnson.)

hampered if the patella is too thick and the joint can become unstable if the resection is too thin. Many systems now offer methods to measure and resect the patellar surface so that patellar height can be restored.

Maintenance of Soft Tissue Tension

The concept of soft tissue balancing is one of the most important advances in total knee arthroplasty surgery. In addition to replacing painful and diseased surfaces, prostheses can be adjusted by sizing the components to place soft tissues about the knee at tensions appropriate to their function. Conversely, without equal tension of the soft tissue structures, abnormal forces are created that either disrupt the kinematics of the replaced surfaces or lead to abnormal stresses on the devices and underlying bone, ultimately producing clinical and mechanical failure. The release of soft tissue to allow for equal tensioning of the ligaments in both extension and flexion was a concept introduced by Freeman and coworkers[11] and Insall[14, 15] in the early 1970s. Since then, many long-term successes have demonstrated the concept to be sound.[21, 22, 29]

Release for severe fixed varus deformity includes removal of medial osteophytes and release of the deep and superficial fibers of the medial collateral ligament, the semimembranosus insertion, and the tendinous insertion of the pes anserine tendons. Although some controversy exists, release of the posterior cruciate ligament may also be needed to correct severe fixed varus deformities. The degree to which these structures are released depends upon the individual knee.[13, 15, 17] In our experience, few knees require extensive release of all structures. Each case must be considered individually, however. Surgeons must have instruments available to help them judge the adequacy of the releases performed.

The structures released for correction of severe fixed valgus deformities include the popliteus tendon, the iliotibial band, the lateral head of the gastrocnemius muscle, the posterolateral capsule, and the lateral collateral ligament. Rarely, the biceps femoris will need to be released. These releases are usually accompanied by lateral retinacular release of the patella. Substantial disruption of the lateral blood supply will be encountered, and the patella can be substantially compromised. Great care must be taken to avoid injury to the peroneal nerve.[24]

Posterior capsular release may be necessary when there is significant fixed flexion deformity in an arthritic knee. Although several different methods of dealing with fixed flexion deformity are

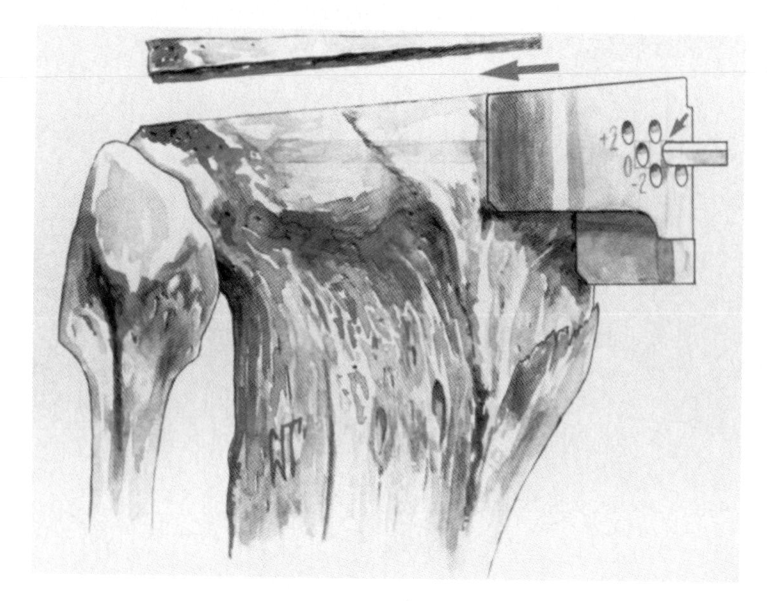

FIGURE 28–8. When the posterior cruciate ligament is retained and is too tight, it will tend to tilt the tibial component or to inhibit flexion. When tension in extension is already proper, the tight flexion may be corrected by increasing the angle of anteroposterior resection. (Courtesy of Johnson & Johnson.)

available, some, such as additional distal femoral resection and posterior cruciate ligament sacrifice, may require acceptance of kinematic alterations the surgeon does not wish to make. Posterior release is performed by removing osteophytes and stripping the capsule off the posterior condyles of the distal femur. If release is inadequate and not improved by resection of the posterior cruciate ligament, formal capsulotomy must be performed under direct visualization.[15] (See Chapter 30, *Primary Total Knee Replacement.*)

Alignment systems allow the surgeon to check soft tissue balance in different ways. Early knee instrument systems put strong emphasis on an apparatus that would produce tension in the ligaments—the tensor.[11, 13, 15] Coupled with alignment jigs, tensors were employed to determine whether equal tension was applied to the medial and lateral collateral ligaments and, if so, whether it placed the knee surfaces in the correct alignment. If alignment was incorrect, ligament releases were required.

Current popular approaches separate the bone resection steps from the ligament release steps. With alignment jigs, the surgeon resects the distal femur and proximal tibia perpendicular to their respective axes. Trial implants help determine if stability has been achieved in the proper alignment. If stability is equal but overall limb alignment is not, it means either that the bones were inaccurately resected or that additional ligament release is required, usually supplemented by a thicker tibial component. This approach is more often employed with systems that retain the posterior cruciate ligament. One can safely assume that flexion and extension gaps are equal if the implant exactly replaces the amount of bone resected from the distal and posterior condyles of the femur.

With devices that retain the posterior cruciate ligament, the surgeon must also judge the tension of the ligament. The surgeon must determine first that the knee is stable against posterior displacement and then that the ligament is not too tight. When the ligament is overly tight, flexion will tend to tilt the tibial component anteriorly or inhibit flexion. This problem must be corrected by either selectively releasing the posterior cruciate ligament[23] or increasing the angle of anteroposterior resection (Fig. 28–8).

Restoration of Patellofemoral Alignment

Despite the excellent results of total knee arthroplasty in general, patellofemoral articulation remains a continued source of problems for surgeon and patient. Until the past several years, very little research had been done to investigate this aspect of total knee arthroplasty.[3, 7, 9, 27] Now it has become apparent that improved flexion obtained with present implant designs and techniques has been achieved at a price—the stresses on patellar surfaces place both the polyethylene portion of the component and the fixation interfaces at significant risk. This problem is influenced by several factors related to both the design and the techniques employed to implant femoral and patellar components. Clearly, however, alignment of the patellar mechanism is important and must be assessed accurately intraoperatively. Judgments that affect patellar mechanism function and are directly controlled by the surgeon include rotational alignment of tibial and femoral components, position of the patellar implant, size of the patellar implant, and release of the lateral retinaculum. The "no thumb" rule of patellar tracking (proper patellar tracking at surgery without any pressure against the patella) is of assistance when judging the accuracy of restoration of the patellofemoral mechanism.

References

1. Abbott, L. C. and Carpenter, W. F.: Surgical approaches to the knee joint. J. Bone Joint Surg. 47A:277–310, 1945.
2. Bartel, D. L., Burstein, A. H., Santavilla, E. A., et al.: Performance of the tibial component in total knee replacement. Conventional and revision designs. J. Bone Joint Surg. 64A:1026, 1982.
3. Bayley, J. C., Scott, R. D., Ewald, F. C., et al.: Failure of metal-backed patellar component after total knee replacement. J. Bone Joint Surg. 70A:668, 1988.
4. Behrens, J. C., Walker, P. S., and Shoji, H.: Variation in strength and structure of cancellous bone at the knee. J. Biomech. 7:201, 1974.
5. Coonse, K. and Adams, J. D.: A new operative approach to the knee joint. Surg. Gynecol. Obstet. 77:344–347, 1943.
6. Craig, S. M.: Soft Tissue Considerations. Total Knee Revision Arthroplasty. Edited by W. N. Scott. Orlando, Grune & Stratton, 1987.
7. deSwart, R. J., Stulberg, B. N., Gaisser, D. M., et al.: The fate of polyethylene patellar components: An analysis of 41 components retrieved at revision total knee arthroplasty. Transactions of the 35th Annual Meeting of the Orthopedic Research Society, Las Vegas, 1989.
8. Fahny, N. F., Chandler, H. P., Danylchuk, K., et al.: Blood gas and circulatory changes during total knee replacement. Role of the intramedullary alignment rod. J. Bone Joint Surg. 72A:19–26, 1990.
9. Figgie, M. P., Wright, T. M., Santner, T., et al.: Performance of dome-shaped patellar components in total knee arthroplasty. Transactions of the 35th Annual Meeting of the Orthopedic Research Society, Las Vegas, 1989.
10. Fitzgerald, R. H. and Ilstrup, D. M.: A prospective study of unidirectional airflow operating rooms. American Academy of Orthopaedic Surgeons, New Orleans, 1990.
11. Freeman, M. A. R., Swanson, S. A. V., and Todd, R. C.: Total replacement of the knee using the Freeman-Swanson knee prosthesis. Clin. Orthop. 94:153, 1973.
12. Goldberg, V. M., Figgie, H. E., and Figgie, M. P.: Technical considerations in total knee surgery: Management of patella problems. Orthop. Clin. North Am. 20(2):189, 1989.
13. Hungerford, D. S., Krackow, K. A., and Kenna, R. V.: Total Knee Arthroplasty: A Comprehensive Approach. Baltimore, Williams & Wilkins, 1984.
14. Insall, J. N.: Surgical Approaches to the Knee. Surgery of the Knee. New York, Churchill Livingstone, 1984.
15. Insall, J. N.: Total Knee Replacement. Surgery of the Knee. New York, Churchill Livingstone, 1984.
16. Krackow, K. A.: Surgical Procedure. The Technique of Total Knee Arthroplasty, pp. 168–196, St. Louis, C. V. Mosby Company, 1990.
17. Krackow, K. A.: Surgical Procedure. The Technique of Total Knee Arthroplasty, pp. 249–372, St. Louis, C. V. Mosby Company, 1990.
18. MicroLoc Porous Coated Knee System. Surgical Technique Manual. New Brunswick, NJ, Johnson & Johnson.
19. PCA Modular Total Knee System. Surgical Technique Manual. Rutherford, NJ, Howmedica.
20. PFC Modular Total Knee System with Specialist Instruments. Surgical Technique Manual. New Brunswick, NJ, Johnson & Johnson.
21. Ranawat, C. S.: Surgical Technique of Total Condylar Knee Arthroplasty. Total Condylar Knee Arthroplasty—Technique, Results and Complications. Edited by C. S. Ranawat, New York, Springer-Verlag, 1985.
22. Ranawat, C. S. and Boachie-Adjei, O.: Survivorship analysis and results of total condylar knee arthroplasty—eight- to eleven-year follow-up period. Clin. Orthop. 226:6, 1988.
23. Ritter, M. A., Faris, P. M., and Keating, E. M.: Posterior cruciate ligament balancing during total knee arthroplasty. J. Arthroplasty 3(4):323–326, 1988.
24. Rose, H. A., Hood, R. W., Otis, J. C., et al.: Peroneal nerve palsy following total knee arthroplasty. A review of the hospital for special surgery experience. J. Bone Joint Surg. 64A:347, 1982.
25. Salvati, E. A., Robinson, R. P., Zeno, S. M., et al.: Infection rates after 3175 total hip and total knee replacements performed with and without a horizontal unidirectional filtered airflow system. J. Bone Joint Surg. 64A:525, 1982.
26. Scott, R. D. and Siliski, J. M.: The use of a modified V-Y quadricepsplasty during total knee replacement to gain exposure and improve flexion in the ankylosed knee. Orthopedics 8:45–48, 1985.
27. Stulberg, S. D., Stulberg, B. N., Hamati, Y., et al.: Failure mechanisms of metal-backed patellar components. Clin. Orthop. 236:88, 1988.

28. Tooms, R. E.: Arthroplasty of Ankle and Knee. Campbell's Operative Orthopaedics. St. Louis, C. V. Mosby Company, 1987.
29. Vince, K. G., Insall, J. N., Kelly, M. A., et al.: Total condylar knee prosthesis: Ten to twelve year follow-up and survivorship analysis. American Academy of Orthopaedic Surgeons, Atlanta, 1988.
30. Weinzweig, N., Dowden, R. V., and Stulberg, B. N.: The use of tissue expansion to allow reconstruction of the knee. A case report. J. Bone Joint Surg. 69A:1238, 1987.
31. Whiteside, L. A. and Ohl, M. D.: Tibial tubercle osteotomy for exposure of the difficult total knee replacement. Scientific presentation, American Academy of Orthopaedic Surgeons, New Orleans, 1990.
32. Whiteside, L. A.: Surgical Procedure for the Whiteside Ortholoc Modular Knee System. Arlington, TN, Dow Corning Wright, 1990.
33. Wolff, A. M., Hungerford, D. S., Krackow, K. S., et al.: Osteotomy of the tibial tubercle during total knee replacement. J. Bone Joint Surg. 71A:848–852, 1989.

CHAPTER 29

Indications and Preoperative Planning for Total Knee Arthroplasty

BERNARD STULBERG
TIMOTHY HUPFER

Before total knee arthroplasty is performed, the surgeon must evaluate the causes and progression of the disease in the knee, the degree to which pain and functional compromise contribute to the patient's disability, and the likelihood that pain relief and functional improvement will be sufficient to warrant surgery. As more long-term results are reported from various medical centers,[28, 29, 37, 44] it is clear that total knee arthroplasty has gained a prominent place in the armamentarium of surgeons who deal with arthritis and other afflictions of the knee joint. Given the success of total knee replacements, the limits of its application are likely to be pushed. It remains for investigators, however, to provide proof of the efficacy of less common applications before they are widely adopted.

INDICATIONS

The general indications for total knee arthroplasty are end-stage joint destruction due to osteoarthritis; degenerative arthritis due to primary synovial conditions, such as osteochondromatosis and pigmented villonodular synovitis; arthritis due to crystal deposition diseases, such as gout and pseudogout; rheumatoid arthritis and other inflammatory arthritides, such as systemic lupus erythematosus and juvenile rheumatoid arthritis; osteonecrosis; and post-traumatic arthritis. Total knee arthroplasty may also be done for the patient with failure of a high tibial or supracondylar osteotomy and for the elderly patient with advanced and disabling patellofemoral osteoarthritis.[15]

Post-traumatic arthritis can be related to either intra-articular fracture or ligament disruption with subsequent instability (Fig. 29–1). For patients, many of whom are young, with this instability, the surgeon may be reluctant to proceed with total knee replacements and may wish to consider alternatives. Possible alternatives to knee replacement should also be carefully considered for younger patients with osteoarthritis. These alternatives include arthroscopy with or without debridement, osteotomy, and arthrodesis. In a patient with varus deformity, osteotomy should be done at the proximal tibia. For valgus deformity, osteotomy is usually performed at the distal femur. These alternatives are discussed briefly.

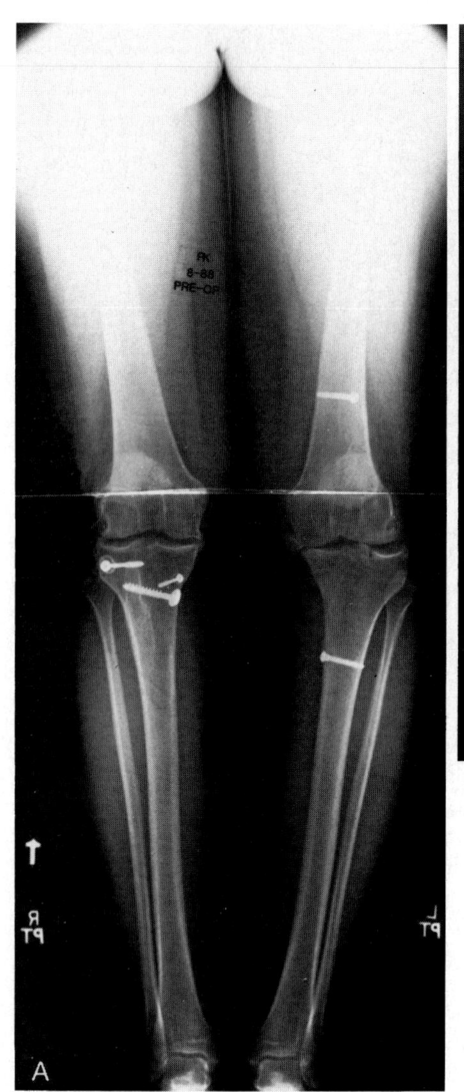

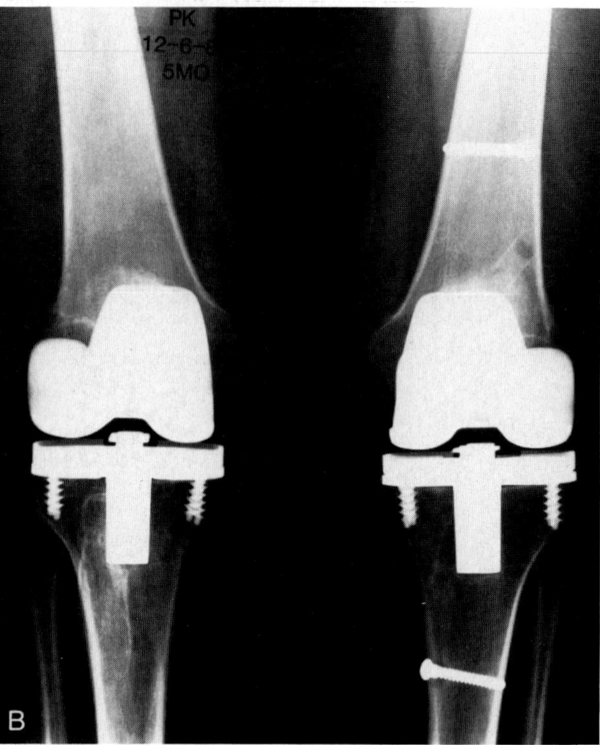

FIGURE 29–1. *A,* This 32-year-old patient had undergone more than ten ligament reconstruction procedures in each knee for problems related to anterior and posterior cruciate deficiencies. The patient was wheelchair-bound with persistent pain. *B,* Postoperative radiograph of this patient at 5 months postoperatively showing bilateral uncemented implants with cruciate substitution capabilities. The patient remained asymptomatic, walked without aids, and returned to her job.

ARTHROSCOPY[17, 18, 30, 32, 33]

Many patients with advanced knee pain and disability have objective clinical and radiographic findings that do not suggest end-stage arthritic involvement of the knee joints. In such cases, conservative management is appropriate: activity modification, muscle-strengthening program, and anti-inflammatory medication. In the occasional patient for whom this approach is unsuccessful, arthroscopic assessment, lavage, and debridement may prove useful. However, patients should be selected carefully. In addition, such an intervention should be preceded by extensive nonoperative management and thorough evaluation. The goals of intervention are pain relief and decreased disability from moderately advanced arthritis. Treatment should not be regarded as curative. Moreover, outcome tends to be unpredictable. Although functional and symptomatic improvement can last a long time in properly selected patients, in those with mechanical malalignments, such approaches have limited success.

HIGH TIBIAL OSTEOTOMY[1, 5, 12, 16, 19]

Proximal tibial osteotomy deserves a place in the armamentarium of every orthopaedic surgeon who treats arthritic conditions of the knee (Fig. 29–2). Long-term success can be achieved in a high percent-

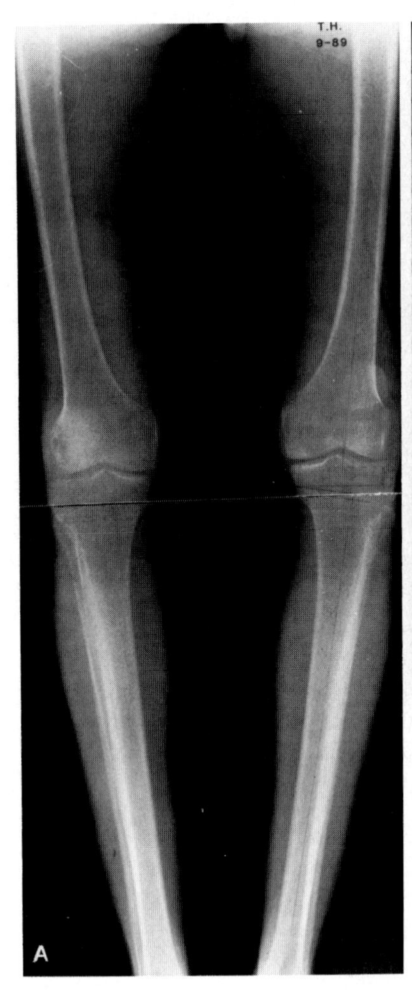

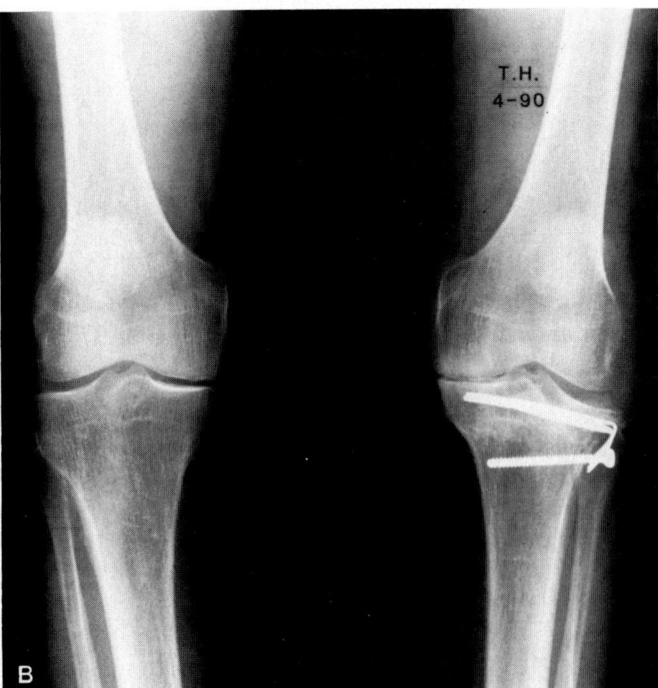

FIGURE 29–2. *A*, Radiograph of a 56-year-old man with evidence of medial osteoarthritis. As a handyman, he is on his feet constantly. This patient had symptoms entirely consistent with medial joint arthritis. Arthroscopic debridement provided symptomatic relief for 18 months. *B*, Postoperative radiograph of this patient following high tibial osteotomy. Patient returned to full activities with only mild symptoms.

age of patients if they are carefully selected, if the procedure is performed meticulously, and if correct postoperative management is observed. We agree with Scott and Rubinstein[36] that this procedure is particularly appropriate for the younger patient, but that the indications for high tibial osteotomy are related more to conditions of documented unicompartmental mechanical overload (weightbearing pain) than to age in the patient with functional goals and activity levels that put substantial demand on the knee joint. Thus, high tibial osteotomy is just as appropriate for the 60- to 70-year-old who wishes to play tennis, jog, or perform other high impact activities as it is for younger individuals whose symptoms and signs point to largely unicompartmental disease. Most investigators believe that patellofemoral arthritis is not in itself a contraindication to high tibial osteotomy, although the disadvantages should be considered.

SUPRACONDYLAR OSTEOTOMY[13, 20]

As for tibial osteotomy for medial compartment disease, unicompartmental overload of the lateral compartment of the knee may be suitably addressed by osteotomy of the distal femur. For knees with valgus deformities, we prefer supracondylar osteotomies that place the knees in 0 to 2 degrees of valgus (Fig. 29–3). Such an intra-articular procedure requires internal fixation and early postoperative mobilization. The technical details are important, and overcorrection into varus is to be avoided. Patellofemoral mechanics can be substantially improved by osteotomy.

ARTHRODESIS

Many experienced orthopaedic surgeons believe that primary arthrodesis of the

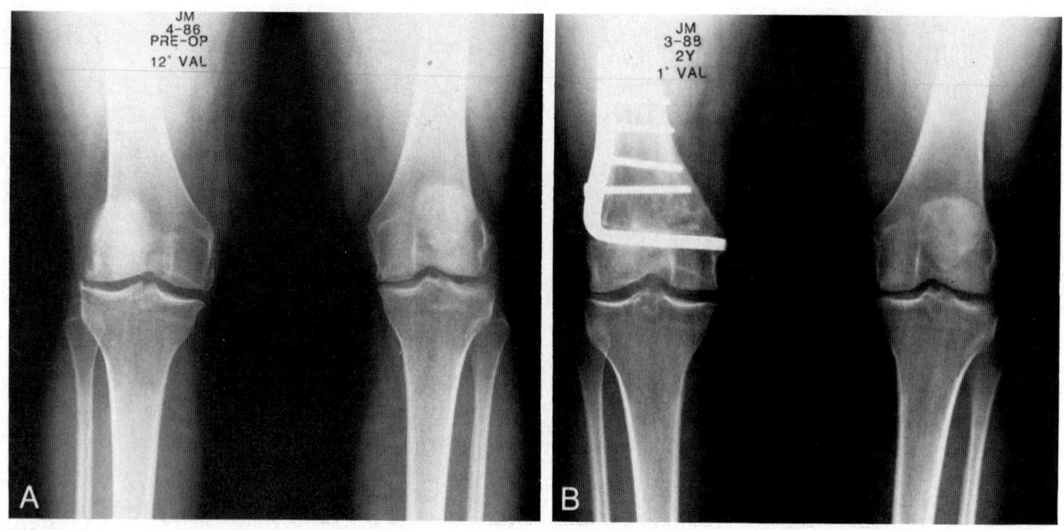

FIGURE 29–3. *A,* Supracondylar osteotomy in a 28-year-old woman with advanced lateral joint pain and evidence of lateral osteoarthritis. *B,* Postoperative radiograph showing supracondylar osteotomy with blade plate fixation of this patient.

knee is rarely indicated for end-stage arthritis. These surgeons prefer to consider arthrodesis as the second procedure to be performed when prosthetic arthroplasty fails.[40] Although this approach may be appealing, strong consideration of arthrodesis is warranted in some patients. These include young patients with unilateral post-traumatic arthritis, diminished knee mobility, and widespread articular surface disruption; patients with neuromuscular incompetence for whom stability and pain relief are the primary goals; and patients with either locally persistent or contiguous infection for whom the further risk of infection is unacceptably high. Treatment requires careful individualization and a good physician-patient relationship. A number of satisfactory techniques are available to achieve arthrodesis. References are available for in-depth discussions of the technical aspects of this procedure.[11, 39, 40] (See Chapter 36, *Knee Anthrodesis for Failed Total Knee Arthroplasty.*)

CONTRAINDICATIONS

In the past, absolute contraindications to total knee arthroplasty have included infection, neuropathic arthropathy, and prior knee arthrodesis. However, as surgeons gain increasing skill and understanding of total knee arthroplasty, each of these indications has become less absolute, especially when the forefront of the technique is being pushed in certain medical centers. For example, infection associated with advanced arthritis destruction can often be treated successfully by radical surgical debridement and antibiotic therapy. Once cleared of infection, the knee usually has enough bone and ligamentous support to allow reconstruction with arthroplasty techniques (Fig. 29–4). However, multidisciplinary management and extensive prosthetic inventories are often required. Therefore, such a patient may be managed more appropriately at those institutions with adequate expertise and facilities.

Neuropathic arthropathy at the knee may be subtle or dramatic. Insall and colleagues (see Soudry[38]) have shown that patients with this condition can be treated by total knee replacements with a high degree of success. A nonlimiting but highly conforming style of implant, such as the posterior stabilized total condylar prosthesis, has allowed for correction of deformity and stability through constraint and ligament balancing. Late loosening has not proven a problem. The results of these investigators provide encouragement to surgeons who wish to consider the benefits of arthroplasty for this disabled patient population.

Other forms of neuropathy continue to be contraindications to total knee arthro-

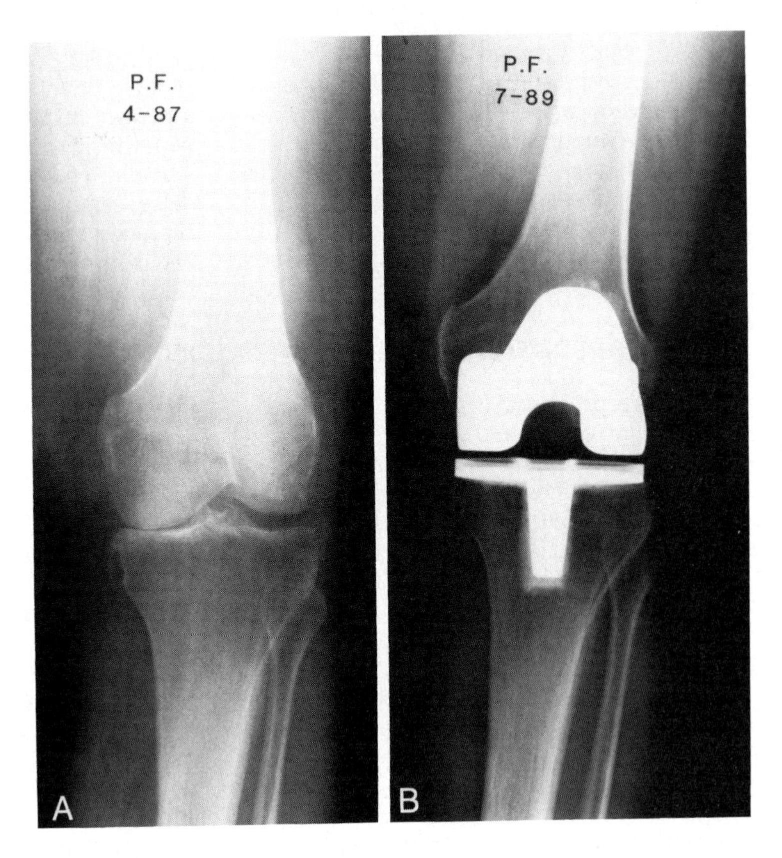

FIGURE 29–4. *A,* Radiograph of a 61-year-old woman with postarthroscopy infection. The patient had persistent mild synovitis, erythema, and marked symptoms consistent with advanced osteoarthritis. A radical synovectomy and debridement were performed, and the knee was rendered infection free. *B,* Postoperative radiograph of this patient demonstrating successful total knee replacement after eradication of infection. This patient was asymptomatic at 2-year follow-up.

plasty. Absence of sufficient neuromuscular control of the quadriceps or hamstring musculature may necessitate long-term bracing for functional purposes. This may make total knee arthroplasty less desirable than arthrodesis for the patient.

Despite the availability of better methods to clear infection within the joint so that knee replacement can be performed, persistent infection in other anatomic areas should lead the surgeon to proceed with great caution. Recurrent urinary tract infection and serious distal extremity neurovascular compromise with intermittent infection are particularly worrisome. All potential sources of sepsis should be fully evaluated and treated before total knee arthroplasty is planned.

Experience with total hip arthroplasty inevitably led to attempts to perform arthroplasty in patients with previous arthrodesis of the knees. Although technically possible and perhaps in rare cases advisable, we find this application of knee replacement to be particularly hazardous. Muscle integrity about the knee joint is likely to be compromised significantly, and it is unclear whether the shortening of musculoskeletal structures that one encounters allows restoration of enough function to make arthroplasty worthwhile for the patient. Both the surgeon and patient should consider the magnitude of the undertaking fully before deciding to proceed with this type of surgery. Their goals should be realistic and the consequences of failure appreciated.

PATIENT SELECTION

The decision to treat the patient with a painful, arthritic knee by total knee arthroplasty can be difficult. Pain in the knee joint has many possible sources, and it is not uncommon to find very little correspondence between the severity of pain and the objective findings of arthritic involvement, whether clinical or radiographic. Total knee replacement must be recommended with great caution in these cases. Also, patient compliance during the rehabilitation period is often difficult to ensure, even in well-motivated patients. Misinterpretation of a patient's level of pain and disability may lead to significant unhappiness for both surgeon and patient regarding the outcome of an arthroplasty. Almost every surgeon who performs this procedure regularly can describe at least one such case. Thus, an awareness of the limitations of arthroplasty is an important element in the decision-making process, especially when revision of a painful total knee arthroplasty is being considered.[22]

PREOPERATIVE PLANNING

Although preoperative templating is less likely to be performed for total knee arthroplasty than for total hip arthroplasty, planning for knee arthroplasty prior to surgery is particularly useful. In the past, some workers[27] have suggested that preoperative anteroposterior radiographs are needed to determine the amount of bone resection required to align the knee satisfactorily and lateral radiographs to select the correct size femoral component. Preoperative planning is discussed here in a broader sense. As techniques and prosthetic choices have multiplied, so have the range of problems that can be addressed through total knee arthroplasties, including management of complex deformities in primary and revision circumstances. Substantive preoperative planning is necessary in these situations. The surgeon must decide whether any of the patient's problems are related to medical or psychologic factors, or to both, making total knee replacement a hazardous undertaking. In addition, the surgeon may need to consider the problems of bone deformity, deficiency, or both; the status of normal stabilizing structures; the amount of soft tissue coverage; and the potential sources of infection. These considerations affect how the surgeon applies an instrument system, the choice of incisions and approaches to the knee, and the selection of prosthetic devices. These considerations also influence the decision to perform soft tissue procedures that will provide satisfactory wound healing, mobility, and function after arthroplasty.

MEDICAL AND PSYCHOLOGIC REQUIREMENTS

As a major surgical procedure, total knee arthroplasty is associated with major surgical risks. The list of potential complications of such surgery is long. Both surgeon and patient need to weigh the risks and benefits of proceeding with elective intervention. Although anesthesia is technically simpler to perform for total knee replacement than for total hip replacement because of the patient's position, the limited blood loss, and the nature of peripheral limb surgery, the population for whom this procedure is appropriate includes many individuals with substantial medical problems. Indeed, the decreased activity level occasioned by the arthritic knee can mask an otherwise borderline cardiac or respiratory reserve. In such a patient, the stress of surgery can lead to serious complications in the intraoperative or early postoperative period. Consequently, surgeons who regularly treat geriatric patients with questionable cardiac and pulmonary status must exercise particular caution. By identifying risk factors that can increase morbidity and mortality well before the surgical procedure is performed, the surgeon has time to lower the chances of complications. In addition, the patient can be given a clear idea of the activity level he or she can expect after surgery.

The psychologic requirements for successful total knee arthroplasty must also be weighed. Surgeons who deal with afflictions of the knee occasionally have patients who report substantial pain and disability but have no objective findings that justify total knee arthroplasty. Total knee arthroplasty is done to correct specific alterations of the articular surface and ligamentous structures that result in pain and disability. If the procedure is utilized to treat pain and disability when these alterations are not present, the likelihood of a successful result is diminished, causing much frustration to both the patient and surgeon. For this reason, other alternatives should be exhausted for this small, but usually persistent, subset of patients before total knee arthroplasty is planned.

PREOPERATIVE ASSESSMENT: CLINICAL AND RADIOGRAPHIC

Certain aspects of the routine clinical and radiographic evaluation of the arthritic knee should alert the observant surgeon to the need for a more thorough assessment. Of specific concern are signs of bone deficiency or deformity, ligament insufficiency, and soft tissue compromise that might require the application of devices, procedures, or techniques beyond that of routine standard devices, procedures, or techniques.

The clinical examination should focus on evidence for skin incisions or soft tissue injuries that might hamper satisfactory wound closure over a properly aligned prosthesis. The surgeon may need to consider a modified standard skin incision,[21, 34] soft tissue expansion,[10, 45] or soft tissue transfer. A transfer procedure usually requires coordination with a colleague in plastic surgery.[6] In patients who are undergoing revision arthroplasties or in those who are being considered for two-stage reimplantations due to infections, such procedures and their timing assume great importance. Other factors in the clinical examination include the status of the musculature about the knee; the evidence of peripheral vascular disease or peripheral neuropathy; and the evidence of joint instability in the medial-lateral, anteroposterior, and rotational planes. Each of these assessments can influence the decision to proceed with arthroplasty, the selection of prosthetic device most appropriate for the patient (see subsequent discussion), and the estimation of what can reasonably be expected from successful surgical intervention. Other factors that can affect the surgical procedure and morbidity risk include the patient's nutritional status, weight, and activity level and the stiffness of the knee joint and subsequent difficulty in exposure of the knee.[10, 14, 24]

An important and often difficult judgment in the assessment of the patient with an arthritic knee is the degree to which the patellofemoral joint affects pain and functional disability. Isolated patellofemoral arthritis is rarely considered a major indication for total knee arthroplasty. This patient is usually best managed by such approaches as arthroscopic debridement and retinacular release, realignment, or tibial tubercle elevation. When tibiofemoral involvement is present, however, the degree of patellofemoral involvement may influence the decision to consider other surgical procedures, such as high tibial osteotomy or unicompartmental replacement.[35] A thorough history and physical examination help establish the contribution of patellofemoral arthritis sufficiently to provide a basis for discussion of appropriate treatment options between physician and patient.

For the patient being evaluated for possible revision of a painful knee arthroplasty, the clinical examination must focus on factors related to the preoperative and postoperative states. The surgeon must establish the degree of disability before and after arthroplasty. The temporal relationship of impending failure of the arthroplasty to its initial implantation, the evidence for infectious causes of failure, and the clinical features that suggest mechanical abnormalities of implant fixation or function must be identified. Particular attention should be paid to issues of delayed wound healing and persistent pain or instability following arthroplasty that would suggest a less than desirable early outcome.[34]

The initial radiographic evaluation is performed to give the surgeon a clear idea of the degree of deformity of the lower extremity and the extent to which bony deformity contributes to malalignment. Anteroposterior radiographs made during weightbearing are a necessary part of the examination. Lateral and patellar views are taken to determine the extent of patellofemoral joint involvement and patellofemoral articulation alignment. They also allow the surgeon to judge implant sizing for the femur. The long (i.e., whole limb) standing radiograph in both the anteroposterior and lateral planes is important to have available when certain styles of instrumentation systems are employed.[23, 26] We believe that the surgeon performing total knee arthroplasty must have a clear idea of where the mechanical axis is located in the anteroposterior plane if longevity of the arthroplasty is to be assured. This ability requires knowledge of where the center of the femoral head is situated. Such a determination can be made only through the use of a long radiograph that includes the hip and knee joint or through the use of hip markers placed preoperatively under fluoroscopy. If a standard length radiograph is employed, the angle between the anatomic axis of the femur and mechanical axis can be calculated and the intramedullary alignment system adjusted accordingly. If an externally placed hip marker is selected, extramedullary adjustment of rods allows the surgeon to judge the mechanical axis at the time of surgery. Increasing evidence suggests that the margin for error is less when intramedullary systems are used for this important judgment.[8, 42] In addition, these radiographs allow the surgeon to determine abnormalities of distal femoral or proximal tibial anatomy that will affect the utilization of an intramedullary alignment rod.[23, 25]

If the initial radiographic assessment provides inadequate information regarding the bony deformity or deficiency, additional studies may be necessary, particularly in knees with post-traumatic changes, arthritis related to childhood knee abnormalities, or previous surgical procedures (Figs. 29–5 and 29–6). Studies may include magnification-marked radiographs, aspiration/arthrograms, tomograms, or computerized axial tomography (CAT) scans. We have found CAT scans with bone modeling particularly helpful in isolated cases of severe bony abnormality and three-plane deformity (see Fig. 29–6).[4] The goal of supplemental studies is to determine bone abnormalities or deficiencies that affect the support for the implants, and therefore the need for any special implants or techniques. Both routine and special radiographic studies can identify cases of bone deficiency that need to be dealt with at the time of knee arthroplasty. Advances in arthroplasty devices and techniques are also addressing those deficiencies in several ways. Modular devices help the surgeon deal with major bone deficiencies of both femur and tibia. Intramedullary stems, altered fixation surfaces, and modular spacers are features of these systems. Because standard surgical techniques and instrumentation may be modified, the surgeon needs a sound understanding of the technical and theoretic aspects of these approaches before using them. The surgeon and operating team should also be thoroughly familiar with the prosthesis system before actually performing the procedure.[2, 3]

An alternative method of dealing with bone deficiency is bone grafting.[46] The surgeon and team should have a thorough understanding of the sources of bone graft and the planned technique for application. A carefully planned surgical intervention expedites the actual procedure and allows for optimal restoration of the kinematics of the knee.

In many revision knee arthroplasties and in some primary arthroplasties, the history and physical examination suggest the possibility of infection within the joint. In these cases, special studies must be performed to help the surgeon determine and recommend the best form of therapeutic intervention. Aspiration of the knee joint, with or without arthrogram, bone scanning, and blood tests, may be performed to help the surgeon gather evidence regarding the presence or absence of infection. Occasionally, enough doubt will exist to make open biopsy, debridement, or both advisable before proceeding with an arthroplasty (Fig. 29–7). The surgeon must remember that the primary goal is to give the patient a pain-free functional arthroplasty. Every potential cause of failure must be identified and addressed appropriately if success is to be achieved.

SOFT TISSUE INSUFFICIENCY

Although the routine assessment of prior incisions and vascular and neurologic structures is critical,[24] two areas of soft tissue assessment play particularly important roles in the success of a knee arthroplasty and therefore require special mention.

First, the soft-tissue coverage of the knee wound must be visualized after the arthroplasty has been completed. In most knees, no problem exists and the surgeon can proceed with confidence. However, this may not be the case in the severely deformed, previously operated, or infected knee. The nutritional status of the tissues about the knee can be severely compromised by prior trauma or surgical intervention, and special techniques may be needed to allow the surgeon to perform total knee arthroplasty safely. We have applied soft tissue expansion techniques when the compromise was related primarily to skin coverage.[45] In these techniques, healthy skin and subcutaneous tissue are expanded to cover a limited area of deficiency (Fig. 29–8). When tissue compromise includes the deeper tissues, muscle

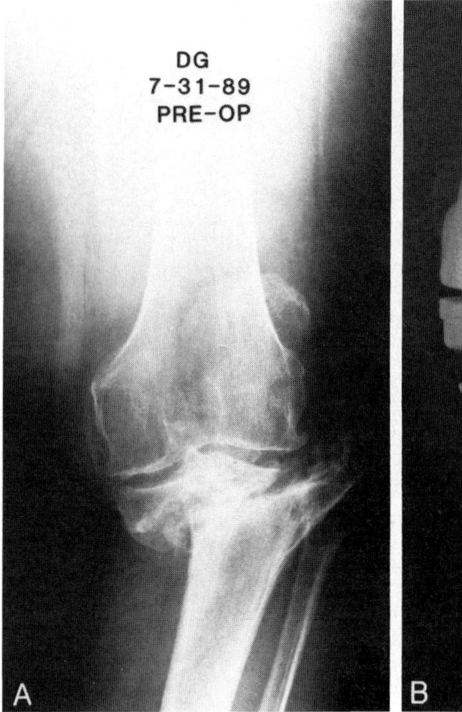

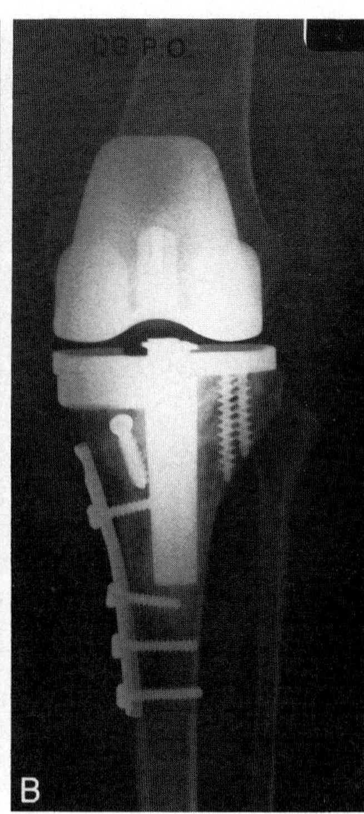

FIGURE 29–5. *A,* Patient with nonunion of a tibial condylar fracture with extensive varus deformity. The full extent of the deformity could not be appreciated on routine radiographs. Computerized tomographic scanning with bone modeling was performed to allow for better definition of deformity. *B,* Postoperative radiographs demonstrating the use of an augmented customizable implant with supplemental screw fixation, medial buttress plating, and bone grafting. The patient remained clinically asymptomatic at 12-month follow-up.

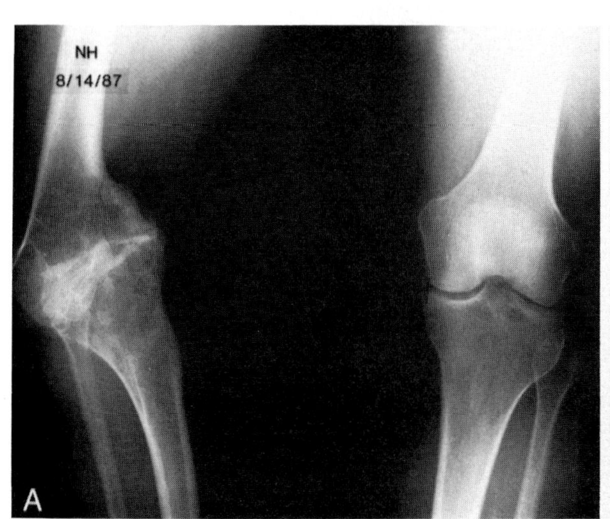

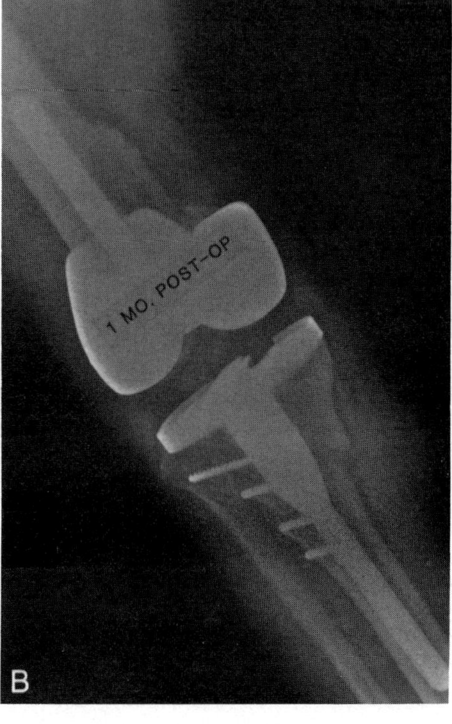

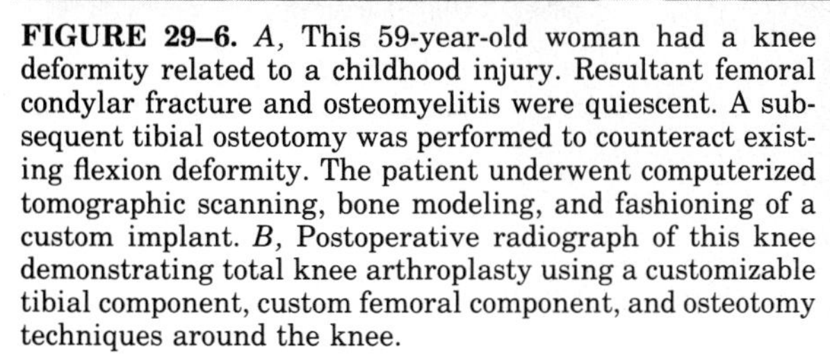

FIGURE 29–6. *A,* This 59-year-old woman had a knee deformity related to a childhood injury. Resultant femoral condylar fracture and osteomyelitis were quiescent. A subsequent tibial osteotomy was performed to counteract existing flexion deformity. The patient underwent computerized tomographic scanning, bone modeling, and fashioning of a custom implant. *B,* Postoperative radiograph of this knee demonstrating total knee arthroplasty using a customizable tibial component, custom femoral component, and osteotomy techniques around the knee.

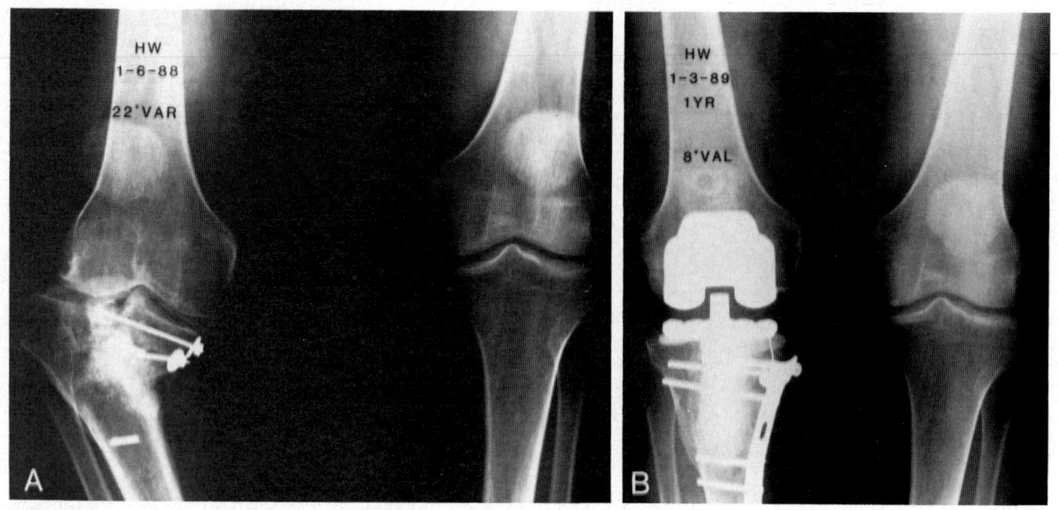

FIGURE 29–7. *A,* Radiograph of a patient with bicondylar tibial fracture treated by open reduction and internal fixation. Partial union of the lateral plateau was achieved, but the medial plateau remained ununited. A soft tissue wound suggested the possibility of deep infection. This patient underwent removal of hardware and biopsy of soft tissues prior to total knee arthroplasty. *B,* The same patient 1 year after cemented total knee arthroplasty with posterior stabilized components. Buttress plate fixation of the condylar nonunion and soft tissue releases allowed for restoration of alignment.

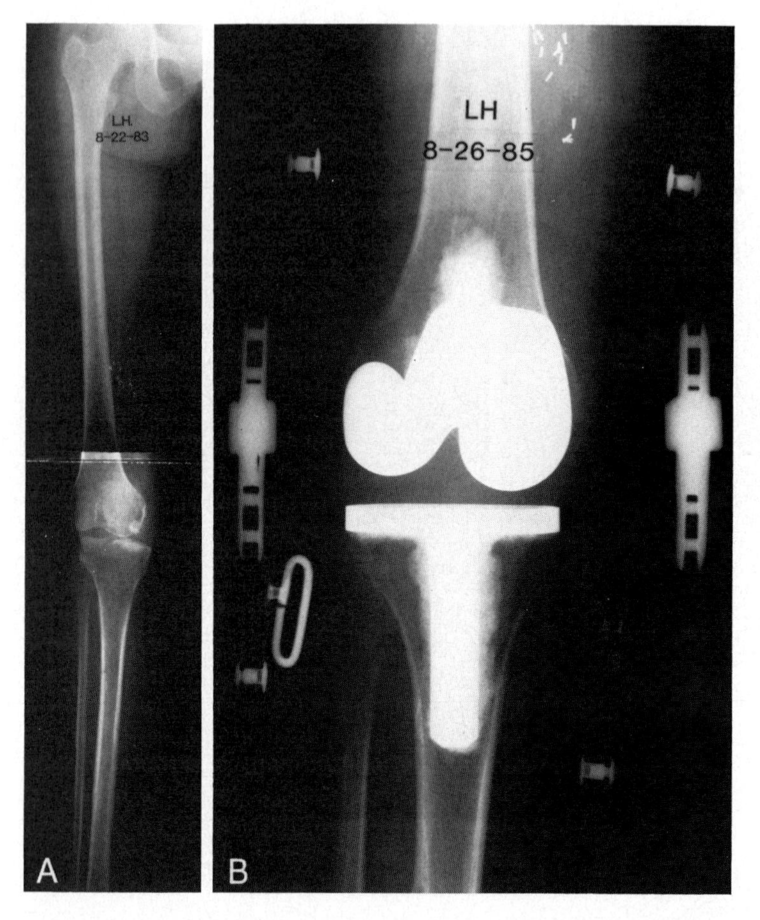

FIGURE 29–8. *A,* Radiograph of a woman with dislocation of the right knee and loss of popliteal fossa soft tissue. The patient had suffered amputation of the opposite knee at mid thigh. Soft tissue loss did not allow for routine approaches to total knee arthroplasty. Severe pain and stiffness of the knee made function difficult, even in a wheelchair. *B,* Same patient after constrained total condylar replacement with cemented components through a modified Coonse-Adams approach. Soft tissue expanders were utilized to obtain sufficient skin coverage; therefore, additional soft tissue procedures were not necessary. At 5-year follow-up, the patient successfully functioned with ankle/foot orthosis on the right and above-knee prosthesis on the left.

tissue transfer and skin grafting are advisable. The proximal medial tibia is a site where tissue loss occurs most frequently. Gastrocnemius rotation flaps are particularly useful.[6] The assistance of a plastic surgeon is also valuable in this case. In the rare case of salvage arthroplasty or arthrodesis, a transfer of vascularized free muscle tissue may be required. Part of the preoperative planning must include a thorough, straightforward discussion with the patient and family, as the morbidity following these procedures can be substantial and the goals of intervention are more limited.

The second area of soft tissue insufficiency is related to the status of the normal stabilizing structures of the knee. Deformity and injury either can lead to the loss of the usual ligamentous support available for knee arthroplasty or can require sacrifice of such structures to correct the deformity and to balance the ligamentous structures about the knee. Knee systems have lacked until lately the flexibility to change the degree of prosthetic constraint intraoperatively without switching knee devices and systems. Thus, the surgeon who routinely uses knee devices requiring retention of the posterior cruciate ligament might need to use a different type of knee implant in a patient who requires sacrifice of this ligament. Making the decision to sacrifice the ligament preoperatively can avoid redundant instruments and systems intraoperatively. Modular systems that allow separate judgments regarding the bone-prosthetic interface and the degree of prosthetic constraint between tibial and femoral component address this problem, and their popularity is likely to grow.

In this chapter, it was not our intent to discuss the pros and cons of different styles of knee devices or the philosophies behind their designs. Many detailed descriptions are available to surgeons who wish to study current devices more thoroughly.[7, 41, 43] We do believe that modular devices offer substantial flexibility to surgeons who perform total knee arthroplasty frequently. The ability to move from minimally constrained to substantially constrained geometry without altering bony anatomy offers distinct advantages.

FIXATION

Substantial controversy surrounds the subject of implant fixation for total knee arthroplasty. The advantages and disadvantages of cemented or uncemented fixation are beyond the scope of this discussion. We believe that the controversy will continue for many years without resolution. Surgeons must make their own decisions regarding which approaches they prefer for the joint surfaces to be replaced. Their patients are entitled to a thorough discussion of the risks and benefits of each approach. In addition, surgeons must make certain that the devices and techniques they plan to use are available and understood by their operating teams before procedures are performed. This planning will provide the best environment for technically successful arthroplasty.

References

1. Bauer, G. C. H., Insall, J. N., and Koshino, T.: Tibial osteotomy in gonarthrosis (osteoarthritis of the knee). J. Bone Joint Surg. 51A:1545, 1969.
2. Brand, M. G., Daley, R. J., Ewald, F. C., and Scott, R. D.: Tibial tray augmentation with modular metal wedges for tibial bone stock deficiency. Clin. Orthop. 248:71, 1989.
3. Brooks, P. J., Walker, P. S., and Scott, R. D.: Tibial component fixation in deficient tibial bone stock. Clin. Orthop. 184:302, 1984.
4. Cella, J. P. and Stulberg, B. N.: Customization in total knee arthroplasty. Am. J. Knee Surg. 2:93–100, 1989.
5. Coventry, M. B.: Current concept review: upper tibial osteotomy for osteoarthritis. J. Bone Joint Surg. 67A:1136, 1985.
6. Craig, S. M.: Soft Tissue Considerations. Total Knee Revision Arthroplasty. Edited by W. M. Scott. Orlando, Grune & Stratton, 1987.
7. Dorr, L. D., Ochsner, J. L., and Leffers, D.: Prospective comparison of posterior cruciate retained versus cruciate sacrificed total knee surgery. Presented at the Open Scientific Meeting of The Knee Society, New Orleans, February 7, 1988.
8. Engle, G. A. and Petersen, T. L.: Comparative experience with intramedullary and extramedullary alignment in total knee arthroplasty. J. Arthroplasty 5:1–8, 1990.
9. Ewald, F. S., Hsu, H. P., and Walker, P. S.: Is kinematic total knee replacement better than total hip replacement? Orthop. Clin. North Am. 20(1):79, 1989.
10. Greene, K. A., Wilde, A. H., and Stulberg, B. N.: Preoperative nutritional status of total joint patients. Relationship to postoperative wound complications. American Academy of Orthopaedic

Surgeons Poster Presentation, Las Vegas, Nevada, 1989.
11. Insall, J. N.: Miscellaneous items: arthrodesis, the stiff knee, synovectomy, and popliteal cysts. Surgery of the Knee, pp. 729–733. New York, Churchill Livingstone, 1984.
12. Insall, J. N.: Osteotomy. Surgery of the Knee, p. 551. New York, Churchill Livingstone, 1984.
13. Insall, J. N.: Osteotomy. Surgery of the Knee, p. 579. New York, Churchill Livingstone, 1984.
14. Insall, J. N.: The stiff knee. Surgery of the Knee, p. 7. New York, Churchill Livingstone, 1984.
15. Insall, J. N.: Total knee replacement. Surgery of the Knee, pp. 618–620. New York, Churchill Livingstone, 1984.
16. Insall, J. N., Joseph, D. M., and Msika, C.: High tibial osteotomy for varus gonarthrosis: a long-term follow-up study. J. Bone Joint Surg. 661:1040, 1984.
17. Jackson, R. W. and Rouse, D. W.: The results of partial meniscectomy in patients over 40 years of age. J. Bone Joint Surg. 64B:481, 1982.
18. Johnson, L. L.: Arthroscopic abrasion arthroplasty. Arthroscopy 2:54, 1986.
19. Koshino, T., Morii, T., Wada, J., et al: High tibial osteotomy with fixation by a blade plate for medial compartment osteoarthritis of the knee. Orthop. Clin. North Am. 20(2):227, 1989.
20. Krackow, K. A.: Patient selection: indications, assessment and alternatives. The Technique of Total Knee Arthroplasty, pp. 20–37. St. Louis, C. V. Mosby Company, 1990.
21. Krackow, K. A.: Surgical procedure. The Technique of Total Knee Arthroplasty, pp. 168–169. St. Louis, C. V. Mosby Company, 1990.
22. Krackow, K. A.: The Technique of Total Knee Arthroplasty, pp. 16–48. St. Louis, C. V. Mosby Company, 1990.
23. Laskin, R. S.: Alignment of total knee components. Orthopaedics 7(1):62–72, 1984.
24. Lotke, P.: Soft tissue problems. Presentation at *Controversies of Total Knee Arthroplasty: Issues for the 90s.* Scottsdale, Arizona, November, 1989.
25. Marmor, L.: Marmor modular knee in unicompartmental disease. J. Bone Joint Surg. 61A:347, 1979.
26. Moreland, J. R., Hungerford, D. S., Insall, J. N., et al: Symposium: Total Knee Instrumentation. Contemp. Orthop. 17(5):93–126, 1988.
27. Ranawat, C. S.: Preoperative planning for total knee arthroplasty. Total Condylar Knee Arthroplasty—Technique, Results and Complications, pp. 26–30. Edited by C. S. Ranawat. New York, Springer-Verlag, 1985.
28. Ranawat, C. S. and Boachie-Adjei, O.: Survivorship analysis and results of total condylar knee arthroplasty—eight- to eleven-year follow-up period. Clin. Orthop. 226:6, 1988.
29. Ranawat, C. S. and Hausraj, K. K. Effect of posterior cruciate sacrifice on durability of the cement-bone interface: a nine-year survivorship study of 100 total condylar arthroplasties. Orthop. Clin. North Am. 20(1):63, 1989.
30. Rand, J. A.: Degenerative meniscal tears. Arthroscopy 1:253, 1986.
31. Rosenberg, A. G., Barden, R., and Galante, J. O.: A comparison of cemented and cementless fixation with the Miller-Galante total knee arthroplasty. Orthop. Clin. North Am. 20(2):97–111, 1989.
32. Salisbury, R. B., Nattage, W. N., and Gardner, V.: The effect of alignment on results in arthroscopic debridement of the degenerative knee. Clin. Orthop. 198:268, 1985.
33. Schonholtz, G. J.: Arthroscopic debridement of the knee joint. Orthop. Clin. North Am. 20(2):257, 1989.
34. Scott, R. D.: The decision to operate. Total Knee Revision Arthroplasty, pp. 51–78. Edited by W. M. Scott. Orlando, Grune & Stratton, 1987.
35. Scott, R. D.: Robert Brigham unicondylar knee surgical technique. Techn. Orthop. 5(1):15–23, 1990.
36. Scott, W. N. and Rubinstein, M. P.: Total condylar arthroplasty: indications. Total Condylar Knee Arthroplasty. Edited by C. S. Ranawat. Springer-Verlag, New York, 1985.
37. Scuderi, G. R. and Insall, J. N.: The posterior stabilized knee prosthesis. Orthop. Clin. North Am. 20(1):71, 1989.
38. Soudry, M., Binazzi, R., Johanson, N. A., et al: Total knee arthroplasty in Charcot and Charcot-like joints. Clin. Orthop. 208:199, 1986.
39. Stewart, M.: Arthrodesis. Operative Orthopaedics, pp. 1100–1141. Edited by A. Edmonson and A. Crenshaw. St. Louis, C. V. Mosby Company, 1980.
40. Stulberg, S. D.: Arthrodesis in failed total knee replacements. Orthop. Clin. North Am. 13(1):213, 1982.
41. Stulberg, S. D. and Stulberg, B. N.: The biological response to uncemented total knee replacements. Total Arthroplasty of the Knee—Proceedings of the Knee Society, 1985–1986, pp. 143–172. Edited by J. A. Rand and L. D. Dorr. Rockville, MD, Aspen Publishers, 1987.
42. Tillet, E. D., Engle, G. A., and Petersen, T. L.: A comparative study of extramedullary and intramedullary alignment systems in total knee arthroplasty. Clin. Orthop. 230:176, 1988.
43. Vince, K. G., Insall, J. N., and Kelley, M. A.: Posterior stabilized and total condylar knee arthroplasties: Comparative long-term survivorship analysis. American Academy of Orthopaedic Surgeons, Atlanta, Georgia, 1988.
44. Vince, K. G., Insall, J. N., Kelly, M. A., and Silva, M.: Total condylar knee prosthesis: Ten- to twelve-year follow-up and survivorship analysis. American Academy of Orthopaedic Surgeons, Atlanta, Georgia, 1988.
45. Weinzweig, N., Dowden, R. V., and Stulberg, B. N.: The use of tissue expansion to allow reconstruction of the knee. A case report. J. Bone Joint Surg. 69A:1238, 1987.
46. Windsor, R. E., Insall, J. N., and Sculco, T. P.: Bone grafting of tibial defects in primary and revision total knee arthroplasty. Clin. Orthop. 205:132, 1986.
47. Wong, R. Y., Lotke, P. A., and Rothman, R. H.: Bilateral total knee arthroplasty: a comparison of paired total condylar and posterior stabilized prostheses. Total Arthroplasty of the Knee—Proceedings of The Knee Society, 1985–1986, pp. 274–278. Edited by J. A. Rand and L. D. Dorr. Rockville, MD, Aspen Publishers, 1987.

CHAPTER 30

Primary Total Knee Replacement

THOMAS P. SCULCO

The success and durability of total knee arthroplasty, now a commonplace orthopaedic procedure, has been demonstrated by an abundant literature.[3, 7, 12, 16, 17, 28, 29, 33, 42, 43, 49, 53–55, 60, 67] Approximately 100,000 total knee arthroplasties are performed in the United States each year, primarily to reconstruct knee joints ravaged by osteoarthritis or rheumatoid arthritis. Knee replacement surgery was initially approached with apprehension of early mechanical failure. Certainly these fears were not groundless as evidenced by early hinge designs. However, improvements in implant design, surgical technique, and rehabilitation have resulted in consistently excellent long-term functional results.

Previous chapters of this text have described bioengineering concepts, anatomy, surgical approaches, indications, and preoperative planning. This chapter focuses first on surgical considerations, including (1) surgical exposure, (2) soft tissue balancing, (3) femoral and tibial bone cuts, (4) management of bone deficits, and (5) the patellofemoral joint. Management of the more complex reconstructions in total knee arthroplasty are discussed, including (1) the stiff knee, (2) the severe flexion contracture, (3) the biplane and triplane deformity, and (4) the grossly unstable knee.

PREOPERATIVE EVALUATION

When a patient complains of knee pain, in addition to the evaluation of the knee, a thorough general history and physical examination are essential. These are especially important in elderly patients who often have other medical problems (see Chapter 10, *Anesthesia for Joint Replacement Surgery* and Chapter 16, *Total Hip Arthroplasty: Preoperative Evaluation*). Knee evaluation includes a history of previous injuries or operations. It is essential to determine if the patient has any chronic infections (e.g., dental and urinary) that require treatment prior to joint replacement surgery.

Knee range of motion is important to determine as a prognostic indicator for postoperative motion and for special considerations before surgery. For example, the surgeon must specifically plan for correction of flexion contracture or other deformity. Stability may be impaired by ligamentous deficiency or bone loss. If a deformity can be corrected to anatomic position with a good end point, the ligament is stable. The apparent instability is due to bone deficiency that allows the knee to collapse into a deformed position. If the knee goes beyond the anatomic position and stops with a good end point, instability may be due either to bone deficiency or to an elongated ligamentous complex that has structural integrity. The cause can be differentiated usually by correlating the radiograph with the physical examination findings. If a soft end point to varus or valgus stress is evident, the ligament is deficient but the bone may be deficient as well.

Patellar tracking is evaluated. Although final determination of patellar tracking and the need for lateral retinacular release will be made during the operation, lateral patellar tracking noted preoperatively suggests release may be required. Lateral release is more likely to be required in association with valgus deformity.

The plain radiograph is the most valuable imaging study for patients with knee disease. In certain instances, bone scans, plain or computerized tomography, and magnetic resonance imaging are helpful. Computerized tomography is especially helpful in evaluating severe bony deformity (see Chapter 11, *Imaging of Total Joint Replacement*). A routine chest radiograph is made as part of an elderly patient's general examination.

All patients scheduled for surgery undergo hemograms and urinalyses. Urine cultures are done if any suspicion exists of urinary tract infections. Some patients should also undergo laboratory tests for electrolyte levels, liver function, and renal function (see Chapter 10, *Anesthesia for Joint Replacement Surgery*).[52]

PREOPERATIVE PREPARATION

The patient is oriented to the hospital environment, the plans for the operation, and the postoperative protocol. Brochures, videotapes, and illustrated books may all be helpful, but discussion with the physicians, nurses, and therapists providing an opportunity for the patient to ask questions is invaluable for setting the stage for a successful result and in allaying anxiety. Orientation is especially important for the patient who will be admitted to the hospital the day of surgery. The patient showers or bathes with an antibacterial soap the night before and the morning of surgery. Preventive antibiotics are given in the operating room just before the procedure.

SURGICAL EXPOSURE

The difficulty of surgical exposure of the knee joint depends on the preoperative deformity and range of motion. If possible, incisions from previous procedures should be used. Large skin flaps should be avoided, as undermining of the subcutaneous tissue leads to impaired blood flow to skin margins. Either a gentle medial parapatellar incision may be made, extending just below the tibial tubercle,[31] or a straight incision[30] may be made (Fig. 30–1). However, the straight incision has two disadvantages: (1) because the incision extends over the patella where subcutaneous tissue is reduced, undermining is required to reach the interval between the vastus medialis and the quadriceps tendon, and (2) because the incision rests directly over the patella, kneeling may later be painful.

Once the skin has been incised, the dissection is continued directly to the interval between vastus medialis and quadriceps tendon. At this point, the surgeon must resist the temptation to undermine flaps. The quadriceps tendon is incised sharply with a scalpel in one layer, and lamination of the tendon and multiple cuts into its substance are avoided. Several millimeters of quadriceps tendon are left attached to the vastus medialis. This step allows tendon-to-tendon closure rather than a tendon-muscle repair that is less secure and may fail, as knee flexion increases during rehabilitation (Fig. 30–2). The capsular incision extends just medial and distal to the tibial tubercle.

The medial capsular investment along the tibial face is elevated free subperiosteally (Fig. 30–3). This dissection continues posteriorly beneath the superficial me-

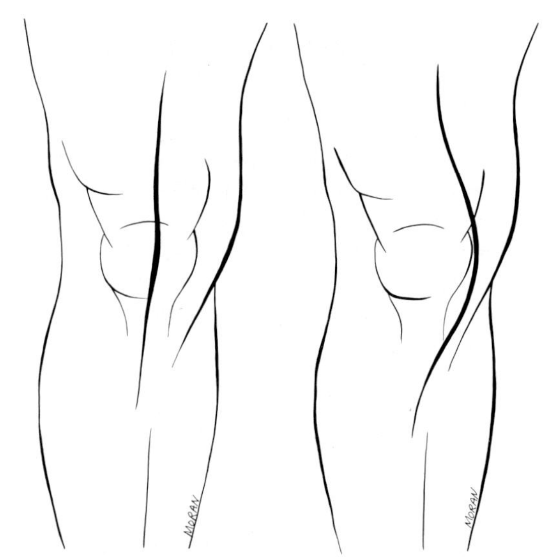

FIGURE 30–1. Skin incisions for total knee arthroplasty. *First example,* Straight vertical incision. *Second example,* Gentle medial parapatellar incision.

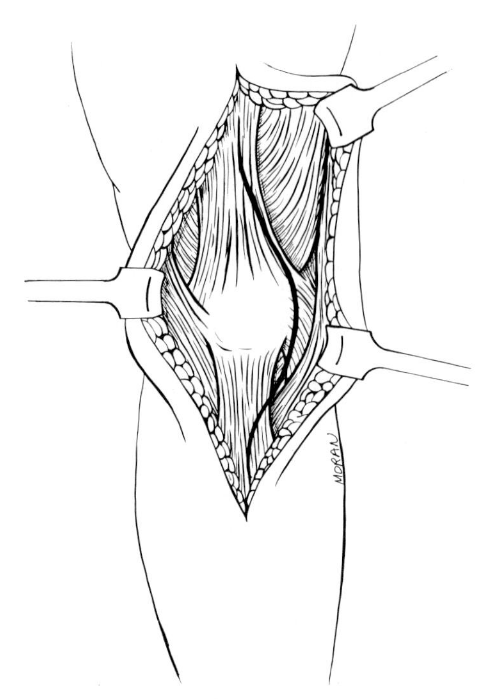

FIGURE 30–2. Capsular incision extends proximally within the substance of the quadriceps tendon to provide secure repair during closure.

dial collateral ligament to the posterior quadrant of the tibia medially and remains just below the joint line. The dissection is facilitated by external rotation of the tibia. The tibia can be subluxed anteriorly when the knee is flexed, allowing excellent exposure for femoral and tibial bone cuts.

The patella is dislocated laterally and everted, and the knee is flexed. Most patients have intact patellofemoral ligaments that prevent complete lateral subluxation of the patella. These ligaments must be released sharply (Fig. 30–4). The dissection extends to the posterior border of the lateral collateral ligament, allowing the surgeon to place a narrow-angled Hohmann retractor lateral to the tibia. By lateral retraction, the patella is held behind the narrow-angled Hohmann and away from the surgical area.

The surgeon must take care to monitor the tension at the insertion of the patellar tendon and to make a generous proximal incision into the quadriceps tendon if excessive tension is generated distally during knee flexion. In a tight knee, the patellar tendon insertion may be elevated sharply several millimeters if it tends to avulse with knee flexion. Avulsion of the patellar tendon insertion must be avoided, because repair involves placing metallic fixation devices (e.g., wires and screws) in a minimally covered area below the knee joint where skin breakdown may occur. In patients with significant contractures of the quadriceps mechanisms, a proximal inverted V-Y quadricepsplasty may be performed (see subsequent discussion.)

If the infrapatellar fat pad is redundant, it may be partially removed to improve exposure to the lateral compartment of the knee joint. The blood supply to the inferior pole of the patella will not be compromised if resection is not excessive (Fig. 30–5).

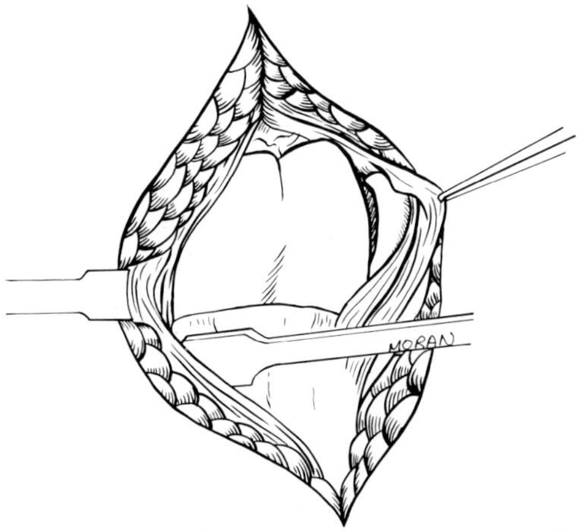

FIGURE 30–3. Elevation of the medial capsular investment along the tibial face.

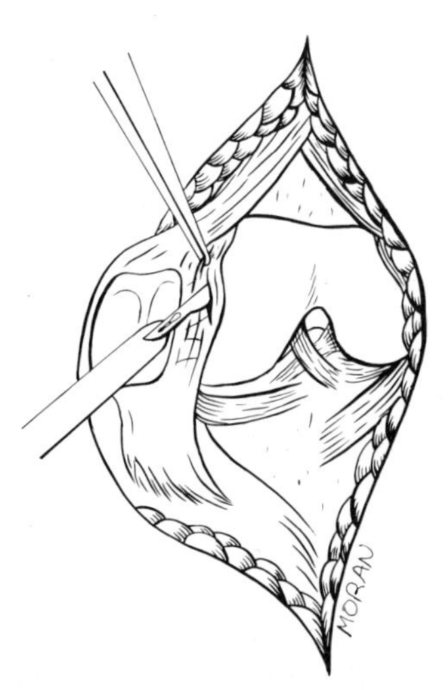

FIGURE 30–4. An intact patellofemoral ligament may prevent complete lateral subluxation of the patella unless it is released.

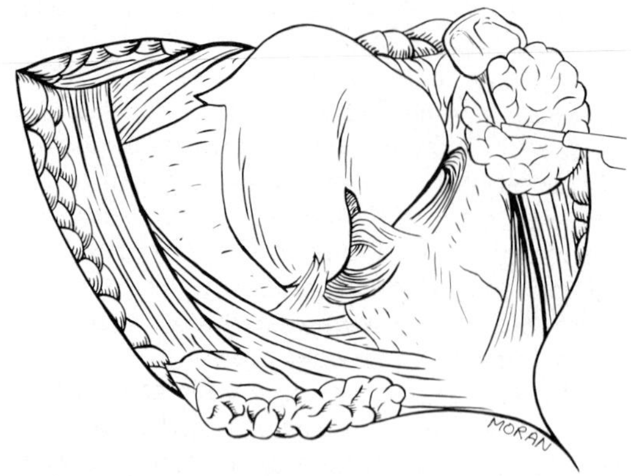

FIGURE 30–5. Excision of redundant fat pad (the portion adjacent to the joint after patellar eversion). This step maintains a protective fat pad covering beneath the patellar tendon and allows maintenance of a larger portion of the blood supply to the patellar tendon.

After the knee has been flexed to 90 degrees, the anterior cruciate ligament, if still intact, should be resected. At this point, exposure on the medial side of the knee may be continued posteriorly to allow the tibia to be dislocated anteriorly without difficulty. This maneuver greatly helps the surgeon remove more remnants of the meniscus and allows complete visualization of the upper tibial surface when the proximal tibial bone is cut. Once the knee has been exposed and fully flexed, attention should be paid to balancing of contracted soft tissue about the investment of the joint.

SOFT TISSUE BALANCING

A fundamental precept in total knee arthroplasty is that soft tissue asymmetry across the knee joint must be balanced before the prosthetic knee is implanted.[9] At what point this important step is performed varies among surgeons, but it should be done adequately to prevent later joint deformity or instability. As a rule, soft tissues should be balanced before bone cuts are made. Further adjustment can follow bone cuts during trial reduction. The pathologic features of the soft tissues investing the knee joint in angular deformity are such that contracture occurs on the concave side of the deformity and soft tissue is relatively lax on the convex side. In the varus knee, the soft tissues are usually contracted on the medial side of the joint as the result of medial collapse and deformity. The lateral structures become relatively lax as the knee shifts into varus. In the valgus knee, the opposite is true; the soft tissues are contracted on the lateral side of the joint and are lax medially. Contractures associated with valgus deformity tend to be worse than those associated with varus deformity. Not uncommonly, complex soft tissue asymmetries are present with biplane and triplane deformities. For example, posterior contractures may occur in combination with medial or lateral contractures in patients who have flexion contractures. Rotational contractures may also be observed along with flexion and medial or lateral deformities, further complicating the soft tissue management of these knees. The management of biplane and triplane deformities is discussed subsequently in more detail.

Varus Knee Deformity

To correct the soft tissue contracture on the medial side of the deformity in a varus knee, the surgeon must perform careful and progressive subperiosteal elevation medially. Elevation begins distally above the insertion of the superficial medial collateral ligament and is carried sharply along the tibial plateau surface. From anterior to posterior, the contracted tissues are released from their bony insertion. The surgeon must not transect these structures horizontally. To avoid this, a periosteal elevator may be utilized. The phrase "soft tissue release," commonly used to describe this aspect of the procedure, is a misnomer, as no release or transection is actually performed. Rather, the contracted structures are incised at their bony insertion and peeled free from the underlying bone.

In severe deformities, more extensive dissection must be performed distally and posteriorly. In a patient with severe varus deformity, it may be necessary to elevate the insertion of the superficial medial collateral ligament (Fig. 30–6). If severe posterior contracture is evident, the insertion of the semimembranosus tendon into the tibia must be freed sharply. Once these releases have been performed, the knee may be stressed medially and laterally. An equal degree of laxity should be present on both sides of the joint.

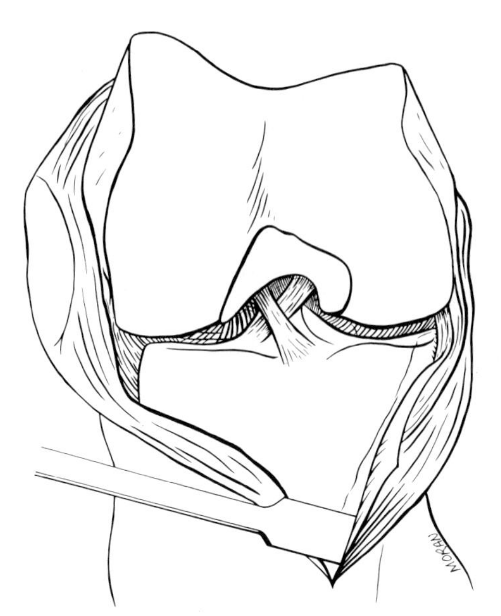

FIGURE 30–6. In the patient with severe varus deformity, it may be necessary to elevate the insertion of the superficial medial collateral ligament.

Valgus Knee Deformity

The valgus knee deformity presents more complex soft tissue problems than the varus. Commonly, the deformity has a rotational component, and the patella often tracks laterally. The patella may be subluxed because of contracted lateral parapatellar soft tissues and a tight, severely contracted patellofemoral ligament.

Initial exposure of the knee is similar to that of the varus knee. A medial parapatellar incision is preferred. Soft tissue is first released along the proximal tibial surface extending proximally to distally. All contracted soft tissues must be released from the upper tibia. The proximal portion of the insertion of the patellar tendon is often elevated several millimeters from its tibial insertion to better expose the proximal tibia. The insertion of the iliotibial band is released as it inserts into the tibia. Further dissection is continued posteriorly until the fibula is encountered. In valgus deformities of less than 15 degrees, release along the tibial surface is adequate to balance the soft tissues laterally and to effect symmetric soft tissue tension across the joint.

For more severe deformities, especially those with flexion and rotational components, it may be necessary to release the origin of the lateral collateral ligament subperiosteally from its bony insertion into the posterior aspect of the femur (Fig. 30–7). Extensive release of these soft tissues may be necessary. The lateral femoral condyle may be completely exposed after thorough release of the ligament origin. These soft tissues also must not be transected but released subperiosteally from anterior to posterior. If soft tissues remain contracted after tibial and femoral release, the iliotibial band should be transected about 2.5 cm above the joint surface. The iliotibial band can be palpated proximal to the knee joint. When a varus force is exerted on the joint, it will be quite taut. Tissues may then be released without difficulty. Release continues through the band until the knee becomes lax laterally and is balanced with the medial side. Iliotibial band release is generally the last element in the radical lateral release for the severely affected valgus knee.

Because of the contracted patellofemoral ligament and lateral retinaculum in the valgus knee, the surgeon must be prepared to do a liberal lateral retinacular release of the patella to ensure proper patellar tracking.

FEMORAL AND TIBIAL BONE CUTS

The technique of making femoral and tibial bone cuts varies from one knee implant design to another and is based on

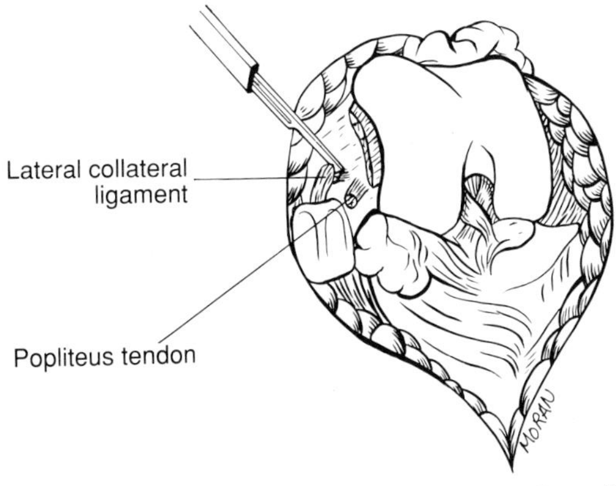

FIGURE 30–7. Release of the origin of the lateral collateral ligament for severe lateral knee contracture.

the accompanying instrumentation. However, the principles are the same regardless of what knee prosthesis is inserted. Mild variations in implant placement do occur, but with many of the currently available designs marked similarities exist and necessarily the bone cuts must be performed in a related fashion. Depending on the instrument system, either distal femoral or proximal tibial osteotomies may be made first. Most instrument systems include blocks or guides to help the surgeon make accurate cuts. The surgeon should keep an eye on the block and cutting blade to be sure that the blade follows the guide block. An assistant should watch the bone cut itself, warning the surgeon if the blade begins to go astray.

Proximal Tibial Osteotomy

The proper orientation of the proximal tibia cut in knee replacement surgery is a matter of debate. Hungerford and coworkers[24, 25] advocate maintaining the osteotomy at the same angle as the normal knee—approximately 3 degrees of varus. Theoretically, there is much to support this concept, although in practice an osteotomy at right angles to the long axis of the tibia is less difficult and more reproducible. Rand and Bryan[44] found that when they attempted a 3-degree varus cut, the varus inclination of the tibial cut averaged 4.6 degrees. Several studies have documented an increased incidence of interface radiolucencies associated with tibial cuts in varus of 4 to 5 degrees.[13, 17, 18, 45] The angulation of the joint raises the shear stress, predisposing the patient to earlier prosthesis loosening. In addition, the varus inclination of the tibial component requires greater valgus placement of the femoral component to properly align the limb. This maneuver may contribute to lateral subluxation or dislocation of the patella.

The jig device is placed parallel to the long axis of the tibia, and the osteotomy is made perpendicular to the axis. With many systems, the alignment instrument provides for placement of a cutting block held with pins. This is the osteotomy guide. The alignment rod should bisect the ankle joint—the true distal landmark for the tibial bone cut. The center of the ankle joint is located by palpating the interval between the extensor hallucis longus and the extensor digitorum longus. Finding the center is particularly important if any degree of tibial bowing is present. If the surgeon fails to make a precise cut when trying to achieve a varus orientation to the proximal tibia osteotomy, excess varus tilting of the proximal tibial osteotomy may occur, possibly causing the prosthesis to be inserted in a sloped fashion. This effect, in turn, may lead to asymmetric loading and possible failure on the lateral tibial side, as tension forces rise on the lateral tibial implant with a tendency for prosthetic lift-off and loosening.

The surgeon should perform the osteotomy carefully, taking into consideration the amount of bone being resected and remembering that the further distal into the tibia the bone cut is made, the lower the quality of bone that is available to support the implant. This factor is due to the trumpet-like character of the tibia and the greater exposure of weaker cancellous bone farther into the distal tibia (Table 30–1).[6] The tendency to resect to the base of bone deficits must be resisted when the proximal tibial osteotomy is made. As a

Table 30–1. INDENTATION STRESSES AT FOUR LEVELS OF SECTION IN ONE TIBIA

Area Indented	Number of Indentations	Average Indentation Stress (MN/m^2) at Given Depth (mm) from Articular Surface			
		5	*15*	*25*	*35*
Medial	6 total	4.4	3.3	3.5	1.6
Central	6 total	3.1	2.5	2.4	—
Lateral	7 total	4.2	4.3	2.4	1.6
Average for level of section		3.9	3.4	2.7	1.6

Bargren, J. H., Day, W. H., Freeman, M. A. R., and Swanson, S. A. V.: J. Bone Joint Surg. 60B:256–261, 1978. By permission. (MN/m^2 = meganewtons per square meter.)

rule, about 6 to 10 mm of bone should be resected. Procedures to augment these deficits are discussed subsequently.

To facilitate the bone cut, the tibia should be subluxed completely anterior to the femur to expose its entire upper surface. After the osteotomized tibial bone is removed, peripheral osteophytes can be removed. These often tent the soft tissues on the contracted side of the knee and contribute to the soft tissue contracture on the concave side of the deformity. Removal will help produce ligamentous symmetry.

After osteotomy, the tibial surface should be prepared to accept the implant. A central peg hole or multiple holes, screws, or both may be employed for fixation, depending on the type of total knee system and whether the components are cemented or noncemented. Areas of hard eburnated bone on the tibial surface should be fenestrated with a small drill bit to expose trabecular bone and to allow better penetration of cement or improved vascularity for ingrowth of a noncemented component.

Femoral Bone Osteotomy

Femoral bone cuts should achieve five objectives: (1) restoration of the knee to a physiologic degree of valgus, permitting loadbearing along the mechanical axis; (2) placement of the femoral component in proper anteroposterior orientation, providing as nearly normal kinematics as possible; (3) close coaptation of the femoral implant to bone by careful shaping of bone cuts (directed by the jig system); (4) resection of a proper amount of femur to allow full extension of the knee; and (5) achievement of proper rotation of the femoral component. Various methods for achieving these goals have been developed, utilizing instrumentation guides of different designs. Currently, all five objectives are best achieved with intramedullary instrument systems, although Tillett and colleagues[64] have demonstrated little difference between intramedullary and extramedullary systems. Extramedullary systems use the anterior superior iliac spine as an objective marker. The position of the femoral head is then estimated based on its being 2 to 3 cm medial to the anterior superior iliac spine. These systems are somewhat inaccurate, however, as it may be difficult to locate the anterior iliac crest and spine exactly by palpation after draping. Also, because of the differences in pelvic breadth, particularly in women, aiming the axis of the distal femoral cut 2 to 3 cm medial to the anterior iliac spine may be inaccurate. Intraoperative radiographs locate the femoral head more precisely but are time consuming. Radiography also increases operating room traffic and the resulting danger of wound contamination. Another method for locating the femoral head when using an extramedullary alignment system is to place a radiopaque marker that can be palpated through any draping and ascertain its relation to the center of the femoral head with a preoperative radiograph.

The loadbearing axis across the prosthetic knee joint should simulate that in the normal knee. Therefore, the axis of the load should be along a line extending from the femoral head through the knee joint just medial to the midline. The axis should pass distally to bisect the ankle joint (Fig. 30–8). Minor variations in this load vector

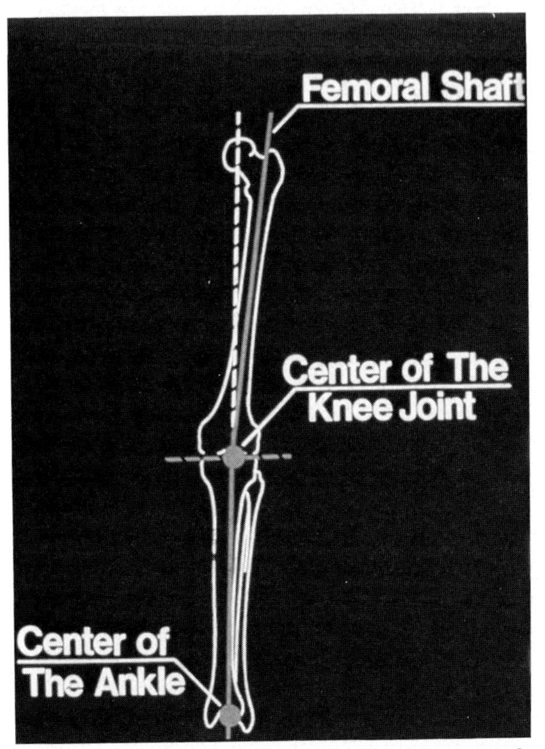

FIGURE 30–8. The loadbearing axis of the normal knee.

are compatible with excellent function as in the varied alignment of nonpathologic knees. However, it is of paramount importance to approximate this referenced mechanical axis of weightbearing in the prosthetic joint.

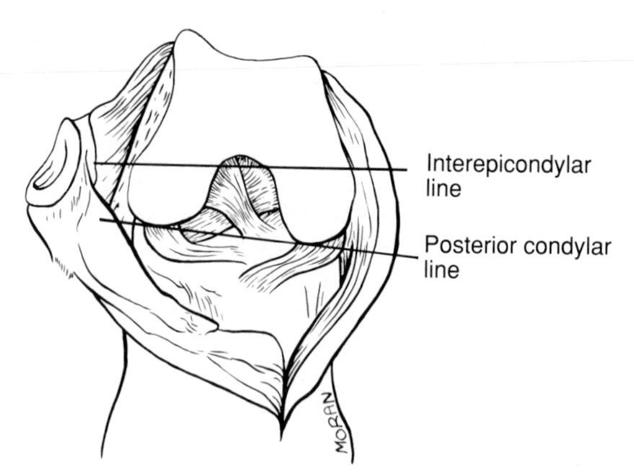

FIGURE 30–10. Rotation of the femoral component should be based on the femoral interepicondylar line. Relying on the posterior condyles to establish rotation may result in malrotation that will create abnormal kinematics of the femorotibial articulation and maltracking of the patella.

Intramedullary guides are most commonly selected to position the femoral component in valgus orientation and to align the resultant load along the mechanical axis. The entry hole into the femoral canal must be along the center line of the intramedullary canal. Otherwise, orientation of the rod and the femoral cuts will be out of alignment. The starting hole is centered in the femoral trochlea immediately anterior to the edge of the articular surface. These intramedullary guides must pass into the femoral canal at least 15 to 20 cm to ensure that they are along the long axis of the femur. If a previous femoral fracture has occurred or if femoral angulation is excessive, intramedullary systems may be inaccurate. Under these circumstances, extramedullary instruments should be used, with the femoral head serving as the guide for the osteotomy. Any one of various cutting blocks or guides is then placed to allow the surgeon to cut the distal femur into the degree of valgus desired. As a rule, the distal femur is cut in 5 to 7 degrees of valgus. The distal femoral bone cut should be made perpendicular to the mechanical axis but should be in valgus orientation to the anatomic axis of the femur (Fig. 30–9).

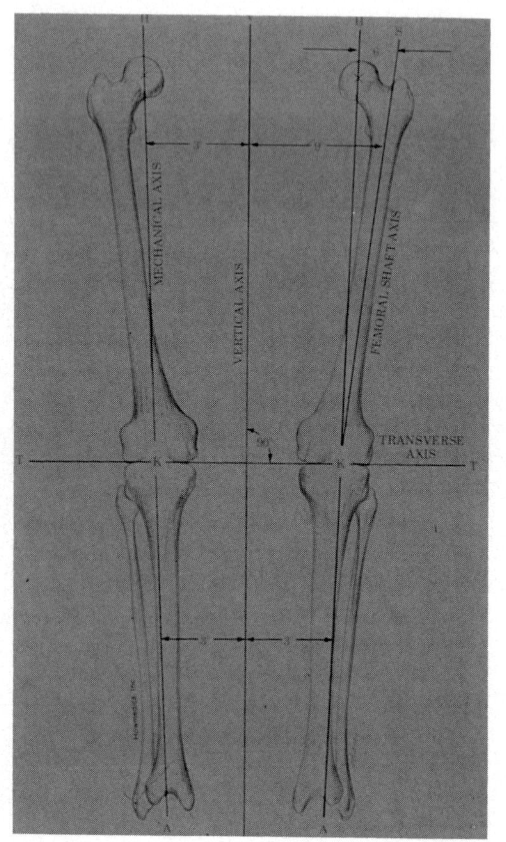

FIGURE 30–9. The relationship of the mechanical axis of the limb and the anatomic axis of the femur.

Proper rotational alignment is important to proper femorotibial kinematics and extensor mechanism function. It is best to establish rotation based on the interepicondylar line. Relying on the posterior condyles to establish rotation may cause malrotation due to anatomic variation or bone deficit. The medial posterior condyle is often more prominent than the lateral. If rotation is based on the posterior condyles, it may result in placement of the femoral component in internal rotation and cause maltracking of the patella (Fig. 30–10).

Once alignment has been achieved in both the medial lateral and anterior posterior planes, the remaining bone resection on the femoral side is done to allow accurate coaptation of the implant to the distal femur. Care must be taken to apply the cutting guides accurately and atraumatically, particularly in osteopenic bone, to prevent imprecise bone cuts.

In a patient with a significant flexion contracture, posterior release must be performed. With more severe flexion contracture, it may be necessary to remove additional bone from the femur so that the knee can be brought into extension.

MANAGEMENT OF BONE DEFICITS

In patients with loss of bone associated with angular deformities, techniques must be utilized to augment the deficient bone. Bone is most often lost on the tibial side of the joint, and deficits are generally more marked in the posterior portion of the tibia. This finding is most likely when a flexion contracture exists in combination with an angular deformity. The floor of the defect is generally flattened, sclerotic, and devoid of cartilage. Because the tibia usually subluxes as the deformity progresses, the peripheral rim of the tibia may be destroyed in more severe deformities (see Fig. 30–15A).

Although significant femoral deficiency is also seen on the affected side of the angular deformity, it is less frequent and usually less severe than tibial deficiency. The condylar design of the distal femur tends to drive it into the proximal tibia and leads to collapse of the tibial bone with an associated bone defect.

The management of bone loss in total knee replacement depends on the location and degree of the bone loss. Measures that have been employed include (1) implantation of bone cement alone,[36] (2) bone cement reinforced with mesh or screws,[44] (3) bone grafting,[5, 15, 69] and (4) custom[65] or modular augmented total knee implants. The surgeon must adopt a basic principle when managing bone defects, i.e., resection of bone from the tibia to the floor of the defect must be avoided except in the slightest of bone deficits (<8 mm). Resecting excessive bone from the proximal tibia will expose the weaker cancellous bone, making loosening and failure more likely.[6, 22, 60] If a revision arthroplasty becomes necessary, valuable bone will have been removed. In total knee surgery, bone stock must be preserved whenever possible. Additionally, when tibial bone is removed to the floor of a large defect, an increased gap in flexion is created, requiring a thicker tibial implant to fill the void. The need for a larger tibial implant leads to further problems in patellofemoral kinematics, as the patella is fixed distally by the patellar tendon and therefore may make contact with this thickened implant as the knee is flexed. Sizing may also be affected because of the reduced cross-sectional area on the upper portion of the tibia now available for implant seating. In summary, resection of the tibia to the floor of but the most trivial deficiency is to be avoided and will potentially jeopardize the quality of the arthroplasty.

For defects 8 to 13 mm and encompassing less than half of one tibial plateau, several techniques are available. About 8 mm of the less-involved portion of the tibia is usually resected, so that the resected bone approaches the level of the bed of the deficit. The floor of the involved side of the tibia will be very sclerotic, making it necessary to fenestrate the surface to ensure penetration of bone cement into tibial subchondral bone. If only a few millimeters of deficit remain, the deficit can be filled with bone cement alone. Unsupported columns of cement in this range have been prone to neither fracture nor loss of implant support. Larger columns of bone cement may be problematic, however. These are a concern particularly when optimal alignment has not been achieved in the arthroplasty.

Where defects of more than 3 to 5 mm are present after resection of the upper tibia, the bone cement may be reinforced with cortical screws (Fig. 30–11). The screws are placed just below the polyethylene or metal tray of the tibial implant, and cement incorporates them to fill the bone defect. If the implant has a tendency to tilt into the defect, the screws may be placed so that their heads are in contact with the prosthesis, thereby acting as a strut and preventing sinking of the implant into the defect. Incompatible metals must be avoided if this technique is employed.

In tibial defects larger than 13 to 15 mm and encompassing more than a third of the tibial surface, other techniques should be utilized. A prosthetic implant may be customized with a wedge to fill the void on the affected tibial side. Although good long-term results have been reported with this technique, problems related to custom fabrication of the tibial implants can occur.

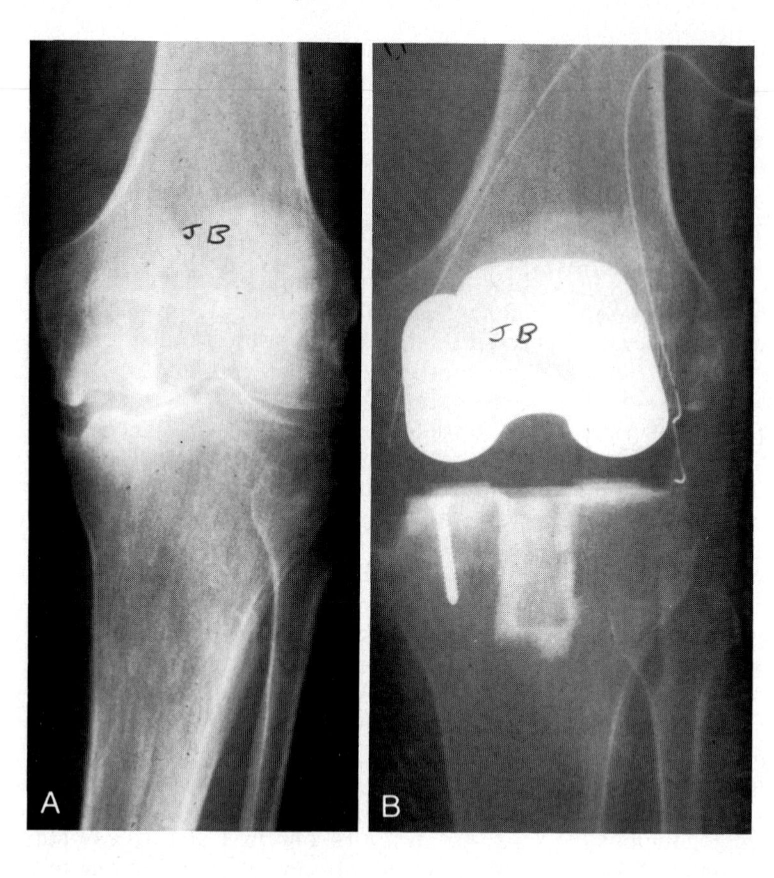

FIGURE 30–11. Management of moderate tibial defect with bone cement reinforced with screws. *A*, Preoperative radiograph shows moderate medial tibial deficiency. *B*, Defect was filled with bone cement reinforced with cortical screws.

If the implant does not fit at the time of surgery, the surgeon is left with little flexibility. Also, these custom implants are expensive and take several weeks to make. Modular implants in varying sizes that augment the undersurface of the tibia have given surgeons the ability to construct whatever implant configuration they require (Fig. 30–12). Bone grafting is an effective and more physiologic method for filling bone defects. Bone grafting allows the flexibility to fashion the graft to fit the defect and preserve the bone stock at the same time.

Bone Grafting for Tibial Deficiency

Bone grafting of the proximal tibia for deficiency in severe angular deformity may be performed employing bone removed during knee arthroplasty.[5, 69] I prefer to fill tibial defects with bone taken from the distal femoral condyles. In this technique, the hard reactive bone is removed from the base of the tibial deficiency in a planar fashion so that the bed is primarily cancellous. Because the defect generally extends through the peripheral rim of the tibia, this cut along the upper tibia leaves a smooth surface as the recipient bed. Bone removed from the distal femoral condyle may be used to fill the bed. Generally, more medial femoral condylar bone is available than lateral bone, so it is selected. The cancellous surface of the femoral condylar bone is apposed to the tibia, and the condyle is rotated until the defect is most fully covered. The graft is held in place with two K-wires. The tibial surface on the more normal side of the joint is a guide, and the overhanging bone graft is removed in line with the upper tibial osteotomy (Fig. 30–13). Two cancellous screws then fix the graft to the bed. At this point, a look at the upper tibial surface reveals that the subchondral rim of the femoral graft acts as a peripheral rim for the tibia and that the upper surface of the tibia has been reconstituted (Fig. 30–13). The tibial peg hole should be made before

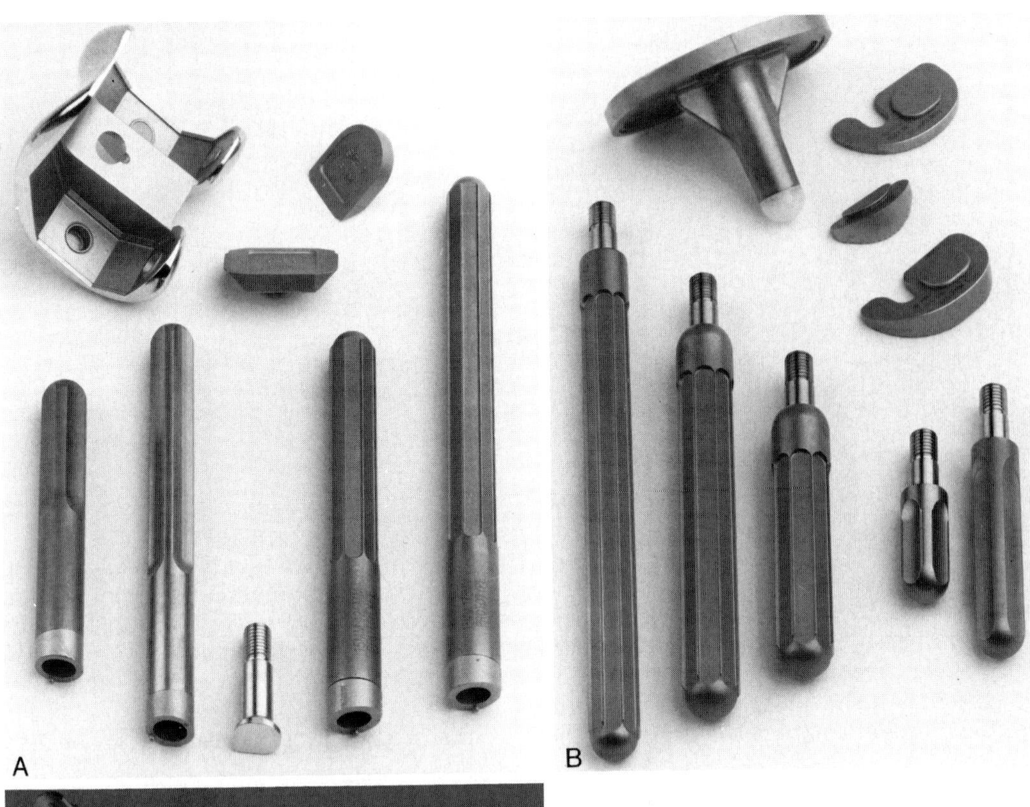

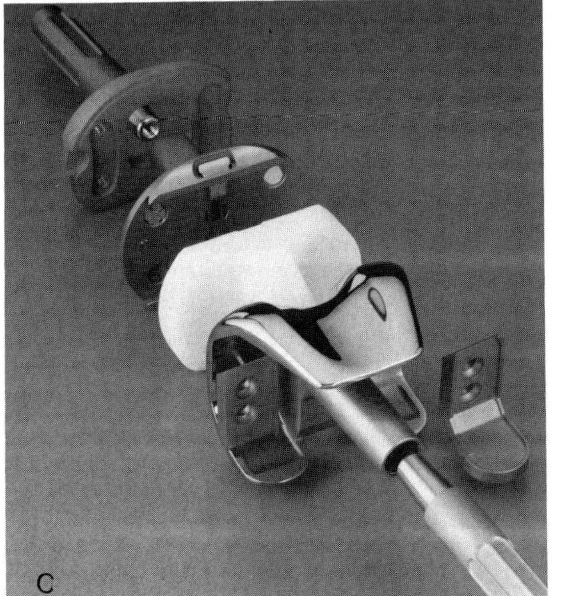

FIGURE 30–12. Examples of augmentation implants available for filling bone defects. *A,* Femoral component augmentation devices. (Courtesy of Johnson & Johnson.) *B,* Tibial component augmentation devices. (Courtesy of Johnson & Johnson.) *C,* Augmentation devices available in a modular implant system. (Courtesy of Zimmer, Inc.)

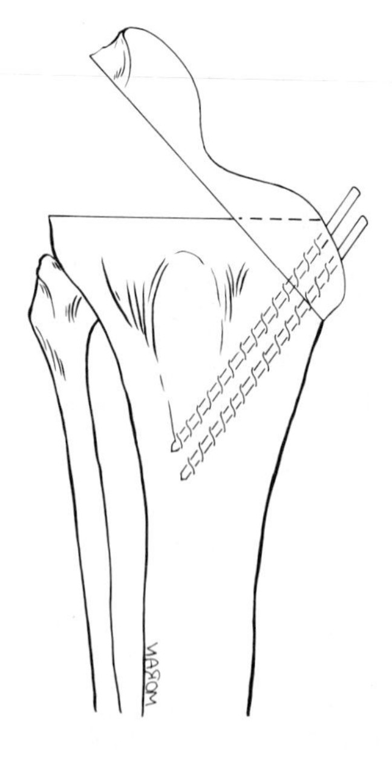

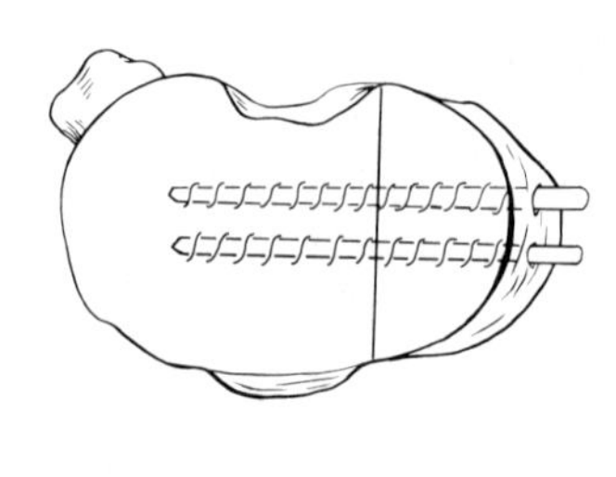

FIGURE 30–13. Technique for filling tibial defect with bone graft from the excised femoral condyle.

grafting. In this way, the screws can be watched and kept from entering the area of the peg hole. Bone cement, from a separate batch, can be made to caulk the interface of the graft and the bed on the tibial surface. This important step prevents cement from entering the bone graft interface when the tibial prosthesis is implanted. Cement between the graft and the recipient bed will prevent healing of the host bone to the bone graft.

Over 30 patients have undergone this procedure in an 11-year period with no evidence of graft resorption, loss of implant position, or other premature implant failures related to the bone graft (Fig. 30–14). All grafts have consolidated. No modifications of postoperative rehabilitation have

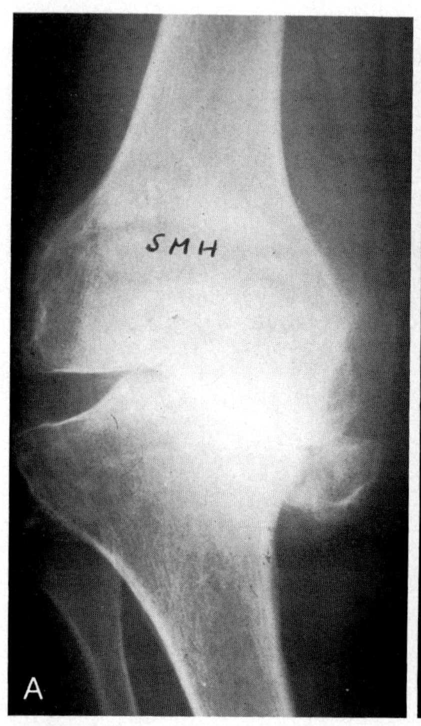

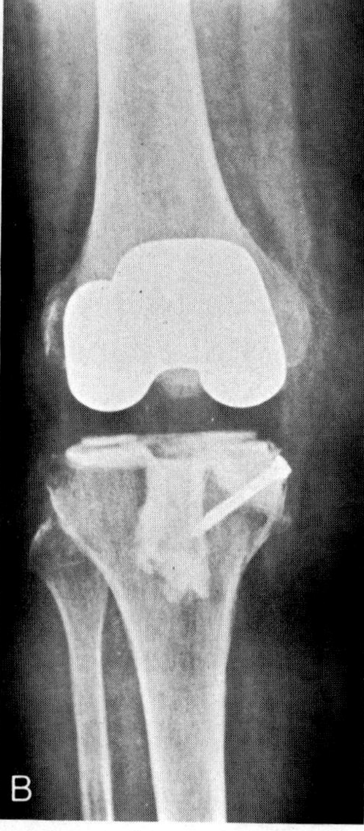

FIGURE 30–14. Filling tibial bone defect with autogenous bone graft from femoral condylar resection. *A,* Preoperative radiograph shows varus deformity with severe medial tibial bone deficiency. *B,* Ten-year follow-up radiograph. The tibial bone defect was filled with an autogenous bone graft from the femoral condyle and fixed with a bone screw. Knee alignment and component fixation are excellent. Graft healed despite cement partially between graft and bed.

been needed in these patients. Another excellent source of autogenous bone graft is the bone resected from the tibial plateau opposite the defect (Fig. 30–15).

Similar bone grafting procedures may be employed for deficiencies of the distal femur. Bone may be shaped to fill voids, with larger grafts held in place by screws. Local bone removed during arthroplasty may be used to fill cystic deficiencies both on the femoral and tibial sides. These deficiencies are more common in patients with rheumatoid arthritis or severe osteopenia. Cancellous bone from the iliac crest may also be utilized if larger deficiencies are present and not enough local bone is harvested during arthroplasty.

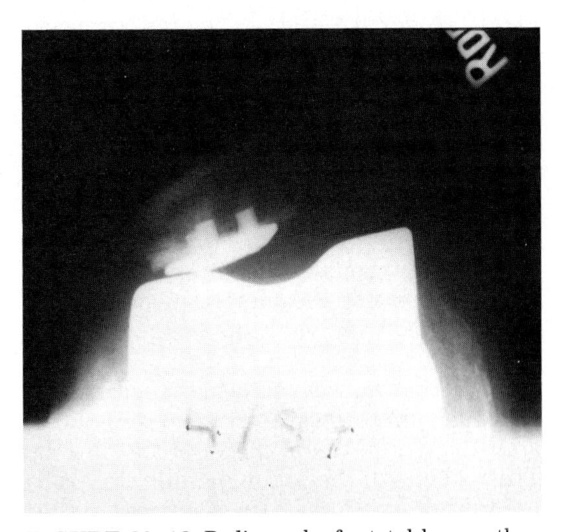

FIGURE 30–16. Radiograph of a total knee arthroplasty with maltracking of the patella. Metal-backed patella is sometimes associated with the complications of component dissociation and wear through of the polyethylene.

PATELLOFEMORAL JOINT

Replacement of the patellofemoral joint continues to be a problem, despite good long-term results in implant fixation and dramatic improvements in technique and instrumentation. Diverse complications are related to the patellofemoral mechanism, compromising the end result of total knee arthroplasty.[20, 21, 23, 26, 27, 35, 37, 38, 40, 41, 51, 63, 66] These complications include (1) malalignment and instability of the patellofemoral joint, (2) fracture, (3) prosthetic loosening, (4) prosthetic failure and metallosis in metal-backed patellar prostheses, and (5) parapatellar pain and crepitus. The worst and most preventable problems are malalignment of the extensor mechanism and mistracking of the patella (Fig. 30–16). Attention to procedural detail while placing the prosthetic patellofemoral joint will reduce these problems. After the patellar surface has been prepared for patella component implantation, a trial implant should be inserted and the knee flexed and extended. If the patella has a tendency to slide or tilt laterally with knee flexion, a lateral retinacular release should be performed. Another method to check patellar tracking is to flex and extend the knee with the thumb just next to the patella. If pressure with the thumb must be applied to stabilize the patella, a lateral release should be performed. In my experience, the lateral release is best performed whenever the patella shows any tendency to lateral subluxation. Release should be done from

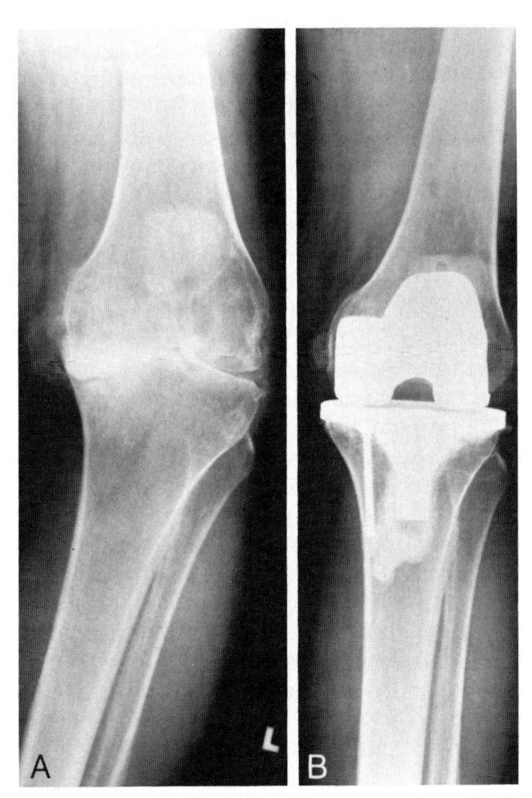

FIGURE 30–15. Patient with severe osteoarthritis of the knee with medial tibial bone loss. *A*, Preoperative radiograph shows marked varus deformity with medial tibial bone loss. *B*, The tibial defect as filled with autogenous bone graft taken from the lateral tibial plateau. The bone graft was fixed with a screw. Alignment and component fixation are excellent.

inside the joint just lateral to the patella. The surgeon should release all tight lateral structures, as well as subcutaneous tissue, if needed (Fig. 30–17). The superior lateral geniculate artery should be avoided if possible. Although the lateral structures may be released from outside the joint, this maneuver requires dissection of the skin and subcutaneous tissues from the patella, a procedure not recommended because of the potential for vascular compromise to the skin.

To further improve patellar tracking, the surgeon may position the prosthesis slightly medial to the center of the patella. This step will help the patella to track appropriately. In the case of severe patellar malalignment seen in marked valgus deformity, patellar instability may persist even after thorough lateral retinacular release. In the most complex case, the insertion of the patellar tendon may be moved medially and a radical proximal release performed. Generally, this maneuver produces enough medialization of the extensor mechanism to allow for adequate patellar tracking. The tendon may be fixed with staples or heavy sutures through tibial bone, or the patellar ligament insertion is transferred with a block of bone that can be firmly fixed with screws. If screws are used, they should be placed to the sides so they are not beneath the skin at the most prominent point of the tubercle.

Aside from patellar tracking, the surgeon must take care to remove the correct amount of patellar bone. The amount of bone resected should approximate the thickness of the patellar prosthesis to be implanted. The patellar bone cut must be horizontal to prevent impingement of a portion of the patella against the femoral component. The patella is best osteotomized by everting it completely, using Kocher clamps or other instruments to hold the tendon above and below the patella, maintaining a horizontal position to the patella parallel to the floor. If the patella is cut with the saw blade perfectly horizontal, a flat resection should result (Fig. 30–18). When a patellar component is too small, exposed patellar bone will remain, increasing the possibility for impingement and pain. If the patellar component is too large, problems with knee flexion will occur and may even compromise wound closure. Excessive resection will weaken the remaining patella, increasing fracture risk.

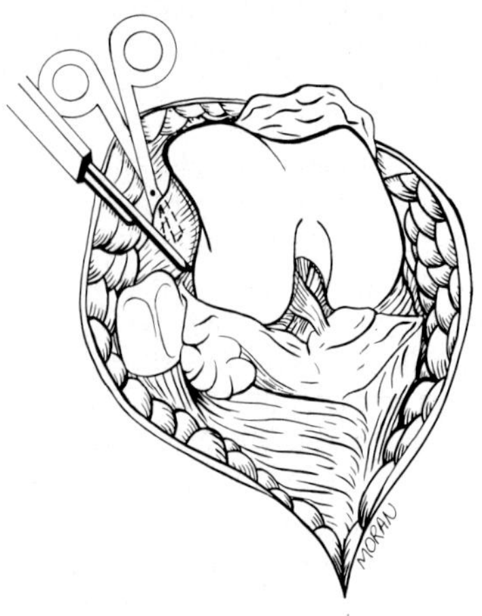

FIGURE 30–17. Lateral retinacular release.

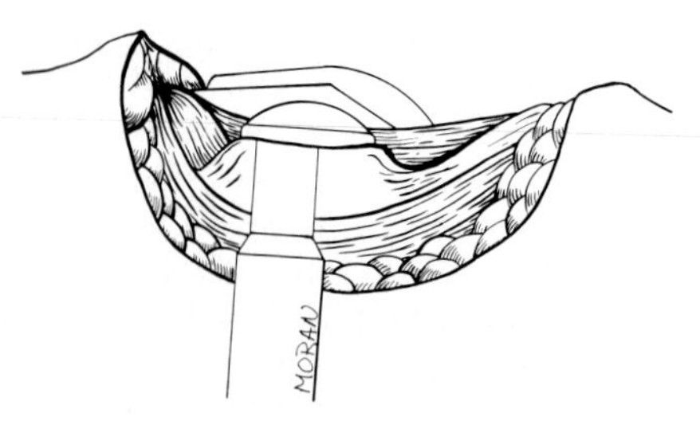

FIGURE 30–18. Osteotomy of the patella. The patella is held in the everted position and parallel to the floor so that a flat, horizontal cut with the saw will be less difficult to make.

Patellar fracture has been reported after total knee arthroplasty in varying degrees ranging from complete absence of fracture to 21 percent.[35] Although the cause has not been clearly defined, it is probably multifactorial. The patient who falls hard on the operated knee may sustain a traumatic fracture, but fracture may also occur with less force if the bony patella has been weakened substantially during replacement. A more common occurrence after total knee replacement is a stress fracture of which the patient may be unaware. It may be discovered only on radiographs at follow-up evaluation. The relatively high incidence of these fractures has been partially attributed to the greater range of motion allowed by current total knee implants and the use of excessively large patellar components.[29] With increasing flexion of the knee, tension forces may be raised across the patella. Fracture may result through the stress riser effect of a patellar peg hole. The surgeon must be aware of the weakening of patellar bone that accompanies operation and remove bone only to the extent that the remaining bone plus prosthesis is equivalent to the normal patellar thickness. The remaining patella should be at least 1 to 1.5 cm thick. The surgeon should avoid removing too much bone from the periphery of the patella. Although overhanging osteophytes may be excised to prevent painful impingement, the peripheral cortex of the patella should be left intact.

Patellar holes should not be drilled deeper than required by the implant. Drilling through the anterior patellar cortex will weaken the patella significantly and heighten the risk of fracture due to the stress riser created by the hole. Care must also be taken to choose the correct size of patellar replacement. Surgeons sometimes tend to choose large patellar replacements that cover the entire exposed patellar bed but increase stress across the patellofemoral joint during flexion. A component should be selected that will prevent significant peripheral patellar bone exposure but not at the expense of an excessively thick patellar component.

Debate continues on the contribution of altered blood supply to patellar fracture. The arterial blood supply to the patella is well documented. Both an extraosseous and intraosseous supply takes origin from a ring of six main arteries: supreme geniculate, medial superior geniculate, medial inferior geniculate, lateral inferior geniculate, lateral superior geniculate, and anterior tibial recurrent.[35] The medial vessels are interrupted by the medial approach to the knee joint. How much the lateral vessels are compromised depends on the extent of lateral patellar release. The remaining blood supply derives primarily from the intratendinous supply and the superior lateral geniculate artery, which should be preserved when lateral release is performed. Kayler and Lyttle[32a] have demonstrated that preservation of the prepatellar vessels and radial intraosseous vessels as well as some of the infrapatellar fat pad is important to patellar viability. Scuderi and associates[56] reported a 57 percent increase in incidence of cold patellae on bone scan after lateral releases, compared with 15 percent without lateral release. However, when Ritter and Campbell[47] compared patients with and without lateral release, they found that the former group had no increase in osteonecrosis, patellar bone-cement radiolucency, or patellar fracture. The surgeon should preserve as much arterial supply to the patella as possible. At least the procedure should spare the prepatellar anastomosis, superior lateral geniculate, and infrapatellar supply through the fat pad, which should not be totally excised.

After noncemented fixation was introduced for total knee replacement, metal backing was added to patellar polyethylene components in an attempt to distribute the load to the patella more evenly. Metal backing is necessary if bone ingrowth is to be promoted through a beaded or sintered surface. In an attempt to improve upon the dome-shaped polyethylene patella, a more anatomic patella with medial and lateral facets has been developed. However, the alterations in patella implant design have met with problems as evidenced by intermediate term follow-up studies.[37, 41, 63] Mainly, the patellar component has disassociated (loosened) from the bone; bead shedding has occurred; polyethylene and metal components have disassociated; and the thin polyethylene has worn through, exposing the metallic substrate and producing extensive debris with severe metallic synovitis of the joint. Although problems with patellar instability are theoretically lessened by a more congruent and constrained patella, greater shear forces may lead to failure at the bone-cement interface and patellar loosening.

The dome patella has proved very successful in long-term studies, with infrequent loosening, mechanical failure or surface damage—the common causes of failure.[43] The data stand on their merits despite experimental evidence reported by Hsu and Walker[27] that susceptibility to deformation is increased and the potential for failure is high. These investigators also found that more anatomic patellae limit normal rotational movements. They theorize that increased torque and shear forces are generated that may compromise patellar fixation. A dome shape to the patellar articular surface may also make right and left femoral components less necessary. Because the dome shape may be inherently less stable than a more anatomic shape, soft tissue balancing is particularly important to reduce problems of instability.

Technique cannot be emphasized too much in any discussion of implanting and balancing the patellar component in total knee surgery. If attention to detail is not meticulous, problems will result due to instability, fracture, or improper fixation.

Prosthetic Selection

When faced with prostheses selection, surgeons who perform total knee arthroplasties have difficulty agreeing on whether or not to preserve the posterior cruciate ligaments. Because the anterior cruciate ligament is often deficient and its removal facilitates prosthetic design and implantation, excision is accepted. With the advent of the total condylar prosthesis its designers advocated removal of both cruciate ligaments. The design provided more congruence to the tibial component to provide knee joint stability. However, studies have demonstrated that gait (walking) characteristics of the normal knee are more clearly simulated, particularly during stair climbing, if the posterior cruciate ligament is retained.[1, 2, 14] Nonetheless, long-term studies of patients with total condylar prostheses have demonstrated 88 percent good or excellent results at 10- to 12-year follow-up evaluations.[67]

To promote greater stability and range of motion, the posterior stabilized or posterior cruciate replacing prosthesis was developed in 1978. Range of motion was increased to an average of 115 degrees,[29] and long-term results were excellent, similar to those with the total condylar prosthesis.[3, 29, 54, 55] However, more patellar problems have been encountered in the posterior stabilized design, which may be attributed to the greater range of motion. In a 2- to 4-year follow-up study of the posterior stabilized prosthesis reported by Insall and associates,[29] fracture of the patella occurred in 11 of 113 replaced knees. Fracture incidence was reduced significantly by alteration of technique and resection of less patellar bone.[54] A later modification of the femoral component to allow improved patellar tracking has also become available.

Retention of the posterior cruciate ligament is commonplace in many current prosthetic designs. The advantage is that the posterior femoral rollback mechanism is maintained, with resulting improvement of the quadriceps lever arm and thereby its power. Because of this femoral rollback, the posterior portion of the tibial implant must be flat to reduce impingement as the knee is flexed and the femoral component slides posteriorly. If the tibial component had a dish-like shape, contact would occur posteriorly creating a wedge effect that would impede flexion and potentiate forces that could loosen the implant. Maintaining proper tension in the posterior cruciate ligament may be technically difficult for the surgeon, however.[48] In a series of ten knees in which Corces and colleagues[11] measured the strain characteristics of the posterior cruciate ligament, only one had a strain pattern consistent with a functioning posterior cruciate ligament. Bone resection must be consistent with the thickness of the tibial implant. If not, the joint line will be moved, usually upward, causing dysfunction of the posterior cruciate ligament. If too little bone is resected, the knee will be tight in flexion (Fig. 30–19). Additionally, with flexion, the implant will tend to open anteriorly in a book-like fashion and the tibia may sublux anteriorly. Range of motion will also be limited if the knee is tight in flexion. If excess bone is resected, the posterior cruciate ligament will be incompetent and nonfunctional. The accuracy of bone resection thickness is less critical when posterior stabilized implants are used. Clinical results with prostheses that retain the posterior cruciate ligaments and those that sacrifice them have been similar.[7, 49]

When complex deformity and contractures are present in the knee, the posterior cruciate ligament may have to be sacrificed to correct the deformity and achieve soft tissue balance. Under these circumstances, a posterior stabilized-type tibial component is necessary.

Cemented Prostheses and Porous Implants

After the success demonstrated in hip arthroplasty, efforts were directed toward studying the applicability of noncemented designs to the knee joint. In long-term studies, the results of cemented total knee

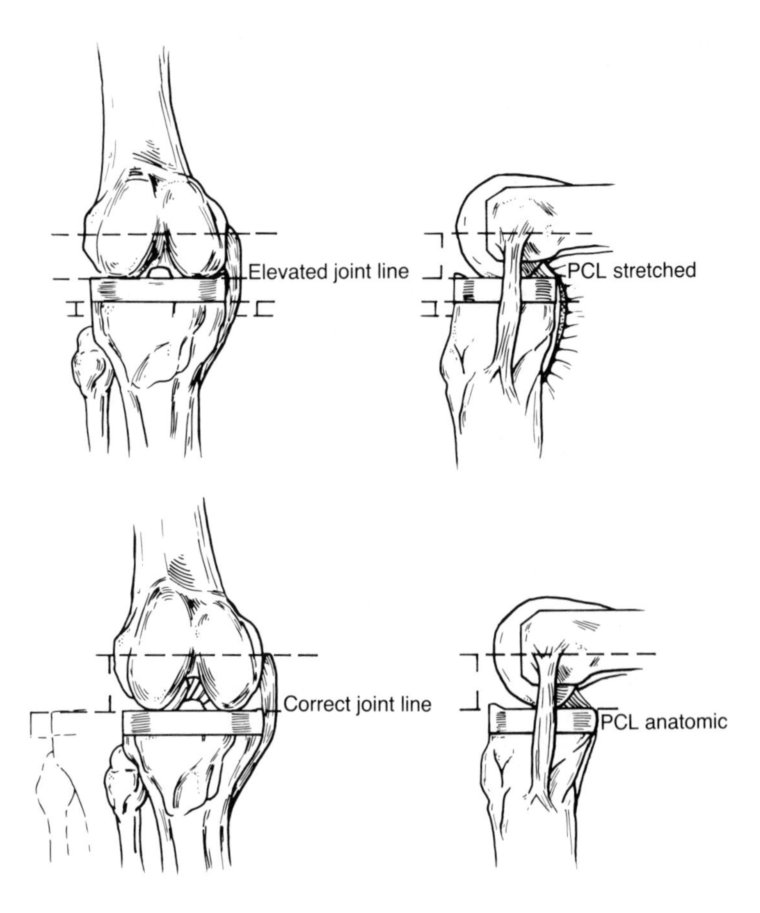

FIGURE 30–19. If the posterior cruciate ligament (PCL) is retained and the amount of bone resection from the tibia is less than the thickness of the implant, the joint line will be moved upward and the posterior cruciate ligament will be tight in flexion.

arthroplasty differed from hip arthroplasty in one major way—fewer mechanical failures.[16, 24, 28, 44, 46, 51] If the arthroplasty is performed well initially, excellent long-term results can be anticipated. Radiolucencies are demonstrable but tend not to progress. Loosening remains uncommon.

Porous implants require careful surgical technique to ensure absolute coaptation of implant to underlying bone. In a cemented total knee replacement, small voids are filled with bone cement and fixation is not impaired. This does not occur in a cementless implant. For bone ingrowth, bone and implant must come into intimate contact. This requires instrumentation that offers a high degree of accuracy and a high degree of surgical skill.

Various types of fixation have been employed for porous systems. Most rely on a press-fit intimate contact for the femur and patella. On the tibial side, pegs and various screw fixation patterns have been employed.

Histologic evaluation has raised concern about whether bone ingrowth occurs in total knee implants. In a histologic and radiographic analysis of 85 porous-coated knee components, Cook and associates[10] found little bone ingrowth. In 52 percent of components there was no evidence of bone ingrowth. In 29 percent it was minimal, and in 12 percent it was moderate. Only 7 percent showed considerable ingrowth. Ingrowth was no greater in the femoral than in the tibial and patellar components—ingrowth being universally poor. What little bone ingrowth occurred was concentrated mainly around fixation pegs or screws. No one design type was superior over another in this respect, nor did porous surface pattern make a difference. Clinical findings have also demonstrated inferior results with noncemented designs,[50] with higher reoperation rate and reduced range of motion.

Because long-term results with various cemented implants continue to be excellent, the surgeon should be cautious about selecting noncemented total knee designs, especially for the tibia and patella. Further basic and clinical research must be done before these implants can be advocated for universal insertion.

COMPLEX RECONSTRUCTIONS IN TOTAL KNEE ARTHROPLASTY

Stiff Knee

Although relatively uncommon, severe degenerative joint disease may be associated with a markedly reduced range of motion. Previous knee sepsis, hemophilia, juvenile rheumatoid arthritis, and posttraumatic arthritic afflictions most commonly lead to major loss of knee flexion. Knee stiffness may also be encountered in revision arthroplasty for intra-articular fibrosis, loosening, posterior cruciate ligament tightness, and removal of a total knee replacement for deep infection. Patients with flexion contractures along with loss of knee motion do not present as onerous a challenge as those with knee stiffness in extension. With flexion deformity, the quadriceps tendon and muscle are somewhat elongated, facilitating exposure and rehabilitation.

The patient with a knee stiff in extension poses an especially difficult technical challenge in total knee arthroplasty.[4, 8, 57] Generally, range of motion is markedly restricted (<20 degrees) and little if any flexion contracture is present. The major problems are exposure of the knee, which is complex because of the shortened extensor mechanism, and removal of the dense intra- and extra-articular fibrosis. Having successfully exposed the knee and implanted the prosthetic knee, the surgeon must then achieve the goal of improved knee motion.

During surgery, radical excision of all periarticular fibrotic tissues must be performed. Dense intra-articular adhesions are removed. If the patellofemoral joint has a fibrous ankylosis, it must be dissected free. The femur and tibia must be freed subperiosteally of all adherent fibrous tissue.

When all contracted peri- and intra-articular scar tissue has been removed, knee flexion should be attempted. Soft tissue contracture must be released further if the knee cannot be flexed. Care must be exercised not to avulse the patellar tendon during attempted knee flexion. If the knee cannot be fully flexed despite this radical release, two options are available to the surgeon for exposing the knee. One is a method advocated by Whitesides,[68] which incorporates an osteotomy of the upper tibia with the tubercle and patellar tendon attached. At the end of the procedure, the tibial bone with attached patellar tendon is reattached with internal fixation. The dilemma confronting the surgeon with this approach is that distal elevation of the patellar tendon does not deal with the source of the problem because the contracture is in the quadriceps mechanism and motion will not be improved because soft tissue contracture remains proximal. Additionally, fixation of the tibial fragment may be troublesome because the area is poorly protected by subcutaneous tissue and is in a location where skin closure is tenuous.

The other option, proximal quadricepsplasty, allows for exposure by permitting the quadriceps to be turned distally as needed. The tendon can then be lengthened at the end of the procedure. An inverted V-Y type quadricepsplasty (Fig. 30–20) may be used. The lateral limb may or may not extend distally to the edge of the patella depending on the degree of mobilization necessary. Once the tendon has been turned down, visualization is improved and further soft tissue can be released as necessary. The knee can then be flexed to 90 degrees, and the knee arthroplasty can be completed.

The final task is adjustment of tension in the quadriceps tendon before closure. This adjustment is done by allowing the tendon to slide distally and suturing it in a lengthened position. If the tendon is lengthened excessively, an extension lag will occur. When the tendon is repaired too tightly, flexion will be impaired. To achieve a proper balance, the tendon should be sutured so that it becomes taut at about 40 degrees of flexion. Most patients obtain further flexion as the extensor mechanism elongates, but an extensor lag is prevented. In seven patients upon whom I operated using this technique, postoperative range of motion was 75 to 80 degrees and extensor lag was absent.[57] Re-

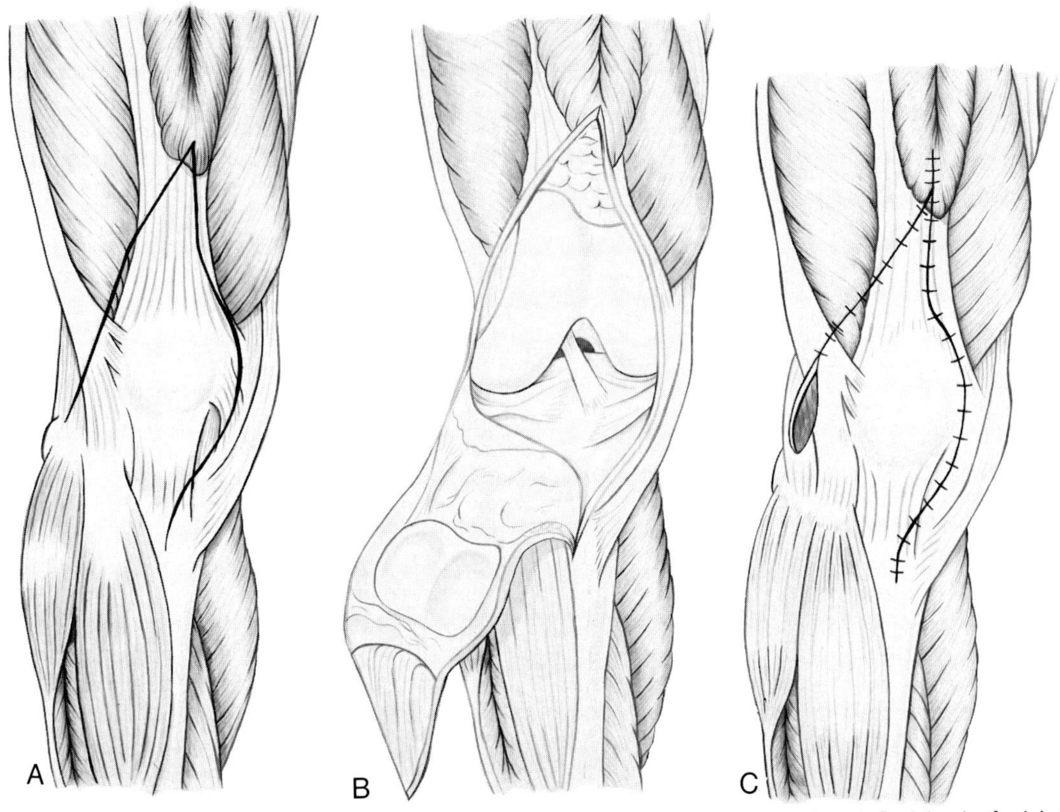

FIGURE 30–20. Proximal quadricepsplasty for exposure of the knee tight in extension. *A,* Incision in the joint capsule and quadriceps tendon. *B,* Exposure afforded by reflecting the patellar and quadriceps mechanism laterally and distally. *C,* The V-Y repair to provide lengthening of the quadriceps mechanism. The tendon should be sutured so that it becomes taut at about 40 degrees of flexion.

habilitation is slow in these patients, and continuous passive motion in the immediate postoperative period should be limited to a 45 degree range. If full flexion is allowed, the extensor mechanism stretches and the patient will have a marked extensor lag and a weak unstable knee.

At about 2 to 3 weeks after surgery, further flexion is allowed under the supervision of a physical therapist. Continuous passive motion is applied at home. If knee flexion at 6 to 8 weeks is poor, manipulation using anesthesia is performed. This step may be repeated several times over the first 6 to 9 months after surgery if progress with motion is slow. The surgeon should expect an extensor lag in the postoperative period that may persist for up to 6 months but generally resolves.

Because of the severe degree of dissection and extensive resection of scar in these patients, wound problems are more common. Care should be taken with closure, and excessive tension should be avoided on skin flaps. Delaying motion until healing has occurred may be necessary if severe swelling, drainage, or worrisome skin flaps are present postoperatively.

Severe Flexion Contracture

The patient with a severe flexion contracture (>45 degrees) presents another soft tissue problem in total knee reconstruction. The extensor mechanism is not contracted but rather may be quite lax once the deformity has been corrected. Also, soft tissue release alone may be insufficient to correct the flexion attitude of the knee, and bone resection may be necessary.[58]

Exposure is performed in the usual fashion, although it may be quite difficult in the posterior aspect of the knee joint. The surgeon must be persistent in resecting

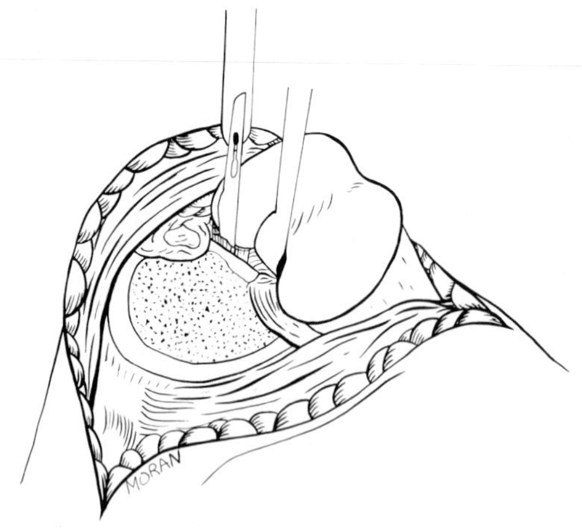

FIGURE 30–21. All soft tissues are released from the proximal tibia subperiosteally extending 1 to 2 cm below the joint surface.

scar from the posterior aspects of the joint to expose the posterior surface of the tibia. Once achieved, further dissection must ensure subperiosteal release of all contracted soft tissues inserting into the posterior tibia. This maneuver is best performed sharply. It should continue at least 1 to 2 cm below the upper surface of the tibia. The gastrocnemius insertion must be released as well (Fig. 30–21). When the contracted posterior capsule and other soft tissues have been released from the tibia, attention is turned to the femoral side. Preserving the posterior cruciate ligament is impossible in these cases because it is often incorporated in the deformity and therefore must be excised. Sharp dissection is continued along the intercondylar notch, releasing all soft tissue attachments (Fig. 30–22A). Once the adherent cruciate ligaments and capsule are removed from the notch, subperiosteal elevation of the femoral soft tissue attachments may be performed extending several centimeters proximally to the origin of the posterior cruciate ligament (Fig. 30–22B). Despite this radical release of all posterior structures, contracture may still be present and prevent knee extension. In this case, transverse release of the posterior capsule can be performed. Release must be done with care, particularly in the midline, to avoid injuring the popliteal vessels and posterior tibial nerve. If soft tissue is released as described, extension will be improved by approximately 30 to 40 degrees. If significant flexion contracture remains, bone resection is necessary to accomplish further knee extension.

Bone resection to more fully extend the knee afflicted with a severe flexion contracture should always be performed from the distal femur rather than the proximal tibia, although resection at either location will lead to greater extension. Bone removed from the femur will alter only the extension gap and not change the flexion gap. If tibial bone is removed both the flexion gap and the extension gap will be affected. The knee will require a thicker tibial implant to achieve stability during flexion. A thicker tibial implant will impair extension, and the flexion contracture will remain. If tibial bone is resected, the alternative is a thinner tibial component to allow greater knee extension. However,

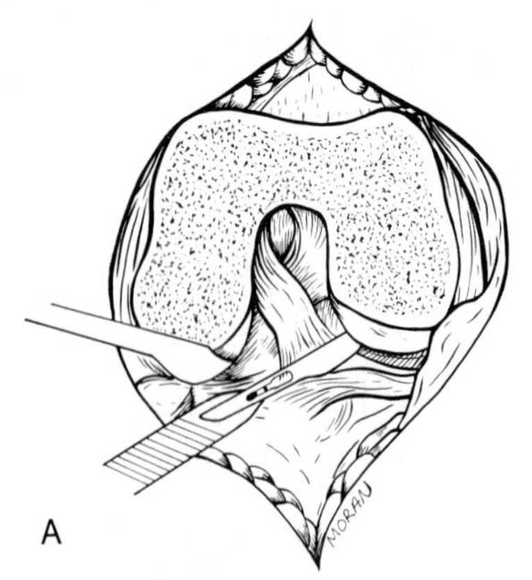

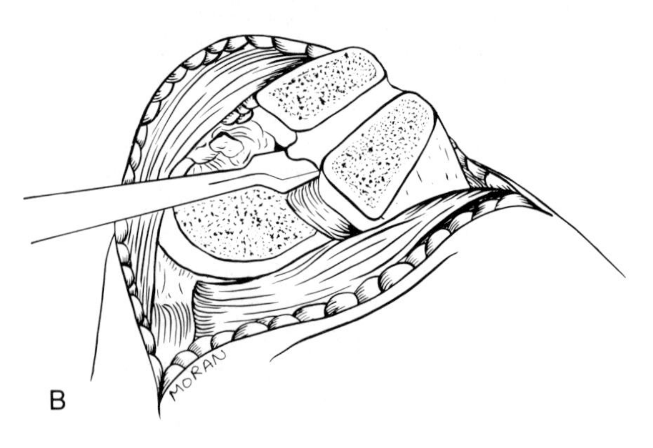

FIGURE 30–22. Posterior femoral release for flexion contracture. *A,* Contracted tissue is released sharply from the posterior aspect of the femur. *B,* Soft tissues are released in the intercondylar notch for 2 to 3 cm proximally.

this effect will lead to an unstable knee in flexion that will be prone to subluxation and dislocation.

When soft tissue and bone resection have led to satisfactory knee extension, the quadriceps mechanism in the most severe cases may be redundant. Although some degree of quadriceps laxity will eventually correct itself, imbrication of the quadriceps tendon should be performed if laxity is excessive. This maneuver can be completed by simply folding a segment of quadriceps tendon on itself in a reef-like fashion to achieve the desired shortening. Postoperatively, the knee is splinted in extension. Rehabilitation is slowed to allow healing of the soft tissues and the imbricated quadriceps mechanism.

With correction of these severe flexion contractures, peroneal nerve function must be observed closely after surgery. Should the peroneal nerve not be functioning while the patient is in the recovery room, the splint should be removed immediately and the knee placed in 30 to 40 degrees of knee flexion. Function generally returns if the neurapraxia is identified and treated early, although some degree of peroneal nerve loss may persist.

Biplane and Triplane Deformity

The management of soft tissue contractures about the medial and lateral sides of the deformed knee was mentioned, but complex deformities and associated soft tissue contractures require additional consideration. In these complex deformities, a significant component of malalignment exists in more than one plane. Malalignment may represent the biplanar severe varus-flexion deformity, the triplanar deformity seen in juvenile rheumatoid arthritis, or the valgus-flexion-external rotation seen in hemophilia. Because these deformities exist in more than one plane, asymmetry may be present in soft tissue contracture and laxity and attempt at release may lead to imbalances in various planes.

The underlying concept is the same as that in the management of less complex soft tissue contractures, i.e., the knee is balanced in all planes so that soft tissue is balanced across the joint. This result may be impossible in more complex contractures in which the flexion or rotational deformity may exceed the angular deformity. If the knee remains more unstable in flexion or extension after soft tissue release of all deformities, an implant must be chosen that has additional constraint or that augments the areas of persistent instability. If, for example, the knee remains unstable in flexion but is well balanced in extension with a particular tibial component, selecting a thicker tibial component to stabilize the knee in flexion will prevent the knee from extending and will produce a persistent flexion contracture. Therefore, a posteriorly augmented femoral component (either modular or custom) must be used. This component stabilizes the flexion gap by augmenting the posterior femur but will not alter the extension fit.

Conversely, if the knee is stable in flexion with a particular tibial component but remains unstable in extension after medial and lateral soft tissue balancing, augmentation must be performed on the distal portion of the femoral prosthesis. This maneuver stabilizes the knee in extension without altering the fit of the implant in flexion.

Where a considerable gap and instability are present in both flexion and extension, the surgeon should resist the tendency to correct them with a thicker tibial implant because patellofemoral tracking problems will result. Because the patellar tendon is fixed distally, when the implant is greater than 15 mm, the patella will descend relative to the femoral component and produce a patella infera. Not only will the kinematics of the knee joint be altered by this malpositioning of the joint line in a more cephalad direction, but the patellar component is likely to articulate against the thickened tibial implant. Where instability is present in flexion and extension, augmentation must be performed on both tibial and femoral sides to avoid this serious abnormality in the patellofemoral joint.

With the advent of modular total knee systems, prostheses can now be augmented as needed either on the femoral or tibial side. In more complicated situations, a custom implant may be necessary.

Because soft tissue release must often be quite radical in more complex deformities, instability may persist in one or another plane despite the use of modular or custom implants; therefore, more constrained devices may be necessary. Results with the Total Condylar III implant for severe deformity and revision surgery have been good to excellent in 77 percent of cases.[12, 59] The Spherocentric prosthesis has also performed well in these difficult cases.[32, 39] The risk of mechanical failure is greater due to more constraint in the implant; the increased shear and rotational stresses at the bone cement interface may lead to earlier loosening.

Grossly Unstable Knee

When the knee is grossly unstable at the outset of reconstruction, the surgeon must first make certain that the underlying diagnosis is not instability secondary to a neuropathic joint. Although successful total knee replacement has been performed in neuropathic joints, the condition should be considered a relative contraindication to knee replacement.[61] The rationale is obvious: the lack of proprioception responsible for joint destruction may produce the same end result in the prosthetic knee.

In knees with severe instability, the cause is usually related to insufficiency or absence of ligament support or to severe bone loss or to both. In the most severe cases, ligament continuity is completely lacking. Despite attempts to balance on the contralateral side of the joint, asymmetric instability persists. This situation is seen most commonly in the severe valgus knee. Almost always, bone loss is severe in the lateral compartment, more markedly so on the tibial side. Although the concepts of reconstruction of the arthritic knee discussed previously apply, with absence of ligament support several options are available to the surgeon. Krackow[34] has advocated a cephalad advancement and fixation of a lax ligament, although he presented no clinical results. In my experience, this technique has not been successful. Instability eventually recurs, as these atrophic tissues become attenuated again.

The reconstruction of these unstable joints after attempts at soft tissue balancing often requires the utilization of a more constrained implant. The Total Condylar III or other constrained devices improve stability in both flexion-extension as well as medially and laterally. However, in my

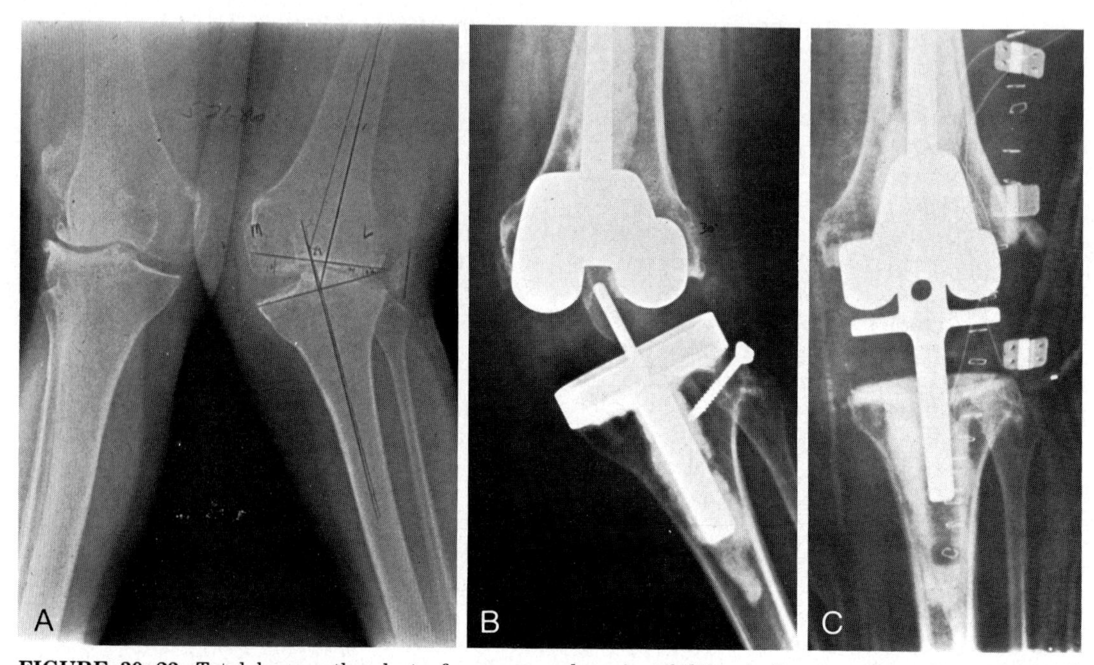

FIGURE 30–23. Total knee arthroplasty for severe valgus instability. *A*, Preoperative radiograph shows marked valgus instability. *B*, Total Condylar III prosthesis was used for reconstruction with resultant continuing instability. *C*, A rotating hinge prosthesis provided stability.

experience they do not compensate for complete absence of a collateral ligament. In the severe valgus knee with total medial incompetence, a rotating hinge device may be necessary to stabilize the joint. Few indications exist in primary knee arthroplasty for these implants, but the degree of stability they provide is needed in these unusual and severely unstable knees. On several occasions, I have relied on a constrained implant of the Total Condylar III type for the valgus knee with an absent medial ligament; recurrent deformity and instability occurred nonetheless (Fig. 30–23).

Bone loss may be so excessive in patients with marked instability that bone grafting or prosthetic augmentation of segmental bone loss is necessary. When instability is symmetric medially and laterally and bone deficiency is the cause, augmented implants on the distal or posterior femur and thicker tibial implants when bone loss of the medial and lateral tibia is symmetric often improve knee stability greatly without the need to proceed to a more constrained implant.

Despite all attempts to produce a stable joint by the conclusion of the arthroplasty, some degree of instability may persist. This should be identified in the operating room. If instability persists despite intraoperative attempts at remedy, bracing should be employed in the postoperative period. A brace that allows flexion and extension but provides medial and lateral support is recommended for 6 or more weeks postoperatively. At first, range of motion of the knee may be partially restricted by the brace and then gradually increased as stability improves. In patients with more severe instability, the knee should be immobilized for 6 weeks. Manipulation is performed if motion is slow after mobilization. If instability persists despite these measures, revision knee replacement may be necessary.

SUMMARY

Total knee replacement is a technically demanding, precise surgical procedure. To provide the patient with a painless functional knee, the surgeon must pay careful attention to the precepts of implantation, including exposure, soft tissue balancing, coaptation of prosthesis to bone, augmentation of bone deficits, restoration of the mechanical axis of weightbearing, and correct patellofemoral tracking. Because most failures in total knee replacement (instability, malalignment, unstable patellofemoral joint) are avoidable by careful technique, the surgeon must be versed in the basic tenets of arthroplasty and capable of producing a mechanically sound result. Uncommon complex deformities should be approached by extending the principles of less-complicated primary knee replacements and by being prepared to modify the selection of the implant based on the characteristics of the knee after soft tissue and bony reconstruction. As these more challenging cases require considerable preoperative planning and surgical expertise, significant clinical experience is recommended before a surgeon attempts knee arthroplasty for these complex problems.

References

1. Andriacchi, T. P., Stanwych, T. S., and Galante, J. O.: Knee biomechanics and total knee replacement. J. Arthroplasty 1:211–216, 1986.
2. Andriacchi, T. P., Galante, J. O., and Fermier, R. W.: The influence of total knee replacement design on walking and stair-climbing. J. Bone Joint Surg. 64A:1328–1335, 1982.
3. Aglietti, P. and Buzzi, R.: Posteriorly stabilized total condylar knee replacement. J. Bone Joint Surg. 70B:211–216, 1988.
4. Aglietti, P., Windsor, R., Buzzi, R., and Insall, J. N.: Arthroplasty for the stiff or ankylosed knee. J. Arthroplasty 4:1–5, 1989.
5. Altchek, D., Sculco, T. P., and Rawlins, B.: Autogenous bone grafting for severe angular deformity in total knee arthroplasty. J. Arthroplasty 4:151–155, 1989.
6. Bargren, J. H., Day, W. H., Freeman, M. A. R., and Swanson, S. A. V.: Mechanical tests on the tibial components of non-hinged knee prostheses. J. Bone Joint Surg. 60B:256–261, 1978.
7. Bourne, M. H., Rand, J. A., and Ilstrup, D. M.: Posterior cruciate condylar total knee arthroplasty. Clin. Orthop. 234:129–136, 1988.
8. Bradley, G. W., Freeman, M. A. R., and Albrektsson, B. E. J.: Total prosthetic replacement of ankylosed knees. J. Arthroplasty 3:179–183, 1987.
9. Boiardo, R. A. and Dorr, L. D.: Surgical approaches for total knee replacement arthroplasty. Contemp. Orthop. 12:60–68, 1986.
10. Cook, S. D., Barrach, R. L., Thomas, D. A., and Haddad, R. J.: Quantitative histologic analysis of tissue growth in porous total knee components. J. Arthroplasty [Suppl]:33–43, 1989.

11. Corces, A., Lotke, P. A., and Williams, J. L.: Strain characteristics of the posterior cruciate ligament in total knee replacement. Proceedings of the American Academy of Orthopaedic Surgeons, Las Vegas, 1989.
12. Donaldson, W. F., III, Sculco, T. P., and Insall, J. N.: The Total Condylar III knee prosthesis, long-term follow-up. Clin. Orthop. 226:22–27, 1988.
13. Dorr, L. D., Conaty, J. P., Schreiber, R., et al.: Technical Factors that Influence Mechanical Loosening of Total Knee Arthroplasty. The Knee. Edited by L. D. Dorr. Baltimore, University Park Press, 1985.
14. Dorr, L. D., Ochsner, J. L., Gronley, J., and Perry, J.: Functional comparison of posterior cruciate retained versus cruciate sacrificed total knee arthroplasty. Clin. Orthop. 238:36–43, 1988.
15. Dorr, L. D., Ranawat, C. S., and Sculco, T. P.: Bone grafting for tibial defects in total knee arthroplasty. Clin. Orthop. 205:153–165, 1986.
16. Ecker, M., Lotke, P. A., Windsor, R. E., and Cella, J. P.: Long-term results after total condylar knee arthroplasty. Clin. Orthop. 216:151–158, 1987.
17. Ewald, F. C., Jacobs, M. A., Miegel, R. E., et al.: Kinematic total knee replacement. J. Bone Joint Surg. 66A:1032–1040, 1984.
18. Ewald, F. C., Walker, P. S., Poss, R., et al.: Uncemented, Press-Fit Total Knee Replacement. Total Arthroplasty of the Knee. Edited by J. A. Rand and L. D. Dorr. Rockville, MD, Aspen Systems, 1986.
19. Goldberg, V. M., Figgie, H. E., and Figgie, M. P.: Technical considerations in total knee surgery. Orthop. Clin. North Am. 20:189–199, 1989.
20. Goldberg, V. M., Figgie, M. P., and Figgie, H. E.: The effect of fracture type on results of patella fracture following condylar total knee replacement. Clin. Orthop. 236:115–122, 1988.
21. Hersh, D. M.: Pain after total knee arthroplasty caused by soft tissue impingement. J. Bone Joint Surg. 71B:591–592, 1989.
22. Hofmann, A. A., Daniels, A. V., and Wyatt, R. Y.: Clinical and laboratory comparison of the tibial cut for total knee arthroplasty. Orthop. Trans. 79, 1987.
23. Hozack, W. J., Rothman, R. H., Booth, R. E., and Balderston, R. A.: The patellar clunk syndrome. Clin. Orthop. 241:203–208, 1989.
24. Hungerford, D. S., Kenna, R. V., and Krackow, K. A.: The porous coated anatomic total knee. Orthop. Clin. North Am. 13:103–122, 1982.
25. Hungerford, D. S. and Krakow, K. A.: Total joint arthroplasty of the knee. Clin. Orthop. 192:23–33, 1985.
26. Hungerford, D. S., Krackow, K. A., and Kenna, R. V.: Cementless total knee replacement in patients 50 years old and under. Orthop. Clin. North Am. 20:131–146, 1989.
27. Hsu, H. P. and Walker, P. S.: Wear and deformation of patellar components in total knee arthroplasty. Clin. Orthop. 246:260–265, 1989.
28. Hvid, I., Kjaersgaard-Anderson, P., Wethelund, J., and Sneppen, O.: Knee arthroplasty in rheumatoid arthritis. J. Arthroplasty 2:233–239, 1987.
29. Insall, J. N., Lachiewicz, P. F., and Burstein, A. H.: The posterior stabilized condylar prosthesis: A modification of the total condylar design. J. Bone Joint Surg. 64A:1317–1326, 1982.
30. Insall, J. N.: A midline approach to the knee. J. Bone Joint Surg. 53A:1584–1588, 1971.
31. Johnson, D. P.: Midline or parapatellar incision for knee arthroplasty. J. Bone Joint Surg. 70B:656–658, 1988.
32. Kaufer, H. and Matthews, L. S.: Spherocentric arthroplasty of the knee. Clinical experience with an average four-year follow-up. J. Bone Joint Surg. [Am] 63A(4):545–559, 1981.
32a. Kayler, D. E. and Lyttle, D.: Surgical Interruption of Patellar Blood Supply by Total Knee Arthroplasty. Clin. Orthop. 229:221–227, 1988.
33. Kjaersgaard-Anderson, P., Hvid, I., Wethelund, J., and Sneppen, O.: Total condylar knee arthroplasy in osteoarthritis. Clin. Orthop. 238:167–173, 1989.
34. Krackow, K.: Management of collateral ligament incompetence at revision total knee arthroplasty. Tech. Orthop. 3:15–33, 1988.
35. Leblanc, J.: Patella complications in total knee arthroplasty. Orthop. Rev. 3:296–304, 1989.
36. Lotke, P. A., Wong, R., and Ecker, M. L.: The management of large tibial defects in primary total knee replacement. Proceedings of the American Academy of Orthopaedic Surgeons, Las Vegas, 1985.
37. MacCollum, M. S. and Karpman, R. R.: Complications of the PCA anatomica patella. Orthopaedics 12:1423–1428, 1989.
38. Marmor, L.: Technique of patellar resurfacing in total knee arthroplasty. Clin. Orthop. 230:166–173, 1988.
39. Matthews, L. S., Goldstein, S. A., Kolowich, P. A., and Kaufer, H.: Spherocentric arthroplasty of the knee. A long-term and final follow-up evaluation. Clin. Orthop. 205:58–66, 1986.
40. Merkow, R. L., Soudry, M., and Insall, J. N.: Patellar dislocation following total knee replacement. J. Bone Joint Surg. 67A:1321–1327, 1985.
41. Moreland, J. R.: Mechanisms of failure in total knee arthroplasty. Clin. Orthop. 226:49–64, 1988.
42. Ranawat, C. S. and Boachie-Adjei, O.: Survivorship analysis and results of total condylar knee arthroplasty, eight to eleven years follow-up period. Clin. Orthop. 226:6–13, 1988.
43. Ranawat, C. S. and Hansraj, K. K.: Effect of posterior cruciate sacrifice on durability of the cement-bone interface. A nine year survivorship study of 100 total condylar knee arthroplasties. Orthop. Clin. North Am. 20:63–70, 1989.
44. Rand, J. A. and Bryan, R. S.: Alignment in Porous Coated Anatomic Total Knee Arthroplasty. The Knee. Edited by L. D. Dorr. Baltimore, University Park Press, 1985.
45. Rand, J. A., Bryan, R. S., Chao, E. Y. S., and Ilstrup, D. M.: A Comparison of Cement Versus Cementless Fixation in Porous Coated Anatomic Total Knee Arthroplasty. Total Arthroplasty of the Knee. Edited by J. A. Rand and L. D. Dorr. Rockville, MD, Aspen Systems, 1986.
46. Ritter, M. A.: Screw and cement fixation of large defects in total knee arthroplasty. J. Arthroplasty 1:125–129, 1986.
47. Ritter, M. A. and Campbell, E. D.: Posteroperative patellar complications with and without lateral release during total knee arthroplasty. Clin. Orthop. 219:163–168, 1988.
48. Ritter, M. A., Faris, P. M., and Deating, M. E.: Posterior cruciate ligament balancing during to-

tal knee arthroplasty. J. Arthroplasty 3:323–326, 1988.
49. Ritter, M. A., Gioe, T. J., Stringer, E. A., and Littrell, D.: The posterior cruciate condylar total knee prosthesis. Clin. Orthop. 184:264–269, 1984.
50. Rorabeck, C. H., Bourne, R. B., and Nott, L.: The cemented Kinematic II and the non-cemented porous coated anatomic prosthesis for total knee replacement. J. Bone Joint Surg. 70A:483–490, 1988.
51. Rosenberg, A. G., Barden, R., and Galante, J. O.: Cemented and cementless fixation with the Miller-Galante total knee arthroplasty. Orthop. Clin. North Am. 20:97–111, 1989.
52. Sanders, D. P., McKinney, F. W., and Harris, W. H.: Clinical evaluation and cost effectiveness of preoperative laboratory assessment on patients undergoing total hip arthroplasty. Orthopaedics 12:1449–1453, 1989.
53. Scott, R. D. and Volatile, T. B.: Twelve years experience with posterior cruciate retaining total knee arthroplasty. Clin. Orthop. 205:100–107, 1986.
54. Scott, W. N., Rubinstein, M., and Scuderi, G.: Results after knee replacement with a posterior cruciate substituting prosthesis. J. Bone Joint Surg. 70A:1163–1170, 1988.
55. Scuderi, G. and Insall, J. N.: The posterior stabilized knee prosthesis. Orthop. Clin. North Am. 20:71–77, 1989.
56. Scuderi, G., Scharf, S. C., Meltzer, L. P., and Scott, W. N.: The relationship of lateral release to patella viability in total knee arthroplasty. J. Arthroplasty 2:209–214, 1987.
57. Sculco, T. P. and Faris, P.: Total knee replacement in the stiff knee. Techn. Orthop. 3:5–10, 1988.
58. Sculco, T. P.: Technique of Correction of Flexion Contracture during Total Knee Arthroplasty. Total Condylar Knee Arthroplasty: Techniques, Results and Complications. Edited by C. S. Ranawat. New York, Springer-Verlag, 1985.
59. Sculco, T. P.: Total Condylar III prosthesis in ligament instability. Orthop. Clin. North Am. 20:221–227, 1989.
60. Sneppen, O., Christensen, P., and Larsen, H.: Mechanical testing of trabecular bone in knee replacement. Int. Orthop. 5:251–255, 1981.
61. Soudry, M., Binazzi, R., Johanson, N. A., et al.: Total knee arthroplasty in Charcot and Charcot-like joints. Clin. Orthop. 208:199–204, 1986.
62. Stuart, M. J. and Rand, J. A.: Total knee arthroplasty in young adults who have rheumatoid arthritis. J. Bone Joint Surg. 70A:84–87, 1988.
63. Sutherland, C. J.: Patellar component dissociation in total knee arthroplasty. Clin. Orthop. 228:178–181, 1988.
64. Tillet, E. D., Engh, G. A., and Peterson, T.: A comparative study of extramedullary and intramedullary alignment systems in total knee arthroplasty. Clin. Orthop. 230:176–181, 1988.
65. Urs, W., Binazzi, R., Insall, J. N., et al.: Custom total knee arthroplasty. Proceedings of the American Academy of Orthopaedic Surgeons, Atlanta, 1988.
66. Vernaci, F. V., Rothman, R. H., Booth, R. E., and Balderston, R. A.: Arthroscopic management of the patellar clunk syndrome following posterior stabilized total knee arthroplasty. J. Arthroplasty 4:179–182, 1989.
67. Vince, K. G., Insall, J. N., and Kelly, M. A.: The total condylar prosthesis, 10-12 year results of a cemented knee replacement. J. Bone Joint Surg. 71B:793–797, 1989.
68. Whitesides, L.: Proximal Osteotomy for Total Knee Replacement in the Stiff Knee. Presented at the Knee Society, New Orleans, 1990.
69. Windsor, R. E., Insall, J. N., and Sculco, T. P.: Bone grafting of tibial defects in primary and revision total knee arthroplasty. Clin. Orthop. 205:153–165, 1986.

CHAPTER 31

Total Knee Arthroplasty: Postoperative Care and Rehabilitation

WILLIAM PETTY

Knee replacement requires a more intense program of rehabilitation than hip replacement. A well-designed program that emphasizes the central role of the patient in carrying out a rehabilitation regimen results in a more rapid and complete recovery. Both preoperative and postoperative patient education should be supported and encouraged by all members of the health care team. They should emphasize to the surgical candidates that those who follow guidelines closely achieve the best treatment outcomes.

IMMEDIATE POSTOPERATIVE CARE

Management of the patient in the immediate postoperative period has many facets. Preventive care is important: precautions must be taken against infection and thromboembolism. If blood loss after surgery is significant, transfusions may be needed. These topics are discussed in other chapters.

Postoperative drains can usually be removed after 24 hours without increasing the risk of hematoma formation. When drains remain in place too long, contamination of the drain site by skin organisms is more likely. Also drain removal permits more comfortable early movement of the knee.[25] The patient should be given appropriate analgesic agents. Patient-controlled analgesia offers the benefits of improved comfort and greater alertness. Epidural analgesia or nerve block is recommended by some surgeons for pain control in the early postoperative period (see Chapter 10, *Anesthesia for Joint Replacement Surgery*). In one study, cold therapy was demonstrated to reduce swelling and pain after total knee replacement but had no effect on achievement of motion.[15a]

REHABILITATION

Physical Therapy

Actually, rehabilitation begins before surgery, as the patient gives the physical therapist information about home and work environments. The therapist responds by planning a postoperative rehabilitation program tailored to the patient's environment and needs. Education of the patient includes instructions about gait (walking), exercises, and precautions for protection of the newly operated knee.

The home environment of most patients is satisfactory for rehabilitation if someone can stay with them when they leave the hospital. Generally, patients can participate in basic activities of daily living without assistance. Even though many patients who undergo knee replacements for unilateral knee disease achieve independence rapidly, they should not be expected to prepare meals or do housework right after returning home. For patients with extensive disability due to multiple musculoskeletal problems or those with severe medical illness, planning should begin early so that appropriate arrangements can be set in motion. The patient may need to go home with a family member or friend, get household help, or stay in an extended care facility.

By learning about the home environment, the therapist can tailor a basic postoperative program to the specific needs of that patient. For example, a patient with stairs to climb requires extra instruction and practice in stair climbing. The therapist should inquire about any safety hazards present in the patient's environment (e.g., loose rugs) so they can be removed before and not after an accident. Preoperative evaluation should include consideration of and planning for vocational and avocational activities during recovery.

The therapist's physical evaluation includes assessment of both the knee to be operated on and the opposite knee. Both lower extremities should be assessed for strength, range of motion, and presence of contractures. The therapist must also evaluate the patient's upper extremities for strength and look for any contractures or other deformities that might make using a walking aid difficult.

When patients know how to use a cane, crutch, or walker, their skill must be assessed. Frequently, patients utilize walking aids incorrectly and require more instruction than if they had no experience at all. Regardless of previous experience, patients approach early postoperative walking more confidently when they master the aids preoperatively. The therapist provides instruction, demonstrates transfer techniques, outlines precautions, and describes the sequence of progression of the postoperative program.

Postoperative Care

After surgery, a bulky cotton dressing with or without plaster splints or a lighter dressing and a knee immobilizer may be applied. Early aggressive motion exercises may increase the incidence of wound complications, especially in patients who have rheumatoid arthritis or those who have been on steroid therapy (see Chapter 32, *Local Complications in Total Knee Replacement*). Some surgeons prefer to apply a light dressing and to start continuous passive motion immediately. The extremity can be elevated by raising the foot of the bed.

As soon as patients recover consciousness, nursing personnel should remind them to begin the exercises practiced preoperatively: ankle dorsi and plantar flexion, ankle circles, and quadriceps sets. When the quadriceps muscles are strong enough, straight leg raising may be done. Neuromuscular stimulation of the quadriceps muscles may be helpful initially in patients with weak muscle activity. However, its use has not been found to significantly improve contraction force or motion in extension in most patients.[14] Extension exercises performed with the knee over a bolster help speed the gain in quadriceps strength (Fig. 31–1). Both active and active-assisted flexion exercises are performed (Fig. 31–2).

Most patients may sit up the day of surgery or the day after surgery and are able to stand the day after surgery. Transfers, if practiced preoperatively, can usually be done readily with help at first and then without help. Patients who can stand comfortably are assisted in taking a few steps the first or second time they stand with walkers or crutches. Most feel somewhat uncomfortable moving about until drains, urinary catheters (if placed), and intravenous lines are removed.

For cemented arthroplasty, the prosthesis fixation is probably as strong at 24 hours as it will ever be. From this standpoint, full weightbearing may begin immediately. Some surgeons express concern about bone necrosis adjacent to the implant and advocate guarded weightbearing. However, remodeling of this necrotic bone takes months: therefore, no logical reason exists to avoid weightbearing for a few weeks.[5, 9] No evidence is available to indicate that early weightbearing jeopardizes long-term durability of the knee replacement. Weightbearing is gradually started mainly for patient comfort and to allow muscles time to recover from the trauma

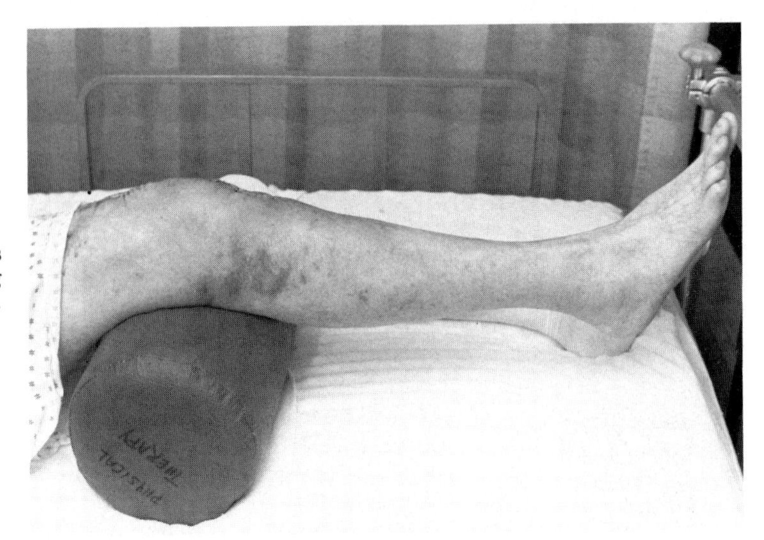

FIGURE 31–1. Quadriceps strength is gained by performing extension exercises over a bolster.

of surgery and regain strength that was lost owing to protracted knee disease. For the patient with poor balance and other disabilities, walking aids offer added protection. Early weightbearing as tolerated may help in achieving full knee extension.

When gait training is begun, the goal is to help the patient achieve a normal pattern. Patients commonly walk with a shortened or half stride and may tend to walk on tiptoe on the operated side. Walking on tiptoe may result in continuing knee flexion contracture. They are taught to walk with equal stride length, placing the

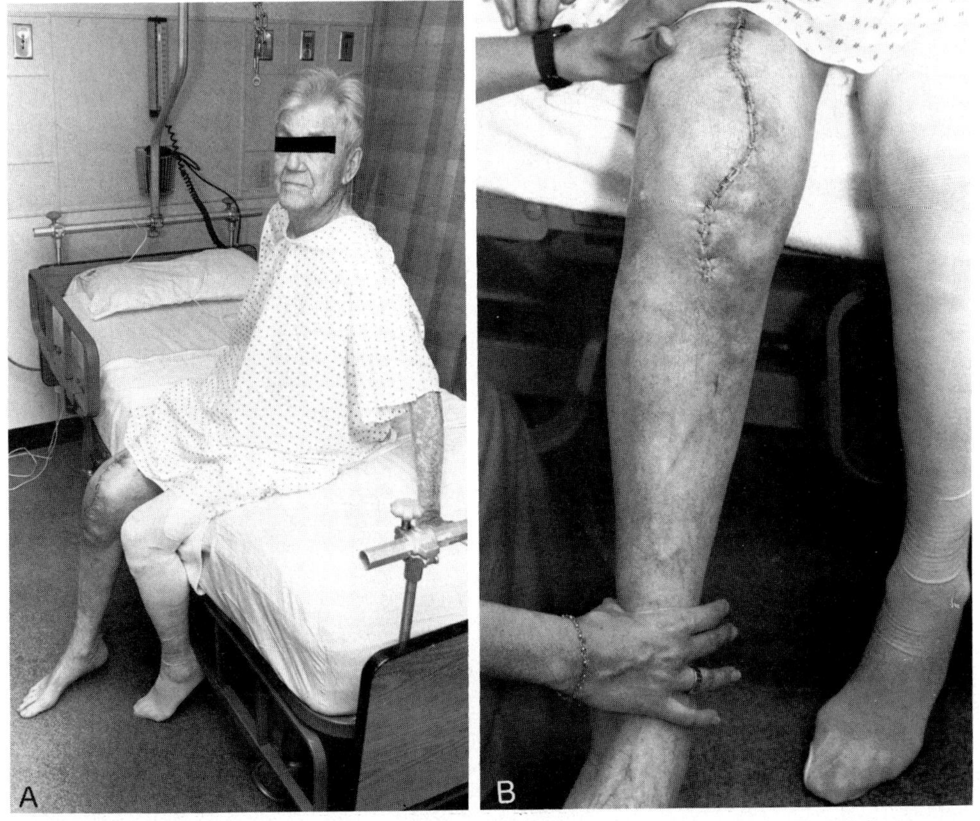

FIGURE 31–2. Flexion exercises. *A,* Active flexion 6 days postoperatively. *B,* Active-assisted flexion exercises.

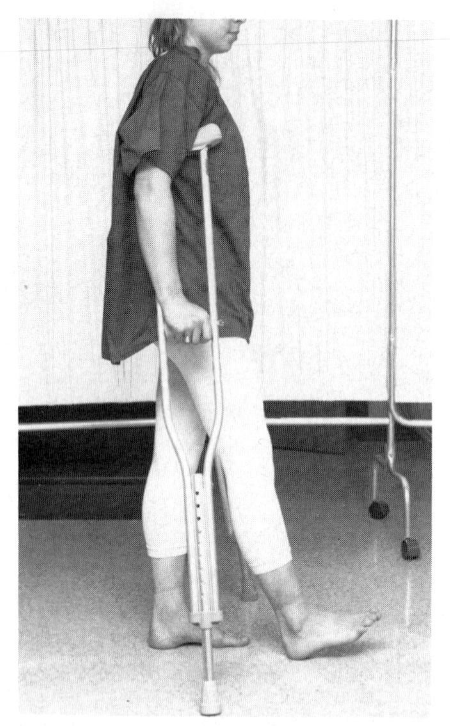

FIGURE 31–3. After total knee arthroplasty, the patient is taught to walk with equal stride length, placing the heel firmly with full extension during stance.

heel firmly with full knee extension during stance (Fig. 31–3). Some patients must be reminded to keep their heads up and look where they are going. A full-length mirror often helps patients develop normal gait.

Patients who have undergone bilateral total knee arthroplasties under the same anesthetic or with a short interval between operations should use the four-point alternating gait. This technique is difficult to master and requires patience to teach. When patients have developed confidence in their walking, they can begin stair climbing, going up with the unaffected leg first, then with the operated leg, then with the crutches. Going down, the crutches come first, then the operated leg, then the unaffected leg. With this technique, the patient raises and lowers the body with the unaffected leg and crutches. After bilateral operations, the stronger limb is considered the unaffected limb.

Patients with good balance may prefer elbow crutches. These devices do not reduce weightbearing as much as regular crutches but are less difficult to use unilaterally and allow a less difficult transition to a cane. Normally, this transition takes 3 to 6 weeks postoperatively in patients who have no other disabilities. The speed of the transition depends on the patient's strength and balance. A therapist or physician should supervise the transition for at least one session to be sure the patient uses the cane properly and safely. Although holding a cane in the contralateral hand does not have the same biomechanical leverage effect for the knee that it does for the hip, holding a cane in the contralateral hand has been shown to reduce floor reaction force and increase both stride length and cadence when compared with a cane in the ipsilateral hand (Fig. 31–4).[6] Balance may also be better with the cane held in the contralateral hand. When the patient has achieved full knee extension and the quadriceps are strong, the cane may be put aside.

No evidence exists that prolonged supported weightbearing makes a difference in patients with porous-coated knee prostheses, but most surgeons recommend

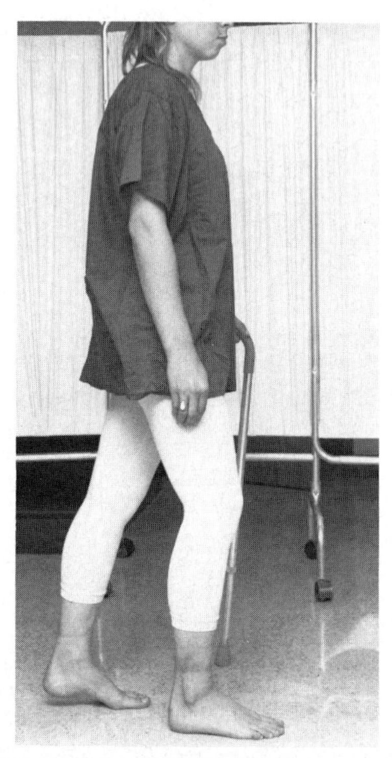

FIGURE 31–4. During rehabilitation for total knee arthroplasty the use of a cane, in the contralateral rather than ipsilateral hand, reduces floor reaction force and tends to increase both stride length and cadence.

more gradual progression of weightbearing when total knee arthroplasty is performed with press-fit fixation, especially when a porous-coated prosthesis is involved. This conservative approach is based on data from animal studies demonstrating that early bone ingrowth requires 2 to 3 weeks and that the increase in strength of bone ingrowth fixation plateaus at about 12 weeks.[3, 13, 19, 22] Although tissue ingrowth in humans probably differs from that of experimental animals and may be more fibrous than osseous, restriction of motion between bone and prosthesis during early biologic attachment of the prosthesis seems logical. When only the femoral component of a total knee arthroplasty is placed without cement, less support is provided for increased protection from weightbearing because the component has a broad base of bone support around the distal femur that makes significant micromotion less likely.

Manipulation

Some surgeons recommend manipulation of a knee with the patient under anesthesia when progress in gaining flexion is poor, although this practice seems less popular than it was in the early years of total knee replacement. Fox and Poss[7] reported an immediate increase in flexion from 71 to 108 degrees with manipulation, but the flexion was reduced to 88 degrees 1 week after manipulation. At 1 year, the manipulated knees had motion similar to that of their unmanipulated counterparts. These workers concluded that preoperative motion and diagnosis were the major determinants of ultimate flexion. In my practice, manipulation is rarely done after total knee replacement and is reserved for special problems.

Continuous Passive Motion

Although the efficacy of continuous passive motion in rehabilitation after total knee arthroplasty is controversial, many hospitals use it (Fig. 31–5). Many investigators report that flexion is gained more rapidly when continuous passive motion is applied.[10, 11, 24] Others find that such motion offers no benefit.[18, 20] Early follow-up results suggest no difference. Patients who gained flexion more rapidly with continuous passive motion had no better motion 2 to 3 months after surgery than those who did not.[10, 11, 24] Some investigators have reported shorter hospital stays in patients who have undergone continuous passive motion,[1, 11] whereas others have reported no significant difference in length of hospital stay.[20, 21] The suggestion has been made that continuous passive motion may reduce deep vein thrombosis.[24] However, a carefully controlled study by Lynch and colleagues[8] failed to confirm this effect.

Complications have been reported with the utilization of a continuous passive motion machine after total knee arthroplasty. Peroneal nerve palsy has occurred because of pressure of the apparatus against the nerve at the fibular neck; reduced knee extension has occurred; and extensor lag has occurred.[1, 16, 20] Problems with extension can be reduced by using the machine for shorter periods of time each day (5 to 12 hours rather than 15 to 20 hours).[1]

Continuous passive motion may allow more rapid gains in flexion, often at the expense of delayed gains in extension and quadriceps strength. If applied, it should be limited to no more than 10 to 12 hours per day to reduce its adverse effect on extension. Ultimate range of motion is unchanged. Reductions in deep vein thrombosis are unlikely.

After Hospitalization

The first postoperative follow-up evaluation should be scheduled with the surgeon about 6 weeks after operation. Additional follow-up visits are usually scheduled at 3, 6, and 12 months. The surgeon should give the patient telephone numbers to call if any problems or questions arise.

Patients who have undergone total knee replacements can expect to resume a normal life unless their preoperative vocational or avocational activities involved high activity levels (e.g., running and jumping). Although no conclusive evidence is available to demonstrate that activities placing high impact loads on the prosthetic knees lead to earlier failures, it seems reasonable to warn patients with knee replacements to avoid such activities.

Many patients with sedentary occupations may return to work within 6 weeks or less after total knee replacements. Those

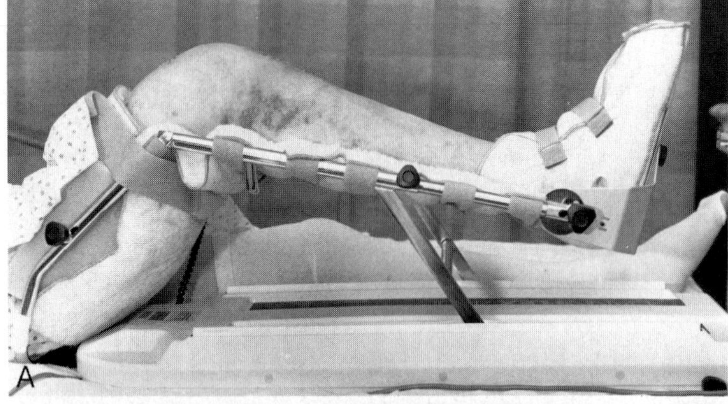

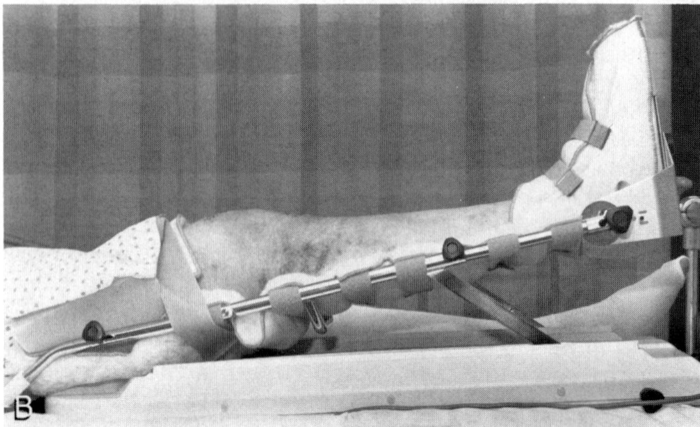

FIGURE 31–5. Use of continuous passive motion. *A*, Continuous passive motion may provide for more rapid gains in flexion but is unlikely to improve ultimate flexion range. *B*, When continuous passive motion is used, it is important to provide full extension in the machine and to limit use of the machine to no more than 10 to 12 hours per day to avoid impairing extension range and strength.

who must lift and carry objects in their jobs may have to delay returning to employment for 3 to 4 months, perhaps longer. Age and sex and whether the knee replacement is unilateral or bilateral have no effect on restoration of function, although bilateral operations may prolong convalescence. Many patients consider their recoveries complete by 3 months after surgery and most by 6 months. Postoperative total motion may be little or no better than preoperative range of motion, but flexion contractures are usually eliminated so that motion takes place in a more functional range.[12]

Patients are generally able to stop using their walking aids by 3 months after operation. Exceptions are patients with arthritis involving multiple joints (most commonly rheumatoid arthritis) who often need both walking aids and other devices to assist them in the activities of daily living.[15] Patients should be encouraged to walk outdoors in good weather. When pavements are icy or wet, exercise should be taken indoors. Gentle swimming and water exercises are excellent.

Patients are encouraged to progress toward living as normally as possible when they go home. Patients who have assumed responsibility for their rehabilitation generally need no supervised physical therapy after leaving the hospital. Patients with multiple problems (e.g., inflammatory arthritis with widespread involvement) often need further therapy, either in a special rehabilitation facility or at home with a therapist.

NONAMBULATORY PATIENTS

Patients with severe functional disabilities, especially those who cannot walk preoperatively, have special requirements for rehabilitation both before and after total joint replacement surgery. Patients with severe bilateral knee disease may have simultaneous replacement.[2, 4, 12, 17, 23] Ultimate function is not impaired and may be improved. Moreover, if both knees must be replaced, simultaneous procedures may be more cost-effective.[4] If three or four major joints require surgery, patients need greater physical and psychologic stamina along with the encouragement and support of the entire health care team involved in their care. Total hip arthroplasty usually precedes total knee arthroplasty. If the destruction and deformity are such that two joints can be reconstructed during one hospitalization and the others can be done 2 to 3 months later, this schedule should be arranged. It allows for both physical and psychologic recovery of the patient. When substantial flexion contracture or severe pain is present in either the hips or knees, the operations should be scheduled as close together as medically and psychologically feasible. Otherwise, unoperated joints will impair ambulation and the patient will experience an inferior result, often developing a recurrence of flexion contracture in the hip or knee. Some patients must have three or four joints reconstructed during the same hospitalization owing to severe pain, deformity, or both.

References

1. Basso, D. M. and Knapp, L.: Comparison of two continuous passive motion protocols for patients with total knee implants. Phys. Ther. 67(3):360–363, 1987. [Published erratum appears in Phys. Ther. 67(6):979, 1987.]
2. Berman, A. T., Zarro, V. J., Bosacco, S. J., and Israelite, C.: Quantitative gait analysis after unilateral or bilateral total knee replacement. J. Bone Joint Surg. [Am] 69(9):1340–1345, 1987.
3. Bobyn, J. D., Pilliar, R. M., Cameron, H. U., and Weatherly, G. C.: Osteogenic phenomena across bone-implant spaces with porous-surfaced intramedullary implants. Acta Orthop. Scand. 52:145–153, 1981.
4. Brotherton, S. L., Roberson, J. R., de Andrade, J. R., and Fleming, L. L.: Staged versus simultaneous bilateral total knee replacement. J. Arthroplasty 1(4):211–228, 1986.
5. Charnley, J.: Low Friction Arthroplasty of the Hip. Berlin, Springer-Verlag, pp. 304–305, 1979.
6. Edwards, B. G.: Contralateral and ipsilateral cane usage by patients with total knee or hip replacement. Arch. Phys. Med. Rehabil. 67(10):734–740, 1986.
7. Fox, J. L. and Poss, R.: The role of manipulation following total knee replacement. J. Bone Joint Surg. [Am] 63A(3):357–362, 1981.
8. Lynch, A. F., Bourne, R. B., Rorabeck, C. H., et al.: Deep-vein thrombosis and continuous passive motion after total knee arthroplasty. J. Bone Joint Surg. [Am] 70(1):11–14, 1988.
9. Gebauer, D. and Blumel, G.: Extreme loading as cause of aseptic loosening of the total hip endoprosthesis socket and the resultant therapeutic consequences. Aktuel. Traumatol. 13(4):154–159, 1983. (Published in German.)
10. Goletz, T. H. and Henry, J. H.: Continuous passive motion after total knee arthroplasty. South. Med. J. 79(9):1116–1120, 1986.
11. Gose, J. C.: Continuous passive motion in the postoperative treatment of patients with total knee replacement. A retrospective study. Phys. Ther. 67(1):39–42, 1987.
12. Gradillas, E. L. and Volz, R. G.: Bilateral total knee replacement under one anesthetic. Clin. Orthop. 140:153–158, 1979.
13. Harris, W. H. and Jasty, M.: Bone Ingrowth into Porous Coated Canine Acetabular Replacements: The Effect of Pore Size, Apposition, and Dislocation. The Hip. St. Louis, C. V. Mosby Company, pp. 214–234, 1985.
14. Haug, J. and Wood, L. T.: Efficacy of neuromuscular stimulation of the quadriceps femoris during continuous passive motion following total knee arthroplasty. Arch. Phys. Med. Rehabil. 69(6):423–424, 1988.
15. Haworth, R. J.: Use of aids during the first three months after total hip replacement. Br. J. Rheumatol. 22(1):29–35, 1983.

15a. Hecht, P. J., Bachmann, S., Booth, R. E., Jr., and Rothman, R. H.: Effects of thermal therapy on rehabilitation after total knee arthroplasty. A prospective randomized study. Clin. Orthop. 178:198–201, 1983.

16. James, S. E. and Wade, P. J.: Lateral popliteal nerve palsy as a complication of the use of a continuous passive motion knee machine—a case report. Injury 18(1):72–73, 1987.
17. Marks, J. S.: Benefits of multiple joint replacement in rheumatoid arthritis. Scand. J. Rehabil. Med. 16(1):43–46, 1984.
18. Nielsen, P. T., Rechnagel, K., and Nielsen, S. E.: No effect of continuous passive motion after arthroplasty of the knee. Acta Orthop. Scand. 59(5):580–581, 1988.
19. Pilliar, R. M.: Porous-surfaced metallic implants for orthopedic applications. J. Biomed. Mater. Res. 21(A1 Suppl):1–33, 1987.
20. Ritter, M. A., Gandolf, V. S., and Holston, K. S.: Continuous passive motion versus physical therapy in total knee arthroplasty. Clin. Orthop. 244:239–243, 1989.
21. Romness, D. W. and Rand, J. A.: The role of continuous passive motion following total knee arthroplasty. Clin. Orthop. 226:34–37, 1988.
22. Sandborn, P. M., Cook, S. D., Spires, W. P., and Kester, M. A.: Tissue response to porous-coated implants lacking initial bone apposition. J. Arthroplasty 3(4):337–346, 1988.
23. Suman, R. K. and Freeman, P. A.: Bilateral hip and knee replacement in rheumatoid arthritis. J. Arthroplasty 1(4):237–240, 1986.
24. Vince, K. G., Kelly, M. A., Beck, J., and Insall, J. N.: Continuous passive motion after total knee arthroplasty. J. Arthroplasty 2(4):281–284, 1987.
25. Willet, K. M., Simmons, C. D., and Bentley, G.: The effect of suction drains after total hip replacement. J. Bone Joint Surg. [Br] 70(4):607–610, 1988.

CHAPTER 32

Local Complications in Total Knee Replacement

THOMAS P. SCULCO

Although systemic complications after total knee replacement may threaten the life of the patient, local complications more often threaten the success of the implant and impair the functional outcome of the arthroplasty. Local complications generally consist of interruptions in the orderly progress of wound healing. They can occur in any soft tissue from the skin surface to the knee joint capsule, with the potentially catastrophic results of prosthesis exposure and deep infection. Accumulations of blood or serous fluid may also delay healing and slow the patient's ability to move the joint. Ultimately, the range of motion may be reduced. If the increased fluid volume creates enough intra-articular pressure, wound dehiscence may result. Prevention depends on meticulous surgical technique, including gentle handling of tissues, maintenance of adequate vascularity at wound edges, judicious retraction of tissues, adequate hemostasis, and careful closure of tissues. Any wound complication that does occur after total knee arthroplasty is cause for serious concern, requiring prompt and aggressive treatment to avoid a disastrous outcome.

Many reports are available on the long-term results of total knee arthroplasty, but few deal with the incidence, cause, and treatment of local complications. The publications that are available on long-term outcome indicate an incidence of wound problems in the range of 4 to 10 percent.[2, 3, 7, 8] The most common are hematoma, seroma, dehiscence, delayed healing and tissue necrosis, cellulitis, and superficial infection. In this chapter, local complications and their causes are described, preventive measures are discussed, and information about management is provided.

HEMATOMA

Causative Factors

Hematoma within the prosthetic joint occurs in some form in every total knee arthroplasty because bone surfaces are exposed and numerous vessels are interrupted. Tourniquets are routinely applied during surgery. Many surgeons deflate the tourniquets before wound closure to obtain better hemostasis. Controversy exists over whether tourniquet deflation and hemostasis attempts reduce overall bleeding and intra-articular hematoma formation. One study suggests that intraoperative tourniquet release results in more postoperative blood loss than tourniquet release after application of pressure dressings.[4]

When the tourniquet is released intraoperatively, the vessels are cauterized and the tourniquet is reinflated for wound closure. If a hypotensive anesthetic agent is administered, the patient's blood pressure should be allowed to recover during tourniquet deflation to facilitate adequate hemostasis. No matter when the tourniquet is released, the surgeon should exercise caution in cauterizing all vessels from which there is significant bleeding, especially the geniculate vessels, which have a tendency to hemorrhage briskly (Fig. 32–1).

Because bleeding does persist after wound closure and tourniquet release, suction drainage is used to remove the collecting hematoma. Faulty placement of drainage tubes or malfunction of the suction drainage system, especially in the early postoperative period, almost always results in significant hematoma formation. If a hematoma remains tense, rehabilitation will be seriously delayed for two reasons: (1) the patient will avoid joint flexion owing to severe pain, and (2) the swollen joint will not move easily owing to increased intra-articular pressure. If the hematoma decompresses through the wound, sanguineous drainage may persist.

Factors other than failure to control intraoperative bleeding and to remove bloody drainage may also lead to hematoma formation after knee replacement. One contributing factor is interference with normal coagulation resulting from prior administration of nonsteroidal anti-inflammatory agents. Another is the presence of a coagulopathy. If the patient's history suggests a coagulation disorder, this possibility should be investigated preoperatively. If possible, the defect should be corrected prior to surgery.

Replacement of arthritic knees in patients with severe deformities requires additional dissections to correct soft tissue imbalances. These, too, may increase the probability of hematoma formation owing to more extensive bleeding—especially if a lateral patellar retinacular release is performed and the superior lateral geniculate artery is transected. However, the vessel can often be preserved with lateral release if careful technique is employed (see Fig. 32–1). If the vessel is transected, it is cauterized. Another cause of large hematoma formation is marked proliferative vascular synovitis in some patients with rheumatoid arthritis, who tend to bleed more after surgery.

Noncemented arthroplasty may predispose a patient to hematoma formation because cut vessels on bone surfaces are not

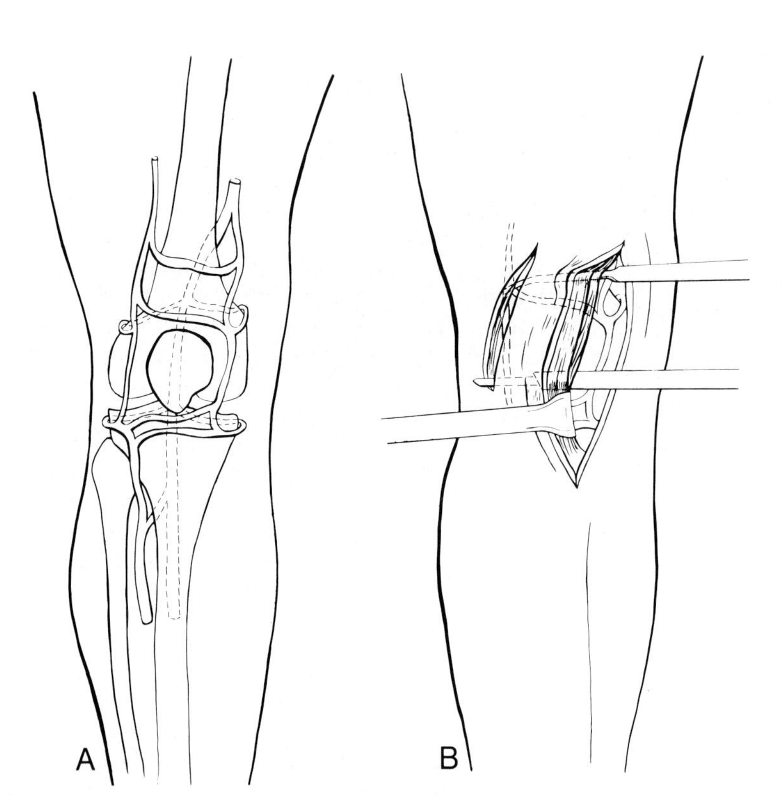

FIGURE 32–1. Geniculate vessels should be preserved when possible during total knee arthroplasty. *A,* Location of geniculate vessels and their anastomoses about the knee. *B,* Special care is taken during lateral retinacular release to preserve the superior lateral geniculate artery.

compressed by bone cement tamponade but remain exposed. Therefore, the surgeon who implants noncemented prostheses must be especially meticulous about hemostasis and must ensure that drainage systems are correctly placed and functioning well.

Anticoagulant therapy is another cause of hematoma development postoperatively. For this reason, patients on warfarin or heparin must be monitored carefully so that intra-articular hemorrhage and severe hematoma development can be prevented. Prothrombin time should be maintained at or below 16 seconds (control, 12 seconds). Bleeding that occurs in patients receiving anticoagulant drugs must be attended to immediately and physical therapy delayed because the hematoma may be severe. If possible, surgical evacuation of the hematoma should be delayed until the anticoagulated state is corrected. If rapid evacuation is indicated, vitamin K should be administered parenterally.

Treatment

When a postoperative hematoma is small and not tense or draining, postoperative rehabilitation can generally proceed unhindered. In fact, resolution of knee joint hematoma after replacement is often promoted by continuous passive motion and accompanying physical therapy. In the patient with marked hematoma formation and severely swollen knee joint, rehabilitation is both painful and severely limited. Unless the hematoma can be resolved rapidly by local treatment (cold compresses and elastic bandages and splint immobilization in severe cases), surgical decompression will be required, with evacuation of the hematoma, irrigation, and wound closure. If large collections of nonclotted blood or fluid are present, the area is first cleansed in the same manner as that for open surgery to reduce the risk of intra-articular bacterial contamination. After this procedure, physical therapy may begin.

Some hematomas decompress and begin to drain spontaneously. When this occurs, sterile dressings must be kept over the drainage site and motion of the joint delayed. A knee immobilizer provides rest for the knee and often reduces draining. Small hematomas with scant drainage often resolve after several days. When resolution fails and drainage persists, the hematoma should be evacuated surgically, the joint irrigated, the bleeding vessels cauterized, and the wound closed primarily. After wound closure, the knee joint may be treated in the same manner as a recently performed arthroplasty and physical therapy may commence routinely.

The surgeon managing a patient who has a tense hematoma or a persistently draining hematoma must act decisively. Either clinical situation, if not treated rapidly by surgical intervention, will lead to a compromised knee arthroplasty with diminished range of motion. More worrisome in the patient with a draining hematoma is the chance of sterile bloody drainage changing to contaminated drainage with secondary periprosthetic infection. If the surgeon has any doubt, the preferred course of action is early hematoma evacuation and wound closure. The surgeon who attempts expectant treatment, while awaiting hematoma resolution when significant hemarthrosis occurs, is likely to obtain an inferior result.

SEROMA

Causative Factors

When serous drainage occurs after total knee arthroplasty, it usually begins later than hematoma drainage. Drainage may be minimal, occurring around the exit portals for the catheter. In this case, it will resolve with dressing changes and mild compression. Obese patients are more prone to serous drainage, which represents fluid from the liquefaction of fat with or without fat necrosis. In patients with rheumatoid arthritis who are on steroid medication, subcutaneous fat is often atrophic and poorly vascularized. The fat and soft tissues often possess an edematous quality, and exuberant synovium is present within the knee joint. Consequently, after knee replacement the patient so affected tends to have more drainage of either a serous or serosanguineous nature—a worrisome sign. In a long-term follow-up study of patients with rheumatoid arthritis who underwent total knee replacements, we found a 40 percent incidence of deep wound infections associated with significant drainage postoperatively.[9] Because serous drainage may represent a late stage of hematoma formation, any etiologic factor that promotes hematoma will increase the chances of seroma formation.

Treatment

A seroma may be treated much the same as a hematoma. The patient with minimal drainage may be managed with repeated changes of sterile dressings and a compression bandage around the knee. Dressings should be changed often and whenever they have become saturated. The knee should be rested with an immobilizer, which also lessens drainage. Except for walking, physical therapy should be delayed until drainage stops. If drainage persists for more than a few days, the patient should be returned to the operating room, the joint irrigated, and the wound closed over suction drainage tubes.

Antibiotics should not be started just because a hematoma or seroma develops. Initially, the wound is treated locally. If drainage persists, open irrigation and closure are performed. The danger of instituting antibiotics prior to re-exploration is that cultures taken at the time of debridement will be useless. If early infection is present in the joint, the opportunity to isolate the causative organism will be lost. Once intraoperative cultures have been obtained, antibiotics can be given parenterally and continued for 48 hours, or until the culture results are available.

After the wound has been irrigated and closed, the continuous passive motion machine can be utilized again and physical therapy begun.

DEHISCENCE

Causative Factors

Frank wound dehiscence, with or without exposure of the implant, is unusual after total knee replacement. When it does occur, contributing factors may include prolonged administration of steroid therapy; several previous operations on the knee with many incisions and poor soft-tissue coverage; and severely limited range of motion preoperatively, especially when the knee was stiff in extension. If previous quadricepsplasty was inadequate, wound closure may be difficult and the deep soft tissues may be under considerable tension during closure. If the patient tries to flex the knee too vigorously in the postoperative period, complete wound dehiscence may result. It may begin just proximal to the patella and extend distally into the area of the tibial tubercle. In rare cases, severe deep infections produce complete wound dehiscence and exposure of the implant (Fig. 32–2).

Treatment

Complete wound dehiscence after total knee replacement is a surgical emergency. The patient must be returned to the operating room immediately for exploration of the wound and an attempt at closure. If tension on the wound is excessive and

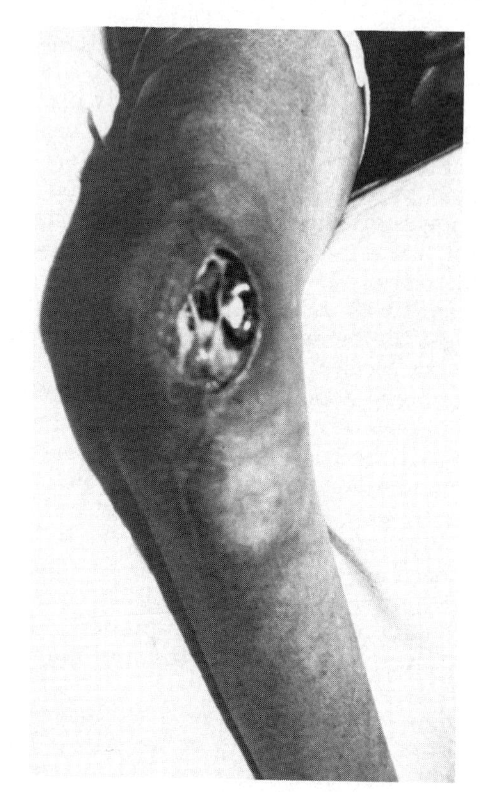

FIGURE 32–2. Wound dehiscence after total knee arthroplasty with exposure of the prosthesis.

closure is not secure, relaxing incisions may be placed to facilitate wound closure. Often, plastic surgery consultation is useful in these situations.

The knee should be immobilized postoperatively and knee flexion held until primary wound healing has occurred. If knee stiffness develops, gentle manipulation of the knee with the patient under anesthesia can be performed several weeks after surgery. The surgeon's primary concern must be stable soft-tissue coverage over the implant. All other functional considerations must be postponed until this has been accomplished. If the dehiscence is secondary to deep infection, the implant must usually be removed and knee joint debridement performed.

DELAYED HEALING AND TISSUE NECROSIS

Causative Factors

Wound-healing problems after total knee replacement may range from minor areas of skin necrosis to severe full-thickness loss of varying sizes. Many of the factors that contribute to draining and dehiscence may also play a role in delayed wound healing. The patients most at risk are those with rheumatoid arthritis who are taking steroid or immunosuppressive medications.[1, 5, 9] The quality of skin in these patients is poor. Often, the skin is quite thin and lacking subcutaneous fat. Patients with severe inflammatory arthritis frequently have associated vasculitis, which further compromises blood flow to the skin margins.

Patients who are obese or have severe deformities are also prone to wound-healing problems, because they require more dissection and retraction of the soft tissues to visualize the joint. The increased tension on the tissues and the vigorous manipulation necessary to mobilize the joint may traumatize the skin and subcutaneous tissue and devascularize skin flaps, causing marginal necrosis. The surgeon must be particularly careful to avoid elevating large skin flaps to expose the joint in these patients. When the skin and subcutaneous tissue are elevated from the underlying knee joint retinaculum, further devascularization is produced. As discussed in Chapter 30, *Primary Total Knee Replacement,* the incision should be made in one plane from the skin to the joint. If the patella is released laterally from the inside of the joint, soft tissues will not have to be elevated from the anterior patellar surface. If release is performed from outside the joint, these anterior soft tissues must be dissected free to allow visualization of the tight lateral peripatellar soft tissues—possibly producing severe devascularization of the lateral skin flap (Fig. 32–3).

Placement of the skin incision itself may influence wound healing. Whenever possible, the surgeon should use previous incision lines in the patient who has had past knee surgery. When the patient has several incisions, the surgeon should choose the one that provides the least difficult access and the least soft-tissue damage. In the previously unoperated knee, a straight or gentle medial parapatellar incision is preferable (see Chapter 28, *Surgical Approaches for Total Knee Replacement* and Chapter 30, *Primary Total Knee Replace-*

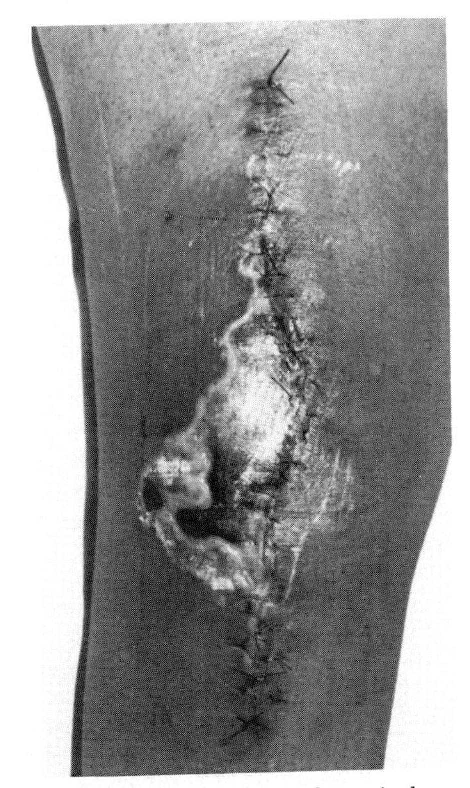

FIGURE 32–3. Extensive lateral marginal necrosis after elevation of a lateral skin flap for lateral retinacular release in an obese patient.

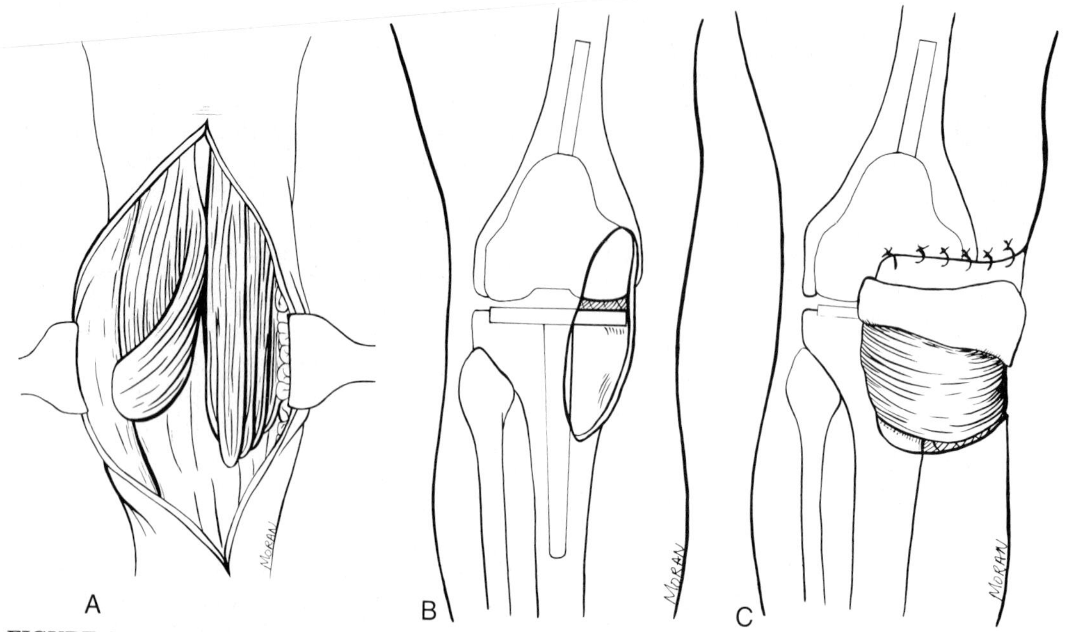

FIGURE 32–4. Technique of muscle flap coverage for full-thickness tissue loss after total knee arthroplasty. *A,* The medial gastrocnemius is mobilized posteriorly. *B,* The medial gastrocnemius is tunneled subcutaneously to the defect anteriorly. *C,* The muscle flap is sutured in place, and a split-thickness skin graft applied.

ment). Evidence has been reported that the gentle parapatellar incision has less tension on it during knee flexion.[6] This factor may lessen the likelihood of wound-healing complications.

In general, these devastating wound complications can be greatly reduced by avoidance of undue tension on skin and soft-tissue margins, preservation of blood flow to skin margins by careful dissection, and thoughtful choice of incision in the previously operated knee.

Treatment

The extent and depth of wound necrosis influence the treatment of areas of delayed wound healing and frank sloughing. Local wound care is sufficient in a patient with an area of marginal necrosis only a few millimeters wide along skin edges and with involvement limited to the subcutaneous layer. These marginal areas will epithelialize beneath the layer of superficial necrosis, after which the surface will slough and be replaced by the healthy tissue underneath. When the zones of necrosis are limited, postoperative rehabilitation usually need not be modified.

When a larger area is involved, extending as much as 1 cm under the skin surface and into the subcutaneous layer, a more formal eschar forms, with a definite level of demarcation. These eschars need not be debrided. They may be left in place. Eventually, they slough and are replaced by the fresh epithelial tissue lying underneath. The key to determining whether a "watch-and-wait" approach is justified is absence of evidence of drainage or cellulitis in the bed. If the eschar progresses to a shell-like appearance without concomitant wound inflammation, a conservative course of action is appropriate. If cellulitis develops, debridement is required. When coverage of a debrided area is extensive or difficult, a plastic surgeon should be consulted.

Whenever wound slough exceeds 1 to 2 cm in length and width, extension is often present through the subcutaneous layer and capsule. In these cases, management must be aggressive if the implant is to be saved. The entire necrotic area is debrided, and the defect is repaired with a flap of gastrocnemius muscle (Fig. 32–4).[3, 10] A split-thickness graft can then be placed over the flap. The surgeon should be alert to the possibility of contamination of the implant with deep periprosthetic infection in these patients due to the precarious nature of the soft tissue in the presence of extensive necrosis. In patients with larger wound sloughs, the orthopaedic surgeon should collaborate with a plastic surgeon, proceeding rapidly and definitely to avoid the catastrophic combination of deep infection and inadequate soft-tissue coverage of the implant.

CELLULITIS

Causative Factors

An uncommon but ominous development after knee replacement surgery is cellulitis in the area of the wound. This seldom occurs in the immediate postoperative period, but when it does, the skin around the wound may feel hot and the patient may have a fever. Sometimes drainage occurs from the knee joint. The patient may complain of pain, which worsens upon movement of the joint, especially in flexion. This constellation of signs and symptoms is usually evidence of deep infection. In some cases, cellulitis occurs at a distance from the wound and suggests a diagnosis of local inflammatory bursitis. Unfortunately, antibiotic treatment masks the underlying problem and makes isolation of the infecting organism difficult. Therefore, antibiotics should not be administered until intra-articular cultures have been obtained.

Treatment

When a patient has cellulitis in the area of a recent knee replacement, the joint should be aspirated and cultures performed to diagnostically eliminate deep infection as the source. Aspiration must be done through a portal, away from the area of cellulitis to avoid inoculating the joint with organisms if, in fact, the process is confined to the superficial tissues. Until culture results are available, treatment should be local, consisting of compresses to the knee and immobilization with a splint.

SUPERFICIAL INFECTION

Causative Factors

Any of the predisposing factors for the previously discussed local complications may also increase the patient's risk of superficial wound infection after total knee arthroplasty. In addition, superficial wound infection is likely in cases of wound drainage, hematoma, or loss of integrity of wound closure, either in the form of a dehiscence or delayed wound healing. Patients at particular risk are those taking corticosteroid or immunosuppressive medication. Diabetic patients also appear to have a greater risk of local wound infections.

Treatment

When purulent drainage from the wound is evident, it may simply represent a reaction to suture material. In this case, suture removal, local cleansing with antiseptics, and debridement are performed. Specific antibiotic therapy is provided if indicated. When purulent drainage emanates from the knee wound itself, the patient should be returned to the operating room for debridement of the wound. Parenteral antibiotic treatment alone is inadequate. If the infection extends below the capsule into the knee joint, cultures of the affected tissues are obtained, and the soft tissues are irrigated copiously. Primary closure of the wound is performed. If the infection is superficial to the joint, the surgeon must take care not to introduce contamination into the joint. The wound should be closed and not left open to granulate secondarily. Multiple cultures should be obtained and Gram stains performed. After the results of intraoperative cultures are known, appropriate antibiotics may be started parenterally. Antibiotics should be continued for 10 to 14 days, until the wound has healed uneventfully and all evidence of infection has disappeared. If the wound has healed completely by the time the patient is discharged from the hospital, oral antibiotics are not needed. Infections that cannot be cleared and are accompanied by persistent drainage usually involve the joint itself.

If the surgeon finds at the time of wound exploration that what was presumed to be a superficial infection has actually extended into the joint, debridement of the joint may be performed with copious irrigation and wound closure. Parenteral antibiotics should be started immediately and continued for 4 to 6 weeks. Parenteral administration of antibiotics is sometimes successful in the management of deep infection if the bone-cement interface has not become involved and if the infection is detected in the early postoperative period. When the surgeon has considered superficial infection but symptoms continue, suggesting deep infection, debridement may be attempted, but the need for implant removal must be considered.

SUMMARY

Local complications may prove to be the undoing of an otherwise successful total knee arthroplasty. To avoid these complications, the surgeon must be knowledgeable about their etiology. Care must be exercised when soft tissues are handled and skin flaps are created to facilitate exposure. The knee joint must be manipulated gently to lessen trauma to the skin and soft tissues. Surgeons who practice meticulous technique are more likely to prevent many of these local complications. Nonetheless, problems are inevitable in some patients. When local complications do arise, the surgeon must identify their presence promptly and treat them rapidly and aggressively. Whenever significant soft tissue is lost, a plastic surgeon should be consulted. An unstable wound should be converted into a more viable one, even if further surgery is required and the patient would prefer a more conservative approach. Failure to take prompt, definitive action may jeopardize the arthroplasty and lead to a severely compromised knee.

References

1. Aglietti, P. and Buzzi, R.: Posterior stabilized total condylar knee replacement. J. Bone Joint Surg. 70B:211–215, 1988.
2. Attenborough, C. G.: The Attenborough total knee replacement. J. Bone Joint Surg. 60B:320–326, 1978.
3. Bengtson, S., Carlsson, A., Relander, M., et al.: Treatment of the exposed knee prosthesis. Acta Orthop. Scand. 58:662–665, 1987.
4. Faralli, V. J., Lotke, P., and Orenstein, E.: Blood loss after total knee replacement: effects of tourniquet release and early motion. Proceedings of the American Academy of Orthopaedic Surgeons, Atlanta, 1988.
5. Hvid, I., Kjaersgaard-Andersen, P., Jon-Oddvar, W., and Sneppen, O.: Knee arthroplasty in rheumatoid arthritis. J. Arthroplasty 2:233–239, 1987.
6. Johnson, D. P.: Midline or parapatellar incision for knee arthroplasty. J. Bone Joint Surg. 70B:656–658, 1988.
7. Kjaersgaard-Andersen, P., Hvid, I., Jon-Oddvar, W., and Sneppen, O.: Total condylar knee arthroplasty in osteoarthritis. Clin. Orthop. 238:167–173, 1989.
8. Rand, J. A., Chao, E. Y. S., and Stauffer, R. M.: Kinematic rotating hinge total knee arthroplasty. J. Bone Joint Surg. 69A:489–497, 1987.
9. Rosa, R., Sculco, T. P., Inglis, A., and Ranawat, C.: Total knee arthroplasty in rheumatoid arthritis: a long term follow-up. Proceedings of the American Academy of Orthopaedic Surgeons, New Orleans, 1986.
10. Sanders, R. and O'Neill, T.: The gastrocnemius myocutaneous flap used as a cover for the exposed knee prosthesis. J. Bone Joint Surg. 63B:383–386, 1981.

CHAPTER 33

Results of Total Knee Arthroplasty

WILLIAM PETTY

Historically, the results of total knee arthroplasty can be divided into three phases. Early procedures performed in the 1970s, providing the early clinical results, used prostheses such as the polycentric, the geometric (or geomedic), the University of California at Irvine (UCI), and the Marmor. In the late 1970s, condylar prostheses were introduced, including the total condylar and kinematic prostheses. The second phase of prosthetic development produced the greatest improvements in clinical results, as one piece components for the femur and tibia were introduced. These designs allowed for more normal kinematics of the knee joint. During this period, patellar resurfacing was also introduced. Later, prostheses have been developed that improve stress transfer to the tibia owing to the metal backing of their components. Hinged prostheses and unicompartmental systems are separate categories and therefore are considered as such in this chapter. Also, cementless application of total knee replacement is compared with cemented replacement.

RATING SYSTEMS

Rating systems for total knee arthroplasty are not as sophisticated as those for total hip replacement, nor have they been as widely used. The most popular rating scale is the Hospital for Special Surgery Knee Rating Scale (HSS) introduced in 1976 (Table 33–1).[25] Another rating system employed in some reports was developed at the University Hospitals of Cleveland (Table 33–2).[18] In 1989, the Knee Society introduced a new total knee rating system (Table 33–3).[28] Important features include separation of the knee rating from functional assessment, 50 points each for pain and function, and deduction of points for walking aids and deformity. The Knee Society developed a separate scoring system for radiographic evaluation (see Chapter 11, *Imaging of Total Joint Replacement*).[17] If these new scoring systems are widely utilized, as the Knee Society hopes, surgeons will be able to make more valid comparisons of reports of total knee arthroplasty results from different centers.[17]

FIRST GENERATION TOTAL KNEE ARTHROPLASTY

In 1971, Gunston[21] described polycentric knee arthroplasty and reported his preliminary results. The prosthesis designed by Gunston was modified slightly by Bryan and Peterson, who reported their 5- to 7-year follow-up results in 101 knees. Of 43 out of an original 64 arthroplasties evaluable after 7 years, 83 percent had good results at 5 years and 64 percent had good

Table 33–1. KNEE RATING SCALE—HOSPITAL FOR SPECIAL SURGERY

Item	Points
Pain (30 points)	
No pain at any time	30
No pain on walking	15
Mild pain on walking	10
Moderate pain on walking	5
Severe pain on walking	0
No pain at rest	15
Mild pain at rest	10
Moderate pain at rest	5
Severe pain at rest	0
Function (22 points)	
Walking and standing unlimited	12
Walking distance of 5–10 blocks and standing ability intermittent (<½ hr)	10
Walking 1–5 blocks and standing ability up to ½ hr	8
Walking less than 1 block	4
Cannot walk	0
Climbing stairs	5
Climbing stairs with support	2
Transfer activity	5
Transfer activity with support	2
Range of Motion (18 points)	
1 point for each 8 degrees of arc of motion to a maximum of 18 points	18
Muscle Strength (10 points)	
Excellent: cannot break the quadriceps power	10
Good: can break the quadriceps power	8
Fair: moves through the arc of motion	4
Poor: cannot move through the arc of motion	0
Flexion Deformity (10 points)	
No deformity	10
Less than 5 degrees	8
5–10 degrees	5
More than 10 degrees	0
Instability (10 points)	
None	10
Mild: 0–5 degrees	8
Moderate: 5–15 degrees	5
Severe: more than 15 degrees	0
Subtraction	
One cane	1
One crutch	2
Two crutches	3
Extension lag of 5 degrees	2
Extension lag of 10 degrees	3
Extension lag of 15 degrees	5
Each 5 degrees of varus	1
Each 5 degrees of valgus	1

Insall, J. N., Ranawat, C. S., Aglietti, P., et al.: J. Bone Joint Surg. 58A:754–765, 1976. By permission.

results at 7 years. Among the 20 knees from an original 37 knees with osteoarthritis, 92 percent had good results at 5 years and 63 percent had good results after 7 years.[11] Lewallen and colleagues,[38] reporting on the same group of patients after 10 years, estimated joint survivorship to be 66 percent. Actual results showed 42 percent of the arthroplasties in patients still alive to be successful after 10 years. Another 10 percent had been successful before death or at last follow-up. Some 34 percent were defined as failures, e.g., reoperation for any reason, unacceptable pain, or loss of function. The most common causes of failure were instability (13 percent), loosening (7 percent), patellofemoral pain (4 percent), and infection (3 percent). Prior knee surgery or axial malalignment increased the incidence of failure.[38]

Riley and Woodyard[49] reported 8-year follow-up results in 71 geometric total knee replacements. Pain relief was good but the failure rate was 18 percent. Torisu and colleagues[60] followed 55 geometric knee replacements from an original group of 70 knees in 56 patients for a mean of 6 years; whereas 81 percent had little or no pain, only 20 percent had no bone-cement lucency and 37 percent had progressive radiolucent zones. Ivarsson and colleagues,[29] following 85 of an original 122 geometric knee replacements for a mean of 5 years, found that 10 knees (12 percent) required revision. Of the remaining knees, 93 percent were considered good or excellent.

Rand and Coventry[48] evaluated 102 knees from patients with osteoarthritis treated with geometric prostheses after a mean of 11 years. Of the 193 knees, 38 (20 percent) required revision procedures: geometric prostheses were implanted in 12 knees, condylar prostheses in 11, and hinged prostheses in 11. The remaining four had arthrodesis. In 24 cases, revision operations were necessary because of component loosening (20 of the tibial component and four of both components). Other causes of failure were axial malalignment in seven cases, infection in four, instability in three, fracture in two, and implant failure (tibial component fracture) in one. Some knees had more than one reason for revision. Of the 102 knees available for follow-up, mild or no pain was present in 83 percent. Estimated retention of prostheses after 10 years was 78 percent. If revision or moderate or severe pain was the end point, success dropped to 69 percent. Lucent lines wider than 1 mm were

Table 33–2. UNIVERSITY HOSPITALS OF CLEVELAND KNEE RATING FORM

Item	Points
A. Pain:	
None/ignores	44
Slight, occasional, no compromise in activity	40
Mild, no effect on ordinary activity, pain after unusual activity, uses aspirin	30
Moderate, tolerable, makes concession, uses codeine occasionally	20
Marked, serious limitations	10
Totally disabled	0
B. Function:	
1. Gait (walking maximum distance):	
a. Limp:	
None	3
Slight	2
Moderate	1
Serious	0
Unable to walk	0
b. Support:	
None	11
Cane, long walks	7
Cane, full time	5
Crutch	4
2 canes	2
2 crutches or walker	0
Unable to walk	0
c. Distance walked:	
Unlimited	11
6 blocks	8
2–3 blocks	5
Indoors only	2
Bed and chair	0
2. Functional activities:	
a. Stairs:	
Ascends and descends normally	6
Ascends normally, has difficulty descending	4
Uses banister at all times	2
Not able	0
b. Ability to get out of chair:	
Able with ease	5
Able with difficulty	3
Unable	0
c. Sitting:	
No difficulty sitting in car or theater	1
Difficulty sitting in car or theater	0
C. Absence of deformity:	
None	2
Varus or valgus, 10°	0
Flexion contracture, 10°	0
D. Range of motion:	
Add each segment of arc to determine total score. Do not add point if any portion of arc is missing.	
Flexion:	
0–15°	2
15–45°	2
45–90°	2
90° or greater	1
Total motion points	
E. Stability:	
Never locks or gives way	7
Rarely locks or gives way	5
Frequently locks or gives way	0
F. Effusion or hemarthrosis:	
Never has an effusion	3
Occasionally has an effusion	1
Frequently has an effusion	0
G. Total knee function rating	

Goldberg, V. M., Heiple, K. G., Ratnoff, O. D., et al.: J. Bone Joint Surg. 63A:695, 1981. By permission.

present in 38 percent of knees and had progressed in 34 percent. The lines were associated mainly with varus axial alignment and varus placement of the tibial component.[48]

Kolstad and Wigren[33] reported 4- to 6-year follow-up evaluations of 66 knee arthroplasties in which the Marmor prosthesis was implanted. Revision was required in five of 52 knees (10 percent) treated for rheumatoid arthritis and one of 18 treated for osteoarthritis. None of the remaining patients had more than mild pain. Marmor,[41] reporting the results of 249 knee replacements, found that 23 had failed by 5 years of follow-up and 14 more failed between 5 and 8 years, for a total failure rate of 15 percent. Follow-up data for 147 of these patients between 5 and 8 years showed good or excellent results in 103 knees (72 percent) and fair results in 27 knees (18 percent).[41]

Hamilton[22] reported the results in 100 UCI knees (80 patients) 5 to 8 years after surgery. Of these, 27 knees (25 patients) were designated failures and required reoperations. Malalignment and thin tibial components (5.0 and 7.5 mm) were the most common causes of failure.[22]

These first generation total knee replacements provided substantial pain relief and functional improvement in most patients. However, the failure rate over time was high, partly because of the limited knowledge about normal knee kinematics and the relatively unsophisticated surgical techniques used during this pioneering era. However, these early knee replace-

Table 33–3. KNEE SCORE—THE KNEE SOCIETY

Patient category
A. Unilateral or bilateral (opposite knee successfully replaced)
B. Unilateral, other knee symptomatic
C. Multiple arthritis or medical infirmity

	Points
Pain	
None	50
Mild or occasional	45
Stairs only	40
Walking and stairs	30
Moderate	
Occasional	20
Continual	10
Severe	0
Range of motion	
(5 degrees = 1 point)	25
Stability (maximum movement in any position)	
Anteroposterior	
<5 mm	10
5–10 mm	5
10 mm	0
Mediolateral	
<5 degrees	15
6–9 degrees	10
10–14 degrees	5
15 degrees	0
Subtotal	___
Deductions (minus)	
Flexion contracture	
5–10 degrees	2
10–15 degrees	5
16–20 degrees	10
>20 degrees	15
Extension lag	
<10 degrees	5
10–20 degrees	10
>20 degrees	15
Alignment	
5–10 degrees	0
0–4 degrees	3 points each degree
11–15 degrees	3 points each degree
Other	20
Total deductions	___
Knee score	___
(If total is a negative number, score is 0.)	

Function	Points
Walking	
Unlimited	50
>10 blocks	40
5–10 blocks	30
<5 blocks	20
Housebound	10
Unable	0
Stairs	
Normal up and down	50
Normal up; down with rail	40
Up and down with rail	30
Up with rail; unable down	15
Unable	0
Subtotal	___
Deductions (minus)	
Cane	5
Two canes	10
Crutches or walker	20
Total deductions	___
Function score	

Insall, J. N., Dorr, L. D., Scott, R. D., et al.: Clin. Orthop. 248:13–14, 1989. By permission.

ment procedures laid the foundation for the improvement that followed in subsequent years.

SECOND GENERATION TOTAL KNEE REPLACEMENT

The total condylar and Townley designs were the first knee prostheses to replace the entire articulation of the knee joint. Insall and Kelly[27] have reported the results of 40 total condylar knee replacements from an original 60 operations in 50 patients 10 years after their operation. Some patients (involving 13 knees) had died, and another seven patients were lost to follow-up evaluations. Although the operations were performed with relatively unsophisticated instruments and techniques and utilized single size components, 35 knees (88 percent) were functioning well after 10 years; none of the 40 knees had loose components or complete radiolucent lines.[27] Of the five failures, all but one (an infection) were due to errors in technique or patient selection.

Goldberg and colleagues[19] evaluated 109 total condylar knee replacements in 82 patients 7 to 11.5 years (mean 9 years) after operation. Of these, ten required revision (9 percent). When the surviving knees were rated by the University Hospitals of Cleveland 100-point scale, the overall mean score was 82, compared with 90 when the same knees were evaluated 4 years earlier. Investigators attributed this decrease in score largely to deterioration in function with advancing age. The average range of motion was 95 degrees; at least 90 degrees of motion was found in 89 percent of knees. Osteoarthritic knees (n = 66) had a lower average score than that for rheumatoid knees (n = 43): 79 versus 85. Knees with patellar resurfacing had better scores than those that did not, especially those treated for osteoarthritis. Although 31 (44 knees) of the original 113 patients died or were lost to follow-up, 38 were evaluated for at least 2 years and none required revision.[19]

Ranawat and Boachie-Adjei,[45] performing survivorship analysis of 112 total condylar knee replacements in 87 patients, predicted survivorship of 94 percent at 11 years. In this series, two patients had component loosening, one of the patella and one of the tibia. In a study of 160 knee replacements 9 years after operation, Aglietti and colleagues[2] found a prosthesis survivorship of 96 percent based on revision and 90 percent based on mechanical and radiologic failures of total condylar prostheses. Scuderi and colleagues[54] reviewed 1430 knee replacements over a 15-year period: survivorship of 224 total condylar prostheses was 91 percent at 15 years; survivorship of 289 posterior stabilized prostheses was 97 percent at 10 years; and survivorship of 917 posterior stabilized prostheses with a metal backed tibial component was 99 percent at 7 years. These groups are not comparable, however, because of improvements in instrumentation and technique over time as well as other factors. These investigators found that age, sex, body weight, and diagnosis did not affect the results.[54] In contrast, Tauber and associates[59] reported inferior results associated with the diagnoses of rheumatoid arthritis, obesity, and preoperative flexion contracture greater than 30 degrees in their study of 71 knee replacements.

In a review of 123 total condylar replacements, Ecker and colleagues[16] found radiolucent lines in 65 percent of knees. Lines were less than 2 mm wide under either the medial or lateral plateau in 36 percent of cases, less than 2 mm under both tibial plateaus in 22 percent, and greater than 2 mm under the plateaus and around the peg in 7 percent. Poor results were associated with only the thickest lines (> 2 mm). In a 2- to 11-year follow-up study of 532 cemented Townley Anatomic Total Knee replacements, Townley[61] judged 89 percent of knees to be good or excellent. The primary mechanical problems were related to the patella and loosening of the tibial component, although tibial loosening requiring revision occurred in only 2 percent of cases; loosening was usually related to axial malalignment.[61]

Bourne and coworkers[9] reviewed 5-year follow-up data for 164 knee replacements in 131 patients with posterior cruciate condylar prostheses (posterior cruciate retaining procedures). The average preoperative knee score (HSS) improved from 57 to 86 after surgery. The average preoperative motion was 102 degrees; postoperatively it was 100 degrees. Three knees (2 percent) required revision. Lucent lines wider than 1 mm occurred in 6 percent of knees, progressing in 3 percent.

Scott and associates[53] evaluated the 2- to 8-year follow-up of 119 knees in 80 patients who had been treated with posterior cruciate substituting prostheses. The average knee score (HSS) improved from 47.5 to 90; the average range of motion improved from 88 to 107 degrees. Radiolucencies of 1 mm or less were observed in 76 percent, of 2 mm in 7 percent, and of 3 mm in 3 percent. The infection rate was 2 percent. Patients with osteoarthritis had better scores than those with rheumatoid arthritis. Those with bilateral procedures had as good a result as those with unilateral procedures.[53]

Aglietti and Buzzi,[1] reviewing 85 knees in 71 patients treated with the posterior stabilized prosthesis after an average of 5 years, found good or excellent results in 90 percent. Four failures (5 percent) were reported: two were due to infection, one to patellar dislocation, and one to loosening. Four other knees (5 percent) showed radiographic signs of tibial loosening. Lucent lines were more common with varus malalignment and tilt of the tibial component of more than 2 degrees.[1]

Knutson and colleagues[32] performed a multicenter study of 8000 total knee replacements, 4505 for osteoarthritis and 3495 for rheumatoid arthritis. They analyzed data after 1, 3, and 6 years. In patients with osteoarthritis, prosthesis survival was 65 percent for hinged prostheses, 87 percent for tricompartmental replacements, and 90 percent for medial compartment replacements. In patients with rheumatoid arthritis prosthesis, survival was 72 percent for unicompartmental replacements and 90 percent for bicompartmental and tricompartmental replacements. Loosening was the most common cause of failure. The second most common cause was infection, occurring in 2 percent of knees with osteoarthritis and 3 percent of those with rheumatoid arthritis.[32]

RESULTS IN YOUNG PATIENTS

Ranawat and colleagues[46] reviewed the results of 93 total knee replacements in 62 patients younger than 55 years of age (mean age 48.7 years) at the time of arthroplasty. The average follow-up interval was 6 years. The preoperative diagnosis was rheumatoid arthritis in 76 knees and osteoarthritis in 17 knees. The average knee rating (HSS) was 87 for the entire group and both subgroups; 30 percent of knees had bone-cement interface lucencies, and two were loose. The predicted survivorship at 10 years was 96 percent.[46] Stuart and Rand[56] followed 44 knee replacements in 26 patients with rheumatoid arthritis for 2 to 8 years. The patients were between 19 and 39 years old at the time of surgery. No pain was reported in 39 knees. In five cases mild weightbearing pain was reported at the follow-up evaluation. The average knee score (HSS) had improved from 52 points preoperatively to 84 points postoperatively; results were good or excellent in 38 cases, fair in six, and poor in none.[56]

RESULTS IN PREVIOUSLY INFECTED KNEES

In a review of 65 knees replaced for previous infections, Jerry and coworkers[30] reported that deep infections occurred in three of 20 cases in which infections involved both joint and bone but in only two of 45 cases in which infection involved the joint only. Subsequent revisions were required in 18 knees (28 percent). The investigators concluded that the failure rate due to both infectious and noninfectious causes was significantly higher in knees with previous infections, especially when infections extended into the bone.

CEMENTLESS KNEE REPLACEMENT

In a report of 2- to 8-year follow-up of 108 ICHL cementless total knee replacements, Albrektsson and Herberts[3] found that 11 tibial components (10 percent) had failed owing to aseptic loosening.

Rorabeck and coworkers[50] compared the results of 110 Kinematic-II cemented and 50 uncemented porous coated anatomic (PCA) knee replacements. After 2 years, patients with the cemented kinematic knee had an average HSS score of 88 and motion of 106 degrees. Those with PCA knees had an average score of 79 and motion of 97 degrees. The reoperation rate was 12 percent for PCA knees and 4 percent for kinematic knees. The investigators attributed the difference in results to the cement and the different prosthetic designs. In his comparison of cementless and cemented total knee replacements, Laskin[36] found comparable results after 2 years.

With the introduction of porous coated knee prostheses, metal backing of patellar components became popular. Unfortunately, many further reports indicate greater incidence of complications with these devices compared with that found for all-polyethylene components, whether cemented or not.[5, 6, 14, 39, 51, 52, 57, 58] Complications have included wearing of the thin polyethylene with subsequent metallosis and synovitis, separation of the polyethylene from the metal back, and failure of the metal backing or porous coating.

MENISCAL BEARING KNEE REPLACEMENT

The New Jersey, Oxford, and Minns total knee prostheses incorporate a polyethylene "meniscus" in an attempt to provide improved metal-polyethylene contact while allowing for rotation and rollback of the femoral on the tibial component. Several reports of short-term to intermediate-term follow-up data indicate results comparable to those of other knee replacements.[12, 13, 20, 44] In a comparison of 67 Oxford knees and 66 kinematic knees, the failure rate was markedly higher with the Oxford knees (30 versus 5 percent for the kinematic knees) after a follow-up interval of

5 to 8 years.[8] The incidence of "meniscal" dislocation requiring reoperation has ranged from 0.7 to 9.3 percent.[7, 13]

HINGED TOTAL KNEE REPLACEMENT

Among the numerous early models of hinged total knee replacements, the most popular were probably the GUEPAR, Shiers, and Walldius prostheses. Although the early results with these prostheses were usually satisfactory, the incidence of severe complications and failure was unacceptably high after even relatively short-term follow-up periods of 2 to 5 years.[4, 15, 23, 24, 31, 37, 55, 63] Frequent complications included sepsis, prosthetic loosening, patellar tendon rupture, patellar dislocation, and component failure. Although many of the knees treated with these prostheses had severe deformity and instability, the results have been too poor to warrant continued implantation.

In an effort to improve the results of total knee replacements in severely deformed or unstable knees, later models of constrained prostheses have introduced rotating bearings or other features to provide stability while reducing the marked transmission of forces to the interface. In an evaluation of the kinematic rotating hinge 2 to 5 years after surgery, Rand and colleagues[47] reported results based on the HSS knee score. The indication for use of the prosthesis was instability or bone loss. Good or excellent results were found in 26 cases, fair results in five, and poor results in another five. Lucent lines were wider than 1 mm in 25 percent of femoral and 50 percent of tibial components. In 13 knees (34 percent) the lines were progressive, and five knees (13 percent) showed probable loosening radiographically. Sepsis occurred in 16 percent, patellar instability in 22 percent, and component failure in 6 percent. The investigators recommended that the prosthesis be considered only for instability that could not be corrected by soft tissue repair.[47]

The spherocentric knee was designed to allow triaxial rotation while providing intrinsic stability. Matthews and coworkers[43] evaluated 48 knees after an average follow-up period of 8 years, using 5-point scales (0 to 4) for pain and function. The average score for pain was 1 (0 designated no pain); for function it was 2.26 (moderate restriction). These workers found that function had deteriorated compared with a previous review but believed this finding was due to advancing age. The infection rate was 5 percent and the reoperation rate 15 percent.[43] Wigren and Amici[62] also reported satisfactory results with no serious complications in short-term follow-up evaluations of 18 procedures employing the spherocentric prosthesis. All patients had severe deformity or instability.

UNICOMPARTMENTAL KNEE REPLACEMENT

Some surgeons recommend unicompartmental replacement as an alternative to tibial osteotomy for some knees with arthrosis limited mostly or entirely to the medial or lateral compartments. However, two reports on unicondylar knee arthroplasty have indicated a high failure rate. Insall and Aglietti[26] reported 22 of 32 unicondylar arthroplasties 5 to 7 years after surgery. At the time of review, one knee was rated excellent, seven good, four fair, and ten poor. Seven knees (28 percent) had been revised. The major reason for failure was progression of arthritis in the unreplaced compartments.[26] Laskin[35] reported that only eight of 22 knees with unicompartment arthroplasty had good or excellent results 5 to 7 years after surgery. Of these knees, 18 had patellectomy at the time of arthroplasty. Later reports describe better results. Marmor[42] reported an average 11-year follow-up (minimum 10 years) of 60 unicompartmental knee replacements that were evaluable from a group of 87 consecutive operations. Knee scores (HSS) were good or excellent in 38 cases (63 percent), fair in four (7 percent), and poor in 18 (30 percent). Failures were associated with thin tibial components (nine knees), disease not limited to one compartment (six knees), degeneration of the uninvolved compartment (two knees), and patellar impingement against the femoral prosthesis (one knee).

Mackinnon and colleagues[40] followed 115 knees in 100 patients for 2 to 12 years after replacement with the St. George sledge prosthesis. They reported good or excellent ratings in 86 percent of knees. Seven revisions (6 percent) for deterioration in the opposite compartment took place.

Broughton and coworkers[10] compared unicompartment arthroplasty in 42 knees with upper tibial osteotomy in 49 knees 5 to 10 years after operation. Good or excellent results were found in 76 percent of knees having arthroplasty compared with only 46 percent of knees having upper tibial osteotomy. Three arthroplasties (7 percent) and ten osteotomies (20 percent) had been revised.

Kozinn and colleagues[34] reported the results of 50 unicompartment arthroplasties performed with modern design prostheses. After an average follow-up time of over 5.5 years, 92 percent of the knees were rated good or excellent, and none required revision.

Many of the reviews of unicompartmental knee arthroplasty indicate that the procedure results in more rapid rehabilitation than does tricompartmental arthroplasty.

SUMMARY

Total knee arthroplasty has evolved over the past two decades into a successful and durable treatment for the severely arthritic knee. Although short-term results with early techniques and designs were generally good, the failure rate was fairly high with longer-term follow-up. Second generation prostheses and improvements in instrumentation and surgical techniques have yielded results at least as good as those reported for total hip arthroplasty. The surgeon who employs modern prostheses and techniques can anticipate good or excellent results in over 90 percent of patients having total knee arthroplasties and can expect these results to last at least 10 to 15 years. In the limited reports available, results in young patients appear comparable to those in older patients, although this finding should not be misinterpreted to suggest that total knee arthroplasty performed in young patients can be expected to last their lifetime.

Results of cementless knee arthroplasty have shown no advantages in clinical result or durability over those of cemented arthroplasty to date. In fact, some reports indicate inferior results in cementless tibial components. Short-term results suggest that cementless femoral components perform as well as those that are cemented. According to many reports, the complication rate with metal backed patellar components, whether cemented or not, is considerably higher than that seen with all-polyethylene cemented patellar components.

The results of unicompartmental knee arthroplasty have improved. Thus, it may be considered as one treatment alternative for the patient with arthrosis limited to the medial or lateral compartment, especially the older patient.

References

1. Aglietti, P. and Buzzi, R.: Posteriorly stabilised total-condylar knee replacement. Three to eight years' follow-up of 85 knees. J. Bone Joint Surg. [Br.] 70(2):211–216, 1988.
2. Aglietti, P., Scrobe, F., Gaudenzi, A., et al.: An analysis of the survival rate of total-condylar total knee prostheses with posterior stability. Ital. J. Orthop. Traumatol. 14(4):419–428, 1988.
3. Albrektsson, B. E. and Herberts, P.: ICLH knee arthroplasty. A consecutive study of 108 knees with uncemented tibial component fixation. J. Arthroplasty 3(2):145–156, 1988.
4. Bargar, W. L., Cracchiolo, A., 3d, and Amstutz, H. C.: Results with the constrained total knee prosthesis in treating severely disabled patients and patients with failed total knee replacements. J. Bone Joint Surg. [Am.] 62(4):504–512, 1980.
5. Bayley, J. C., Scott, R. D., Ewald, F. C., et al.: Failure of the metal-backed patellar component after total knee replacement. J. Bone Joint Surg. [Am.] 70(5):668–674, 1988.
6. Bayley, J. C. and Scott, R. D.: Further observations on metal-backed patellar component failure. Clin. Orthop. 236:82–87, 1988.
7. Bert, J. M.: Dislocation/subluxation of the meniscal bearing elements following New Jersey LCS total knee arthroplasty. American Academy of Orthopaedic Surgeons, Atlanta, 1988.
8. Bourne, R. B., Rorabeck, C. H., Finlay, J. B., et al.: Kinematic I and Oxford knee arthroplasty. A 5- to 8-year follow-up study. J. Arthroplasty 2(4):285–291, 1987.
9. Bourne, M. H., Rand, J. A., and Ilstrup, D. M.: Posterior cruciate condylar total knee arthroplasty. Five-year results. Clin. Orthop. 234:129–136, 1988.
10. Broughton, N. S., Newman, J. H., and Baily, R. A.: Unicompartmental replacement and high tibial osteotomy for osteoarthritis of the knee. A comparative study after 5-10 years' follow-up. J. Bone Joint Surg. [Br.] 68(3):447–452, 1986.
11. Bryan, R. S. and Peterson, L. F.: Polycentric total

knee arthroplasty: a prognostic assessment. Clin. Orthop. 145:23–28, 1979.
12. Buechel, F. F. and Pappas, M. J.: The New Jersey Low-Contact-Stress Knee Replacement System: biomechanical rationale and review of the first 123 cemented cases. Arch. Orthop. Trauma Surg. 105(4):197–204, 1986.
13. Buechel, F. F. and Pappas, M. J.: New Jersey Low-Contact-Stress Knee Replacement System. Ten-year evaluation of meniscal bearings. Orthop. Clin. North Am. 20(2):147–177, 1989.
14. Clayton, M. L. and Thirupathi, R.: Patellar complications after total condylar arthroplasty. Clin. Orthop. 170:152–155, 1982.
15. Duquennoy, A., Decoulx, J., Epinette, J. A., et al.: Hinge prosthesis of the knee. Apropos of 185 cases. Rev. Chir. Orthop. 69(6):465–474, 1983. (Published in French.)
16. Ecker, M. L., Lotke, P. A., Windsor, R. E., et al.: Long-term results after total condylar knee arthroplasty. Significance of radiolucent lines. Clin. Orthop. 216:151–158, 1987.
17. Ewald, F. C.: The Knee Society Total Knee Arthroplasty Roentgenographic Evaluation and Scoring System. Clin. Orthop. 248:9–12, 1989.
18. Goldberg, V. M., Heiple, K. G., Ratnoff, O. D., et al.: Total knee arthroplasty in classic hemophilia. J. Bone Joint Surg. 63A:695–701, 1981.
19. Goldberg, V. M., Figgie, M. P., Figgie, H. E., 3d, et al.: Use of a total condylar knee prosthesis for treatment of osteoarthritis and rheumatoid arthritis. Long-term results. J. Bone Joint Surg. [Am.] 70(6):802–811, 1988.
20. Goodfellow, J. W. and O'Connor, J.: Clinical results of the Oxford knee. Surface arthroplasty of the tibiofemoral joint with a meniscal bearing prosthesis. Clin. Orthop. 205:21–42, 1986.
21. Gunston, F. H.: Polycentric knee arthroplasty. J. Bone Joint Surg. 53B:272–277, 1971.
22. Hamilton, L. R.: UCI total knee replacement. A follow-up study. J. Bone Joint Surg. [Am.] 64(5):740–744, 1982.
23. Hoikka, V., Vankka, E., Eskola, A., et al.: Results and complications after arthroplasty with a totally constrained total knee prosthesis (GUEPAR). Ann. Chir. Gynaecol. 78(2):94–96, 1989.
24. Hui, F. C. and Fitzgerald, R. H. Jr.: Hinged total knee arthroplasty. J. Bone Joint Surg. [Am.] 62(4):513–519, 1980.
25. Insall, J. N., Ranawat, C. S., Aglietti, P., et al.: A comparison of four models of total knee-replacement prostheses. J. Bone Joint Surg. 58A:754–765, 1976.
26. Insall, J. and Aglietti, P.: A five- to seven-year follow-up of unicondylar arthroplasty. J. Bone Joint Surg. [Am.] 62(8):1329–1337, 1980.
27. Insall, J. N. and Kelly, M.: The total condylar prosthesis. Clin. Orthop. 205:43–48, 1986.
28. Insall, J. N., Dorr, L. D., Scott, R. D., et al.: Rationale of the Knee Society Clinical Rating System. Clin. Orthop. 248:13–14, 1989.
29. Ivarsson, I., Myrnerts, R., and Tkaczuk, H.: Long-term follow-up of patients with geomedic prostheses. Arch. Orthop. Trauma Surg. 105(6):353–358, 1986.
30. Jerry, G. J. Jr., Rand, J. A., and Ilstrup, D.: Old sepsis prior to total knee arthroplasty. Clin. Orthop. 236:135–140, 1988.
31. Kenesi, C.: The "caviar" madreporic knee prosthesis. Clin. Orthop. 145:94–100, 1979.
32. Knutson, K., Lindstrand, A., and Lidgren, L.: Survival of knee arthroplasties. A nation-wide multicentre investigation of 8000 cases. J. Bone Joint Surg. [Br.] 68(5):795–803, 1986.
33. Kolstad, K. and Wigren, A.: Marmor knee arthroplasty. Clinical results and complications during an observation period of at least 3 years. Acta Orthop. Scand. 53(4):651–661, 1982.
34. Kozinn, S. C., Marx, C., and Scott, R. D.: Unicompartmental knee arthroplasty. A 4.5–6-year follow-up study with a metal-backed tibial component. J. Arthroplasty 4 Suppl:S1–10, 1989.
35. Laskin, R. S.: Unicompartmental tibiofemoral resurfacing arthroplasty. J. Bone Joint Surg. 60A:182–185, 1978.
36. Laskin, R. S.: Tricon-M uncemented total knee arthroplasty. A review of 96 knees followed for longer than 2 years. J. Arthroplasty 3(1):27–38, 1988.
37. leNobel, J. and Patterson, F. P.: Guepar total knee prosthesis. Experience at the Vancouver General Hospital. J. Bone Joint Surg. [Br.] 63B(2):257–260, 1981.
38. Lewallen, D. G., Bryan, R. S., and Peterson, L. F.: Polycentric total knee arthroplasty. A ten-year follow-up study. J. Bone Joint Surg. [Am.] 66(8):1211–1218, 1984.
39. Lombardi, A. V. Jr., Engh, G. A., Volz, R. G., et al.: Fracture/dissociation of the polyethylene in metal-backed patellar components in total knee arthroplasty. J. Bone Joint Surg. [Am.] 70(5):675–679, 1988.
40. Mackinnon, J., Young, S., and Baily, R. A.: The St. Georg sledge for unicompartmental replacement of the knee. A prospective study of 115 cases. J. Bone Joint Surg. [Br.] 70(2):217–223, 1988.
41. Marmor, L.: The Marmor knee replacement. Orthop. Clin. North Am. 13(1):55–64, 1982.
42. Marmor, L.: Unicompartmental knee arthroplasty. Ten- to 13-year follow-up study. Clin. Orthop. 226:14–20, 1988.
43. Matthews, L. S., Goldstein, S. A., Kolowich, P. A., et al.: Spherocentric arthroplasty of the knee. A long-term and final follow-up evaluation. Clin. Orthop. 205:58–66, 1986.
44. Minns, R. J.: The Minns meniscal knee prosthesis: biomechanical aspects of the surgical procedure and a review of the first 165 cases. Arch. Orthop. Trauma Surg. 108(4):231–235, 1989.
45. Ranawat, C. S. and Boachie-Adjei, O.: Survivorship analysis and results of total condylar knee arthroplasty. Eight- to 11-year follow-up period. Clin. Orthop. 226:6–13, 1988.
46. Ranawat, C. S., Padgett, D. E., and Ohashi, Y.: Total knee arthroplasty for patients younger than 55 years. Clin. Orthop. 248:27–33, 1989.
47. Rand, J. A., Chao, E. Y., and Stauffer, R. N.: Kinematic rotating-hinge total knee arthroplasty. J. Bone Joint Surg. [Am.] 69(4):489–497, 1987.
48. Rand, J. A. and Coventry, M. B.: Ten-year evaluation of geometric total knee arthroplasty. Clin. Orthop. 232:168–173, 1988.
49. Riley, D. and Woodyard, J. E.: Long-term results of Geomedic total knee replacement. J. Bone Joint Surg. [Br.] 67(4):548–550, 1985.

50. Rorabeck, C. H., Bourne, R. B., and Nott, L.: The cemented kinematic-II and the non-cemented porous-coated anatomic prostheses for total knee replacement. A prospective evaluation. J. Bone Joint Surg. [Am.] 70(4):483–490, 1988.
51. Rosenberg, A. G., Andriacchi, T. P., Barden, R., et al.: Patellar component failure in cementless total knee arthroplasty. Clin. Orthop. 236:106–114, 1988.
52. Scott, R. D., Turoff, N., and Ewald, F. C.: Stress fracture of the patella following duopatellar total knee arthroplasty with patellar resurfacing. Clin. Orthop. 170:147–151, 1982.
53. Scott, W. N., Rubinstein, M., and Scuderi, G.: Results after knee replacement with a posterior cruciate-substituting prosthesis. J. Bone Joint Surg. [Am.] 70(8):1163–1173, 1988.
54. Scuderi, G. R., Insall, J. N., Windsor, R. E., et al.: Survivorship of cemented knee replacements. J. Bone Joint Surg. [Br.] 71(5):798–803, 1989.
55. Shindell, R., Neumann, R., Connolly, J. F., et al.: Evaluation of the Noiles hinged knee prosthesis. A five-year study of seventeen knees. J. Bone Joint Surg. [Am.] 68(4):579–585, 1986.
56. Stuart, M. J. and Rand, J. A.: Total knee arthroplasty in young adults who have rheumatoid arthritis. J. Bone Joint Surg. [Am.] 70(1):84–87, 1988.
57. Stulberg, S. D., Stulberg, B. N., Hamati, Y., et al.: Failure mechanisms of metal-backed patellar components. Clin. Orthop. 236:88–105, 1988.
58. Sutherland, C. J.: Patellar component dissociation in total knee arthroplasty. A report of two cases. Clin. Orthop. 228:178–181, 1988.
59. Tauber, C., Bar-On, E. B., Ganel, A., et al.: The total condylar knee prosthesis: a review of 71 operations. Arch. Orthop. Trauma Surg. 104(6):352–356, 1986.
60. Torisu, T., Morita, H., and Kamo, Y.: Geometric total knee arthroplasty—follow-up for an average of six years. Nippon Seikeigeka Gakkai Zasshi 58(10):975–987, 1984. (Published in Japanese.)
61. Townley, C. O.: The anatomic total knee resurfacing arthroplasty. Clin. Orthop. 192:82–96, 1985.
62. Wigren, A. and Amici, F., Jr.: The spherocentric knee prosthesis (long-term results in 18 cases). Ital. J. Orthop. Traumatol. 8(1):53–58, 1982.
63. Wilson, F. C., Fajgenbaum, D. M., and Venters, G. C.: Results of knee replacement with the Walldius and geometric prostheses. A comparative study. J. Bone Joint Surg. [Am.] 62(4):497–503, 1980.

CHAPTER 34

Revision Total Knee Arthroplasty

KENNETH A. KRACKOW

Pain is usually but not always the major complaint of the patient dissatisfied with total knee arthroplasty. A wide variety of other problems also account for the decision to undertake revision total knee surgery. However, the orthopaedic surgeon should view revision as only one of several options and should appreciate what these options are. Careful preoperative evaluation allows intelligent selection from the choices available. For example, would the patient's knee benefit from a revision total knee arthroplasty or would the patient's knee be better left alone? Should fusion be considered? Would a planned pseudoarthrosis be the best course? When choosing one of these options for any of our patients, we consider the patient's ability to undergo future operations, the implications of continued loss of bone stock, and the potential impossibility of future fusion if revision fails.

INDICATIONS FOR REVISION

Complications for which revision total knee arthroplasty may be indicated include infection, pain, prosthetic loosening, component failure, malalignment, ligamentous laxity, subluxation or dislocation, patellofemoral instability, and limited range of motion.

Infection

Acute and subacute perioperative infection as well as late hematogenous infection is one of the most common indications for revision today.[3, 14] Although infection is discussed elsewhere in this text, it needs to be mentioned briefly here as well (see Chapter 35, *Treatment of Infected Total Knee Arthroplasty*). In fact, infection must usually be considered as an underlying etiologic factor in almost any unsatisfactory total knee replacement. This consideration is especially true for any patients with persistent pain, limited range of motion, and loosening, especially loosening that appears to be premature. For these reasons, imaging studies, joint fluid aspirations, cell counts, cultures, and even biopsies should be considered for many patients in whom revision total knee replacement is contemplated.

Patients with obvious infections, especially those suspected on the bases of acute inflammatory changes, open drainage, and so on, pose no special problems. For these patients, treatment possibilities are clear, including incision, drainage, synovectomy, removal, delayed exchange, and fusion. In this chapter, the focus primarily is on patients with stiff, painful knees and early development of lucent lines at bone-cement-prosthesis interfaces.

Pain

When a patient has significant persistent pain, infection as a cause must be excluded before other causes are explored. The surgeon must make sure that an appropriate work-up has been done. If infection is ruled out, the causes of pain that remain for consideration include synovitis (part of the original disease, a reaction to some aspect of the implant, or idiopathic); inapparent loosening; inapparent component tightness secondary to soft tissue factors, leading to stiffness and pain; stiffness; and unrealistic expectations of the patient.

Early in the patient's evaluation, radiographs made prior to the original arthroplasty should be reviewed. The clinical course of the patient should be studied in detail, including the entire history of knee symptoms and prior surgical interventions and their results.

Possibly, treatable causes of postarthroplasty knee pain that we simply do not understand do exist. Nevertheless, clinical experience with patients who had borderline indications for an initial total knee replacement suggests that these patients are in a special class. Most have had no substantial cartilage degeneration to begin with, and their knee pain is usually not relieved much by total knee components. For these patients, revision arthroplasty may not be a good alternative. As one follows and evaluates the patient with pain of unclear origin, it may be a good idea to consider exploratory arthrotomy. This procedure allows the surgeon to investigate more specifically the possibility of inapparent loosening, unusual signs of synovitis, perhaps wear particle reaction, polyethylene wear, and so on. Alternatively, arthroscopy may be considered, although it can be a difficult examination because of limited synovial space secondary to scar tissue. Also, the prosthetic bone interface can almost never be exposed in multiple places while simultaneously stressing the components to elicit the appearance of significant loosening.

When offering the patient an exploratory arthrotomy, the surgeon must make certain points clear. First, there is always a possibility of introducing infection where none existed. Second, one can only "fix" (i.e., revise or replace) what is already "broken" (i.e., loose or worn). Finally, simply revising and exchanging all of the components in the absence of detectable abnormalities cannot reasonably be expected to alter the painful state. In fact, a bigger operation is only superimposed on an already unsatisfactory one, typically causing more stiffness and pain.

Loosening

The most common reason for revision arthroplasty of the knee is loosening. With improvements in prosthetic design and operative technique, problems with the patella and extensor mechanism have become more common. Correction of extensor mechanism complications may or may not require surgery or revision of prosthetic components. Severe prosthetic loosening can be corrected only by revision arthroplasty, arthrodesis, or possibly resection arthroplasty in selected cases. The major symptom of loosening is pain that occurs primarily with weightbearing; it is often worst when the patient first rises after a period of rest. The plain radiograph is the most valuable diagnostic tool for detecting loosening of the prosthetic components. Many total knee arthroplasties have minimal radiolucent lines at the bone-cement interface or, in the case of cementless components, at the bone-prosthesis interface. These lines, most common at the tibial and patellar components, do not indicate a loose prosthesis.[6, 7, 13, 17, 31, 37] However, lucencies that are continuous around the entire implant or are wide ($\geq$2 mm) and progressive on serial radiographs do suggest loosening.

Definite signs of loose components include migration and demonstrated movement. Migration is apparent on serial radiographs or, when these are unavailable, may often be suggested by an abnormal position of a component on a single radiograph. Image intensification fluoroscopy may be employed to detect prosthetic motion during motion and stress examinations. Rarely, relative component movement may be seen at the interface, especially in uncemented prostheses, when interface abnormalities are not otherwise apparent. Arthrography and other imaging studies may also be helpful in the diagnosis of loosening (see Chapter 11, *Imaging of Total Joint Replacement*).

Prosthetic Component Failure

Prosthetic failure may occur in the body of the component or on its articular surfaces. Usually, failure in the body of the component involves fracture of hinged prostheses, polyethylene tibial components, or metal trays of modular tibial components. Fracture of femoral total knee components is rare.[21,29] Because fixed hinge prostheses are employed in cases of severe instability, component fracture is usually a catastrophic event of which the patient is immediately aware because of acute instability and pain. Often severe material wear produces substantial metallic or other debris within the joint. Failure of hinge prostheses is often associated with substantial bone loss.

Fracture of a tibial resurfacing component, whether polyethylene or metal, is generally more subtle. The patient's primary complaint is pain. Deformity may also result from the failure and from the associated fracture or collapse of the involved tibial plateau. Although a first look at the radiograph may not reveal the problem, it can be detected with careful examination.[22,23,30,32,36] Fracture of patellar components may also occur. Since the advent of the metal backed patella, dissociation and breakage of metal pegs have been reported for many different designs.[1,2,9,18,26,33,34,38]

Loosening of the porous coating of all three components of total knee prostheses has been reported. Except for loosening of the patella, no symptomatic failures have been reported. However, loose porous coatings are often associated with prosthesis-bone lucency. In addition, loose beads or wire mesh particles may contribute to substantial third body wear if interposed between the articulating surfaces.[8,27]

Articular surface damage involves the polyethylene components, with wear or deformation of patellar components often noted during secondary surgery of total knee arthroplasty. Changes are seldom associated with symptoms or other apparent problems, although significant production of wear particles might predispose the patient to component loosening. Although wear of the tibial polyethylene component has not been a common problem, with longer-term follow-up and modifications of material and design, the polyethylene surface may be susceptible to failure (Fig. 34–1)[12,42,43] (see Chapter 3, *Polymers,* and Chapter 27, *Design of Total Knee Replacements*). Concern has been increasing about failure of articulating surfaces made of titanium alloy, especially when they have undergone no special treatment to reduce wear.[20]

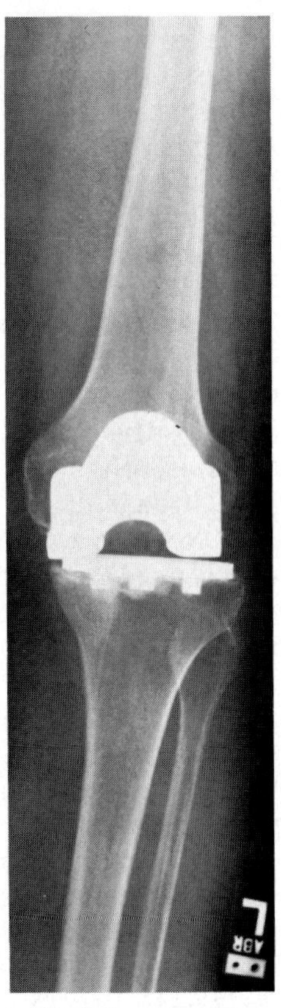

FIGURE 34–1. Medial subluxation of the femoral component on the tibial component with severe wear of the medial articular polyethylene surface, resulting in articulation of the femoral component with the metal tibial tray.

Malalignment

When malalignment occurs, either the anatomic or mechanical axis is incorrect or the femoral and tibial components are malaligned so that the joint line is not level. Malalignment of either type results in increased shear and tension forces on the prosthetic components. Severe malalignment may increase the tension on either the medial or lateral ligaments enough to stretch these ligaments and produce instability. Malalignment is defined as a variation of more than 3 degrees from normal in either direction or a variation of less than 4 degrees or more than 10 degrees of valgus. This fairly strict definition of malalignment certainly does not indicate that revision should be considered for most knees aligned outside this range. Many knees with moderate malalignment function very well. However, it is well established that malalignment, especially varus malalignment, leads to an increased incidence of interface lucency and long-term loosening.[6, 13, 19, 31, 37]

Surgeons who manage patients with more severe malalignment need to ask themselves whether revision should be undertaken. Usually, the issue is not pain but anticipated loosening as a consequence of eccentric weightbearing on malaligned components.[16, 25] We have no rigid guidelines for such cases. One of our patients had postoperative varus deformity that was considered intolerable not only because of its degree but because the patient was younger than 30 years old. Although we decided that action in his case was warranted, we decided upon distal femoral osteotomy rather than revision arthroplasty (Fig. 34–2). This case raises an important point regarding the condition of the capsular ligamentous (soft tissue) sleeve about the knee with respect to collateral ligament stability. Symmetrically tight medial and lateral aspects in the presence of actual deformity imply that if revision were undertaken for such a presumably major deformity, a substantial amount of soft tissue release and balancing would be necessary. In comparison, if ligaments were very lax on the concave side of the deformity, the soft tissues might be better balanced and actually in a nondeformed state. Thus, revision of one or both components into more proper alignment could be the best course. If realignment were accomplished by osteotomy instead, the laxity of the concave side might only seem to be brought into a more noticeable position, its manifestation having been relatively protected while on the concave side of the deformity.

Ligamentous Laxity

The discussion that follows is limited to laxity or ligamentous "sloppiness" unaccompanied by subluxation and dislocation (Fig. 34–3). The patient may express concern about problems related to ligamentous laxity in terms of medial opening on valgus or lateral opening on varus stress and increased anteroposterior drawer sign. Naturally, concern increases with the extent of instability. Careful questioning and examination by the surgeon are necessary in these cases, as many patients with very great amounts of specific or even global ligamentous instability function quite well.

Actually, in one report, the functional outcome in patients with relatively lax knees was better than that of patients with normal tight stability.[10] If the ligamentous laxity appears to be serious enough to warrant surgical intervention, its nature must be understood as well as possible. Surgeons who treat these patients must ask themselves a number of questions. Is the laxity global, that is, of equivalent degree in the four standard directions: medial, lateral, anterior, and posterior? This finding implies that the laxity is equivalent in flexion and extension. Is there full extension or, instead, any tendency to flexion contracture or recurvatum? If the ligamentous instability is primarily collateral, is it more medial than lateral, or vice versa? Is it more evident in flexion or extension? If the instability is anteroposterior, is it functionally significant to the patient in the absence of specific subluxation events, that is, without pivot shift and without posterior (posteromedial or posterolateral) subluxation?

The answers to these questions can be used as the surgeon considers the following points.

1. Revision or plastic spacer change, which simply makes the tibial component thicker, will decrease extension somewhat.
2. Global instability might, to some degree, be addressed by such a move, i.e., simply a thicker tibia, if extension is not restricted. Otherwise, a flexion contracture would be induced by thickening the tibial component.
3. Relatively symmetric collateral instability in extension only would theoretically be addressed by re-establishing the femoral component in a more distal position.
4. Symmetric instability (collateral and possibly anteroposterior) in flexion would theoretically be addressed by moving the femoral component more posterior or by using a thicker tibial component in combination with a similar type of femoral component moved more cephalad.

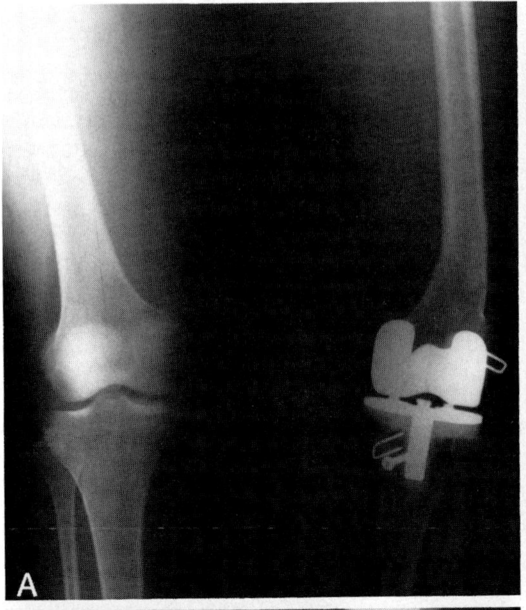

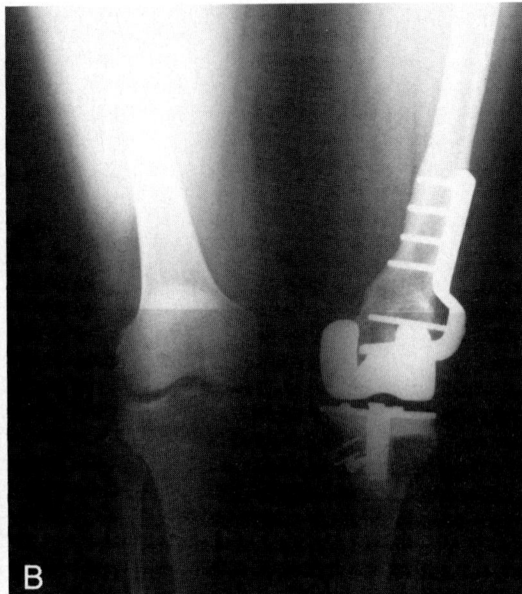

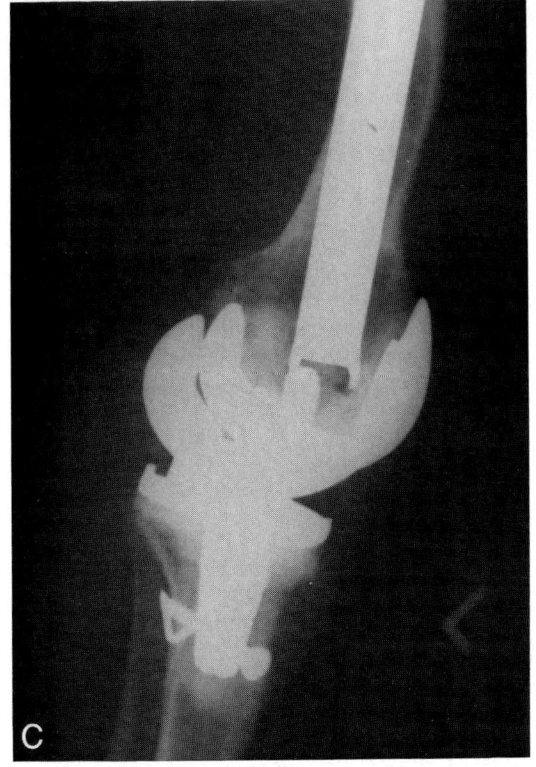

FIGURE 34–2. Standing preoperative and postoperative radiographs of a patient less than 30 years old with a major varus deformity after total knee arthroplasty. A decision was made to correct this deformity to proper alignment by osteotomy rather than by revision. *A,* Preoperative radiograph. *B,* Postoperative anteroposterior radiograph. *C,* Postoperative lateral radiograph.

5. Symmetric anteroposterior instability will, to some degree, be addressed by having more closely conforming femoral and tibial tray geometry, as in the original total condylar design, in combination with proper tensioning of the collateral ligaments in flexion.

6. Asymmetric instability might theoretically be addressed by either tightening the lax ligament (i.e., performing a primary ligamentous reconstruction) or revising the components and performing the necessary soft tissue release at the "tight" side, so that the soft tissue is "elongated" enough to balance the laxity of the other side.

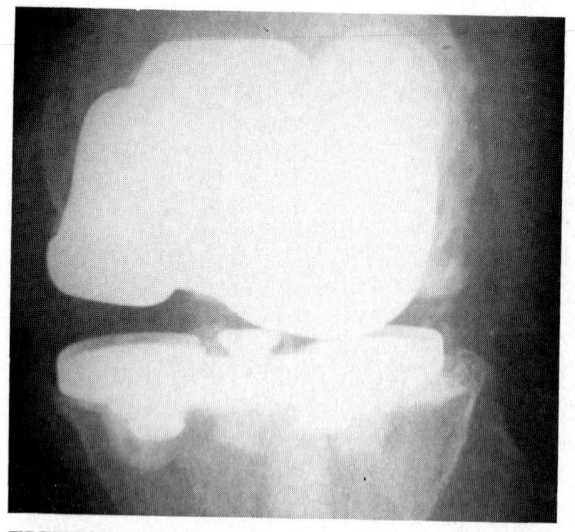

FIGURE 34–3. Postoperative radiograph showing obvious ligamentous laxity but not frank component subluxation.

Before a primary ligament reconstruction is undertaken, the surgeon must recognize that a good outcome from this approach is impossible if the laxity is present on the convex side of a deformity. In fact, this option of reconstruction might most comfortably be considered if the laxity existed on the concave side of an acceptable amount of deformity. One must, however, wonder if such a situation would be adequately symptomatic to warrant this surgery.

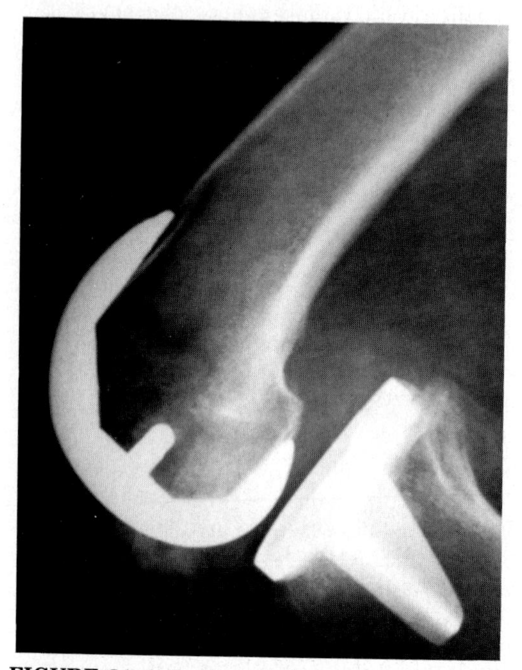

FIGURE 34–4. Radiograph demonstrating a condylar type prosthesis that subluxed posteriorly.

In general, the options for treating ligamentous laxity are primary ligament surgery; revision with care to proper ligament balance, and possibly use of a more stabilized prosthesis or even single component change; and watching and waiting. Fortunately, ligamentous instability alone is not a common indication for surgical intervention.

Subluxation or Dislocation

Although ligamentous instability short of the amount necessary to produce subluxation is an infrequent reason for revision, frank subluxation or dislocation patterns will probably be tolerated poorly and will almost surely necessitate revision (Fig. 34–4). The patient's clinical situation and the results of physical examination and radiographic findings must be studied carefully to understand the cause of the problem. Specific conditions to look for include apparent rupture of posterior cruciate ligament that originally provided adequate stability; generally inadequate soft tissue balancing for fairly severe *a priori* deformity; spastic conditions with overactive knee flexors (normally hamstrings pulling the tibia posteriorly); specific errors in either component sizing or component placement; and rupture or attenuation of collateral ligamentous soft tissue, usually in combination with some other aspect of laxity in the soft tissue sleeve. An understanding of these problems permits a more intelligent approach to management, possibly with a minimally constrained prosthesis. Caution is important when a knee has remained subluxed or dislocated in a fixed attitude. Rarely can this situation be managed just by ligamentous repair, reconstruction, or simple balancing together with placement of a thicker tibial component. Most of these patients require revisions to at least a central stemmed tibial pegged component that prevents side-to-side and posterior translation. In some cases, special care must be taken to protect neurovascular structures when correcting dislocation.

Patellofemoral Instability

Patellofemoral instability may be a concern in overall component revision if subluxation is secondary to significant aberrance in femoral and tibial component positioning. The possibilities include an overall excessive valgus alignment; abnormal femoral component rotation; and grossly abnormal tibial component rotation leading to a markedly increased Q angle, which, in selected cases, may be better approached by altering the tibial component's position than medializing the tibial tubercle (see Chapter 30, *Primary Total Knee Replacement*).

Limited Range of Motion

The patient whose main complaint is poor range of motion after total knee arthroplasty in many ways resembles the patient with excessive pain: the poor range of motion may simply be a manifestation of not well-understood postoperative pain. Of course, the argument can become circular when one considers that poor range of motion can also be a cause of pain, as the patient continually tries to stretch through the subcapsular scar. However, more objective considerations of component position may be related to range of motion.

At least five basic causes of decreased flexion can be attributed to problems with prosthetic components. The first is an excessively thick patella. In some patients, a patellar component that is relatively thick compared with the amount of patellar bone resected can lead to an extensor mechanism tenodesis, which blocks flexion. Second, placement of a femoral component that provides substantially more metal at the anterior and anterodistal chamfer area than bone which was removed does the same thing—it increases the requisite excursion of the extensor mechanism, often leading to an identical tenodesis effect. Third, the flexion space or flexion gap may be too tight owing to either a femoral component that was positioned too posteriorly or an inadequate tibial resection, possibly in combination with a distal femoral resection, that was adequate or more than adequate. Here the extension space is greater than the flexion space. If the extension space is more "normal" and the flexion space is tight, flexion is decreased.

In addition, flexion space may be too tight if the tibia slopes downward anteriorly and up posteriorly and if the distal femoral cut is placed too far proximally, with the posterior cruciate ligament attached at the femur too close to the joint line. In the first situation, if femoral rollback is attempted, the tightness of the higher tibial surface posteriorly blocks flexion (Fig. 34–5). In the second situation, the posterior cruciate ligament tightens with flexion. It draws the tibia forward, and the point may be reached where either the tibia dislocates anteriorly or further flexion is blocked (see Fig. 30–19).

Flexion contracture that is seen immediately after surgery and fails to resolve during early rehabilitation is usually due to an extension space that is too tight. When contracture is noted during the primary knee replacement procedure, the femoral component should be moved more proximally by additional bone resection to achieve correction. When one is performing a revision and the modular tibial component is thick, the temptation is to replace it with a thinner tibial insert. This maneuver may improve extension, but it may create instability in flexion. The best correction is achieved by femoral component revision, placing the femoral component more proximally. If limited motion is caused by components that are tight in both flexion and extension, the tibial component can be moved distally by placing a thinner tibial tray or by revising of the entire tibial component.

PROSTHESIS SELECTION

When selecting revision prosthetic components, choices include everything from a minimally constrained, three ligament type of total knee prosthesis to a fixed hinge prosthesis or a rotating hinge prosthesis. In between are the more constrained roller-in-trough, two ligament prostheses, "revision" components with specific femoral buildup, and prostheses with tibial intercondylar pegs that provide posterior and translational stability and sometimes varus-valgus stability.

A basic point of component selection and

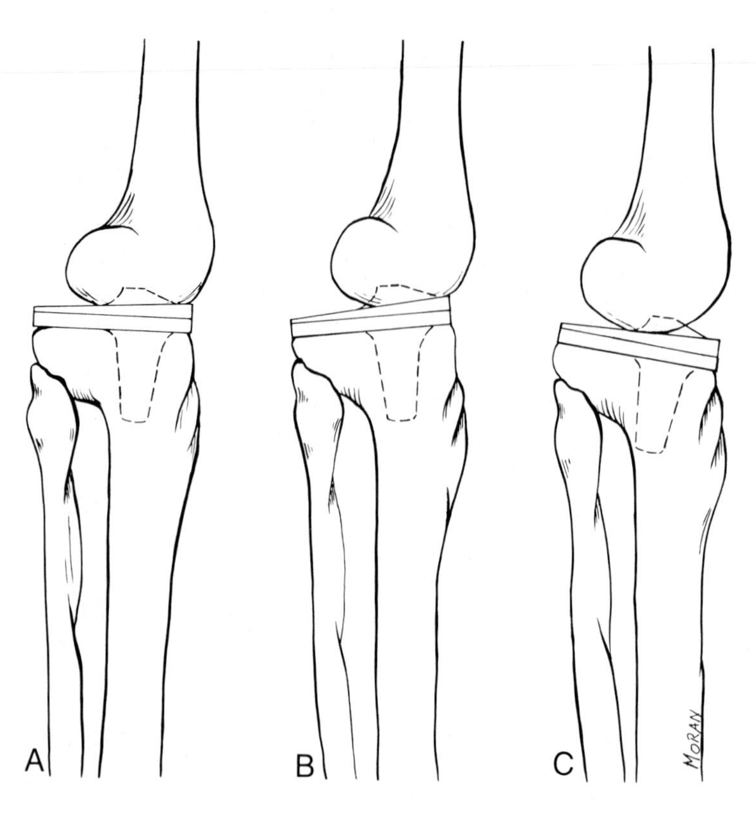

FIGURE 34–5. Influence of tibial component slope on knee motion. *A* and *B,* Tibial component perpendicular to the long axis of the tibia or sloping downward from anterior to posterior, with a flexion gap sufficient to allow knee flexion. *C,* Impingement of the femoral condyles against the tibial component when the tibial component slopes downward anteriorly and up posteriorly, as the knee is flexed. Tibial component slopes upward posteriorly, resulting in a block to flexion.

resulting prosthetic stability needs to be appreciated, even in the absence of major bone loss, deformity, or apparent ligamentous imbalance. In the first decade of total knee replacement surgery, the specific implications of femoral bone loss versus tibial loss were largely disregarded in revision cases. General bone loss was addressed only on the tibial side, utilizing femoral components of conventional dimensions in combination with thicker and thicker tibial pieces. This practice tends to move the prosthetic joint line closer to the femoral epicondyles, which are the collateral ligament origins. It results in a number of instability patterns. Newer prostheses (Fig. 34–6) address femoral bone loss on the femoral side with specifically designed femoral revision components that have thicker surfaces that employ the dimensionality of the tibial component to address only tibial bone loss. Specific revision femoral components, providing for bone loss directly on the femoral side, preserve the flexion-extension ligament length patterns. In most cases, satisfactory overall stability can be achieved without resorting to increased levels of prosthetic constraint, such as intercondylar pegs or hinges. This concept has been extended to some posterior stabilized systems and other systems, in the form of both fixed femoral buildup and attachable "modular" femoral buildup elements.

When components are selected, the problem of excessive bone loss must be considered. The options for managing bone loss include autogenous or allogeneic bone graft (solid or cancellous), addition of modular spacers available with some prosthetic systems, custom buildup, and specially designed prostheses for large bone deficiencies or custom prostheses.[28, 41]

Bone Grafting

The advantage of bone graft for filling deficiencies is that if the graft heals well, bone stock is improved. This may provide better force distribution to the bone. Also, if later surgery is required, the extra bone stock may make it easier. The principles used for treating bone defects about the

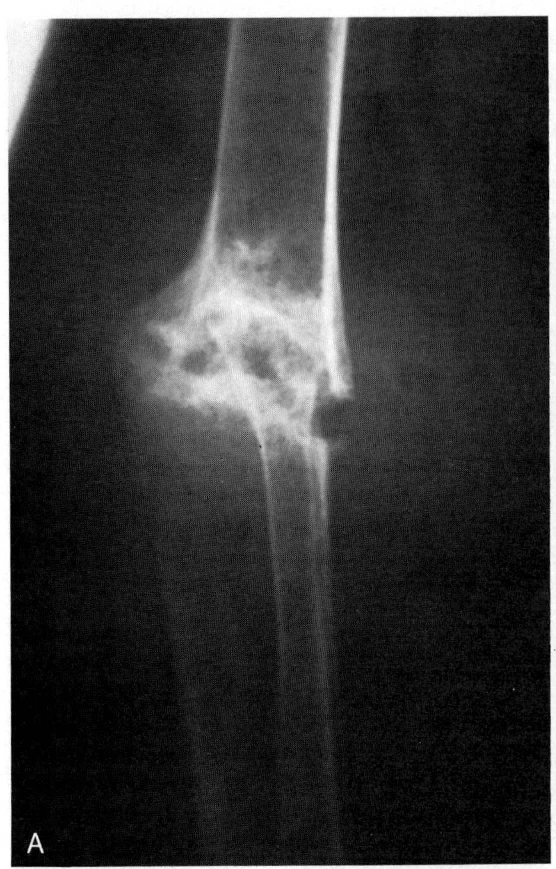

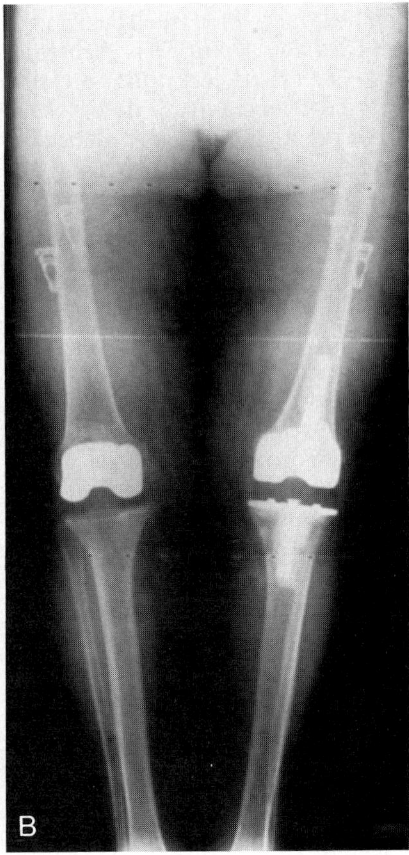

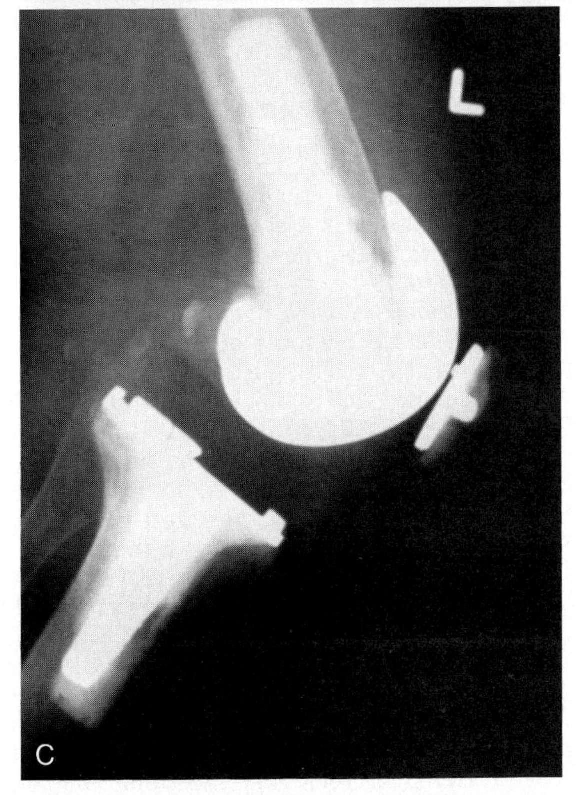

FIGURE 34–6. Prosthetic components specifically designed for revision arthroplasty. The femoral component has distal as well as posterior buildup to substitute for bone loss. *A,* Preoperative radiograph. *B,* Standing, postoperative radiograph. Patient's left knee has the revision component. Note the longer stem on the tibial side, with a relatively larger polyethylene space. *C,* Lateral view. Thicker anterior, posterior, and distal aspects to the femoral component compensate for bone loss and maintain the joint line at the appropriate level.

hip may be adapted for the knee (see Chapter 23, *Revision Total Hip Arthroplasty*) (Fig. 34–7). Any defect that is contained within the cortex (cavitary defect) and still allows for prosthesis support against existing bone can be repaired with particulate bone, either autograft or allograft.[39] If a defect involves major areas of the cortex or if a graft is expected to provide initial stability to the prosthesis, the strength required can be supplied only by structural graft that includes cortex. Tricortical iliac crest graft may be sufficient for some defects; allograft may be necessary for others. The best source for structural allograft is the distal femur or proximal tibia, although other sources including the femoral head have been employed successfully. Although structural grafts may be fixed with screws, in many instances plate fixation is better.

Modular Spacers

Some modular total knee systems provide modular buildup spacers that permit filling of both distal femoral and proximal tibial defects. Some have wedges for filling in wedge-shaped defects of either the medial or lateral tibial plateau.[5] Advantages include intraoperative flexibility and ease of use. Disadvantages include the limitation to certain type and size defects and the theoretic concern about metal-metal corrosion *in vivo*.

Cement Buildup

Bone cement can fill cavitary defects of various sizes. The advantages are ease of use, excellent distribution of forces to the remaining bone, and long-term experience. Disadvantages include the presence of a large volume of implant material when defects are large, no rebuilding of bone stock, and the potential for further bone stock loss if loosening recurs.

Prostheses Designed for Major Bone Defects

Long stem prostheses of the fixed and modular types and custom-designed prostheses for individual patients may be chosen for revision total knee arthroplasty when bone deficiencies are severe. In some circumstances, they may be combined with major structural allograft that provides for improved soft tissue repair (see Chapter 43, *Joint Reconstruction After Tumor Resection*).

SURGICAL TECHNIQUE

Although surgical technique is influenced by the selection of the prosthesis and the nature of the bone defect, certain aspects of exposure, component removal, and alignment are common to all procedures.

Exposure

In virtually all cases, the surgeon must utilize the incision placed for the primary procedure. Although it may be extended proximally, distally, or both, taking an alternative path would create a dangerous skin bridge. After identification of the capsular level and the surface of the quadriceps musculature and tendon, in the more proximal aspect of the wound, arthrotomy and component exposure are undertaken.

The difficulty of achieving adequate exposure is best predicted by the patient's existing range of motion. Other factors include any thickening of the capsule and subcapsular synovial tissues and whether the patient is obese. Stiff knees that do not flex to 90 degrees are especially difficult to expose.

Before embarking on total knee revision, the surgeon should be thoroughly familiar with the techniques of tibial tubercle osteotomy and quadriceps turndown (Figs. 34–8 and 34–9) (see also Figs. 28–4 and 30–20). In addition to the need for meticulous attention to detail, four points should be considered as the surgeon plans and performs the procedure. First, is there base tibial bone remaining for reattachment of the osteotomized tibial tubercle? Tibial tubercle osteotomy is riskier if the tibia in this area is just a cortical shell. Second, the tibial tubercle osteotomy provides better exposure and greater ease of anterior displacement of the tibia. It is especially useful for removing the tibial component

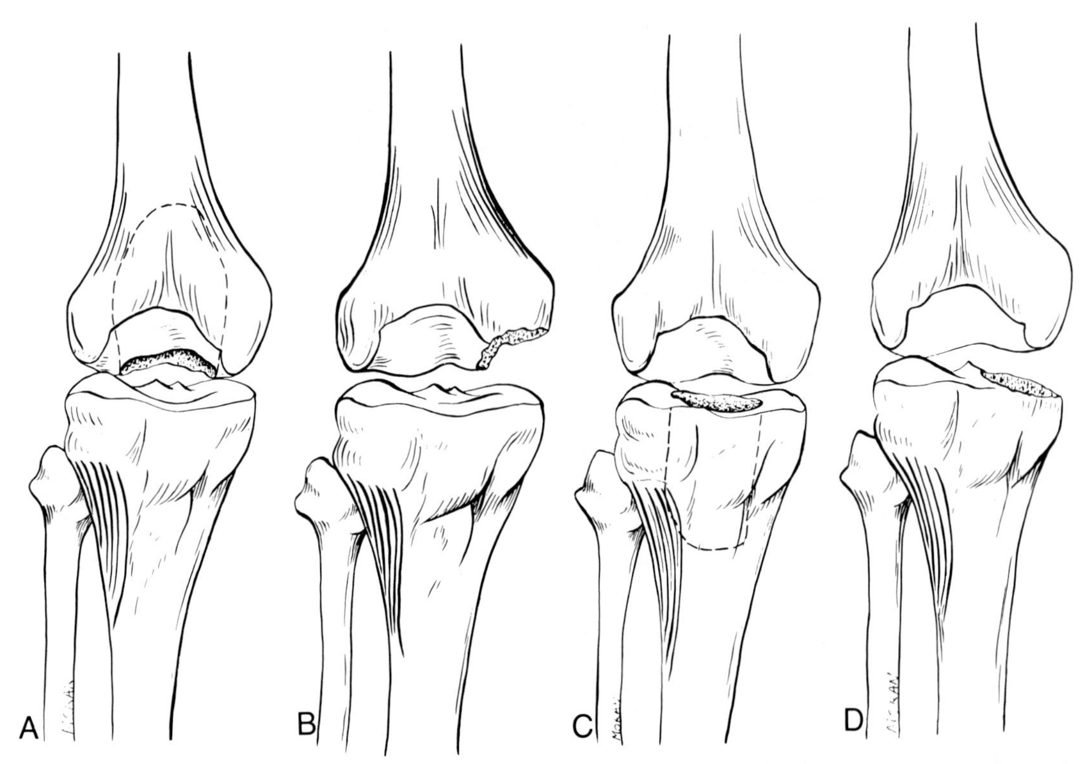

FIGURE 34–7. Examples of bone deficiency that may be encountered in revision total knee arthroplasty. *A,* A cavitary deficiency in the femur that may result from removal of a cemented femoral component with a stem. *B,* Segmental bone loss of the medial femoral condyle. *C,* Cavitary bone deficiency in the proximal tibia. *D,* Segmental deficiency of the medial tibial plateau.

Cavitary deficiencies in either the femur or tibia may be filled with autogenous or allogeneic bone graft, cement, or prosthesis. Bone grafting has the advantage of rebuilding bone stock. Segmental defects (*B* and *D*) may be filled with structural autogenous or allogeneic bone graft, custom prosthesis, or modular prosthetic spacers.

without first removing the femoral prosthesis. Third, the patellar tendon attachment must not be avulsed because secure reattachment may not be possible. Fourth, if quadriceps turndown must be performed to improve exposure (e.g., in particularly stiff knees), a significant lateral patellar release will probably be required, leaving an isolated peninsula of patella and patellar tendon together with inferior lateral capsular tissue.

In most cases, total or near total synovectomy is necessary, not to eliminate "inflammatory" tissue but to develop a capsule that is sufficiently thin and pliable to permit adequate patellar eversion and knee flexion. Synovectomy includes tissue all around the margin of the tibial, femoral, and patellar components. The surgeon must not only assess the margins to free the interfaces but must inspect them for loosening in questionable cases, to effect the bone cuts, to clear nearby fibrous tissue, and to position retractors safely.

In performing adequate exposure and debridement during revision knee arthroplasty, the surgeon must be even more cautious than in primary cases about damaging the main posterior vasculature, the geniculate vessels close to their origins, and the peroneal nerve.

Component Removal

When revision is performed for gross component loosening, removal of the "loose components" is seldom a major problem. Rigid components are another matter. Particular problems are posed by (1) metal-backed tibial trays, (2) securely fixed stems, (3) long femoral stems or stems below metal-backed tibial components, (4) stems that are porous coated and ingrown

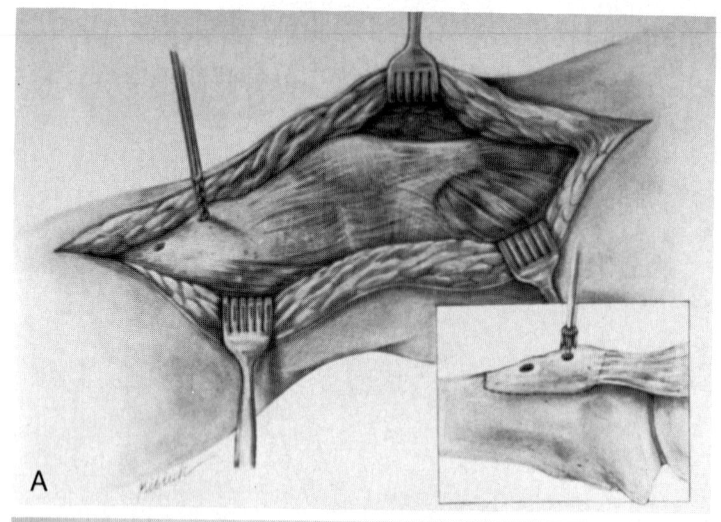

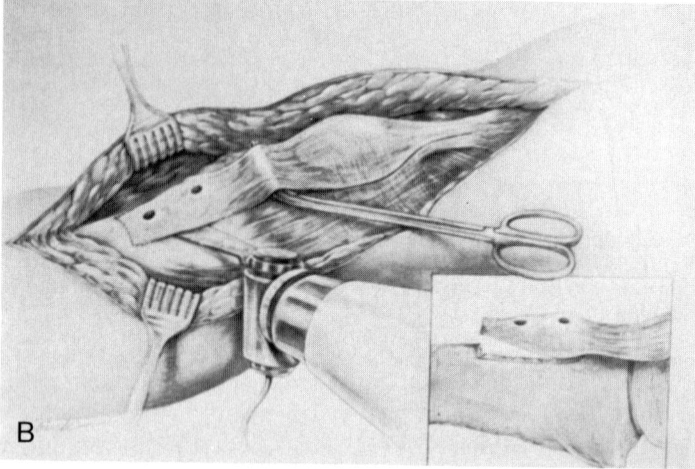

FIGURE 34–8. Tibial tubercle osteotomy for improved exposure. *A*, Predrilled fixation holes prepared with countersink instrument. *B*, Osteotomy performed with saw, including proximal contouring when possible, so that proximal migration could occur only with anterior displacement.

or cemented or that have a surface configuration that precludes simple pullout extraction from cement, and (5) undercut pegs or porous pegs that are fixed well with cement or ingrown with bone.

The surgeon must have an accurate and intimate knowledge of the topography of the interface of the piece. It is especially helpful to have a sample prosthesis available in the operating room. The surgeon can have it held up to see where the removal "hangups" will originate.

Femoral Component

Before removing the femoral component, the surgeon must assess the accuracy of its rotational position. The new component may be placed largely or partly in relation to the propriety of the current orientation. Correct position is important for achieving the proper axis of flexion, particularly as it relates to patellar tracking and ligamentous stability.

The interface of a well-fixed femoral component may be broken with osteotomes, high speed burrs, and saws (Fig. 34–10). We prefer to free the interface of most components by some form of sawing maneuver. For a well-fixed component, and especially one that is well cemented, a useful technique involves dividing the interface with a Gigli saw (Fig. 34–11). If the surgeon uses care, virtually the entire interface, except for that involving the pegs and stem, can be approached in most modern knee prostheses having no large intercondylar housing (i.e., the femoral cutout that envelopes an upward protruding tibial polyethylene peg). The interface can also be well freed over some areas by utilizing an oscillating saw and some form of totally toothed reciprocating saw. Approaching the interface with an osteotome,

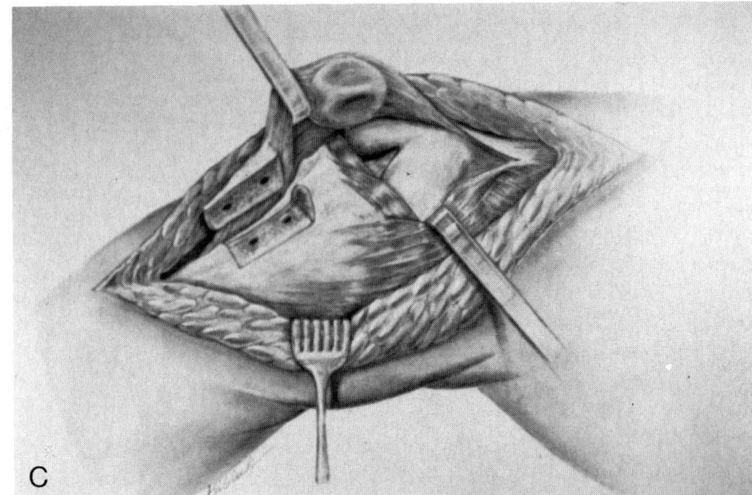

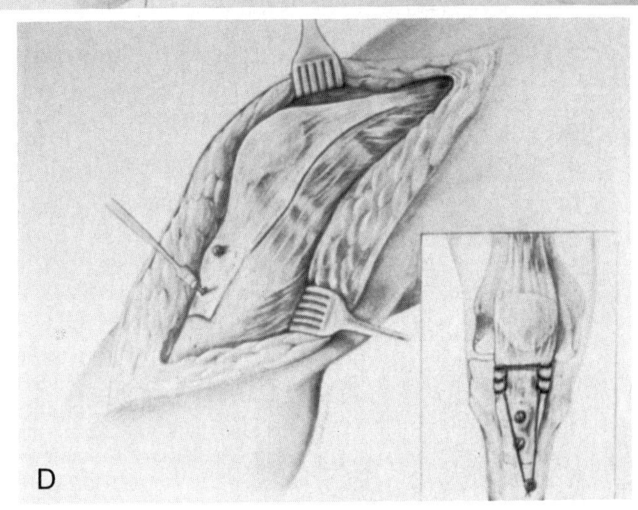

FIGURE 34–8 *Continued C,* General exposure after removal of tibial tubercle. *D,* Tubercle fixed with screws after replacement. *Inset,* After screw fixation, reinforcing ligament suture was placed in the edges of the patellar tendon. These sutures can be tied to a screw, staple, or any other distally secure structure. (Krackow, K. A.: Technique of Total Knee Arthroplasty. C. V. Mosby Co., 1990. By permission.)

especially in cemented cases, has two disadvantages: the osteotome blade becomes quickly dulled, damaged, and essentially ruined, and the blade usually deflects "deep" to the cement, resulting in greater bone loss by compression of what is typically osteoporic cancellous structure.

Tibial Component

All-polyethylene tibial components pose relatively few removal problems. If necessary, the base can be amputated from a securely fixed stem, which then can be removed in a second stage. Securely fixed metal-backed tibial components of any type (precluding simple cephalad pullup) may be another matter, often requiring high-speed metal cutting instruments. They can be employed to separate the base plate from its stem.

If a securely fixed stem simply will not yield and the base plate cannot be separated, "deep" tibial tubercle osteotomy to the level of the stem may be considered (Fig. 34–12). The technique involves removing the bone anterior to the stem, providing access to the medial and lateral aspects. Usually some degree of access to the posterior interface of a rectangular or rounded stem may be obtained from above via the tibial tray cutout for the posterior cruciate ligament. If access is impossible or if ingrowth or cement fixation texture precludes pulling the tibial component forward upon removal of the anterior bone plug and freeup described so far, component metal cutting may be imperative.

Patellar Component

A solidly fixed patellar component, especially one that is solidly porous ingrown,

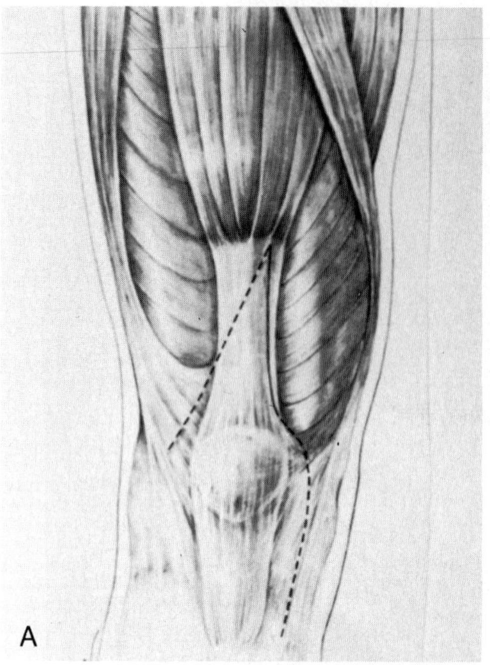

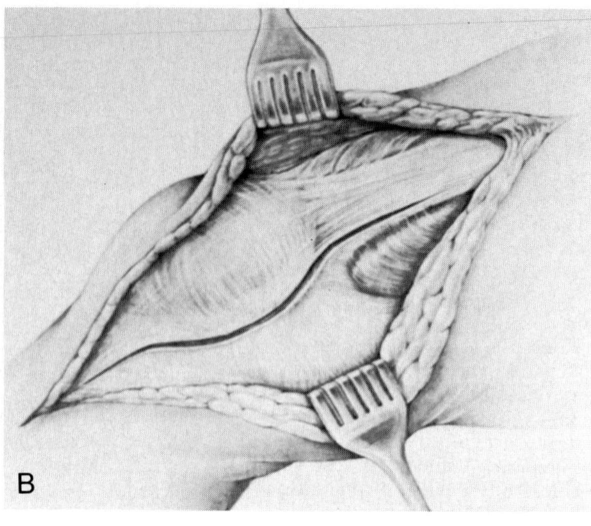

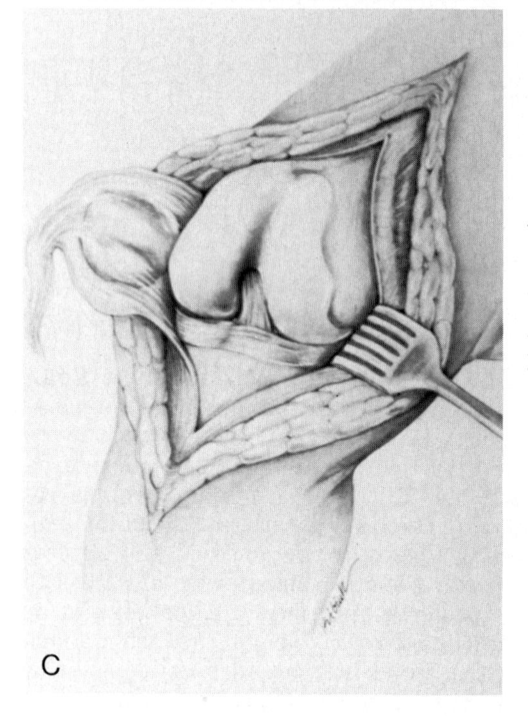

FIGURE 34–9. Lateral quadriceps turndown technique. *A*, Diagrammatic relationship between main medial capsulotomy and proximal lateral oblique incision. *B*, Anteromedial capsulotomy shown with minimal dissection necessary to achieve proximal lateral incision. *C*, Exposure after proximal lateral turndown. (Krackow, K. A.: Technique of Total Knee Arthroplasty. C. V. Mosby Co., 1990. By permission.)

can be difficult to remove. Our discussion of the patella appears after that of removal of the femoral and tibial pieces because we feel it should be removed last. If the exposure is very difficult and the patella is vigorously manipulated each time the joint is flexed and extended, prior removal may weaken the patellar bone, possibly leading to fracture. A saw may be appropriate when the fixation is rigid, especially at the patella-prosthesis interface. An osteotome small enough to work around or between pegs may have a wedging effect, leading directly to fracture.

Deformity Management

Management of varus, valgus, flexion contracture or even recurvatum deformity

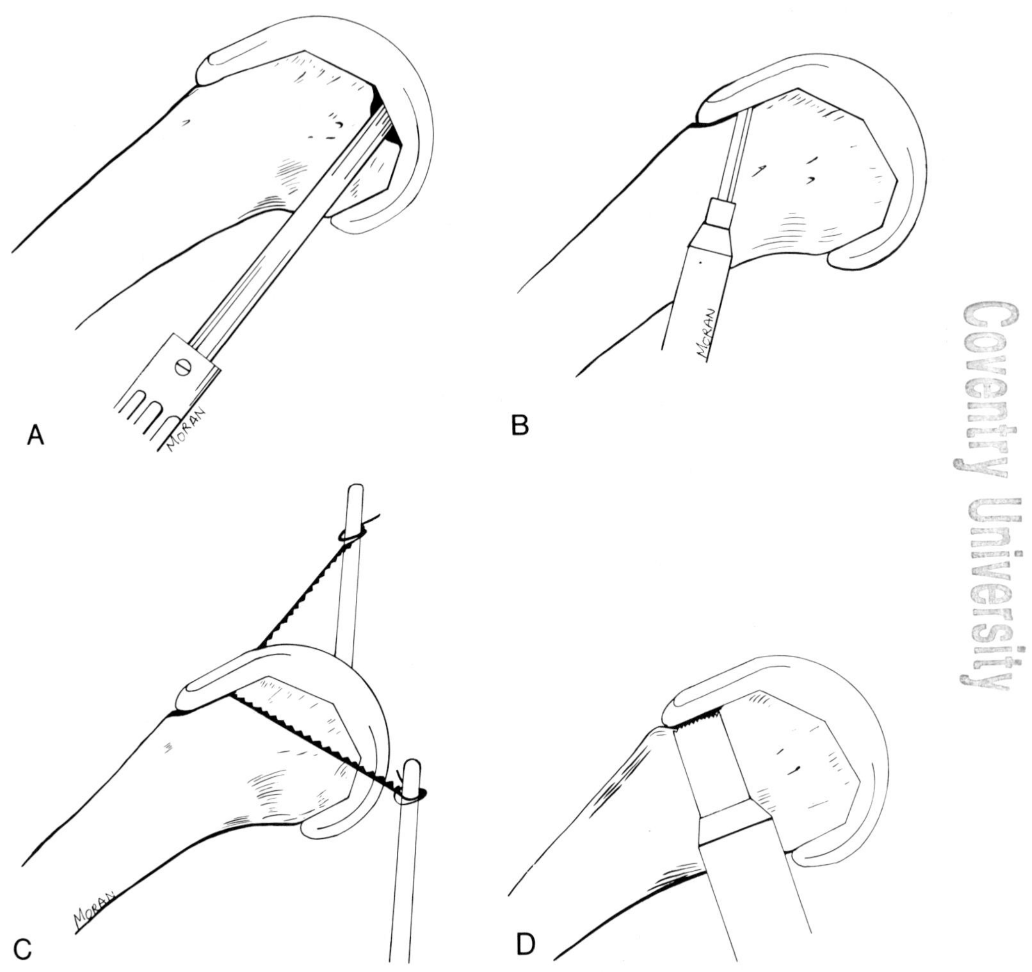

FIGURE 34–10. Methods for freeing well-fixed femoral component. *A,* Osteotome. Great care must be taken to avoid removal of valuable bone stock when using an osteotome. *B,* A high-speed burr, if small, will remove a minimal amount of bone, but care must be taken to avoid loss of valuable bone stock. In addition, the use of high-speed burrs often results in the generation of a large amount of metallic debris. *C* and *D,* A Gigli or other type saw may be utilized to cut the interface between prosthesis and bone.

is particularly important in revision total knee replacement, especially if any of these conditions is related to the cause of initial failure. The principles are identical to those enumerated for primary total knee replacements. They involve surgical release or stripping of the capsular ligamentous sleeve on the tight concave side of the contracture in varus and valgus cases, typically the tibia in varus knees and the femoral aspect in valgus knees. The overall management may be made more difficult by the general thickening of tissues and their subsequent lack of pliability and distensibility.

Major flexion contraction deformity is relatively uncommon in cases of revision for a number of reasons. Management usually consists simply of careful attention to the relative size of the flexion extension gaps and, when necessary, moving of the femoral component a bit more proximal. Because of typical distal femoral bone loss, though, such additional proximal movement is rarely necessary.

Recurvatum occasionally results from component instability and bone loss rather than from posterior capsular attenuation. For this reason, simply re-establishing prosthetic integrity and fixation and filling the gap between femur and tibia usually solves the back knee problem.

When deformity is more severe and adequate ligament balance appears impossi-

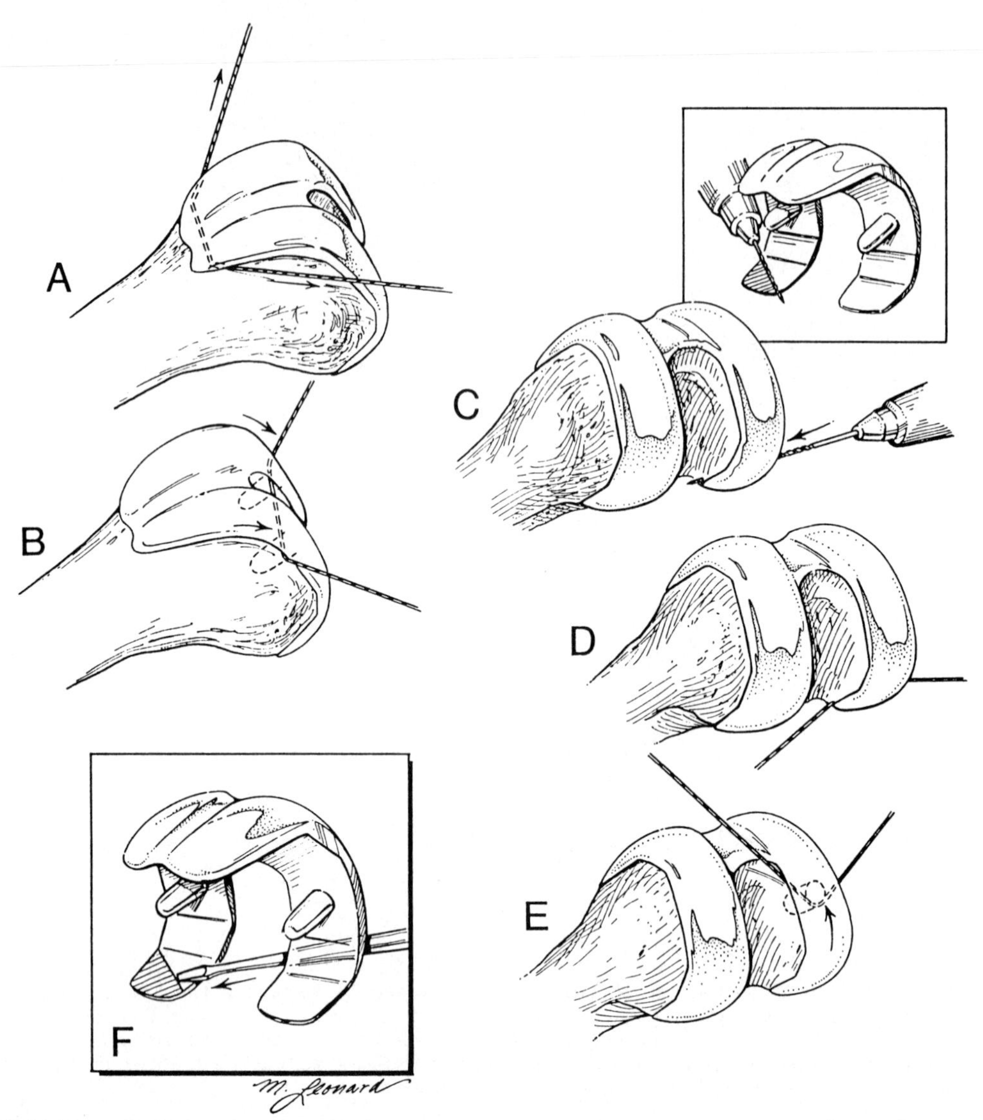

FIGURE 34–11. Technique for efficient and conservative removal of solidly fixed femoral component at revision total knee arthroplasty. Technique is applicable to bone ingrowth as well as cemented components. The Gigli saw cuts through cement. *A,* Gigli saw placed under the anterior flange. The saw is advanced to divide the interface at the anterior flange progressing to the anterior chamfer and distal surface as in *B*. *C,* A drill point is placed from the peripheral aspect at the posterior cut surface, directed along that cut surface in a proximal cephalad direction to exit at the posterior mesial corner. (Also see inset.) *D,* Gigli saw placed through the hole as shown in *C*. *E,* Gigli saw brought up in a back-and-forth and anterior direction to divide the interfaces at the proximal half of the posterior cut for that condyle, the entire posterior chamfer, and the posterior half of the distal cut for that condyle. An analogous process as that in *C, D,* and *E* is repeated for the opposite condyle. *F,* Division of the remaining posterior peripheral interface with an osteotome, working from the intercondylar area outward toward the posterior periphery of the posterior condylar interfaces.

ble, a more constrained prosthesis must be selected or intraoperative ligament tightening procedures must be performed. Attempts at ligamentous reconstruction to improve stability in unstable total knee arthroplasty have not been very effective.[24] Nonetheless, in rare and selected cases, surgeons who are knowledgeable about techniques for ligamentous reconstruction in the midst of total knee revision can find them helpful. An example is when the next degree of constraint in prosthetic design is not readily available intraoperatively or when the ligament balance instability dictates a fixed or rotating hinge in a patient too young or too active for that approach.

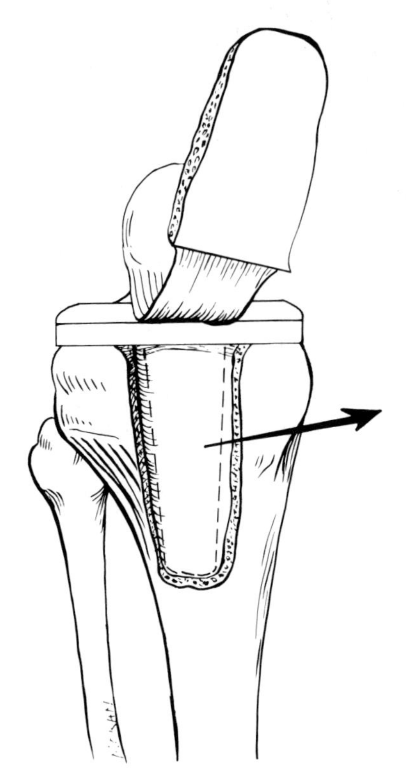

FIGURE 34–12. Removal of a well-fixed tibial stem. When impossible by other means, the stem may be removed by performing a deep tibial tubercle osteotomy to the level of the stem.

Bone Cuts and Preparation

After exposure is achieved, the surgeon may be tempted to remove prosthetic components and proceed immediately with debridement of the resulting bony surfaces. Although it seems too obvious to mention, such debridement and preparation are more wisely performed after the desired bone cuts have been made so that less bone surface will have to be prepared. Bone is less difficult to cut and prepare after all of the intruded cement has been removed. Temporarily, the fibrous tissue can remain.

The general goal of alignment and prosthetic placement is to establish an anatomically positioned joint line with components that are properly positioned with regard to the various directions of displacement and malrotation. The best way to achieve this depends upon the prosthesis and instrumentation system. After the prior rotational attitude of the femoral component has been noted and judged for accuracy, one has an approximate reference. The interepicondylar axis can also be employed to the degree that it is evident. Its relationship to the normal anatomic posterior condylar axis is one of external rotation. The epicondylar axis may also be used as a basic reference with respect to the level of the joint line. It is important to be aware of when the joint line is moving too far proximal or cephalad.

The surgeon can usually make use of the intramedullary axis of the femur to assist with varus-valgus and flexion-extension orientation of the femoral component.

On the tibial side, the desired joint line position may be deduced by determination of the true tibial tubercle position, by gauging the level of some aspect of the fibula, or by both methods. Generally, intraoperative radiographs are not required.

The tibia has three rotational references: the general rotational position assumed by the tibia when traction is placed across the excised joint space, the position of the tibial tubercle, and the orientation of the ankle malleoli and the foot. This last reference assumes that the knee is held in extension and that the foot is examined in a weight-bearing position, with the sole held at a right angle to the leg by pressure against the palm of the surgeon or assistant's hand.

After the primary bone cuts are planned and executed, the surgeon may face the problem of managing substantial tibial or femoral bone loss, or both. The options include autograft/allograft, cement, standard and stock prosthesis buildup features, prosthesis modular features, and custom components with varying prosthetic build-up, together with some substantial intramedullary stem support. In my opinion, the adequacy and accuracy of fit of augmented intramedullary stem supports are probably the most important considerations. Without them, it is hard to imagine any of the aforementioned materials holding up well.

Even without major bone loss, in most cases prosthetic dimensions have to be adjusted relative to the commonly used ones for primary total knee replacements. Selecting thicker tibial components generally poses no problems. However, the surgeon does not always have femoral components available that address analogous problems of bone loss on the femoral side. In many revision total knee arthroplasties, femoral components are utilized that make no special provision for the typical uniform bone loss encountered here. Employing components that do substitute for bone loss (see Fig. 34–6) allows the orthopaedic surgeon to reposition the femoral joint line in a more anatomic location and preserve proper flexion-extension ligament balance. With such systems, trial components are generally provided that have a useful degree of stability against the respective bones, and meaningful trial reductions can be obtained.

The rest of the revision procedure resembles that of primary arthroplasty. The tourniquet must almost always be deflated even if the surgeon does not do this routinely at primary total knee arthroplasty. The reason is simply time; it is unlikely that an entire revision can be performed in less than 2 hours.

Final placement of components follows hemostasis, whether the prosthesis is cemented or noncemented. In our routine, the bone surface is meticulously prepared and cement in a relatively low viscosity state is used. Cement restrictors of bone or cement or polymers similar to those for total hip arthroplasty should be utilized to improve cementation and to avoid extension of the cement in the intramedullary canal (see Chapter 17, *Total Hip Arthroplasty: Operative Technique*).

In revision cases, the surgeon must be particularly careful to check patellar tracking and passive range of motion, because dimensions and joint line positions can change significantly despite one's best efforts, impacting on both these aspects of knee performance. Patellar stability needs to be assessed. In some cases, one may be surprised at the initial tightness of the quadriceps mechanism creating an extensor tenodesis and limited range of flexion. We do not perform V-Y lengthening of the quadriceps mechanism for fear that it will create an extension lag. Also, the gradual improvement in range of motion seen in these patients can be substantial.

The wound is closed and drained with closed suction systems. Prophylactic antibiotic administration and deep venous thrombosis prophylaxis are similar to those recommended for primary total knee arthroplasty (see Chapter 8, *Prevention of Postoperative Infections*, and Chapter 9, *Thromboembolic Disease*). In my practice, perioperative parenteral antibiotics are continued for at least 5 to 7 days, until intraoperative cultures are reported. Although a positive culture result does not necessarily indicate clinical infection, it may influence the surgeon to continue antibiotic treatment for 10 to 14 days.

POSTOPERATIVE CARE

Postoperative management of the total knee revision patient varies with the complexity of the individual case. Surgeons must ask themselves questions that do not necessarily apply to routine cemented primary total knee replacements. Does the extensor mechanism need protection because of a tibial tubercle osteotomy or a quadriceps turndown? Are there porous-coated uncemented components that should be protected from unrestricted weightbearing for a longer period of time? Should large bone grafts be protected from weightbearing? Are there any ligament reattachments that should be protected in case of untoward varus-valgus moments or extremes of range of motion and possibly weightbearing?

When modifying conditions are present, the surgeon must make certain that provisions are made for weightbearing, range of motion, and protection of muscles and ligaments. We allow at least 6 weeks for tendon repair, ligament reattachment, or both. We recommend 6 weeks of nonweightbearing or partial weightbearing to protect uncemented prostheses, especially at the tibia, followed by 6 weeks of progressive weightbearing to a status of full weightbearing. The intervals needed to protect sizable grafts for bone defects depend on how much the bone graft is expected to contribute to initial prosthesis stability.

With tibial tubercle osteotomy or quadriceps turndown, 6 weeks of protection against forceful passive flexion and active extension is advisable. Any form of collateral ligament reattachment should be protected for at least 6 weeks in a knee brace without restriction of range of motion.

RESULTS OF REVISION TOTAL KNEE ARTHROPLASTY

The results of early revisions of total knee arthroplasty were comparable to those of revisions of total hip arthroplasty. In a 1982 report of 2- to 11-year follow-up data for 78 knee revision arthroplasties, Cameron and Hunter[7] stated that results were good or excellent in 37 percent and fair or poor in 60 percent; 3 percent had failed. Successes were dependent on prosthesis type; in 48 percent of semiconstrained prostheses, results were good or excellent; the same was true for 24 percent of unlinked hinges and 21 percent of linked hinges. That same year, Thornhill and associates[35] reported 2- to 5-year follow-up evaluations of 65 revisions for failed noninfected total knee arthroplasty: 53 knees (82 percent) were improved, with an average knee score of 80 points; eight knees (12 percent) required further surgery. Insall and Dethmers[14] reported the results of 72 revisions followed for 2 to 7 years involving the following prostheses: total condylar, total condylar III, posterior stabilized, and custom. The preoperative knee scores (HSS) improved from 49 to 83 points, with 89 percent rated good or excellent. Although these results were almost as good as those reported by the same investigators for primary knee replacement, extensor mechanism problems were more frequent and pain relief was not as good.

In a report of 20 knees with severe bone loss revised with uncemented long-stem prostheses and particulate bone graft, Whiteside[39] reported that all patients achieved full weightbearing by 6 months and all but two walked without aids by 1 year. Three patients continued to have pain, two mild and one severe. This last patient also had severe pain before revision of prostheses that were not loose.

Goldberg and colleagues,[11] reporting 2- to 10-year follow-up of 59 revision knee arthroplasties, found that 46 percent of knees were rated good or excellent and 42 percent were rated fair or poor. The infection rate was 4.5 percent. The lowest failure rate was with the total condylar III prosthesis and the highest with the total condylar and kinematic rotating hinge.

Jacobs and coworkers,[15] following 24 patients with 28 porous coated anatomic (PCA) primary or revision prostheses, found that 68 percent had good or excellent results 2 to 4 years after revision. Of those with definable mechanical problems before revision, 83 percent achieved good or excellent results. Patients who had revisions for unexplained pain did not improve.

In a follow-up study of 52 revision arthroplasties done with the Stannmore hinged prosthesis, Karpinski and Grimer[16] reported good results in 23 percent, fair results in 48 percent, and poor results in 29 percent; mean follow-up was 45 months. The infection incidence was 4 percent.

Rand and Bryan[25] reported ratings of good or excellent in 76 percent of knee revisions with condylar prostheses (n = 50) after an average follow-up interval of 4.8 years. Few complications were found: one postoperative hematoma, one loose piece of cement that had to be removed, and three loose prostheses.

In a comparison of the results of the kinematic stabilizer prosthesis in 26 primary and 53 revision arthroplasties after a mean of 3 years, Hanssen and Rand[12a] reported good or excellent results in 92 percent of the primary and 81 percent of the revision arthroplasties.

Bertin and associates[4] evaluated the results of stemmed, cementless prostheses in 49 knee revisions after 6 to 48 months postoperatively. Four failed owing to early complications—one infection and three lateral patellar dislocations. In the remaining 45 patients, 91 percent had successful pain relief, 84 percent had at least 90 degrees of motion, and 80 percent could walk for over 30 minutes at a time.

Fortunately, the number of revision procedures required in patients with total knee arthroplasty has not been as great as originally anticipated. Overall results suggest that the quality of revision total knee replacements is almost as good as that of primary total knee arthroplasty, although there appear to be fewer "excellent" results and less improvement of motion. Also, pain relief may not be quite as good. A successful outcome would be one with none to mild instability, none to mild pain, and flexion to 90 degrees. Although overall the failure rate of revision total knee arthroplasty appears to be only slightly higher than that of primary knee replacement, rerevision is another matter. In re-revision arthroplasty cases, the infection rate is higher and one often sees such additional problems as extensor mechanism complications, troublesome radiolucent lines, and overall instability.

In a review of the results according to

mechanisms of failure, Rand and Bryan[25] reported that revision for failure by fixation was associated with 75 percent good to excellent results. Ligamentous laxity, component malposition, and patellar alignment problems were revised with 90 percent good to excellent results. Few good to excellent results were reported in patients whose revision procedures were done for pain; we have obtained the same results.[15]

CONCLUSION

Revision total knee arthroplasty is a challenging procedure that requires careful patient selection and meticulous planning. Fortunately, the percentage of satisfactory results is high. However, good outcomes are not uniform, stressing the importance of patient selection, planning, and attention to detail at the time of initial arthroplasty.

References

1. Bayley, J. C. and Scott, R. D.: Further observations on metal-backed patellar component failure. Clin. Orthop. 236:82–87, 1988.
2. Bayley, J. C., Scott, R. D., Ewald, F. C., et al.: Failure of the metal-backed patellar component after total knee replacement. J. Bone Joint Surg. [Am.] 70(5):668–674, 1988.
3. Bengtson, S., Knutson, K., and Lindgren, L.: Treatment of infected knee arthroplasties. Clin. Orthop. 245:173–178, 1989.
4. Bertin, K. C., Freeman, M. A., Samuelson, K. M., et al.: Stemmed revision arthroplasty for aseptic loosening of total knee replacement. J. Bone Joint Surg. [Br.] 67(2):242–248, 1985.
5. Brand, M. G., Daley, R. J., Ewald, F. C., et al.: Tibial tray augmentation with modular metal wedges for tibial bone stock deficiency. Clin. Orthop. 248:71–79, 1989.
6. Bryan, R. S. and Rand, J. A.: Revision total knee arthroplasty. Clin. Orthop. 170:116–122, 1982.
7. Cameron, H. U. and Hunter, G. A.: Failure in total knee arthroplasty: mechanisms, revisions, and results. Clin. Orthop. 170:141–146, 1982.
8. Cheng, C. L. and Gross, A. E.: Loosening of the porous coating in total knee replacement. J. Bone Joint Surg. [Br.] 70(3):377–381, 1988.
9. Conway, W. F., Gilula, L. A., and Serot, D. I.: Breakage of the patellar component of a kinematic total knee arthroplasty. A case report. Orthopedics 9(4):532–534, 1986.
10. Edwards, E., Miller, J., and Chan, K. H.: The effect of postoperative collateral ligament laxity in total knee arthroplasty. Clin. Orthop. 236:44–51, 1988.

10a. Engh, G. A.: Failure of the polyethylene bearing surface of a total knee replacement within four years. A case report. J. Bone Joint Surg. [Am.] 70(7):1093–1096, 1988.

11. Goldberg, V. M., Figgie, M. P., Figgie, H. E. 3d, et al.: The results of revision total knee arthroplasty. Clin. Orthop. 226:86–92, 1988.
12. Graham, D. R.: Polyethylene wear: a cause of failure of the variable-axis total knee prosthesis. A report of three cases. J. Bone Joint Surg. [Am.] 70(6):942–943, 1988.

12a. Hanssen, A. D. and Rand, J. A.: A comparison of primary and revision total knee arthroplasty using the kinematic stabilizer prosthesis. J. Bone Joint Surg. 70:491–499, 1988.

13. Hvid, I. and Nielsen, S.: Total condylar knee arthroplasty. Prosthetic component positioning and radiolucent lines. Acta Orthop. Scand. 55(2):160–165, 1984.
14. Insall, J. N. and Dethmers, D. A.: Revision of total knee arthroplasty. Clin. Orthop. 170:123–130, 1982.
15. Jacobs, M. A., Hungerford, D. S., Krackow, K. A., et al.: Revision total knee arthroplasty for aseptic failure. Clin. Orthop. 226:78–85, 1988.
16. Karpinski, M. R. and Grimer, R. J.: Hinged knee replacement in revision arthroplasty. Clin. Orthop. 220:185–191, 1987.
17. Ladkin, R. S.: Total condylar knee replacement in patients who have rheumatoid arthritis. J. Bone Joint Surg. 72A:529–535, 1990.
18. Lombardi, A. V. Jr., Engh, G. A., Volz, R. G., et al.: Fracture/dissociation of the polyethylene in metal-backed patellar components in total knee arthroplasty. J. Bone Joint Surg. [Am.] 70(5):675–679, 1988.
19. Marmor, L.: Unicompartmental arthroplasty of the knee with a minimum ten-year follow-up period. Clin. Orthop. 228:171–177, 1988.
20. Milliano, M. T., Whiteside, L. A., Kaiser, A. D., et al.: Evaluation of the effect of articular surface material on a metal backed patellar component. Trans. Orthop. Res. Soc. 15:279, 1990.
21. Moreland, J. R.: Fracture of a unicompartmental knee replacement femoral component. Clin. Orthop. 206:166–168, 1986.
22. Morrey, B. F. and Chao, E. Y.: Fracture of the porous-coated metal tray of a biologically fixed knee prosthesis. Report of a case. Clin. Orthop. 228:182–189, 1988.
23. Mowery, C., Botte, M., and Bradley, G.: Fracture of polyethylene tibial component in a total knee replacement. A case report. Orthopedics 10(2):309–313, 1987.
24. Pritsch, M., Fitzgerald, R. H. Jr., and Bryan, R. S.: Surgical treatment of ligamentous instability after total knee arthroplasty. Arch. Orthop. Trauma. Surg. 102(3):154–158, 1984.
25. Rand, J. A. and Bryan, R. S.: Results of revision total knee arthroplasties using condylar prostheses. A review of fifty knees. J. Bone Joint Surg. [Am.] 70(5):738–745, 1988.
26. Rosenberg, A. G., Andriacchi, T. P., Barden, R., et al.: Patellar component failure in cementless total knee arthroplasty. Clin. Orthop. 236:106–114, 1988.
27. Rosenqvist, R., Bylander, B., Knutson, K., et al.: Loosening of the porous coating of bicompartmental prostheses in patients with rheumatoid arthritis. J. Bone Joint Surg. [Am.] 68(4):538–542, 1986.

28. Samuelson, K. M.: Bone grafting and noncemented revision arthroplasty for the knee. Clin. Orthop. 226:93–102, 1988.
29. Sandborn, P. M., Cook, S. D., Kester, M. A., et al.: Fatigue failure of the femoral component of a unicompartmental knee. Clin. Orthop. 222:249–254, 1987.
30. Scott, R. D., Ewald, F. C., and Walker, P. S.: Fracture of the metallic tibial tray following total knee replacement. Report of two cases. J. Bone Joint Surg. [Am.] 66(5):780–782, 1984.
31. Scuderi, G. R., Insall, J. N., Windsor, R. E., et al.: Survivorship of cemented knee replacements. J. Bone Joint Surg. [Br.] 71(5):798–803, 1989.
32. Skinner, H. B., Mabey, M. F., Paganelli, J. V., et al.: Failure analysis of PCA revision total knee replacement tibial component. A preliminary study using the finite element method. Orthopedics 10(4):581–584, 1987.
33. Stulberg, S. D., Stulberg, B. N., Hamati, Y., et al.: Failure mechanisms of metal-backed patellar components. Clin. Orthop. 236:88–105, 1988.
34. Sutherland, C. J.: Patellar component dissociation in total knee arthroplasty. A report of two cases. Clin. Orthop. 228:178–181, 1988.
35. Thornhill, T. S., Dalziel, R. W., and Sledge, C. B.: Alternatives to arthrodesis for the failed total knee arthroplasty. Clin. Orthop. 170:131–140, 1982.
36. Tjornstrand, B. and Lidgren, L.: Fracture of the knee endoprosthesis. Report of three cases of tibial component failure. Acta Orthop. Scand. 56(2):124–126, 1985.
37. Vince, K. G., Insall, J. N., and Kelly, M. A.: The total condylar prosthesis. Ten- to 12-year results of a cemented knee replacement. J. Bone Joint Surg. [Br.] 71(5):793–797, 1989.
38. Wasilewski, S. A. and Frankl, U.: Fracture of polyethylene of patellar component in total knee arthroplasty, diagnosed by arthroscopy. J. Arthroplasty 4:S19–S22, 1989.
39. Whiteside, L. A.: Cementless reconstruction of massive tibial bone loss in revision total knee arthroplasty. Clin. Orthop. 248:80–86, 1989.
40. Wilde, A. H., Sweeney, R. S., and Borden, L. S.: Hematogenously acquired infection of a total knee arthroplasty by *Clostridium perfringens*. Clin. Orthop. 229:228–231, 1988.
41. Windsor, R. E., Insall, J. N., and Sculco, T. P.: Bone grafting of tibial defects in primary and revision total knee arthroplasty. Clin. Orthop. 205:132–137, 1986.
42. Wright, T. M., Astion, D. J., Bansal, M., et al.: Failure of carbon fiber-reinforced polyethylene total knee-replacement components. A report of two cases. J. Bone Joint Surg. [Am.] 70(6):926–932, 1988.
43. Wright, T. M., Rimnac, C. M., Faris, P. M., et al.: Analysis of surface damage in retrieved carbon fiber-reinforced and plain polyethylene tibial components from posterior stabilized total knee replacements. J. Bone Joint Surg. [Am.] 70(9):1312–1319, 1988.

CHAPTER 35

Treatment of Infected Total Knee Arthroplasty

WILLIAM PETTY

The causes of infection after total knee arthroplasty are intraoperative contamination, failure of wound healing (see Chapter 32, *Local Complications in Total Knee Replacement*), and hematogenous seeding of bacteria. Hematogenous infection of total knee replacement is more common in patients with rheumatoid arthritis. The management of an infected total knee arthroplasty resembles that of a knee arthroplasty that has failed for other reasons, but it differs in some ways. Several surgical treatment options are available. Treatment always includes appropriate antibiotic therapy.

PATIENT EVALUATION

Evaluation begins with a thorough history of the patient's previous knee operations. If problems with wound healing have occurred at any previous operation, the surgeon should be alert to the possibility of infection. The surgeon should also ask about current or previous infections elsewhere in the body that could have affected the knee by hematogenous spread. Symptoms usually include pain and sometimes warmth, swelling, and fever. Active drainage from the knee almost always indicates infection.

Physical examination may reveal knee stiffness, painful motion, and antalgic limp. Erythrocyte sedimentation rate and C-reactive protein level elevations are usually present during infection. Although these indicators are not as helpful in patients with inflammatory arthritis, marked elevations may still suggest infections. Plain radiographs may or may not show signs of loosening of the components or bone destruction or both (Fig. 35–1A). Aspiration of the knee for culture is the most valuable test. Results can establish the diagnosis and provide valuable information for treatment. In difficult cases, special imaging studies may help (see Chapter 11, *Imaging of Total Joint Replacement*).

SURGICAL TREATMENT

Options for surgical treatment include (1) debridement with retention of the prostheses, (2) one- or two-stage debridement and revision arthroplasty, (3) resection arthroplasty, and (4) knee arthrodesis.

Debridement

Debridement may clear infections that occur within 4 to 6 weeks postoperatively. The earlier the infection is diagnosed, the more likely it is that debridement will be successful. However, if extensive synovitis has developed, the method is likely to fail.

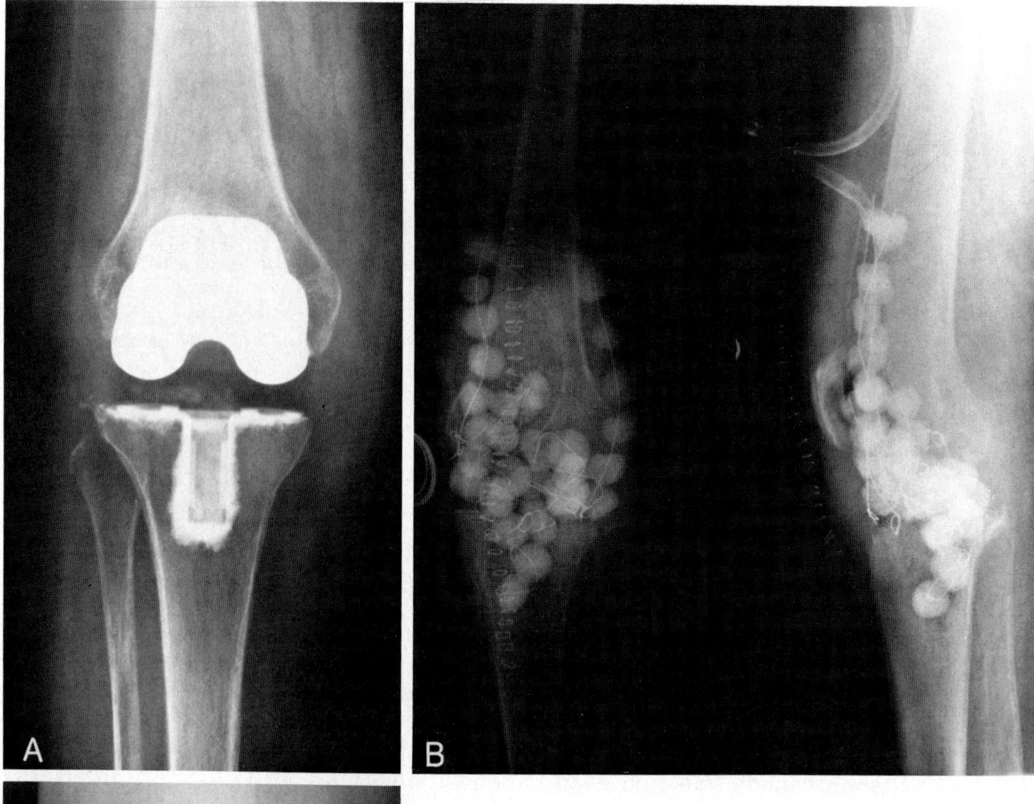

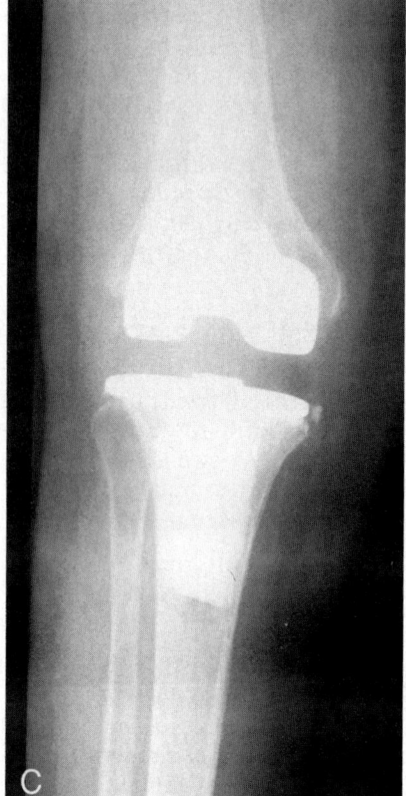

FIGURE 35–1. Two-stage revision arthroplasty. *A,* Preoperative radiograph shows excellent fixation of components with no evidence of bone destruction. However, the patient had pain, swelling, and warmth of the knee. Erythrocyte sedimentation rate was 82, and joint fluid aspiration revealed positive culture findings for *Staphylococcus aureus*. *B,* All implant material was removed and thorough debridement performed. Bone cement beads containing tobramycin were implanted. Aspiration of the joint 2 weeks later revealed negative culture findings. *C,* At 3 weeks after initial debridement, revision total knee arthroplasty was done.

A thorough synovectomy is impossible to perform, especially posteriorly, with the components in place. If a cementless total knee arthroplasty was performed, it is better to remove the prostheses before bone or fibrous ingrowth occurs and to treat the infection with one- or two-stage revision. Component removal allows for better debridement.[1, 3, 7, 15]

All purulent material, granulation tissue, and inflamed synovium are debrided. Either closed suction-irrigation or drainage systems are placed, although the closed suction-irrigation system has become less popular because of the concern of secondary bacterial contamination. However, the problem is unlikely if either closed suction-irrigation or drainage is limited to 48 to 72 hours. After debridement, wound closure is performed carefully in layers. Synthetic monofilament and braided absorbable sutures are best for wound closure because they are the most resistant to infection.[5, 17] Wire sutures or staples may also be used. In comparison, natural suture materials are less resistant to infection.

Postoperatively, motion of the patient's knee should be limited completely or to 20 to 30 degrees initially. If the wound is healing well after several days, the knee may be rehabilitated in the usual fashion.

One-Stage Revision Arthroplasty

In the patient with either early or late infection, one-stage revision arthroplasty may be performed. In the case of acute infection, the procedure is preferable to debridement without component removal because more complete debridement is possible. Success is less likely with one-stage revision when the infection is caused by highly virulent organisms (gram-negative bacilli or group D streptococci).[3, 7, 14] The operative technique requires extensive debridement of the prosthesis, all cement, and all necrotic bone and soft tissue. When debridement is complete, there must be no visible evidence that infection was ever present. If the new prosthesis is to be cemented, adding antibiotic to the cement may reduce the likelihood of persistent infection.[4, 12, 13, 19] Techniques for adding antibiotics are described in Chapter 7, *Fixation Methods*. Reimplantation of a prosthesis without cement may also reduce the risk of infection.[7] Postoperative management is similar to that for debridement only.

Two-Stage Revision Arthroplasty

Two-stage revision arthroplasty of the total knee is more likely to eradicate infection than either debridement or one-stage revision (Fig. 35–1).[1, 3, 8, 16] However, the interval between stages is less than that for the hip—normally 6 weeks or less. Longer periods result in excessive scarring of soft tissue, causing an inferior functional result.[8, 16] The first stage consists of thorough debridement of all prostheses and cement, granulation tissue, inflamed synovium, and necrotic bone or soft tissue. An excellent method to deliver antibiotic locally is placing bone cement spacer or beads that contain the antibiotic. This method also maintains soft tissue length and space for the prosthesis.[2, 6]

The preoperative planning and the surgical procedure for a second-stage revision are similar to those for a revision arthroplasty in which infection is not involved (see Chapter 34, *Revision Total Knee Arthroplasty*). Evaluation for persistent infection is especially important, including determination of erythrocyte sedimentation rate, C-reactive protein levels, and knee aspiration findings. At surgery, materials for histologic examination and culture are taken from several areas of the wound before any antibiotics are given. Tissue that arouses suspicion may be sent for frozen-section examination. Microabscesses indicate continued infection. If more than a few polymorphonuclear leukocytes are present, infection is likely.

Resection Arthroplasty

Resection arthroplasties may be indicated for patients with septic total knee arthroplasties who have difficulty walking due to multiple joint arthritis or other systemic disease. For resection arthroplasty, debridement must be thorough and include all implant material. Steinmann

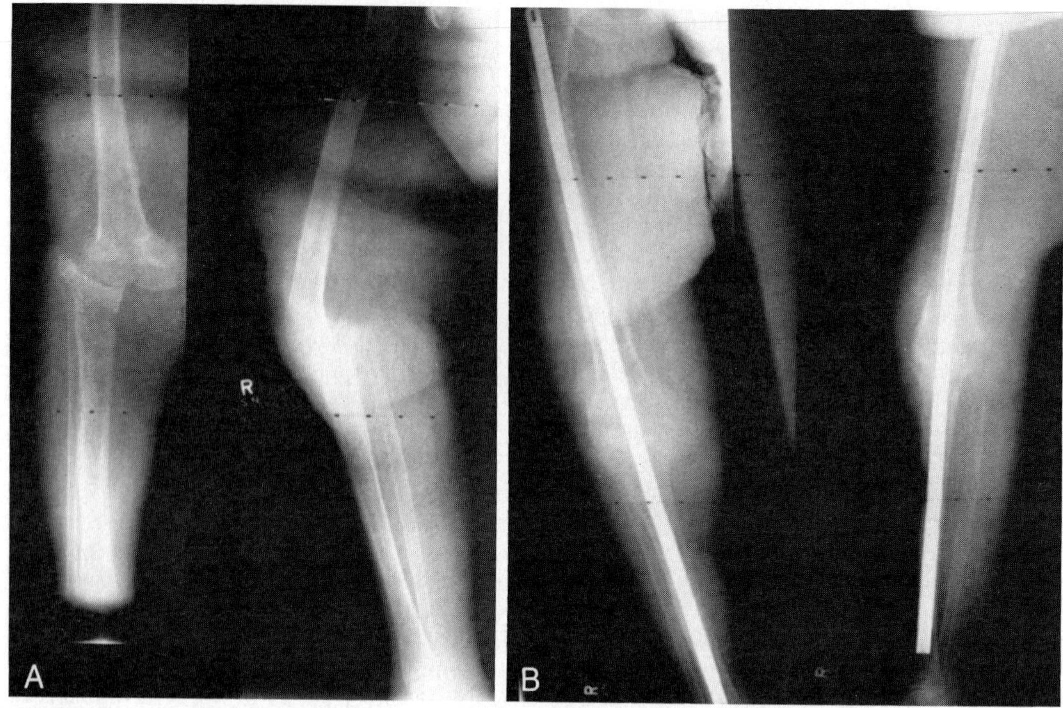

FIGURE 35–2. Unsuccessful resection arthroplasty that had been performed for treatment of an infected total knee arthroplasty was converted to knee arthrodesis. *A,* Preoperative radiograph shows substantial bone loss. The patient had marked knee instability. She also continued to have drainage of purulent material, which was treated with thorough debridement and muscle flap transfer. *B,* Three months after the wound had healed, knee arthrodesis was performed employing a long intramedullary rod and an allograft to make up for 6 cm of bone loss.

pins may be placed across the joint to hold its position temporarily. In 1 to 3 weeks after satisfactory wound healing and cast application, the pins may be removed. Postoperatively, the knee is immobilized in a long leg cast or brace for 6 to 9 months to achieve a strong fibrous ankylosis. The knee is immobilized in 7 degrees valgus and 15 degrees flexion, utilizing correct rotation to provide for the best function of the resection arthroplasty. Weightbearing is allowed as tolerated in the cast.[9, 18] Resection arthroplasty is an excellent method for eradicating sepsis. The major problem with this treatment is instability of the knee, which may require continued use of a brace. Also, the knee may cause the patient continued pain. If resection arthroplasty is unsatisfactory, it may be converted to arthrodesis (Fig. 35–2) or a second-stage revision arthroplasty may be considered.[9, 10, 18]

Arthrodesis

When arthrodesis is performed because of a total knee replacement that is a failure due to infection, the techniques are similar to those for failures due to other causes (see Chapter 36, *Knee Arthrodesis for Failed Total Knee Arthroplasty*). External fixators may be applied after initial debridement. If an intramedullary rod or plates are employed for fixation, the infection should be cleared before the definitive fusion operation is performed. This practice avoids extension of the infection proximally in the femur or distally in the tibia (see Fig. 35–2). If cortical autograft or allograft is needed to regain length, the definitive fusion should be delayed until the infection is cleared. Arthrodesis may be accomplished successfully using the Papineau technique of cancellous bone grafting combined with external fixation.[11]

ANTIMICROBIAL THERAPY

Antimicrobial therapy is an essential part of the management of infection after total knee arthroplasty. The same principles applied in the treatment of infection after total hip arthroplasty are also applied (see Chapter 23, *Revision Total Hip Arthroplasty*).

References

1. Bliss, D. G. and McBride, G. G.: Infected total knee arthroplasties. Clin. Orthop. 199:207–214, 1985.
2. Booth, R. E., Jr. and Lotke, P. A.: The results of spacer block technique in revision of infected total knee arthroplasty. Clin. Orthop. 248:57–60, 1989.
3. Borden, L. S. and Gearen, P. F.: Infected total knee arthroplasty. A protocol for management. J. Arthroplasty 2(1):27–36, 1987.
4. Buchholz, H. W., Elson, R. A., Englebrecht, E., et al.: Management of deep infection of total hip replacement. J. Bone Joint Surg. 63B:342–353, 1981.
5. Chu, C. C. and Williams, D. F.: Effects of chemical configuration and chemical structure of suture materials on bacterial adhesion: A possible link to wound infection. Am. J. Surg. 147:197–204, 1984.
6. Cohen, J. C., Hozack, W. J., Cuckler, J. M., and Booth, R. E., Jr.: Two-stage reimplantation of septic total knee arthroplasty. Report of three cases using an antibiotic-PMMA spacer block. J. Arthroplasty 3(4):369–377, 1988.
7. Freeman, M. A., Sudlow, R. A., Casewell, M. W., and Radcliff, S. S.: The management of infected total knee replacements. J. Bone Joint Surg. [Br] 67(5):764–768, 1985.
8. Insall, J. N., Thompson, F. M., and Brause, B. D.: Two-stage reimplantation for the salvage of infected total knee arthroplasty. J. Bone Joint Surg. [Am] 65(8):1087–1098, 1983.
9. Kaufer, H. and Matthews, L. S.: Spherocentric arthroplasty of the knee. Clinical experience with an average four-year follow-up. J. Bone Joint Surg. 63A:545–559, 1981.
10. Kaufer, H. and Matthews, L. S.: Resection arthroplasty: an alternative to arthrodesis for salvage of the infected total knee arthroplasty. Instr. Course Lect. 35:283–289, 1986.
11. Lortat-Jacob, A., Lelong, P., Benoit, J., and Ramadier, J. O.: Infected total knee prostheses treated by Papineau's technique and arthrodesis. (Author's transl.) Rev. Chir. Orthop. 65(8):461–468, 1979. (Published in French.)
12. Lynch, M., Esser, M. P., Shelley, P., and Wroblewski, B. M.: Deep infection in Charnley low-friction arthroplasty. Comparison of plain and gentamicin-loaded cement. J. Bone Joint Surg. [Br] 69(3):355–360, 1987.
13. Petty, W., Spanier, S., and Shuster, J. J.: Prevention of infection after total joint replacement. Experiments with a canine model. J. Bone Joint Surg. [Am] 70(4):536–539, 1988.
14. Rand, J. A. and Bryan, R. S.: Reimplantation for the salvage of an infected total knee arthroplasty. J. Bone Joint Surg. [Am] 65(8):1081–1086, 1983.
15. Rand, J. A., Bryan, R. S., Morrey, B. F., and Westholm, F.: Management of infected total knee arthroplasty. Clin. Orthop. 205:75–85, 1986.
16. Rosenberg, A. G., Haas, B., Barden, R., et al.: Salvage of infected total knee arthroplasty. Clin. Orthop. 226:29–33, 1988.
17. Sharp, W. V., Belden, T. A., King, P. H., and Teague, P. C.: Suture resistance to infection. Surgery 91:61–63, 1982.
18. Stulberg, S. D.: Arthrodesis in failed total knee replacement. Orthop. Clin. North Am. 13:213–224, 1982.
19. Tripple, S. B.: Antibiotic-impregnated cement in total joint arthroplasty. J. Bone Joint Surg. [Am] 68(8):1297–1302, 1986.

CHAPTER 36

Knee Arthrodesis for Failed Total Knee Arthroplasty

WILLIAM PETTY

Successful knee arthrodesis, the major alternative to revision arthroplasty for failed total knee arthroplasty, provides a stable extremity that allows excellent function and usually produces no pain. However, the patient must live with the limitation of a stiff knee joint thereafter. No absolute indications exist for arthrodesis in preference to revision arthroplasty, but factors to consider include the general health of the patient, status of the adjacent joints, integrity of the muscles that control knee movement, integrity of the stabilizing ligaments, condition of the bone about the knee, virulence and sensitivity of any infective organisms, and functional requirements of the patient.[12, 19]

SURGICAL TREATMENT

Before operation, the surgeon should evaluate how much bone stock has been lost as well as that anticipated from implant removal. The possibility of infection must be considered, and if present how it will be treated (see Chapter 35, *Treatment of Infected Total Knee Arthroplasty*). Total knee cutting guides are helpful in preparing the bone surfaces to achieve appropriate alignment of slight valgus and flexion of the arthrodesis. The surgical methods for achieving arthrodesis are external fixation, intramedullary rod fixation, and fixation with plates.

Bone Grafting

Whether deficient bone must be replaced for arthrodesis depends primarily on the type of implanted prosthesis and whether additional bone destruction resulted from septic or aseptic failure. Loss of circumferential bone from the tibia, femur, or both determines whether the surgeon must consider measures for re-establishing limb length. If limb shortening is less than 5 cm, a shoe lift may be all that is needed, especially if the knee is fused. When greater shortening is expected, the surgeon should consider restoring length.

The degree of circumferential bone loss depends mainly on the longitudinal space occupied by the knee arthroplasty components. If a previous primary or revision arthroplasty has required thick tibial or femoral components, or both, to achieve stability, bone loss may be substantial. A patient who has been treated with attempted arthrodesis or resection arthroplasty for failed knee arthroplasty may have considerable bone loss, especially when continuing sepsis has been a problem (see Fig. 35–2). Deficiencies causing unacceptable limb shortening are best managed by circumferential allograft obtained from the distal femur or proximal tibia. However, infection must be cleared before placement of these grafts.

The surface contact area of bone available for arthrodesis may be reduced dramatically by bulky femoral or tibial stems or prosthesis protrusions into trabecular bone to accommodate stabilizing features of the prosthesis.[8] Although this bone deficiency does not affect limb length if the peripheral cortices remain intact, healing of the arthrodesis may be compromised. The deficiency may be treated with cancellous or cortical grafts or combinations of the two, and they may be autogenous or allogeneic. Whereas cortical grafting, either autogenous or allogeneic, should be avoided until all sepsis is cleared, the Papineau technique of cancellous grafting has been utilized successfully within 2 weeks of initial debridement for infection.[13]

External Fixation

In early attempts at arthrodesis for failed total knee arthroplasty, surgeons used uniplanar external fixation methods. In some series, failure rates were high.[11, 15] *In vitro* studies of external fixation devices have indicated that biplanar pin placement makes the fixation more rigid than uniplanar pin placement.[2, 6, 10] Some investigators have reported higher success rates with these newer techniques, whereas others have reported no improvement over earlier uniplanar fixation.[1, 12, 16–18, 20] These differences suggest that other factors influence outcome, including quality of bone, adequacy of grafting, and presence or absence of sepsis. One advantage of external fixation over other methods is that, because the pins can be placed away from the knee joint, excellent fixation can be achieved immediately after debridement of a septic joint. This immediate rigid immobilization is helpful in treating the infection (Fig. 36–1).

The surgical procedure for external fixation requires careful planning and application of the device. Multiplanar pin application is preferable. Initially, the surgical wound may be treated by open or closed means. Time to fusion varies, but the average duration of external fixation is about 4 months. After the external fixation device is removed, the limb is further protected with a cast or brace until solid healing can be demonstrated radiographically and until defects left by the fixation pins have had time to heal.

The major complication of external fixation is pin tract infection. Because infection is more likely when pins are placed through retained cement, all cement should be removed.[16] Pin tract infections are treated with pin removal and pin replacement at another site, local debridement, antibiotic administration, or combinations of these methods.

Intramedullary Rod Fixation

Intramedullary rod fixation for knee arthrodesis usually provides secure fixation and a high degree of success for fusion. Moreover, little or no supplemental external immobilization is generally required in the form of a cast or brace (Fig. 36–2).[4, 7, 9, 12, 21, 22] Only when infection is cleared can the technique be used, however. If infection recurs after placement of a long rod, it may well involve the full extent of the femur and tibia. Careful surgical technique, including careful sizing of the rod for both length and diameter, is essential to provide adequate fixation while avoiding the complication of fracture.

Both curved and straight rods of many designs have been employed for arthrodesis. Curved rods allow the knee to be positioned in modest flexion, which is desirable. The most effective surgical technique is retrograde placement of the rod into the femur through the knee joint, reduction of the bone surfaces, and impaction of the rod into the tibia. If cortical graft is needed to regain length, it is placed between the femoral and tibial surfaces. The rod is driven across the joint. Proper rotation is established before impacting the rod into the tibia.

If fixation is secure, partial weightbearing can begin the day after surgery. A major advantage of this method of knee arthrodesis is that weightbearing provides compression of the bone surfaces to promote early healing. If the surgeon has any reservations about the stability of fixation or the patient's compliance, external im-

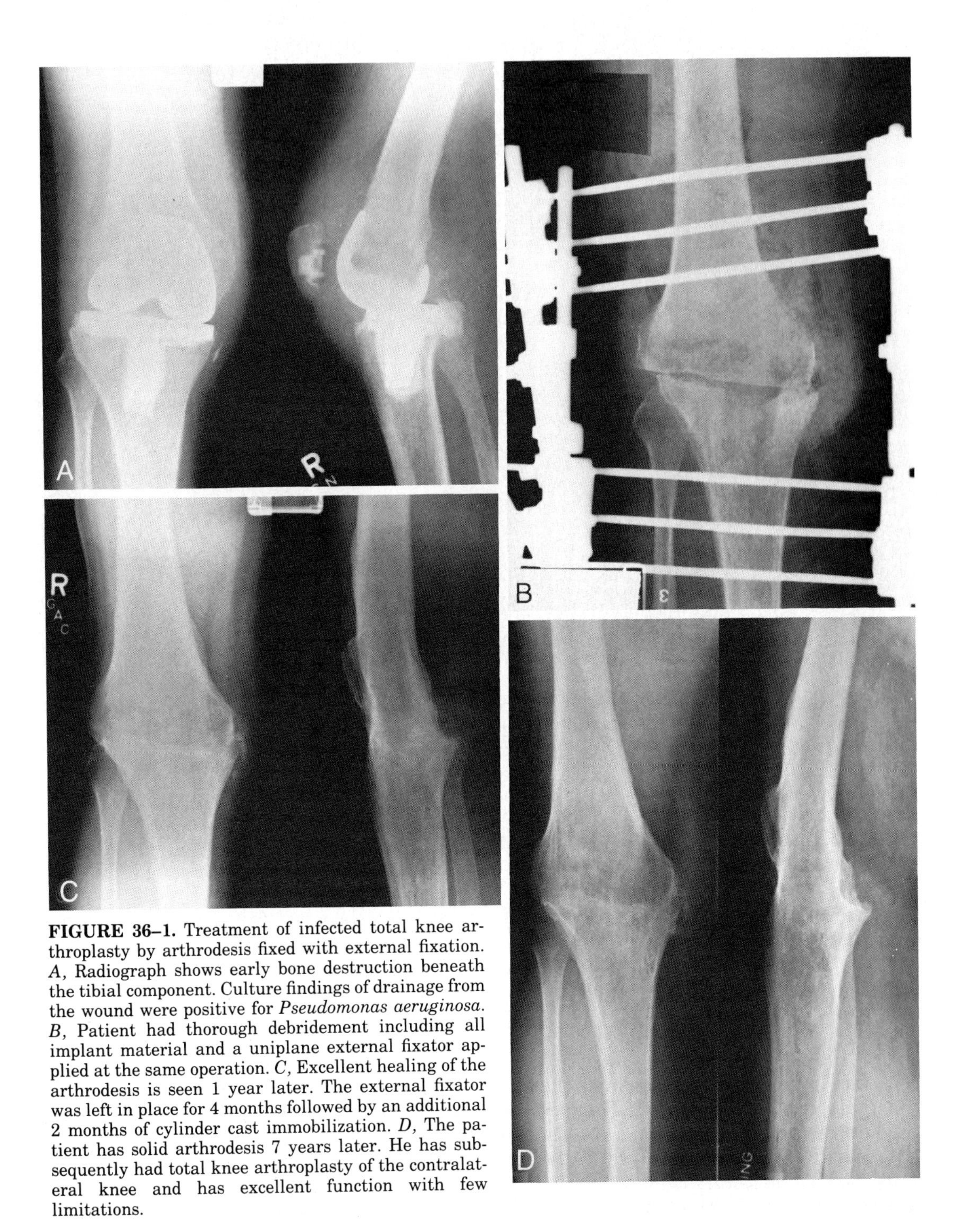

FIGURE 36–1. Treatment of infected total knee arthroplasty by arthrodesis fixed with external fixation. *A,* Radiograph shows early bone destruction beneath the tibial component. Culture findings of drainage from the wound were positive for *Pseudomonas aeruginosa.* *B,* Patient had thorough debridement including all implant material and a uniplane external fixator applied at the same operation. *C,* Excellent healing of the arthrodesis is seen 1 year later. The external fixator was left in place for 4 months followed by an additional 2 months of cylinder cast immobilization. *D,* The patient has solid arthrodesis 7 years later. He has subsequently had total knee arthroplasty of the contralateral knee and has excellent function with few limitations.

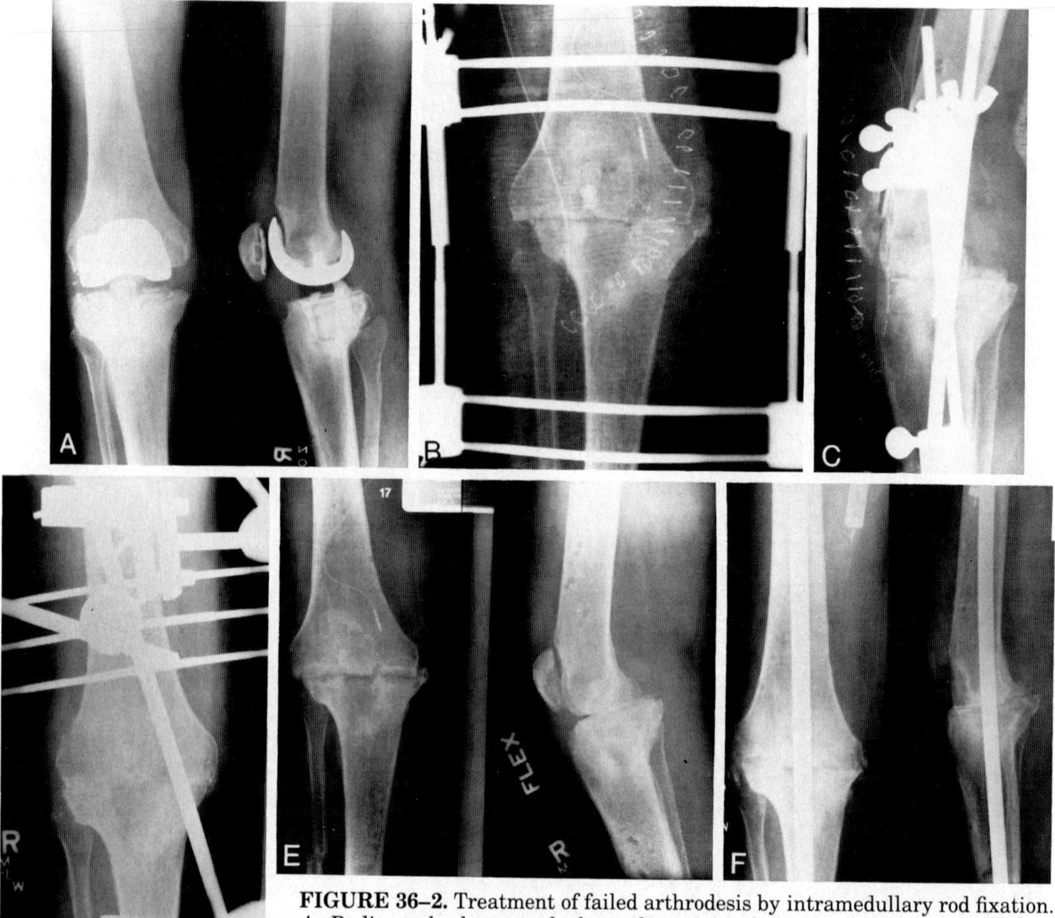

FIGURE 36–2. Treatment of failed arthrodesis by intramedullary rod fixation. *A,* Radiograph shows early bone destruction beneath all three components. Culture and drainage from the wound provided positive findings for *Pseudomonas aeruginosa. B* and *C,* Patient had thorough debridement including all implant material. A uniplane external fixator and bone growth stimulator were applied at the same operation. *D,* Arthrodesis was not achieved and was reattempted with a multiplane external fixator. *E,* The arthrodesis was judged to be solid, but after removal of the external fixation device, the patient again developed painful motion at the knee joint. *F,* Solid arthrodesis was obtained after internal fixation with an intramedullary rod.

mobilization in the form of a cast or brace may be provided for the first 4 to 6 weeks.

Plate Fixation

The third method of fixation for knee arthrodesis after failed total knee arthroplasty is the use of plates. Their major advantages are secure fixation and lack of external pins.[14] However, an infection must be cleared before the procedure. Disadvantages of the method include the bulkiness of the plates, which may impair wound closure, and the potential stress shielding over time, which may weaken the bone. Because of the potential for stress shielding, many surgeons recommend plate removal after bone healing, necessitating a relatively major additional operation.

Plates must be bent to conform to the bone contours. Because of the large lever arm of the limb and the weakened bone stock, four or more bicortical screws should be applied both proximally and distally to the fusion site: compression is applied through the plates. Two plates are normally placed, either medially and laterally or on one side and anteriorly. An anterior plate may make wound closure more difficult and the patient more susceptible to painful minor trauma postoperatively.[5]

RESULTS

Success of Fusion

In a multicenter study, Knutson and coworkers[11] achieved fusion in 50 percent of 108 attempted fusions in 91 failed total knee arthroplasties. Three conditions were associated with better results after failed knee replacements: (1) failed unicompartment arthroplasty, (2) use of biplanar external fixation or intramedullary rod fixation, and (3) control of infection before or at the time of the arthrodesis procedure.

Rand and Bryan[15] reported successful fusion in 56 percent of failed hinge arthroplasties and 81 percent of resurfacing arthroplasties utilizing a uniplanar external fixator. Biplane fixation failed to raise their success rate, with 85 percent of resurfacing and 43 percent of failed hinge implants achieving arthrodesis. These investigators now prefer intramedullary fixation for aseptic failure or quiescent infection.[16] Harris and Froehlich[9] achieved fusion in seven of eight knee arthrodeses with intramedullary rods for especially complex problems associated with failed knee replacements. These problems included obesity, segmental fracture, and severe bone loss. Knutson and associates[12] reported successful arthrodesis with an intramedullary nail in four patients in whom fusion had not been achieved by initial treatment with external fixation.

Munzinger and coworkers[14] attempted arthrodesis for failed total knee arthroplasty in 44 knees: 34 with compression plates and ten with external fixation. Fusion occurred within 6 months in 100 percent of those treated with plates and 60 percent treated with external fixation.

Figgie and coworkers[5] evaluated the function of 23 patients with rheumatoid arthritis who had undergone attempted knee arthrodeses for failed knee replacements. Four patients had bilateral arthrodeses. Twenty knees were solidly fused. Knees in a position of 7 ± 5 degrees of valgus and 0 to 30 degrees of flexion were most likely to have solid fusion. They also had the lowest rate of problems with surrounding joints and functioned best. Persistent sepsis and severe bone loss were associated with higher rates of failure.

Knee arthrodesis is most likely to be successful when infection is controlled and rigid fixation is achieved at the time of the procedure. I prefer the use of a curved, fluted rod for arthrodesis—it is strong, the knee can be placed in slight flexion, and postoperative management is less complicated. If external fixation is done, rigid fixation with a biplanar system is preferred.

References

1. Behr, J. T., Chmell, S. J., and Schwartz, C. M.: Knee arthrodesis for failed total knee arthroplasty. Arch. Surg. 120(3):350–354, 1985.
2. Briggs, B. T. and Chao, E. Y. S.: The mechanical performance of the standard Hoffman-Vidal external fixator apparatus. J. Bone Joint Surg. 64A:566–573, 1982.
3. Broderson, M. P., Fitzgerald, R. H., Peterson, L. F. A., et al.: Arthrodesis of the knee following failed total knee arthroplasty. J. Bone Joint Surg. 61A:181–185, 1979.
4. Fern, E. D., Stewart, H. D., and Newton, G.: Curved Kuntscher nail arthrodesis after failure of knee replacement. J. Bone Joint Surg. [Br] 71(4):588–590, 1989.
5. Figgie, H. E., 3d, Brody, G. A., Inglis, A. E., et al.: Knee arthrodesis following total knee arthroplasty in rheumatoid arthritis. Clin. Orthop. 224:237–243, 1987.
6. Fischer, D. A.: Skeletal stabilization with a multiplane external fixation device. Design rationale and preliminary clinical experience. Clin. Orthop. 180:50–62, 1983.
7. Goldberg, J. A., Drummond, R. P., Bruce, W. J., et al.: Huckstep nail arthrodesis of the knee: a salvage for infected total knee replacement. Aust. N. Z. J. Surg. 59(2):147–150, 1989.
8. Hankin, F., Louie, K. W., and Matthews, L. S.: The effect of total knee arthroplasty prostheses design on the potential for salvage arthrodesis: measurements of volumes, lengths and trabecular bone contact areas. Clin. Orthop. 155:52–58, 1981.
9. Harris, C. M. and Froehlich, J.: Knee fusion with intramedullary rods for failed total knee arthroplasty. Clin. Orthop. 197:209–216, 1985.
10. Knutson, K., Bodelind, B., and Lidgren, L.: Stability of external fixators used for knee arthrodesis after failed knee arthroplasty. Clin. Orthop. 186:90–95, 1984.
11. Knutson, K., Hovelius, L., Lindstrand, A., and Lidgren, L.: Arthrodesis after failed knee arthroplasty. A nationwide multicenter investigation of 91 cases. Clin. Orthop. 191:202–211, 1984.
12. Knutson, K., Lindstrand, A., and Lidgren, L.: Arthrodesis for failed knee arthroplasty. A report of 20 cases. J. Bone Joint Surg. [Br] 67(1):47–52, 1985.
13. Lortat-Jacob, A., Lelong, P., Benoit, J., and Ramadier, J. O.: Infected total knee prostheses treated by Papineau's technique and arthrodesis. (Author's transl.) Rev. Chir. Orthop. 65(8):461–468, 1979. (Published in French.)

14. Munzinger, U., Knessl, J., and Gschwend, N.: Arthrodesis following knee arthroplasty. Orthopade 16(4):301–309, 1987. (Published in German.)
15. Rand, J. A. and Bryan, R. S.: The outcome of failed knee arthrodesis following total knee arthroplasty. Clin. Orthop. 205:86–92, 1986.
16. Rand, J. A., Bryan, R. S., and Chao, E. Y.: Failed total knee arthroplasty treated by arthrodesis of the knee using the Ace-Fischer apparatus. J. Bone Joint Surg. [Am] 69(1):39–45, 1987.
17. Rothacker, G. W., Jr. and Cabanela, M. E.: External fixation for arthrodesis of the knee and ankle. Clin. Orthop. 180:101–108, 1983.
18. Rudolph, F., Fengler, F., and Hein, W.: Arthrodesis as an alternative in infected knee arthroplasty. Beitr. Orthop. Traumatol. 36(8):374–380, 1989. (Published in German.)
19. Thornhill, T. S., Dalziel, R. W., and Sledge, C. B.: Alternatives to arthrodesis for the failed total knee arthroplasty. Clin. Orthop. 170:131–140, 1982.
20. Vahvanen, V.: Arthrodesis in failed knee replacement in eight rheumatoid patients. Ann. Chir. Gynaecol. 68(2):57–62, 1979.
21. Wilde, A. H. and Stearns, K. L.: Intramedullary fixation for arthrodesis of the knee after infected total knee arthroplasty. Clin. Orthop. 248:87–92, 1989.
22. Zucman, J., Lemerle, R., Moati, J. C., and Montagliari, C.: Knee arthrodesis using tibio-femoral rods following ablation of the septic total prosthesis. Rev. Chir. Orthop. 75(6):415–419, 1989. (Published in French.)

CHAPTER 37

Prostheses for Total Knee Arthroplasty

WILLIAM PETTY

A wide array of knee prostheses is available to the orthopaedic surgeon. The selection of a prosthesis for a specific patient depends on many factors, including the surgeon's familiarity with the device and its placement, the surgeon's preference, and the patient's condition. Fortunately, over two decades of careful evaluation of patients with total knee arthroplasties have yielded much knowledge about the requirements for success. Surgeons performing total knee replacement surgery can use this knowledge to provide the best possible reconstruction for their patients.

Descriptions of the prostheses and the illustrations included in this chapter were supplied by the manufacturers of these various prostheses. An attempt was made to include prostheses based on their popularity, either past or present, or on their unique design features. Some prostheses could not be included because the manufacturers were unable to supply the information requested.

ANATOMICALLY GRADUATED COMPONENTS (AGC) TOTAL KNEE SYSTEM

The Anatomically Graduated Components (AGC) Total Knee System (Biomet, Inc.) was introduced in March, 1983 (Fig. 37–1). The original design included a one-piece metal-backed component, a universal cobalt-chromium femoral component, and a metal-backed or an all-polyethylene patellar button. All femoral and tibial components had a porous coating of titanium alloy plasma spray or a roughened interlocking finish for enhanced cement fixation. Five femoral and tibial dimensions are provided and are interchangeable, permitting independent sizing of each bone. The sizing rationale was based upon a morphologic study by Mensch and Amstutz, which predicted variations in the dimensions of the bones composing the knee.

The current AGC system has both universal and left-right specific femoral components, as well as modular tibial components with optional screw fixation and modular stems. Revision and posterior-stabilized options, as well as a unicondylar system, can be implanted employing common intramedullary or extramedullary instrumentation.

GENESIS TOTAL KNEE SYSTEM

Genesis (Richards, Inc.) is a modular system with parts and sizes that fit each other and interchange with each other, allowing the surgeon to select and assemble implants at the time of surgery (Fig. 37–2). The tibial component consists of an

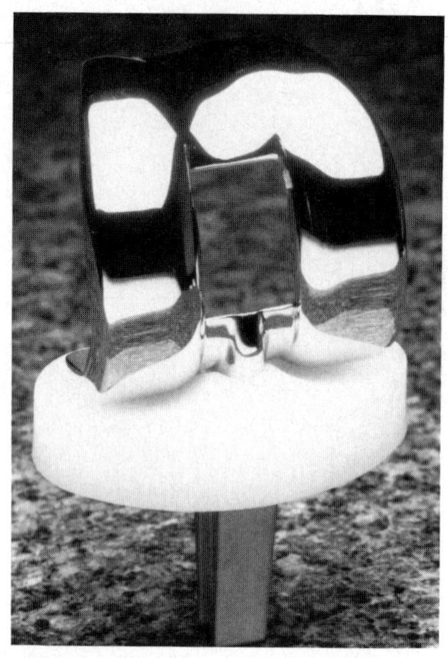

FIGURE 37–1. The Anatomically Graduated Components (AGC) Total Knee System (Biomet, Inc.).

asymmetric, titanium-alloy tray to improve bone coverage on the proximal tibia and a variety of articular surface types to address different requirements for knee joint stability. The femoral components are manufactured from cobalt-chromium alloy because of its hardness and wear resistance to microfretting against polyethylene when compared with titanium alloy. The anterior lateral flange on the femoral component is raised to reduce the risk of patellar dislocation and to minimize femoral-patellar wear. The modular system provides implants for both primary and revision cases.

INSALL/BURSTEIN II MODULAR KNEE SYSTEM

The Insall/Burstein II Modular Knee System (Zimmer, Inc.) is an updated design of the Insall/Burstein Total Knee System (Fig. 37–3). A posterior design offers stability with additional range of motion. A condylar design gives added constraint to partially restricted varus/valgus and rotational movement. Biomechanical and kinematic function are improved over the old design, and the surgeon is provided with a number of options during the procedure.

The cruciate-substituting design of the new system makes implantation less difficult and provides good stability and kinematics. Particular attention has been paid to stress and wear resistance relative to the tibial articular surface. The femoral components are cobalt-chromium alloy. The tibial trays are titanium alloy (Ti-6Al-4Va) for biocompatibility with optimal fatigue and yield strength. The Zimmer Intramedullary Instrumentation System helps to make the surgical procedure more accurate and reproducible.

LACEY TOTAL KNEE SYSTEM

The Lacey Total Knee System (Dow Corning Wright) is a press-fit, cementless system (Fig. 37–4) with the femoral component manufactured from cobalt-chrome alloy. Fixation is achieved by a three-sided fin design with small cleats on the internal anteroposterior dimensions. The internal design loads the bone in compression and reduces stress shielding. The tibial component is cast from titanium alloy, a material providing good stress distribution to the bone. Ultrahigh molecular weight polyethylene inserts of an unconstrained rotational design are snapped into the titanium tray. Fixation is dependent upon the fin configuration for a press-fit. To improve range of motion, the tibial inserts are sloped posteriorly. Titanium patellar components are made of ultrahigh molecular

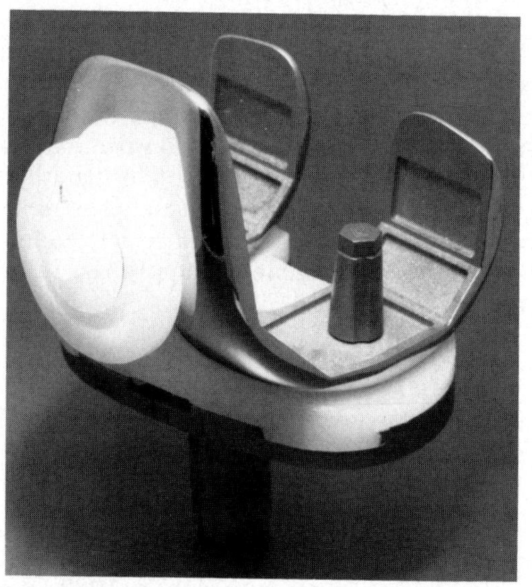

FIGURE 37–2. The Genesis Total Knee System (Richards, Inc.).

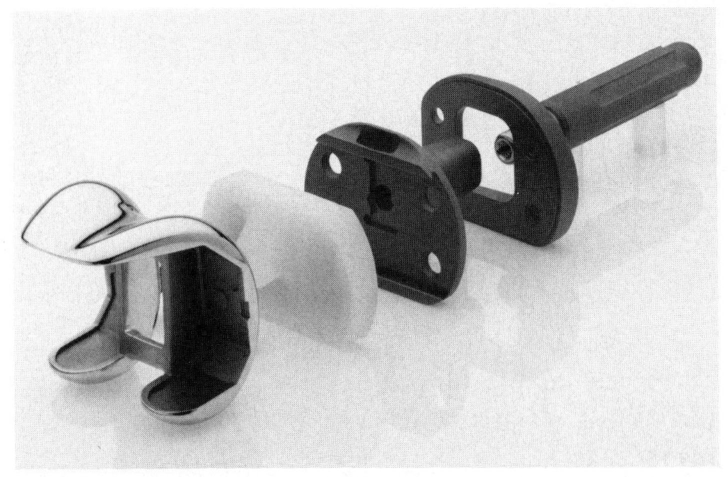

FIGURE 37–3. The Insall/Burstein II Modular Knee System (Zimmer, Inc.).

weight polyethylene mechanically locked to a titanium backing. The dome-shaped patella component "floats" in the groove of the femoral component.

LCS TOTAL KNEE SYSTEM

The mobile meniscal bearings of the LCS Total Knee System (DePuy, Inc.) are designed to simulate the biomechanics of a normal knee (Fig. 37–5). Greater component congruency and less constrained axial rotation help decrease contact stresses at the femoral-tibial bearing interface and eliminate torque loads, improving the chances for long-term implant performance and fixation. Multicenter clinical trials conducted over a 5-year period have shown the system to be successful in treating osteoarthritis, rheumatoid arthritis, and revisions of failed prostheses.

MILLER/GALANTE (MG) II KNEE SYSTEM

The Miller/Galante (MG) Knee System (Zimmer, Inc.) has eight femoral anteroposterior sizes to accommodate to most patients' dimensions with an accuracy of ±2 mm (Fig. 37–6). Any of the femoral sizes can be utilized with any of the MG II tibial component sizes. The MG II femoral component is wider mediolaterally to give full bone coverage and better distribution of stress in the femoral and tibial components. Proper patellofemoral articulation was a major consideration in the design of the MG II components. The depth of the patellar groove allows more anatomic tracking, thereby reducing shear forces and lateral subluxing tendencies. Contact between the patellar and femoral components is maximized throughout the range of motion, and gradual femoral radius allows smooth patellar movement. The metal-backed patella is made of titanium fiber-metal. The all-polyethylene patella has a textured surface, islands, and undercuts to improve fixation. The MG II fixation plate was designed to cover the resected tibial surface completely, resulting in uni-

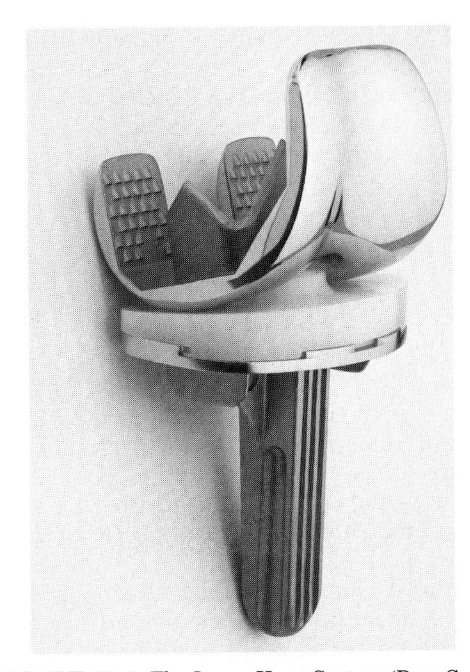

FIGURE 37–4. The Lacey Knee System (Dow Corning Wright).

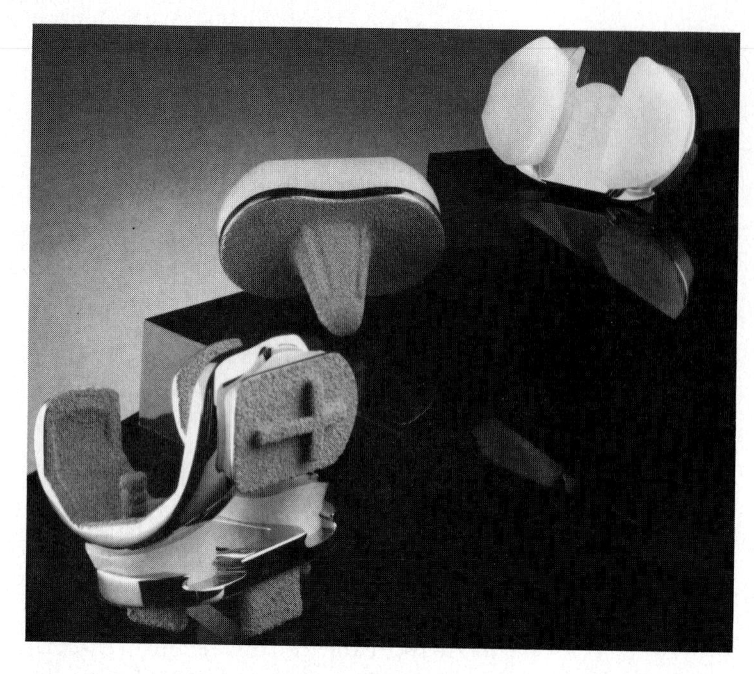

FIGURE 37–5. The LCS Total Knee System (DePuy, Inc.).

form distribution of forces. This plate also takes advantage of the strongest bone and lowers the chances of subsidence or bone resorption around the implant periphery. Pegged or stemmed tibial fixation plate designs are available. Bone screws can be angled up to 10 degrees through pegs and 15 degrees through anterior screw holes on stemmed components. The femoral, tibial, and metal-backed patellar components have titanium fiber-metal pads on all fixation surfaces. The system uses nitrogen-ion implantation on the femoral articular surface to increase surface hardness and thereby improve wear resistance.

PRESS-FIT CONDYLAR MODULAR TOTAL KNEE SYSTEM

The P.F.C. Modular Total Knee System (Johnson & Johnson Orthopaedics) is a metal-to-plastic, resurfacing tricompartmental knee prosthesis (Fig. 37–7). Its femoral and tibial components are designed for retention of the posterior cruciate ligament (PCL). Others are designed specifically for cruciate ligament substitution. A modular tibial component permits assembly of any one of four different plastic insert topographies to a universal metal tray. The cruciate-retaining femoral component articulates with either a posterior-lipped or a curved tibial insert, providing two levels of constraint in PCL-retaining cases. The cruciate-sacrificing femoral component articulates with either a stabilized tibial insert for PCL substitution or a constrained insert for collateral ligament instability.

Femoral components are made of cast cobalt-chromium alloy. Tibial inserts and patellar components are machined ultra-high density polyethylene, and tibial trays are machined Ti-6Al-4Va. Femoral and tibial components are available with and

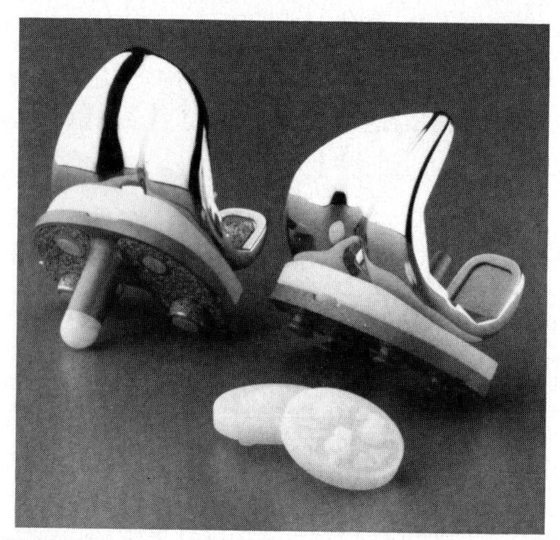

FIGURE 37–6. The Miller/Galante Knee System (Zimmer, Inc.).

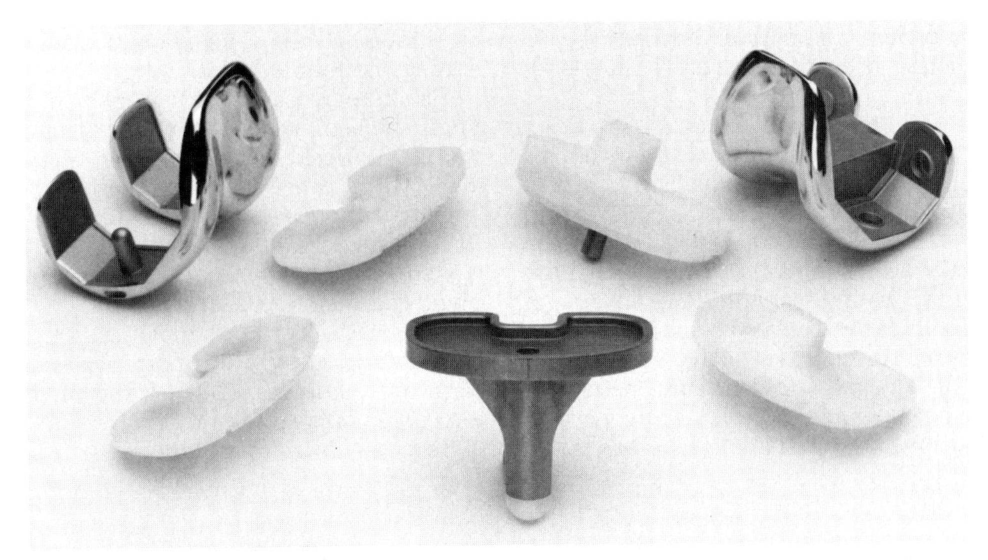

FIGURE 37–7. The P.F.C. Modular Total Knee System (Johnson & Johnson Orthopaedics).

without porous coating. The porous coating method is a high-temperature, gravity-sintering process in which a layer of beads is applied to the component. Average pore size is 350 μm.

For revision surgery, femoral and tibial components can be modified with modular wedges and stem extensions. Femoral modularity includes distal and posterior condylar augmentation and a bolt and stem assembly for either cemented stems or press-fit fluted rods. Condylar augmentation is secured mechanically with a peg and snap-ring design that engages into a cavity on the femoral component. Tibial modularity consists of metal wedges for restoration of proximal bone loss, cemented stem extensions, and press-fit fluted rods. Femoral and tibial stems are secured with Spiralock threads, which are self-locking, vibration-resistant fasteners used extensively in both aerospace technology and orthopaedic surgery.

WHITESIDE ORTHOLOC MODULAR KNEE SYSTEM

The Whiteside Ortholoc Modular Knee System (Dow Corning Wright) combines the features of all previous Ortholoc knee designs (Fig. 37–8). The standard IM Rod System approach is used in instrumentation, and the implants have been designed to address complications associated with patellar problems and tibial component fixation.

The femoral component is made of cobalt-chromium alloy. The patellar flange is in a right-and-left design with a raised lateral condyle. The patellar groove is extended deeper into the notch than in other prostheses to enhance tracking. The femo-

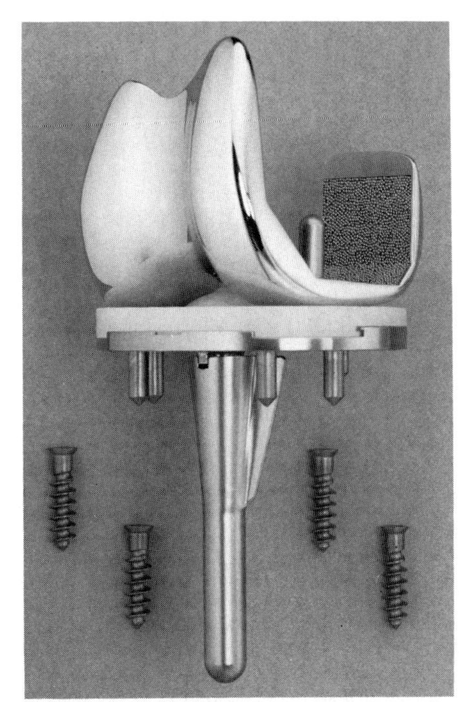

FIGURE 37–8. The Whiteside Ortholoc Modular Knee System (Dow Corning Wright).

ral component has porous coating only on the surfaces that receive compression loading.

The tibial component maintains fixation by means of titanium cortical screws, small smooth pegs located peripherally, and a variety of centralized stems in several lengths. Porous coating is located on the undersurface of the tibial tray. Ultrahigh molecular weight polyethylene inserts of various thicknesses can be snapped into a variety of tibial tray widths. A posterior slope of 3 degrees and an unconstrained surface make up the articulating portion of the tibial insert. Tibial trays are made of titanium alloy for weight reduction, strength, and biocompatibility.

The patellar component is made of ultrahigh molecular weight polyethylene mechanically locked to a titanium metal undersurface, consisting of a porous coating and smooth fixation pegs. Recessed into the natural patella, a dome-shaped component articulates on the femoral component and seeks its own tracking.

A variety of sizes, stems, and implant options including a unicompartmental design are available. All of the components are keyed off a single IM Rod System using precision cutters and planers.

SECTION VIII

UPPER EXTREMITY REPLACEMENT

CHAPTER 38

Shoulder Replacement Arthroplasty

JAMES A. TURNER

Since Charles Neer II, a pioneer in the development of modern shoulder arthroplasty, designed his first humeral head prosthesis in 1951, there has been increasing interest in shoulder replacement arthroplasty.[77, 100, 124] Cofield[34] reports that about 100 total shoulder joint replacements are done each year at the Mayo Clinic, ranking this arthroplastic procedure third in frequency after hip and knee replacements.

Proper performance of shoulder arthroplasty depends on a knowledge of normal shoulder anatomy and biomechanics, topics that are reviewed in the beginning of this chapter. Indications for total shoulder replacement, hemiarthroplasty, and arthroplasty to treat acute fractures and dislocations are then discussed. The types of shoulder prostheses available are examined in some detail before surgical techniques are reviewed. Shoulder arthroplasty is usually performed through an anterior approach, but the posterior approach and surgical technique for repair of fractures are also discussed. Special problems facing orthopaedic surgeons performing shoulder replacement arthroplasty include deficiencies in rotator cuff or bone and malunion and nonunion of fractures. Like any surgical procedure, shoulder arthroplasty may not be successful. Reasons for complications and failures of shoulder replacements, which are closely linked, are explored. The chapter concludes with a discussion of the surgeon's role in rehabilitation of the patient with a prosthetic shoulder joint.

THE NORMAL SHOULDER

Anatomy

The ultimate function of a shoulder arthroplasty is dependent on the restoration of the shoulder anatomy to as close to normal as possible.

Skeletal Anatomy

The design of the shoulder allows the hand to be positioned within a large hemisphere in front of the body and in a more limited area to the side and back. This function requires a joint designed for skeletal mobility. Thus, the glenoid is small and shallow, and less than 25 percent of the humeral head is in contact with it at any one time (Figs. 38–1 to 38–3).[19, 63, 102] Skeletal mobility also is dependent on five articulations: (1) the sternoclavicular joint, (2) the acromioclavicular joint, (3) the subacromial joint (bursa is the joint cavity here), (4) the glenohumeral joint itself, and (5) the scapulothoracic joint (Fig. 38–4).[67] Malfunction of any of these articulations can limit shoulder motion.

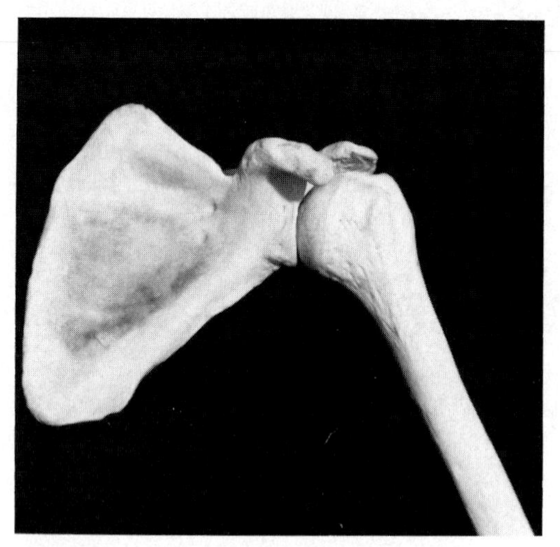

FIGURE 38–1. Anterior view of the scapula and glenoid, articulating with the humeral head. Note how little of the humeral head is in contact with the glenoid.

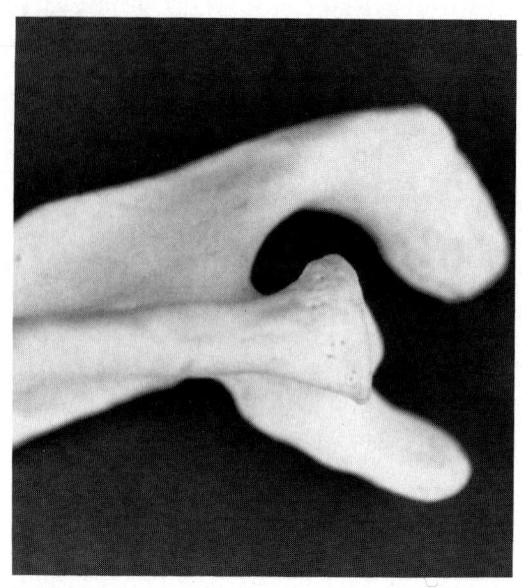

FIGURE 38–3. Inferior margin of the glenoid viewed superiorly toward the acromion and coracoid process.

To achieve prosthetic stability in the humeral head replacement, the surgeon must take into consideration the rotational relationships or version of both the humeral head and glenoid. The humeral head is retroverted approximately 30 degrees relative to the humeral condyles, and the glenoid is retroverted 7 to 10 degrees relative to the body of the scapula (Figs. 38–5 and 38–6).

Ligamentous Anatomy

Because the skeletal structure of the shoulder is designed primarily for mobility, shoulder stability must be provided by ligaments and muscles. The ligaments are classified as intrinsic and extrinsic.

The intrinsic ligaments—the more important ones for providing stability—in-

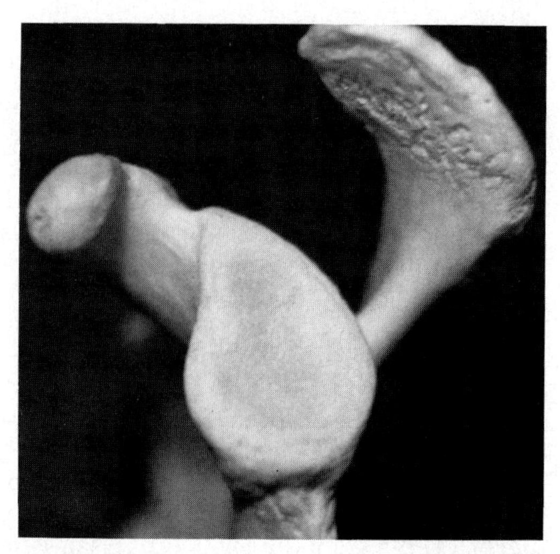

FIGURE 38–2. Articular surface of the glenoid. Note that it is somewhat pear-shaped and wider at its inferior surface. The thick base of the coracoid provides some anterior-superior reinforcement.

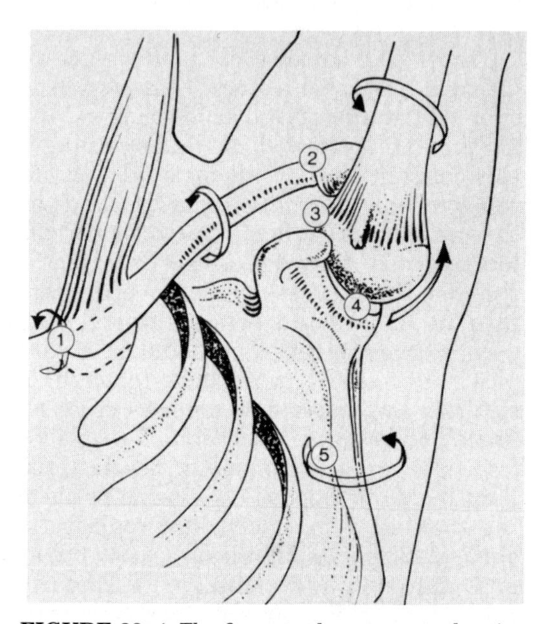

FIGURE 38–4. The five actual or conceptual articulations of the shoulder joint complex. (Kessel, L.: Clinical Disorders of the Shoulder. New York, Churchill Livingstone, 1982. By permission.)

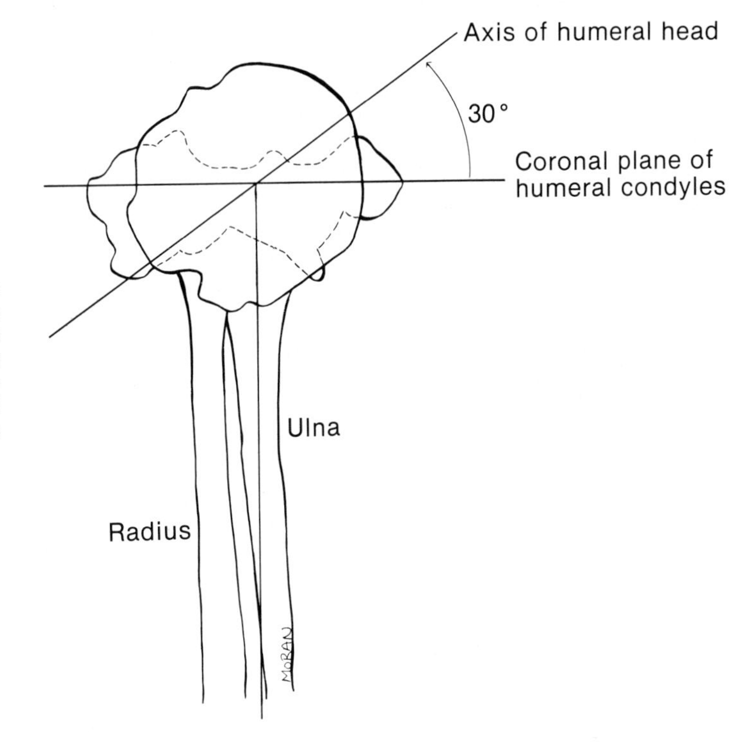

FIGURE 38–5. Retroversion of the humeral head with the shoulder in neutral position. The axis of the humerus is superimposed on the humeral condyles. Note the 30-degree retroversion of the humeral head in relation to the coronal plane of the humeral condyles.

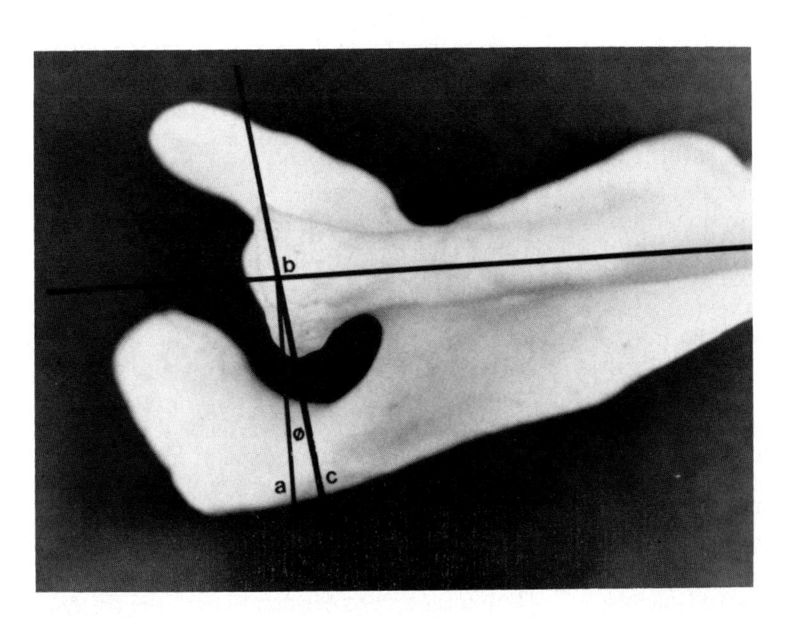

FIGURE 38–6. Normal retroversion of the glenoid at 7 to 10 degrees, with respect to the body of the scapula. Line *bc* demonstrates the retroversion of the glenoid described by angle ϕ with respect to line *ab*, which is perpendicular to the body of the scapula.

clude the glenohumeral ligaments (inferior, middle, and superior) and the glenoid labrum. The capsule of the glenohumeral joint, attaching to the humeral head at the anatomic neck and at the margins of the glenoid as it becomes continuous with the labrum, thickens in its anterior portion to form the glenohumeral ligaments. The strongest and most important of these is the inferior ligament. The glenohumeral ligaments add stability to the joint as the arm is moved, and they become taut in different positions of the arm.[113, 131] The glenoid labrum, which serves to deepen the glenoid socket, is a fibrocartilaginous thickening of the capsule around the margins of the joint. The glenoid labrum is continuous with the ligaments of the joint.

The five extrinsic ligaments are the acromioclavicular, coracoacromial, coracohumeral, conoid, and trapezoid. The extrinsic ligaments stabilize the clavicle and help suspend the scapula from the clavicle.

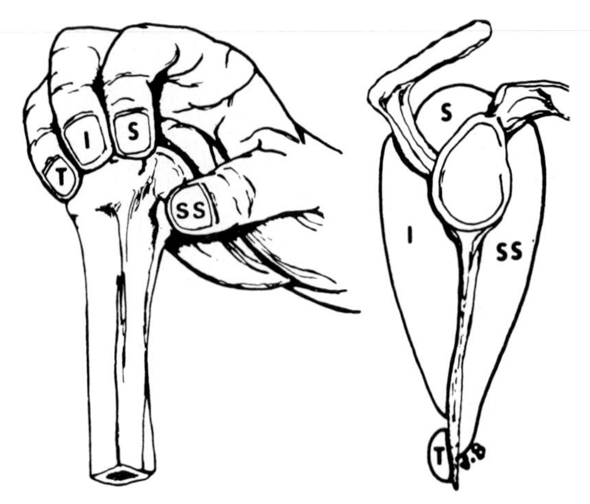

FIGURE 38–7. Encompassment of the humeral head by the rotator cuff mechanism. (S = supraspinatus; I = infraspinatus; T = teres minor; SS = subscapularis.) (Grant, J.C.B.: Grant's Atlas of Anatomy, 8th ed. Edited by J. E. Anderson. Baltimore, Williams & Wilkins, 1983. By permission.)

Musculature

Stability and positional control of the shoulder are dependent on both intrinsic and extrinsic shoulder muscles. The intrinsic muscles originate on the scapula and clavicle and insert on the upper humerus. They include the deltoid, subscapularis, supraspinatus, infraspinatus, teres minor, and teres major. The main motor muscles of the glenohumeral joint constitute the intrinsic muscles. The rotator cuff muscles—the subscapularis, supraspinatus, infraspinatus, and teres minor—encompass the humeral head (Fig. 38–7).[54] Stabilization of the humeral head in the glenoid is to a large degree dependent on these important rotator cuff muscles. Without a functioning rotator cuff, prosthetic stability and function are compromised. Therefore, the orthopaedic surgeon should maintain or, when necessary, mobilize and repair the rotator cuff.

The extrinsic shoulder motors originate from the neck and thorax and insert on the scapula or humerus. They include the trapezius, levator scapulae, rhomboids, latissimus dorsi, pectoralis major and minor, and serratus anterior. The extrinsics change the position of the scapula as the arm is raised or lowered. In addition, the pectoral muscles and the latissimus dorsi are powerful adductors and internal rotators of the arm.[60, 75]

From a functional point of view, the rotator cuff muscles stabilize the humeral head in the glenoid as the deltoid begins elevation of the arm. Then both of these muscle groups become responsible for further elevation. Because the teres minor and infraspinatus are the only external rotator muscles of the arm, their loss severely compromises positioning of the hand.[94] The subscapularis, pectoralis major, latissimus dorsi, and teres major internally rotate the arm. The trapezius, levator scapulae, rhomboids, and serratus anterior all rotate the scapula to position the glenoid under the humeral head as the arm is raised and lowered.[75]

The biceps brachii, coracobrachialis, and triceps do not fit into either the intrinsic or extrinsic muscle category. The biceps and triceps act as flexors and extensors, respectively, of the elbow. If the elbow is fixed, these muscles can act as flexors or extensors of the arm at the shoulder. In addition, the biceps and triceps function to support the humerus in the glenoid. When their tone is lost, as often occurs after fracture about the upper humerus, the humeral head may sublux downward (Fig. 38–8).

The long biceps tendon, which originates at the supraglenoid tubercle, stabilizes the humeral head by acting as a head depres-

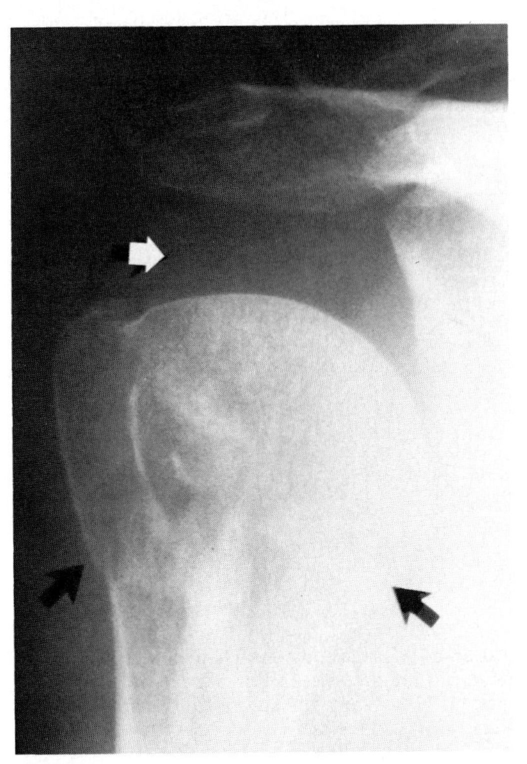

FIGURE 38–8. Impacted fracture of the surgical neck of the humerus (two lower arrows). Muscle tone is often lost in association with fractures of the upper humerus, especially in the elderly, allowing inferior subluxation of the humeral head (upper arrow). Isometric exercises for the biceps and triceps can help alleviate this problem.

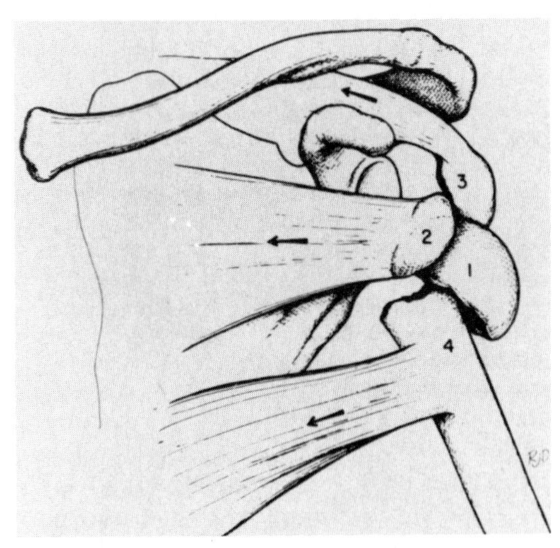

FIGURE 38–9. Muscle attachments to the fragments of a four-part fracture of the humerus and the directions of muscle pull. Muscles are the pectoralis major on the shaft, the subscapularis on the lesser tuberosity, and the supraspinatus and infraspinatus/teres minor on the greater tuberosity. (Neer, C. S., II: Part 1: Fractures about the Shoulder. Fractures in Adults, 2nd ed., vol. I. Edited by C. A. Rockwood, Jr. and D. P. Green. Philadelphia, J. B. Lippincott Company, 1984. By permission.)

sor.[91] It also serves as an excellent landmark for the surgeon working on a fractured or scarred shoulder.[104] When the anatomy is distorted by trauma, the biceps tendon can be found deep to the insertion of the pectoralis major tendon in the bicipital groove. From here, it can be followed up to the interval between the greater and lesser tuberosities. The short head of the biceps and the coracobrachialis join after their origins at the coracoid process and form the conjoined tendon, running directly anterior to the subscapularis muscle and the axillary nerve. These tendons, as well as the pectoralis major, are enveloped in the clavipectoral layer of fascia.[75] This fascia must be incised to expose the conjoined tendon. It and the underlying musculocutaneous nerve can be retracted medially to expose the front of the shoulder.

In analyzing and treating fractures about the upper end of the humerus, the surgeon should keep in mind how the muscles attach to each fragment and their direction of pull (Figs. 38–9 and 38–10).

Neuroanatomy

Neuromotor control of the shoulder is transmitted through the nerve roots C4–T1 and the brachial plexus. The roots and trunk of the brachial plexus are in the interscalene area, the divisions between the clavicle and first rib, and the cords deep to the pectoralis minor.

All of the intrinsic muscles derive their innervation from either cords or trunks (Table 38–1). Of the extrinsic muscles, only the latissimus dorsi and the pectoralis major and minor derive their innervation from cords. The other extrinsic muscles are innervated from roots or the spinal cord.[40]

Of the motor nerves to the shoulder, the axillary, musculocutaneous, and suprascapular nerves are most at risk during surgical procedures.

The axillary nerve arises from the posterior cord and courses downward across the subscapularis, coming dangerously close to the glenohumeral joint as it passes beneath the joint capsule to the quadrangular space (Fig. 38–11).[71] Here it inner-

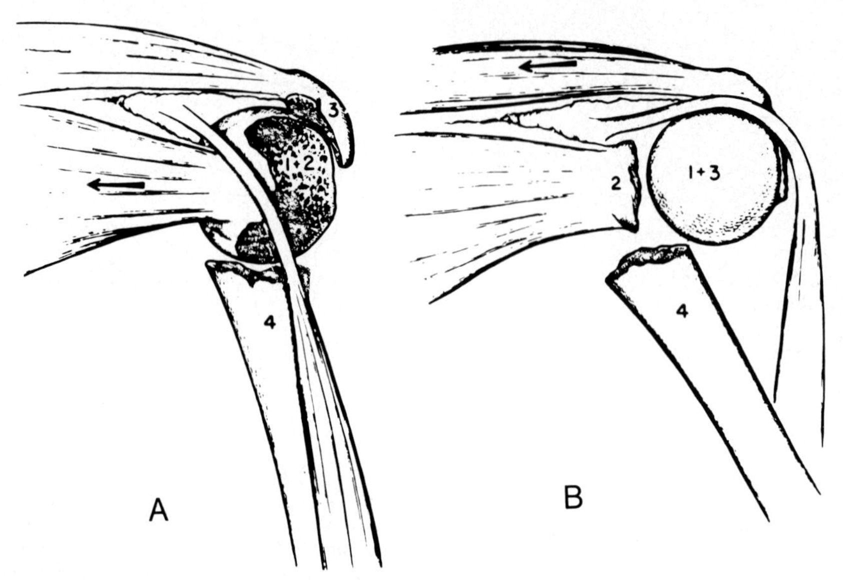

FIGURE 38–10. *A*, A three-part fracture with the lesser tuberosity remaining attached to the head. This allows the subscapularis to internally rotate the humeral head so that the articular surface faces posteriorly. *B*, A three-part fracture in which the greater tuberosity is intact. This allows the supraspinatus and external rotators to externally rotate the humeral head so that the articular surface faces anteriorly. (Neer, C. S., II: Part 1: Fractures About the Shoulder. Fractures in Adults, 2nd ed., vol. I. Edited by C. A. Rockwood, Jr. and D. P. Green. Philadelphia, J. B. Lippincott Company, 1984. By permission.)

Table 38–1. INNERVATION OF THE SHOULDER MUSCLES

Motor	Nerve	Cord	Root
Deltoid			
Anterior	Axillary	Posterior	C5, C6
Middle	Axillary	Posterior	C5, C6
Posterior	Axillary	Posterior	C5, C6
Supraspinatus	Suprascapular	Upper trunk	C5, C6
External Rotators			
Infraspinatus	Suprascapular	Upper trunk	C5, C6
Teres minor	Axillary	Posterior	C5, C6
Internal Rotators			
Subscapularis	Subscapular	Posterior	C5, C6
Pectoralis major	Lateral and medial pectoral nerves	Lateral and medial	C5, C6, C7 C6, C7, C8, T1
Latissimus dorsi	Thoracodorsal	Posterior	C6, C7, C8
Teres major	Lower subscapular	Posterior	C5, C6
Serratus Anterior	Long thoracic		C5, C6, C7
Trapezius			
Upper	Spinal accessory		C3, C4
Middle	Spinal accessory		C3, C4
Lower	Spinal accessory		C3, C4
Levator Scapulae	Dorsal scapular		C3, C4, C5
Rhomboids	Dorsal scapular		C4, C5

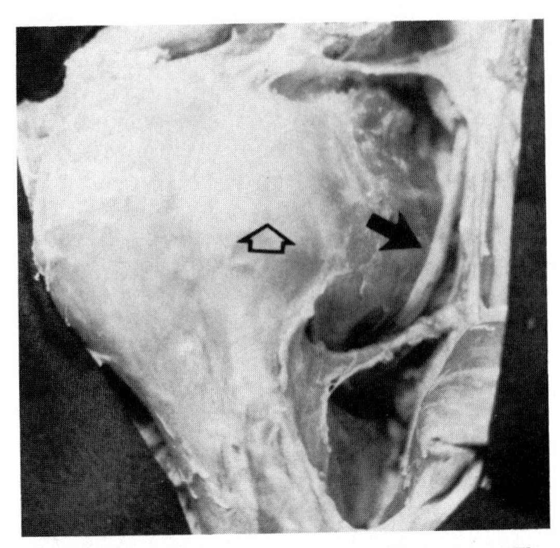

FIGURE 38–11. Dissection of the axillary nerve. The black arrow points to the axillary nerve crossing the subscapularis; the white arrow points to the insertion of the subscapularis into the lesser tuberosity.

vates the teres minor, an important fact to bear in mind with posterior approaches to the shoulder. The axillary nerve then passes posterior to the glenoid neck to reach the undersurface of the deltoid, which it innervates (Fig. 38–12). With any surgical approach to the shoulder, it is important to remember that the axillary nerve traverses the underside of the deltoid, approximately 5 cm distal to the edge of the acromion. Because of this neuroanatomy, the deltoid should never be split more than 4 cm distal from the acromion.

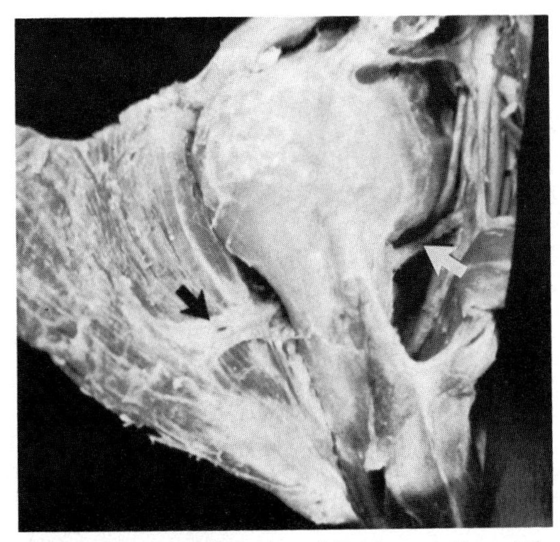

FIGURE 38–12. Dissection of the innervation of the deltoid. The deltoid has been laid back, exposing its undersurface. The arrow points to the axillary nerve and vessels.

The musculocutaneous nerve, originating from the lateral cord, innervates the coracobrachialis, biceps, and brachialis muscles. The branch to the coracobrachialis enters the muscle 2 to 5 cm distal to the tip of the coracoid process.[46] Leaving the coracoid and attached conjoined tendon in place during surgery allows the muscle belly to protect the musculocutaneous nerve during retraction.

The suprascapular nerve, which derives directly from the upper trunk of the brachial plexus in the C5–C6 distribution, enters the supraspinous fossa through a small notch in the superior border of the scapula near the base of the coracoid (Fig. 38–13). The nerve then courses around the lateral margin of the spine of the scapula to enter the infraspinous fossa. The suprascapular nerve innervates both the supraspinatus and infraspinatus muscles. The motor branches to the supraspinatus arise within 1 cm of the suprascapular notch, and the terminal motor branches to the infraspinatus arise within 1 cm of the base of the scapular spine.[7] The suprascapular nerve comes very close to the posterior rim of the glenoid as it passes around the base

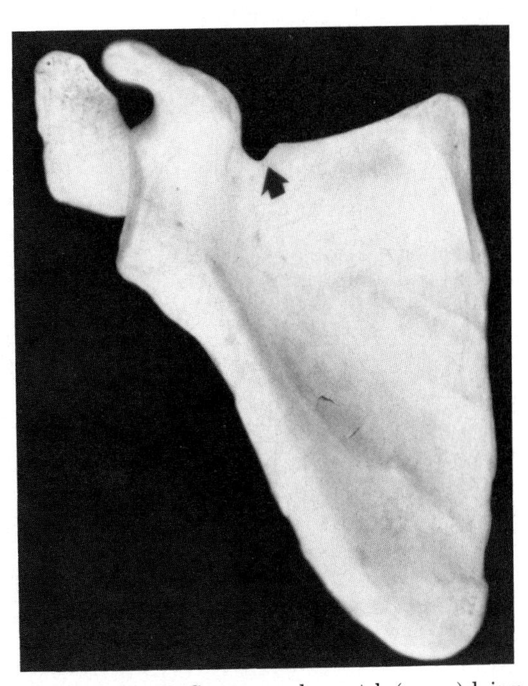

FIGURE 38–13. Suprascapular notch (arrow) lying close to the glenoid.

of the spine of the scapula. Freeing the infraspinatus muscle when repairing a large or massive rotator cuff tear might jeopardize this nerve.

Vascular Anatomy

The anterior and posterior circumflex vessels course laterally from the axillary artery and anastomose around the surgical neck of the humerus (Fig. 38–14). In 1956, Laing[69] demonstrated that the humeral head receives its blood supply from the circumflex vessels as they enter the bone from the bicipital groove area. Later, Gerber and associates[53] demonstrated that the humeral head is supplied with blood through an anterolateral ascending branch of the anterior circumflex artery, which runs along the lateral aspect of the long biceps tendon and enters the humeral head laterally and proximally to the bicipital groove. This arcuate artery supplies blood to almost the entire humeral head, as the posterior circumflex artery supplies only the inferolateral aspect of the humeral head and the greater tuberosity (see Fig. 38–14). If this ascending branch is injured close to the humeral head, the blood supply to the head is likely to be interrupted.

Fractures through the anatomic neck region of the humerus usually separate the humeral head from its blood supply, resulting in osteonecrosis.[82] Because of this, many such fractures are treated by prosthetic replacement.

The blood supply to the supraspinatus tendon near its insertion is sparse, contributing to cuff disruption in this area.[83, 91]

If a neurovascular structure medial to the glenohumeral joint should be injured, exposure and control can be safely achieved in a stepwise fashion. Bleeding initially is controlled by packing off the vessel. Exposure with safe, definitive control is gained by first taking down the conjoined tendon or the tip of the coracoid with tendon attached and, if necessary, the pectoralis major. This maneuver exposes the pectoralis minor with the underlying neurovascular bundle. The pectoralis minor can be taken down without difficulty for further exposure. If even more exposure is necessary, appropriate muscles can be taken down subperiosteally from the clavicle to expose the neurovascular structures deep to the clavicle and in the supraclavicular fossa.

Biomechanics

Forces

The mobility and stability of the shoulder are dependent not only on the anatomy

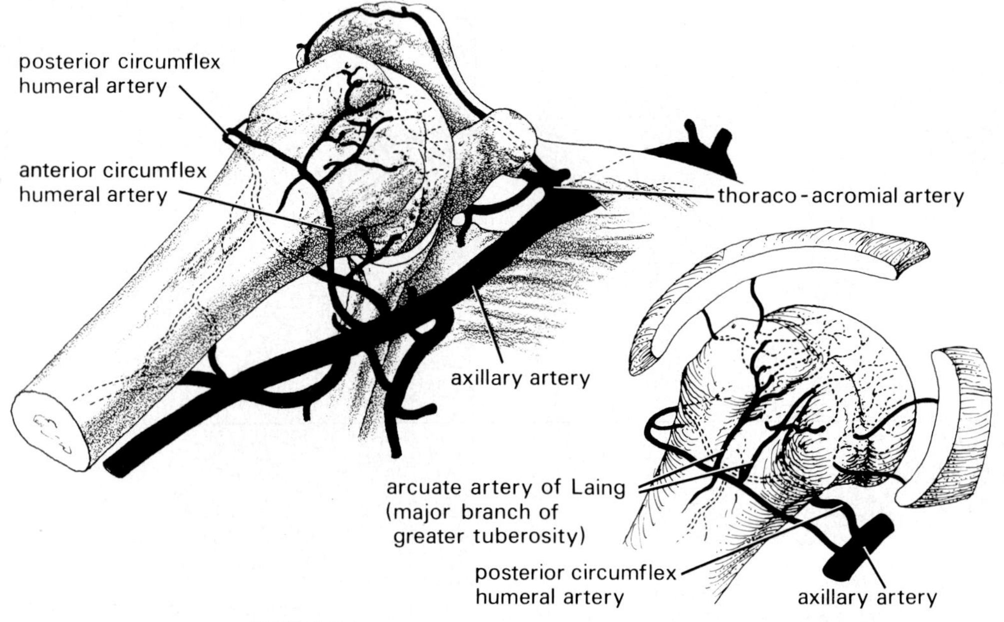

FIGURE 38–14. Vascular anatomy of the shoulder.

Table 38–2. FORCE CAPABILITY OF MUSCLE

Muscle	Area (cm^2)	Force (kg)
Middle deltoid	12	48
Anterior deltoid	9	36
Posterior deltoid	9	36
Supraspinatus	6	24

The cross-sectional area of a muscle multiplied by the force produced per square cm (4 kg/cm^2) will give the force that the whole muscle is capable of producing.

but also on the forces acting about the shoulder joint. The force that any muscle is capable of exerting depends on its cross-sectional area.[41, 112] Perry[112] suggests a force of 4 kg/cm^2. Thus, the middle deltoid, with an area of 12 cm^2, exerts a force of 48 kg, whereas the anterior deltoid, at 9 cm^2, has a force of 36 kg. The smaller supraspinatus, which is 6 cm^2 in area, is capable of exerting a force of 24 kg (Table 38–2).

The force that a muscle exerts also depends on its leverage, i.e., the perpendicular distance between the muscle's line of pull and the center of motion. For muscles with broad areas of attachment, such as the deltoid, leverage changes as arm position changes.[111]

Forces acting on the shoulder joint tend to produce motion around an instant center of rotation in the humeral head. Poppen and Walker[114, 115] demonstrated that this center lies close to the geometric center of the humeral head in normal shoulders but not necessarily in pathologic shoulders, such as those with previous glenohumeral dislocations or rotator cuff tears.[114, 115] These forces can either enhance or detract from the function of the musculoligamentous structures in providing stability.

Thus, forces about the shoulder can be thought of as either destabilizing forces, producing shear, or stabilizing forces, producing compression. Combined forces produce both shear and compression (Fig. 38–15). Shear is directed parallel to the glenohumeral joint and tends to produce upward or downward displacement of the humeral head or prosthetic components. Compression forces, in contrast, are directed toward the joint surface, promoting stability of the joint. The compression forces are particularly important in the shoulder because it has so little inherent skeletal stability. Most muscles about the shoulder produce combined forces to varying degrees, depending on their anatomic alignment in the resting position with respect to the glenohumeral joint and on the position of the arm.[72]

Inman and colleagues[65] in 1944 analyzed the force contributed by the weight of the arm acting at its center of gravity, the force contributed by the abducting musculature, and the result of these two forces acting through the center of rotation of the shoulder. They calculated that the maximum force exerted against the glenoid was about 90 percent of body weight at 90

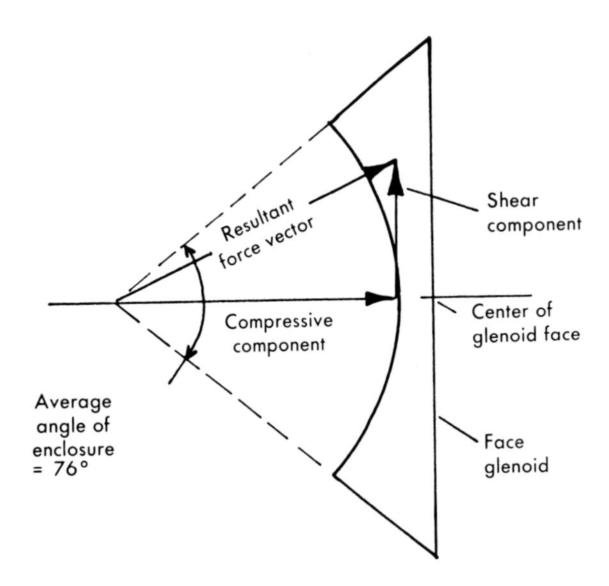

FIGURE 38–15. Compressive and shear components of the resultant force between the humeral head and the glenoid in the scapular plane. The resultant force vector becomes more compressive as the arm is elevated toward 90 degrees. (Walker, P. S.: Some Bioengineering Considerations of Prosthetic Replacement for the Glenohumeral Joint. Symposium on Total Joint Replacement of the Upper Extremity. Edited by A. E. Inglis. St. Louis, C.V. Mosby, 1982. By permission.)

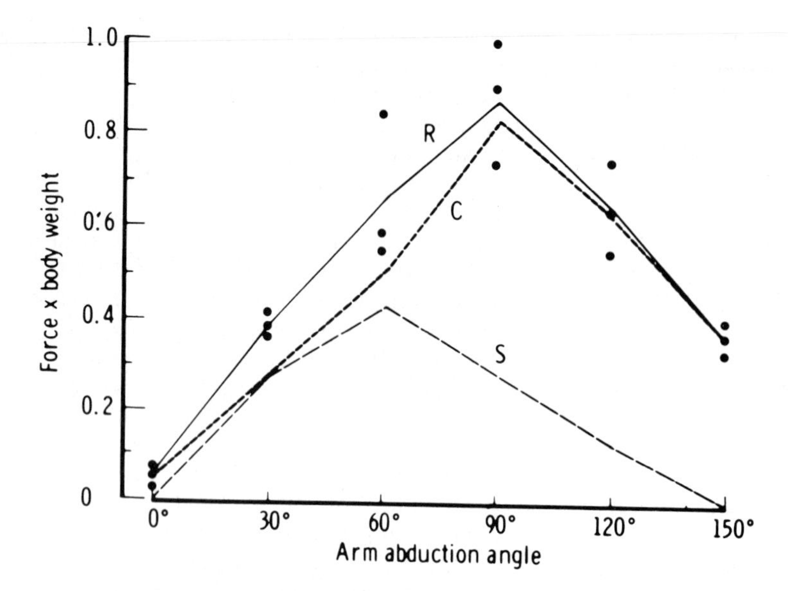

FIGURE 38–16. The resultant force (R) at the glenohumeral joint, the compressive component (C) perpendicular to the face of the glenoid, and the shear force (S) up the face of the glenoid. The three points at each angle are the results for three specimens. (Poppen, N. K. and Walker, P. S.: Forces at the glenohumeral joint in abduction. Clin. Orthop. 135:69, 1978. By permission.)

degrees of abduction and that the corresponding maximum force producing elevation was 8.2 times the weight of the extremity. In 1978, Poppen and Walker[115] demonstrated that the joint reaction force increases linearly with the degree of abduction. At 90 degrees of abduction, when the arm is perpendicular to the face of the glenoid, the force across the joint reaches a maximum of 0.89 times body weight (52 kg in a 70-kg man) (Fig. 38–16). This force is essentially the same magnitude proposed by Inman and coworkers.[65]

Poppen and Walker[115] also found that the shearing force along the face of the scapula becomes maximal at 60 degrees of abduction, when it reaches 0.42 times body weight. It then decreases linearly, reaching zero at 150 degrees of abduction. Therefore, the balance between shear and compression depends on arm position relative to the glenoid joint.

Most analyses of shoulder forces have been two dimensional. Morrey and Chao,[76] however, performed three-dimensional analysis, determining a medial contact force, an inferior shear force, an anterior shear force, and a joint resultant force. With the arm at 90 degrees of abduction and 90 degrees of external rotation, the unloaded shoulder demonstrated an anterior shear force of 12 kg. By comparison, the anterior shear force was 42 kg when the shoulder was abducted 90 degrees, externally rotated 90 degrees, and extended 30 degrees. With the arm in this position, the joint resultant force against the glenoid reached 222 kg. The prosthetic shoulder has to be capable of withstanding these high forces.[48]

Kinematics

Three types of surface motion may take place in any given plane at the glenohumeral joint: rotation, rolling, and translation or gliding.[134] During rotation—the main type of surface motion at this joint—the contact point on the glenoid remains constant, whereas the contact point on the humeral head changes. During rolling, the contact point on each joint surface changes by an equal amount. During gliding, the contact point on the humeral head remains constant, whereas that on the glenoid changes.

Poppen and Walker,[115] in their study of normal and abnormal motion of the shoulder, demonstrated some superior translation of the humeral head. It moved upward on the glenoid about 3 mm as the arm was abducted from 0 to 60 degrees in the plane of the scapula, probably a result of shear forces in early abduction. After 60 degrees of abduction, the maximum translation was 2 mm up or down with each successive position of the arm. Harryman and colleagues[58] found in cadaver studies that 5 mm of anterior translation was normal when the capsule was intact. If the capsule had been excised, no anterior translation occurred. In human volunteers, an obligate anterior translation of 2 to 5 mm could not be prevented.

INDICATIONS FOR SHOULDER ARTHROPLASTY

Total Shoulder Arthroplasty

The primary indication for total shoulder arthroplasty is pain from pathologic conditions of the glenohumeral joint that result in incongruity of the joint surfaces.[1–3, 18, 27, 39, 43, 44, 88] Relief of this pain is most important, whereas improvements in range of motion and function are secondary goals.

Specific conditions for which total shoulder arthroplasty is indicated, some of which are discussed in more detail hereafter, include the following:[22, 31, 36, 39, 45, 88, 94, 100, 106]

1. Osteoarthritis
2. Post-traumatic arthritis
3. Old fractures and fracture-dislocations
4. Rheumatoid arthritis
5. Nonrheumatoid inflammatory arthroses (e.g., ankylosing spondylitis, lupus)
6. Osteonecrosis
7. Arthritis of dislocation
8. Failed reconstructive shoulder surgery
    a. Humeral head replacement
    b. Proximal humeral head resection arthroplasty
    c. Shoulder arthrodesis
    d. Total shoulder replacement
9. Old sepsis
10. Some three-part and four-part fractures in which the glenoid has been damaged significantly
11. Proximal humeral neoplastic disease.

Total shoulder replacement should not be considered under certain circumstances. Contraindications include the following: (1) insufficient symptoms or pathology[25]; (2) recent active infection[25, 88, 100]; (3) neuropathic joint[25, 100]; (4) extensive paralysis, with loss of deltoid and rotator cuff function[20, 88, 100]; (5) extreme osteoporosis, with a flexible, insufficient glenoid[25]; and (6) marked medial resorption of the glenoid, leaving only a small scapular neck to articulate with the humeral head.[25, 100] In the last two conditions, the surgeon may have to be satisfied with implanting only a humeral head prosthesis, but a bone graft may occasionally allow a glenoid prosthesis.

Osteoarthritis

In osteoarthritis of the glenohumeral joint, cartilage on both articular surfaces is lost to variable degrees.[100, 105, 111, 123] The articular cartilage of the humeral head is thinnest in the area that articulates with the glenoid between 60 and 100 degrees of abduction. This is the area of maximum joint reactive force.[76, 115] The underlying bone becomes sclerotic and polished, and degenerative cysts develop.[39, 88, 100] Marginal osteophytes develop around the head, especially at the inferior margins (Fig. 38–17).[79, 100]

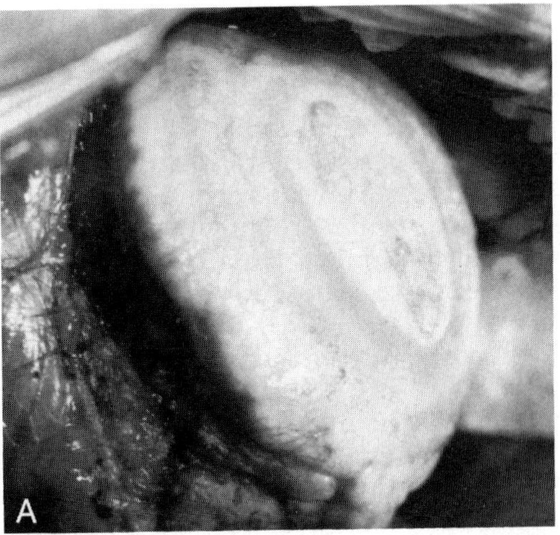

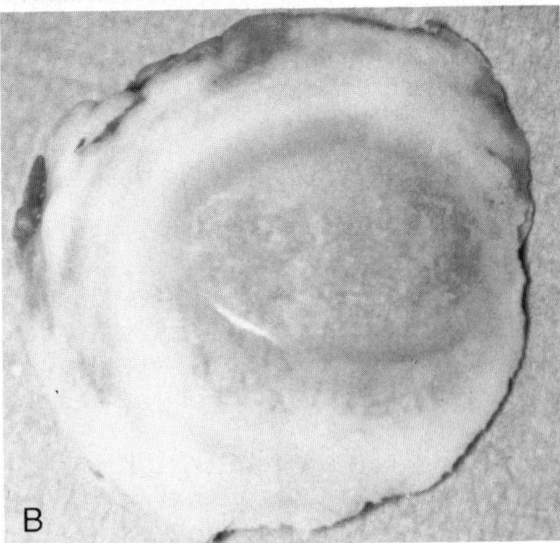

FIGURE 38–17. *A, In situ* view of an osteoarthritic humeral head at surgery. Note the central erosion of articular cartilage and the marginal osteophyte formation. *B,* The same humeral head removed at surgery, with a direct view of the area of central cartilage erosion.

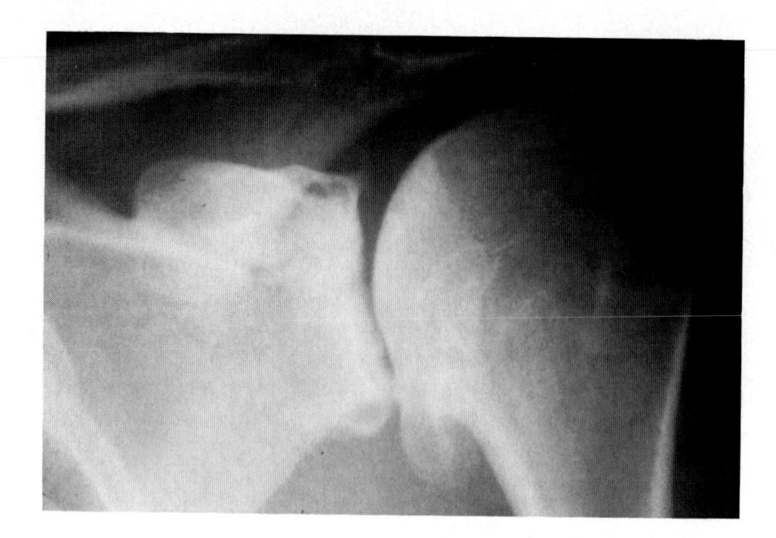

FIGURE 38–18. Radiograph showing changes typical of osteoarthritis of the glenohumeral joint, including narrowing of the joint cartilage, sclerosis, and typical teardrop type of inferior humeral head osteophyte.

The glenoid becomes flattened and demonstrates some of the same subchondral eburnation as the humeral head. The glenoid tends to wear posteriorly, causing the surface to slope in that direction.[39, 84] This deficit, which also can occur in arthritis of dislocation and rheumatoid arthritis, sometimes requires bone grafting to provide adequate seating for the glenoid prosthesis.[84]

In osteoarthritis, the rotator cuff is often intact.[26, 88] The cuff tears that are present are usually small or moderate in size.

Radiographs show typical reactive bone formation, subchondral cyst formation, narrowing of the joint cartilage, and marginal osteophytes (Fig. 38–18). Asymmetric glenoid wear is sometimes seen on the axillary view.[39]

Rheumatoid Arthritis

This disease process involves varying degrees of destruction of both skeletal and soft tissue components of the joint.[79, 87, 100, 106] In the more acute phases, when synovial proliferation is common, synovectomy is a necessary part of the surgical procedure.

The quality of the rotator cuff tissue in rheumatoid arthritis is often poor.[26, 39, 66, 73, 87, 88] In a series of 69 shoulders afflicted with rheumatoid arthritis, Neer[87] found that thinning of the rotator cuff was common. Complete thickness tears of the cuff of varying severity were seen in 42 percent of the cases. Most of the tears could be repaired, but 12 patients demonstrated massive disruption of the cuff.[87] Cofield[26, 28] found rotator cuff tears of varying sizes in 27 percent of 66 shoulders affected by rheumatoid arthritis. The bone is almost invariably osteoporotic and the glenoid often deficient (Fig. 38–19).

Because the acromioclavicular joint is often involved in the disease process, excision of this joint concomitantly with total shoulder arthroplasty is often wise. Continuing disease in this joint could impede a satisfactory outcome following replacement arthroplasty.[88]

As the disease becomes less acute, secondary degenerative changes can be superimposed on the rheumatoid destruction. It is in this inactive stage that total shoulder replacement is often most successful.

Secondary Degenerative Arthritis

Conditions that produce changes in the articular cartilage, the bone structure, or both promote the development of secondary degenerative arthritis. Such conditions include trauma, osteonecrosis, infection, nonrheumatoid inflammatory arthritis, metabolic disease affecting articular cartilage such as gout, instability or dislocations, massive long-standing cuff tears (cuff tear arthropathy), and radiation necrosis.

In arthritis of dislocation, secondary degenerative changes result from damage to the glenohumeral joint produced by instability and recurrent dislocation or sublux-

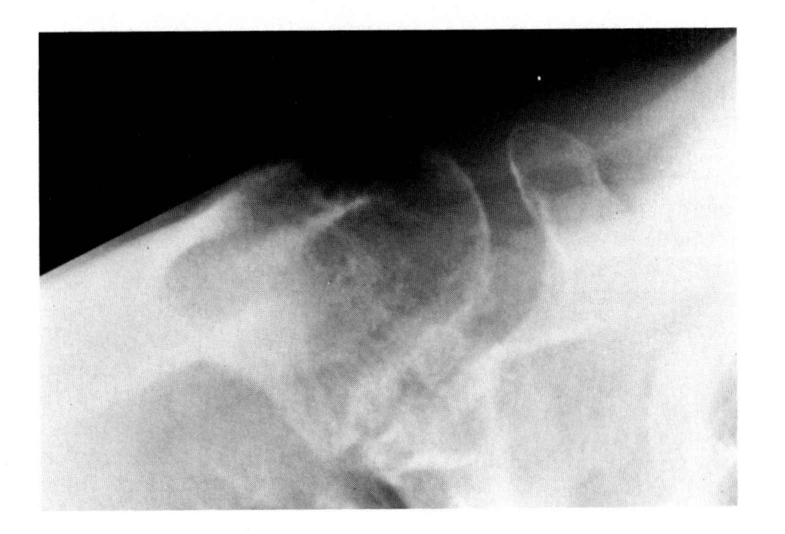

FIGURE 38–19. Radiographic changes characteristic of rheumatoid arthritis, including osteopenia and destruction of the humeral head as the disease progresses.

ation. Arthritis of dislocation also can result from an incorrectly performed repair procedure that produces fixed subluxation in a direction opposite that of the dislocation.[39, 88, 122, 125, 126] Special surgical techniques may be required not only because of the secondary degenerative changes but also because of significant erosion of the posterior and sometimes anterior glenoid. The high side of the glenoid or the version of the humeral component may need to be altered. Sometimes bone grafting of the glenoid is necessary.[36, 97, 100, 102] Shoulders in which severe degenerative changes are associated with multidirectional instability may require posterior capsule tightening to prevent posterior dislocations of the prostheses.

The term cuff tear arthropathy applies to a type of degenerative arthritis that develops because of longstanding, massive rotator cuff tear.[90] Cuff tear arthropathy is thought to result from loss of synovial fluid pressure and, therefore, loss of nutrition of the articular cartilage in association with instability of the humeral head. The humeral head eventually migrates superiorly, causing erosion of the glenoid and acromion. A characteristic radiologic feature is collapse of the proximal portion of the articular surface of the humeral head. In most patients, superior migration of the humeral head is quite evident (Fig. 38–20). Associated subluxations or dislocations are common. The articular cartilage becomes completely denuded on both sides

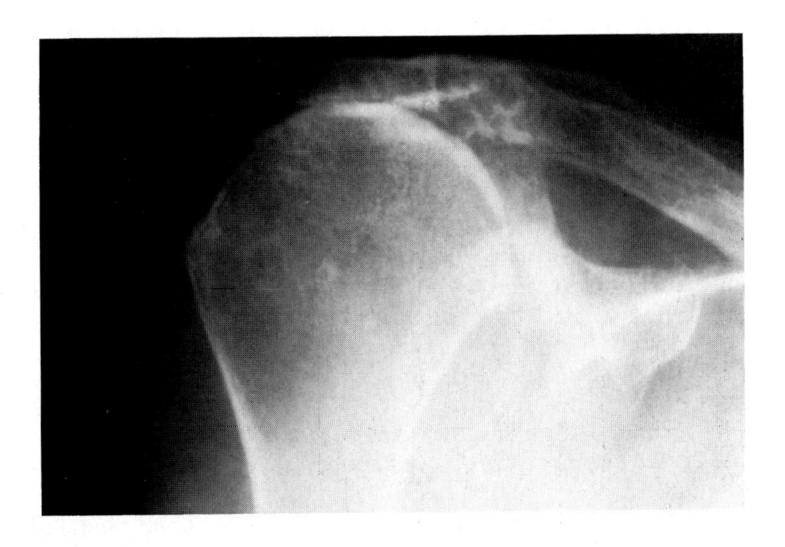

FIGURE 38–20. Radiographic changes typical of cuff tear arthropathy. Note the superior migration of the humeral head with impingement on the acromion and the superiorly oriented degenerative changes.

at points of contact between the humeral head and glenoid. All of these pathologic changes make treatment of cuff tear arthropathy difficult.

Trauma to the shoulder can result in nonunion and malunion of fractures, osteonecrosis, and secondary degenerative changes involving both sides of the joint. Associated scarring and contracture of soft tissue about the joint make reconstruction difficult.[39, 88, 106]

Hemiarthroplasty

If the glenoid is in good condition, it need not be replaced. Hemiarthroplasty with a humeral head prosthesis alone can be quite satisfactory, but results are not as predictable as those when both surfaces are replaced.[22, 39, 84, 133] Indications for hemiarthroplasty include the following:

1. Four-part fractures and fracture-dislocations in which the glenoid remains undamaged.[22, 32, 80, 82, 93, 95, 104, 108, 128, 129]
2. Some three-part fractures in elderly or debilitated patients.[82, 93, 104, 108]
3. Any other fracture of the proximal humerus with complete separation of the head fragment from the humeral shaft and soft tissues.[25, 80, 93, 104, 108]
4. Nonunions of the upper humerus in elderly or debilitated patients with poor bone stock.[25, 93, 105, 132]
5. Such severe deficiencies of the glenoid bone stock that not enough remains for secure fixation of the glenoid prosthesis. This can occur, for example, in some patients with rheumatoid arthritis.[22, 24, 31, 73, 100]
6. Certain fractures of the humeral head and neck associated with fracture of the humeral shaft. Both fracture sites can be treated with the prosthesis, with the stem serving as a transfracture intramedullary rod.
7. Splitting fractures of the humeral head.[82, 93, 104, 108]
8. Malunions of the proximal humerus in which the glenoid remains intact but the humeral articular surface has been damaged.[11, 24, 100, 104, 129]
9. Osteonecrosis with an intact glenoid.[22, 25, 93, 104]
10. Some benign or malignant tumors of the upper humerus that do not involve the glenoid.[10, 64, 100]
11. Chronic dislocations of the shoulder in which the humeral head has become soft and osteoporotic. These might occur, for example, with longstanding anterior dislocations of the humeral head.[25, 99, 100, 122, 125]

Acute Fractures and Fracture Dislocations

In a study on displaced proximal humeral fractures published in 1970, Neer[81] analyzed 300 such fractures treated with either closed reduction or surgery (open reduction or prosthetic replacement). Those patients with fracture fragment displacement of less than 1 cm or angulation of less than 45 degrees between the fragments had good clinical results. The fractures could be treated most satisfactorily with short-term immobilization and early rehabilitation. Neer[81, 85] classified displaced fractures and fracture-dislocations as two-, three-, and four-part fractures.

In a separate report, Neer[82] analyzed 117 consecutive patients with three-part and four-part proximal humeral fractures treated by closed reduction, open reduction, or prosthetic replacement of the proximal humerus. Closed reduction produced satisfactory results in only three of 77 shoulders. Open reduction produced satisfactory results in 19 of 30 three-part fractures (63 percent) but in none of the 13 four-part fractures. Osteonecrosis developed in six of eight four-part fractures in which the head of the humerus was retained at open reduction (75 percent). A proximal humeral prosthesis was utilized to treat 11 patients with three-part injuries, and eight of them had satisfactory results (73 percent). A prosthesis was also applied in the treatment of 32 four-part injuries, and 31 of these had satisfactory results (97 percent). Neer concluded that the preferred treatment for four-part fractures was prosthetic humeral head replacement, whereas that for three-part fractures was open reduction. Further experience has shown that replacement arthroplasty can be beneficial in certain three-part fractures in which satisfactory reduction cannot be maintained.[104, 129]

Four-part fractures are associated with a notoriously high incidence of osteonecrosis of the humeral head (75 to 80 percent) if they are treated by closed or open reduction. If the fracture separates the head from all soft tissue attachments, osteonecrosis is virtually assured. The appropriate treatment of four-part fractures is prosthetic arthroplasty with repair of the rotator cuff and tuberosities.[82, 104, 129]

Ideally, three-part fractures and fracture-dislocations should be treated by open reduction and internal fixation. Stable fixation can be achieved with such techniques as tension band suture combined with Ender intramedullary rods.[82, 100, 104, 108] Because screws and plates are avoided, earlier rehabilitation can be carried out. In the patient with good bone stock, these techniques work well. In the older or debilitated patient, prosthetic arthroplasty and early rehabilitation are sometimes more appropriate.[104] Some of these patients have such poor bone stock that fixation that would allow early rehabilitation is impossible. In other cases, the fractures come apart with rehabilitation, and nonunion subsequently develops. These patients tolerate prolonged immobilization poorly. Such immobilization always has an adverse effect on the soft tissues about the shoulder. Scarring and contracture ultimately lead to poor results.

Acute fractures appropriately treated by prosthetic arthroplasty thus include the following:

1. Four-part fractures and fracture-dislocations
2. Three-part fractures that are unstable or fail after open reduction
3. Head splitting fractures
4. Impression fractures of the humeral head involving 50 percent or more of the articular surface
5. Fractures of the anatomic neck of the humerus in which the humeral head is deprived of soft tissue attachments and blood supply.

Rarely, prosthetic arthroplasty might be appropriate to treat a severely comminuted fracture of the proximal end of the humerus associated with a fracture of the midhumeral shaft. Prostheses with long stems, which can serve as transfracture intramedullary rods, are used in these cases.

PREOPERATIVE EVALUATION

The first step in preoperative evaluation is to analyze the patient's shoulder problem clinically and radiographically. A complete general history and physical examination are performed (see Chapter 10, *Anesthesia for Joint Replacement Surgery*, and Chapter 16, *Total Hip Arthroplasty: Preoperative Evaluation*). Both active and passive range of motion of the shoulder are evaluated, paying special attention to rotator cuff function. Neurovascular status is determined.

The radiographic studies include true anteroposterior views of the glenohumeral joint with the arm first in internal rotation, then in external rotation; a lateral scapular view; and an axillary view (Fig. 38–21).[81, 93, 104] Other specialized views can be made as necessary. Little movement or positioning of the patient's arm is required to obtain these radiographs. This situation is especially helpful when evaluating acute injuries.

Other specialized studies that might be helpful in preoperative assessment include arthrography, computerized tomography, magnetic resonance imaging, electromyography, and nerve conduction studies.[107]

After analyzing the patient's shoulder problem, the clinician should define it in terms of its component parts so that each can be addressed properly at surgery, if indicated. For example, the definition of a painful shoulder might include degenerative arthritis involving both joint surfaces, some wear of the posterior glenoid, and associated symptomatic disease in the acromioclavicular joint. Having thus defined the problem, the surgeon can address each aspect to optimize the results.

Cofield[32] proposed a stepwise analysis for fractures of the proximal end of the humerus. Before obtaining radiographs, the clinician should conduct a thorough physical examination that includes a neuromotor assessment. The ability of the shoulder and upper arm muscles to contract isometrically should be evaluated. Nerve injury is not uncommon with comminuted proximal humeral fractures, and a peripheral examination determines whether all nerves are intact (Table 38–3).[68] Peripheral reflexes should also be evaluated (Table 38–4). When denervation patterns begin to appear, 2 to 3 weeks after the injury, electromyographic evaluation of the muscles about the shoulder may be helpful.[8] Peripheral vasculature should also be as-

TRAUMA SERIES—THREE "PAINLESS" VIEWS

X-RAY EVALUATION IN THREE
RIGHT-ANGLE PLANES IS ESSENTIAL

AP in scapular plane.

Arm supported
in sling.

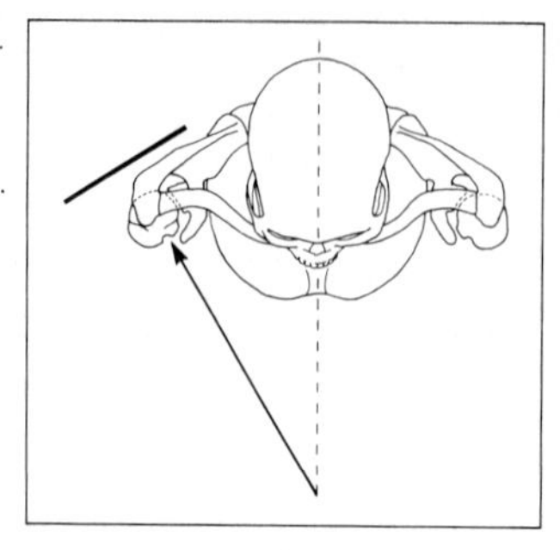

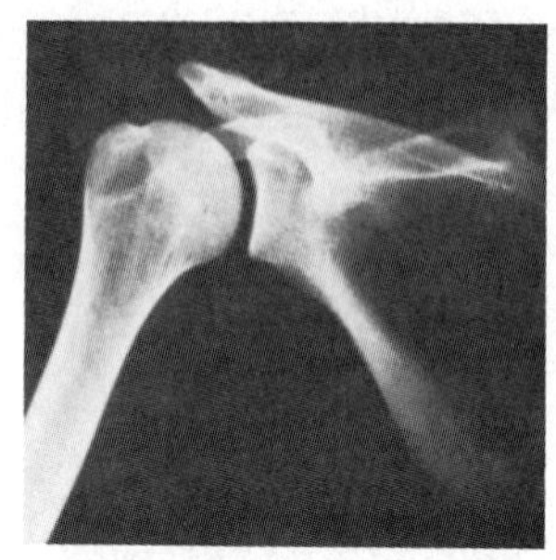

No overlap of head
and glenoid.

Lateral in
scapular plane.

Arm supported
in sling.

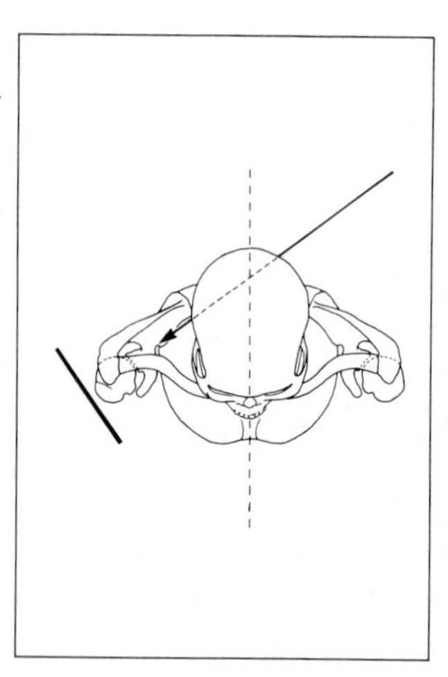

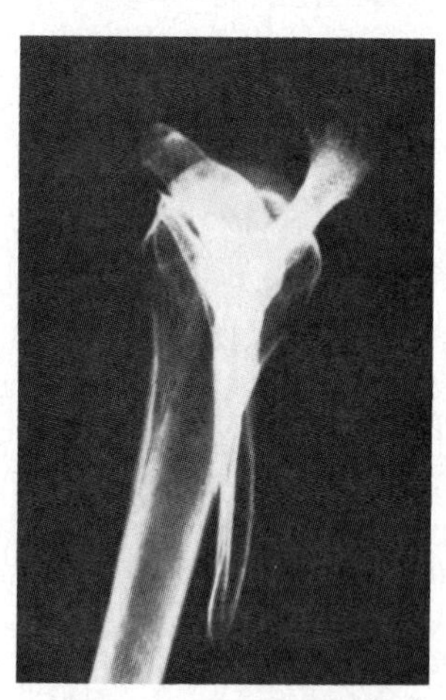

90° to AP.

Head in center of Ɏ.

Identify anterior and
posterior displacement.

Identify greater
tuberosity displacement.

Evaluate shape of
acromion for etiology of
impingement or cuff
tears.

Emergency axillary.

Arm is gently
abducted.

Tube at the hip.

Involved shoulder
supported on pad.

Arm holds I.V. pole
or supported
by assistant.

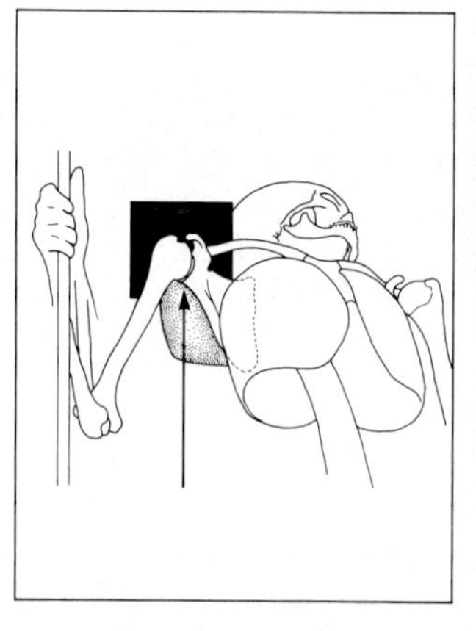

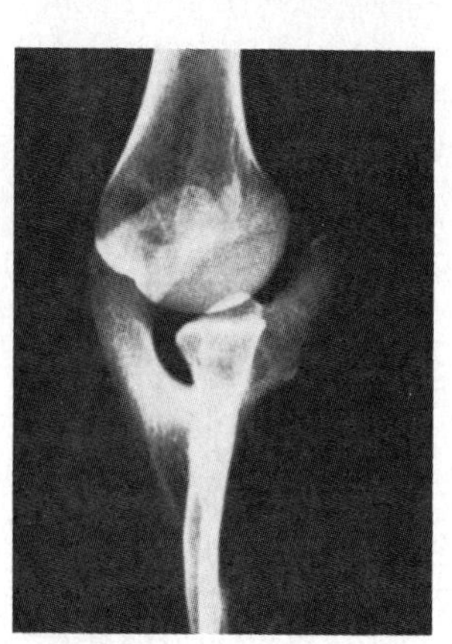

Evaluate glenoid
for uneven wear or rim
fractures.

Identify anterior and
posterior dislocation.

Identify displaced
tuberosities.

Identify unfused
acromial epiphysis.

ALL VIEWS MAY BE MADE WITH THE
PATIENTS STANDING—SITTING—SUPINE

FIGURE 38–21. Three basic views for evaluating the shoulder. (Adapted from Norris, T. R.: Fractures and Dislocations of the Glenohumeral Complex. Operative Orthopaedics, vol. 1. Edited by M. Chapman. Philadelphia, J. B. Lippincott Company, 1988. By permission.)

Table 38–3. COMMON MOTORS OF THE ARM, HAND, AND WRIST THAT CAN BE QUICKLY TESTED FOR NERVE DEFICIT[40, 60, 75]

Root	Motor	Nerve	Cord
C5–C6	Biceps	Musculocutaneous	Lateral
C6–C7–C8	Triceps	Radial	Posterior
C6–C7–C8	Wrist extensors ECRL and ECRB (C6–C7) ECU (C7–C8)	Radial	Posterior
C7–C8	Finger extensors EDC	Radial	Posterior
C7–C8–T1	Finger flexors		
	FDP, index, long	Median	Medial
C8–T1	FDP, ring, little	Ulnar	Medial
C6–C7–C8–T1	Wrist flexors		
	FCR (C6, C7)	Median	Medial
	FCU (C7–C8–T1)	Ulnar	Medial
C8–T1	Finger abductors 1st DI Abductor digiti quinti	Ulnar	Medial

sessed, although injury to the axillary vessels is infrequent.[32]

The first step in the analysis of radiographs for proximal humeral fractures is to identify the position of the humeral head in relation to the articular surface of the glenoid.[32] This identification determines whether an anterior, lateral, or posterior dislocation or subluxation is present. The next step is to define the relationship of the head and shaft fragments to each other. Lastly, the greater and lesser tuberosities are identified, and their relationship to the humeral head is determined. This analysis enables the surgeon to identify and determine the position of all four segments of the humeral head. If there is any question about identification of fragments on plain radiographs, a computerized tomogram is obtained.[104] If there is a question about the length of the humerus, scanograms may be obtained.[104] Having defined the fracture fragments and determined the fracture type, the surgeon can develop the treatment plan.

All evaluations should be recorded in a standardized format. Reports in the literature from different centers thereby become comparable and more meaningful. The format devised by the American Shoulder and Elbow Surgeons is recommended (Table 38–5). It is designed to evaluate, grade, and record pain, range of both active and passive motion, strength, stability, and function.

Table 38–4. COMMONLY TESTED REFLEXES IN THE UPPER EXTREMITY WITH THEIR ROOT INNERVATIONS[40, 60]

Reflex	Root
Biceps	C5–C6
Brachioradialis	C5–C6
Triceps	C7
Extensor carpi ulnaris	C8

PROSTHESES FOR SHOULDER ARTHROPLASTY

Design

Three basic types of prosthetic shoulder designs are available: (1) unconstrained, such as the Neer prosthesis; (2) constrained, such as the Michael Reese prosthesis; and (3) semiconstrained, an example being the Gristina prosthesis (Fig. 38–22).[57] In the unconstrained prosthesis, stability depends on an intact, functioning rotator cuff mechanism. The totally constrained prosthesis is not dependent on the musculoligamentous tissues for stability. The semiconstrained prosthesis is primarily dependent on the cuff mechanism, but some constraint is built into its design.[37] Most commonly, the glenoid component of a semiconstrained prosthesis is shaped so that it roofs over the superior aspect of the humeral component, thus resisting the upward shear force produced when the arm is elevated.[56]

Table 38–5. AMERICAN SHOULDER AND ELBOW SURGEONS EXAMINATION DATA FORM

Evaluation Date:
Name: Chart# Dominance:
List findings as Involved/Uninvolved: (R/L) (L/R) Bilateral?
Diagnosis:
Previous surgery:
Number of steroid injections:

I. Pain: *(5 = none, 4 = slight, 3 = after unusual activity, 2 = moderate, 1 = marked, 0 = complete disability)*
II. Shoulder Motion:
  A. Patient sitting:
    1. Active total elevation of arm: / degrees
    2. Active external rotation with arm at side: / degrees
    3. Active rotation—90 degrees abduction: / degrees
    4. Passive internal rotation (segment reached): /*

**1 = Less than trochanter*	*5 = L5*	*9 = L1*	*13 = T9*	*17 = T5*
2 = Trochanter	*6 = L4*	*10 = T12*	*14 = T8*	*18 = T4*
3 = Gluteal	*7 = L3*	*11 = T11*	*15 = T7*	*19 = T3*
4 = Sacrum	*8 = L2*	*12 = T10*	*16 = T6*	*20 = T2*

  B. Patient supine:
    1. Passive total elevation of arm: / degrees
    2. Passive external rotation with arm at side: / degrees
    3. Passive external rotation—90 degrees abduction: / degrees
    4. Passive internal rotation—90 degrees abduction: / degrees
    **Total elevation of arm measured by viewing patient from side and using goniometer to determine angle between arm and thorax.*
  C. Impingement:
    1. Painful arc of motion: /
    2. Relieved by subacromial xylocaine injection: /
    3. Crepitus: /
III. Strength: *(5 = normal, 4 = good, 3 = fair, 2 = poor, 1 = trace, 0 = paralysis)*
  A. Anterior deltoid: /
  B. Middle deltoid: /
  C. External rotation: /
  D. Internal rotation: /
  E. Trapezius /
  F. Triceps /
  G. Biceps /
IV. Stability: *(5 = normal, 4 = apprehension, 3 = rare subluxation, 2 = recurrent subluxation, 1 = recurrent dislocation, 0 = fixed dislocation)*
  A. Anterior: /
  B. Posterior: /
  C. Inferior: /
  D. Superior: /
V. Function: *(4 = normal, 3 = mild compromise, 2 = difficulty, 1 = with aid, 0 = unable)*
  F1. / Use back pocket
  F2. / Rectal hygiene
  F3. / Wash opposite underarm
  F4. / Eat with utensil
  F5. / Comb hair
  F6. / Use hand/arm @ shoulder
  F7. / Carry 10–15 lb/arm at side
  F8. / Dress
  F9. / Sleep on shoulder
  F10. / Pulling
  F11. / Use hand overhead
  F12. / Throwing
  F13. / Lifting
  F14. / Do usual work
  F15. / Do usual sport
VI. Patient Response: / *(3 = much better, 2 = better, 1 = same, 0 = worse)*

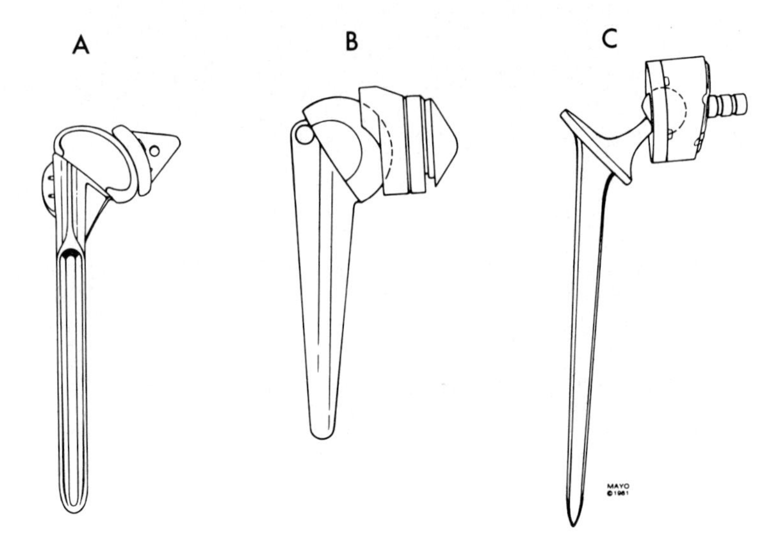

FIGURE 38–22. Three basic types of shoulder prostheses. *A*, Unconstrained (Neer). *B*, Semiconstrained (Gristina). *C*, Constrained (Michael Reese). (Cofield, R. H.: The Shoulder and Prosthetic Arthroplasty. Surgery of the Musculoskeletal System. Edited by C. M. Evarts. New York, Churchill Livingstone, 1983. By permission from the Mayo Foundation.)

Neer Prosthesis

Neer conceived and designed the humeral head prosthesis in response to the poor results of standard treatment of fracture-dislocation of the shoulder.[78, 80] The original prosthesis replaced only the articular surface of the humeral head. The design enabled the tuberosity fragments, with attached rotator cuff, to be secured to the prosthesis through a hole in the neck of the prosthesis. Variation in the diameter of the medullary canal was addressed by three different stem diameters. Early results demonstrated good pain relief and reasonably good function.

In 1973, Neer redesigned the original humeral head prosthesis, changing the flattened head and overhanging edges so that it could be used with a polyethylene glenoid prosthesis. The latter conformed to the radius of curvature of the articulating surface of the glenoid. Neer[80, 88] reviewed his experience in 1982 in a series of 273 shoulders with metal-to-plastic glenohumeral units. Whereas pain relief was good and predictable, function was dependent on the quality of the rotator cuff and deltoid muscles. The nearly normal anatomic design of the Neer-type prosthesis allows maximum return of function. A minimal amount of bone must be removed, preserving the soft tissue attachments, especially the rotator cuff. The design avoids mechanical blocking of prosthetic movements and emphasizes reconstruction and rehabilitation of the soft tissues about the prosthesis.[88]

The radius of the curvature of all the humeral head prostheses is 26 mm. Two head thicknesses are available: 23 mm, or the large head, and 15 mm, or the small head. Each head thickness comes with three different stem diameters: 6.3, 9.5, and 12.7 mm. The stems are slightly thicker proximally for better press-fit (Fig. 38–23). Special drills and tapered reamers, corresponding to each diameter, enable proper shaping and sizing of the stem channel (Fig. 38–24). Different stem lengths are available.

Glenoid Prostheses

Two Neer glenoid prostheses are available: the standard polyethylene prosthesis and the metal-backed modification. A modification of the Neer II glenoid component incorporates two screws and a porous coating on the metal tray (Fig. 38–25).

The porous-coated glenoid component requires minimal removal of bone stock. Fixation depends on a precise fit and screws, with the potential for bone ingrowth, although the prosthesis can be fixed with bone cement.[35, 36] The metal glenoid prosthesis is fixed to the glenoid first. The polyethylene articular surface is then press-fit into the metal tray.

Constrained Prostheses

On occasion, a fully constrained shoulder prosthesis may be indicated as a salvage procedure in a patient who has continued

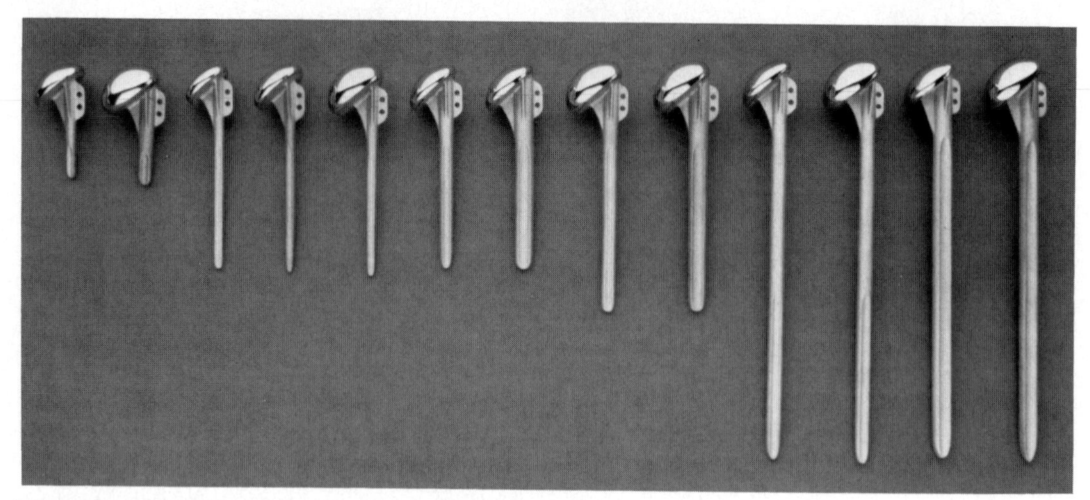

FIGURE 38–23. Neer II System humeral head prostheses. Special sizes are not pictured. (Courtesy of Kirschner Medical Corporation.)

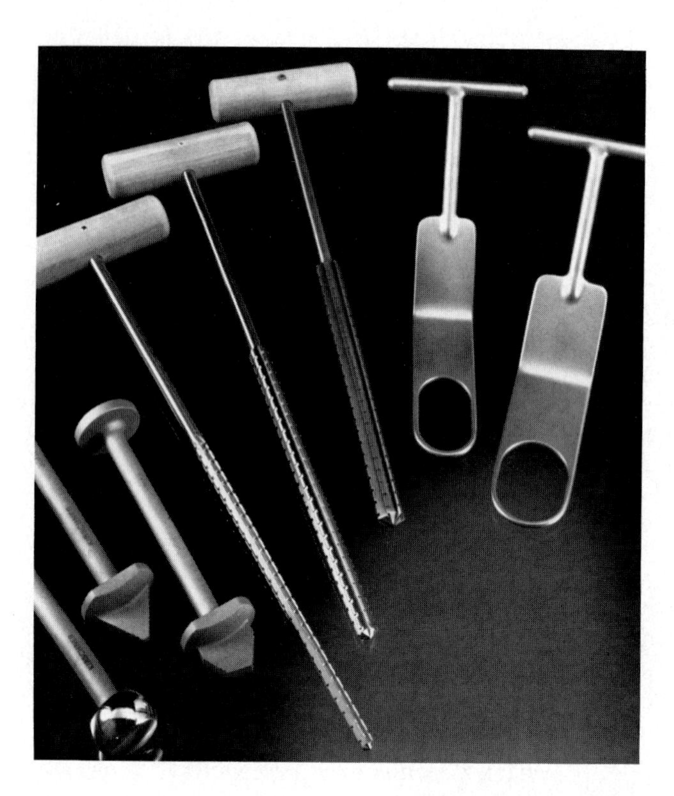

FIGURE 38–24. Instrumentation available for the Neer II system. From left to right are an impactor, a keel broach for the Neer polyethylene glenoid, a keel broach for the Neer metal-backed glenoid, the three sizes of tapered reamer for the three stem sizes for the humeral head prostheses, and two Fukuda retractors. (Courtesy of Kirschner Medical Corporation.)

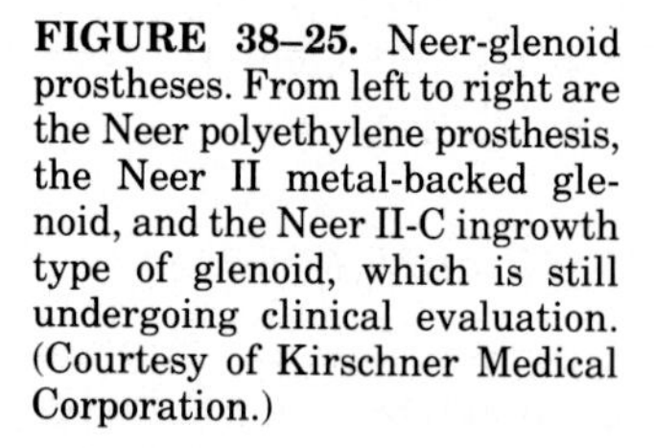

FIGURE 38–25. Neer-glenoid prostheses. From left to right are the Neer polyethylene prosthesis, the Neer II metal-backed glenoid, and the Neer II-C ingrowth type of glenoid, which is still undergoing clinical evaluation. (Courtesy of Kirschner Medical Corporation.)

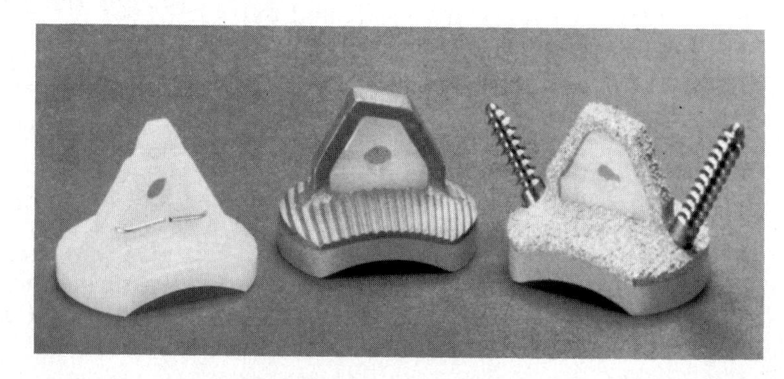

severe pain in an unstable shoulder without a rotator cuff. Sometimes, a constrained prosthesis may be implanted as a replacement in resection surgery for malignancy. The Michael Reese, Stanmore, and Trispherical prostheses may be used in these circumstances.[55, 70, 116–121]

By nature of the design of any completely constrained prosthesis, stresses at the bone-implant interface are increased. This finding is especially true in the glenoid, making loosening of the component more likely.[50, 121] Dislocation of the implants and instability have also been reported.[36]

Constrained total shoulder arthroplasty should be done only when unconstrained arthroplasty with its relatively low risk and greater durability cannot be performed.[119, 121] Perhaps in some instances shoulder arthrodesis might be a better choice.[21]

Modular shoulder systems have been introduced of late. These allow the surgeon to change the humeral head size without removing the stem of the humeral component from the bone. Thus, tension of the rotator cuff can be adjusted. Unfortunately, *in vivo* dissociation of modular heads has occurred.

Prosthesis Loading

Glenoid Prosthesis

The shear and compression forces that load the shoulder joint make the design of a glenoid prosthesis challenging.[110] Neer's[88] basic design of the glenoid prosthesis included a triangular keel. Metal backing was added later to improve stress distribution. Stresses on constrained shoulder prostheses are especially critical, and the main point of failure often is the glenoid fixation.

Fukuda and colleagues[52] analyzed the stability and fixation strength of four different types of glenoid prostheses: the Neer I (polyethylene only), the Neer II (polyethylene with a metal backing), the Cofield, and the Gristina models. One objective was to determine the shear force or load required to sublux the humeral head component on the glenoid prosthesis under varying compressive loads. A linear relationship was found between the subluxation force and the compressive load on the articulating surface (Fig. 38–26). The larger curvature of the Gristina glenoid created the greatest resistance to subluxation. The investigators suggested that in

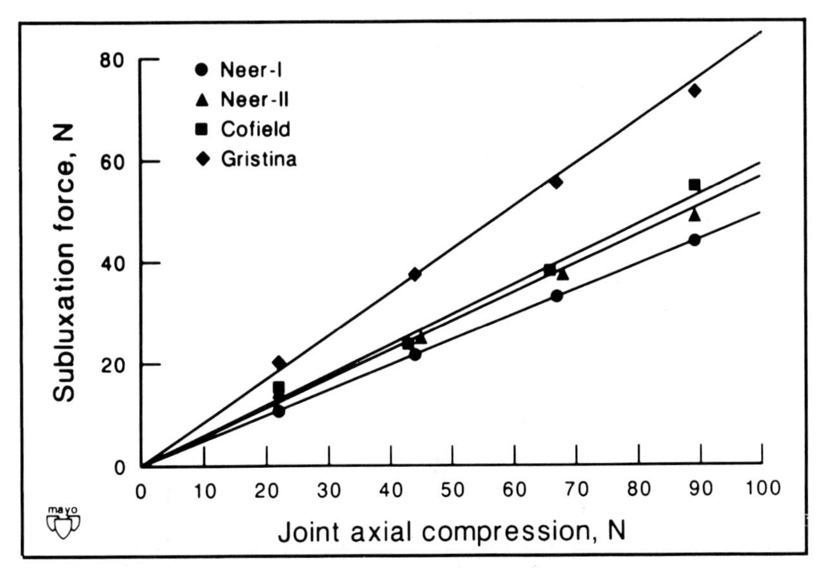

FIGURE 38–26. Linear relationship between anteroposterior subluxation forces of the humeral prosthetic components on the different glenoids used in Fukuda's study and increasing compressive loads. Superior subluxation forces followed the same pattern but the forces were greater.[65] (Fukuda, K., Chen, C., Cofield, R. H., and Chao, E. Y. S.: Biomechanical analysis of stability and fixation strength of total shoulder prostheses. Orthopedics 2:141–149, 1988. By permission from the Mayo Foundation.)

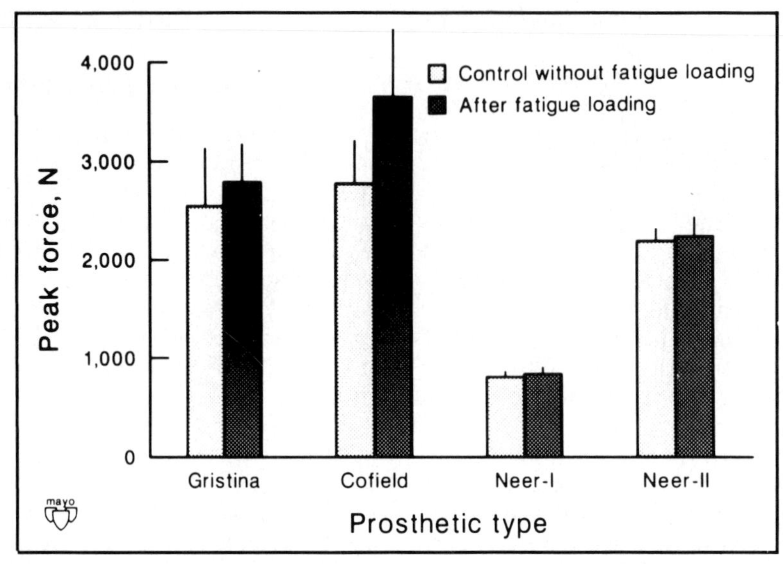

FIGURE 38–27. Comparison of the peak distraction force of the glenoid components used in Fukuda's study before and after fatigue-loading of 1 million cycles.[65] The Cofield and Gristina glenoids demonstrated the highest peak distraction forces. (Fukuda, K., Chen, C., Cofield, R. H., and Chao, E. Y. S.: Biomechanical analysis of stability and fixation strength of total shoulder prostheses. Orthopedics 2:141–149, 1988. By permission from the Mayo Foundation.)

cases in which superior subluxation is a clinical problem, a prosthesis with a greater curvature might be indicated. Proper placement of the humeral head in relation to the glenoid, these workers concluded, would prevent eccentric loading and thereby reduce subluxation and wear.[52]

These investigators also sought to define the loading directions and conditions that might contribute to loosening of the glenoid. The tests showed that the Cofield design resisted pull-out best, whereas the Neer I prosthesis could be pulled out most easily (Fig. 38–27). The Neer I failed by fracture through the serrated grooves in the keel. The other three glenoid designs studied had sufficient fixation strength to resist normal shoulder joint forces.[52]

Orr and coworkers[110] performed finite element stress analyses on two keel geometries. One design was a triangular configuration, implanted in the center of the glenoid cavity. The other, a rectangular design, was implanted so that the stem rested at an angle on the inferior wall of the glenoid. Stress patterns in the natural glenoid corresponded with the trabecular patterns. With an all-plastic component, the load was transmitted centrally. Bone stresses near the edges of the component were less than those for the natural joint. Stress distributions with the metal-backed component were similar to those with the all-plastic glenoid, but the magnitude of bone stresses was slightly less, except directly beneath the metal tray. Metal backing, therefore, may improve the transfer of stress to cortical bone. The rectangular keel, angled to rest on the inferior cortex, was found to counteract the bending moments produced by joint loading. However, the investigators cautioned that surgeons might have difficulty inserting this type of stem in a confined space.[110]

In addition, Orr and coworkers[110] tested a glenoid prosthesis with a superior constraint to prevent upward shear displacement. Tensile stresses at the prosthetic interface were increased inferiorly, and compressive forces were increased superiorly. These forces might contribute to loosening of such constrained designs.[110]

The bony anatomy of the scapula plays an important role in securing fixation of the prosthesis to the glenoid. Studying sections of glenoids, Post and associates[116] noted that the vault was covered with cortical bone around a mass of cancellous bone (Fig. 38–28). The greatest cancellous density was just beneath the thin cortical plate. Inept surgical technique or disease

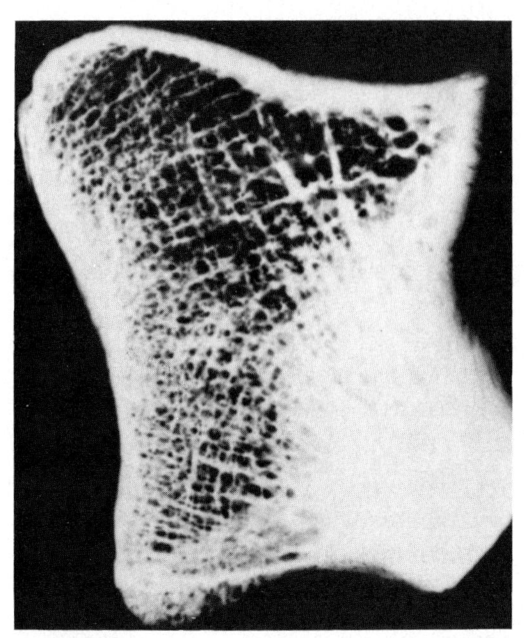

FIGURE 38–28. Frontal section of the glenoid. Note the thickened subchondral bone and the trabecular pattern. (Orr, T. E., Carter, D. R., and Schurman, D. J.: Stress analysis of glenoid component designs. Clin. Orthop. 232:217–224, 1988. By permission.)

that destroys the cortical vault cover or the subchondral glenoid plate or that decreases the cancellous bone mass weakens the glenoid and predisposes to loosening.[116]

Humerus

Orr and Carter[109] did a similar stress analysis of the upper humerus with and without a prosthesis implanted. The loading cases tested were 0, 45, and 90 degrees of abduction. The design geometries tested included prosthetic-bone interfaces that were convex, flat, and concave. The analysis showed that in the normal humerus, compressive joint forces are transmitted from the articular surface through the cancellous bone to the inferior cortical shell. The stress patterns corresponded with the trabecular morphologic patterns of the humeral head. With a fully porous coated prosthesis, stresses in the proximal humerus changed significantly. However, when only the undersurface of the prosthetic head was porous coated, the stress distribution was similar to that of the normal humerus. Orr and Carter[109] concluded that implantation of uncemented smooth stems reduces adverse bone remodeling and creates more normal stress fields.

Prosthesis Motion

Studying glenohumeral and scapulothoracic motion after total shoulder replacement, Friedman[49] found little translation or excursion of the humeral prosthesis on the glenoid, less than 2 mm superiorly or inferiorly during the entire arc of motion. He concluded that this meant a higher degree of conformity and stability between the prosthetic components than in the normal glenohumeral joint. In patients with total shoulder arthroplasties, the ratio of glenohumeral to scapulothoracic motion was normal between 90 and 120 degrees of abduction. Between 0 and 90 degrees of abduction, however, each degree of glenohumeral motion was associated with two degrees of scapulothoracic motion. Friedman[49] concluded that from 0 to 90 degrees of abduction, less motion occurs between the prosthetic components than in a normal joint, but the scapulothoracic motion remains unchanged.

Biomechanical analysis of 14 hemiarthroplasties performed for four-part fractures suggested a direct relationship between the "humeral offset" and the patient's ability to abduct the humerus (Fig. 38–29).[123] Humeral offset was defined as the distance between the geometric center of the humeral head and the lateral aspect of the greater tuberosity. Reduction of the distance between the geometric prosthetic center and the greater tuberosity reduced the lever arm for both the supraspinatus and the deltoid. This finding emphasizes the biomechanical advantage of restoring anatomy to normal. Proper placement and design of the prosthesis help the surgeon create a satisfactory lever arm for these two abductors.

SURGICAL TECHNIQUE

The basic surgical technique for replacement arthroplasty of the shoulder is the anterior approach. Occasionally, a posterior approach may be necessary.

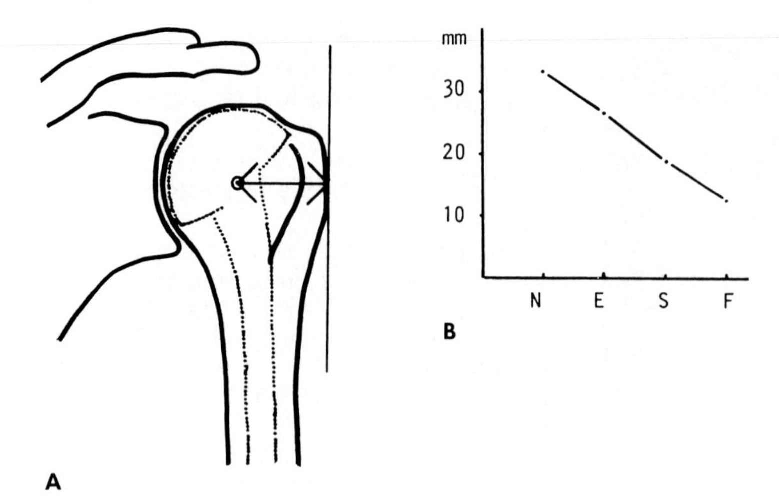

FIGURE 38–29. *A,* Humeral offset as measured from the geometric center of the humeral head to the lateral edge of the greater tuberosity. *B,* A graphic representation of the mean humeral offset related to the clinical result in the study by Rietveld. N = normal shoulder, 33 mm (nine cases); E = excellent result, 26.5 mm (two cases); S = satisfactory result, 19 mm (three cases); and F = failure, 12.5 mm (four cases). (Rietveld, A. B. M., et al: The lever arm in glenohumeral abduction after hemiarthroplasty. J. Bone Joint Surg. 70B:561–565, 1988. By permission.)

Anterior Approach

Incision and Exposure

A neurosurgical head rest allows more room about the shoulder (Fig. 38–30). Foam padding is used as necessary to protect exposed areas, such as the heels and malleoli, the ulnar nerve at the elbow of the unoperated arm, and the ears. The operating table is moved into the beach chair position, with the patient semisitting and the knees slightly flexed. The shoulder protrudes over the edge so that the surgeon has access all around it. Access to the posterior aspect of the shoulder is important should an additional approach be required. The shoulder is then draped. The arm is covered with a stockinette and wrapped with an elastic bandage so that it can be positioned freely.

An anterior incision is made, beginning at the clavicle just medial to the acromioclavicular joint and extending straight distally 15 to 17 cm to the anterior border of the insertion of the deltoid (Fig. 38–31).[59]

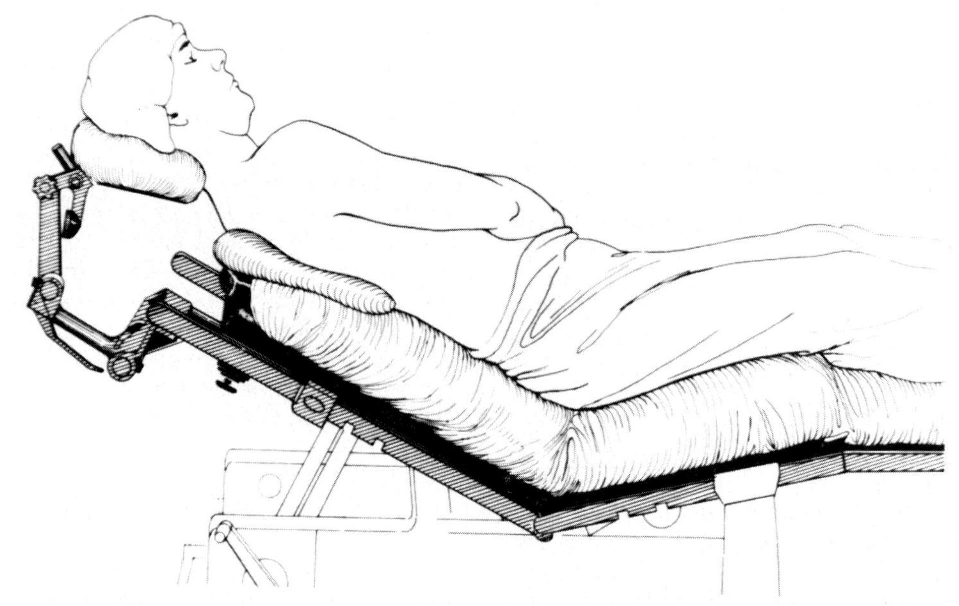

FIGURE 38–30. The usual beach chair–type position for shoulder surgery. The neurosurgical headrest allows the surgeon more room around the shoulder. (Norris, T. R.: Fractures and Dislocations of the Glenohumeral Complex. Operative Orthopaedics, vol. 1. Edited by M. Chapman. Philadelphia, J. B. Lippincott Company, 1988. By permission.)

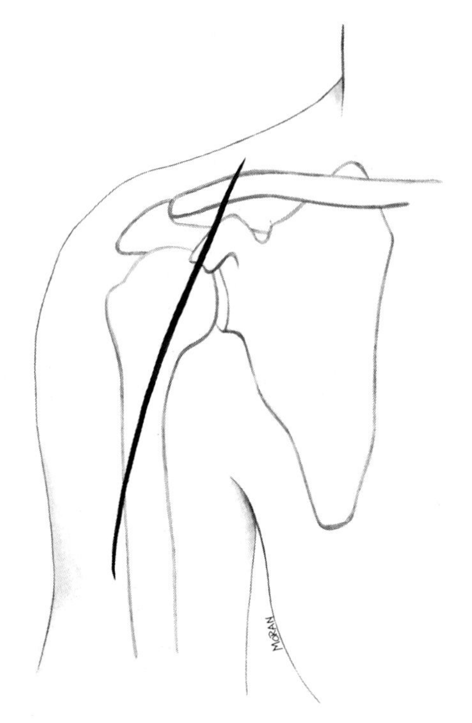

FIGURE 38–31. Anterior skin incision for shoulder arthroplasty.

Skin margins are undermined medially to expose the deltopectoral interval (Fig. 38–32). Dissection begins proximally between these two muscles at the infraclavicular triangle. The cephalic vein is usually preserved. Acromial branches of the thoracoacromial artery are cauterized proximally as they are encountered.

Dissection is continued distally, with the deltoid retracted laterally as branches to the cephalic vein are cauterized and transected. As the deltoid is retracted laterally, the clavipectoral fascia is exposed (Fig. 38–33). This fascial layer, which covers the conjoined tendons of the short head of the biceps and coracobrachialis, is incised. Retraction of the conjoined tendon and the underlying musculocutaneous nerve medially exposes the subscapularis and front of the shoulder joint. The axillary nerve crosses the subscapularis and courses along the inferior capsule of the shoulder joint. In a previously operated or traumatized shoulder, distorted anatomy and abundant scar tissue may conceal the nerve. When retracting the deltoid, care should be taken not to retract directly on the axillary nerve.

After retraction of the deltoid, the arm is abducted 20 to 30 degrees and is rested on a padded, sterile-draped stand adjacent to the operating table. The shoulder is then

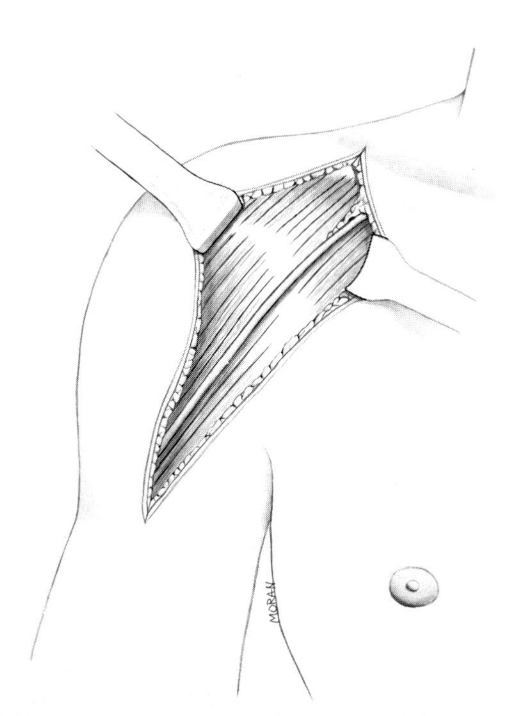

FIGURE 38–32. Medial undermining of skin margins to expose the deltopectoral interval.

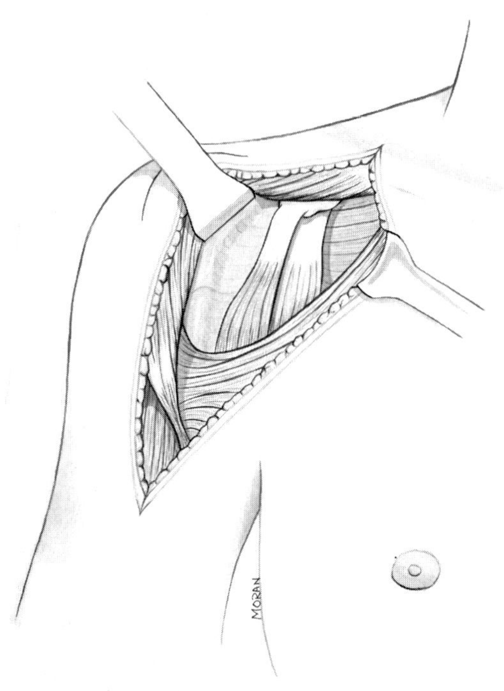

FIGURE 38–33. Continuation of dissection distally, with retraction of the deltoid laterally. This maneuver exposes the clavipectoral fascia overlying the conjoined tendons of the short head of the biceps and coracobrachialis.

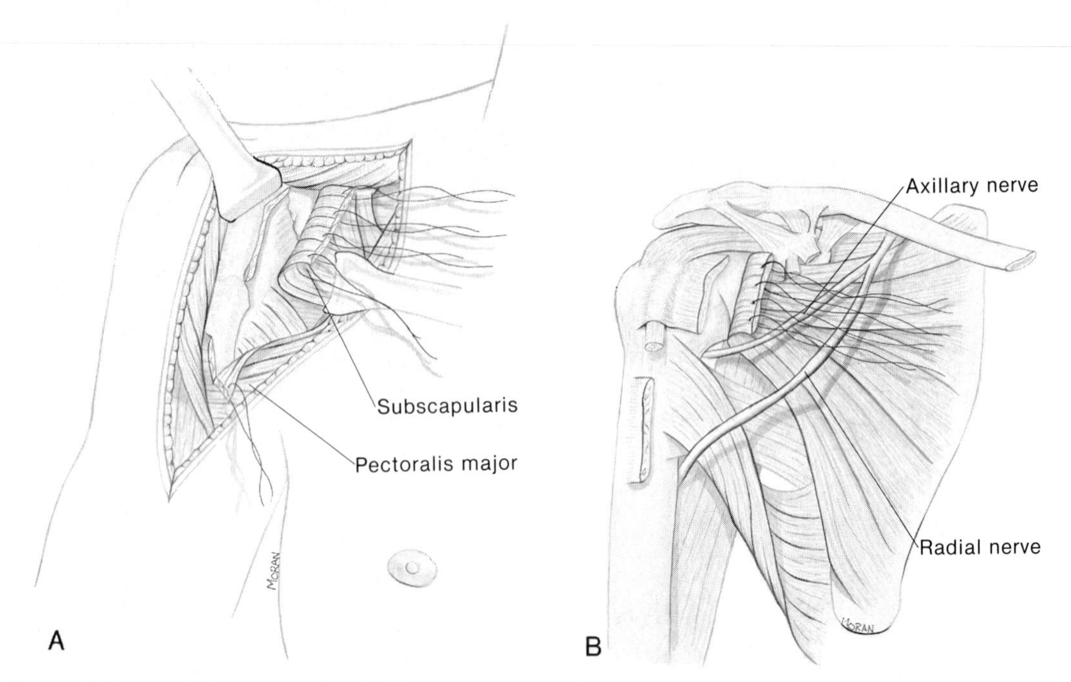

FIGURE 38–34. *A*, Entry into the shoulder joint via an incision in the subscapularis and the capsule near its insertion into the lesser tuberosity. Tagging sutures are placed in the subscapularis to prevent it from retracting medially. A portion of the pectoralis major insertion may be released as necessary. *B*, Relationship of the radial and axillary nerves to the anterior shoulder exposure.

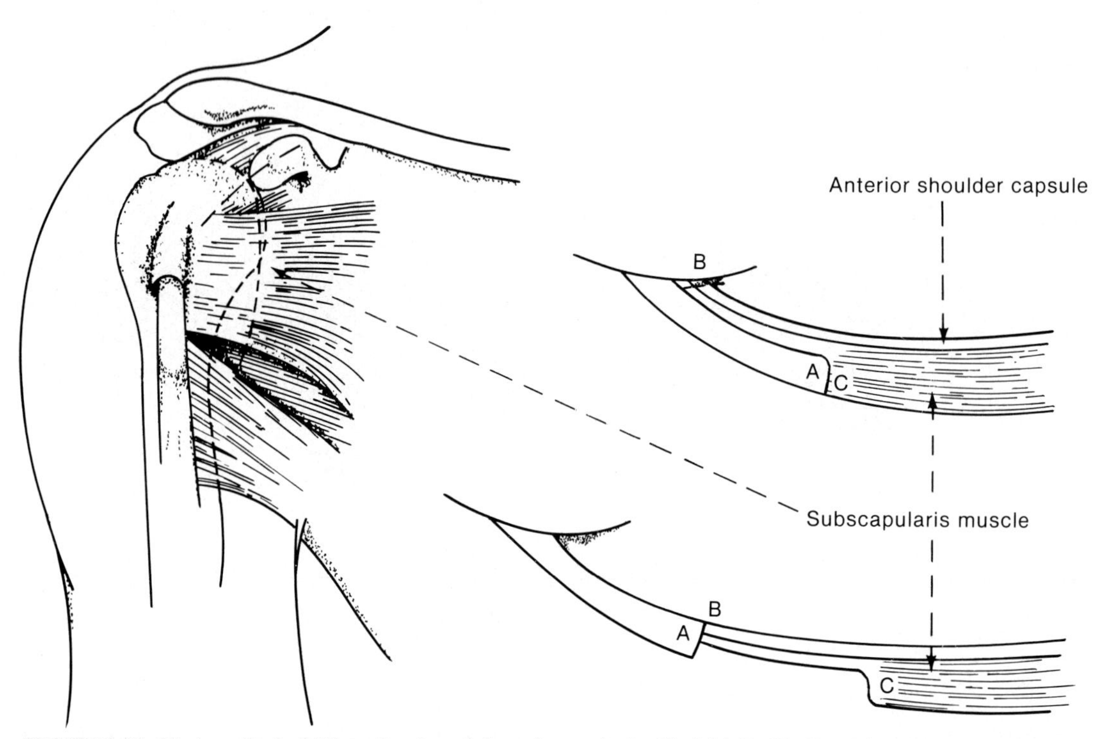

FIGURE 38–35. A method of Z-lengthening of the subscapularis. (Cofield, R. H.: Total Shoulder Arthroplasty. American Academy of Orthopaedic Surgeons Course: Shoulder Surgery—Current Techniques. Los Angeles, September, 1987. By permission.)

tested for any tightness that limits external rotation. The coracoacromial ligament is usually transected at this time. Further exposure and additional external rotation may be gained by releasing the proximal portion of the insertion of the pectoralis major.

If 40 degrees of external rotation can be easily attained, the shoulder joint is entered by incising the subscapularis and the capsule near its insertion into the lesser tuberosity after the anterior circumflex vessels at the inferior border of this muscle are cauterized or ligated. The incision in the muscle and capsule is continued upward slightly anterior to the biceps tendon. Enough tissue must be left at the insertion into the tuberosity to allow later repair of the subscapularis. Tagging sutures should be placed in the subscapularis to prevent it from retracting medially (Fig. 38–34). If external rotation is limited to less than 40 degrees by a tight capsule and subscapularis, they may be lengthened by Z-plasty (Fig. 38–35).[31]

The joint is freed of any adhesions by extending, abducting, and externally rotating the arm. The humeral head can now be dislocated (Fig. 38–36).

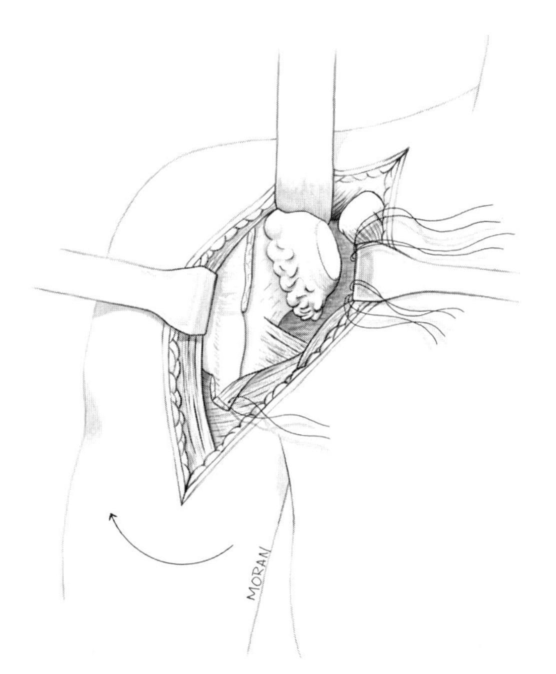

FIGURE 38–36. Dislocation of the humeral head by extending, abducting, and externally rotating the arm.

Osteotomy

Osteotomy and removal of the head then can be accomplished. The head is not removed in line with its anatomic neck. The osteotomy is started just inside the attachment of the supraspinatus and extended downward 50 degrees in a medial direction. A trial prosthesis is laid over the upper humerus as a guide. The line of the osteotomy, a 50-degree lateral-to-medial slope, is determined and marked on the humerus. Usually, only a small amount of bone is removed from the head of the humerus. More can be removed later if necessary (Fig. 38–37).

The osteotomy should be made so that the prosthesis will be in the normal 30 to 40 degrees of retroversion with respect to the humeral condyles (Fig. 38–38).[24, 97, 100, 102] This maneuver can be accomplished by positioning the forearm, with the elbow flexed to 90 degrees, as if it were one arm of a goniometer. To place the prosthesis in 30 degrees of retroversion, the arm and forearm are rotated outward 30 degrees. With the blade of the saw or the osteotome held vertically, the osteotomy is made at the mark. When the prosthesis is later placed flush with this osteotomy, it will lie in 30 degrees of retroversion. Less retroversion might sometimes be indicated, for instance, to compensate for excessive retroversion of the glenoid due to posterior marginal wear.

The osteotomy can be made with either an oscillating saw or osteotome. Care should be taken to avoid amputating the insertion of the external rotators by removing too much head or performing the osteotomy in too much retroversion. The biceps tendon should be protected with an elevator or other retractor while the osteotomy is made.

Preparing for the Humeral Prosthesis

Once the osteotomy has been completed and the head removed, marginal osteophytes are trimmed from the neck. Attention is then turned to the joint itself, which can be better visualized once the head has been removed. Joint debridement and synovectomy are carried out as necessary. The glenoid is inspected, and the rotator cuff is

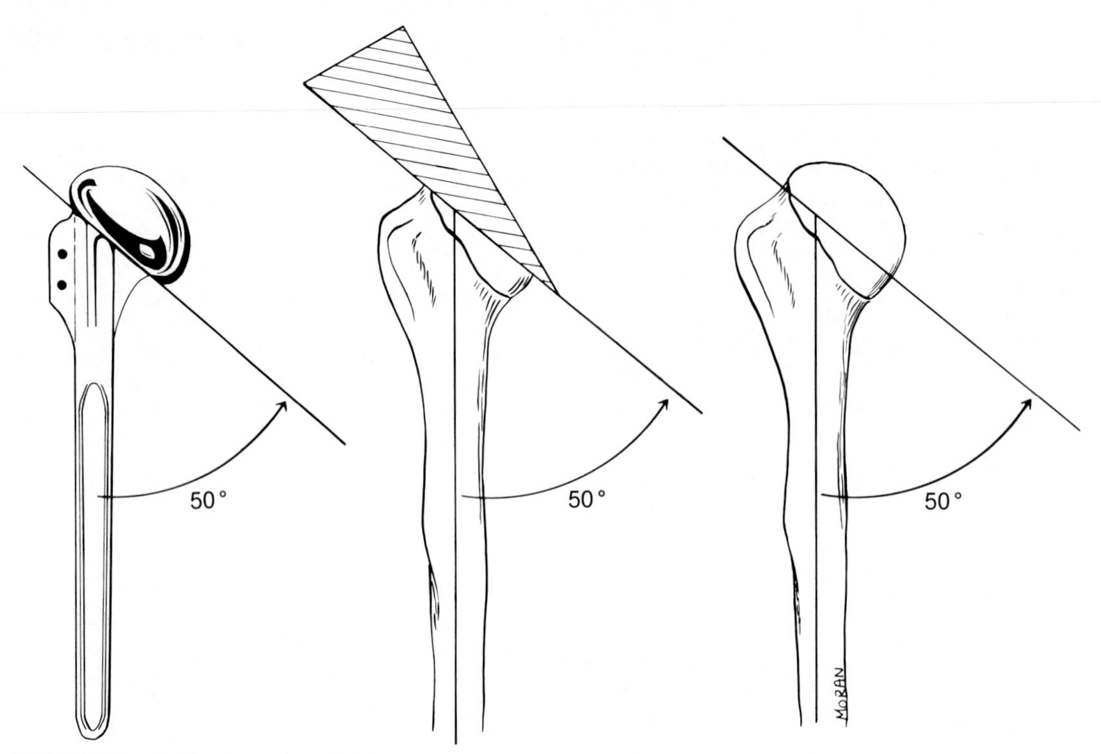

FIGURE 38–37. Trial prosthesis laid over the upper humerus as a guide for the osteotomy. The osteotomy has a 50-degree lateral-to-medial slope. The osteotomy line is marked on the humerus.

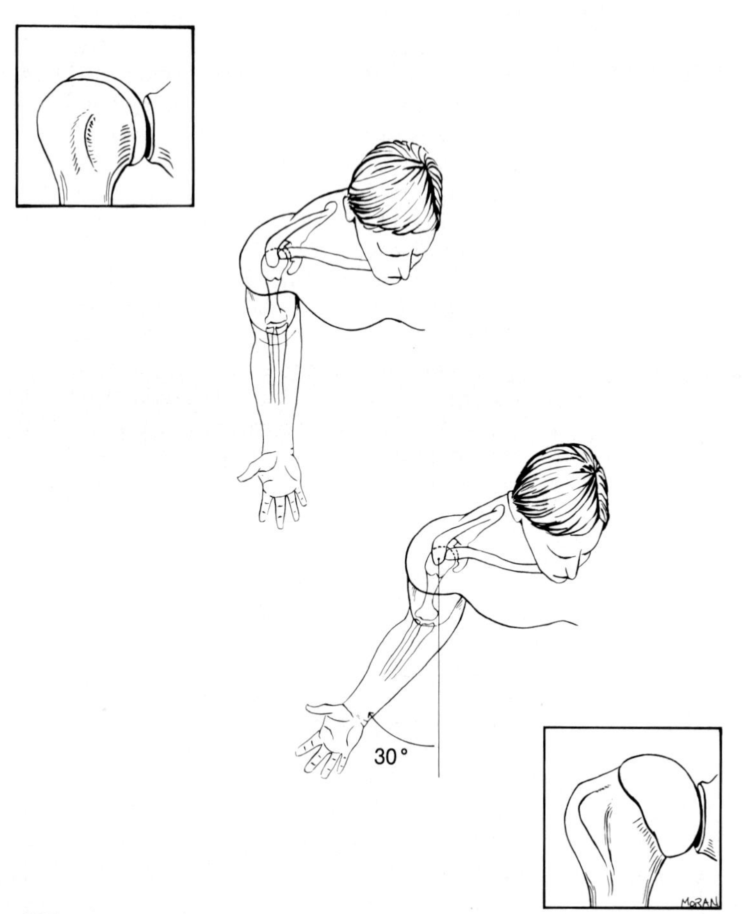

FIGURE 38–38. Osteotomy placed so that the prosthesis is in 30 to 40 degrees of retroversion with respect to the humeral condyles. The forearm can be used as a goniometer placing it in 30 degrees of external rotation. The saw blade or osteotome is then held vertically and the osteotomy made. This measure will result in the amount of retroversion in which the forearm was held while externally rotated.

further evaluated. The acromioclavicular joint and undersurface of the acromion are palpated for pathology. Any necessary surgical correction, for example, acromioplasty and removal of inferior osteophytes at the acromioclavicular joint, or resection of the distal clavicle, is completed.

The upper humerus is further prepared. Evaluation of the medullary canal on the radiograph will help in estimating the stem size. With a drill point, a curette, or a stem of a small prosthesis, the medullary canal is located just posterior to the bicipital groove. Tapered reamers are employed to prepare the medullary canal for the prosthesis (Fig. 38–39). Toggling the reamers is avoided so as not to enlarge the upper canal, making a good press-fit less likely.

The selected trial prosthesis is inserted (Fig. 38–40). It is not placed to engage the prosthetic flanges in the bone until the surgeon is certain that the version and position are correct (Fig. 38–41). Once the flange channels are established, the position of the prosthesis should not be altered; doing so will compromise the press-fit. The trial prosthesis is seated (Fig. 38–42). If

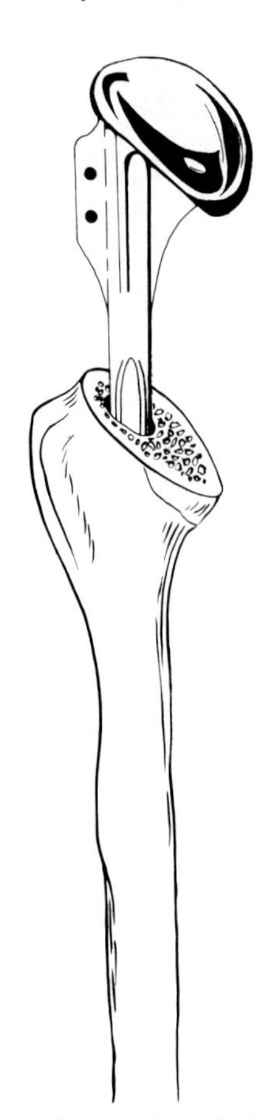

FIGURE 38–40. Insertion of trial prosthesis.

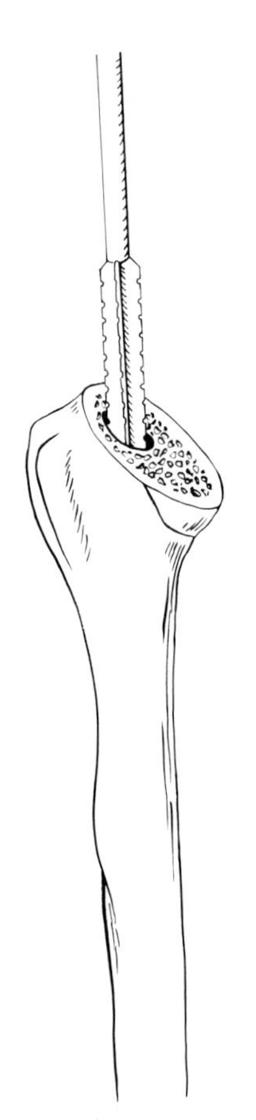

FIGURE 38–39. Tapered reamers for preparing the medullary canal for the prosthesis.

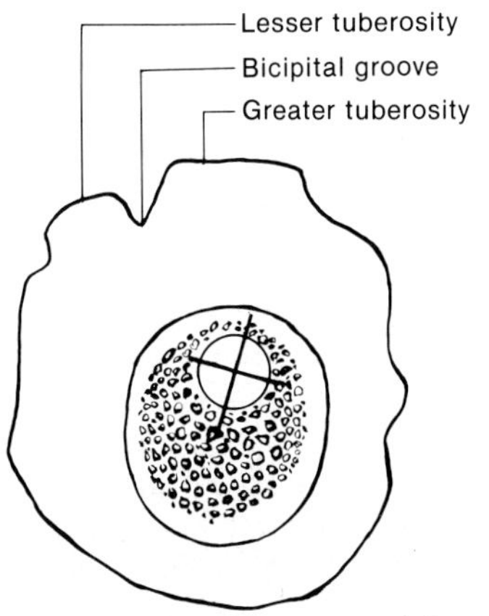

FIGURE 38–41. Proper placement of the prosthetic flanges before the trial prosthesis is driven. Normally, the lateral flange should point just posterior to the bicipital groove.

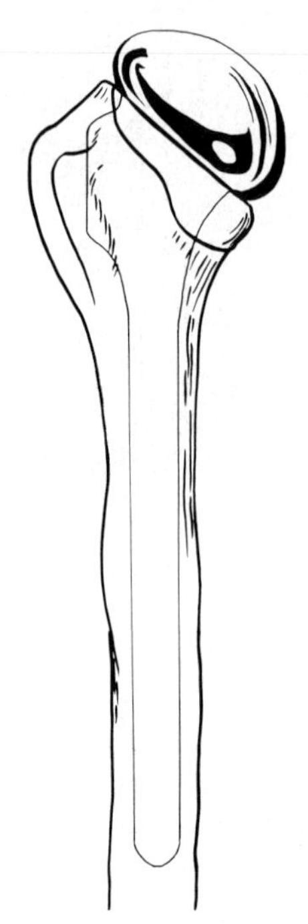

FIGURE 38–42. The trial prosthesis is seated after correct version is assured.

the bone is very osteoporotic or is shortened owing to fracture or nonunion, the prosthesis may have to be cemented at the proper height later in the procedure. Preoperative scanograms can be useful in determining the proper height.[106]

Glenoid Preparation

At this point, if the patient needs a glenoid prosthesis, the trial humeral prosthesis is removed. The upper humerus is carefully retracted posteriorly with a Fukuda or other shoulder retractor, exposing the glenoid.

Prosthetic preparation entails placement of a slot or channel for the keel of the prosthesis and preparation of the articular surface of the glenoid. All redundant tissue is first removed from the margins of the glenoid. To help direct the channel properly and to avoid penetrating the wall of the scapula, the labrum is excised along the anterior edge of the glenoid so that a finger may be inserted to palpate the anterior neck of the glenoid. Should the glenoid wall be accidentally penetrated with instruments, the defect is grafted with bone from the previously removed humeral head to prevent cement from escaping.

Any remaining areas of articular cartilage and fibrous tissue are removed with curettes. The subchondral bone is then roughened with an air-driven burr. However, subchondral bone is not removed, as its support is vital for the prosthesis. The guide or template is placed, and the subchondral bone is marked with inferior and superior holes to indicate the ends of the slot or channel (Fig. 38–43). The channel is created with a dental burr the same width as the prosthetic keel, beginning just below the base of the coracoid process and ending just above the infraglenoid tubercle inferiorly (Fig. 38–44). The slot thus favors a slightly superior position. The margins of the slot are undermined and deepened with straight and angled curettes to provide for better cement fixation (Fig. 38–45). A glenoid rasp may be used to size the channel (Fig. 38–46).

The trial glenoid prosthesis is placed (Fig. 38–47). If the glenoid has been prepared properly, the prosthesis will not rock but will fit the contour of the glenoid almost perfectly. If the prosthesis does rock despite adequate preparation of the channel, a high spot exists on the prepared

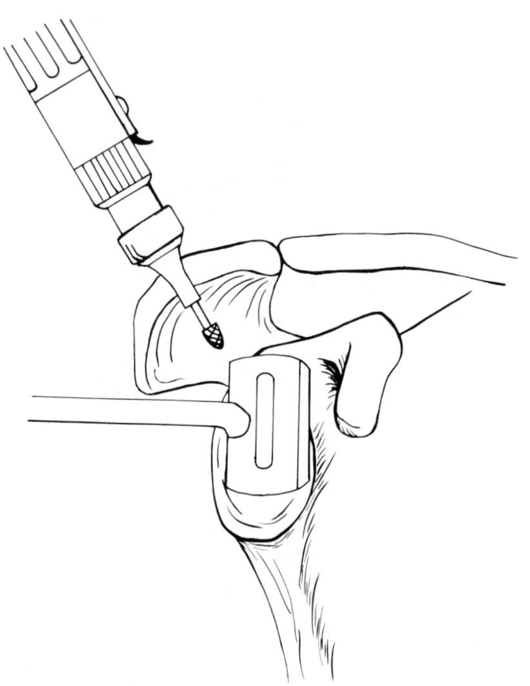

FIGURE 38–43. Extension of the channel for the glenoid component from just below the base of the coracoid process to just above the infraglenoid tubercle. A template may help in marking the channel.

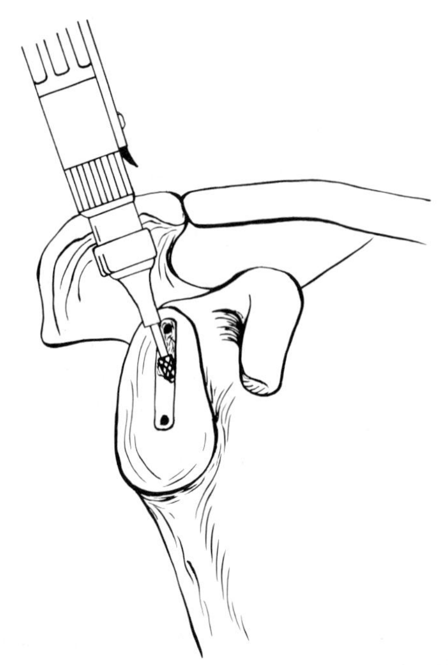

FIGURE 38–44. Creation of the channel with a dental burr the same width as the prosthetic keel.

glenoid surface. The effect is similar to a table with one leg slightly longer than the other three. This problem is corrected by carefully lowering the high area with a dental burr. Attempting to compensate for

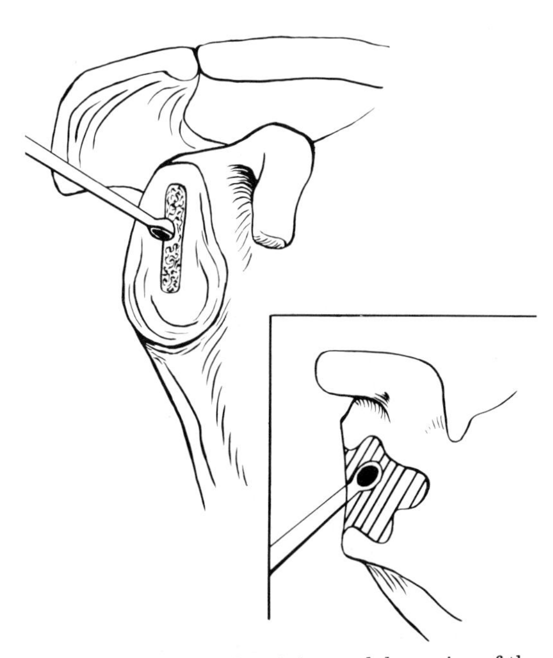

FIGURE 38–45. Undermining and deepening of the slot with curettes.

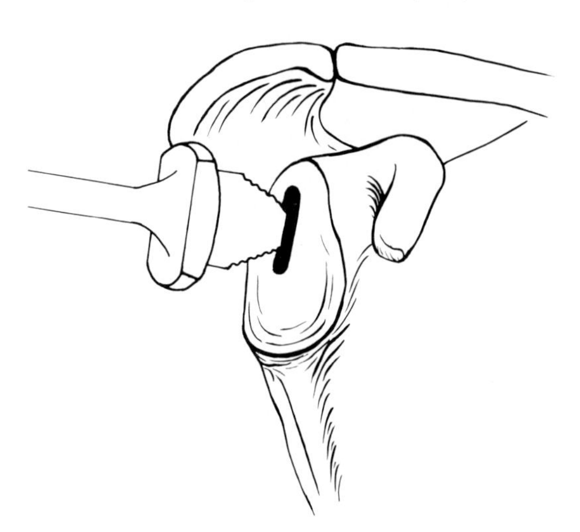

FIGURE 38–46. Use of a glenoid rasp to size the channel.

the defect by applying extra cement will increase the chances of prosthetic loosening. Good subchondral support of the entire prosthesis is essential to absorb the forces on the prosthesis evenly.

Either metal-backed or nonmetal-backed prostheses may be used (Fig. 38–48). The metal-backed prosthesis was designed for better stress distribution to prevent loosening. At times, however, a nonmetal-backed prosthesis is the only one that will fit.

The trial glenoid prosthesis is left in place, and the trial humeral prosthesis is inserted (Fig. 38–49). The margins of the humeral neck around the prosthesis are

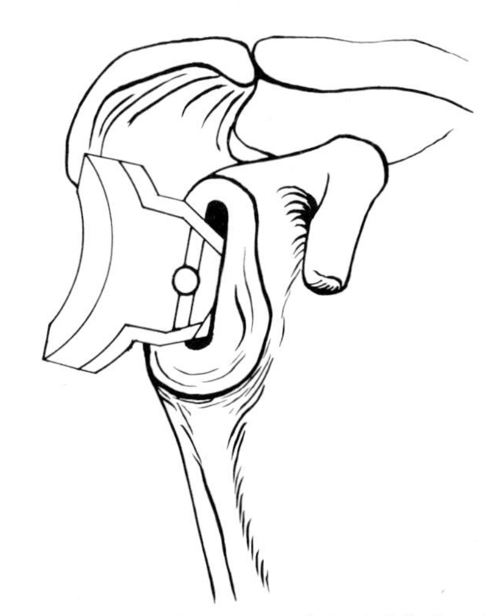

FIGURE 38–47. Placement of the trial glenoid prosthesis.

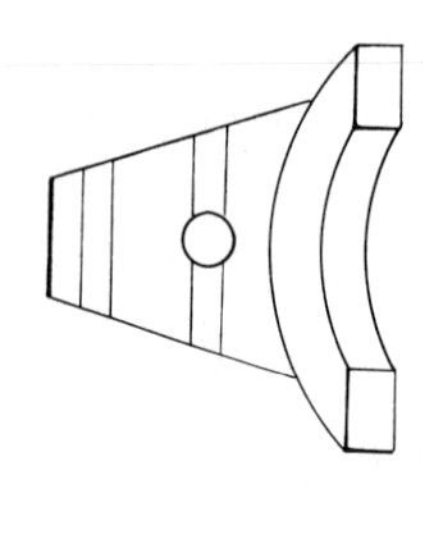

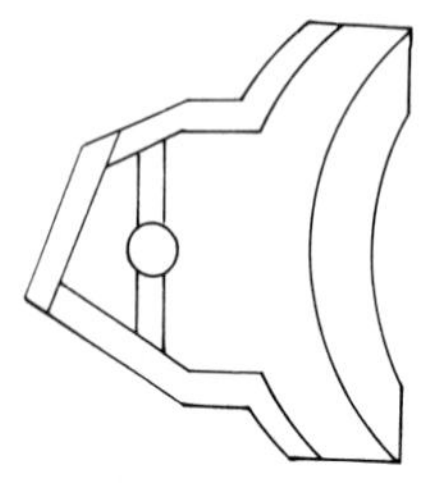

FIGURE 38–48. Metal-backed (below) and nonmetal-backed (above) prostheses.

trimmed. A trial reduction is accomplished. Stability and range of motion are evaluated. Correct head size selection is confirmed by proper tension of the rotator cuff and adequate external rotation, which is tested with the subscapularis held at the proposed repair site.

Prosthesis Placement

Once satisfactory fit, stability, and motion have been obtained, the trial prostheses are removed. The upper humerus is once again retracted to expose the prepared glenoid for cementing. If the glenoid surface is very hard and eburnated, small holes may be drilled to improve cement fixation (Fig. 38–50). To be sure that the cement fills all the interstices in the glenoid channel, blood and debris are cleaned from the glenoid and the channel with a pulsed irrigation system.

Cement is first introduced into the channel with a syringe and is packed in thoroughly with a sponge to force it into the interstices. Excess cement is wiped out, and the channel is filled with more cement by syringe. A small amount of cement is placed on the underside of the tray of the prosthesis. The prosthetic glenoid is inserted, gently impacted, and held firmly in place with the impactor while the cement sets. Excess cement is carefully removed from around the margins of the prosthesis while still soft. Care is taken not to undermine the edges of the prosthesis.

When the cement has set and the glenoid is stable, attention is turned to the humerus. The humeral prosthetic channel is irrigated clear of debris, and the humeral prosthesis is inserted for a press-fit. If the humeral prosthesis must be cemented, the technique described for the glenoid is applied, assuring that the cement is forced into bone interstices. Usually, a bone plug obtained from the humeral head or another type of cement restrictor is introduced into the medullary canal 1 to 2 cm distal to the tip of the prosthesis. The plug prevents the

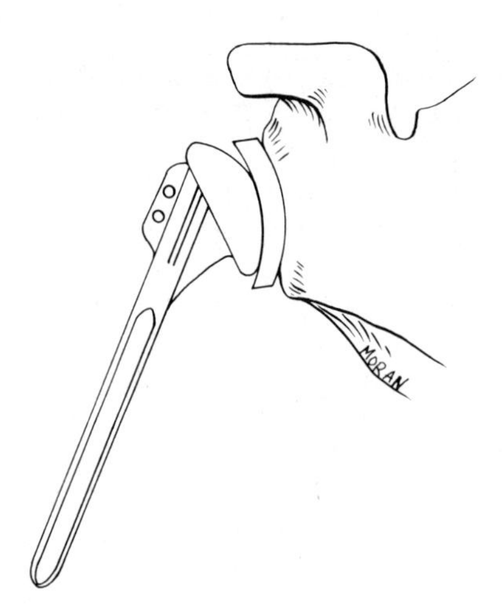

FIGURE 38–49. Trial reduction with both glenoid and humeral prostheses. Stability and range of motion are evaluated.

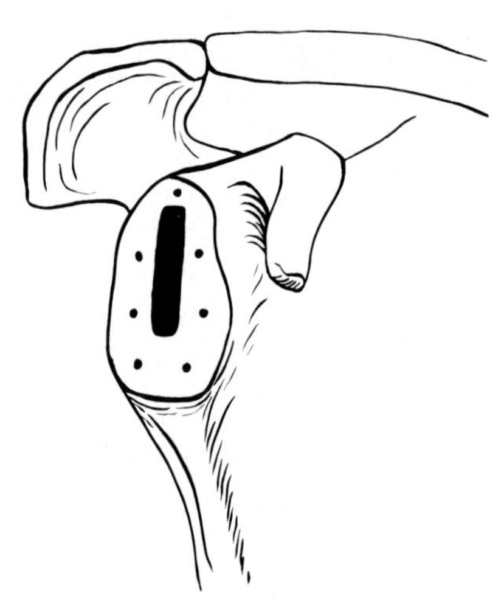

FIGURE 38–50. Small drill holes placed to enhance fixation. This may be done if the surface of the glenoid is especially hard and eburnated.

escape of cement and allows pressure to force the cement into the interstices of the medullary canal. After cement is introduced retrograde by syringe, the prosthesis is inserted.

After the cement has set, the prosthetic shoulder is reduced. Fit, stability, and motion are given a final check. The arm is positioned and the previously placed sutures utilized to repair the subscapularis. A drain may be placed, and the subcutaneous tissue and skin are closed.

Posterior Approach

The surgeon may sometimes need to make a posterior approach to the shoulder in addition to the anterior approach. This step might be necessary, for instance, to attain proper reduction of a malunited greater tuberosity fracture in conjunction with a replacement arthroplasty. The posterior approach may also be necessary to mobilize and repair the posterior rotator cuff. Therefore, the patient should be positioned and draped so that the back of the shoulder as well as the front will be accessible at surgery.

Anatomic Considerations

The axillary nerve, after emerging from the quadrangular space at the inferior border of the teres minor between the long and lateral heads of the triceps, immediately supplies a branch to the teres minor. The nerve continues around the lateral head of the triceps to the undersurface of the deltoid, follows it laterally to innervate the deltoid, and courses to the anterior aspect of the muscle at the level of the surgical neck of the humerus, approximately 5 cm below the tip of the acromion (see Fig. 38–12). This nerve must be protected when taking down the deltoid.

The posterior approach involves the more important of the only two external rotators, the infraspinatus. Repair of this muscle must be carefully and meticulously performed to preserve adequate function. The suprascapular nerve is located in the infraspinous fossa, deep to the infraspinatus, about 1.8 cm medial to the posterior edge of the glenoid.[7] Great care must be taken to avoid damage to this nerve's innervation of the infraspinatus when taking down this muscle and retracting it medially to expose the posterior glenohumeral joint (Fig. 38–51F).

The tissues at the back of the shoulder joint are not as substantial as those at the front. Because they are more delicate, appropriate care must be taken when working with these structures.

Technique (Fig. 38–51)

The posterior deltoid is exposed and its origin removed from the spine of the scapula (Fig. 38–51B). Enough tissue is left on the bone for later repair. The deltoid is then retracted inferiorly as it is split. While splitting the muscle laterally along the posterior edge of the middle deltoid, the surgeon must be careful not to damage the axillary nerve. Retraction of the posterior deltoid exposes the infraspinatus lying over the posterior glenoid (Fig. 38–51C). Posterior inferior acromioplasty may provide better exposure of the infraspinatus insertion. The infraspinatus tendon and posterior capsule are incised along the insertion of the tendon into the posterior aspect of the greater tuberosity (Fig. 38–51D). The tendon, muscle, and capsule are retracted medially along the interval between the supraspinatus and teres minor, exposing the glenohumeral joint (Fig. 38–51E). Retraction of these tissues must be performed gently so as not to damage the suprascapular nerve (Fig. 38–51F).

In cases involving a retracted and malunited greater tuberosity that cannot be adequately reduced from the front, the surgical approach has to be modified. Because of this distortion in anatomy, the infraspinatus and teres minor will be retracted with the greater tuberosity and supraspinatus. Particular care must be given in identifying and protecting the nerves in this situation.

Replacement Arthroplasty

Although quite unusual, replacement arthroplasty can be done through a posterior approach. The humeral head is dislocated by flexing, adducting, and internally rotating the arm. The articular surface of the humeral head is removed, and version is corrected, just as in the anterior approach.

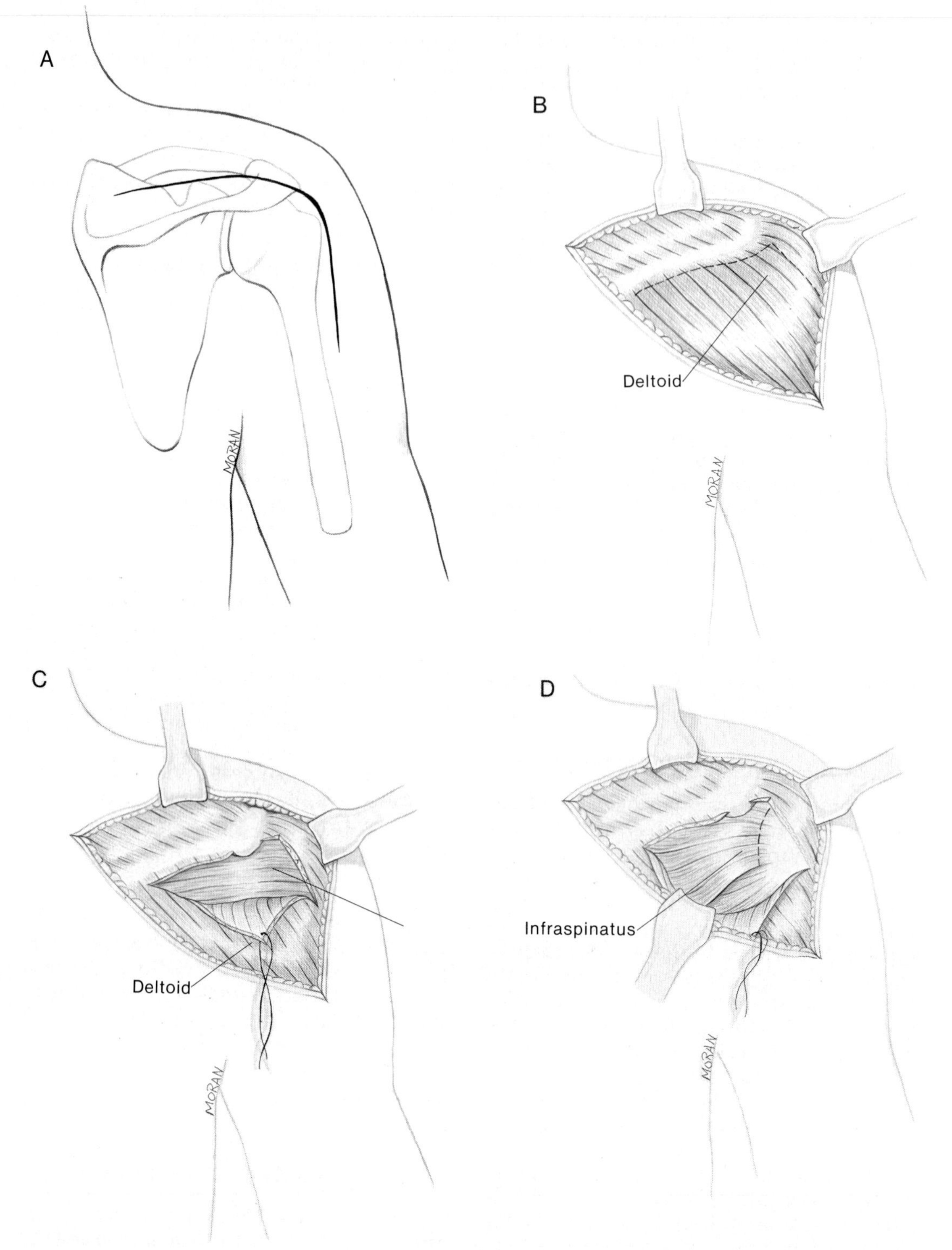

FIGURE 38–51. Posterior approach to the shoulder joint. *A,* Skin incision. *B,* Exposure of the posterior deltoid and the origin that will be removed from the spine of the scapula (marked). *C,* Removal of the posterior deltoid origin from the spine of the scapula to expose the infraspinatus. *D,* Incision in the infraspinatus tendon and posterior capsule along the insertion of the tendon into the posterior aspect of the greater tuberosity.

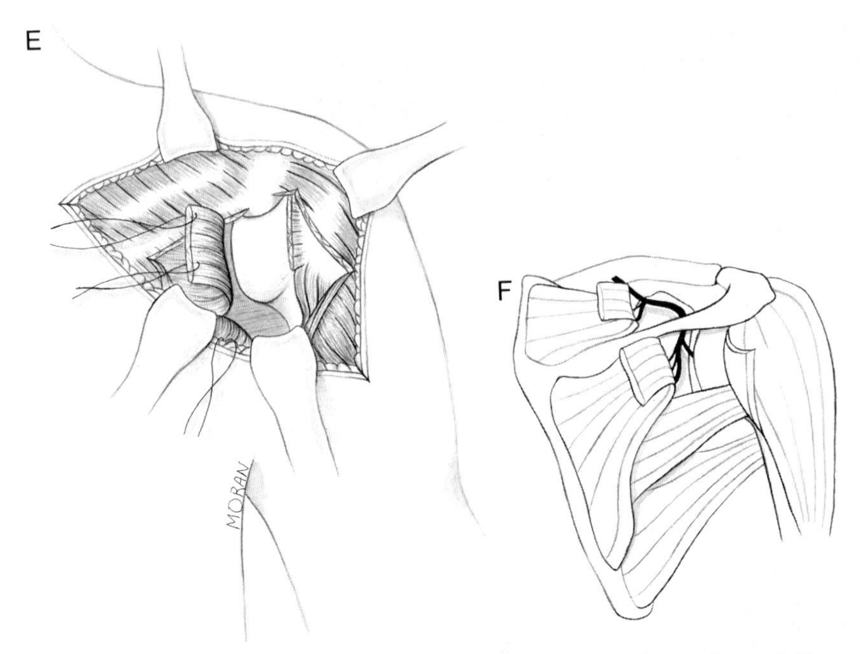

FIGURE 38–51 *Continued E,* Retraction of the infraspinatus tendon and capsule medially to expose the glenohumeral joint. *F,* Gentle retraction done to avoid damage to the suprascapular nerve.

The joint is thus exposed. After it is cleaned of debris, the glenoid is inspected and prepared. Secure repair of the infraspinatus is important when closing.

Technique for Fractures

The fracture is approached anteriorly through a long deltopectoral incision. Better exposure may be obtained by transecting the upper 1 cm of the pectoralis major insertion into the humerus. The clavipectoral fascia is incised. The conjoined tendon with the musculocutaneous nerve is carefully retracted medially, whereas the deltoid is retracted laterally with a smooth retractor. Blood and clot are irrigated from the wound.

The biceps tendon serves as a guide into the fracture site between the greater and lesser tuberosities. Found deep to the pectoralis major tendon, the biceps tendon is exposed at that point and followed into the fracture site by palpation. Number-5 sutures are placed into the supraspinatus tendon at its insertion into the greater tuberosity and into the subscapularis tendon at its insertion into the lesser tuberosity. These sutures are tagged and used as traction sutures to control and mobilize the rotator cuff, with its attached bone segments. The defect in the rotator cuff between the supraspinatus and the subscapularis is developed in a proximal direction, and the loose head fragment is exposed and removed. The arm is rotated and positioned to expose the fractured upper end of the humeral shaft.

A trial prosthesis is utilized primarily to determine which head size will allow closure of the rotator cuff with the tuberosities reduced to the flange of the prosthesis and to the shaft. The tuberosities should be below the level of the articular surface of the prosthesis to avoid impingement.[104] The trial prosthesis selected is inserted into the shaft by hand, in 30 degrees of retroversion. A trial reduction of the tuberosities is made to be sure the cuff will close properly. Wobbling the prosthesis during trial reduction will compromise the stem channel in the shaft. If closure of the rotator cuff is difficult, a prosthesis with a smaller head should be selected.

Before the real prosthesis is inserted, #5-nonabsorbable sutures are placed through the two holes in the keel for suturing and securing the tuberosities to the flange. The two tuberosities form the upper 3 cm of the humeral shaft, and the humeral head prosthesis needs to be inserted proud

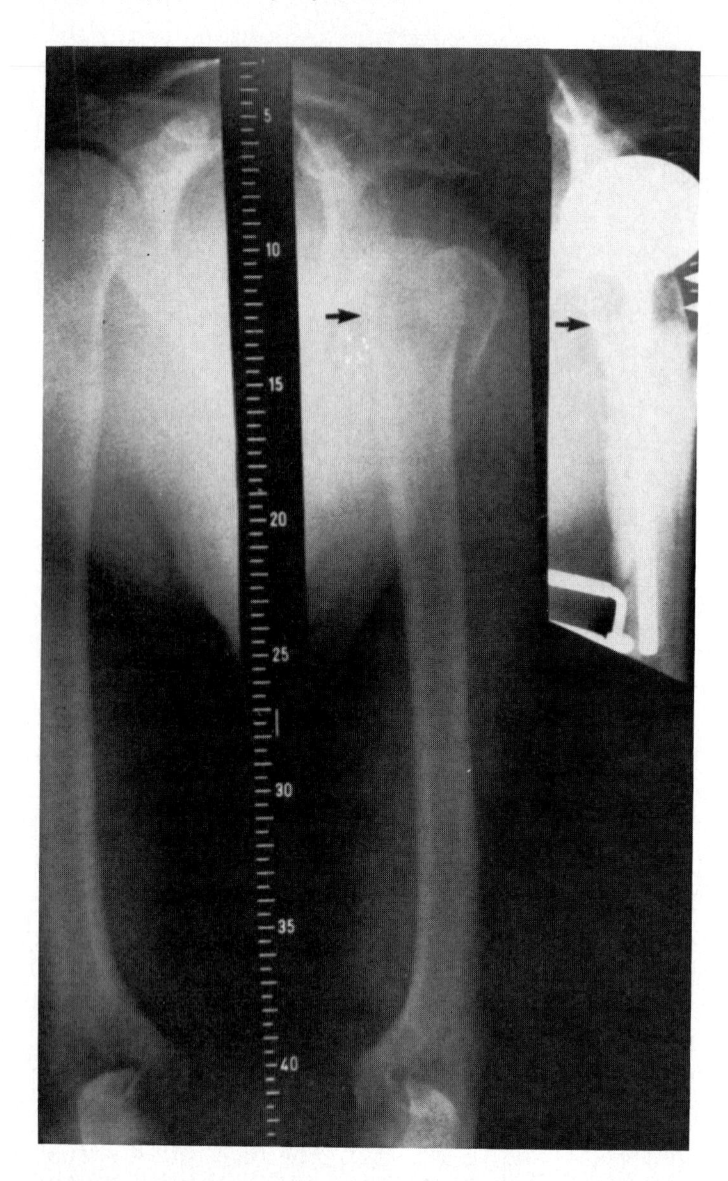

FIGURE 38–52. Scanograms can be very helpful in determining and restoring length relationships in proximal humeral fractures. It is most important to restore length when treating fractures with a prosthesis. Sometimes this means cementing a prosthesis as illustrated here. (Norris, T. R.: Fractures and Dislocations of the Glenohumeral Complex. Edited by M. Chapman. Philadelphia, J. B. Lippincott Company, 1988. By permission.)

enough to accommodate these structures at the flange.[129] Referring to the preoperative scanograms, the surgeon selects a point on the humeral shaft that can be employed as a reference for measuring how high above the fractured end of the humeral shaft the prosthesis should sit to restore arm length (Fig. 38–52).[104]

The prosthesis is then inserted. If bony support is adequate and arm length maintained, the prosthesis need not be cemented. Otherwise, cement is used to ensure security, height, and position of the prosthesis.

The next step is to reduce the tuberosities to the upper shaft and the flange of the prosthesis. A small amount of bone may have to be removed from the tuberosities to fit them to their reduced position at the prosthetic flange. If too much bone is removed from the tuberosities, they may not heal to the shaft.[32] The tuberosities are repaired and sutured to each other, the prosthetic keel, and the shaft (Fig. 38–53).[104] The wound is then irrigated. A drain is placed, and the wound is closed. Occasionally, grafts may be necessary around the proud prosthetic stem, as in Figure 38–54.[88]

SPECIAL PROBLEMS

Posterior glenoid erosion is often seen in patients with osteoarthritis, whereas soft tissue destruction, osteopenia, and medial

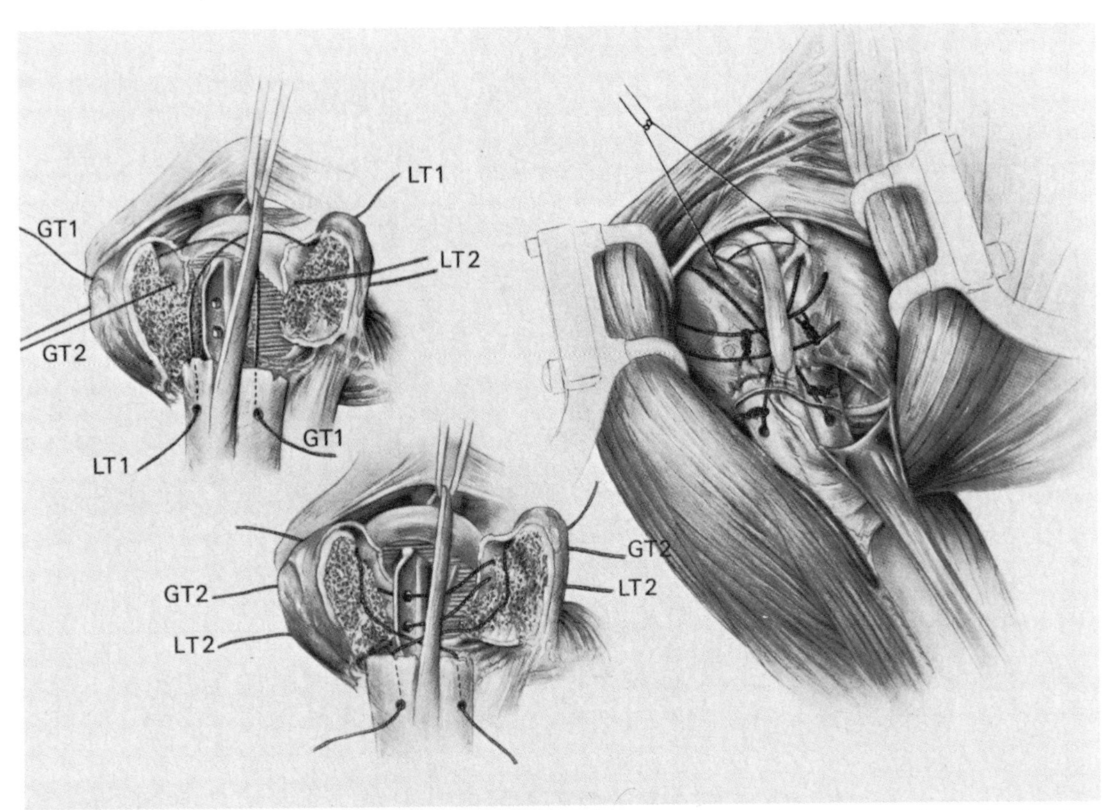

FIGURE 38–53. Appropriate technique for bringing fractured tuberosities back into position and attaching them to the prosthesis. (GT = greater tuberosity suture; LT = lesser tuberosity suture.) (Norris, T. R.: Fractures and Dislocations of the Glenohumeral Complex. Operative Orthopaedics, vol. 1. Edited by M. Chapman. Philadelphia, J. B. Lippincott Company, 1988. By permission.)

glenoid erosion are seen in those with rheumatoid arthritis. Loss or deformity of bone is a special problem in trauma cases.[27] Chronic subluxation or dislocation or an overly tight instability repair can lead to posterior or anterior glenoid wear, soft tissue deficiency, or a soft, deformed humeral head.[97, 102, 126] Trauma may result in malunited fractures or disruption of the anterior or posterior glenoid because of acute dislocations.[88, 102]

Rotator Cuff

The most important principles when repairing the torn rotator cuff are adequate exposure and careful freeing of retracted and contracted rotator cuff tissue.[23, 29, 42, 74] Most rotator cuff tears can be repaired, but not all repaired rotator cuffs function satisfactorily.

Sometimes, part of the subscapularis must be transferred superiorly to help in the repair of a deficient supraspinatus. Rarely, fascial grafts or other transfers, such as transfer of the pectoralis major or latissimus dorsi, are indicated.

Cuff tear arthropathy presents the combined problem of loss of the rotator cuff and loss of bone.[15, 17, 36, 88, 90, 100] Often, the tear of the rotator cuff is massive, involving both the supraspinatus and the infraspinatus. Repair of the rotator cuff in this circumstance is very difficult. Continuing deficiencies in tissue and function demand realistically limited postoperative goals. Patients with cuff tear arthropathy are often older, may not be suited for spica cast immobilization, and have soft deficient scapular bone. Because they may be unsuitable candidates for arthrodesis or constrained arthroplasty, Neer[90] recommends replacement arthroplasty with repair of the rotator cuff.

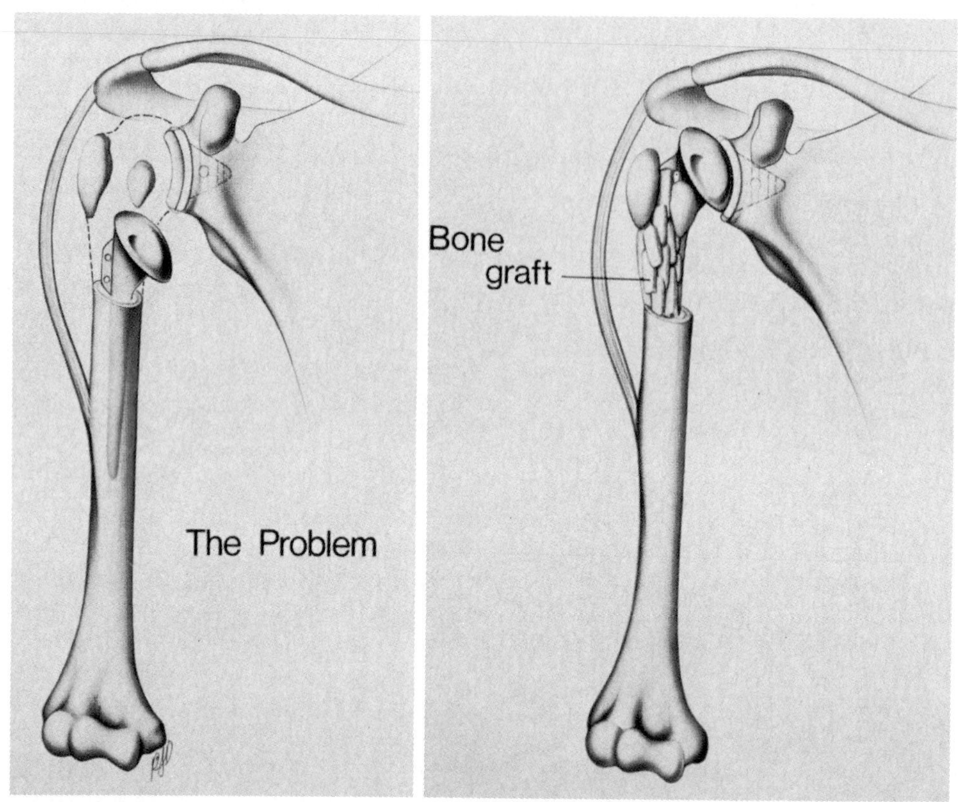

FIGURE 38–54. The problem of restoring length to maintain deltoid tone and mechanical advantage and to prevent dislocation sometimes requires cementing the prosthesis proud, using scanograms as guides, then bone grafting the deficit between the upper shaft and the tuberosities. (Neer, C. S., II, Watson, K. D., and Stanton, F. J.: Recent experience in total shoulder replacement. J. Bone Joint Surg. 64A:319–337, 1982. By permission.)

Bone Deficiency

Uneven wear and deficiency of the glenoid are present to some degree in most patients with pathologic conditions of the shoulder.[27, 73, 88, 89, 101, 102] Computerized tomography is the best way to evaluate the glenoid deformity.[102] If the surgeon does not recognize glenoid erosion, the glenoid prosthesis may be malpositioned. Cementing the glenoid prosthesis in a malposition may cause subluxation or dislocation of the humeral head prosthesis, as it tends to slide out in the direction in which the glenoid is tilted (Fig. 38–55).

In most cases, altering the degree of retroversion to compensate for slight posterior or anterior wear on the glenoid is acceptable.[24, 97, 100, 102] If adequate support and stability of the glenoid component cannot be attained by reshaping or molding the glenoid surface, glenoid bone grafting may be necessary.[63, 97] Cortical-cancellous bone for the glenoid graft usually is harvested from the previously resected humeral head. If this graft is inadequate, iliac crest may be used. In 1988, Neer and Morrison[97] reported the necessity of employing large, internally fixed glenoid grafts in 20 of 463 total shoulder arthroplasties, an incidence of 4.4 percent. Although the incidence is not high, the surgeon must recognize the indications and be familiar with techniques of glenoid bone grafting.

A total of 80 percent of the surface of the metal-backed prosthesis and the entire back of the polyethylene prosthesis should be well supported by bone.[97] Anything less is inadequate and would be considered an indication for bone grafting. Without bone support, loosening is much more likely. In the past, glenoid prostheses augmented on one side to compensate for the glenoid bone defect were occasionally used. These are no longer recommended. Support by bone

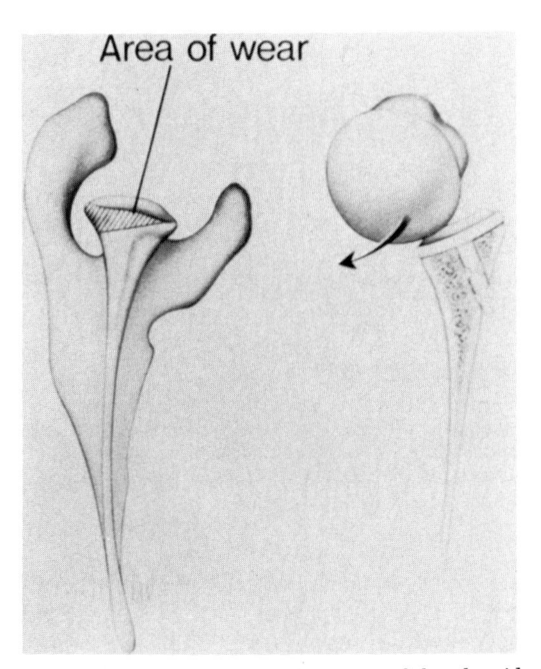

FIGURE 38–55. Improper placement of the glenoid, allowing the humeral head to slide off the angled glenoid and sublux or dislocate. To avoid this problem, the surgeon must be cognizant of malversion of the glenoid and correct for it. (Neer, C. S., II and Morrison, D. S.: Glenoid bone grafting in total shoulder arthroplasty. J. Bone Joint Surg. 70A:1154–1162, 1988. By permission.)

stock is preferable to support by thicker polyethylene. The bone graft is shaped to fit the defect, thereby supplying the missing bony support for the prosthesis (Fig. 38–56).[97, 102]

The technique for bone grafting in cases of anterior wear and deficiency in the glenoid is shown in Figure 38–57.[102] Insufficient bone at the posterior neck prohibits this procedure posteriorly. An osteotome is employed to lever out a wedge of cortical bone at the anterior glenoid neck. The bone graft can then be keyed into the wedged space between the anterior cortex of the glenoid and the remaining posterior body. Whenever possible, the graft should be fixed to the glenoid with screws. The screws should not interfere with the channel for the glenoid prosthetic keel and should not be in contact with the glenoid component. If screws would block placement of the glenoid prosthesis, the graft can be keyed into position and held with sutures sewn through the graft and the glenoid bone. A double cementing technique, as described in *Surgical Technique,* assures good fixation of the prosthesis.[99]

Loosening is more likely if the surgeon attempts to compensate for glenoid wear by building up the low side with cement. Fragments of cement may fracture into the joint.[102]

If the erosion is not recognized and the surgeon attempts to place the prosthesis flush with a malpositioned glenoid surface, the channel for the keel will become angled in relation to the anterior or posterior glenoid cortical wall. The wall will be penetrated as the channel is deepened. The direction of the channel must be corrected and the hole in the cortical wall packed with bone graft from the humeral head so that cement will not escape when the prosthesis is placed.

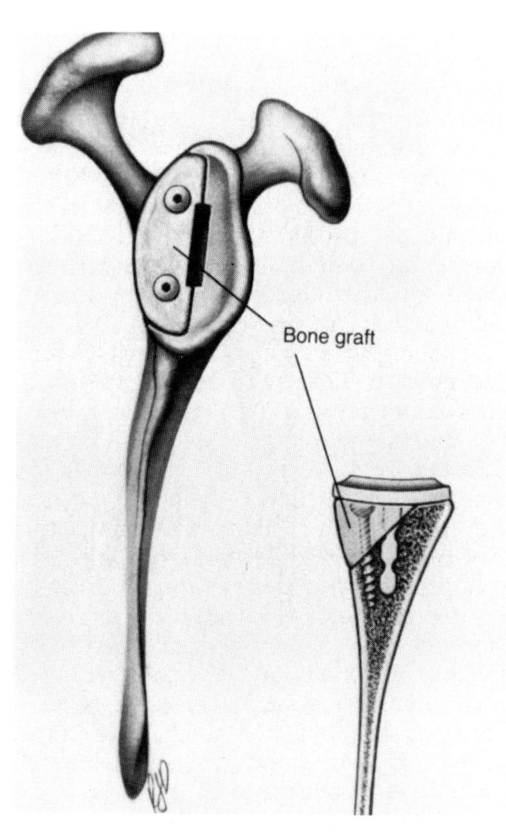

FIGURE 38–56. Graft is shaped to fit the defect. Such grafts are usually fixed with screws that are countersunk to avoid interference with the prosthesis. (Neer, C. S., II and Morrison, D. S.: Glenoid bone grafting in total shoulder arthroplasty. J. Bone Joint Surg. 70A:1154–1162, 1988. By permission.)

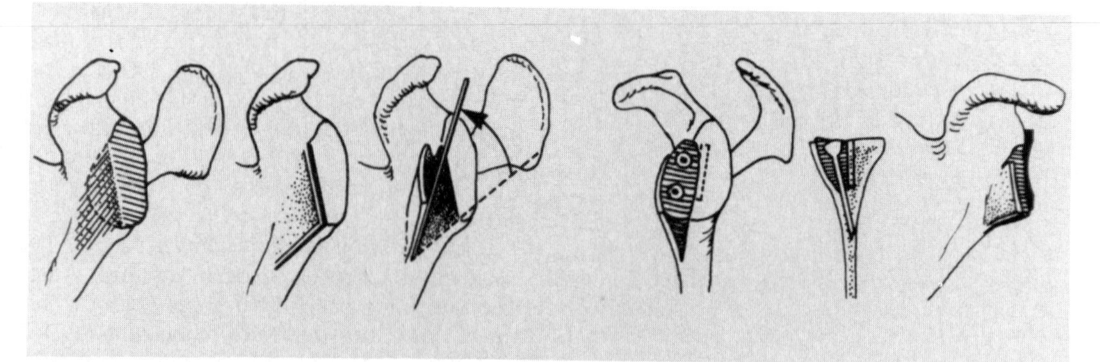

FIGURE 38–57. Method of bone grafting the anterior glenoid. The anterior cortex of the glenoid is osteotomized as shown and gently pried anteriorly to open a space for the graft. The graft is then inserted and fixed with countersunk screws. (Norris, T. R.: Bone Grafts for Glenoid Deficiency in Total Shoulder Replacements. In Proceedings of the Third International Conference on Surgery of the Shoulder. Professional Postgraduate Services, Fukuoka, Japan, 1986, pp. 373–376. By permission.)

Malunions

Chronic fracture problems for which prosthetic arthroplasty is indicated as definitive treatment include malunion with incongruity of the articular surface of the humeral head and osteonecrosis associated with fracture.[129] Often, patients with chronic fracture problems have had one or more previous surgical procedures. Failed closed reduction may have resulted in significant malposition of the united fracture fragments. The anatomy is frequently distorted, and the rotator cuff may be scarred and inelastic. Excessive amounts of scar tissue may be present. The surgeon may also have to deal with the remnants of failed internal fixation, such as screws, pins, wires, and plates.

Postoperative results are variable. In the series of Tanner and Cofield,[32, 129] motion and function in patients with malunited fractures were related to the presence of a rotator cuff and capsule of good quality as well as to tuberosities that were in nearly anatomic position or that could be repositioned and healed without displacement. If the repair was tenuous because of poor tissue or tuberosity positioning and required support of the arm in abduction, the postoperative range of abduction and external rotation were not as good.

The surgical approach and operative technique for these problems are basically the same as for any shoulder arthroplasty. Of special importance is the often difficult task of developing the subdeltoid and subacromial spaces, which are frequently obliterated by scar, so that the deltoid can be retracted adequately. The retraction must be done carefully to avoid damage to the axillary nerve, which lies on the undersurface of the deltoid.[129] Should the nerve be damaged, paralysis of the anterior deltoid could result. The biceps tendon is a helpful guide to the intertubercular area where the anatomy has been distorted by fracture and scar. The axillary nerve should also be identified and protected, as it courses around the edge of the subscapularis and lies adjacent to the inferior capsule of the glenohumeral joint at the humeral neck.

Sometimes, the surgeon must osteotomize malunited tuberosities and attempt to reposition them more normally, a task that is not always simple and may even be impossible owing to a scarred and contracted rotator cuff. The goal is still the restoration of the cuff. Radiographs made in multiple planes should be analyzed preoperatively to determine the relationship of the tuberosities to the shaft and to plan the osteotomy.[129] In general, the osteotomy of the lesser tuberosity can be in one plane, but the osteotomy of the greater tuberosity is biplanar because of the attachments of the supraspinatus and the external rotators. After the osteotomy, the tuberosities are repositioned against the flange of the prosthesis and the upper humeral shaft. The head in this instance is exposed by retracting the osteotomized tuberosities and attached rotator cuff.

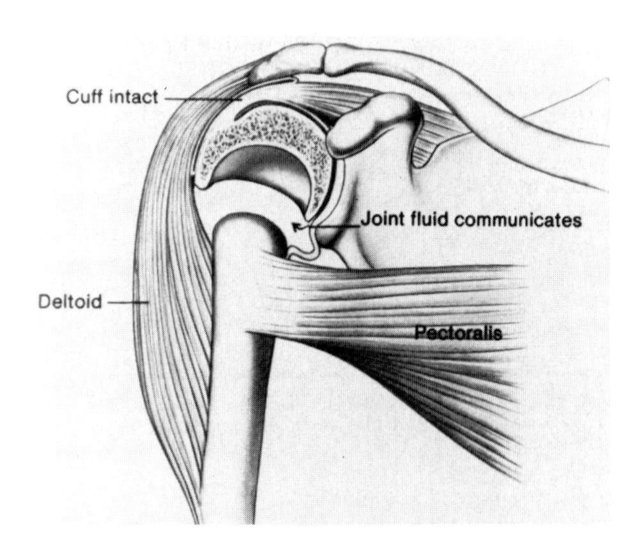

FIGURE 38–58. Proximal humeral nonunion demonstrating the synovial pseudoarthrosis that develops at the nonunion site because of communication with the adjacent glenohumeral joint. Also shown are the resorption and cavitation of the humeral head that often occurs. (Neer, C. S., II: Part 1: Fractures About the Shoulder. Fractures in Adults, 2nd ed., Vol. 1. Edited by C. A. Rockwood, Jr. and D. P. Green. Philadelphia, J. B. Lippincott Company, 1984. By permission.)

Nonunions

The most common cause of nonunion in fractures of the upper humerus above the deltoid insertion is inadequate immobilization, often combined with traction on the fracture site from the weight of the arm or cast.[132] Accumulation of joint fluid at the fracture site promotes nonunion and synovial pseudoarthrosis. Softening, resorption, cavitation of the head, and soft tissue interposition contribute to nonunion. In some cases, lack of cancellous bone of good quality is a factor (Fig. 38–58).[92, 93, 105, 132] Nonunion itself can result in problems that make successful treatment difficult. For example, resorption and superior migration of the shaft produce relative lengthening and consequent weakness of the deltoid. Inferior subluxation of the head also complicates treatment.[132]

Patients with surgical neck nonunions who may be best treated by prosthetic arthroplasty include patients who have developed a small atrophic head fragment,[104, 129] patients who have experienced more than one failed attempt at surgical repair, and elderly or debilitated patients with poor bone stock.[132] The last-mentioned patients tolerate prolonged immobilization poorly, and the quality of their bone often prohibits adequate fixation and healing.[104, 132]

Measurement on scanograms is helpful in providing the information necessary to restore proper length. Cement stabilizes the humeral component at the correct height. Proper prosthetic version and reconstruction of the tuberosities and cuff are important. Bone graft can be taken either from the remains of the humeral head or from the iliac crest.[132]

COMPLICATIONS AND FAILURE

Complications may result in the failure of prosthetic arthroplasty, making revision necessary.[51, 98] Because of the close relationship between complications, failure, and revision of shoulder arthroplasty, these problems are addressed together.

In a review of the literature, Cofield[36] reported complications of Neer hemiarthroplasty in 8 percent of cases, of Neer total shoulder arthroplasty in 12 percent, and of shoulder arthroplasty with various other implant designs in 17 percent (Tables 38–6 and 38–7). He estimated that perhaps half of the complications with the Neer

Table 38–6. COMPLICATIONS OF 229 NEER HEMIARTHROPLASTIES

Infection	2
Intraoperative fracture	1
Nerve injury	3
Ectopic ossification	2
Instability	6
Rotator cuff tear, tuberosity malunion, nonunion	4
Total	18 (8%)

Modified from Cofield, R. H.: The Shoulder. Edited by C. A. Rockwood, Jr. and F. A. Matsen, III. Philadelphia, W. B. Saunders Co., 1990.

Table 38–7. COMPLICATIONS OF 586 NEER TOTAL SHOULDER ARTHROPLASTIES

Infection	3 (0.51%)
Intraoperative fracture	8 (1.4%)
Nerve injury	4 (0.68%)
Ectopic ossification	1 (0.17%)
Instability	11 (1.9%)
Impingement	6 (1.0%)
Rotator cuff tear, tuberosity malunion, nonunion	20 (3.4%)
Glenoid loosening	15 (2.6%)
Humeral loosening	2 (0.34%)
Total	70 (12.0%)

Modified from Cofield, R. H.: The Shoulder. Edited by C. A. Rockwood, Jr. and F. A. Matsen, III. Philadelphia, W. B. Saunders, Co., 1990.

prosthesis will need revision.[34] Neer[100] reported 22 complications (3 percent) requiring further surgery in his series of 776 unconstrained arthroplasties (Table 38–8).

A list of reported complications is provided in Table 38–9. Obviously, some complications can occur irrespective of the skill of the surgeon, whereas others are due to errors in surgical technique. Technical errors are particularly common in the treatment of fractures of the upper humerus. For example, the surgeon may fail to restore humeral length or may not accurately place, replace, or secure fractured tuberosities.[89, 106, 129]

To treat complications effectively and salvage failed arthroplasties, the surgeon should accurately define the problem and elucidate the cause.[33, 89, 100] Only in this way can revision surgery be accomplished with any reasonable hope of success. Bone loss, muscle loss, scar tissue, threat of fracture, and increased risk of infection make revision the most difficult of shoulder arthroplasties.[33, 89, 100]

Table 38–8. COMPLICATIONS THAT REQUIRED REOPERATION IN NEER'S PERSONAL SERIES OF 776 NONCONSTRAINED ARTHROPLASTIES

	No. Patients
Infection	2
Fracture out of bone	2
Repair of cuff	3
Late breakage of tuberosity wire	2
Excess anteversion	2
Nonunion of greater tuberosity	2
Broken stem of glenoid component	5
Loosening of glenoid component	2
Unexplained pain	2
	22

(Neer, C. S., II: Shoulder Reconstruction. Philadelphia, W. B. Saunders Company, 1990. By permission.)

Table 38–9. REPORTED COMPLICATIONS OF PROSTHETIC ARTHROPLASTY OF THE SHOULDER

Infection	Acute (early)
	Acute (late)
	Delayed
Fracture	Intraoperative
	Postoperative
Nerve injury	Contusion
	Stretching
	Laceration
	Thermal injury (from extruded cement)
Ectopic ossification	
Instability	Superior
	Posterior
	Anterior
	Inferior
Impingement	Failure to correct acromion
	Humeral prosthesis below greater tuberosity
Rotator cuff tear	
Deltoid dehiscence	
Tuberosity nonunion	
Tuberosity malunion	
Glenoid loosening	
Humeral loosening	
Penetrating cortex of humerus or glenoid	
Protrusion of glenoid or humeral stem through bone	
Broken glenoid stem	
Medial subsidence of glenoid	
Errors of version	
Errors of length (height)	
Complications of cement	Extrusion
	Cement particles in joint
Wound healing problems	Dehiscence
	Hematoma
Transection external rotators osteotomizing humeral head	
Postoperative stiffness	
Reflex sympathetic dystrophy	

(Data from refs. 1, 4, 9, 12, 14, 18, 22, 25, 27, 33, 34, 36, 39, 47, 51, 88, 89, 98, 100, 127, 133.)

Surgical Errors

Nerve Injuries

Any of the nerves about the shoulder are in danger of injury because of their anatomic proximity to the glenohumeral joint. The axillary nerve is dangerously close to the inferior capsule and neck of the humerus (see Fig. 38–12).

We have treated referred patients with lacerated axillary nerves that were not discovered until after surgery. We have also explored referred patients with deltoid paralysis and found that a suture had been placed inadvertently around the nerve during capsular repair. In one patient referred with deltoid paralysis after a Bristow procedure, we found that the conjoined tendon had been wrapped around the axillary nerve when the coracoid tip was transferred inferiorly.[103]

Partial denervation of the deltoid can occur if the muscle is split too far distally when the shoulder joint is exposed. In these cases, the nerve is lacerated as it lies on the undersurface of the muscle, coursing laterally and anteriorly. To avoid the nerve, the surgeon should not split the muscle any farther than 4 cm from the edge of the acromion.[83] Placing a suture at the distal end of the muscle split will remind the surgeon not to split past this point.

The suprascapular nerve is also in danger because of its proximity to the joint. This nerve can be injured during arthroscopy, while freeing up the infraspinatus during cuff repair or while making a posterior approach to the shoulder.

A thorough knowledge of anatomy and constant awareness of the location of nerves as well as vessels will prevent most neurovascular complications. In doing revision arthroplasty complicated by scar tissue and distorted anatomy, normal nerves should be identified away from the shoulder and then followed into the surgical field.

Fractures

Fractures sometimes occur during arthroplasty procedures, especially revision surgery, and they greatly complicate the procedure. The humeral shaft is most often involved, but fracture of the glenoid or glenoid neck occurs on occasion.[130] Fractures are most common in osteoporotic bone, owing to age or disuse because of the chronic shoulder problem. Fractures are usually caused by excessive torque on the humeral shaft, which occurs when the surgeon attempts to dislocate the head, reduce a prosthetic head that is too large, or reduce a prosthesis when not enough head has been resected. If the channel for the prosthetic stem is too tight, the humeral shaft can fracture as the prosthesis is being inserted.

A full complement of prosthetic sizes, including long stems, will help in solving the problem of inadvertent fracture during arthroplasty. Treatment may include a long-stem prosthesis as an intramedullary rod across the fracture site. Comminuted fragments can be held in a reduced position around the stem of the prosthesis with cerclage wires or screws. Sometimes, cement will be necessary. Bone grafting, employing the resected portion of the humeral head, is often wise. A fractured greater tuberosity should be reduced and secured well.[104, 108]

Disruption of Deltoid Repair

As a general rule, it is best not to detach the origin of the anterior deltoid from the clavicle or acromion.[86, 130] An intact deltoid is important for early rehabilitation, and detaching it subjects it to the possibility of dehiscence. Disruption can also result from retraction that is too vigorous. If more exposure is needed (e.g., during revision), it is better to detach part of the insertion of either the deltoid or the pectoralis major. If disruption does occur, it must be repaired.

Postoperative Complications

Rotator Cuff Tears

Acute tear of the rotator cuff occurs occasionally after arthroplasty.[12, 36] Barrett and coworkers[4, 5] and Franklin and associates[47] reported an increased incidence of glenoid loosening associated with rotator cuff tears, presumably because of eccentric loading of the glenoid prosthesis. It would therefore make sense to repair these tears, even though the patient may not seem disabled enough to want to undergo another operation.

Atrophic rotator cuff tissue may disrupt after surgery. Rather than repair, symptomatic treatment may be the only reasonable approach. Goals for postoperative results may have to be more limited in patients with atrophic rotator cuffs.

Instability

Superior migration of the prosthesis may signal rotator cuff disruption.[13] Posterior dislocation or subluxation may occur if the humeral head was placed in too much retroversion or if posterior wear of the glenoid was not corrected. Anterior instability also may be due to malposition of the prosthetic components (e.g., too much humeral anteversion). However, anterior instability is more often due to disruption of the subscapularis, and it must be repaired.[33] Inferior subluxation may simply be due to muscle atony, and in this case it will respond well to isometric exercises for the biceps, triceps, and deltoid.[33] However, inferior subluxation could be caused by nerve injury. Failure to restore length when doing arthroplasty may also result in an unstable prosthesis.[88]

Infections

Infections are rare after prosthetic arthroplasty, the incidence being less than 1 percent.[36, 88] However, the infections that do occur can be disastrous. Infections are usually late in onset and are most often due to *Staphylococcus aureus*.[36]

Drainage and debridement are important in acute and delayed infections. Antibiotics initially are administered intravenously and are continued orally for a prolonged period.[36] Chronic infections may require a "clean-out procedure," in which all prosthetic components and cement are removed.[112] Neer[89] suggests that after removal of the prosthesis, antibiotics be given for 3 months or longer and a sling be applied for 3 to 6 months, followed by active use as tolerated. If pain and loss of function are severe, Neer would consider fusion. Based on experience with infections in total knee and hip arthroplasties, delayed replantation of a prosthesis after the infection is cleared may be considered in some cases.

Stiffness

Postoperative stiffness may be the result of periarthritis, heterotopic bone formation, or reflex sympathetic dystrophy. A mechanical problem with the prosthesis may be to blame. An inadequate rehabilitation program or a noncompliant patient may contribute to the problem.[31, 33]

Fractures

Fractures of the humerus have occurred when an elderly or a debilitated patient attempted to force a shoulder beyond its postoperative limits. Usually, the humeral shaft is fractured just below the stem of the prosthesis. The fracture may be transverse or oblique. Revision of the humeral prosthesis to a long stem that will serve as an intramedullary rod will stabilize the fracture and allow early resumption of motion.

We treated a patient with this type of fracture conservatively, because revision of the humeral prosthesis would have been very difficult. She had had five previous operative procedures on the shoulder, and the humeral component was cemented. We treated the arm with longitudinal plaster slabs about the humeral shaft and a shoulder immobilizer. After a prolonged period, the bone united.

Failures Necessitating Revision

Neer and Kirby[89] analyzed the causes of failure and treatment of 40 unsatisfactory humeral head and total shoulder arthroplasties (Table 38–10). In 34 of the 40 cases, treatment consisted of implantation of a Neer II unconstrained total shoulder system. The other revision surgeries were removal of the implant and cement in two cases, arthrodesis in three, and implant of a Neer fixed-fulcrum prosthesis in one case. Reasons for failure of unconstrained arthroplasties are similar for both humeral head arthroplasties and total shoulder arthroplasties, except for glenoid problems.[89, 100]

Many patients develop an internal rotation contracture from a tight subscapularis, the result of holding the arm turned in against the chest to diminish pain.[89] Neglecting to address this problem at revision dooms the procedure to failure. The subscapularis must be freed, and often it must be lengthened.

The effect of detaching the deltoid to expose the shoulder at arthroplasty has already been discussed. The deltoid had been weakened by such detachment in all but 3 of the 40 revisions reported by Neer and Kirby.[89] In five patients, the deltoid had been denervated.

Scarring is always a problem once a shoulder has been operated on. Scarring and adhesions are frequently found in the subacromial space, between the deltoid and

Table 38–10. SUMMARY OF CAUSES OF FAILURE OF HUMERAL HEAD AND TOTAL SHOULDER PROSTHETIC ARTHROPLASTIES

General	
Psychological	Lack of motivation, alcoholism
Nerve injury or cervical root defect	Electromyograms, etc.
Arthritis	Acromioclavicular or sternoclavicular joints
Scapulothoracic mechanism	Weakness or deformity
Local	
Infection	Aspiration and cultures, scans, frozen section during surgery
Instability	Dislocations
Heterotopic bone	Delay revision if active
Deltoid defects	Detached, retracted, scarred
Cuff defects	Contractures, adhesions, detached
Bone defects	Bone loss, bony prominence, nonunion, impingement, retracted tuberosity, retained head, too long, loss of length, glenoid slope, "centralization," pannus erosion
Contractures and adhesions	Always present
Implant	
Humeral component	Version, height, head length, stability, stem size, loosening, breakage, cement
Glenoid component	Version, face upward, height, loosening, breakage, wear, cement

(Neer, C. S., II: Shoulder Reconstruction. Philadelphia, W. B. Saunders Company, 1990. By permission.)

the rotator cuff, and between the rotator cuff and underlying capsule. The gliding planes of these muscles must be freed at revision and kept free through a rehabilitation program. Indeed, a main point in doing revision shoulder arthroplasty surgery is to free up the deltoid and subacromial space while gaining exposure for revision.[89]

Either a retracted or a prominent tuberosity can cause failure.[89] Placing the prosthetic head below the level of the greater tuberosity makes the tuberosity relatively prominent, and it will impinge against the acromion when the arm is elevated. Acromioplasty will not correct the problem. If a fractured and retracted greater tuberosity is not repositioned adequately at initial surgery, it can interfere with both external rotation and elevation. This problem can be especially difficult to correct at revision surgery. The surgeon may have to choose an additional posterior approach to expose the retracted bone adequately and free it for advancement to the correct position.

A common cause of arthroplasty failure is neglecting to restore the length of the fractured humerus. The result is an unstable prosthesis and weakness of the deltoid muscle. In the series of Neer and Kirby,[89] 27 of the failed arthroplasties had been performed for fractures, and 18 of them developed such problems. The prosthesis had to be removed and a new one inserted so that the myofascial sleeve was at normal tension and length.

If uneven glenoid wear is not corrected at the initial surgery, the prosthesis will likely sublux or even dislocate. Slight posterior wear of the glenoid might be compensated for by setting the humeral head prosthesis in less retroversion. The unevenness can sometimes be corrected by lowering the high side of the glenoid. Occasionally, a glenoid bone graft will be required.[88, 98, 100, 102] Building up with cement is an inappropriate way to correct the abnormal slope, as this practice predisposes the patient to loosening and cement fragmentation.

Central wear of the glenoid allows the head to migrate medially (arthrokatadysis).[36, 87] If the joint space is too large, the prosthesis will be unstable.[88] The failure is corrected by the employment of a thick humeral head or possibly by a bone graft or special glenoid component.

Radiolucent Lines and Loosening

Over the long run, loosening of the glenoid component may be the most frequent problem associated with replacement arthroplasty of the shoulder. In a review of nine series of shoulder arthroplasties, Cofield[36] noted that the incidence of glenoid loosening was 2.6 percent. Humeral component loosening is not common, occurring in only 0.34 percent of cases.

Brenner and colleagues[16] reported the presence of radiolucent lines in 57 percent of the Neer prostheses in their series of 38 arthroplasties. Despite the high incidence of radiolucent lines reported by some workers, the overall revision rate for glenoid loosening is less than 1 percent.[100] Seeing lucent lines in patients referred for revisions, Neer[100] expected to find loose glenoid components at surgery. However, no demonstrable loosening was found in some cases. In his review of 273 patients with total shoulder replacement, Neer[100] did not find any evidence of clinical loosening of the glenoid, although lucent lines were present at some part of the bone-cement interface in 30 percent of cases.

Settergren and Cofield,[127] in a 5- to 10-year follow-up of 71 Neer total shoulder arthroplasties, found a complete lucent line of 1.5 mm or greater or a shift in position of one third of the glenoids. Revision surgery was necessary for three of the five patients who had loose glenoids. The earliest revision was 4 years after surgery. These investigators suggested that glenoid loosening is the most frequent of the potential complications of Neer total shoulder arthroplasty. As length of follow-up increases, more revisions become necessary.[127]

Barrett and associates[6] reviewed 140 total shoulder replacements in patients with polyarticular rheumatoid arthritis. Average follow-up was 4.9 years. The incidence of lucent lines was 80 percent, but only 5 percent of the glenoids were loose; 3 percent of these were revised. The relatively high incidence of glenoid loosening may reflect the quality of bone found in patients with rheumatoid arthritis.

Bonutti and coworkers[9] reported their experience in revising eight loose glenoid and three loose humeral components following total shoulder arthroplasties. The average time from the initial procedure to the revision was 3.1 years. Pain associated with "clunking" caused these patients to seek medical attention. Most of the revisions were to metal-backed glenoids.

Boyd and colleagues[12] reviewed failures among 313 total shoulder arthroplasties and 123 humeral head arthroplasties. Five humeral components and seven glenoids were grossly loose. Only four of these were associated with lucent lines greater than 2 mm in width. This suggests that loosening can be present even with small lucent lines.

In reviewing experience with 50 total shoulder replacements, Barrett and associates[4] found an association between rotator cuff disease and glenoid loosening. Four of the six painful shoulders had loosening of the glenoid and massive tearing of the rotator cuff. Subsequently, three other patients were found to have glenoid loosening associated with rotator cuff tears. In all of these patients, radiographs demonstrated that the humeral component had migrated proximally on the glenoid and the glenoid component had tipped superiorly. Massive rotator cuff defects apparently altered the kinematics of the shoulder. With the upward force of the deltoid being unopposed, eccentrically applied compressive forces at the glenoid caused rocking of the glenoid component on the underlying osseous glenoid and increased the stress at the bone-cement interface. A complete or incomplete radiolucent line was associated with 74 percent of the glenoid components in this series. Radiolucent lines about the flange were not associated with loosening. These investigators reported a 36 percent incidence of radiolucent lines about the keel and expressed concern about the 10 percent glenoid loosening rate over a relatively short time.[4]

Reviewing eight different series of total shoulder arthroplasties, Cofield[36] found that the incidence of radiolucent lines varied from 30 to 93 percent. The median incidence of radiolucent lines identified about the keel of the prosthesis in these series was 36 percent. In the series reported in 1984, Cofield[27] found that in some cases lucent lines developed over time. He expressed concern that in his series and that of Barrett and coworkers, serial radiographs demonstrated a shift in glenoid position relative to its immediate postoperative position, even in some cases without lucent lines, strongly suggesting loosening.[36, 100]

Brems and colleagues[14] studied glenoid lucent lines on the radiographs of 69 Neer II total shoulder replacements. Although 69 percent of the patients had radiolucent lines before leaving the hospital after initial arthroplasties, only six shoulders demonstrated further widening or progression of the lucent lines at an average 5-year follow-up. None was symptomatic. The workers concluded that variability in surgical technique was the factor most responsible for the high incidence of lucent lines.[14]

Surgical technique and expertise as factors in glenoid loosening have been implicated by other investigators as well. Barrett and associates[4] suggested that loosening might be decreased by careful contouring of the osseous glenoid to match the glenoid prosthesis and by use of a metal-backed component. Neer and coworkers[88] noted that the incidence of radiolucent lines about the glenoid was lower in those shoulders operated on later in their series, suggesting that experience might have made for better cementing technique.

Summary

It would seem that some complications of prosthetic arthroplasty could be reduced by a thorough understanding of anatomy and careful surgical technique. Of particular importance are the following: (1) proper cementing technique, (2) restoration of humeral length when treating fractures, (3) adequate replacement of displaced tuberosities, (4) proper version of the humeral head prosthesis, (5) correct height relationships between the humeral head and greater tuberosity, (6) correction for glenoid deterioration, and (7) restoration of the rotator cuff.

REHABILITATION

Postoperative rehabilitation is just as important as the surgery itself; in fact, the two are codependent. The surgeon's role does not stop when the operation is over; he or she must be directly involved in patient rehabilitation. Only the surgeon knows precisely what was done in the operating room and is aware of the quality of the tissue repaired and, therefore, the limits of the postoperative exercise program. The rehabilitation program needs to be individualized by the patient's surgeon.

Patient cooperation is crucial to the success of the postoperative program. Patients must understand that they are their own best therapists. Although the surgeon and the physical therapist can assist them, the real work can be done only by the patients themselves. Patient understanding and cooperation are particularly important in this age of medical cost containment, when long hospital stays for postoperative rehabilitation can no longer be justified. Furthermore, in a prolonged hospital situation, the patient may become overdependent on the surgeon and the therapist rather than independent.

Patients generally work harder and cooperate best if they are provided with a written and illustrated rehabilitation program and a precise schedule that they must follow each day. The instructions must clearly state the daily number of exercise sessions and the number of repetitions of each exercise. I have found that without such instructions, patients often do their program in a haphazard fashion, not accomplishing as much as they could if they were better organized. The goal toward which the patient strives might be the range of motion of the opposite, unoperated shoulder, provided it is free of pathology and the surgery does not contraindicate this degree of motion.

Phases of Rehabilitation

Hughes and Neer[61] have described an excellent basic postoperative rehabilitation program, which is divided into three phases.

The first phase consists of passive exercises to prevent adhesions and postoperative stiffness. The program begins with pendulum exercises (Fig. 38–59). Then,

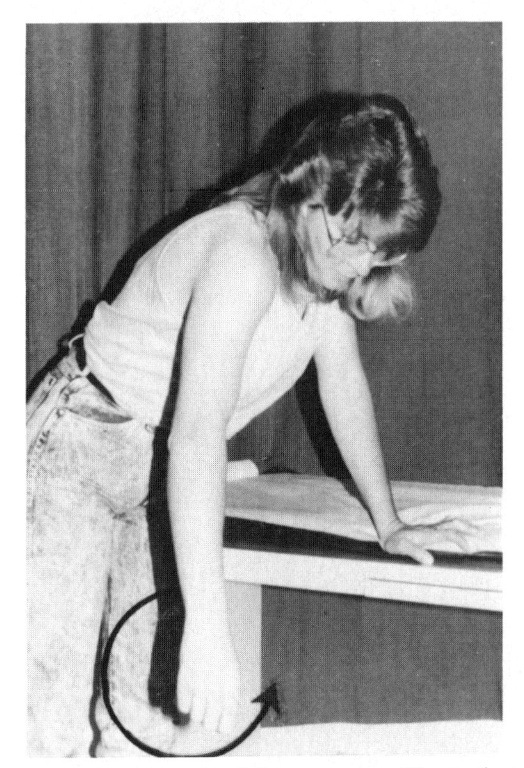

FIGURE 38–59. Pendulum exercise. The patient bends forward at the waist, first circling the operated arm inward with the palm facing backward, then circling the arm in an outward direction with the palm facing forward.

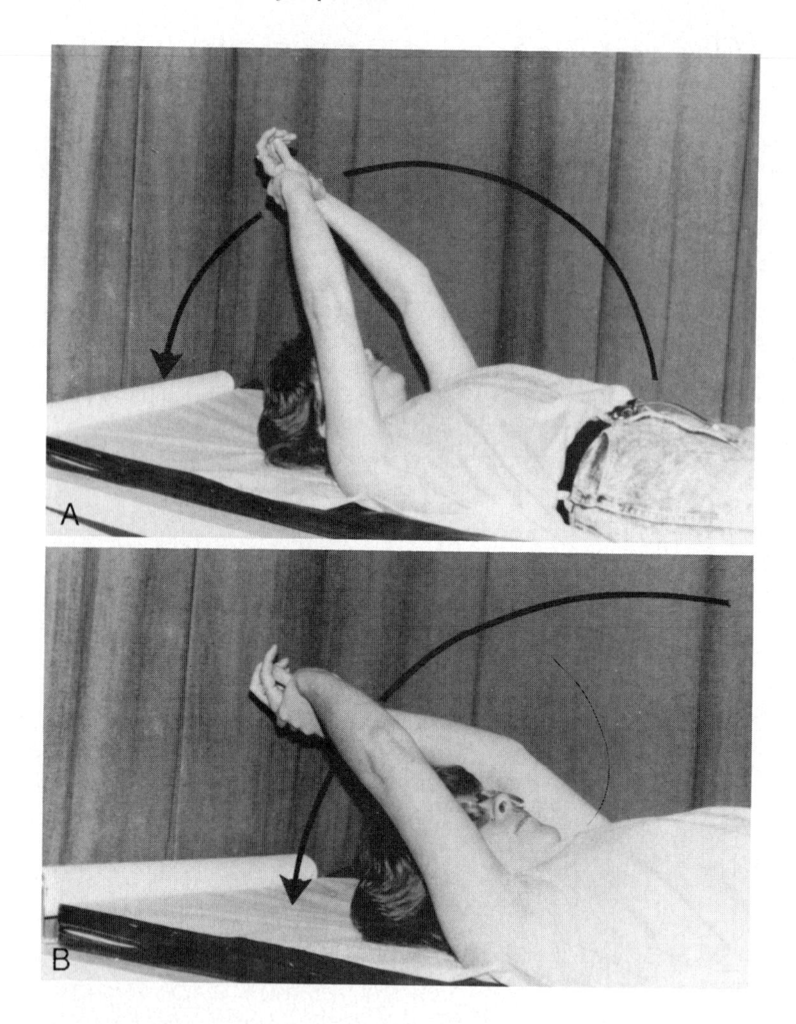

FIGURE 38–60. *A,* Assisted (passive) forward elevation. With the arms lying on the abdomen, the patient grasps the wrist of the operated arm (in this case, the left) with the opposite hand, then uses the unoperated arm to passively elevate the other arm. Gradual stretching is accomplished until the operated arm can be brought into a fully elevated position above the head and close to the table top (arrow). *B,* Assisted (passive) forward elevation is shown, as the arm approaches the fully elevated position above the head.

passive forward elevation and external rotation done in the supine position are added (Figs. 38–60 and 38–61). Range of motion is gradually increased as the patient becomes more comfortable. As the patient progresses during the next 6 to 8 weeks, pulley exercises, passive internal rotation behind the back, and external rotation with the hands placed behind the neck are added (Figs. 38–62 and 38–63).

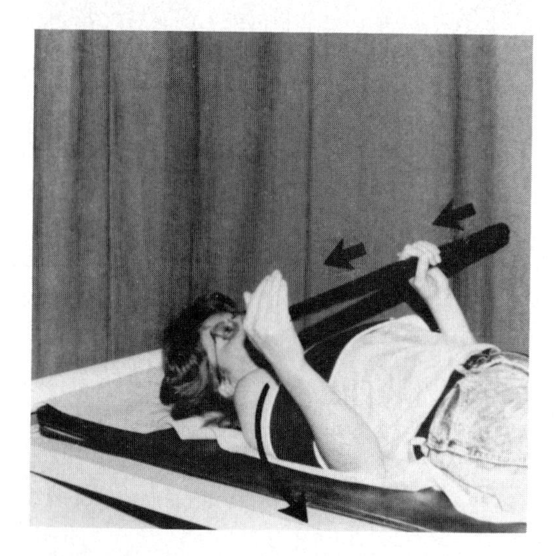

FIGURE 38–61. Assisted external rotation using the "broomstick." With elbows kept at the patient's side and at right angles, the forearm and hand of the operated side (right) point directly toward the ceiling. The opposite hand and broomstick are then used to rotate the operated arm into external rotation (arrows). A Velpeau chest strap from a shoulder immobilizer is utilized to help hold the operated arm to the chest wall so that any force will be concentrated on external rotation and not dissipated by abducting the arm.

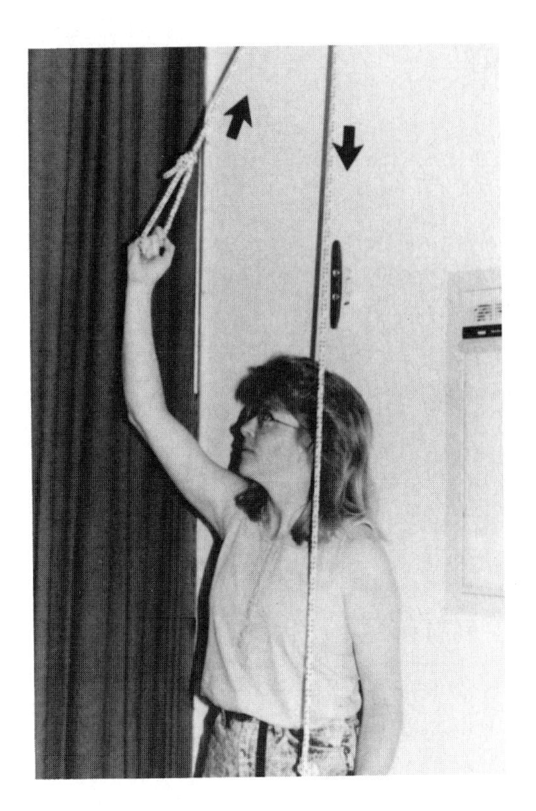

FIGURE 38–62. Pulley exercises. These exercises are used to passively elevate the operated arm (in this case the right arm) to stretch out adhesions and to promote gliding of the soft tissue planes past one another. The unoperated arm is used to pull the operated arm upward in the plane of the scapula as shown. The exercise is best done with the patient's back supported flat against a wall or door surface. This practice prevents the patient from raising the arm by bending the spine backward at the waist as the operated shoulder becomes uncomfortable with further elevation. If that happens, proper gradual stretching of the shoulder tissues cannot occur. As the patient's tissues become accustomed to the exercise, the initial discomfort of stretching will pass.

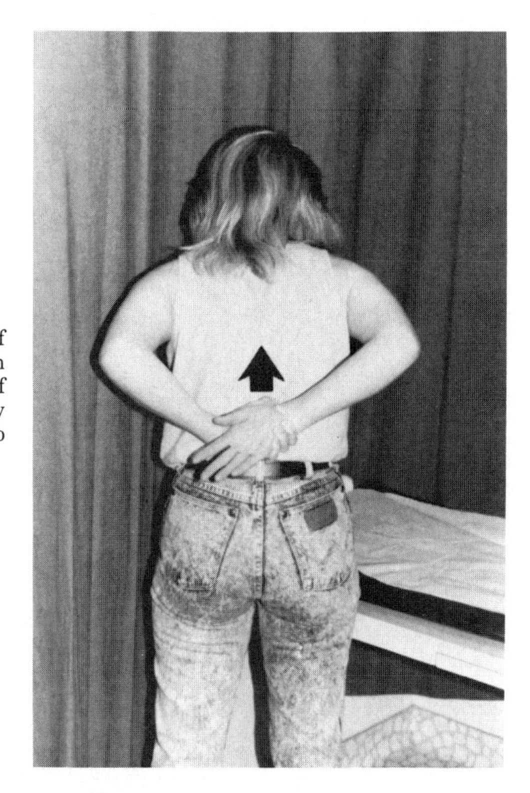

FIGURE 38–63. Assisted internal rotation. The hand of the unoperated arm grasps the wrist of the operated arm on the ulnar side, with the hands initially at the level of the sacrum. The unoperated arm is then used to gradually push the operated arm (in this case the right arm) into internal rotation (arrow).

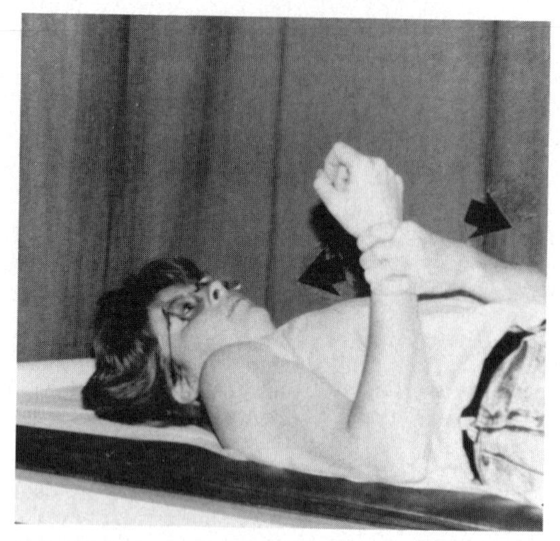

FIGURE 38–64. Isometric strengthening of the external rotators. The operated arm (right) is kept from rotating outward by the resisting opposite hand that prevents movement of the operated arm as the external rotators contract isometrically. The patient can contract the muscles, hold for a few seconds, and then relax. The sequence is repeated for the number of repetitions recommended by the surgeon or therapist.

At the third postoperative week, isometric muscle strengthening should begin. The isometric exercises are done for the internal and external rotators as well as for the forward elevators, abductors, and extensors (Figs. 38–64 through 38–70).

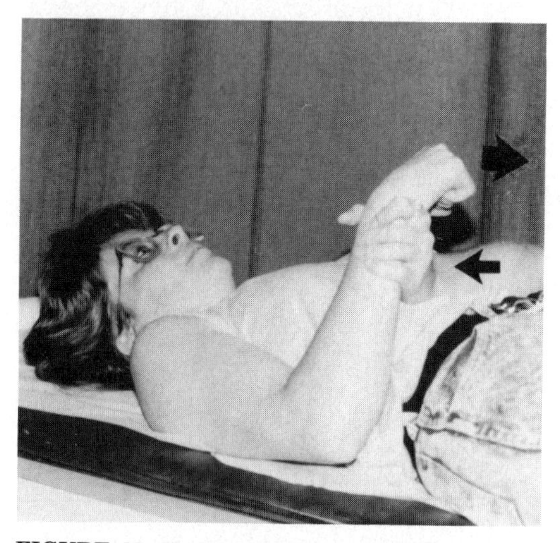

FIGURE 38–65. Isometric strengthening of the internal rotators. The operated arm (right) is kept from rotating inward by the opposite hand as the internal rotator muscles isometrically contract against the resistance provided. The patient can contract the muscles, hold for a few seconds, and then relax. The sequence is repeated for the number of repetitions recommended by the surgeon or therapist.

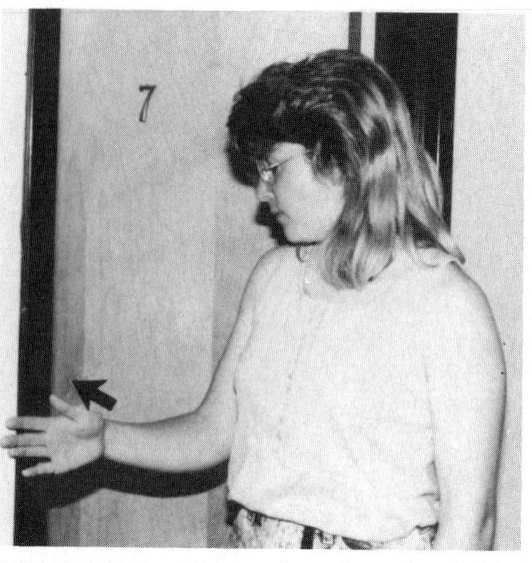

FIGURE 38–66. Isometric strengthening of the external rotators. The back of the hand and wrist is placed against a door frame with the elbow at a right angle. The hand is then pushed against the surface by isometrically contracting the external rotators. The elbow should be kept close to the patient's body during the exercise so that the force exerted is mainly that of the external rotators.

The second phase begins 4 to 6 weeks after surgery and is designed for more active muscle participation. New exercises involve unassisted forward elevation in the supine position and active-assisted forward elevation while sitting or standing (Figs.

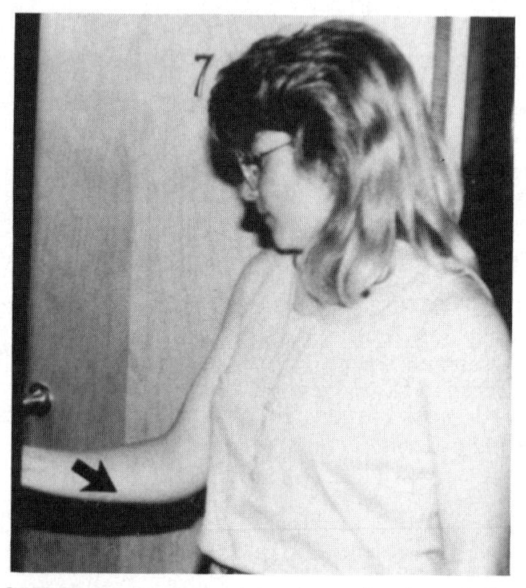

FIGURE 38–67. Isometric strengthening of the internal rotators. The hand and wrist of the operated arm are placed on the opposite side of a door frame, with the elbow at a right angle close to the body. The hand and wrist are then pulled against the door frame (arrow) toward the torso. The force is exerted by isometrically contracting the internal rotators the number of prescribed repetitions.

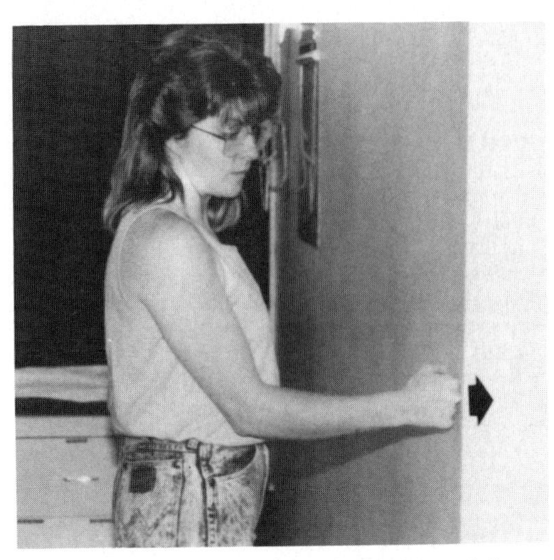

FIGURE 38–68. Isometric strengthening of the anterior deltoid. The hand of the operated side pushes against a wall while the deltoid is contracted isometrically. This exercise is repeated for the recommended number of times.

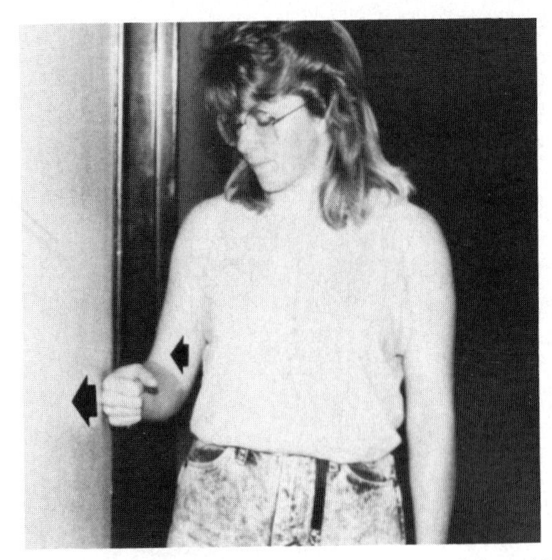

FIGURE 38–70. Isometric strengthening of the middle deltoid. The elbow is flexed to a right angle and the forearm placed against the wall or frame surface. The forearm is then pushed against the surface by isometrically contracting the middle deltoid. This exercise is repeated for the recommended number of times.

38–71 and 38–72). The previous mobilization exercises are continued also. As the patient progresses, resistance exercises are started. Rubber tubing of different grades of elasticity is useful for this part of the program. The patient begins using tubing with the least elastic resistance and progresses to more resistive tubing as strength improves (Figs. 38–73 through 38–76).

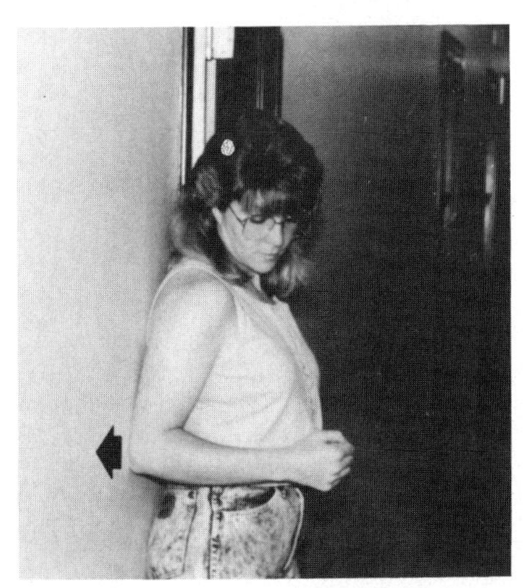

FIGURE 38–69. Isometric strengthening of the posterior deltoid. The back of the flexed elbow is placed against a wall. The patient pushes backward against the wall by isometrically contracting the posterior deltoid for the prescribed number of repetitions.

The third phase begins after about 3 months. This is a program of progressive stretching and strengthening (Figs. 38–77 through 38–79).

Neer[88] divides postoperative patients into two groups. One group of patients is able to pursue the normal postoperative rehabilitation program just described. The other group of patients have bone and soft tissue deficiencies that cannot be completely corrected. Neer assigns these patients limited goals for rehabilitation. Their program is directed at preserving stability of the shoulder and achieving a more limited range of motion.

Continuous passive motion has lately been employed in the early rehabilitation period.[38] It must be used judiciously and carefully directed by the operating surgeon.[96] Obviously, this apparatus is not safe for every reconstructed shoulder.

Special Concerns for Patients With Fractures

A carefully planned postoperative rehabilitation program is most important in patients with acute and chronic fracture problems and nonunions. Tanner and Cofield[129] noted that active forward eleva-

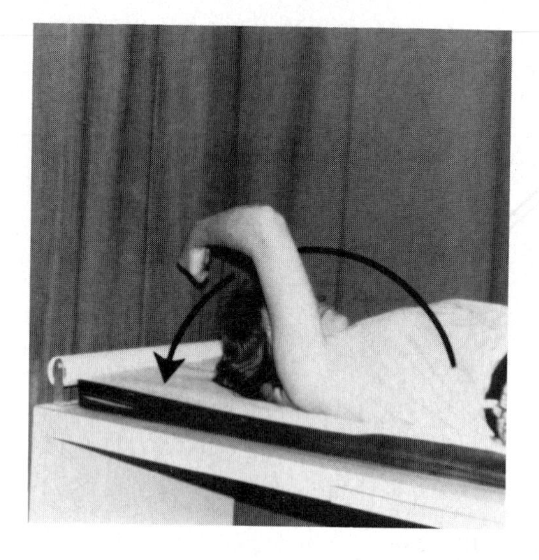

FIGURE 38–71. Unassisted active forward elevation of the operated arm. The patient begins with the elbow and upper arm on the table at the side, the elbow at about a right angle. The arm is then actively elevated in the direction of the arrow by contracting the deltoid and rotator cuff muscles. This exercise is easier to do if started in a supine position. As the muscles become stronger, the same exercise can be done in the standing position, first working just against gravity, then adding light weights and increasing these as strength improves. Weights can be used in the supine position in a similar way. Repetitions are done as prescribed.

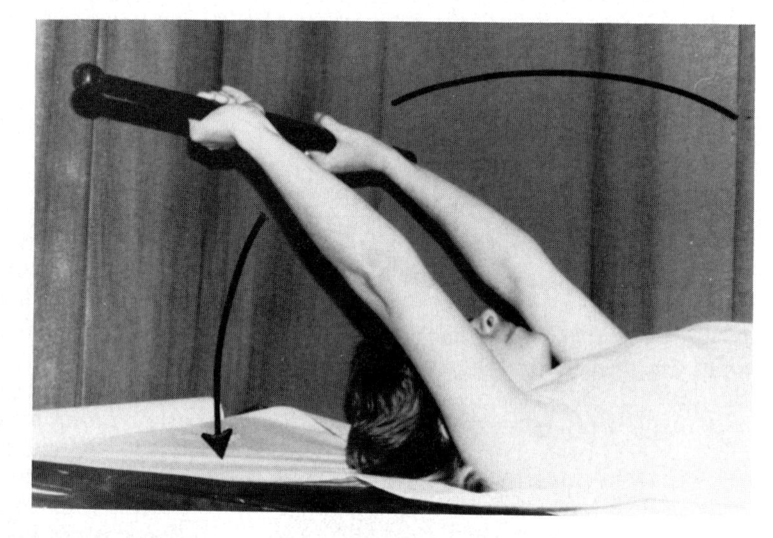

FIGURE 38–72. Active assistive strengthening of the anterior deltoid. The "broomstick" is grasped with two hands as it lies transversely across the thighs. The exercise begins with the arms down at the sides—elbows held almost straight. The arms are then raised (arrow) with the unoperated arm assisting the operated one. This early strengthening exercise for the deltoid is first done in a supine position. As the muscle becomes stronger, the patient can stand, doing more work against gravity. The goal is full elevation, if possible. This exercise also helps maintain range of motion.

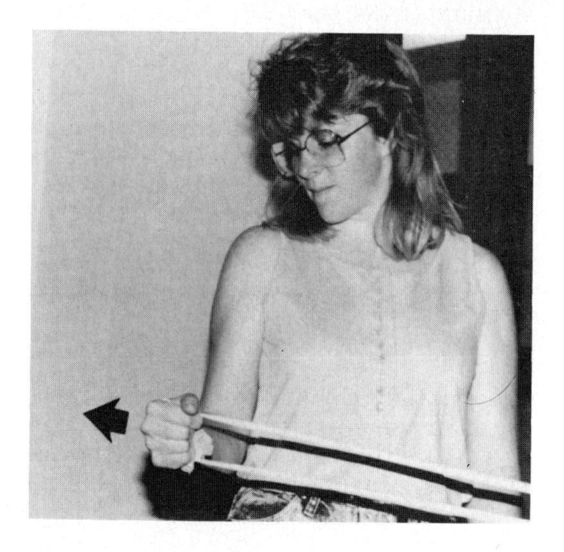

FIGURE 38–73. Active strengthening of the external rotators using the resistance of elastic tubing (dental dam). The elbow of the operated arm is placed at a right angle next to the body. It is held there as the forearm and hand are rotated outward (arrow) by the external rotator muscles. The forearm should not drift out of the right-angle position or use of the external rotators will not be maximized.

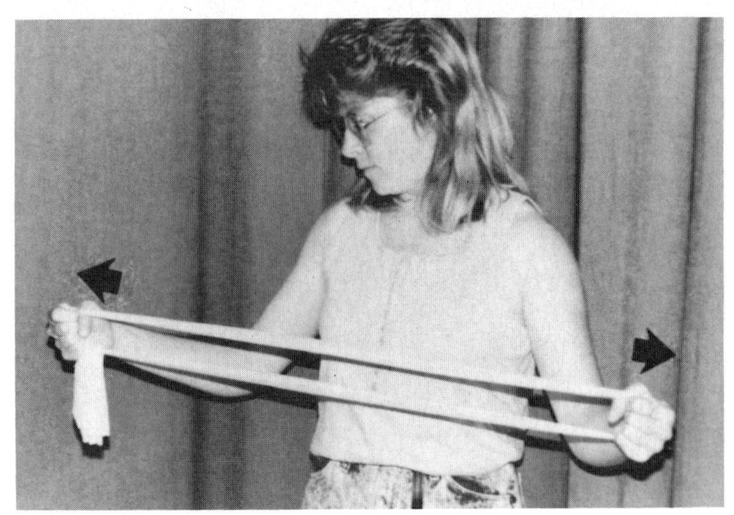

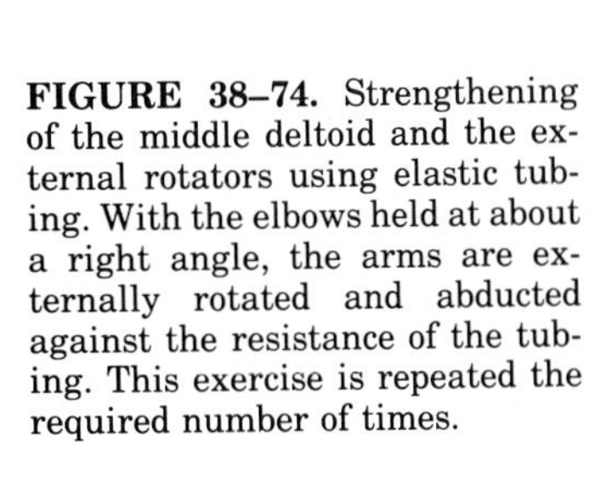

FIGURE 38–74. Strengthening of the middle deltoid and the external rotators using elastic tubing. With the elbows held at about a right angle, the arms are externally rotated and abducted against the resistance of the tubing. This exercise is repeated the required number of times.

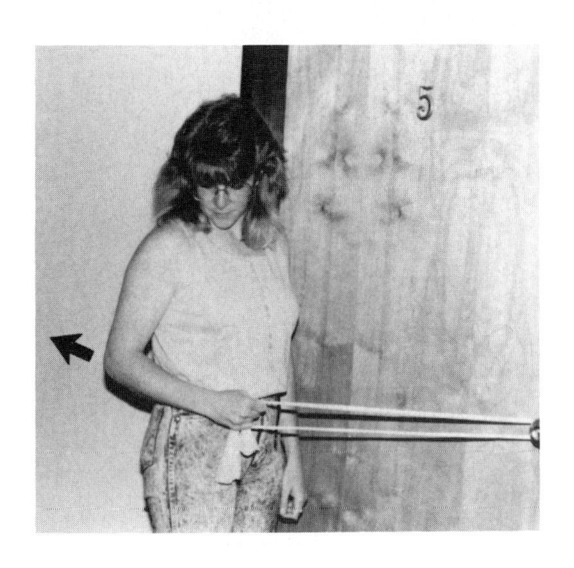

FIGURE 38–75. Active strengthening of the posterior deltoid using the resistance of varying grades of elastic tubing. The elbow is placed by the side at a right angle and moved backward (arrow), pulling against the resistance.

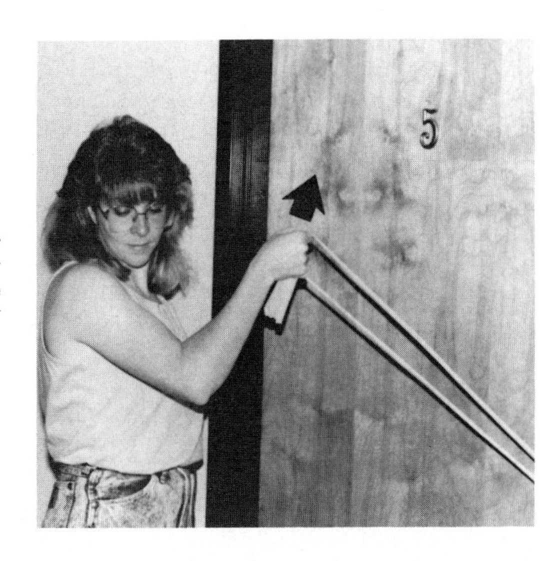

FIGURE 38–76. Active strengthening of the anterior deltoid. The arm is lifted upward in front of the body (arrow) against the resistance of elastic tubing. The elbow is kept at a right angle. The lifting is done by the shoulder muscles not by the biceps to flex the arm.

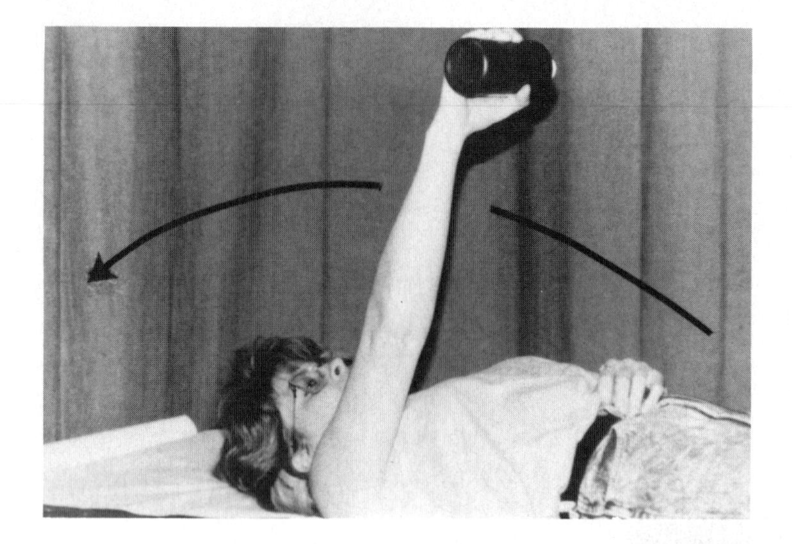

FIGURE 38–77. Active forward elevation with weight. This exercise is first done without weight until strength and tolerance improves. It is most easily performed in the supine position. As strength increases, the patient changes to the standing position, elevating the arm against only gravity to begin with, progressing to weights.

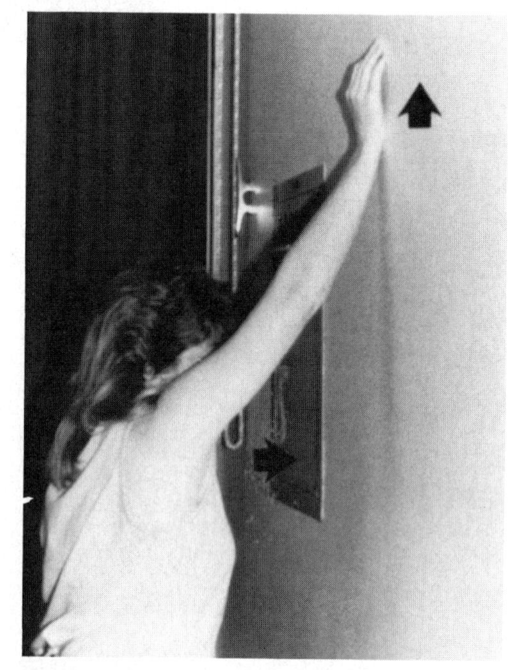

FIGURE 38–78. Stretching exercise to attain and maintain forward elevation. This late stretching exercise obviously cannot be done until the patient is able to attain approximately the position shown. The hand of the operated arm is placed against the wall, and the patient stands away from the wall but leans toward it. As the body is allowed to lean more toward the wall, the hand slides upward (arrow), stretching the tissues gradually into more forward elevation.

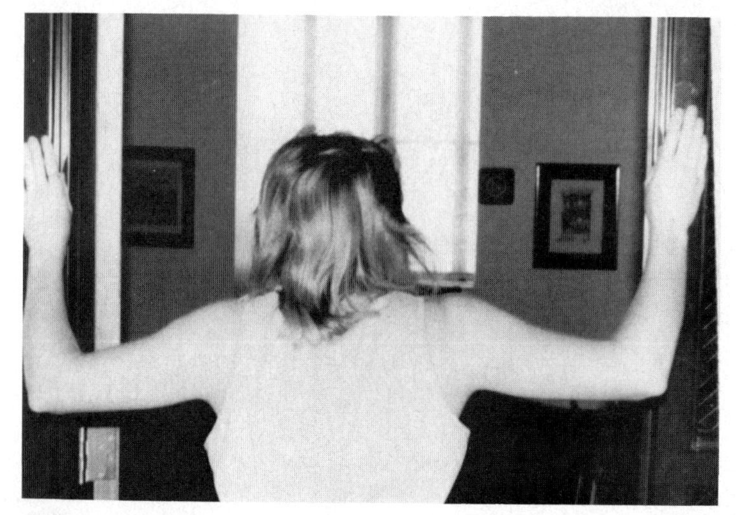

FIGURE 38–79. Stretching to achieve more external rotation. As the patient stands in a doorway with the elbows abducted to about shoulder level, the forearms are placed on the door jamb on either side. The patient then leans forward, gradually stretching the arms into more external rotation.

tion in patients with chronic fractures was better if motion was begun within 2 weeks after surgery and was supervised for more than 2 months.

The quality of tissue and the repair dictates the extent of the rehabilitation program. The surgeon would not want to stress a tenuous repair, protected by an arm held in postoperative abduction. In this case, passive forward elevation could be carried out from the abducted position, with the splint acting as the stopping point on returning the arm toward the side.

At the completion of surgery, the tension-free limits of the cuff repair are known. Passive motion can be carried out within the tension-free "safe zone" above the level of the protective splint.[129] The surgeon can determine the safe limits of passive external rotation in the same way. A passive motion program within these tension-free limits usually can begin within the first week after surgery. Active-assisted range of motion exercises and isometric strengthening are started in 4 to 6 weeks, after early healing has begun.[129]

It often takes 1 to 2 years for the patient to reach maximum improvement. The rehabilitation program should be carried out conscientiously during this time. Discontinuing a therapy program prematurely is certain to compromise results.

If the repair is secure, it may be advantageous to place the patient into a continuous passive motion apparatus after surgery.[108] The apparatus can be applied in the operating room as the patient is transferred to the bed. The equipment holds the arm in neutral rotation and can also be set to hold the arm in a desired degree of forward elevation. The arm is automatically elevated through a 30-degree arc of motion with each cycle. Use of this apparatus in the first 2 days after surgery seems to make it easier for the patient to begin passive range of motion exercises. The goal of early motion is to prevent the development of strong adhesions by gentle range of motion exercises that do not stress fracture fixation.

References

1. Adams, M. A., Weiland, A. J., and Moore, J. R.: Nonconstrained shoulder arthroplasty: an eight year experience. Orthop. Trans. 10(2):232, 1986.
2. Amstutz, H. C., Hoy, A. L., and Clarke, I. C.: UCLA anatomic total shoulder arthroplasty. Clin. Orthop. 155:7–20, 1981.
3. Amstutz, H. C., Thomas, B. J., Kabo, J. M., et al.: The Dana total shoulder arthroplasty. J. Bone Joint Surg. 70A:1174–1182, 1988.
4. Barrett, W. P., Franklin, J. L., Jackins, S. E., et al.: Total shoulder arthroplasty. J. Bone Joint Surg. 69A:865–872, 1987.
5. Barrett, W. P., Jackins, S. E., Wyss, C. R., et al.: Total shoulder arthroplasty: the University of Washington experience. Orthop. Trans. 100(2):232, 1986.
6. Barrett, W. P., Thornhill, T. S., Thomas, W. H., et al.: Nonconstrained total shoulder arthroplasty for patients with polyarticular rheumatoid arthritis. Orthop. Trans. 11(2):238, 1987.
7. Bigliani, L. U., McCann, P. D., and Dalsey, R. N.: An anatomic study of the suprascapular nerve. Presented at the American Shoulder and Elbow Surgeons 5th Open Meeting, Las Vegas, 1989.
8. Blom, S. and Dahlback, L. O.: Nerve injuries in dislocations of the shoulder joint and fractures of the neck of the humerus. A clinical and electromyographical study. Acta Chir. Scand. 131:461, 1970.
9. Bonutti, P. M., Hawkins, R. J., and Pepper, P.: Component loosening following total shoulder arthroplasty. Presented at American Shoulder and Elbow Surgeons 6th Open Meeting, New Orleans, 1990.
10. Bos, G., Sim, F. H., Pritchard, D. J., et al.: Prosthetic Proximal Humeral Replacement: The Mayo Clinic Experience. Limb Salvage. Edited by W. F. Enneking. New York, Churchill Livingstone, 1987.
11. Bovill, D. and Norris, T. R.: Common problems with proximal humeral fractures leading to malunions: a review of 27 cases. Presented at the American Shoulder and Elbow Surgeons 5th Open Meeting, Las Vegas, 1989.
12. Boyd, A. D., Washington, D. C., Thomas, W. H., et al.: Failed shoulder arthroplasty. Presented at the American Shoulder and Elbow Surgeons 6th Open Meeting, New Orleans, 1990.
13. Boyd, A. D., Jr., Thornhill, T. S., Thomas, W. H., et al.: Post-operative proximal migration in total shoulder replacement: incidence and significance. Presented at the American Shoulder and Elbow Surgeons 5th Open Meeting, Las Vegas, 1989.
14. Brems, J. J., Wilde, A. H., Borden, L. S., et al.: Glenoid lucent lines. Orthop. Trans. 10(2):231, 1986.
15. Brems, J. J. and Wilde, A. H.: Surgical management of cuff tear arthropathy. Orthop. Trans. 12(3):729, 1988.
16. Brenner, B. C., Ferlic, D. C., Clayton, M. L., et al.: Survivorship of unconstrained total shoulder arthroplasty. J. Bone Joint Surg. 71A:1289–1296, 1989.
17. Brownlee, R. C. and Cofield, R. H.: Shoulder replacement in cuff tear arthropathy. Orthop. Trans. 10(2):230, 1986.
18. Clayton, M. L., Ferlic, D. C., and Jeffers, P. D.: Prosthetic arthroplasties of the shoulder. Clin. Orthop. 164:184–191, 1982.
19. Codman, E. A.: The Shoulder. Boston, Thomas A. Todd, Co., 1934.
20. Cofield, R. H.: Total joint arthroplasty: the shoulder. Mayo Clin. Proc. 54:500–506, 1979.

21. Cofield, R. H.: Glenohumeral arthrodesis. J. Bone Joint Surg. 61A:673, 1979.
22. Cofield, R. H., Post, M., Wilde, A. H., et al.: Symposium: shoulder joint replacement. Contemp. Orthop. 5:99–127, 1982.
23. Cofield, R. H.: Subscapularis muscle transposition for repair of chronic rotator cuff tears. Surg. Gynecol. Obstet. 154:667–672, 1982.
24. Cofield, R. H.: Personal communication, 1987.
25. Cofield, R. H.: The Shoulder and Prosthetic Arthroplasty. Surgery of the Musculoskeletal System. Edited by C. M. Evarts. New York, Churchill Livingstone, 1983.
26. Cofield, R. H.: Unconstrained total shoulder prosthesis. Clin. Orthop. 173:97–108, 1983.
27. Cofield, R. H.: Total shoulder arthroplasty with the Neer prosthesis. J. Bone Joint Surg. 66A:899–906, 1984.
28. Cofield, R. H.: Total shoulder arthroplasty: associated disease of the rotator cuff, results and complications. Surgery of the Shoulder. Edited by J. E. Bateman and R. P. Welsh, Philadelphia. B. C. Decker, Inc., 1984.
29. Cofield, R. H.: Rotator cuff disease of the shoulder—current concepts review. J. Bone Joint Surg. 67A:974–979, 1985.
30. Cofield, R. H.: Preliminary experience with bone ingrowth total shoulder arthroplasty. Orthop. Trans. 10(2):217, 1986.
31. Cofield, R. H.: Total shoulder arthroplasty. American Academy of Orthopaedic Surgeons Shoulder Surgery—Current Techniques. Los Angeles, 1987.
32. Cofield, R. H.: Comminuted fractures of the proximal humerus. Clin. Orthop. 230:49–57, 1988.
33. Cofield, R. H.: Management of complications of shoulder arthroplasty. American Academy of Orthopaedic Surgeons Instructional Course Lectures, Las Vegas, 1989.
34. Cofield, R. H.: Symposium. How serious are our complications? Presented at the Fourth International Conference on Surgery of the Shoulder, New York, 1989.
35. Cofield, R. H.: Uncemented total shoulder arthroplasty. Presented at the American Shoulder and Elbow Surgeons 6th Open Meeting, New Orleans, 1990.
36. Cofield, R. H.: Degenerative and arthritic problems of the glenohumeral joint. The Shoulder. Edited by C. A. Rockwood, Jr. and F. A. Matsen, III. Philadelphia, W. B. Saunders Company, 1990.
37. Coughlin, M. J., Morris, J. M., and West, W. F.: The semiconstrained total shoulder arthroplasty. J. Bone Joint Surg. 61A:574–581, 1979.
38. Craig, E. V.: Continuous passive motion in the rehabilitation of the surgically reconstructed shoulder. Orthop. Trans. 10(2):233, 1986.
39. Craig, E. V.: Total shoulder replacement. Orthopedics 2:125–136, 1988.
40. DeGroot, J. and Chusid, J. G.: Correlative Neuroanatomy, 20th ed. East Norwalk, CT, Appleton and Lange, 1988.
41. DeLuca, C. J. and Forrest, W. J.: Force analysis of individual muscles acting simultaneously on the shoulder during isometric abduction. J. Biomechanics 6:385–393, 1973.
42. DeOrio, J. K. and Cofield, R. H.: Results of a second attempt at surgical repair of a failed initial rotator cuff repair. J. Bone Joint Surg. 66A:563–567, 1984.
43. Engelbrecht, E. and Heinert, K.: More than Ten Years' Experience with Unconstrained Shoulder Replacement. Shoulder Replacement. Edited by R. Kilbel, B. Helbig, and W. Blauth. Berlin, Springer-Verlag, 1987.
44. Faludi, D. D. and Weiland, A. J.: Cementless total shoulder arthroplasty: preliminary experience with thirteen cases. Orthopedics 6:431–437, 1982.
45. Figgie, H. E., III, Inglis, A. E., Goldberg, V. M., et al.: An analysis of factors affecting the long-term results of total shoulder arthroplasty in inflammatory arthritis. J. Arthroplasty 3(2):123–130, 1988.
46. Flatow, E. L., Bigliani, L. U., and April, F. W.: An anatomic study of the musculocutaneous nerve and its relationship to the coracoid process. Clin. Orthop. 244:166–171, 1989.
47. Franklin, J. L., Barret, W. P., Jackins, S. E., et al.: Glenoid loosening in total shoulder arthroplasty: association with rotator cuff deficiency. J. Arthroplasty 3:39–46, 1988.
48. Friedman, R. J.: Biomechanics of the shoulder following total shoulder replacement. Presented at the Fourth International Conference of Surgery of the Shoulder, New York, 1989.
49. Friedman, R. J.: Glenohumeral and scapulothoracic motion following total shoulder replacement. Presented at the American Shoulder and Elbow Surgeons 5th Open Meeting, Las Vegas, 1989.
50. Friedman, R. J., Brookings, M. S., and Dooley, R. L.: Finite element analysis of glenoid component design. Presented at the American Shoulder and Elbow Surgeons 6th Open Meeting, New Orleans, 1990.
51. Fukuda, H.: Symposium: how serious are our complications? Presented at the 4th International Conference in Surgery of the Shoulder, New York, 1989.
52. Fukuda, H., Chen, C., Cofield, R. H., et al.: Biomechanical analysis of stability and fixation strength of total shoulder prostheses. Orthopedics 2:141–149, 1988.
53. Gerber, C., Schneeberger, A., and Vinh, T.: The arterial vascularization of the humeral head. Presented at the American Shoulder and Elbow Surgeons 6th Open Meeting, New Orleans, 1990.
54. Grant, J. C. B.: Grant's Atlas of Anatomy, 8th ed. Edited by J. E. Anderson. Baltimore, William & Wilkins, 1983.
55. Gristina, A. G. and Webb, L. X.: The Trispherical Total Shoulder Replacement. Shoulder Surgery. Edited by I. Bayley and L. Kessel. New York, Springer-Verlag, 1982.
56. Gristina, A. G., Romano, R. L., Kammire, G. C., et al.: Total shoulder replacement: biomechanics, technique and results. Surg. Rounds Orthop. 2(10):17–29, 1988.
57. Gristina, A. G., Kammire, G. C., Webb, L. X., et al.: Total shoulder replacement: Biomechanics, technique and results. Surg. Rounds for Orthop 2(10):17–26, 1988.
58. Harryman, D., Sidles, J., McQuade, K., et al.: Glenohumeral translations: a three dimensional

analysis. Presented at the Fourth International Conference of Surgery of the Shoulder, New York, 1989.
59. Henry, A. K.: Extensile Exposure, 2nd ed. Edinburgh, E & S Livingstone, Ltd., 1966.
60. Hollinshead, W. H.: Anatomy for Surgeons, Vol. 3. New York, Harper and Brothers, 1958.
61. Hughes, M. and Neer, C. S., II: Glenohumeral joint replacement and postoperative rehabilitation. Physical Med. 55:850–858, 1975.
62. Huiskes, R. and Chao, E. Y. S.: A survey of finite element analysis in orthopedic biomechanics: the first decade. J. Biomech. 16:385–409, 1983.
63. Husely, R. E. and Norris, T. R.: Bone grafts for glenoid deficiency in total shoulder replacement. Presented at the American Shoulder and Elbow Surgeons 6th Open Meeting, New Orleans, 1990.
64. Imbriglia, J. E., Neer, C. S., II, and Dick, H. M.: Resection of the proximal one-half of the humerus in a child with chondrosarcoma. Preservation of function using fibular graft and a Neer prosthesis. J. Bone Joint Surg. 60A:262–264, 1978.
65. Inman, V. T., Saunders, J. B. deC. M., and Abbott, L. C.: Observations on the function of the shoulder joint. J. Bone Joint Surg. 26A:1–30, 1944.
66. Kelly, I. G., Foster, R. S., and Fisher, W. D.: Neer total shoulder replacement in rheumatoid arthritis. J. Bone Joint Surg. 69B:723–726, 1987.
67. Kessel, L.: Clinical Disorders of the Shoulder. New York, Churchill Livingstone, 1982.
68. Knight, R. A. and Mayne, J. A.: Comminuted fractures and fracture-dislocations involving the articular surface of the humeral head. J. Bone Joint Surg. 39A:1343, 1957.
69. Laing, P. G.: The arterial supply of the adult humerus. J. Bone Joint Surg. 38A:1105, 1956.
70. Lettin, A. W. F., Copeland, S. A., and Scales, J. T.: The Stanmore total shoulder replacement. J. Bone Joint Surg. 64B:47, 1982.
71. Loomer, R. and Graham, B.: Anatomy of the axillary nerve and its relationship to inferior capsular shift. Clin. Orthop. 243:100–105, 1989.
72. Lucas, D. B.: Biomechanics of the shoulder joint. Arch. Surg. 107:425–432, 1973.
73. Marmor, L.: Hemiarthroplasty for the rheumatoid shoulder joint. Clin. Orthop. 122:201–203, 1977.
74. McLaughlin, H. L.: Lesions of the musculotendinous cuff of the shoulder. The exposure and treatment of tears with retraction. J. Bone Joint Surg. 26:31–51, 1944.
75. Moore, K. L.: Clinically Oriented Anatomy. Baltimore, Williams & Wilkins, 1985.
76. Morrey, B. F. and Chao, E. Y. S.: Recurrent anterior dislocation of the shoulder. Clinical Biomechanics. Edited by J. Black and J. H. Dumbleton. New York, Churchill Livingstone, 1981.
77. Neer, C. S., II, Brown, T. H., and McLaughlin, H. H.: Fracture of the neck of the humerus with dislocation of the head fragment. Am. J. Surg. 85:252–258, 1953.
78. Neer, C. S., II: Articular replacement for the humeral head. J. Bone Joint Surg. 37A:215–228, 1955.
79. Neer, C. S., II: Degenerative lesions of the proximal humeral articular surface. Clin. Orthop. 20:116–124, 1961.
80. Neer, C. S., II: Follow-up notes on articles previously published in the journal. Articular replacement for the humeral head. J. Bone Joint Surg. 46A:1607–1610, 1964.
81. Neer, C. S., II: Displaced proximal humeral fractures. Part I. J. Bone Joint Surg. 52A:1077–1089, 1970.
82. Neer, C. S., II: Displaced proximal humeral fractures. Part II: Treatment of three and four-part displacement. J. Bone Joint Surg. 52A:1090–1103, 1970.
83. Neer, C. S., II: Anterior acromioplasty for the chronic impingement syndrome in the shoulder. A preliminary report. J. Bone Joint Surg. 54A:41–50, 1972.
84. Neer, C. S., II: Replacement arthroplasty for glenohumeral arthritis. J. Bone Joint Surg. 56A:1–13, 1974.
85. Neer, C. S., II: Four segment classification of displaced proximal humeral fractures. American Academy of Orthopaedic Surgeons Instructional Course Lectures. St. Louis, C. V. Mosby Company, 1975.
86. Neer, C. S., II and Marberry, T. A.: On the disadvantages of radical acromionectomy. J. Bone Joint Surg. 63A:416–419, 1981.
87. Neer, C. S., II: Reconstructive surgery and rehabilitation of the shoulder. Textbook of Rheumatology, Vol. II. Edited by W. N. Kelley, E. D. Harris, Jr., S. Ruddy, and C. B. Sledge. Philadelphia, W. B. Saunders Company, 1981.
88. Neer, C. S., II, Watson, K. C., and Stanton, F. J.: Recent experience in total shoulder replacement. J. Bone Joint Surg. 64A:319–337, 1982.
89. Neer, C. S., II and Kirby, R. M.: Revision of humeral head and total shoulder arthroplasties. Clin. Orthop. 170:189–195, 1982.
90. Neer, C. S., II, Craig, E. V., and Fukuda, H.: Cuff tear arthropathy. J. Bone Joint Surg. 65A:1232–1244, 1983.
91. Neer, C. S., II: Impingement lesions. Clin. Orthop. 173:70–77, 1983.
92. Neer, C. S., II: Nonunions of the surgical neck of the humerus. Orthop. Trans. 7(3):389, 1983.
93. Neer, C. S., II: Part I: Fractures about the shoulder. Fractures in Adults. Edited by C. A. Rockwood, Jr. and D. P. Green. Philadelphia, J. B. Lippincott Company, 1984.
94. Neer, C. S., II: Unconstrained shoulder arthroplasty. Surgery of the Shoulder. Edited by J. E. Bateman and R. P. Welsh, Philadelphia, B. C. Decker, Inc., 1984.
95. Neer, C. S., II and McIlveen, S. J.: Recent results and technique of prosthetic replacement for 4-part proximal humeral fractures. Orthop. Trans. 10(3):475, 1986.
96. Neer, C. S., II, McCann, P. D., MacFarlane, E. A., et al.: Earlier passive motion following shoulder arthroplasty and rotator cuff repair. Orthop. Trans. 11(2):231, 1987.
97. Neer, C. S., II and Morrison, D. S.: Glenoid bone grafting in total shoulder arthroplasty. J. Bone Joint Surg. 70A:1154–1162, 1988.
98. Neer, C. S., II: Symposium: how serious are our complications? Presented at the 4th International Conference in Surgery of the Shoulder, New York, 1989.

99. Neer, C. S., II, Miller, S. R., and Flatow, E. L.: Chronic unreduced anterior dislocation of the shoulder. Presented at the American Shoulder and Elbow Surgeons 6th Open Meeting, New Orleans, 1990.
100. Neer, C. S., II: Shoulder reconstruction. Philadelphia, W.B. Saunders Company, 1990.
101. Norris, T. R.: Analysis of failed repair of shoulder instability. A preliminary report. Surgery of the Shoulder. Edited by J. E. Bateman and R. P. Welsh. Philadelphia, B. C. Decker, Inc., 1984.
102. Norris, T. R.: Bone grafts for glenoid deficiency in total shoulder replacements. Proceedings of the Third International Conference on Surgery of the Shoulder. Professional Postgraduate Services, Fukuoka, Japan, 1986.
103. Norris, T. R. and Bigliani, L. U.: Complications following the modified Bristow procedure for shoulder instability. Orthop. Trans. 11:232–233, 1987.
104. Norris, T. R.: Fractures and Dislocations of the Glenohumeral Complex. Edited by M. Chapman. Philadelphia, J. B. Lippincott Company, 1988.
105. Norris, T. R., Turner, J. A., and Bovill, D.: Nonunion of the upper humerus: an analysis of the etiology and treatment in 28 cases. Presented at the American Shoulder and Elbow Surgeons 5th Open Meeting, Las Vegas, 1989.
106. Norris, T. R.: Unconstrained prosthetic shoulder replacement. The Shoulder. Edited by M. Watson. London, Churchill Livingstone, 1989.
107. Norris, T. R.: History and physical examination of the shoulder. The Upper Extremity in Sports Medicine. Edited by J. A. Nicholas and E. B. Hershman. St. Louis, C. V. Mosby Company, 1990.
108. Norris, T. R.: Fractures of the proximal humerus and dislocations of the shoulder. Skeletal Trauma. Edited by B. D. Browner. Philadelphia, W. B. Saunders Company, 1990.
109. Orr, T. E. and Carter, D. R.: Stress analysis of joint arthroplasty in the proximal humerus. J. Orthop. Res. 3:360–371, 1985.
110. Orr, T. E., Carter, D. R., and Schurman, D. J.: Stress analysis of glenoid component designs. Clin. Orthop. 232:217–224, 1988.
111. Perry, J.: Anatomy and biomechanics of the shoulder in throwing, swimming, gymnastics, and tennis. Clin. Sports Med. 2:247–270, 1983.
112. Perry, J.: Shoulder biomechanics. Presented at the Shoulder Educator's Course, Newport, RI, 1985.
113. Pollack, R. G., Bigliani, L. U., Flatow, E. L., et al.: The mechanical properties of the inferior glenohumeral ligament. Presented at the American Shoulder and Elbow Surgeons 6th Open Meeting, New Orleans, 1990.
114. Poppen, N. K. and Walker, P. S.: Normal and abnormal motion of the shoulder. J. Bone Joint Surg. 58A:195–201, 1976.
115. Poppen, N. K. and Walker, P. S.: Forces at the glenohumeral joint in abduction. Clin. Orthop. 135:165–170, 1978.
116. Post, M., Jablon, M., Miller, H., et al.: Constrained total shoulder joint replacement: a critical review. Clin. Orthop. 144:135–150, 1979.
117. Post, M.: Indications for unconstrained and constrained arthroplasty. American Academy of Orthopaedic Surgeons Instructional Course Lecture, Las Vegas, 1985.
118. Post, M.: Constrained arthroplasty of the shoulder. Orthop. Clin. North Am. 18:455–462, 1987.
119. Post, M.: Constrained total shoulder arthroplasty—long term results. Orthop. Trans. 11(2):238, 1987.
120. Post, M., Haskell, S. S., and Jablon, M.: Total shoulder replacement with a constrained prosthesis. J. Bone Joint Surg. 62A:327–335, 1980.
121. Post, M. and Jablon, M.: Constrained total shoulder arthroplasty. Clin. Orthop. 173:109–116, 1983.
122. Pritchett, J. W. and Clark, J. M.: Prosthetic replacement for chronic unreduced dislocations of the shoulder. Clin. Orthop. 216:89–93, 1987.
123. Rietveld, A. B. M., Daanen, H. A. M., Rozing, P. M., et al.: The lever arm in the glenohumeral abduction after hemiarthroplasty. J. Bone Joint Surg. 70B:561–565, 1988.
124. Rockwood, C. A., Jr.: Development of shoulder surgery in the United States. Orthopedics 2:39–40, 1988.
125. Rowe, C. R. and Zarins, B.: Chronic unreduced dislocations of the shoulder. J. Bone Joint Surg. 64A:494–505, 1982.
126. Samilson, R. L. and Prieto, V.: Dislocation arthroplasty of the shoulder. J. Bone Joint Surg., 65A:456–460, 1983.
127. Settergren, C. R. and Cofield, R. H.: Total shoulder arthroplasty: five to ten year assessment. Orthop. Trans. 11(2):238, 1987.
128. Stableforth, P. G.: Four-part fractures of the neck of the humerus. J. Bone Joint Surg. 66B:101–108, 1984.
129. Tanner, W. and Cofield, R. H.: Prosthetic arthroplasty for fractures and fracture-dislocations of the proximal humerus. CORR 179:116–128, 1983.
130. Thornhill, T. S. and Barrett, W. P.: Total shoulder arthroplasty. The Shoulder. Edited by C. R. Rowe. New York, Churchill Livingstone, 1988.
131. Turkel, S. J., Panio, M. W., Marshall, J. L., et al.: Stabilizing mechanisms preventing anterior dislocation of the glenohumeral joint. J. Bone Joint Surg. 63A:1208–1217, 1981.
132. Turner, J. A. and Norris, T. R.: Surgical treatment of nonunions of the upper humerus shaft fracture in the elderly. Presented at the American Shoulder and Elbow Surgeons 3rd Closed Meeting, Boston, 1984.
133. Zuckerman, J. D. and Cofield, R. H.: Proximal humeral prosthetic replacement in glenohumeral arthritis. Orthop. Trans. 10(2):231, 1986.
134. Zuckerman, J. D. and Matsen, F. A., III: Biomechanics of the shoulder. Basic Biomechanics of the Musculoskeletal System. Edited by M. Nordin and V. H. Frankel. Philadelphia, Lea & Febiger, 1989.

CHAPTER 39

Total Elbow Arthroplasty

MARK P. FIGGIE
ALAN E. INGLIS
HARRY E. FIGGIE, III

Total elbow arthroplasty has improved so that predictable and durable results can be obtained in patients with inflammatory arthritis. Refinements in surgical technique and implant design, as well as recognition of the importance of the restoration of anatomy, have led to better clinical outcomes. However, advances in total elbow arthroplasties have been made more slowly than those in total hip and total knee arthroplasties because fewer of these procedures are performed every year. The purposes of this chapter are to describe the anatomy, biomechanics, and surgical aspects of total elbow surgery and to discuss possible complications.

ANATOMY

Elbow Joint

The elbow joint consists of the articulation among the distal humerus, proximal ulna, and proximal radius. The distal humerus has two condyles: the trochlea on the medial aspect and the capitellum on the lateral aspect (Fig. 39–1). The trochlea articulates with the proximal ulna, whereas the capitellum articulates with the proximal radius. The ulnohumeral articulation acts as a hinged joint (ginglymus) with degrees of freedom only in flexion and extension. The radiohumeral joint and the proximal radioulnar joint allow axial rotation with pronation and supination and thus represent a trochoid joint. Based upon these two articulations, the elbow is a trochoginglymoid joint.[70]

The trochlea itself is a bicondylar, a saddle-shaped, and an asymmetric joint surface between the medial and lateral condyles. Hyaline cartilage covers it in an arc that varies from 300 to 330 degrees.[32, 69, 72] The capitellum is spheroidal, articulating with the concave aspects of the proximal radius.[72] The depression of the radial head is covered by hyaline cartilage as well as the 240-degree arc of circumference that articulates with the ulna, allowing approximately 180 degrees of pronation and supination.

The proximal ulna consists of the olecranon—the site of the attachment for the triceps tendon. The greater sigmoid notch, which articulates with the trochlea at the humerus, is incompletely covered with hyaline cartilage.[72] The anterior aspect of the sigmoid notch consists of the coronoid process. The insertion of the brachialis muscle is distal to the coronoid tip but does not attach to the tip directly. Along the lateral aspect of the proximal ulna, the lesser semilunar notch articulates with the large circumferential margin of the proximal radius. The radius is stabilized by the annular ligament, which circumscribes the neck of the radius.

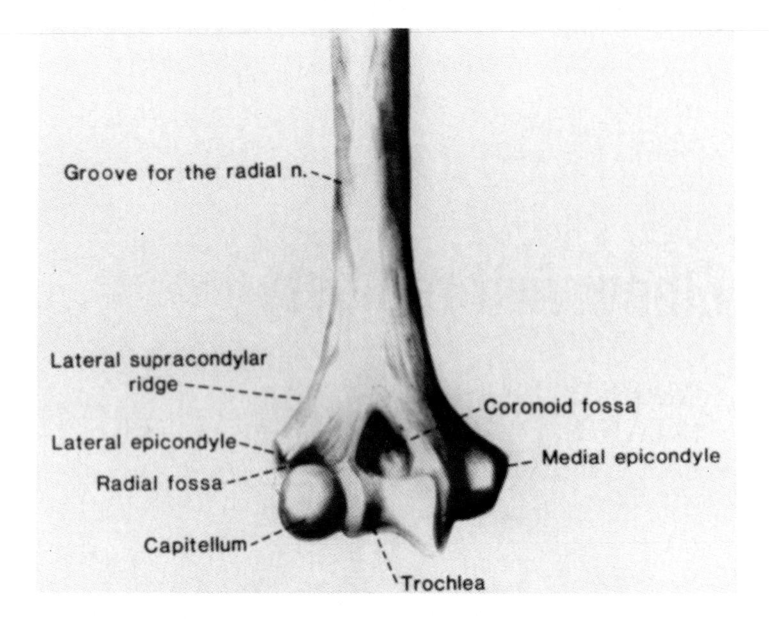

FIGURE 39–1. Representative bony landmarks of the distal humerus.

The extra-articular landmarks of the elbow include the medial and lateral epicondyles of the distal humerus (see Fig. 39–1). The medial epicondyle is more prominent in its site of attachment of the ulnar collateral ligament and the flexor and pronator musculature of the forearm. The lateral epicondyle is the site of attachment of the lateral collateral ligament and the mobile wad of three muscles: brachioradialis, extensor carpi radialis longus, and extensor carpi radialis brevis. The posterior aspect of the lateral epicondyle is the origin of the anconeus muscle. The ulnar nerve lies in a sulcus of the cubital tunnel distal to the medial epicondyle. The distal humerus has three recesses or sulci that allow for the greater range of motion of the elbow. The coronoid fossa accommodates the coronoid process, whereas the radial fossa, which is above the surface of the capitellum, accommodates the radial head in positions of elbow flexion. The olecranon fossa, which is posterior, accommodates the tip of the olecranon in full extension. The coronoid and olecranon fossae are supported by the medial and lateral supracondylar ridges of the distal humerus. The supporting ridges or pillars provide support to most designs of semiconstrained total elbow replacements. In addition, they are important structures in the open reduction and internal fixation of distal humeral fractures. The lateral supracondylar column is larger with a flat posterior surface, whereas the medial supracondylar pillar is smaller.

The orientation of the elbow joint articulation with the shafts of the humerus and ulna must be appreciated in order to properly restore the anatomic relationships

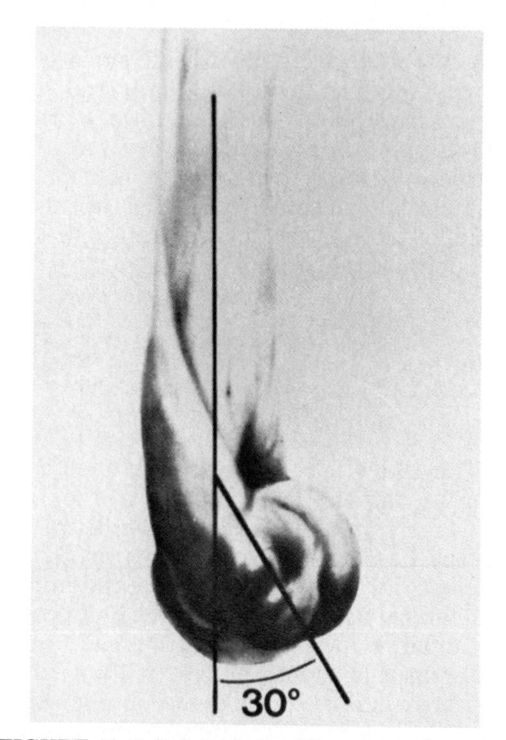

FIGURE 39–2. Relationship of the center of rotation through the capitellum and trochlea angulated anteriorly 30 degrees from the humeral shaft.

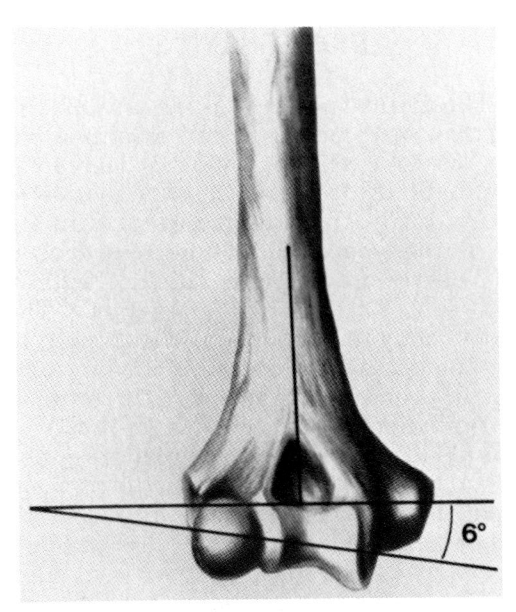

FIGURE 39–3. Angulation of the center of rotation approximately 6 to 8 degrees of valgus orientation with respect to the long axis of the humerus.

with total elbow replacement. The trochlea and capitellum are angulated at 30 degrees anterior to the long axis of the humerus (Fig. 39–2). In addition, the center of rotation of the articulation is approximately 6 to 8 degrees of valgus orientation to the long axis of the humerus (Fig. 39–3).[33] In addition, the axis is internally rotated 5 to 7 degrees from the line bisecting the epicondyles (Fig. 39–4).[37]

There is a 15 degree angle of the neck of the radius with respect to the long axis of the radius[13] compared with a 4 degree valgus angulation of the sigmoid notch of the proximal ulna with respect to the shaft of the ulna (Figs. 39–5 and 39–6).[33]

The valgus angle of the elbow is provided by the valgus angle of the humeral articulation with the long axis of the humerus and the valgus angle of the sigmoid notch with the long axis of the ulna. This angle is the relationship of the long axis of the forearm to the long axis of the humerus with the arm extended. In a patient with multiple joint disease, this angle allows the patient to reach the face more easily than if the axis of the forearm and humerus were parallel.

Soft Tissues

The elbow is supported by the medial and lateral collateral ligament complexes. The medial collateral ligament is more discrete and complex, consisting of three bundles: anterior, posterior, and transverse (Fig. 39–7). The anterior portion extends from the medial epicondyle to the sublimis tubercle of the proximal ulna.[44, 64] The posterior portion is well defined only at 90 degrees of flexion and, like the transverse ligament, provides little stability.

The lateral collateral ligament complex is less discrete (Fig. 39–8). The radiocollateral ligament originates from the lateral epicondyle and terminates in the annular ligament.[32, 52] The radiocollateral ligament appears to be taut throughout the normal range of flexion and extension. The accessory lateral collateral ligament, by comparison, apparently functions only when varus stress is applied to the elbow.

The musculature is described only as it applies to total elbow replacements. The important secondary stabilizers of the elbow joint are the flexor and extensor masses; they attach at the medial and lateral epicondyles, respectively. The flexor mass includes the flexor pronator group: pronator teres, flexor carpi radialis, palmaris longus, and flexor carpi ulnaris.

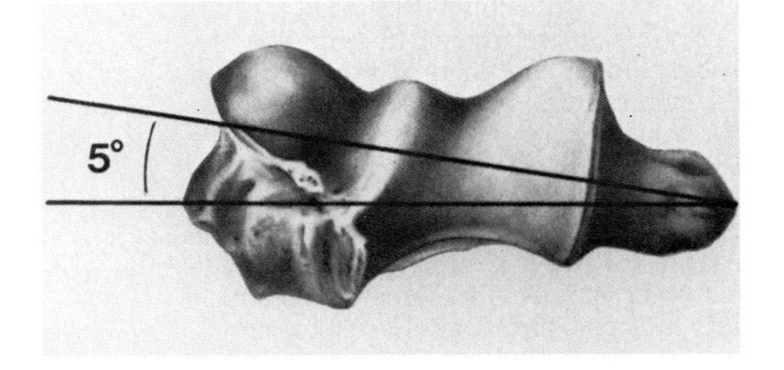

FIGURE 39–4. Center of rotation through the trochlea and capitellum. A 5 to 7 degrees of internal rotation with respect to the reference line through the medial and lateral epicondyle is seen.

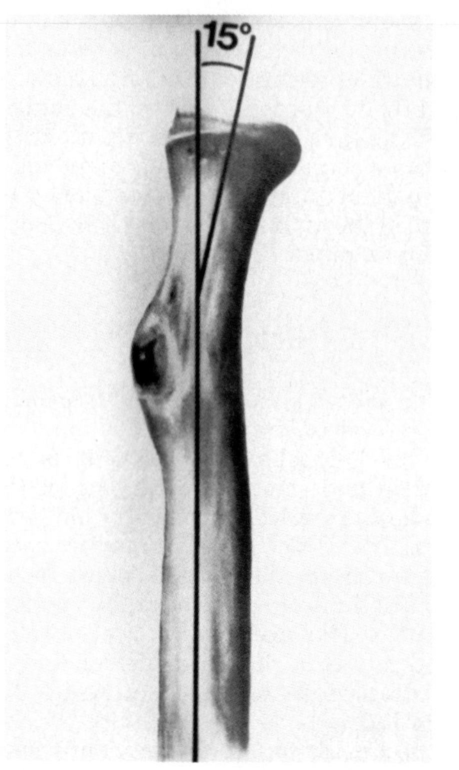

FIGURE 39–5. The 15-degree angle of the radial neck with respect to the long axis of the radius.

The extensor muscles attaching at the lateral epicondyle include the brachioradialis and the extensor carpi radialis brevis and longus. The extensor digitorum communis also originates in the anterior aspect of the lateral epicondyle. One head of the extensor carpi ulnaris originates from the communis extensor group. The anconeus muscle, which aids in elbow extension, originates from the posterior aspect of the lateral epicondyle and inserts into the surface of the proximal ulna. The supinator muscle also has an origin on the lateral epicondyle as well as the lateral collateral ligament in the proximal aspect of the ulna along the crista supinatoris.

The major extensor of the elbow is the triceps brachii. It inserts into the olecranon through a large triceps tendon. This muscle attaches into the periosteum of the proximal ulna. Electromyographic studies have indicated that the major flexor of the elbow is the brachialis, inserting at the base of the coronoid process. Although the biceps brachii aids in forearm flexion, it also acts as a supinator of the forearm.[81]

BIOMECHANICS

The normal elbow has an arc of 160 degrees of flexion from full extension, 80 degrees of pronation, and 85 degrees of supination.[48] However, most activities of daily living can be performed with an arc of flexion from 30 to 130 degrees, with a 100-degree arc of rotation divided equally between pronation and supination.[43] The range of motion of the elbow is thought to be limited by the geometry of the joint surfaces and impingement of the bone on surrounding capsule and muscle. However, the 30-degree anterior angulation of the distal humerus combined with the coronoid and olecranon fossae helps increase the elbow's range of motion.[32] The primary functions of the elbow include positioning the hand in space, providing a stable axis for the forearm as a lever, and functioning as a weightbearing joint. This last function is of help to patients who use assistive devices for walking, such as crutches and canes.[28]

Although the location of the center of

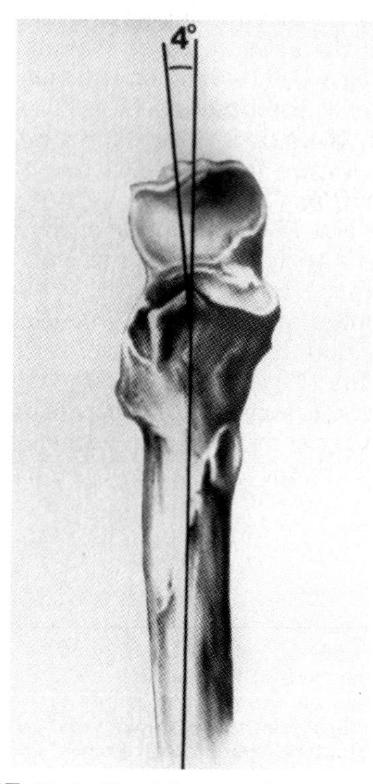

FIGURE 39–6. The 4-degree valgus angulation of the olecranon with respect to the shaft of the ulna, contributing to the valgus-carrying angle.

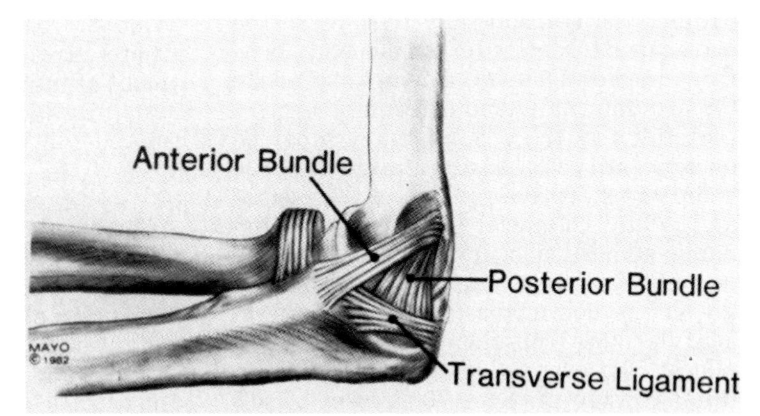

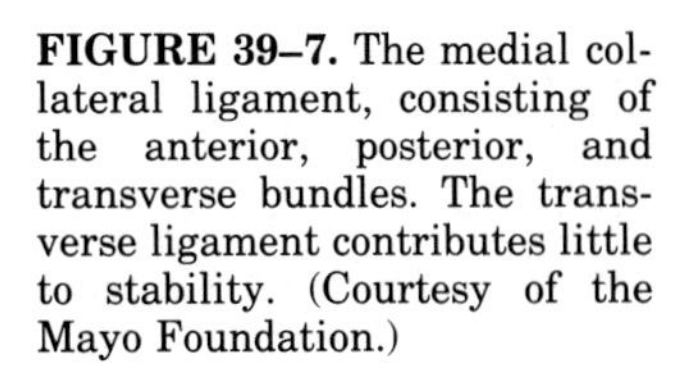
FIGURE 39–7. The medial collateral ligament, consisting of the anterior, posterior, and transverse bundles. The transverse ligament contributes little to stability. (Courtesy of the Mayo Foundation.)

rotation of the elbow has been the subject of numerous investigations, no consensus has been reached on the matter. Youm and colleagues concluded that the axis of rotation does not change with flexion and extension.[81] Morrey and Chao[43] have suggested that the instant centers vary and that the elbow is not a true hinge joint, but that deviations from the centers of rotation are minimal through most of the arc of motion, occurring mainly at the extremes of motion. Thus, the axis of rotation could be assumed to be a single point aligned to the center of the arc formed by the trochlear sulcus and capitellum.[37]

Elbow joint reaction forces of up to two to three times body weight can be generated with normal activities of daily living owing to the movement of the forearm with any lifting activities.[48] Torzilli[73] demonstrated that biceps force must be up to 38 times the static force applied to the extended elbow because of the short moment arm of the muscular attachment with relationship to the relatively long moment arm of the applied force. Dynamic loading—occurring when one lifts an object, rises from a seated position with the aid of the arm, or uses an assistive device to walk—may generate peaks of more than six times body weight. For the purposes of implant design, therefore, the elbow must be considered a weightbearing joint.

Walker,[78] Hui and associates,[26] and Pearson and associates[55] determined that the largest joint reaction forces were directed in a posterior plane at the distal humerus. The forces may result in posterior shifting of a prosthetic humeral component with anterior rotation and stem pressure along the anterior humeral cortex.

Rotational stresses along the total elbow replacement may also be high, especially in the patient with a stiff shoulder. In this

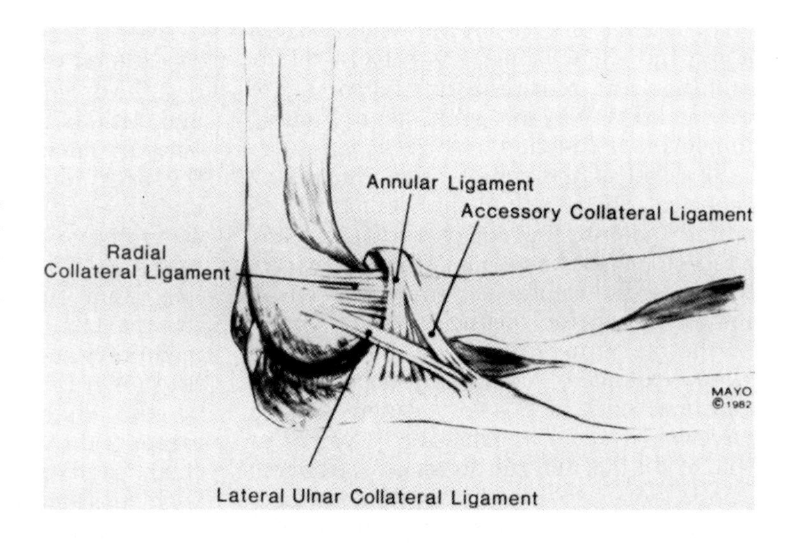

FIGURE 39–8. The complete radial collateral ligament, consisting of the radial collateral, lateral ulnar collateral, annular, and accessory collateral ligaments. (Courtesy of Mayo Foundation.)

patient, the transmission of loads to the bone-cement interface of the elbow replacement increases during attempts to rotate the arm internally and externally.

Stability of the elbow joint is provided by joint surface congruity; static soft tissue stabilization, including that of the medial and lateral collateral ligaments; and dynamic stabilization, including that of the flexor and extensor muscle masses attaching at the epicondyles. The ulnohumeral joint is quite congruous, accounting for almost 50 percent of its stability. The anterior capsule provides 70 percent of soft tissue restraint to distraction in extension, and the medial collateral ligament assumes this function at 90 degrees of flexion. In extension, varus stress is resisted equally by the joint articulation and the soft tissues, including the lateral collateral ligament and capsule. In flexion, the joint congruity provides 75 percent of the resistance to varus stress.

Resistance to valgus stress in extension is divided equally between the medial collateral ligament and the joint congruency in concert with the capsule. Valgus stress with the elbow flexed is primarily stabilized by the medial collateral ligament. A secondary stabilizer is joint congruency. Because the origin of the medial collateral ligament is not at the center of rotation, the anterior portion of the ligament is taut during extension and flexion, and the posterior portion is taut only during flexion.[46, 54, 64] The lateral ligament complex, with its origin at the center of rotation, is taut during flexion and extension. Most activities of daily living are performed with the elbow flexed and result in valgus stress along the elbow. Thus, the medial collateral ligament, providing over 50 percent of the stability for the joint, is extremely important to function.

Removal of the radial head places further demands on the medial collateral ligament as joint congruency is lost, and valgus stress must be resisted almost entirely by the medial collateral ligament. Approximately 60 percent of the stress is shared by the radiohumeral articulation with the elbow extended and axially loaded.[25] In addition, with the elbow flexed, tensile forces may reach two times body weight in the medial collateral ligament, whereas compressor forces on the radial head may reach up to three times body weight.[1] Excision of the radial head may result in greater stress in the medial collateral ligament of up to nine times body weight.

HISTORY

The development of total elbow replacement has paralleled that of other total joint arthroplasties, with its progression from hemiarthroplasty to constrained metal-on-metal hinges, with the use of bone cement fixation, and with its progression to semiconstrained and nonconstrained devices with polyethylene-bearing surfaces. Coonrad has divided the development of total elbow arthroplasty into four eras: biologic repair, hemiarthroplasty and total elbow arthroplasty, bone cement fixation, and semiconstrained and nonconstrained prostheses.[8]

Biologic Repair

The first era (1885–1947) was marked by biologic repair of elbow disease, including arthrodesis, synovectomy, and interpositional arthroplasty. The first indication for resection arthroplasty was ankylosis due to tuberculosis. Because these resections were extra-articular and included the ligaments, they often failed owing to instability.

Hemiarthroplasty and Early Total Prosthetic Arthroplasty

Dissatisfaction with interpositional and resectional arthroplasties led to the second era, the development of hemiarthroplasties and total elbow arthroplasties. In 1937, Virgen[75] developed a metal replacement for the proximal olecranon. In 1947, Mellen and Phalen[41] and, in 1954, McAusland[39] attempted hemireplacement of the distal humerus. These devices were fixed with a long stem. In 1965, Barr and Eaton[2] used two transfixing cortical screws in an intramedullary stemmed replacement of the distal humerus. This technique was followed by the distal humeral replacement by Street and Stevens[71] in 1974, who reported their results in ten patients. Their patients with post-traumatic arthritis had improved results after a follow-up interval of up to 7 years. In 1942, Boerma and de Waard[3] first reported an implant replacing both sides of the joint. In the 1950s, a straight-stemmed metal-hinged total elbow replacement was developed, but poor results were obtained because the device did not allow for restoration of the proper center of rotation.[8] Chatzikakis[7] reported on a hinged prosthesis in 1970, and Driessen[12] reported on a hinged prosthesis in 1972. Unfortunately the devices that emerged in these decades were not well designed, offering unpredictable pain relief and inconsistent function. Many failed owing to rapid loosening caused by poor implant fixation.

Bone Cement Fixation

The next major development in total elbow replacement was the advent of improved fixation techniques using bone cement. Several hinged-type replacements were introduced in the early 1970s, including those designed by Dee (Fig. 39–9),[11] McKee,[40] Gschwend, Scheier, and Bahler (the GSB replacement),[24] and the Stanmore prosthesis.[31] All were metal-to-metal hinged prostheses, and their development paralleled that of the Walldius and GUEPAR metal-to-metal hinged total knee replacements. The early, short-term results for the elbow were similar to those for the knee, showing excellent pain relief with good motion. However, longer-term follow-up data showed significant deterioration secondary to loosening of the prostheses. The problem was due to the constraint of the prosthesis along with the high metal wear debris resulting from metal-on-metal articulation. In addition, several of these designs required complete resection of the distal humerus, including the attachments of the flexor and extensor muscles. Thus, the soft tissue supporting sleeve of the elbow was lost, transferring further stress to the bone-cement interface and causing failure.[22]

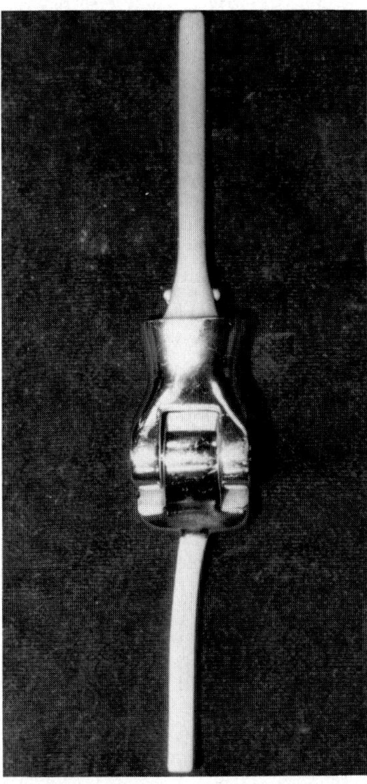

FIGURE 39–9. The Dee total elbow replacement with metal-on-metal hinge.

Semiconstrained and Nonconstrained Prostheses

The next major development in total elbow replacement occurred in the mid 1970s with the development of semiconstrained and nonconstrained prostheses. Semiconstrained prostheses were designed with laxity in the prosthetic joint to allow the soft tissues to share stress and to decrease stress at the bone-cement interface, thereby making loosening less likely. In nonconstrained prostheses, the designs allowed for the soft tissues to provide stability. Several types of semiconstrained prostheses have been designed, including the Mayo,[45, 50] Pritchard-Walker,[57] Coonrad,[8] Volz,[76] triaxial,[27, 28] and Schlein[63] prostheses.

The Mayo implant, first used in 1972, was a three-part semiconstrained device with snap fit of the humeral component and a separate polyethylene radial head replacement. The humeral component was fabricated from stainless steel. Left and right designs were available, with a carrying angle of 7 degrees. Initially, the ulna was all polyethylene but this was revised in 1975 to a metal-backed component. The radial head was all polyethylene.[45, 50] This device is no longer in use.

The Pritchard-Walker implant was a semiconstrained metal polyethylene prosthesis, initially with a polyethylene hu-

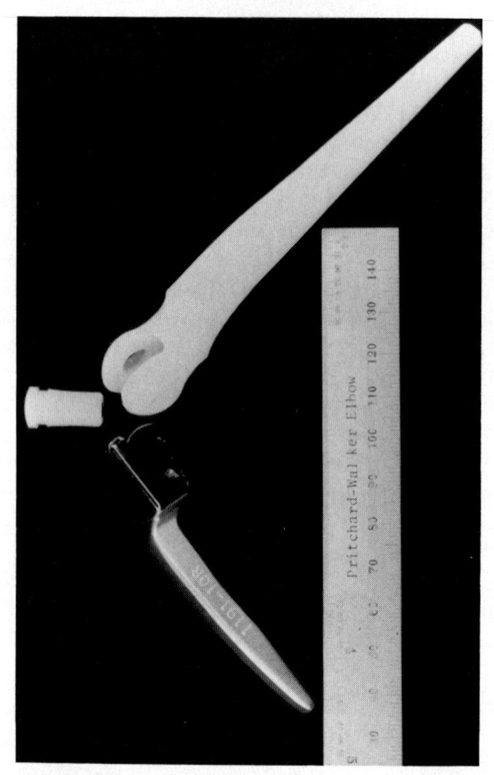

FIGURE 39–10. The Pritchard-Walker type I total elbow replacement designed at the Hospital for Special Surgery. This prosthesis included a polyethylene humeral component that was prone to fracture.

meral component and a metal ulnar component (Fig. 39–10). The polyethylene axle was also utilized for fixation. First implanted in 1974, it was modified (Mark II design) with a metal humeral component having a polyethylene-bearing insert to avoid the high incidence of fractures.[57]

The Coonrad implant is a semiconstrained replacement with metal humeral and ulnar components and polyethylene bushing (Fig. 39–11). The initial design, allowing for 2 to 3 degrees laxity, was modified to the type II design in 1978, allowing for 7 degrees of laxity in both rotary and varus/valgus motion. Since then, a type III design has been introduced that includes an anterior flange to help resist posterior migration (Fig. 39–12). This flange is plasma sprayed for biologic fixation with bone grafting in the coronoid fossa.[9]

The Volz or Arizona radiocapitellar replacement was a three-component semiconstrained metal polyethylene prosthesis with 15 degrees of laxity. The prosthesis had a polyethylene radial head replacement and an accessory capitellum.[76] It is no longer manufactured, however.

The triaxial component, first implanted in 1974, is a "sloppy-fit" semiconstrained device with a snap fit of the ulnar component into a humeral bushing (Fig. 39–13).[27, 28] The triaxial design has been the basis of a newer but as yet unnamed component, which is a sloppy-fit semiconstrained prosthesis having a restraining nonloadbearing constraining axle (Fig. 39–14). This design differs from the triaxial component in several ways, including the shapes of the humeral component and ulnar component and the articulation. The humeral component is shaped to optimize the loadbearing characteristics and to take advantage of optimum bone stock. The ulnar component is designed to better restore the carrying angle of the elbow. The bushing, redesigned to allow for loadbearing in the central portion, offers improved wear characteristics as the load is borne on the concave surface of the polyethylene instead

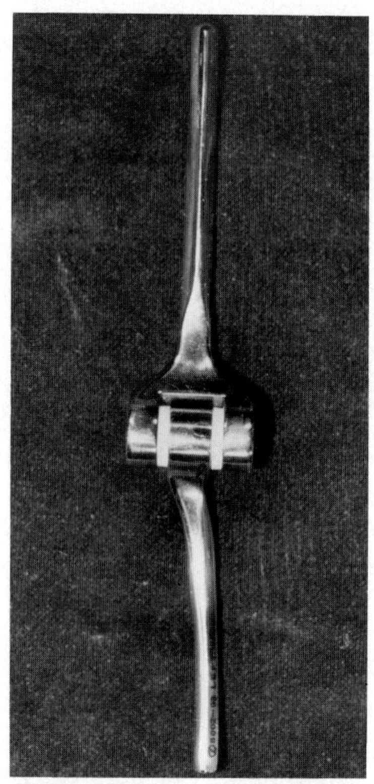

FIGURE 39–11. Original Coonrad total elbow replacement. This semiconstrained implant had little varus and valgus motion. It was later modified to allow more movement in the medial-lateral plane.

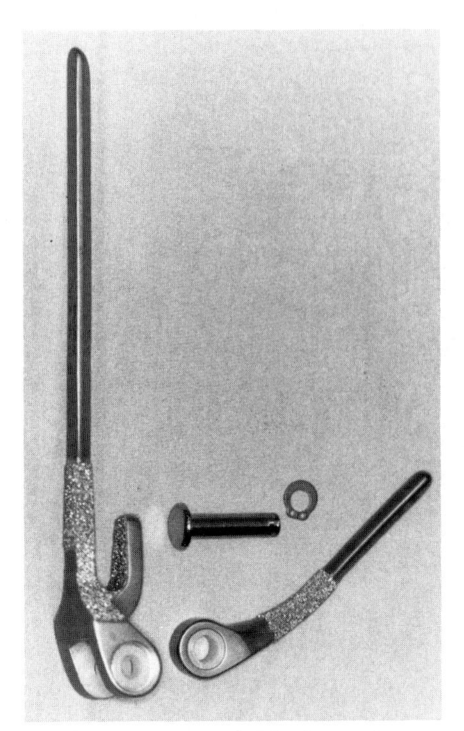

FIGURE 39–12. Coonrad III elbow. An anterior flange with a porous coating was added to help resist rotational and posterior displacement stresses.

of on the convex surface. The restraining axle is nonloadbearing. It was added to prevent late dislocations secondary to polyethylene wear.

The Schlein[63] semiconstrained implant was a loose-fitting snap-hinged component with metal humeral and ulnar components and a snap-fit bushing (Fig. 39–15).

Unconstrained implants are stabilized by joint congruity and soft tissue stability, including that offered by the medial collateral ligament. Available resurfacing devices include the capitellocondylar implant and the Kudo, London, Souter, Wadsworth, ICLH, Liverpool, Ishizuki, and Pritchard implants.[8, 14, 30, 34, 35, 36, 57, 67, 68, 74, 77] The capitellocondylar device, designed by Ewald, was first used in 1974 (Fig. 39–16).[14] Although initially a two-component device, this prosthesis had an optional radial head added. The first design employed a humeral component and an all-polyethylene ulnar component, but this was later reinforced with a metal-backed ulnar component.[14] The London nonconstrained implant was a two-part implant with a metal humeral component and a polyethylene ulnar component.[36] The Pritchard device[57] includes a radial head replacement. Attempts have been made to implant this with porous ingrowth fixation.

Other semiconstrained implants, designed and used outside the United States, include the Kudo and Ishizuki implants from Japan; the Liverpool, ICLH, and Wadsworth implants from England; and the Souter implant from Scotland. The Kudo prosthesis, first implanted in 1971, has a metal distal humeral cuff with a polyethylene ulnar component—there is no stem fixation for the humeral component. The humeral component contours were modified in 1975.[34] The Ishizuki prosthesis resembles the Kudo, with a stemless metal humeral component and a stemmed polyethylene ulnar component. However, the humeral component more closely approximates the contours of the distal humerus.[30] The Liverpool replacement is a two-part nonconstrained elbow prosthesis with bicondylar articulation. The humeral component has an optional stem, and the ulnar component is polyethylene.[67] The Souter replacement is a bicondylar design. The

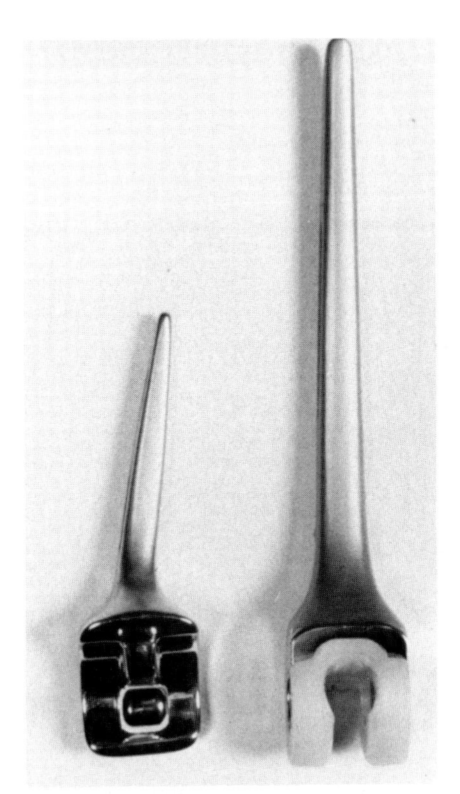

FIGURE 39–13. Triaxial total elbow replacement is a loose-hinged semiconstrained elbow replacement.

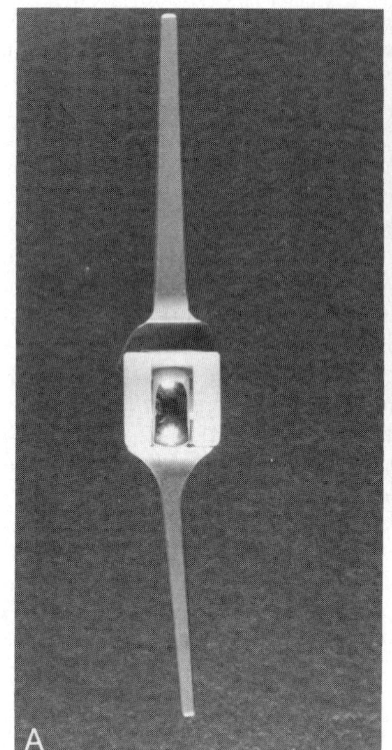

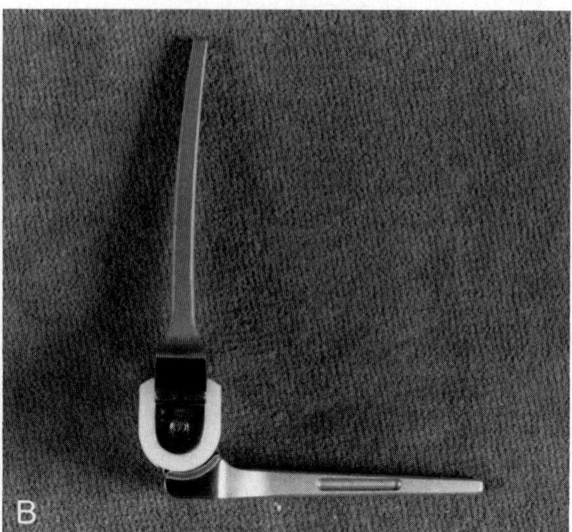

FIGURE 39–14. *A* and *B*, Custom-fit semiconstrained total elbow replacement from the Hospital for Special Surgery. A nonloadbearing linkage is included to prevent dislocation after polyethylene wear has occurred.

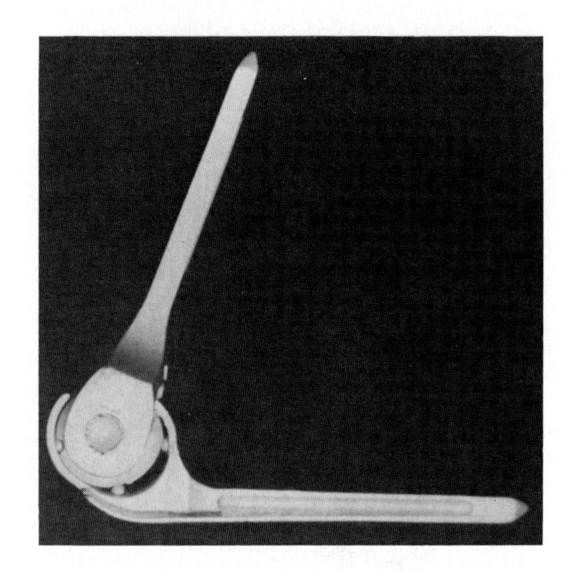

FIGURE 39–15. The Schlein semiconstrained total elbow replacement.

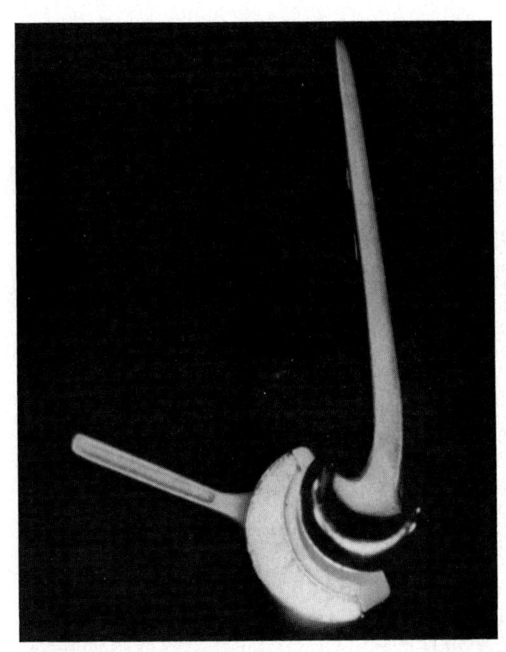

FIGURE 39–16. Capitellocondylar total elbow replacement.

distal humeral component has a flange that inserts into the distal humerus. The ulnar component is polyethylene. The Wadsworth prosthesis has a stemmed humeral component with a polyethylene bushing. The ulnar component is all metal.

INDICATIONS

The indications for total elbow arthroplasty have broadened as improvements in surgical technique and implant design have produced more predictable results. In general, the indications include pain, loss of function, including the inability to perform activities of daily living because of pain or loss of motion at the elbow; and gross instability secondary to a fracture nonunion.

Rheumatoid Arthritis

Rheumatoid arthritis is the most common disease necessitating total elbow replacement (Fig. 39–17). The patient may present with significant pain, loss of motion, and joint destruction resulting in inability to perform certain activities of daily living. In addition, the patient may have incomplete ulnar neuropathy secondary to marked synovitis causing pressure on the ulnar nerve at the cubital tunnel. To be considered a candidate for a total elbow replacement, the patient should have synovitis that is resistant to medical management. Other conservative treatment should have failed, including administration of remittent agents and local cortisone injections. Radiographic class III or IV changes, including marked joint destruction, should be apparent. A patient with intact cartilage and minimal cystic changes may be better treated by open or arthroscopic synovectomy with or without radial head resection.

Before the decision is made to offer total elbow replacement to the patient with rheumatoid arthritis, a comprehensive examination should be performed including evaluation of the patient's functional abilities and needs. A thorough cervical spine examination with neurologic testing should also be performed. Both upper extremities should be evaluated, including range of motion at the shoulders and wrists and hand function. In addition, the lower extremities should be assessed, including walking ability and any requirement for ambulatory aids. If lower extremity surgery is indicated, ideally it should be before elbow replacement in order to reduce the requirement for walker, crutches, or cane after elbow replacement. Exceptions to this exist, however. Some of our patients with class IV rheumatoid arthritis would be unable to use even a platform walker after total hip or total knee replacement because their elbows are so severely diseased. In these patients, we sometimes perform the elbow replacements prior to lower extremity surgery so they can use ambulatory aids after lower extremity joint replacements.

If hand, wrist, or both types of surgery are required, we prefer to do them before elbow replacement to provide a functional hand. This gives the patient the incentive to utilize the hand and provides better motivation for and success with rehabilitation of the elbow. We recommend the surgery for the elbow next—then shoulder surgery if needed. The exception is when the patient has an extremely stiff shoulder with no rotation. In this case, we recommend shoulder surgery first to re-establish

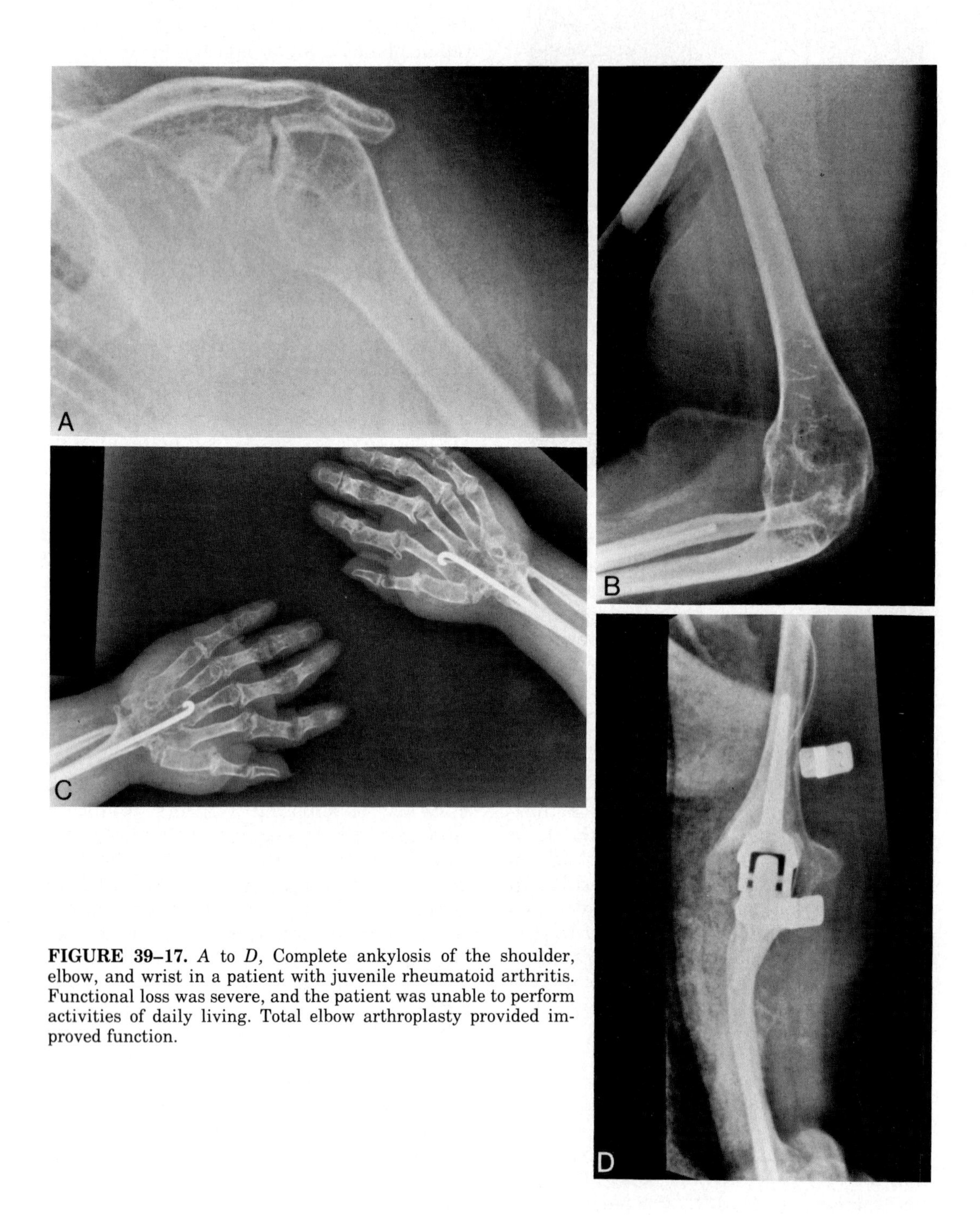

FIGURE 39–17. *A* to *D,* Complete ankylosis of the shoulder, elbow, and wrist in a patient with juvenile rheumatoid arthritis. Functional loss was severe, and the patient was unable to perform activities of daily living. Total elbow arthroplasty provided improved function.

rotary motion before the elbow replacement is done. Otherwise, ankylosis of the shoulder will produce high rotational stress on the total elbow replacement, resulting in loosening or failure of the articulation.

Occasionally, we perform total shoulder and total elbow replacements during one hospitalization, often within 2 weeks of each other. We do this when the patient has so much pain in both the shoulder and the elbow that, if only the elbow is replaced, the shoulder pain will interfere with rehabilitation. In other instances, we stage the ipsilateral upper extremity joint replacements in different hospitalizations, allowing the patient to fully rehabilitate from one operation before having another. Often, the elbow replacement allows the patient to gain enough function and range of motion that shoulder replacement may not be necessary. When shoulder and elbow replacement are performed on the same extremity, a short-stemmed humeral component should be utilized to keep the stems of the humeral component of the shoulder replacement from meeting the humeral component of the elbow replacement within the shaft of the humerus.[4, 5, 10, 19, 35, 38, 58, 59, 60, 61, 62, 79]

Ankylosis

Ankylosis of the elbow results in significant functional loss, often enough to hamper the patient in the activities of daily living, which require a 100-degree arc of flexion at the elbow ranging from 30 degrees of extension to 130 degrees of flexion.[43] Patients typically have difficulties with grooming and personal hygiene, especially in cases of ipsilateral shoulder and elbow ankylosis as in juvenile rheumatoid arthritis. The problem is worse, of course, when both elbows are ankylosed. Although pain is often absent, pronation and supination may be painful owing to arthritis at the radial head. However, the main indication for restoring motion in these patients is to improve function.[17]

Post-Traumatic Arthrosis

Indications for total elbow replacement for post-traumatic arthrosis have broadened with improvements in implant design. Many patients with severe joint destruction accompanied by pain, loss of motion, and loss of function are now candidates for elbow replacements, although they should first be considered for any biologic procedures that may be feasible. Total elbow replacement should be regarded as a salvage procedure, especially in active patients who perform heavy labor.

A patient with post-traumatic arthrosis presents a more significant challenge for several reasons. Alterations in the bony architecture are often accompanied by marked bone loss and soft tissue deformities. Previous operations may have left multiple skin incisions, putting the patient at a higher risk for wound-healing problems and infections. Ulnar nerve entrapment may be present preoperatively. As a result, the patient is more predisposed to infection, loosening, and postoperative ulnar neuropathy. Total elbow replacement may offer an opportunity for salvage, although the surgical technique is challenging and the complication rate is high. Careful preoperative counseling is imperative, with emphasis on the need for compliance with the postoperative regimen.[20, 50]

Supracondylar Nonunion

Supracondylar nonunion of the humerus occurs infrequently, but when it does, the disability may be significant (Fig. 39–18). The patient may have a flail upper extremity and may be unable to reach the face. Although the procedure of choice is an open reduction and fixation of the distal humerus with bone grafting, this may be impractical in some cases because bone in the distal humerus is inadequate to hold fixation. In some patients, periarticular fibrosis of the joint would lead to poor results even if union of the distal humerus were obtained. Thus, total elbow replacement may be a salvage procedure in an older patient with a flail upper extremity secondary to a supracondylar nonunion. In these instances, a semiconstrained device should be implanted, with salvage of the humeral epicondyles and their soft tissue attachments. Because the patient with supracondylar nonunion tends to have a high failure rate after total elbow replacement, it should be considered a salvage procedure

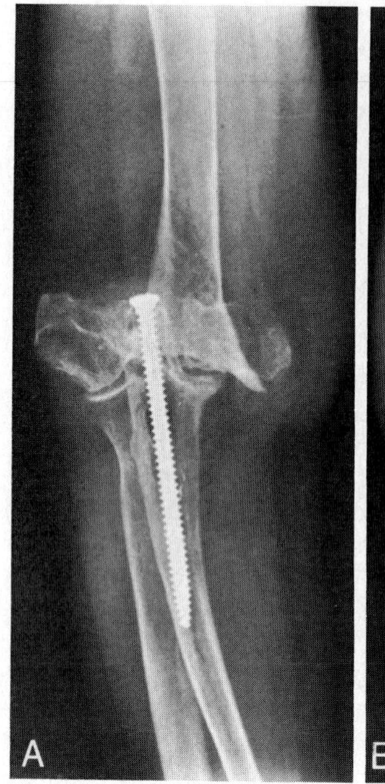

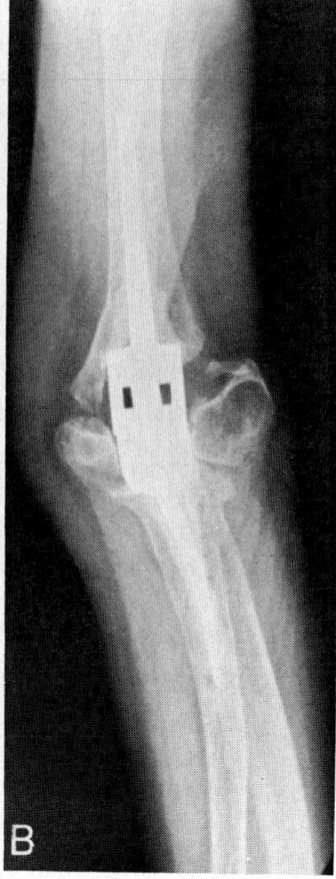

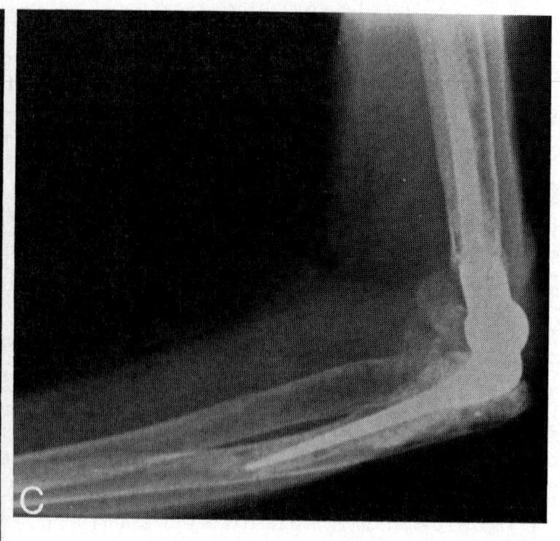

FIGURE 39–18. *A,* Supracondylar nonunion resulting in a flail elbow with gross deformity and inability to position the hand in space. *B* and *C,* Salvage by total elbow replacement. This procedure may be used when no other will suffice.

when no good biologic option is available. These patients are exposed to the same risks as those who have post-traumatic arthritis (e.g., higher rates of loosening, infection, and ulnar nerve dysfunction).[18, 42, 65]

CONTRAINDICATIONS

Contraindications to total elbow arthroplasty include active sepsis, marked loss of bone stock and soft tissue, Charcot joint, and noncompliance. Active infection at the elbow must be treated and a biologic procedure performed to reduce pain and improve function. If infection is present, a prosthesis must not be implanted. Infection in another site in the body must be eradicated before total elbow replacement is considered.

Significant loss of bone from the distal humerus or proximal ulna combined with loss of soft tissue is a relative contraindication. If the distal humerus is absent and the extensor and flexor masses are nonfunctional, all the stress is imposed on the bone-cement interface, causing a prosthesis to undergo rapid loosening. However, loss of the distal humerus with preservation of the muscles may be addressed by a custom-fit total elbow replacement or a distal humeral allograft and a cemented elbow replacement with attachment of the muscle masses. Preservation of the extensor and flexor masses stabilizes the elbow, reducing stress at the bone-cement interface.

A warm erythematous elbow with marked joint destruction and soft tissue calcification, with or without pain, should be evaluated for the possibility of Charcot arthropathy. Because the condition may be secondary to syringomyelia of the cervical spine, a full neurologic examination should be performed. A total elbow replacement in a Charcot joint would loosen rapidly owing to abuse of the implant. In addition, any patient with paralysis of the upper extremity should not undergo elbow replacement, as adequate extensor and flexor muscles are required to power the implant.

Marked skin loss or ulceration about the elbow is also a relative contraindication because of interference with wound healing and the high probability of infection. Before elbow replacement is considered, the problem must be addressed and adequate soft tissue healing must be obtained. Rheumatoid nodules and olecranon bursitis, although not considered contraindications to surgery, do increase the chances of poor wound healing postoperatively and thus raise the risk of infection.

If a patient is likely to be noncompliant

with the rehabilitation regimen, this is another contraindication for surgery. Also, the elbow must not be abused. If any question exists about the patient's ability to comply, surgery should not be performed.

BIOLOGIC OPTIONS

Biologic options include fascial arthroplasty, distraction arthroplasty, and arthrodesis. Fascial arthroplasty gives satisfactory results in certain cases, but outcomes are often unpredictable and instability may ensue. A distraction arthroplasty often gives satisfactory results and maintains the bony architecture, especially with extrinsic ankylosis of the elbow where the bony architecture and cartilage have been relatively spared. Morrey[51] has described distraction arthroplasty as an adequate salvage procedure for the patient with post-traumatic contracture, with the caveat that the technique is demanding and the complication rate is high. In a series of 25 patients, he obtained satisfactory results in 96 percent.[51]

Elbow arthrodesis is seldom recommended, as it is difficult to achieve and may produce significant functional loss, including the inability to perform activities of daily living. The exception is when the patient would otherwise be left with a functionless flail extremity due to resection arthroplasty and a total elbow replacement could not be considered as a salvage procedure.

PREOPERATIVE PLANNING

Preoperative planning is an essential part of successful total elbow replacement. First, the proper implant must be selected: a semiconstrained or a nonconstrained device. Nonconstrained implants are indicated for patients with rheumatoid arthritis who have intact medial collateral ligaments and no marked bone loss or soft tissue contractures. If ligament support is inadequate, a semiconstrained device should be used. Semiconstrained prostheses may be employed for all patients with rheumatoid arthritis whether or not the medial collateral ligament is sufficient (Fig. 39–19). Semiconstrained implants should also be chosen for patients with supracondylar nonunion, post-traumatic arthritis, and ankylosis of the elbow. Those with post-traumatic arthritis and supracondylar nonunion may have marked joint fibrosis, requiring extensive dissection and release of soft tissues including contracted medial collateral ligaments. Nonconstrained im-

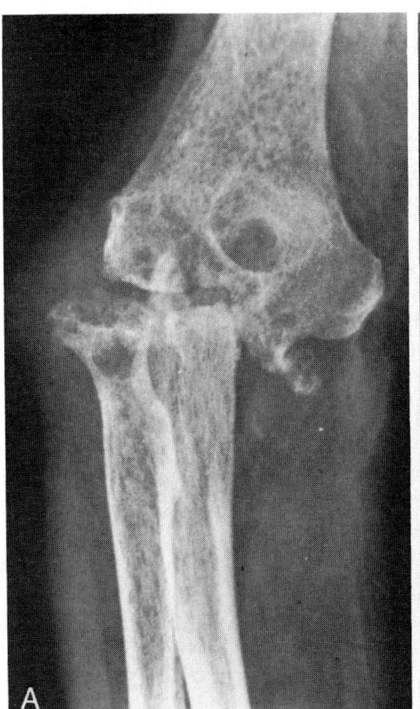

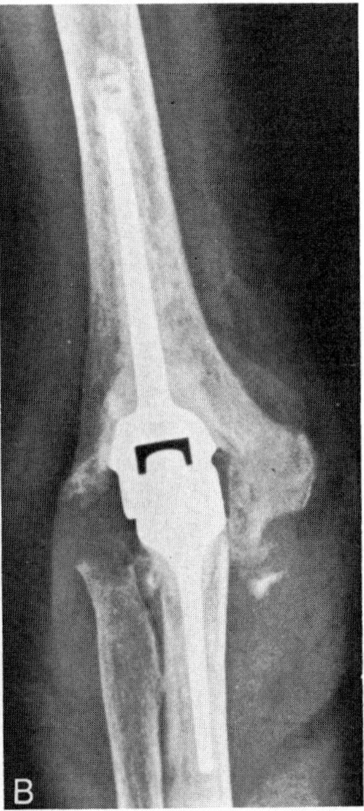

FIGURE 39–19. Marked elbow destruction due to rheumatoid arthritis. *A,* Laxity of the collateral ligaments is seen in addition to cartilage and bone destruction. Because of ligament laxity, this patient was not a good candidate for a nonconstrained total elbow replacement. *B,* Radiographic appearance after replacement with a semiconstrained prosthesis.

plants may be less successful for these patients because they may generate sufficient forces postoperatively to produce dislocation of the implants. In a patient with complete ankylosis of the elbow, the medial collateral ligament is often encased in bone. This ligament must be completely resected, and the elbow supported by a semiconstrained implant.

The surgeon must next size the elbow to determine whether the implant selected will properly restore the anatomy of the distal humerus and recreate the center of rotation in the joint. Restoration of the ulnar center of rotation is also important. In a series of 56 elbows, Figgie and coworkers[15] obtained a statistically significant improvement in results when the elbow was placed so that the center of rotation was restored to within a neutral range. Thus, the planning for elbow replacement should allow restoration of this center of rotation.

The elbow should fit properly within the canals of the humerus and the ulna as determined by preoperative templating. In some patients, custom-fit implants may be required to achieve proper fit and anatomy restoration. These include patients with significant deformities or bone losses secondary to post-traumatic arthritis or those with juvenile rheumatoid arthritis with deformities due to premature closure of the epiphyses. In a patient with complete ankylosis of the elbow, computerized tomography may be required to properly measure the humerus and ulna for fit of the implant, because adequate anteroposterior and lateral radiographs are often difficult to obtain. Computerized tomography may also be helpful in certain other patients with marked bone deformities.

SURGICAL TECHNIQUE

The surgical approaches differ for nonconstrained devices. Nonconstrained devices are implanted using an extensile Kocher approach—a lateral approach using a triceps flap.[53] In this approach, the ulnar nerve is not identified and the medial collateral ligament is left intact.

When a semiconstrained device is selected, the medial collateral ligament may be stripped off to provide greater exposure of the elbow. This maneuver allows the surgeon to employ a posteromedial approach as described by Bryan and Morrey.[6] Almost a mirror image of the extensile Kocher approach, the procedure involves taking down the triceps as a continuous flap posteromedially to laterally, thereby exposing the elbow. In this approach, the ulnar nerve is also identified and isolated. The triceps Z approach and olecranon osteotomy are not recommended as part of the procedure, as they require a large soft tissue flap with detachment of the triceps mechanism. As a result, wound-healing complications often arise and postoperative range of motion may be compromised owing to the prolonged immobilization required after surgery.

Extensile Kocher Approach

In the extensile Kocher approach (Fig. 39–20), the skin incision is made in the lateral aspect of the arm, beginning approximately 8 cm proximal to the joint just posterior to the supracondylar ridge of the lateral epicondyle. The incision curves at the joint line and proceeds distally 6 cm along the anconeus muscle. The interval between the triceps and the muscles in the mobile wad (brachioradialis and extensor carpi radialis longus and brevis) is identified. In addition, the interval between the extensor carpi radialis longus and anconeus muscles is identified and developed. The triceps is then elevated posteriorly along the intramuscular septum and subperiosteally off the proximal ulna. The anconeus muscle is also stripped subperiosteally in a posterior direction. The extensor carpi radialis longus and the extensor carpi ulnaris may be stripped off to provide additional anterior exposure. The radial collateral ligament complex is released subperiosteally from its attachment to the distal humerus. The annular ligament, which supports the proximal radius, must be spared at the attachment to the ulna.

Once the triceps has been reflected subperiosteally, the elbow may be dislocated, hinging along the intact medial collateral ligament. One must be aware that the ulnar nerve is not exposed with this procedure and is vulnerable to sharp instruments. The radial head is routinely re-

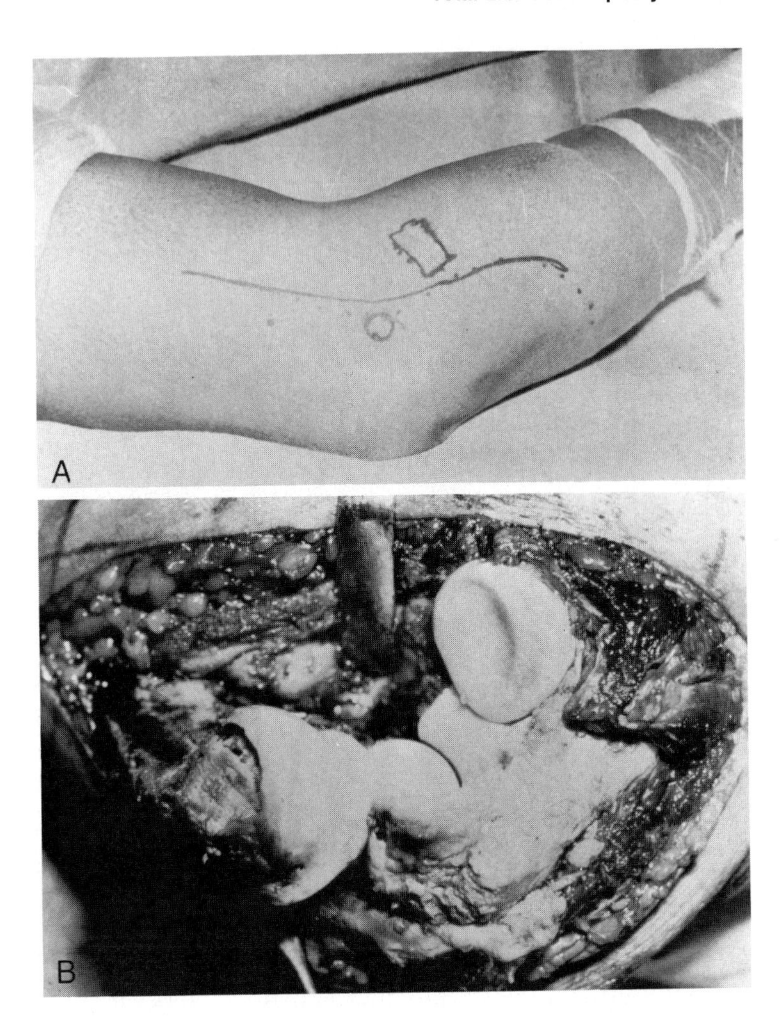

FIGURE 39–20. *A*, The Kocher approach to the elbow. A lateral approach is used, leaving the medial collateral ligament intact. *B*, Excellent exposure may be obtained through this approach.

moved and resurfacing is optional. During exposure and amputation of the radial head, the soft tissues must be protected to avoid injury to the posterior interosseous nerve, which courses anteriorly and distally to the radial head. The distal humerus and proximal ulna are prepared according to the instructions for the prosthesis chosen. The capitellocondylar device uses a stem in the humerus and has an intermedullary guide to help the surgeon resect the proper amount of bone.

Once the bone is resected and trial implants are placed, range of motion and stability are tested in both extension and 90 degrees of flexion. If the elbow is still unstable, a larger polyethylene component may be required. If the elbow remains unstable, a semiconstrained device may be necessary. The elbow components are cemented into place with bone cement that is injected using a syringe and then packed using a finger. While the cement is hardening, the elbow is held in extension and excess cement is trimmed. The tourniquet is deflated, and hemostasis is obtained. The radial collateral ligament is repaired to the distal humerus, and the anconeus and extensor muscles are closed. A suction drain is placed, and closure is completed. The elbow is splinted in extension but it is not forced. The drain is removed at 24 hours if drainage has ceased. Range of motion exercises are begun on postoperative day 3 or 4.

Posteromedial Approach

With the patient in a supine position, the arm is brought up and positioned over the chest for the posteromedial approach (Fig. 39–21).[6] A straight proximal incision is made over the medial border of the

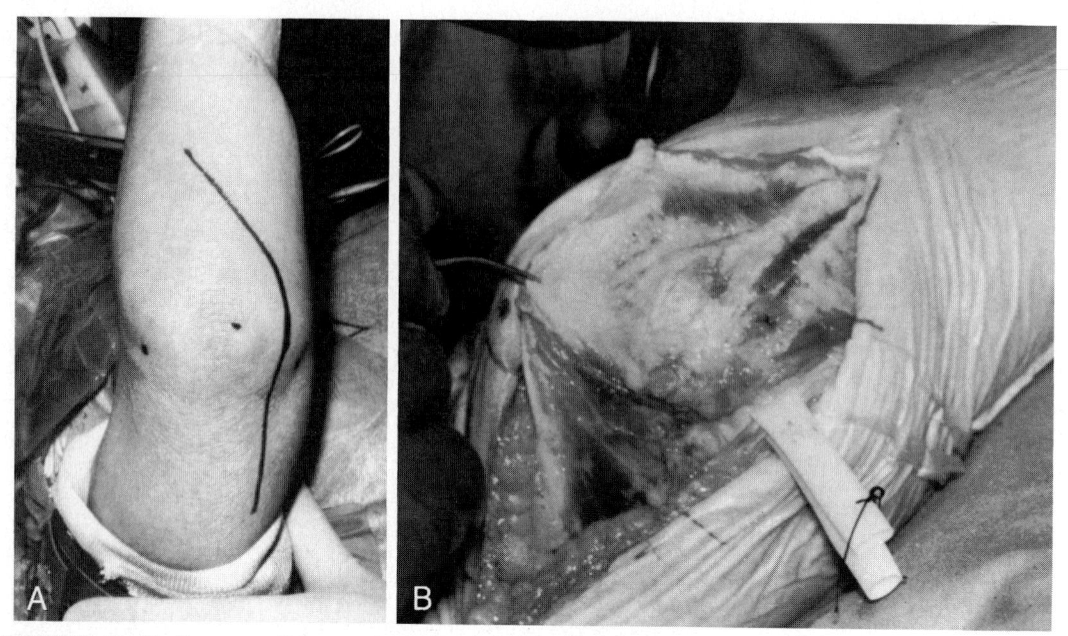

FIGURE 39–21. Posteromedial approach. This approach utilizes a posteromedial based triceps flap. *A*, Skin incision. *B*, Isolation of the ulnar nerve and elevation of the triceps as a single sleeve. This maneuver allows for early rehabilitation after wound healing.

triceps and ulnar nerve and extended to the level of the cubital tunnel. The incision then curves across the proximal third of the ulna.

Subcutaneous tissues are divided, and no subcutaneous flaps are raised. The ulnar nerve is identified at the cubital tunnel and is dissected free along its course proximally and distally. A Penrose drain is placed around the nerve. Sutures are placed through the drain to help maintain positive identification of the nerve. No clamp is placed on the drain to avoid undue tension on the nerve. The nerve is dissected free, creating a passage between the two heads of the flexor carpi ulnaris and allowing the nerve to be translocated anteriorly and protected throughout the operation. The fascia of the flexor carpi ulnaris is divided to the ulna from where the ulnar nerve enters underneath the fascia to its insertion at the proximal third of the ulna. The triceps muscle is also dissected free medially and elevated laterally, with care taken to avoid injuring the ulnar nerve that lies within the fibers of the triceps muscle more proximally.

The posterior capsule of the elbow is left intact at this time. The triceps attachment at the tip of the olecranon is carefully reflected along with the periosteum of the olecranon. The sleeve of the triceps and the forearm fascia remains in continuity. The sleeve is additionally elevated across the lateral epicondyle, exposing the radial head. The anconeus muscle is also reflected.

The capsule and synovium at the radial head are then excised, leaving the annular ligament intact. The radial head is resected with an oscillating saw at the proximal edge of the annular ligament. A rasp is used to smooth the rough edges of the remaining radius.

The proximal ulna is exposed by resecting the capsule laterally to medially. This step involves incising the radial collateral ligament and the posterior capsule and then removing the synovium and the capsule. The medial aspect of the flexor carpi ulnaris is reflected to the sublime tubercle. The medial collateral ligament is dissected subperiosteally from the sublime tubercle. The ulnar nerve must be carefully protected, as it lies extremely close to the sublime tubercle at this point. Once the medial collateral ligament is resected, the elbow can be dislocated, giving good exposure to the proximal ulna. On occasion, an anterior capsulotomy is necessary. This procedure is performed by placing a hemostat anterior to the capsule and incising it. The brachialis muscle protects the anterior structures during the procedure.

After the center of rotation of the olecranon is identified and the appropriate bone cuts made, the semiconstrained implant can be placed. The prosthesis should be aligned so that the centers of rotation of the ulna and the humerus are restored. In addition, when cutting and rasping the distal humerus, one should take care not to invade the supracondylar ridges. Violation of these supracondylar pillars, which provide the main support for the implant, may result in fracture. When the distal humeral cut is made, it is important to remember that the axis of the center of rotation through the trochlea and capitellum is slightly and internally rotated with respect to the epicondyles. This rotation should be restored when placing the implant.

Once the trial components are placed, the elbow should be taken through a range of motion. Full extension and flexion should be obtained. Pronation and supination should also be determined. The radial head should be examined to be sure it does not abut against the implant. In addition, one should check anteriorly to make certain that the coronoid process does not block flexion. If it does, the tip of the coronoid process can be excised to provide further flexion.

After the components are fitted satisfactorily, the bone is prepared for cement. The cement is introduced into the humerus and ulna and pressurized by packing with the finger. The surgeon then inserts the ulna and humeral components, making sure that the proper center of rotation is achieved and that the cement is well pressurized.

The cement should be trimmed before hardening. No cement must extrude anteriorly into the space previously occupied by the radial head. After the cement has set, the tourniquet may be deflated and hemostasis obtained. The arm can then be elevated and the tourniquet reapplied. At this point, the elbow should be articulated. In many cases, it is wise to remove a small amount of the tip of the olecranon to avoid protrusion of the sharp point through the skin. Two drill holes are placed through the olecranon for an absorbable suture. This suture is later employed to help anchor the triceps after it is put back in place. The wound is irrigated, and the elbow is closed in layers by suturing the fascia of the extensor carpi ulnaris and restoring the triceps in continuity. One should make certain that the ulnar nerve is not bound or constricted during closure. Subcutaneous and skin layers are then closed. The patient is provided a well-padded splint with the arm in maximum extension.

RESULTS

Rheumatoid Arthritis

Nonconstrained Prosthesis

(Table 39–1)

In 1980, Ewald and coworkers[14] reported the results of a capitellocondylar prosthesis utilized in 54 total elbow replacements. In this series, 50 patients had rheumatoid arthritis. Satisfactory results were reported for 47 of the 54 elbows during follow-up periods of 2 to 5 years (Fig. 39–22). The average flexion improved 14 to 136 degrees, whereas the postoperative extension remained equal to the preoperative extension of 31 degrees. Average postoperative pronation and supination was 75 degrees and 53 degrees, respectively. Although most of the elbows achieved satisfactory ratings, the complication rate was 39 percent. In total, eight patients required revision of the prostheses—four for dislocation, two for sepsis, one for fracture, and one for humeral component loosening. Three deep infections occurred. Two cases required implant removal, and the third was treated successfully by debridement and suppression. Recurrent dislocation occurred in five elbows—two requiring revision to a semiconstrained prosthesis and one requiring revision of the humeral component. In the fourth patient, an attempt was made to reconstruct the medial collateral ligament, but it failed. Ulnar nerve problems occurred in 11 patients: five had permanent ulnar nerve dysfunction and six had transient ulnar nerve paralysis. No elbows had radiolucent lines at the humeral bone-cement interfaces, but eight

Table 39–1. FOLLOW-UP DATA FOR PATIENTS WITH NONCONSTRAINED ELBOW PROSTHESES

Authors	Year	Prosthesis	No.	Rheumatoid Arthritis	Follow-Up Yrs	Postoperative Extension/ Flexion	Motion Pronation/ Supination	Satis-factory	Revised	Insta-bility	Ulnar Nerve Dysfunction
Ewald, et al.	1980	Capitellocondylar	54	54	2–5	31/136	75/53	47/54	8	8	11
Davis, et al.	1982	Capitellocondylar	30	28	1–5	35/150	79/66	—	2	4	3
Rosenberg, Turner	1984	Capitellocondylar	28	27	1–5.6	33/134	80/72	24/28	3	4	3
Weiland, et al.	1989	Capitellocondylar	40	38	4–12	42/133	67/71	34/40	2	10	9
Simmons, et al.	1990	Capitellocondylar	202	200	2–15	30/138	72/64	—	9	17	42
Kudo, et al.	1980	Kudo	24	24	1–7	42/124	29/49	21/24	0	1	1
Kudo, et al.	1990	Kudo	37	37	1–17	—	33/64	30/37	4	7	4
London	1978	London	16	16	0.5–2	—	—	14/16	—	—	—
Souter	1981	Souter	22	22	0.5–1.5	52/143	65/66	18/22	0	3	5
Tuke	1981	ICLH	27	27	0–3	37/137	62/71	22/27	4	2	0
Wadsworth	1981	Wadsworth	14	11	1–2	24/133	62/74	9/10	1	1	0
Rydholm, et al	1984	Wadsworth	19	19	1.5–4	30/135	65/65	15/19	2	1	3
Pritchard	1983	Pritchard	13	12	3–2.5	15/120	60/45	12/13	1	1	0
Soni, Cavendish	1984	Liverpool	80	69	1–8	32/134	69/62	66/80	14	8	6
Lowe, et al.	1984	Lowe	47	39	1–9	37/135	60/72	22/39	14	8	3
Roper, et al.	1986	Roper-Tuke	60	50	3–9	46/136	69/68	36/51	15	7	4

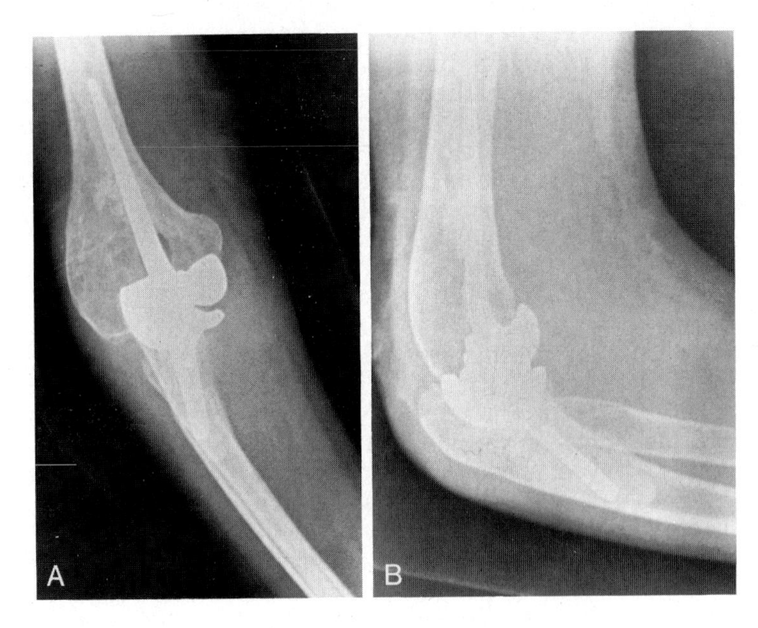

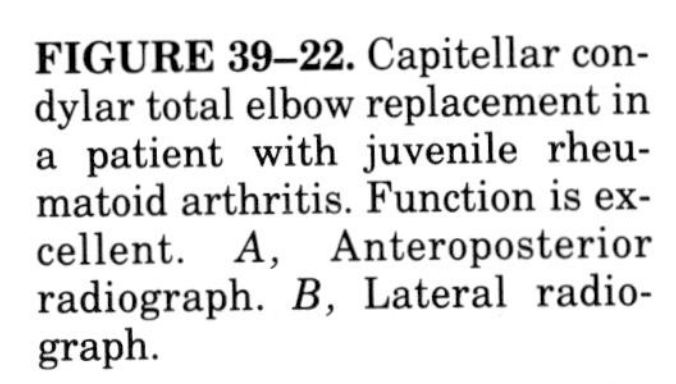
FIGURE 39–22. Capitellar condylar total elbow replacement in a patient with juvenile rheumatoid arthritis. Function is excellent. *A,* Anteroposterior radiograph. *B,* Lateral radiograph.

elbows had radiolucent lines around the ulnar components. In two cases, complete radiolucent lines wider than 2 mm were observed.

In a review of 202 capitellocondylar total elbow replacements with follow-ups from 2 to 15 years, Simmons and colleagues[66] reported an average postoperative range of motion of 30 to 138 degrees with supination of 64 degrees and pronation of 72 degrees. Eight elbows had humeral component radiolucencies and 23 had ulnar radiolucencies. Four elbows underwent revision surgery for aseptic loosening and two for instability. Deep infection occurred in three elbows, whereas 24 had transient ulnar nerve paralysis. In ten other elbows, permanent ulnar nerve paralysis occurred. Instability was evidenced in 17 patients: seven had frank dislocations and ten had subluxations. Despite the high early complication rate, these investigators believed that long-term results were good with low long-term failure rates.

In the first of two studies on the capitellocondylar elbow replacement, Davis and associates[10] reported 2- to 7-year follow-ups for 30 elbow replacements (28 for rheumatoid arthritis). Long-term follow-up data (4 to 12 years) were later reported by Weiland and coworkers[79] for 40 elbow replacements (38 with rheumatoid arthritis). In the initial series, the average postoperative range of motion was 35 degrees of extension to 150 degrees of flexion, with 79 degrees of pronation and 66 degrees of supination. Two elbows required implant removal for deep infection. Of four patients with instability, three were treated with long arm casts, and the fourth required surgical reconstruction of the medial collateral ligament. Ulnar nerve dysfunction occurred in three patients with spontaneous resolution in two. The third patient required neurolysis and anterior transposition of the nerve.

In the second follow-up study reported in 1989, the average range of motion was 42 degrees of extension to 133 degrees of flexion, with pronation of 67 degrees and supination of 71 degrees.[79] Satisfactory results were achieved in 34 of the 40, but ten elbows developed instability—eight with malarticulation and two with frank dislocations. Both dislocations were treated with casts. Seven patients had transient ulnar nerve paralysis and two had permanent ulnar nerve dysfunction. Radiolucent lines were identified in ten prostheses, eight at the ulna and two in the humerus. Six of the ulnar and both of the humeral radiolucencies were incomplete.

In a report of 1-year to 5.6-years follow-up evaluations of 28 capitellocondylar implants (27 performed for rheumatoid arthritis), Rosenberg and Turner[59] found the average postoperative range of motion to be 33 degrees of extension to 134 degrees of flexion, with 80 degrees of pronation and

72 degrees of supination. Results were satisfactory in 24 elbows, but three required revision surgery. The three revisions were performed for late hematogenous infection in one elbow, loosening at 53 months in another, and instability in the third. A fourth patient had loosening secondary to a fracture but declined revision surgery. Four patients had postoperative dislocations. Three of these patients responded to treatment with long arm casts. Three ulnar nerve paresthesias were identified but resolved without treatment. Two infections occurred late in the series. One was treated with debridement and antibiotic suppression and the second with implant removal.

Kudo and associates[34, 35] have reported both early and long-term follow-up studies of patients treated with the Kudo nonconstrained elbow prosthesis, which has undergone three modifications since 1971. Type I, used from 1971 to 1975, had a humeral component shaped like a cylinder. Type II was modified to a saddle shape, with a change in the articular component of the ulna. In 1983, an intramedullary stem was added to the type II Kudo prosthesis—a design that has been used exclusively since then. The first study by this group reported 1- to 7-year follow-ups of 24 elbow replacements for rheumatoid arthritis employing the type I and type II prostheses.[34] The average range of motion was 42 degrees of extension and 124 degrees of flexion, with 29 degrees of pronation and 49 degrees of supination. Of the 24, 21 elbows achieved satisfactory results. No implants were revised, but one patient had painful instability. One ulnar nerve paresis occurred requiring anterior transfer. In four elbows, radiolucent lines were seen at the humeral component, and proximal migration of the humeral component was seen in one.

Kudo's long-term follow-up series included 37 elbow replacements in 36 patients with rheumatoid arthritis (12 type I and 25 type II prostheses).[35] Of the 37 elbows, 30 had satisfactory results, but six had instability. In four of these cases, the patients later underwent revision surgery. Five of the six unstable elbows evidenced gross posterior displacement of the humeral components. Of the four patients who underwent revision of the humeral components, one also had revision of the ulnar component. The two other failures were for persistent subluxation and recurrent ankylosis. Ulnar nerve paralysis occurred in four patients, three of whom had exploration of the nerve. Two had complete resolution of symptoms, whereas two had persistent ulnar nerve symptoms.

Instability occurred in each of the elbows with humeral loosening and in two other elbows. In one case, closed reduction was unsuccessful and subluxation and pain persisted. In a second case, the patient required an open reduction with repair of the medial structures and immobilization in a plaster cast. This elbow was scored as a good result despite the reoperation.

The most disconcerting aspect of the study was the radiologic evaluation, which showed evidence of proximal subsidence of the humeral component in 70 percent of the elbows. Seven ulnar components showed radiolucencies but only two had evidence that suggested loosening of the ulnar components. However, it is uncertain whether this report included the one elbow that required revision for ulnar component loosening. Thus, these workers recommend a stemmed humeral component because of the high rate of proximal subsidence at long-term follow-up in this series.

In 1980, London[36] reported follow-up evaluations of up to 2 years for 16 elbow replacements utilizing a prosthesis of his own design. Good results in 14 of the 16 elbows were reported. However, no further follow-up findings have been published.

In 1981, Souter[68] reported 1- to 1.5-year results in 22 elbows with rheumatoid arthritis. In 18 cases, results were satisfactory. The average postoperative range of motion was 52 to 143 degrees, with pronation of 65 degrees and supination of 66 degrees. No elbows required revision surgery, but three were unstable and five had some postoperative ulnar nerve dysfunction. Ulnar nerve paresis was transitory in three cases but persisted in two. In the unstable elbows, one had recurrent subluxation and two had dislocations. No mention was made of subsequent treatment.

Tuke[74] reported 1- to 3-year follow-up data for 27 ICLH prostheses implanted in patients with rheumatoid arthritis. Of these, 22 achieved satisfactory results. The average motion was 37 to 137 degrees, with 62 degrees of pronation and 71 degrees of supination. Four elbows required revision surgery, three because of infection and one for instability. Tuke found a 20 percent rate of radiolucency at the ulnar component, requiring modification of the design. A stem was added to the humeral component for greater stability.

Two reports have been published regarding the Wadsworth prosthesis in patients with rheumatoid arthritis. In 1981, Wadsworth[77] reported follow-up data on 14 prostheses and, in 1984, Rydholm and colleagues[62] reported on 19 prostheses. Average follow-up interval in the first series was 1 to 2 years, and nine of ten patients achieved satisfactory results. One unstable elbow required revision surgery. In the second study, the follow-up time was 1.5 to 4 years. In this study, 15 of 19 patients achieved satisfactory results. Average motion was 30 to 135 degrees, with 65 degrees each of pronation and supination. Two elbows required revision surgery, one for infection and one for dislocation at 21 months. Three patients had impairment of the ulnar nerve—two cases were transitory and one was permanent. Of the 19 prostheses, ten showed evidence of loosening of the humeral components at follow-up evaluations. Loosening was related to positioning of the humeral component. Rates were lower when proper restoration of anatomy was achieved.

Pritchard[57] reported on 13 elbow replacements with a three-piece nonconstrained implant using a radial head replacement. In 12 of 13 elbows, good to satisfactory results were found at the time of follow-up between 4 months and 2.5 years. One elbow was revised for instability. The average postoperative motion was from 15 to 120 degrees with 60 degrees of pronation and 45 degrees of supination.

In 1984, Soni and Cavendish[67] reported on 80 elbow replacements involving the Liverpool prosthesis. Of these, 55 were done for rheumatoid arthritis. The average length of follow-up was 3.5 years, with a range from 1 to 8 years. Of the 80, 66 achieved satisfactory results. The average range of motion was 32 to 134 degrees of flexion, 69 degrees of pronation, and 62 degrees of supination. Revision surgery was required in 14 elbows: eight for loosening, four for deep infection, one for traumatic dislodgement, and one for loosening of the ulnar component. Nine of these cases occurred in the 55 patients with rheumatoid arthritis; the other five occurred in patients with post-traumatic arthritis or pyknodysostosis. The complication rate was 58 percent. Of the patients with complications, six had ulnar nerve problems, and two of these required anterior transpositions. Some degree of subluxation or postoperative instability was observed in eight elbows.

Lowe and colleagues[38] reported 1- to 9-year follow-up data using the Lowe prosthesis in 47 elbow replacements; 39 were for rheumatoid arthritis. Of 39 elbows studied at follow-up evaluations, 22 had satisfactory results. Average range of motion was 37 to 135 degrees of flexion, with 60 degrees of pronation and 72 degrees of supination. Revision surgery was required for 14 elbows, including 12 of the original 23 condylar prostheses that were revised within 2 years because of loosening. Three other condylar prostheses were loose but not revised. Two of the stemmed prostheses were revised owing to loosening or instability. Three infections were reported in this series: two were suppressed with antibiotics and one required implant removal. Three patients had ulnar nerve lesions postoperatively. Of these patients, two recovered completely but in one the lesion was permanent. Instability occurred in eight elbows, necessitating implant removal in one case.

In 1986, Roper and coworkers reported on the Roper-Tuke elbow.[58] In this series of 60 elbows (50 implanted for rheumatoid arthritis), 36 of the 51 elbows available for study had satisfactory results after 3 to 9 years. The average range of motion was 46 to 136 degrees of flexion, with 69 degrees of pronation and 68 degrees of supination. However, 15 of the elbows required revision surgery, with a 27 percent major complication rate and a 23 percent minor complication rate. Six of the implants were removed because of infections within the first 6 months. Seven revisions were performed for ulnar loosening and two for humeral loosening. There were four cases of transient ulnar nerve paralysis and one transient posterior interosseous nerve paralysis. Detachment of the triceps tendon in one case necessitated reoperation. Instability occurred in seven elbows, four of which were frankly dislocated. Three required revision surgery for dislocation and two others had spontaneous improvement of subluxation.

In summary, nonconstrained implants are indicated only in patients with adequate medial collateral ligament structures. Even then, the surgical technique is demanding and postoperative complications, including subluxation and dislocation, may be high. In addition, ulnar nerve complications may result when the lateral surgical approach is selected because the ulnar nerve is not exposed and visible. Nonstemmed prostheses appear to have higher rates of loosening and migration: a 70 percent subsidence rate occurred with the Kudo prostheses;[35] posterior subluxation occurred with the ICLH prostheses;[74] and loosening occurred with the Liverpool, Lowe, and Roper-Tuke prostheses.[38, 58, 67] The nonconstrained elbow replacement showing the most consistent results is the capitellocondylar prosthesis with its stemmed humeral component. However, even in the most experienced hands, the revision rate as reported by Simmons and colleagues[66] is 4.5 percent, with an instability rate of 8.5 percent and an ulnar nerve dysfunction rate of 20 percent. As reported by Weiland and associates,[79] revision rate is 5 percent, instability rate is 25 percent, and ulnar nerve dysfunction rate is 22 percent.

Semiconstrained Prosthesis

(Table 39–2 and Figure 39–23)

In 1982, Volz[76] reported the results of 15 arthroplasties employing his three-component semiconstrained Arizona Health Science Center (AHSC) prosthesis, of which 13 were performed for rheumatoid arthritis.[76] After 6 months to 3 years, 14 of the 15 had satisfactory results. One patient underwent reoperation for dislocation due to failure of the polyethylene bearing. Only two of the 15 elbows had evidence of radiolucencies at this early follow-up interval. No infections were reported, but two patients partially avulsed the triceps tendons.

Data from this series were again reported in a combined study with Brumfield and the data were identical.[4] No further long-term results for this prosthesis have been reported. Brumfield and Volz[4] also reported 1- to 4.5-year follow-up data for 15 Mayo prostheses implanted for rheumatoid arthritis. Of the 15, 14 achieved satisfactory results. One elbow was revised for loosening at 11 months postoperatively. One ulnar nerve neurapraxia required exploration, and one superficial infection was successfully treated with antibiotics. Of the 15 elbows, five showed evidence of radiolucency at follow-up. Three had fractures of the humeral condyles, which were treated by immobilization.

In 1977, Bryan[5] reported on another series of 41 Mayo prostheses (38 for rheumatoid arthritis) and 34 Coonrad prostheses (21 for rheumatoid arthritis). After 1- to 2-year evaluation of the Mayo prostheses, 29 of the 40 elbows achieved satisfactory results. Two elbows had evidence of radiographic loosening but were not revised. The length of follow-up after Coonrad total elbow replacements ranged from 1 to 3 years. Only 17 of the 34 achieved satisfactory results, and five elbows had evidence of radiolucency. All four reoperations were performed in patients

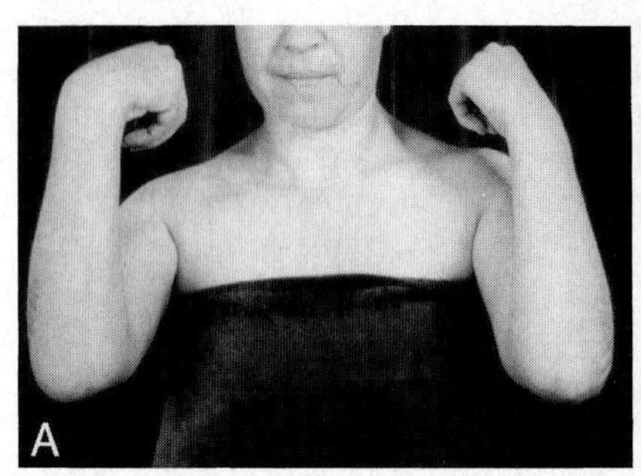

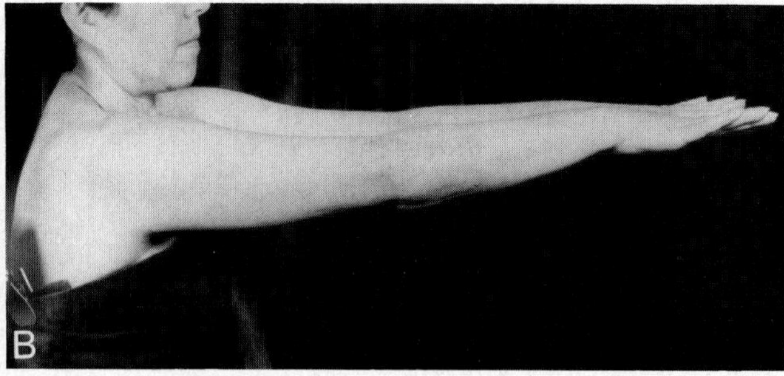

FIGURE 39–23. Bilateral semiconstrained total elbow replacements in a patient with rheumatoid arthritis. The posteromedial approach was used. Rehabilitation was begun on postoperative day 3. This patient has excellent flexion (*A*) and extension (*B*). Her function improved markedly.

Table 39–2. FOLLOW-UP DATA FOR PATIENTS WITH SEMICONSTRAINED PROSTHESES

Authors	Year	Prosthesis	No.	Rheumatoid Arthritis	Follow-Up Yrs	Postoperative Extension/ Flexion	Motion Pronation/ Supination	Satis-factory	Revised	Loosened
Volz	1982	AHSC	15	13	0.5–3	39/135	73/65	14/15	1	3
Brumfield,	1980	AHSC	15	13	0–5.3	40/137	137	14/15	1	0
Volz		Mayo	15	15	1–4.5	28/130	130	14/15	1	1
Bryan	1977	Mayo	41	40	1–2	—	—	29/40	0	2
		Coonrad	34	21	1–3	—	—	17/34	4	5
Morrey, et al.	1981	Mayo	47	44	2–6.5	32/132	57/55	36/47	11	6
		Coonrad	33	15	2–6.5	24/129	67/64	25/33	7	5
Coonrad	1982	Coonrad	150	87	5–7	—	—	85/87	0	1
Pritchard	1981	Pritchard-Walker	269	189	0–5	—	—	75 percent	0	1
Rozenfeld, Anzel	1982	Pritchard-Walker	17	17	1–6	—	—	16/17	3	0
Inglis, Pellicci	1980	Pritchard-Walker	17	26	2–5.5	—	—	29/36	3	2
		Triaxial	19		2–5.5					
Rosenberg	1988	Triaxial	73	62	2–9	28/125	68/60	66/73	2	0
Figgie, et al.	1990	Triaxial	137	137	2–13	103	130	125/137	3	0
		Osteonics			2–13					

with post-traumatic arthritis. One patient with rheumatoid arthritis had loosening, but a fracture of the condyle suffered at the time of surgery may have contributed to this finding. In 1981, a series of Mayo and Coonrad prostheses was reported by Morrey and associates,[45] but it may have included many of the elbows previously reported by Bryan. Morrey's series included 47 Mayo prostheses (44 implanted for rheumatoid arthritis) and 33 Coonrad prostheses (15 implanted for rheumatoid arthritis). The average length of follow-up was 2 to 6.5 years. Satisfactory results were achieved in 36 of the 47 Mayo prostheses and 25 of the 33 Coonrad prostheses. However, 11 of the Mayo prostheses required revision surgery—six for loosening and five for deep infections. In the patients with Coonrad prostheses, seven underwent revision surgery—five for loosening and two for deep infections. Thus, in 18 of 80 cases, revision operations were performed, and 37 other complications were reported, including two permanent and nine transient ulnar neuropathies. Four elbows had delayed wound healing, and ten had significant postoperative triceps weakness. Eleven intraoperative medial/lateral supracondylar pillar fractures and one ulnar fracture occurred. Radiolucency was observed around the humeral component in 25 elbows and around the ulnar component in four others. Of the radiolucencies, ten were nonprogressive, eight were progressive, and eleven developed frank loosening requiring revision. Thus, the radiolucency rate was 29 of 73 elbows (40 percent).

In 1978, results on 150 Coonrad total elbows from several centers were reported, including 39 elbows from the data of the Mayo Clinic.[9] In all, 3- to 7-year follow-up data were available for 87 elbows implanted for rheumatoid arthritis. Satisfactory results were obtained in 85 of these. One elbow had loosened but revision surgery was not required. In the combined series, the overall loosening rate was 13 percent. Complications included triceps rupture in two cases, radial nerve paralysis in one, ulnar nerve paralysis in three, superficial infection in two, and deep infection in three. Two of the patients with deep infections required implant removal. The third was successfully treated with antibiotic suppression.

In 1981, Pritchard[56] reported multicenter data for 269 total elbow replacements using the Pritchard-Walker prosthesis. Of these, 189 were performed for rheumatoid arthritis, and the follow-up interval ranged from 0 to 5 years. Deep infections occurred in six cases, with humeral component loosening in ten and fracture of the humeral component in eight. In addition, a 13 percent rate of postoperative humeral fractures was found with the Mark I polyethylene humeral component. Transient ulnar neuropathy occurred in five of these cases. Overall, good to excellent results were obtained in 75 percent of the cases. However, the average follow-up period was only 2 years.

In 1982, Rosenfeld and Anzel[61] reported on 17 cases employing the Pritchard-Walker prosthesis, with a follow-up interval ranging from 1 to 6 years. In all, 16 of the 17 patients achieved satisfactory results. However, three required revision surgery—two for humeral component fractures and one for two fractures of the humerus. Two other patients also had humeral fractures, and four had ulnar neuropathy, three cases of which resolved.

In 1980, Inglis and Pellicci[27] reported on 35 elbow replacements, 17 with the Pritchard-Walker prosthesis and 18 with the triaxial prosthesis. Of these, 26 were performed for rheumatoid arthritis. After a follow-up period of 2 to 5.5 years, 29 of the 35 elbows had satisfactory results. However, 19 experienced complications. Reoperation was required in eight elbows. One deep infection necessitated implant removal, and one fractured humeral component necessitated revision. Another patient underwent revision because of postoperative fracture of the humerus. Radiographs showed loosening of the Pritchard-Walker ulnar components in two cases, but neither required revision surgery. Postoperatively, one patient had rupture of the triceps and two patients with post-traumatic arthritis had ulnar paresthesias.

In 1986, Rosenberg and coworkers[60] reported the results of 73 elbow replacements with the triaxial component. In all, 62 were performed for rheumatoid arthritis, and follow-up intervals ranged from 2 to 9 years. Satisfactory results were achieved in 66 of the 73 elbows and only two required revision surgery, both in patients

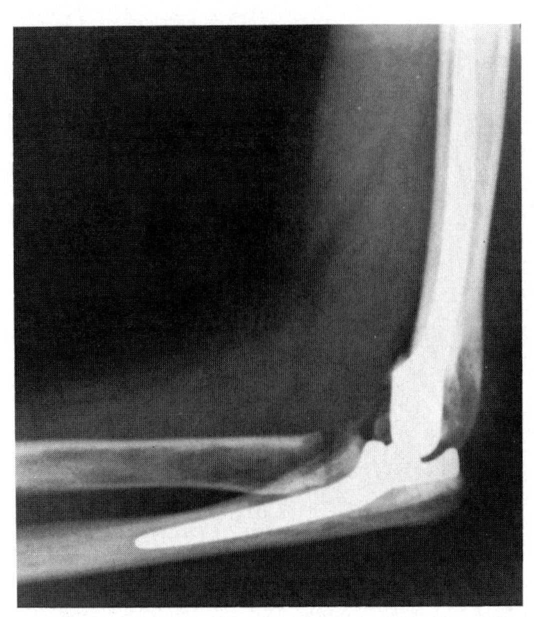

FIGURE 39–24. Triaxial implant in a patient with rheumatoid arthritis. At 12-year follow-up, no evidence of radiolucency was observed.

with post-traumatic arthritis (Fig. 39–24). Among the patients with rheumatoid arthritis, one had deep sepsis and two had superficial infections. Two had persistent nerve paralysis, and three underwent revision for dislocated axle mechanisms and implant dislocations.

In a later follow-up evaluation of 137 semiconstrained total elbow replacements for rheumatoid arthritis, Figgie and colleagues[19] reported follow-up data ranging from 2 to 13 years with the triaxial and custom-fit semiconstrained prostheses. The average postoperative arc of flexion was 103 degrees and rotation was 130 degrees. Of 137 elbows, 125 achieved satisfactory results. Three patients underwent implant removal or revision due to infection. Seven deep infections were reported in this series, three occurring early and four resulting from secondary hematogenous spread. Although no implants were revised for loosening, eight elbows had postoperative dislocations requiring revision of the polyethylene bearing and replacement of the axle component. Other complications included persistent ulnar neuropathy in three elbows and postoperative epicondylar fracture in seven. In two of three elbows with ulnar neuropathy, symptoms resolved over time. One required ulnar nerve transposition and at last follow-up evaluation, the patient had nearly complete recovery. Radiolucency was identified in ten of the 137 elbows, four with evidence of progression.

In summary, the early results with semiconstrained prostheses have been good. The high failure rate for the Pritchard-Walker prosthesis was due to fracture of the polyethylene humeral component. The most successful implants appear to be those with the greatest laxity in the articulation. The Coonrad prosthesis has undergone modification to achieve greater laxity. In the original Coonrad prosthesis, loosening was a problem, but most of the patients so treated had post-traumatic arthritis. Improvements in the articulation have lessened problems with loosening. The triaxial component, with its sloppy-fit articulation, has the most laxity of the semiconstrained prostheses. In a series reported by Figgie and associates,[19] no radiolucency was apparent with up to 13 years of follow-up experience, but eight cases of late dislocations due to polyethylene wear or trauma were seen. Thus, the triaxial component also underwent design modification to improve the articulation and decrease polyethylene wear. The implant was also modified to accept a nonweight-bearing restraining axle to prevent dislocation. No increase in radiolucency has been seen with this design and no dislocations have been observed. Overall, good functional results without increased loosening rates have been found for semiconstrained total elbows. These offer enough laxity to allow the soft tissues to share the stresses and decrease the loads on the bone-cement interface.

Post-Traumatic Arthritis

(Table 39–3)

A patient with post-traumatic arthritis of the elbow presents a significant challenge for reconstruction because of the frequent loss of bone stock, soft tissue deficiency, and high prevalence of failed previous operations. Often the patient has multiple incisions on the elbow with failed internal fixation and he or she may have ulnar nerve entrapment or damage. Frequently, the patient presents with a flail

Table 39–3. FOLLOW-UP DATA FOR PATIENTS WITH NONCONSTRAINED AND SEMICONSTRAINED PROSTHESES IMPLANTED FOR POST-TRAUMATIC ARTHRITIS

Authors	Year	Implant	No.	Follow-Up Yrs	Satis-factory	Revised	Unstable	Infection	Loosened
Nonconstrained									
Lowe, et al.	1984	Lowe	7	1–9	1/7	3	4	1	1
Soni, Cavendish	1984	Liverpool	8	1–8	5/8	3	1	0	3
Roper, et al.	1986	Roper-Tuke	7	3–9	5/7	0	1	0	0
Semiconstrained									
Bryan	1977	Mayo	1	1–2	60 percent	4	0	0	2
		Coonrad	13	1–3					
Morrey, et al.	1981	Mayo	3	2–6.5	2/3	6	0	2	4
		Coonrad	18	2–6.5	12/18				
Coonrad	1982	Coonrad	60	3–7	51/60	6	0	2	4
Inglis, Pellicci	1980	Pritchard-Walker, Triaxial	9	2–5.5	4/9				
Morrey and Bryan	1988	Coonrad	54	2–14.4	47/54	13	0	1	13
Figgie, et al.	1990	Triaxial/Custom	37	2–12	30/37	4	0	3	1

painful elbow and marked functional loss. Biologic options—including open reduction and internal fixation of the supracondylar nonunion and fascial or distraction arthroplasty—may not be suitable. When no other option is acceptable, total elbow arthroplasty may offer a salvage procedure (Fig. 39–25). Because previous incisions may have compromised skin vascularity, the risk of wound dehiscence and deep infection is high in the patient who has undergone total elbow replacement for post-traumatic arthritis. In addition, marked bone loss may lead to inadequate support of the implant and subsequent loosening. Many patients are noncompliant once pain relief is obtained, and they abuse the elbow, also promoting implant failure or loosening. Thus, total elbow arthroplasty should be considered a salvage procedure only in the patient with post-traumatic arthritis.

Total elbow replacements in patients with post-traumatic arthritis have not

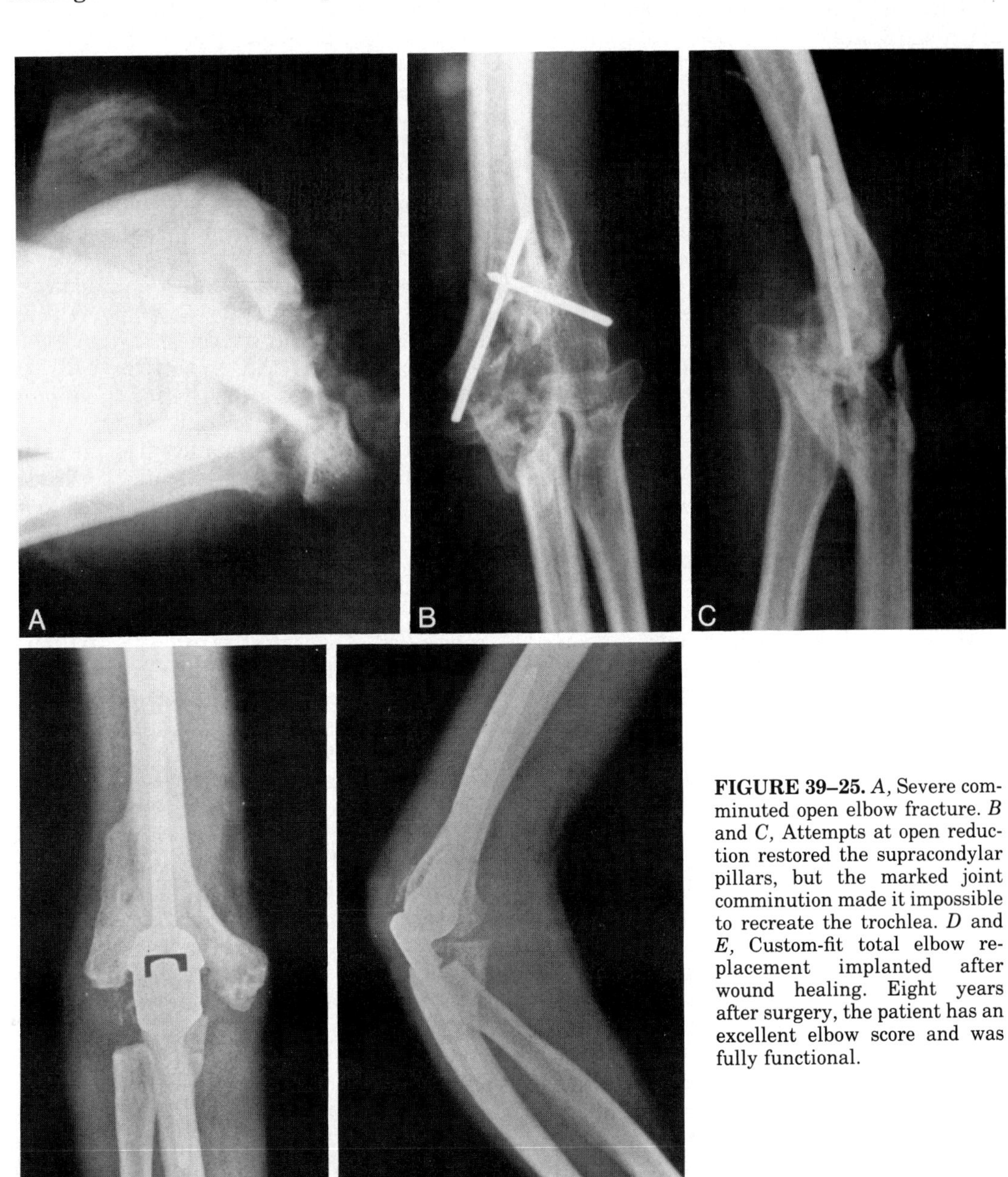

FIGURE 39–25. *A,* Severe comminuted open elbow fracture. *B* and *C,* Attempts at open reduction restored the supracondylar pillars, but the marked joint comminution made it impossible to recreate the trochlea. *D* and *E,* Custom-fit total elbow replacement implanted after wound healing. Eight years after surgery, the patient has an excellent elbow score and was fully functional.

achieved the same satisfactory results as those performed in patients with rheumatoid arthritis. Nonconstrained implants are not generally recommended for patients with post-traumatic arthritis. Indeed, few series have reported on the use of nonconstrained implants for any condition other than rheumatoid arthritis. The only series in which more than two nonconstrained elbow replacements were implanted for post-traumatic arthritis were by Lowe and coworkers,[38] Soni and Cavendish,[67] and Roper and coworkers.[58] Of seven nonconstrained Lowe elbows implanted for post-traumatic arthritis, only one achieved a satisfactory result. Three underwent revision, and four were unstable with one becoming infected and one becoming loose.[38] Soni, reporting on eight Liverpool elbow replacements for post-traumatic arthritis, found satisfactory results in five. However, three underwent revision, one was unstable, and three became loose.[67] Roper and associates,[58] reporting on seven Liverpool elbow replacements, found satisfactory results in five, but one was unstable.

In 1977, Bryan[5] reported on 14 elbow replacements for post-traumatic arthritis utilizing the Coonrad prosthesis in 13 cases and the Mayo prosthesis in one. At 1- to 7-year follow-up examination, 60 percent satisfactory results were obtained, but four patients underwent revision—two for loosening.

Morrey and colleagues[45] later reported on 21 elbow replacements for post-traumatic arthritis, 18 with Coonrad prostheses. Follow-up interval ranged from 2 to 6.5 years, and 14 satisfactory results were achieved. Six underwent revisions, two were infected, and four were loose. Coonrad,[9] reporting on 60 Coonrad total elbow replacements for post-traumatic arthritis with 3- to 7-year follow-up evaluations, found satisfactory results in 51. Six underwent revisions: two were infected and four were loose. Fewer satisfactory results were reported for patients with post-traumatic arthritis than for those with rheumatoid arthritis in this series.

Inglis and Pellicci,[27] in their study of nine patients with Pritchard-Walker and triaxial elbow replacements for post-traumatic arthritis, found satisfactory results in only four elbows. Although pain was relieved in these patients, their ranges of motion and function were less improved than those of patients with rheumatoid arthritis. In addition, the complication rate was higher. The only two series dealing specifically with total elbow replacement for traumatic arthritis were reported by Morrey and Bryan[50] and Figgie and coworkers.[20] In the study reported by Morrey and Bryan, 47 of 54 patients with post-traumatic arthritis who underwent implantation of Coonrad prostheses had satisfactory results. The length of follow-up ranged from 2 to 14.4 years. However, 13 patients required revision, 13 implants were loose, and one was infected. Of the 13 patients who underwent revisions, 11 had satisfactory revisions. The other two patients eventually required resection arthroplasties, including one for infection.

In addition to loosening, a 25 percent complication rate was found. However, when the complication rate was calculated by type of prosthesis, it was 40 percent for the type I Coonrad prosthesis and only 10 to 16 percent for the types II and III implants. This series also stressed the importance of the configuration of the distal humerus and the amount of bone loss. Patients with inadequate bone required a prosthesis with an anterior flange. The flange had a plasma-sprayed surface to allow for bone ingrowth in this region. The flange helps prevent rotation and loosening secondary to torque. These investigators concluded that post-traumatic arthritis could be treated with total elbow replacement but should be reserved for patients over 60 years of age who have no other biologic options.[50]

Figgie and associates[20] followed 37 elbow replacements involving either the triaxial or a custom-fit prosthesis between 2 and 12 years and found 27 good to excellent results and 5 failures. The failures included three patients with deep infections, one with revision for humeral component loosening, and one with revision for dislocation. In this series, the patients were classified as having either adequate or compromised distal humeral bone stock based on the absence or presence of both supracondylar pillars. Of the 37 patients, 24 had loss of one distal humeral pillar. No radiolucencies were seen in the 13 patients with adequate bone stock, whereas eight of the 24 elbows with compromise of the distal humerus had evidence of radiolucencies, including one in the patient who underwent revision surgery for loosening. Four of the radiolucencies showed evidence of progression, including those in two patients who had infections and in one who underwent revision for humeral component loosening.

In summary, the patient with post-traumatic arthritis of the elbow presents a substantial challenge for reconstruction. This patient often has marked loss of soft tissue and bone, and the ulnar nerve may be encased in scar. Biologic procedures should be performed whenever possible, including open reduction and internal fixation of supracondylar nonunion. Distraction arthroplasty may be done for younger, highly active patients.[51] When no viable biologic option is available, total elbow arthroplasty can be considered as a salvage procedure. Nonconstrained implants should not be chosen because of the amount of ligament insufficiency that may be encountered. Semiconstrained implants are recommended. A custom prosthesis may be needed in order to best fit the available bone stock. The other option is to implant a Coonrad III prosthesis with an anterior flange to enhance resistance to rotational stresses. In any case, the surgery must be properly planned and previous incisions must be used. As a result of bone stock deficiency and previous surgery, higher complication rates are observed because of infection, loosening, and ulnar nerve symptoms. The patient must be compliant with the rehabilitation regimen and must not abuse the elbow. Older patients often do better, as they tend to place lower demands on the implants.

Supracondylar Nonunion

Nonunions of fractures of the distal humerus present a challenge for reconstruction. Fortunately, supracondylar humeral fractures occur infrequently in adults; nonunions are rare, and occur at a rate of 2 percent.[65] However, nonunion may leave the patient with an unstable, a painful, and often a useless extremity. The functional disability is profound, as patients with flail extremities are unable to use them for most activities of daily living.

Treatment of supracondylar nonunions in elderly patients is difficult, as patients may have bone with poor osteogenic potential. Thus fixation and healing are likely to be compromised. In addition, high torque is present across the elbow because of the weight of the forearm, and this effect may lead to loosening of any fixation device. Previous immobilization may result in periarticular fibrosis. Thus even a healed supracondylar nonunion may be associated with a poor functional result due to a stiff elbow. This periarticular fibrosis also raises the stress at the nonunion site. Previous operations for the fracture and multiple previous surgical incisions may have compromised the vascular supply to the distal end of the humerus and may lead to poor wound healing and higher infection rates.

The treatment options range from bracing and observation to open reduction and internal fixation with bone grafting, resection arthroplasty, external fixation, and total elbow arthroplasty. Open reduction with internal fixation and bone grafting is preferable when adequate bone of good quality is present. However, satisfactory motion must be present for the joint to have good function after healing. For the patient with a flail, functionless extremity, in whom nonunion is not amenable to open reduction and internal fixation owing to inadequate bone stock or severe periarticular fibrosis, total elbow arthroplasty may offer salvage (Fig. 39–26).

Figgie and coworkers[18] reported on the results of total elbow arthroplasty in 14 patients who had nonunion of a supracondylar humeral fracture. Of these, ten had up to four previous attempts at internal fixation. The average age of these patients at the time of operation was 65 years. Follow-up time after total elbow replacement was 2 to 12 years (mean, 5 years). Semiconstrained prostheses were implanted in all patients: a Pritchard-Walker prosthesis in one, triaxial components in two, and custom prostheses in 11. Good or excellent results were achieved in eight of the patients. Three failures were reported, one due to dislocation, one to loosening of the humeral component, and one to deep infection. The patients with dislocation

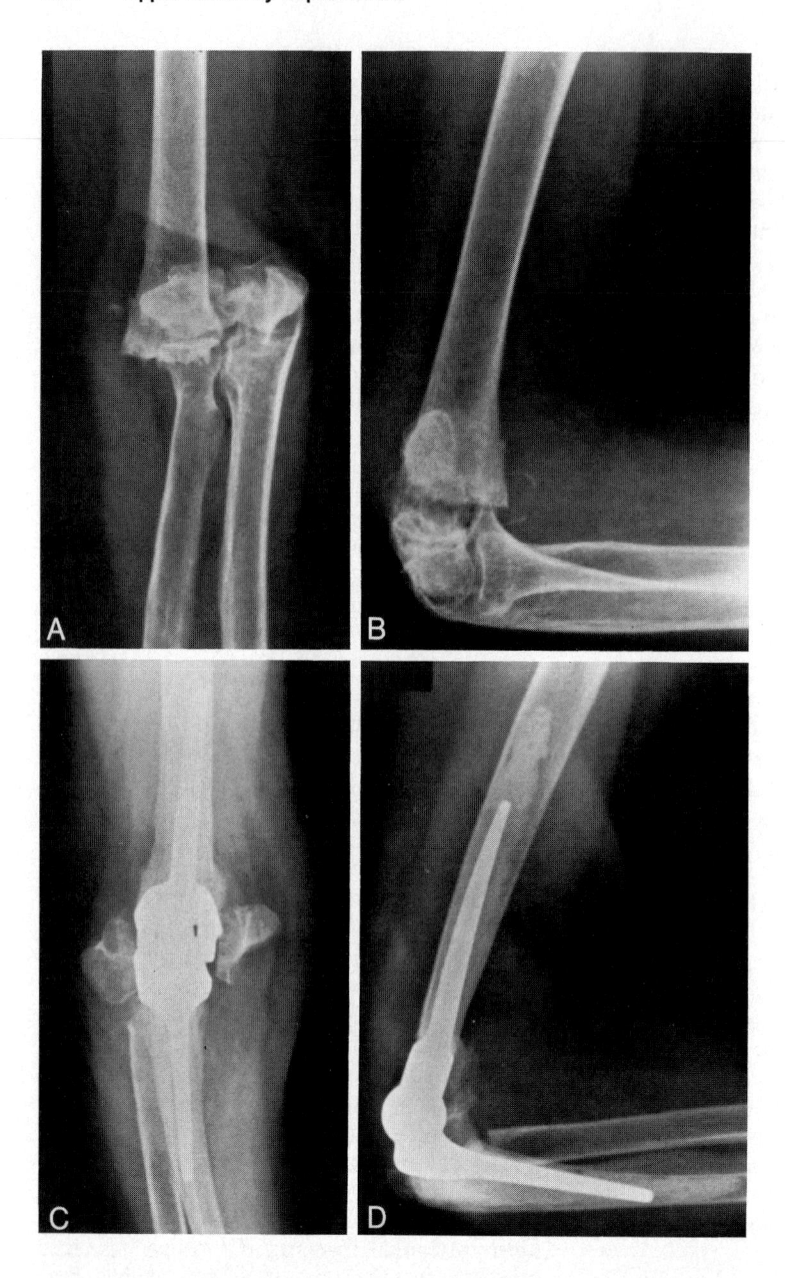

FIGURE 39–26. Supracondylar nonunion of the elbow in a 67-year-old woman treated with total elbow replacement. Several attempts at open reduction and internal fixation were made, but the elbow was flail. In addition, she was unable to position the hand in space. *A* and *B*, Preoperative radiographs. *C* and *D*, Total elbow replacement. The patient had excellent function 8 years after surgery.

and loosening of the humeral component underwent satisfactory revisions, whereas the patient with deep infection required resection arthroplasty.

In patients such as those represented in this series, we recommend the implantation of semiconstrained prostheses owing to inadequate ligamentous structures. In addition, we advise sparing the distal humeral epicondyles, as the flexor and extensor muscle masses attach to them. The epicondyles provide a greater moment arm to the dynamic supports and thus decrease the soft tissue stress in the elbow. This effect reduces the chance of loosening. Another study of total elbow arthroplasty for supracondylar nonunion was published by Mitsunaga and colleagues[42] in a report on condylar nonunions of the distal humerus. These investigators performed total elbow arthroplasties on seven patients for supracondylar nonunions. After excising the distal end of the humerus, they implanted either a Coonrad or Pritchard-Walker prosthesis. Within the first 3 years, two of the seven elbows had reoperations for loosening. The problem occurred because of the loss of the distal humerus and muscle and fascial attachments, which led to greater rotational stresses across the elbow, producing loosening of the humeral stem. To correct this problem, Morrey and Bryan used the Coonrad prosthesis with an anterior flange to resist rotation. However, retention of the humeral epicondyles is also recommended to reduce stress at the bone-cement interface.

Overall, total elbow arthroplasty for salvage of supracondylar nonunion is a technically demanding procedure with a potentially high rate of failure. Patients must be carefully selected and must be compliant with both the rehabilitation regimen and the measures to protect the elbow. The patient should first be considered for open reduction and internal fixation unless inadequate distal humeral bone stock or severe periarticular fibrosis is found. Older patients should generally be selected, because younger active patients usually have enough osteogenic potential to warrant open reduction and internal fixation. In the compliant patient, salvage of supracondylar nonunion with total elbow arthroplasty may produce a satisfactory functional result with good relief of pain. A semiconstrained implant, often a custom fit, is recommended along with the salvage of the humeral epicondyles to maintain the best function of the soft tissues.

Ankylosis

Complete ankylosis of the elbow results in severe disability and functional limitation, especially when other joints in the ipsilateral upper extremity also have limitations of motion. Although complete ankylosis of the elbow usually results in diminished function, pain is seldom a problem. However, because pronation and supination are independent of flexion and extension, pain may be present because of the disease of the radial head. The patient with bilateral ankylosis at the elbows is often severely limited functionally. Function may be improved by total elbow replacement (Fig. 39–27). The patient with functional loss due to unilateral ankylosis may also be a candidate for surgical treatment.

When evaluating the patient, the extent of the ankylosis should be determined. Intrinsic ankylosis involving the joint surfaces themselves should be assessed before total elbow replacement is performed. An extrinsic ankylosis, in which the elbow has intact cartilage surfaces but extra-articular bony block, may be best treated by distraction arthroplasty. Patients who are expected to be compliant with rehabilitation and have marked functional limitations may be considered candidates for surgery.

Figgie and colleagues[17] have reported on 16 patients who underwent 19 semiconstrained total elbow replacements for complete ankylosis. The diagnoses in this series were juvenile rheumatoid arthritis in eight elbows, rheumatoid arthritis in one, post-traumatic ankylosis in five, ankylosis secondary to ankylosing spondylitis in two, and postoperative immobilization ankylosis in three. Semiconstrained prostheses were implanted: four Pritchard-Walker im-

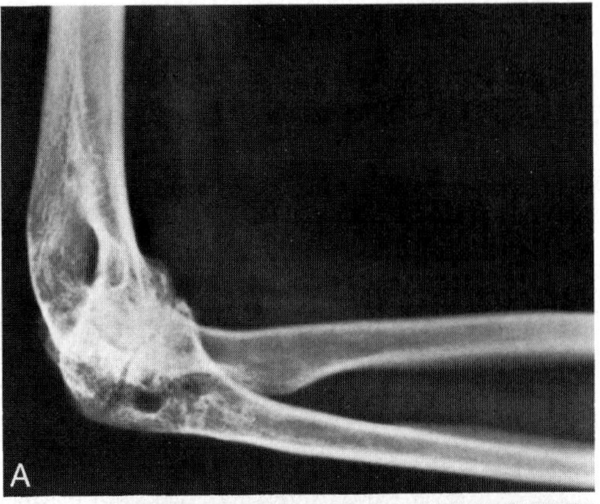

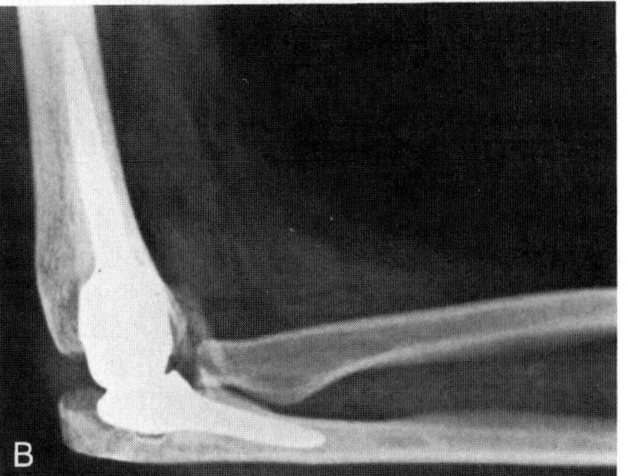

FIGURE 39–27. Juvenile rheumatoid arthritis with ankylosis of both elbows. *A*, Preoperative radiographs. *B*, After total elbow replacement on both sides, the patient had marked improvement in all activities of daily living and was able to feed and dress himself.

plants, seven triaxial implants, and eight custom-fit prostheses. Results were excellent in four cases, good in 11, fair in three, and failed in one. The average arc of postoperative flexion was 80 degrees; the average arc of pronation and supination was 90 degrees. Although none of the implants showed evidence of loosening or migration, five produced complications. One deep infection occurred in a patient with posttraumatic ankylosis that developed after skin slough. The implant was removed, and a fascial arthroplasty was performed. In addition, three postoperative wound problems arose, which were treated conservatively and resolved uneventfully. One patient suffered a fracture at the tip of the olecranon 3 months postoperatively, but the range of motion was not impaired.

In this series, all patients had improved ability to perform their activities of daily living and improved range of motion. The functional improvement was dramatic in many cases, according to the patients.

Although no other series specifically involved total elbow replacements for ankylosis of the elbow, Kudo and Iwano[35] reported nine total elbow replacements in their series for ankylosis—seven patients had bony ankylosis and two had fibrous ankylosis. They reported seven good results, one fair, and one poor. The average range of motion was 75 degrees. In one patient, the replacement failed owing to recurrent ankylosis. Two patients had moderate instability.

Thus, the patient with functional limitations due to ankylosis of the elbow may be a candidate for total elbow replacement. However, the patient must have reasonable expectations and must be willing to comply with the postoperative rehabilitation program. Patients with extrinsic ankylosis may be treated with distraction arthroplasty, while those with intrinsic involvement may be treated with total elbow arthroplasty. Technical considerations are of the utmost importance especially in patients with juvenile rheumatoid arthritis, as they have marked bone deformities due to premature epiphyseal closures. Custom-fit prostheses may be indicated in these patients to properly restore both the anatomy and the center of rotation of the elbows. Semiconstrained prostheses are recommended, as the collateral ligaments are often not functional. Because ligaments are often encased in bone, a nonconstrained prosthesis offers no stability. Although Kudo and Iwano have achieved functional range of motion and good results in seven of nine elbows with nonconstrained prostheses, we believe that semiconstrained prostheses provide more predictable results with better stability in these technically demanding cases. Overall, functional improvement and range of motion are adequate to allow patients to regain the ability to perform activities of daily living.

REVISION ARTHROPLASTY

Revision of a failed total elbow arthroplasty may be an extremely challenging procedure because the size and shape of the humerus and ulna may make removal of the implant difficult. In addition, any bone loss may compromise the reconstruction. Failure of the implant may occur owing to infection, fracture around the implant, material failure of the implant, dislocation, or loosening of the implant. Only revisions for loosening are discussed in this section.

A patient presenting with failure of a total elbow replacement secondary to loosening of the bone-cement interface often reports marked pain with decline in function. Infection must be ruled out in these cases, and an aspiration arthrogram is often recommended. Plain radiographs may reveal marked bone loss with a widening of a radiolucency at the bone-cement interface. Blood tests, including sedimentation rates, are often not helpful because of the high sedimentation rates associated with the patient's disease. Once infection has been ruled out, a one-stage revision operation may be planned. If any question remains unanswered about infection, a staged revision should be performed.

Patients with grossly loose components should have revisions performed before all bone stock has been obliterated. When the surgery is performed, previous incisions should be used. The ulnar nerve should be isolated and protected. If the patient had failure of a nonconstrained component that is being revised to a semiconstrained implant, the posteromedial approach should be chosen to gain adequate exposure. Once the elbow is exposed, the implant can be removed, with care taken to avoid fractures of the distal humerus and proximal ulna. Cement removal is often difficult, even when one uses high-speed drills and head lamps. In fact, the high-speed burrs often cause cortical perforation and make the damaged bone susceptible to fracture. To gain adequate exposure, a trough in the posterior humerus or the ulna may be required before all cement can be removed. Cultures of the bone-cement interface should be taken to check for subclinical infection.

In addition to prosthesis reimplantation, the options for reconstruction include arthrodesis, interpositional arthroplasty, and resection arthroplasty.

Arthrodesis

Arthrodesis is rarely recommended because it leaves the patient with substantial disability (Fig. 39–28). Other options should be considered that provide the patient a mobile functional joint. The only indication for arthrodesis is a flail extremity with implant failure secondary to infection.

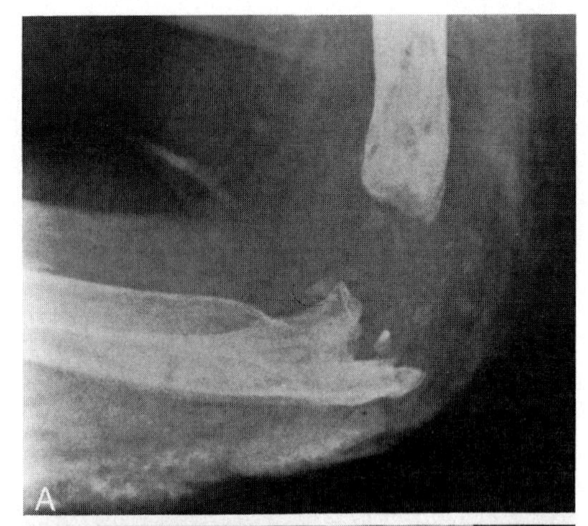

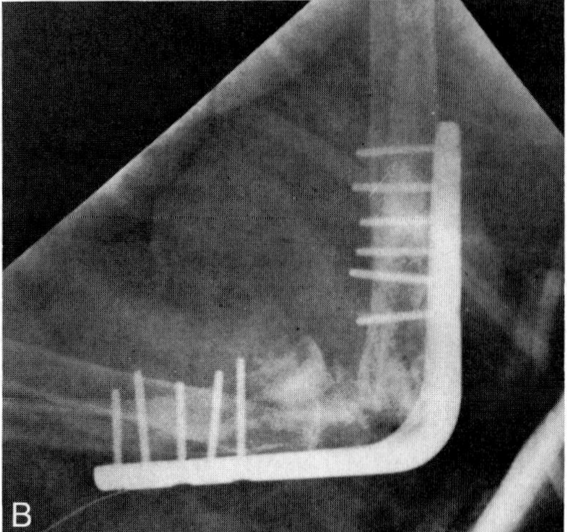

FIGURE 39–28. Removal of a total elbow prosthesis because of infection. *A*, Functionless resection due to inability of the patient to position the arm in space. *B*, After arthrodesis. The patient was unhappy with postoperative function. She could not get her hand to her face and could use the hand only in helping motions.

Interpositional Arthroplasty

Removal of the implant, even though a prosthesis cannot be reinserted, can offer satisfactory salvage when the distal humeral epicondyles are maintained. This leaves the patient with an "anatomic" arthroplasty (Fig. 39–29). In a study by Figgie and associates,[21] 11 patients required implant removal for infection, implant fracture, or recurrent dislocation. Four good, one fair, two poor, and four failed results were reported. Satisfactory results were obtained in seven of the eight arthroplasties in which anatomic containment was achieved. The average arc of motion was 85 degrees with good functional outcome. However, pain was unpredictable, and the patients had mild instability with loss of some triceps power. Placing the patient in a distraction device when the implant is removed sometimes improves range of motion in the salvage of the failed arthroplasty (Fig. 39–30).

Resection Arthroplasty

Removal of the failed elbow prosthesis often involves removal of the complete distal humerus including both supracondylar ridges. This procedure leaves a flail extremity with little reconstructive salvage. Patients have marked functional disabilities because they cannot position their hands in space. An arthrodesis may be required to stabilize the arm adequately. Otherwise, an amputation may be needed.

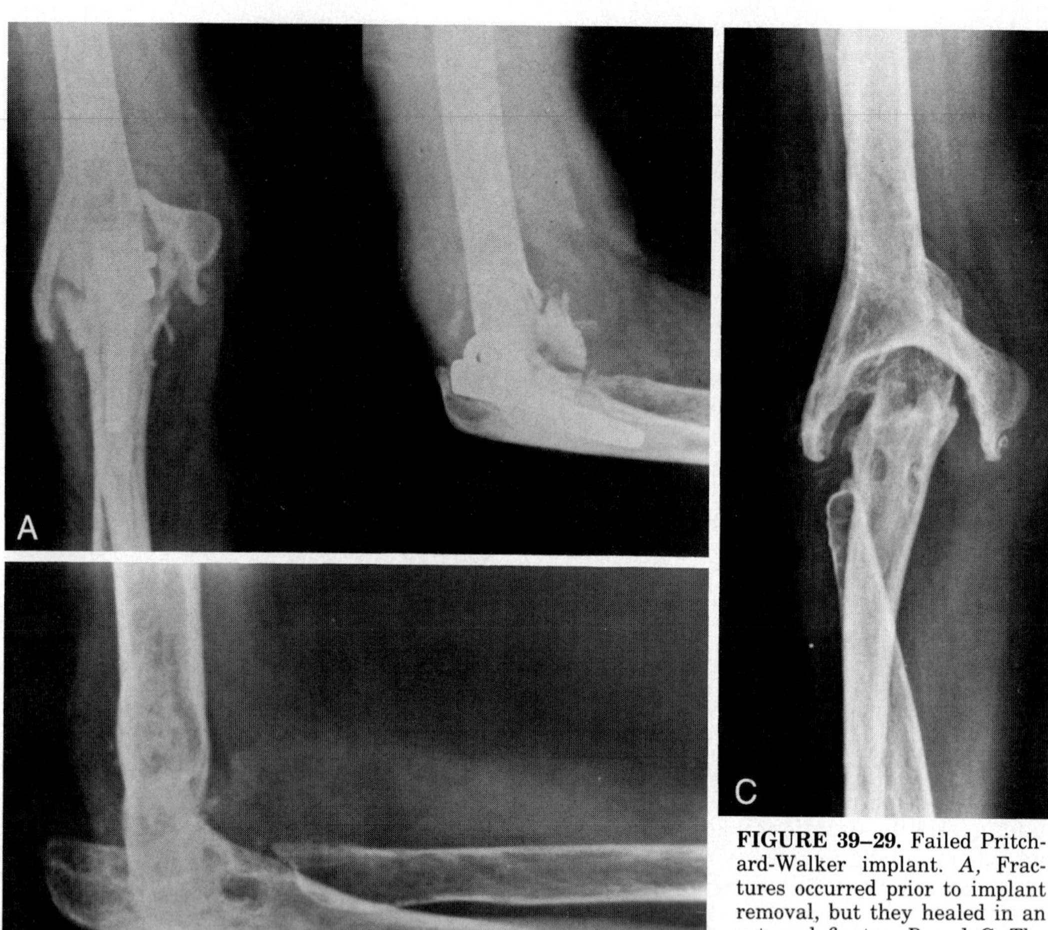

FIGURE 39–29. Failed Pritchard-Walker implant. *A,* Fractures occurred prior to implant removal, but they healed in an external fixator. *B* and *C,* The final result of a resection arthroplasty with containment of the olecranon within the epicondyles. Although the patient subsequently had mild-to-moderate instability, she had excellent function with good range of motion.

Thus, when removing any implant, the surgeon should take care to preserve the supracondylar ridges in order to leave sufficient bone stock for revision arthroplasty.

In some instances, iliac crest bone grafts to form supracondylar pillars as described by Gschwend and coworkers[24] may be indicated. The preferred option for prosthetic loosening is reimplantation with a new device. However, bone stock must be adequate to give the new implant satisfactory support. Often, longer-stemmed implants are required. Custom-fit devices or flanged semiconstrained devices, such as the Coonrad III, may be needed in these difficult cases. Because of the unpredictable status of the soft tissue structures, especially the medial collateral ligaments, semiconstrained implants are recommended. If a cortical fracture or penetration has occurred preoperatively or intraoperatively, the stem of the prosthesis must bypass it by roughly two bone diameters. Bone grafting of fractures or defects may also be needed. In addition, we often recommend the application of antibiotic-impregnated cement during reimplantation of an elbow prosthesis to lower the infection risk.

The results of revision total elbow arthroplasties have been discussed by Morrey and Bryan.[49] In their series of 33 revision total elbow arthroplasties, 28 were revised for loosening, three for implant failure, and two for instability. Moderate

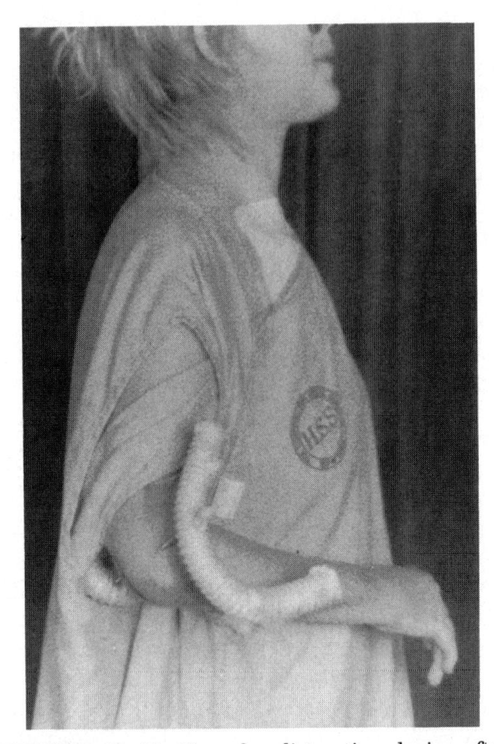

FIGURE 39–30. Use of a distraction device after removal of an elbow prosthesis. An external fixator can be fashioned using half or full pins and anesthesia tubing filled with polymethyl methacrylate. The elbow can be positioned without difficulty. The polymethyl methacrylate added to the tubing provides immediate fixation. This device is left in place for 6 to 8 weeks until wound healing is obtained.

to severe bone loss was found in 29 of the 33 cases. The average length of follow-up after the revision procedure was 5 years. Originally, 22 of the elbows had been replaced for rheumatoid arthritis. The initial implant was a semiconstrained device in 21 cases, a constrained device in seven, a nonconstrained device in two, and a Silastic implant in two. Six different standard prostheses were implanted for 29 of the revision prostheses, and custom prostheses were implanted for four. Six of the prostheses were Coonrad I design, 12 were Coonrad II, and two were Coonrad III. Pritchard-Walker II prostheses were implanted in five elbows, the Mayo long-stemmed device in three, and a long-stemmed capitellocondylar device in one. Good results were reported for 18 of the 33 elbows, whereas poor results were reported for the remaining 15. The poor results were due to infection in three elbows, loosening in six, inadequate motion in two, continued pain in two, and prosthetic failure in two. Each of the 15 patients with poor results required at least one more surgical procedure. Three patients underwent conversion to fascial arthroplasty after removal of the implant for deep infection. In the total series, 32 complications were observed, including ten cases of intraoperative perforation of the cortex of either the ulna or the humerus. Only 13 of the 33 revisions were without complications.

Overall, revision of failed total elbow arthroplasty is a complex and demanding procedure with a high complication rate, even when performed by an experienced surgeon. The patient often presents with marked loosening of the primary total elbow replacement and has significant bone deficiency. Implant removal is difficult, and cortical perforation is frequent. Custom-fit or flanged long-stemmed prostheses may be required to provide sufficient stabilization.

COMPLICATIONS

Infection

The rates of deep infection following total elbow arthroplasty have ranged from 0 to 11 percent. Deep sepsis may produce devastating complications, often requiring prolonged hospital stays and multiple operations, yet still ending in poor functional results. In a study of the risks, complications, and management of deep infections in total elbow arthroplasties, Morrey and Bryan[47] found an overall infection rate of 9 percent. In a similar study, Wolfe and colleagues[80] found an infection rate of 7.3 percent.

Patients who have total elbow replacements may be at high risk for infection for several reasons. First, the soft tissues about the elbow are thin, and the presence of several bony prominences (e.g., the olecranon) may produce pressure on the skin leading to necrosis (Fig. 39–31). Second, the thin subcutaneous tissue will not tolerate hematoma formation, and drainage of a hematoma may make the elbow more susceptible to infection. Third, elbow replacements are often performed under difficult conditions: the patient is likely to have severe rheumatoid arthritis and may

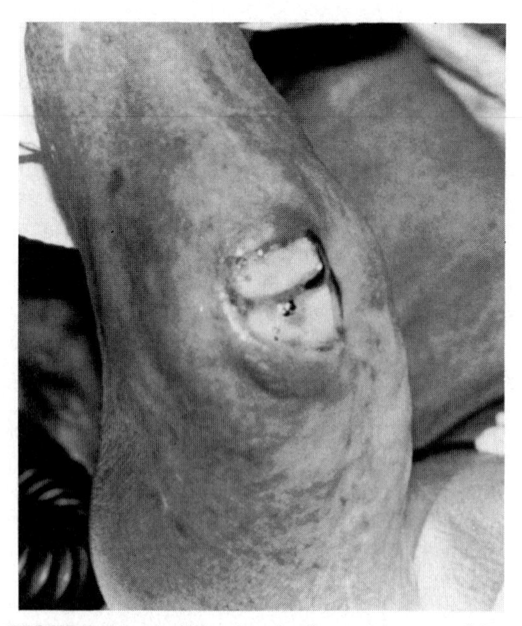

FIGURE 39–31. Skin slough after surgery resulting in deep infection. This patient developed a pressure sore that could not be controlled. Exposure of the implant developed. The prosthesis had to be removed in order to control infection and obtain skin closure.

be taking medications, such as prednisone and methotrexate, so that soft tissue healing is compromised. Steroid therapy may have further thinned the subcutaneous tissue. The patient may also have had previous surgical procedures, with various skin incisions compromising tissue vascularity. In patients with post-traumatic arthritis, previous operations are likely, also raising the risk for infection.

These procedures are often performed on patients with American Rheumatism Association class III and IV disease, who depend upon their arms for weightbearing, as they ambulate with the assistance of walkers, crutches, or canes. The greater stress that this requirement places on the soft tissues may lead to skin slough. Morrey and Bryan[47] identified several predisposing factors in their series. Of the patients whose procedures were performed for rheumatoid arthritis, 11 percent had complications of sepsis. Of 40 patients who had procedures for traumatic arthritis, two had deep infections. The 50 percent of the patients with deep infections were on steroids as opposed to 32 percent of the population receiving total elbow replacements. The 7.5 percent of the patients who had no previous surgery developed deep infections. The rate increased to 12.2 percent in the 49 patients who had previous surgery. In addition, deep infections developed in seven of 34 elbows undergoing subsequent surgery for any reason.

Wolfe and colleagues[80] identified several statistically significant factors that increased the risk for subsequent infection: previous elbow surgery, previous infection in the region of the elbow, psychiatric illness, class IV rheumatoid arthritis, postoperative wound drainage, spontaneous drainage after 10 days, and reoperation for any reason. These workers reported infection in five of 34 patients with traumatic arthritis (15 percent) and in nine of 132 patients with rheumatoid arthritis (7 percent), but the difference was not statistically significant. However, patients with class IV rheumatoid arthritis had a significantly higher infection rate (40 percent) than those with class II or III. In addition, patients who had arthritis in the ipsilateral shoulder had more infections and more frequent problems with wound healing. Of the elbows with early postoperative drainage, 27 percent eventually had deep infections. Nine of the 13 elbows (69 percent) with delayed (more than 10 days postoperatively) spontaneous drainage developed deep infections, as did five of the 23 elbows (22 percent) that were reoperated upon. No significant correlation was found between preoperative nutritional status, sedimentation rate, or any other laboratory value and subsequent infection. In this series, two patients developed acute infections, six developed subacute infections between 3 and 12 months after operation, and six developed late infections. In the series reported by Morrey and Bryan, seven patients had early infections, three had subacute infections, and four had late infections. Altogether, 27 cases of deep infection were reported by Morrey and Bryan and by Wolfe and associates. The responsible bacteria were *Staphylococcus aureus* in 18 elbows, *S. epidermidis* in five, and a different organism in each of the five remaining elbows.

Treatment should include early debridement and bacterial eradication with suppressive antibiotics, if the infection is diagnosed early in an elbow with well-fixed components. Suppression should be tried to avoid, if possible, the difficulty of removing the implant and the subsequent reconstruction. Unfortunately, the success rate appears to be low. In the series reported by Morrey and Bryan, only one of 14 elbows was salvaged by debridement. In the series of Wolfe and coworkers, only three of 13 outcomes were successful. Satisfactory results were found in eight of the ten elbows with resection arthroplasty in Morrey and Bryan's series. Nine were treated by resection arthroplasty in the series of Wolfe, and two required later arthrodesis. In the combined series, three patients underwent delayed reimplantation of total elbow arthroplasty and all had satisfactory function afterward (Fig. 39–32). However, the patients were selected based upon estimates of the ability to adequately eliminate infection as determined by minimum inhibitory concentration levels and the presence of sufficient bone stock and soft tissues to allow for reimplantation of the prosthesis. In general, however, reimplantation is not recommended unless the resection arthroplasty has failed owing to instability.

Several factors must be considered when one assesses the risk of infection. Early infection is related to skin quality, remit-

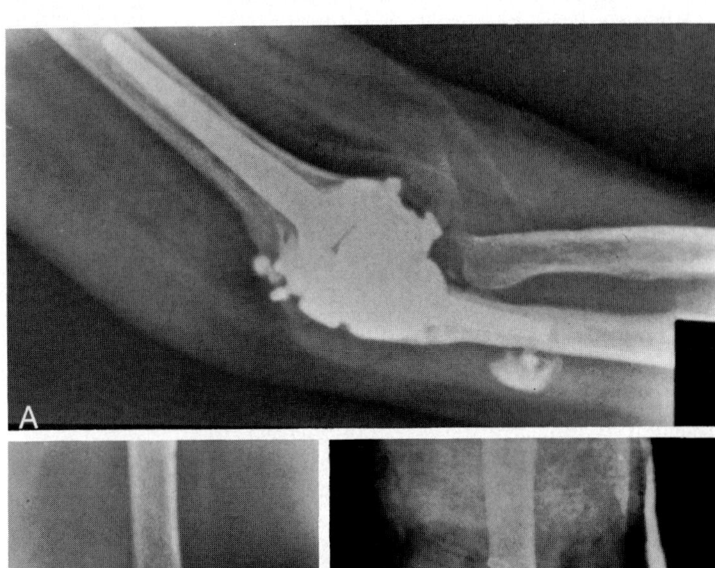

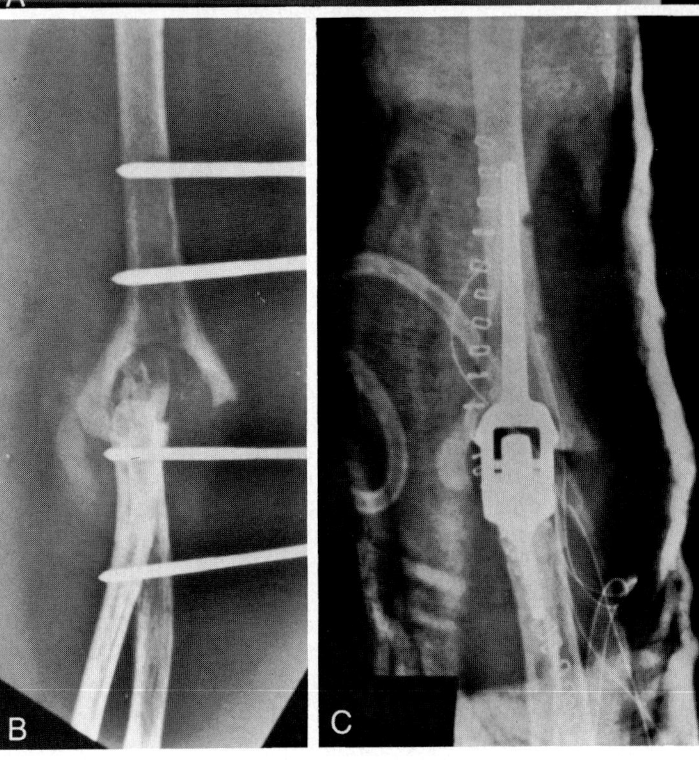

FIGURE 39–32. Revision total elbow replacement for infection. *A*, Hematogenous infection in an elbow after an infection developed at the entry site for brachial artery catheterization. An aspiration/arthrogram was performed that documented the infection. *B*, The implant was removed along with the cement, and the elbow was placed in a distraction device. *C*, Placement of a custom implant after a 6-week course of antibiotics. The patient was doing well at last follow-up 2 years after surgery.

tent agent drug therapy, and prolonged or recurrent postoperative drainage. The triceps flap approach with minimal soft tissue dissection has helped decrease early wound complications and thus the overall deep infection rate. In addition, attention must be given to the patient's functional needs and the amount of weightbearing required by the elbow. If the patient has lost rotation of the shoulder and is likely to place undue pressure on the elbow, rotation of the shoulder should be re-established before the elbow procedure is performed. Postoperatively, the elbow must be well protected to avoid undue pressure on the tip of the olecranon and to prevent skin slough that might result in infection. Patients who have class IV rheumatoid arthritis and those who have had previous surgery should be warned that they are at higher risk for infection. The patients with previous sepsis or psychiatric disorders must be carefully evaluated, and other options must be investigated. Careful consideration of these issues may reduce the chances of early infection.

Late infection is more problematic. Any other infections must be detected and treated vigorously to protect the prosthesis. In addition, the patient must be warned to be careful with the elbow, to reduce the possibility of skin slough. If skin loss does occur, it should be treated aggressively with soft tissue closures and skin rotation flaps in order to prevent a deep infection. Since 1988, we have used gentamicin-impregnated cement in all total elbow replacements and have had no cases of deep infections.

Implant Failure

Failure of total elbow arthroplasty due to fracture occurs rarely except in the Mark I Pritchard-Walker prosthesis. The original Pritchard-Walker implant had an all-polyethylene humeral component, which tended to fracture above the articulation (Fig. 39–33).[8, 60, 61] Fracture of the humeral component leads to gross instability, and implant revision or removal is usually necessary. If the implant is removed, a Mark II–type humeral component can be inserted, obviating the need for revision of the ulnar component. A two-component revision is necessary if a different prosthetic design is selected. The other option is to remove the implant and perform a resection-type arthroplasty, making sure that the supracondylar ridges are preserved.

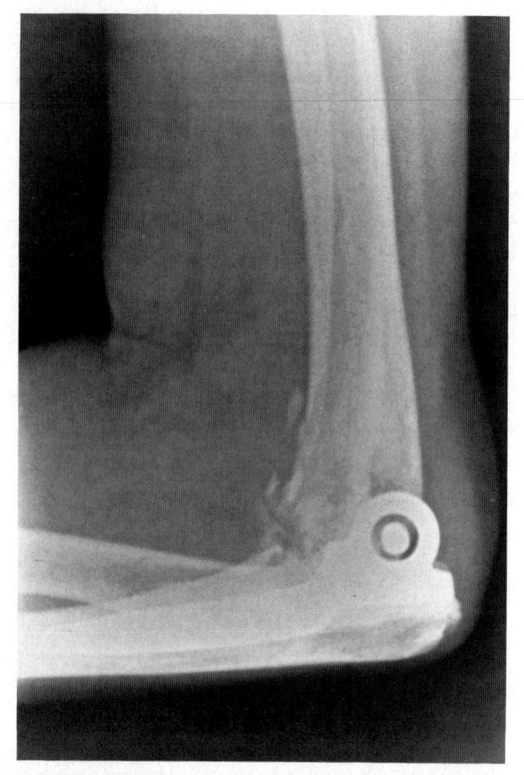

FIGURE 39–33. Original Pritchard-Walker implant with a polyethylene humeral component. This implant was susceptible to fracture as illustrated in this case.

Instability and Dislocation

Instability in nonconstrained prostheses has been reported in 4 to 25 percent of cases (Fig. 39–34).[10, 14, 34, 35, 38, 58, 59, 62, 66, 67, 68, 74, 77, 79] However, instability in nonconstrained devices occurs in various degrees. The elbow may translocate so that the ulna articulates with the radial surface of the humeral component. In addition, transient subluxation may occur with flexion and extension. Frank dislocation may also occur; dislocation may occur in an anterior, posterior, or radial direction, although posterior is most frequent. Weiland and colleagues[79] reported malarticulation in 20 percent of cases and frank dislocations in

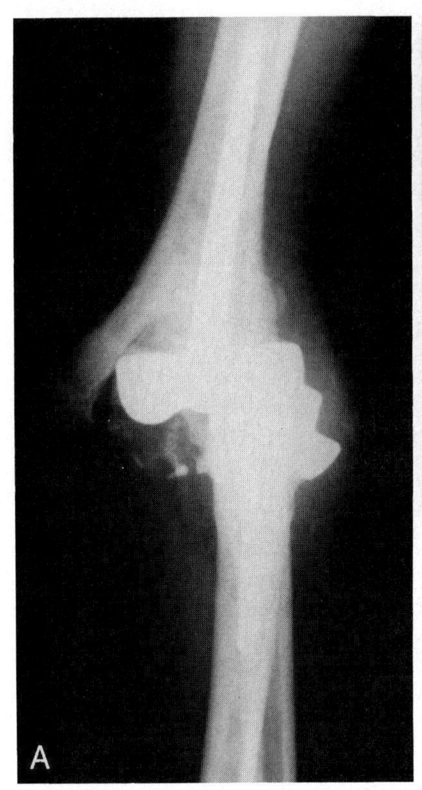

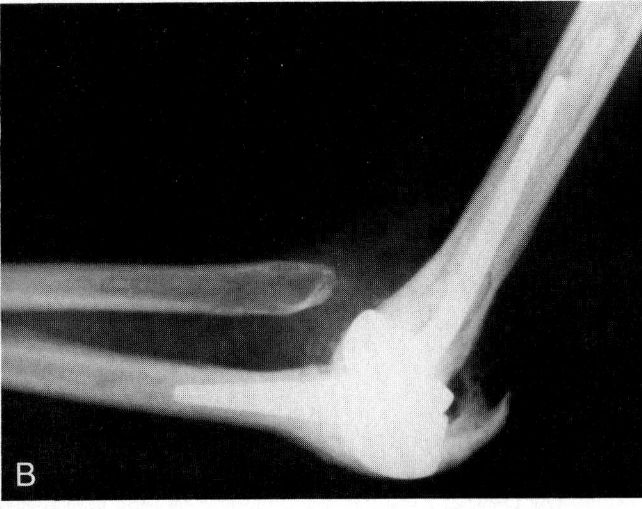

FIGURE 39–34. *A* and *B*, Failure of a capitellocondylar implant in a patient with poor ligamentous stability. The elbow is subluxed. The humeral component has sunk, leaving the patient with an unsatisfactory result.

5 percent. Of the elbows with malarticulation, 75 percent had radial translocation of the ulnar component. When the component translocates radially, malarticulation may be managed simply by observation unless the patient has significant pain or a block to flexion or extension. However, if frank dislocation occurs in either the radial anterior or posterior direction, reduction should be performed, with immobilization in a cast at 90 degrees of flexion in neutral rotation. The patient should wear the cast for 3 weeks and then resume rehabilitation. If the elbow continues to be troublesome, exploration of the medial structures and medial collateral ligament may be required. Revision to a semiconstrained device may be indicated if satisfactory tissues are not available for reconstruction.

Late instability may also occur in semiconstrained snap-fit devices,[19, 27, 76] either secondary to trauma that has dislodged the device from the polyethylene bearing or secondary to late polyethylene wear. This problem was identified by Volz[76] and by Inglis and Pellicci[27] in semiconstrained devices and has tended to increase with time, as noted by Figgie and associates.[19] In their long-term follow-up, eight dislocations occurred with the triaxial implant, one 3 months after trauma and seven from 4 to 6 years after surgery. Two of these dislocations were due to traumatic incidents. In each case, revision of the polyethylene bearing was required. In five cases, an anterior yoke was added to prevent hyperflexion and dislocation of the prosthesis (Fig. 39–35). In a separate study, Figgie and colleagues[15] reported on the higher incidence of dislocation among patients with prosthetic malalignments and shifts in the center of rotation. To prevent dislocation, attention should be paid to restoring the correct anatomic relationships. We no longer use the triaxial component but prefer a semiconstrained prosthesis that has better polyethylene articulation along with improved wear characteristics. In addition, the nonloaded nonweightbearing axle helps prevent dislocations secondary to trauma. With this device, no more radiolucencies have been seen than with the previous triaxial component. In addition, dislocations have been prevented.[16]

With these modifications, dislocation should be reduced. However, if dislocations

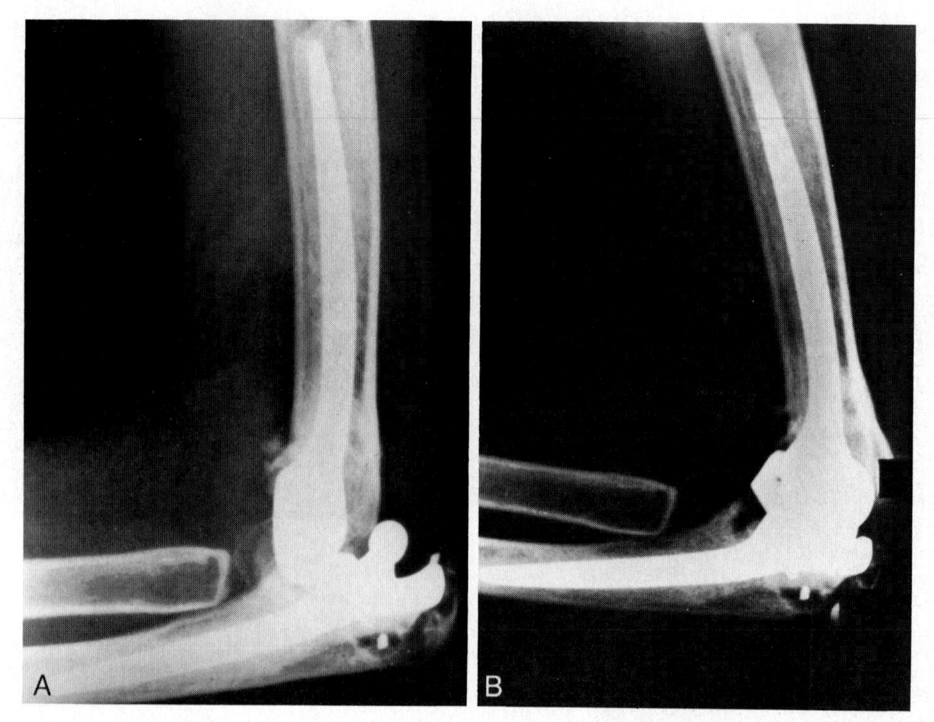

FIGURE 39–35. Dislocation of a semiconstrained device, caused by late polyethylene wear. *A,* A triaxial implant that dislocated 6 years after surgery. *B,* The patient underwent revision with a new bushing and a yoke in order to prevent hyperflexion and recurrent dislocation.

of the triaxial or the semiconstrained devices occur, satisfactory revision can be accomplished with bearing revision and the addition of a yoke device. If a prosthesis is malaligned, however, revision of both components may be required.

Fractures

The most common intraoperative fracture is that of the medial or lateral supracondylar ridge. Often the cause is oversizing or overreaming of the distal humerus when utilizing a semiconstrained device. To avoid this fracture, the prosthesis must be properly aligned and the supracondylar ridges protected. In addition, the implant must be properly selected and sized. If fracture does occur, the supracondylar ridge should be stabilized and incorporated in the cement. The ridges provide resistance to rotation and must be incorporated with the implant replacement. During the period of healing, the prosthesis should be protected with splinting. Early motion may still begin under the direction of a physical therapist. If the fracture is undisplaced, no treatment is required.

The other intraoperative fractures that may occur involve penetration of the cortex of either the ulna or the humerus. They can be prevented with careful reaming using hand instruments rather than power reamers. This practice is especially important in patients with rheumatoid arthritis and thin cortical shells. If the cortex is perforated, the defect should be grafted and bypassed with the stem a distance equal to twice the diameter of the bone. This step helps avoid later fracture at the implant tip.

The most common fracture in the postoperative period is along either of the supracondylar ridges. Figgie's group[19] reported seven such fractures in 151 elbows in which semiconstrained prostheses were implanted. However, in each instance, the cement mantle was not disturbed and the fracture eventually healed with elbow splinting or bracing (Fig. 39–36).

Fracture at the tip of either the humeral or ulnar prosthesis presents a more difficult challenge (Fig. 39–37). The fracture

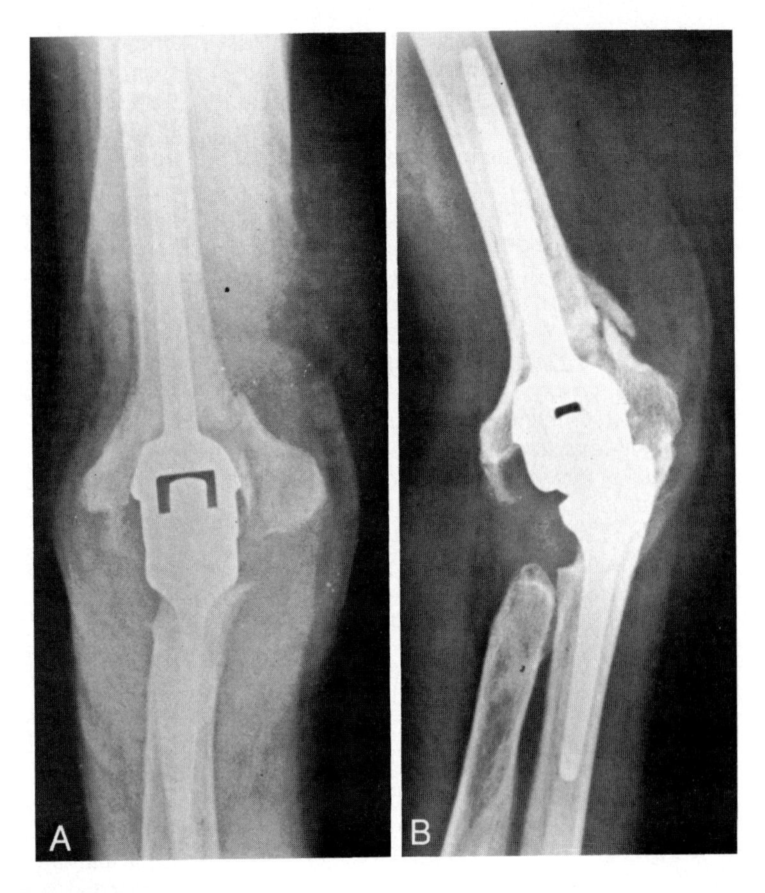

FIGURE 39–36. Fracture of a medial epicondyle postoperatively. *A,* Fracture did not involve the cement mantle and was not associated with loosening. *B,* The patient was treated conservatively. Ultimately full union was obtained.

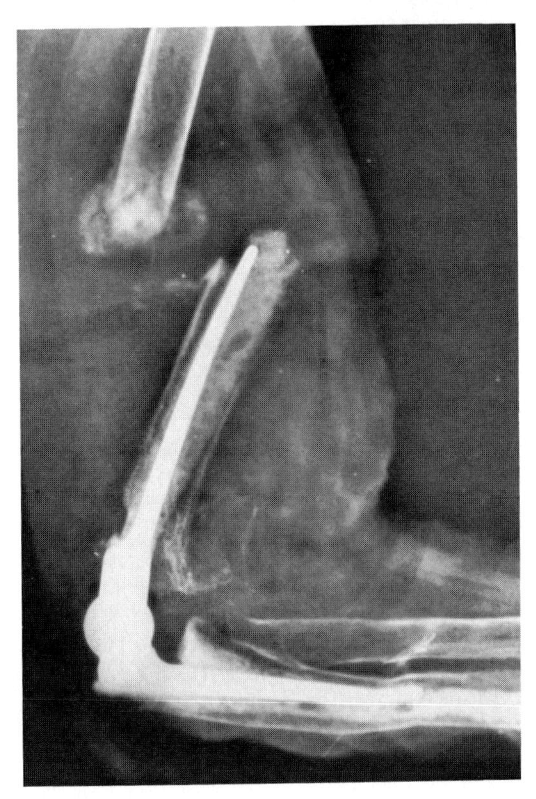

FIGURE 39–37. Fracture at the tip of the humeral stem should be treated much like fracture associated with total hip replacement. If the implant is loose, revision should be performed with fixation of the fracture. If the implant is not loose, an attempt at healing with conservative measures should be made.

should be stabilized with splints or casts, which are kept in place until the fracture heals. The only exception occurs when the implant loosens, and revision is then necessary. The revision can be performed, and a longer stem used for immediate stabilization. However, if the implant is well fixed, revision should not be undertaken owing to the difficulty of preserving the bone stock when removing the prosthesis. Care must be taken during the healing phase to prevent an angular deformity from developing.

Fractures of the distal humerus or proximal ulna that involve the cement mantle are usually treated with immobilization until the bone is healed. Then, revision of the implant can be done if the implant has loosened. Attempts at immediate revision may be extremely difficult as firm fixation and immediate fracture stabilization may be difficult to obtain.

Nerve Injury

Postoperative nerve dysfunction has been reported in 2 to 23 percent of patients in some series.[9, 19, 59] Usually, nerve dysfunction is temporary and resolves. Sometimes, however, the nerve lesion persists and exploration of the nerve is indicated. The ulnar nerve is most often affected. Only rare instances of posterior interosseous or radial nerve involvement have been reported.[9, 38, 45] Many patients present with nerve lesions preoperatively. For example, in post-traumatic arthritis, the nerve may be tethered in the canal and cubital tunnel owing to previous surgery. In rheumatoid arthritis, synovitis in the joint may compress the nerve. This compression may be treated by synovectomy, ulnar nerve transposition, or both.

Hematoma Formation

Initial immobilization aids in primary wound healing. Careful hemostasis and postoperative drainage decrease hematoma formation. Application of a postoperative splint with the elbow in extension lessens pressure on the wound. However, the splint should not cover the tip of the olecranon. The splint must protect the elbow while avoiding pressure on bony prominences.

In the event of early postoperative drainage, the arm should be splinted in extension. Therapy should be discontinued until drainage stops. If a tense wound hematoma occurs, reoperation should be done to evacuate the hematoma and avoid prolonged drainage. A skin slough should be treated immediately with grafting or rotation flaps to avoid deep infection. Exposed triceps tendon or bone must be covered with a flap or graft as soon as possible.

Triceps Insufficiency

Morrey and coworkers[45] reported ten cases of triceps weakness after 80 total elbow replacements. All affected patients had undergone triceps detachment or the Van Gorder approach. Inglis and Pellicci[27] reported on one case in 36 elbow replacements that required reoperation twice for triceps insufficiency following the Van Gorder approach. With the triceps-sparing approaches, such as the posteromedial of Bryan and Morrey and extensile Kocher, the incidence of triceps insufficiency has dropped significantly.[19]

Heterotopic Ossification

In our experience, heterotopic ossification after total elbow replacement is unusual. When it occurs, the functional outcome of surgery does not appear to be compromised. Even in cases of salvage of supracondylar nonunion or ankylosis, only grade I heterotopic ossification is seen postoperatively.[17, 18] Thus, postoperative irradiation or other measures to prevent heterotopic ossification after elbow replacement appear to be unnecessary.

REHABILITATION

Surgical approaches that spare the triceps allow earlier rehabilitation after elbow replacement. With the posteromedial approach, the elbow is splinted in maximum extension for 3 days postoperatively. Range-of-motion exercises are begun if the wound is dry. At night, the patient is

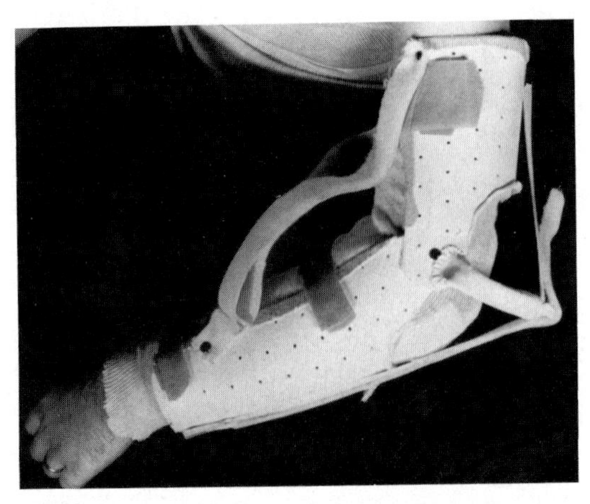

FIGURE 39–38. Elbow splint with straps that can hold the arm in either flexion or extension.

placed in a splint that has straps that maintain the elbow in either flexion or extension, depending upon which motion was lacking (Fig. 39–38). Splinting can usually be discontinued after 6 weeks. A therapist guides the patient through the early rehabilitation stage, but the patient is encouraged to use the arm as much as possible for all activities of daily living. Flexion is usually regained more easily than extension as most activities of daily living require flexion. Pronation and supination should also be stressed during rehabilitation.

The postoperative regimen for nonconstrained implants generally resembles that for semiconstrained implants. The patient is placed in a posterior splint at 90 degrees of flexion and neutral rotation for 3 to 5 days.[59] Passive range-of-motion exercises are begun, and the patient is placed in a resting splint at 90 degrees. At 3 weeks after surgery, active range-of-motion exercises are started. At 2 months postoperatively, active stretching of soft tissues begins. The patient is then encouraged to use the arm for as many activities of daily living as possible.

In either instance, manipulation after surgery is generally not recommended. To date, we have not utilized the continuous passive motion (CPM) machine in the rehabilitation of total elbow arthroplasty.

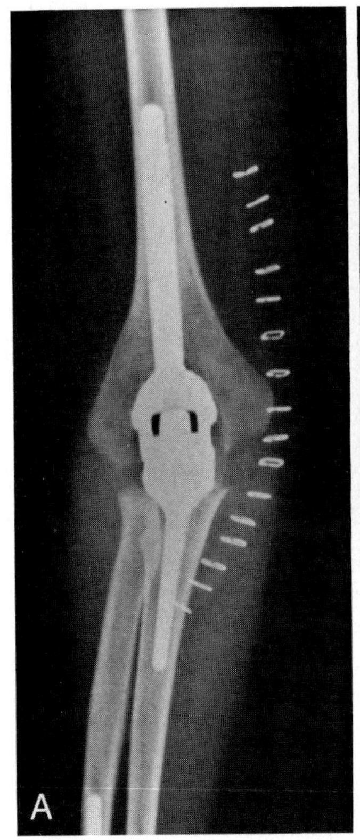

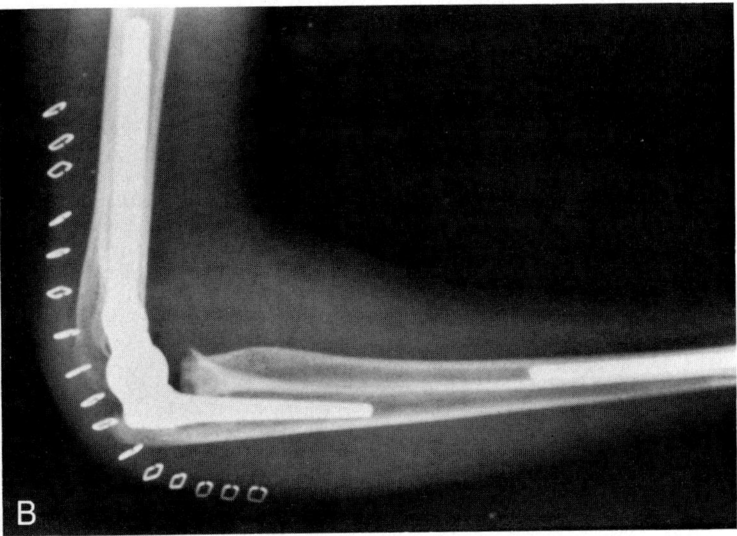

FIGURE 39–39. *A* and *B*, A 23-year-old patient with juvenile rheumatoid arthritis who had a custom-fit noncemented total elbow replacement. The elbow was functioning well at a 2-year follow-up.

SUMMARY

Total elbow replacement provides pain relief and improved function for many patients with severe elbow disease. Complication and failure rates are higher than for hip, knee, or shoulder replacement arthroplasties. Results are best in patients with rheumatoid arthritis because of their lower activity levels. The operation should be considered a salvage procedure for the patient with post-traumatic arthropathy and distal humeral nonunion.

Nonconstrained prostheses, such as the capitellocondylar, have had lower lucency rates than constrained prostheses. Prostheses with stems are less likely to migrate or loosen than those without stems. Although the nonconstrained implants may have lower radiolucency rates due to less constraint, their dislocation rates remain a concern. Indeed, the rates may rise as greater polyethylene wear is encountered, thus reducing joint congruity. A semiconstrained prosthesis seems best for post-traumatic problems, whereas either a nonconstrained or semiconstrained device seems best for the severe damage of rheumatoid arthritis.

Numerous improvements have led to more predictable results for total elbow arthroplasties. However, further investigation is needed in the areas of finite element analysis, joint mechanics, and implant fixation (Fig. 39–39).

References

1. Amis, A. A., Dowson, D., and Wright, V.: Elbow joint force predictions for some strenuous isometric actions. J. Biomechanics 13:765–775, 1980.
2. Barr, J. S. and Eaton, R. G.: Elbow reconstruction with a new prosthesis to replace the distal end of the humerus. J. Bone Joint Surg. 47A:1408, 1965.
3. Boerma, I. and deWaard, D. J.: Osteoplastic Verank-erung von Mettal Prosthesis bei Pseudarthrose und bei Arthroplastic. Acta Chir. Scand. 86:511, 1942.
4. Brumfield, R. H., Jr., and Volz, R. G.: Total Elbow Arthroplasty: A Clinical Review of 30 Cases Employing the Mayo and AHSC Prostheses. Presentation, American Academy of Orthopaedic Surgeons, Atlanta, 1980.
5. Bryan, R. S.: Total replacement of the elbow joint. Arch. Surg. 112:1092, 1977.
6. Bryan, R. S. and Morrey, B. F.: Extensive posterior exposure of the elbow: A triceps-sparing approach. Clin. Orthop. 166:188, 1982.
7. Chatzikakis, C.: Arthroplasty of the elbow joint using a vitalium prosthesis. Int. Surg. 53:119, 1970.
8. Coonrad, R. W.: History of Total Elbow Arthroplasty. Upper Extremity Joint Replacement. Symposium on Total Joint Replacement of the Upper Extremity, 1979. Edited by A. E. Inglis. St. Louis, C. V. Mosby Company, 1982.
9. Coonrad, R. W.: Seven-Year Follow-Up of Coonrad Total Elbow Replacement. Upper Extremity Joint Replacement. Edited by A. E. Inglis. St. Louis, C. V. Mosby Company, 1982.
10. Davis, R. F., Weiland, A. J., Hungerford, D. S., et al.: Nonconstrained total elbow arthroplasty. Clin. Orthop. 171:156, 1982.
11. Dee, R.: Total replacement arthroplasty of the elbow for rheumatoid arthritis. J. Bone Joint Surg. 54B:88, 1972.
12. Driessen, A. P.: Thirty years with a complete elbow prosthesis. Arch. Chir. Neerl. 24(2):87, 1972.
13. Evans, E. M.: Rotational deformity in the treatment of fractures of both bones of the forearm. J. Bone Joint Surg. 27:373–379, 1945.
14. Ewald, F. C., Scheinberg, R. D., Poss, R., et al.: Capitellocondylar total elbow arthroplasty: Two-to-five year follow-up in rheumatoid arthritis. J. Bone Joint Surg. 62A:1259, 1980.
15. Figgie, H. E., Inglis, A. E., and Mow, C.: A critical analysis of biomechanical factors affecting functional outcome in total elbow arthroplasties. J. Arthroplasty 1(3):169–173, 1986.
16. Figgie, M. P., Inglis, A. E., Figgie, H. E., III, et al.: Custom total elbow arthroplasty in traumatic and rheumatoid arthritis. Orthop. Trans. 13:234–235, 1989.
17. Figgie, M. P., Inglis, A. E., Mow, C. S., and Figgie, H. E. III: Total elbow arthroplasty for complete ankylosis of the elbow. J. Bone Joint Surg. 71A:513, 1989.
18. Figgie, M. P., Inglis, A. E., Mow, C. S., and Figgie, H. E., III: Salvage of non-union of supracondylar fracture of the humerus by total elbow arthroplasty. J. Bone Joint Surg. 71A:1058, 1989.
19. Figgie, M. P., Inglis, A. E., Figgie, H. E., III, and Mow, C. S.: Semiconstrained Total Elbow Replacement in Rheumatoid Arthritis. Presentation, The 57th Annual American Academy of Orthopaedic Surgeons, New Orleans, 1990.
20. Figgie, M. P., Inglis, A. E., Figgie, H. E., III, and Mow, C. S.: Total Elbow Arthroplasty in Traumatic Arthritis. Presentation, The 57th Annual American Academy of Orthopaedic Surgeons, New Orleans, 1990.
21. Figgie, M. P., Inglis, A. E., Mow, C. L., et al.: Results of reconstruction for failed total elbow arthroplasty. Clin. Orthop. 253:123, 1990.
22. Garrett, J. C., Ewald, F. C., Thomas, W. H., and Sledge, C. B.: Loosening associated with GSB hinge total elbow replacement in patients with rheumatoid arthritis. Clin. Orthop. 127:170, 1977.
23. Gschwend, N.: Salvage procedure in failed total elbow prosthesis. Arch. Orthop. Trauma Surg. 101:95, 1983.
24. Gschwend, N., Scheier, H., and Bahler, A.: GSB Elbow-, Wrist-, and PIP-Joints. Joint Replacement in the Upper Limb. London, Institution of Mechanical Engineers, 1977.

25. Halls, A. A. and Travill, R.: Transmission of pressures across the elbow joint. Anat. Rec. 150:243, 1964.
26. Hui, F. C., Chao, E. Y., and An, K. N.: Muscle and joint forces at the elbow during isometric lifting. (Abstract.) Orthop. Trans. 2:169, 1978.
27. Inglis, A. E. and Pellicci, P. M.: Total elbow replacement. J. Bone Joint Surg. 62A:1252, 1980.
28. Inglis, A. E.: Tri-Axial Total Elbow Replacement: Indications, Surgical Technique and Results. Symposium on Total Joint Replacement of the Upper Extremity. Edited by A. E. Inglis. St. Louis, C. V. Mosby Company, 1982.
29. Inglis, A. E., Coonrad, R. W., Figgie, H., and Morrey, B. F.: Symposium: Total Elbow Arthroplasty. Contemp. Orthop. 20:529–552, 1990.
30. Ishizuki, M., et al.: Preliminary experiences with hingeless total elbow arthroplasty. Ryumachi 17:4, 1977.
31. John, J. R., Getty, C. J., Mclettin, A. W. F., and Glasgow, M. M. S.: The Stanmore total elbow replacement for rheumatoid arthritis. J. Bone Joint Surg. 66B:732, 1984.
32. Kapandji, I. A.: The Physiology of Joints. Upper Limb, 2nd ed. Baltimore, Williams & Wilkins, 1970.
33. Keats, T. E., Teeslink, R., Diamond, A. E., and Williams, J. H.: Normal axial relationships of the major joints. Radiology 87:904–907, 1966.
34. Kudo, H., Iwano, K., and Watanabe, S.: Total replacements of the rheumatoid elbow with a hingeless prosthesis. J. Bone Joint Surg. 62A:277, 1980.
35. Kudo, H. and Iwano, K.: Total elbow arthroplasty with a non-constrained surface replacement prosthesis in patients who have rheumatoid arthritis: A long-term follow-up study. J. Bone Joint Surg. 72A:355, 1990.
36. London, J. T.: Resurfacing total elbow arthroplasty. Orthop. Trans. 2:217, 1978.
37. London, J. T.: Kinematics of the elbow. J. Bone Joint Surg. 63A:529, 1981.
38. Lowe, L. W., Miller, A. J., Allum, R. L., and Higginson, D. W.: The development of an unconstrained elbow arthroplasty: A clinical review. J. Bone Joint Surg. 66B:243, 1984.
39. MacAusland, A. R.: Replacement of the lower end of the humerus with a prosthesis: A report of four cases. West J. Surg. Obstet. Gynecol. 62:557, 1954.
40. McKee, GC: Total Replacement of the Elbow. Orthopaedic Surgery and Traumatology. Edited by J. Delchef, et al. Proceedings of the 12th Congress of the International Society of Orthopaedic Surgery and Trauma. Amsterdam, Excerpta Medica, 1973.
41. Mellen, R. H. and Phalen, G. S.: Arthroplasty of the elbow by replacement of the distal portion of the humerus with an acrylic prosthesis. J. Bone Joint Surg. 29:348, 1947.
42. Mitsunaga, M. M., Bryan, R. S., and Linscheid, R. L.: Condylar nonunions of the Elbow. J. Trauma 22:787–791, 1982.
43. Morrey, B. F. and Chao, E. Y. S.: Passive motion of the elbow joint. A biomechanical analysis. J. Bone Joint Surg. 58A:501–508, 1976.
44. Morrey, B. F., Askew, L. J., An, K. N., and Chao, E. Y.: A biochemical study of normal functional elbow motion. J. Bone Joint Surg. 63A:872–877, 1981.
45. Morrey, B. F., Bryan, R. S., Dobyns, J. H., and Linscheid, R. L.: Total elbow arthroplasty: A five-year experience at the Mayo Clinic. J. Bone Joint Surg. 63A:1050, 1981.
46. Morrey, B. F. and An, K. N.: Articular and ligamentous contributions to the stability of the elbow joint. Am. J. Sports Med. 11:315, 1983.
47. Morrey, B. F. and Bryan, R. S.: Infection after total elbow arthroplasty. J. Bone Joint Surg. 65A:330, 1983.
48. Morrey, B. F. and An, K. N.: Biomechanics of the Elbow. The Elbow and Its Disorders. Edited by B. F. Morrey. Philadelphia, W. B. Saunders Company, 1985.
49. Morrey, B. F. and Bryan, R. S.: Revision Total Elbow Arthroplasty. J. Bone Joint Surg. 69A:523, 1987.
50. Morrey, B. F. and Bryan, R. S.: Total elbow arthroplasty for post-traumatic arthritis. Orthop. Trans. 12:675, 1988.
51. Morrey, B. F.: Post-traumatic contracture of the elbow operative treatment including distraction arthroplasty. J. Bone Joint Surg. 72A:601, 1990.
52. Morrey, B. F. and An, K. N.: Functional anatomy of the elbow ligaments. Clin. Orthop. (Submitted.)
53. Ocher, T.: Textbook of Operative Surgery, 3rd ed. Translated by H. J. Stiles and C. B. Paul. London, A. & C. Black, 1911.
54. Ogilvie, W. H.: Discussion on minor injuries of the elbow joint. Proc. R. Soc. Med. 23:306–322, 1930.
55. Pearson, J. R., McGinley, D. R., and Butzel, L. M.: A dynamic analysis of the upper extremity. Plantar Motions Hum. Factors 5:59, 1963.
56. Pritchard, R. W.: Long-term follow-up study: Semi-constrained elbow prosthesis. Orthopedics 4:151, 1981.
57. Pritchard, R. W.: Anatomic surface elbow arthroplasty: A preliminary report. Clin. Orthop. 179:223, 1983.
58. Roper, B. A., Tuke, M., O'Riordan, S. M., and Bulstrode, C. J.: A new unconstrained elbow. J. Bone Joint Surg. 68B:566, 1986.
59. Rosenberg, G. M. and Turner, R. N.: Nonconstrained total elbow arthroplasty. Clin. Orthop. 187:154, 1984.
60. Rosenberg, G., Figgie, H. E., III, Ranawat, C. S., et al.: Total elbow replacement for rheumatoid arthritis. Long-term results with a semi-constrained prosthesis. Orthop. Trans. 12:732–733, 1988.
61. Rosenfeld, S. R. and Anzel, S. H.: Evaluation of the Pritchard total elbow arthroplasty. Orthopedics 5:713, 1982.
62. Rydholm, U., Tjornstrand, B., Petterson, H., and Lidgren, L.: Surface replacement of the elbow in rheumatoid arthritis: Early results with the Wadsworth prosthesis. J. Bone Joint Surg. 66B:737, 1984.
63. Schlein, A. P.: Semiconstrained total elbow arthroplasty. Clin. Orthop. 121:222, 1976.
64. Schwab, G. H., Bennett, J. B., Woods, G. W., and Tullow, H. S.: The biomechanics of elbow instability: The role of the medial collateral ligament. Clin. Orthop. 146:42–52, 1980.

65. Sim, F. H.: Nonunion and Delayed Union of Distal Humeral Fractures. The Elbow and Its Disorders. Edited by B. F. Morrey. Philadelphia, W. B. Saunders Company, 1985.
66. Simmons, E. D., Sullivan, J. A., and Ewald, F. C.: Long-Term Review of the Capitellocondylar Total Elbow Replacement. Presentation, The Sixth Open Meeting of the American Shoulder and Elbow Surgeons, New Orleans, 1990.
67. Soni, R. K. and Cavendish, M. E.: A review of the Liverpool elbow prosthesis from 1974 to 1982. J. Bone Joint Surg. 66B:248, 1984.
68. Souter, W. A.: A new approach to elbow arthroplasty. Engin. Med. 10(2):269, 1981.
69. Spinner, M. and Kaplan, E. B.: The quadrate ligament of the elbow—Its relationship to the stability of the proximal, radio-ulnar joint. Acta Orthop. Scand. 41:632–647, 1970.
70. Steindler, A.: Kinesiology of the Human Body, 5th ed. Springfield, Ill., Charles C Thomas, 1977.
71. Street, D. N. and Stevens, P. S.: A humeral replacement prosthesis for the elbow: Results in 10 elbows. J. Bone Joint Surg. 56A:1147–1158, 1974.
72. Tillman, B.: A Contribution to the Function Morphology of Articular Surfaces. Translated by G. Konorza. Stuttgart, Georg Thieme, P. S. G. Publishing, 1978.
73. Torzilli, P. A.: Biomechanics of the Elbow. Symposium on Total Joint Replacement of the Upper Extremity. Edited by A. E. Inglis. St. Louis, C. V. Mosby Company, 1982.
74. Tuke, M. A.: The ICLH Elbow. Engin. Med. 10(2):75, 1981.
75. Virgen (1937): Cited in Schlein, A. P.: Semiconstrained total elbow arthroplasty. Clin. Orthop. 121:223, 1976.
76. Volz, R. G.: Development and Clinical Analysis of a New Semiconstrained Total Elbow Prosthesis. Upper Extremity Joint Replacement. Edited by A. E. Inglis. St. Louis, C. V. Mosby Company, 1982.
77. Wadsworth, T. G.: A new technique of total elbow replacement. Engin. Med. 10(2):69, 1981.
78. Walker, P. S.: Human Joints and Their Artificial Replacements. Springfield, Ill., Charles C Thomas, 1977.
79. Weiland, A. J., Weiss, A., Wills, R. P., and Moore, J. R.: Capitellocondylar total elbow replacement. A long-term follow-up study. J. Bone Joint Surg. 71A:217, 1989.
80. Wolfe, S. L., Figgie, M. P., Inglis, A. E., et al.: Management of infection about total elbow prosthesis. J. Bone Joint Surg. 72A:198, 1990.
81. Youm, Y., Dryer, R. F., Thambyrajah, K., et al.: Biomechanical analysis of forearm pronation-supination and elbow flexion-extension. J. Biomechanics 12:245–255, 1979.

CHAPTER 40

Total Wrist Replacement

LARRY K. CHIDGEY
PAUL C. DELL

The wrist joint extends from the metaphyseal portion of the radius to the carpometacarpal joints distally. Anatomically, the distal radioulnar joint should be considered separately, as its primary function is forearm supination and pronation. However, most diseases that involve the wrist joint also involve the distal radioulnar joint, so both areas must usually be addressed when total joint replacement is considered.

The eight carpal bones are arranged by four in a proximal row (scaphoid, lunate, triquetrum, and pisiform) and four in a distal row (trapezium, trapezoid, capitate, and hamate).[8, 15, 17, 18] The scaphoid acts as a bridge between the proximal and distal rows.[13] The radiocarpal joint refers to the joint between the proximal row and the distal radius, whereas the midcarpal joint refers to that between the proximal and distal carpal rows. The carpal bones are interconnected by a complex network of extrinsic and intrinsic ligaments.[32] The extrinsic ligaments span the radiocarpal and carpometacarpal joints or arise from the triangular fibrocartilage complex covering the ulnar head. The intrinsic ligaments are short structures interconnecting the individual carpal bones. The carpal ligaments, particularly the extrinsic group, blend intimately with the wrist capsule both dorsally and palmarly. Defining a plane between the wrist ligaments and the capsule is difficult. Some of the ligaments actually represent thickenings of the capsule.

A total of 24 tendons cross the wrist.[15] Five can be considered primary wrist-moving tendons, whereas the remainder cross the wrist on their way to the fingers and thumb. The carpal bones are arranged in a transverse arch, defining the carpal tunnel palmarly. This arrangement establishes a well-controlled path for the strong flexor tendons to the fingers. Dorsally, six fibro-osseous tunnels define the path of the wrist, thumb, and finger extensor tendons covered by the dorsal extensor retinaculum. The wrist has no true collateral ligament system. Instead, the extensor carpi ulnaris and the abductor pollicis longus/extensor pollicis brevis tendons act as the dynamic ulnar and the radial collateral ligaments, respectively. Kauer[19] has demonstrated the dynamic collateral ligament function of these muscle-tendon units with electromyography. Although these muscles are active during wrist flexion and extension, measurements in cadavers demonstrate very little excursion of the tendons during these movements. Therefore, these muscle-tendon units are active in an isometric sense and appear to act as dynamic collateral ligaments during pure flexion and extension of the wrist.

BIOMECHANICS

The kinematics of the carpal bones continues to be studied intensively. Different investigators have reported varying contributions of the radiocarpal and midcarpal

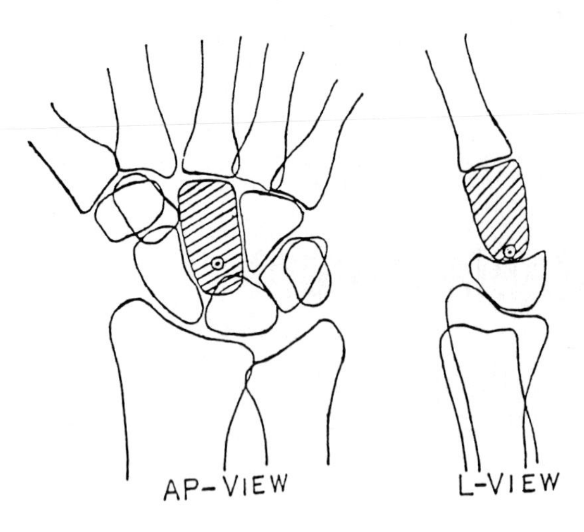

FIGURE 40–1. The center of rotation for composite wrist motion for flexion-extension and radial-ulnar deviation is located in the proximal capitate. The center is located more distally for radial-ulnar deviation. (Modified from Youm, Y. and Yoon, Y. S.: J. Biomechanics 12:613–621, 1979.)

joints to flexion-extension and radial-ulnar deviation. The only safe conclusion is that each joint contributes to each motion.[6, 22, 29, 30] Despite the complex motion of individual carpal bones, Youm and coworkers[37] have shown that the axis of composite wrist motion for both flexion-extension and radial-ulnar deviation passes through a fixed point in the capitate and does not change throughout the range of motion (Fig. 40–1). For radial and ulnar deviation, this point is located distal to the proximal end of the capitate by a distance equal to approximately a fourth of its total length. For flexion and extension, this point is located close to the proximal cortex of the capitate. Youm's study defined points through which the axes pass. However, no one has yet defined the angles these axes make with the wrist as they pass through the points, nor has it been determined whether these angles remain constant throughout the range of motion.

If the radiocarpal joint is disarticulated, the carpal surface resembles that of a section of a torus (a geometric body resembling a doughnut), with a different radius of curvature for flexion-extension than for radial-ulnar deviation (Fig. 40–2). The radius of the curvature for radial-ulnar deviation exceeds that for flexion-extension. The greater radius of curvature provides more stability and a smaller arc of motion in the radial-ulnar deviation plane than that in the flexion-extension plane. Conversely, the smaller radius of curvature in the dorsal-volar plane provides less stability but greater arc of motion. By decreasing the radius of curvature in the radial-ulnar deviation plane, as is done in some total wrist prosthetic designs resembling a ball and socket, it is more difficult maintaining stability in the radial-ulnar deviation plane.

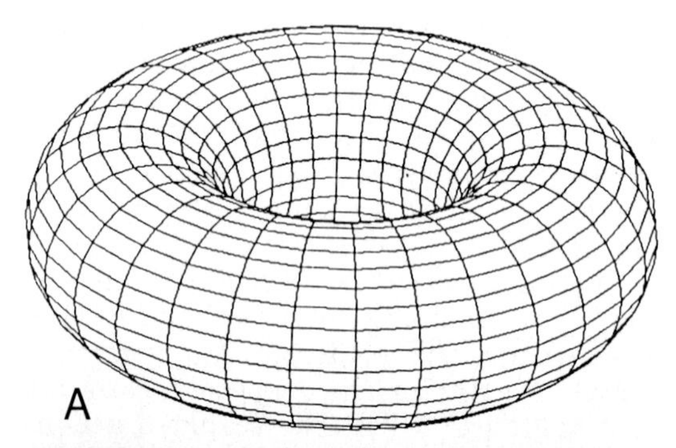

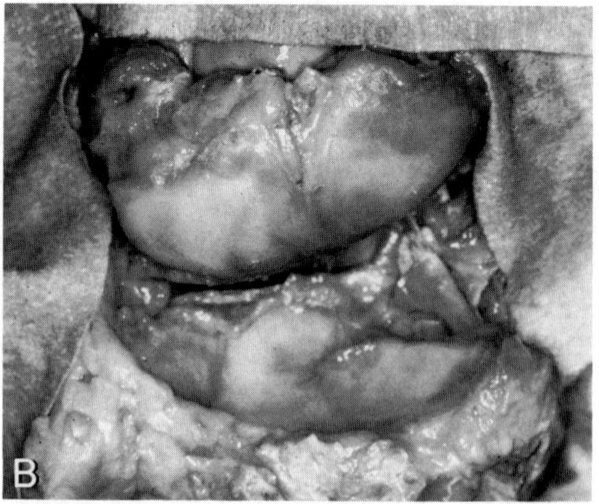

FIGURE 40–2. *A,* Torus (a geometric body resembling a doughnut). *B,* Disarticulated radiocarpal joint (proximal row bones at the top and distal radius at the bottom). The surface of the proximal carpal row is similar to a section of a torus with a larger radius of curvature for radial-ulnar deviation than for flexion-extension.

Agee[1] has discussed the important relationship between the underlying carpal bones and the overlying tendons. The relationship of the tendons to the axes of rotation, and thus the influence of muscle-tendon units on wrist motion, may be modified by the carpal bones throughout the range of motion. He has pointed out how the influence of the strong finger flexors on the wrist is minimized by the anatomy of the carpal tunnel. The carpal tunnel maintains these strong flexors close to the axis of wrist motion, thereby decreasing their moment at the wrist. Agee has also demonstrated how the movement of individual carpal bones can influence the dorsal extensor tendons and adjust their moment arms. A review of the complex interaction between the carpal bones and the overlying tendons makes it obvious that present total wrist prosthetic designs fall far short of duplicating nature.

SURGICAL APPROACHES

The patient is placed supine. The hand is positioned on a table. A pneumatic tourniquet is placed around the upper arm. A dorsal longitudinal incision is made 10 to 12 cm in line with the third metacarpal, extending across the wrist joint (Fig. 40–3A). The superficial radial and ulnar sensory nerves are identified and protected. As many superficial veins as possible are saved by sacrificing only the transverse veins and leaving the longitudinal veins intact and retracting them. The degree of postoperative swelling is proportional to the number of superficial veins that can be saved. The extensor retinaculum is exposed and opened with a step-cut incision over the fifth dorsal compartment containing the extensor digiti quinti (Fig. 40–3B). The extensor retinaculum is elevated both ulnarly and radially, exposing the second

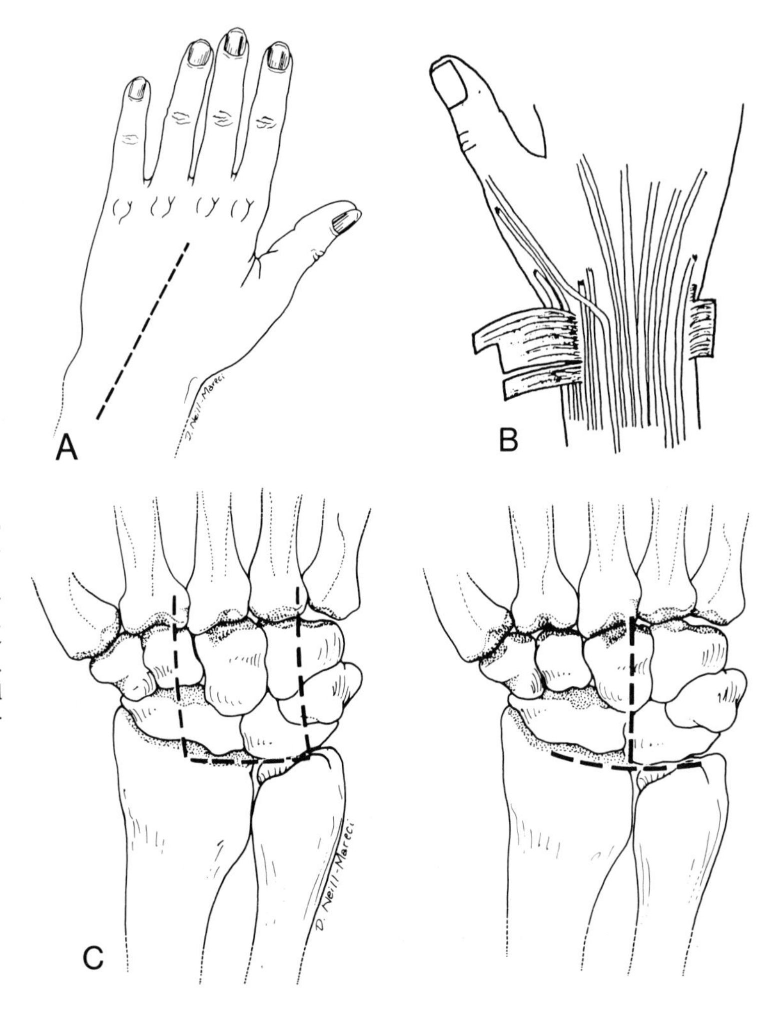

FIGURE 40–3. *A,* Dorsal longitudinal incision for wrist arthroplasty. *B,* Extensor retinaculum opened over the fifth compartment with a step cut. The ulnar portion of the step cut will be used to create a sling for the extensor carpi ulnaris tendon. The radial flap is split into a distal flap to reinforce the dorsal capsule and a proximal flap to reconstruct the extensor retinaculum over the tendons. (Swanson, A. B., de Groot Swanson, G., and Maupin, B. K.: Clin. Orthop. 187:94–106, 1984. By permission.) *C,* The dorsal capsular incision may be elevated as a distally based flap or a T-shaped incision.

through sixth dorsal compartments. The long radial extensor retinacular flap is then divided in line with the collagen direction, creating proximal and distal flaps. The proximal flap is later used to reconstruct the extensor retinaculum over the extensor tendons. The distal flap is utilized to reinforce the capsule palmar to the extensor tendons. The step-cut portion is employed to recreate a sling for the extensor carpi ulnaris tendon. The distal radioulnar joint is then opened through a longitudinal incision. The distal 2 cm of the ulna is exposed by reflecting the capsule and retinaculum subperiosteally. Enough distal ulna is resected to permit clearance of the radial sigmoid notch.

The underlying wrist capsule with accompanying dorsal ligaments is opened and developed in a single layer. This maneuver is done with either of two capsular incisions. The capsular incision recommended by Swanson and coworkers[31] for the insertion of the flexible implant arthroplasty is made by first completing a transverse incision at the radiocarpal joint and extending the incision both radially and ulnarly to the carpometacarpal joint area (Fig. 40–3C). The capsule is then raised sharply from the underlying carpal bones, creating a distally based flap. An alternative capsular incision is a T-shaped incision made by first opening the radiocarpal joint with a transverse incision and completing the T with a second incision, extending to the base of the third metacarpal (Fig. 40–3C). The radial- and ulnar-based flaps are elevated from the underlying carpal bones. On completion of prosthesis insertion, each flap is secured back to the distal radius through drill holes.

INDICATIONS

In selecting treatment for a patient with destructive bony changes in the wrist joint, the surgeon should consider the patient's age; occupation; leisure activities; area of bone and joint involvement; cause and severity of destructive changes; and associated involvement of muscles and tendons, proximal and distal joints, contralateral limb, and lower extremities. When the primary destructive changes are confined to the radiocarpal joint, as in early rheumatoid involvement, excellent results have been reported after radiocarpal fusion.[27] Usually the radius, scaphoid, and lunate are fused and may be fixated by either crossed Kirschner wires or staples. Nalebuff and Millender[27] reported that pain was alleviated in these patients while 30 to 40 degrees of mid row motion was preserved.

When patients have painful destructive changes of both the radiocarpal and midcarpal joints and lesser procedures are no longer useful (e.g., synovectomy, proximal row carpectomy, and limited carpal fusions) essentially three alternatives remain: resection arthroplasty, implant arthroplasty, and total wrist arthrodesis. Resection arthroplasty can be performed without the insertion of an implant, in an attempt to establish a fibrous ankylosis at the wrist joint.[2, 16, 20] Synovectomy, debridement, and temporary Kirschner wire stabilization may be undertaken in an attempt to obtain a stable wrist with restricted motion. A palmar shelf may be created from the distal radius on which the carpus may rest in an effort to improve stability.[2] Although excellent results were reported in 55 percent of a limited series, in general these procedures have been unpredictable. As an alternative to constructing a palmar shelf, an interpositional fascial arthroplasty may be constructed by suturing a flap of dorsal wrist capsule to the volar wrist capsule after resecting the proximal carpal row and proximal half of the capitate. A study in 1989[12] demonstrated satisfactory results in 11 of 14 patients who underwent this procedure. This procedure may be applicable to the patient with a history of septic destruction of the wrist joint who requires some maintenance of motion.

The other two surgical procedures to consider are a total wrist arthrodesis and an implant arthroplasty (either a flexible interpositional implant or a total wrist arthroplasty). Although specific indications and contraindications exist for these procedures, the final decision is often difficult to make and requires a great deal of input from the patient. Patients with rheumatoid arthritis often have involvement of the proximal and distal joints as well as the contralateral limb. Eliminating wrist motion through arthrodesis may significantly add to functional impairment in these patients. In contrast, a young patient who performs heavy manual labor and has monoarticular traumatic arthritis may be better served by a stable, durable arthrodesis. In this situation, we favor an arthrodesis in approximately 20 to 30 degrees of dorsiflexion with an appropriate length of 3.5-mm compression plate (Fig. 40–4). Preoperative placement using a wrist splint of varying positions may help the surgeon select the proper individual position. The patient should be aware that in approximately 50 percent of cases, a second operation is necessary to remove the internal fixation.

A few specific contraindications exist to arthroplasty, such as wrist joint sepsis, loss of wrist extensors,[21] and open physeal plates. However, most of the indications and contraindications are relative. For example, a young musician may require specific wrist motions to continue playing an instrument or an automotive mechanic may require specific wrist motions to repair an engine. In general, arthrodesis should be seriously considered for patients under 50 years old, those who load the wrist repeatedly in their work, or those who must lift more than 10 pounds regularly.[3, 33]

FLEXIBLE IMPLANT ARTHROPLASTY

In 1967, Swanson introduced a flexible hinge implant for use in combination with resection arthroplasty.[23] This implant has a proximal and distal stem with a barrel-shaped midsection, slightly flattened on its dorsal and palmar surfaces (Figs. 40–5A and 40–5B). Initially, the implant was constructed of silicone #372 elastomer, which demonstrated a significantly high tear rate. Since 1974, a higher performance silicone elastomer has been utilized, with additional reinforcement by a Dacron core.[31] The implant is available in five sizes. Also, a wide midsection is now available in addition to the standard midsection. It was introduced to separate the joint space better and to help prevent subsidence of the implant into bone. Because up to 20 percent of implants were found to tear on

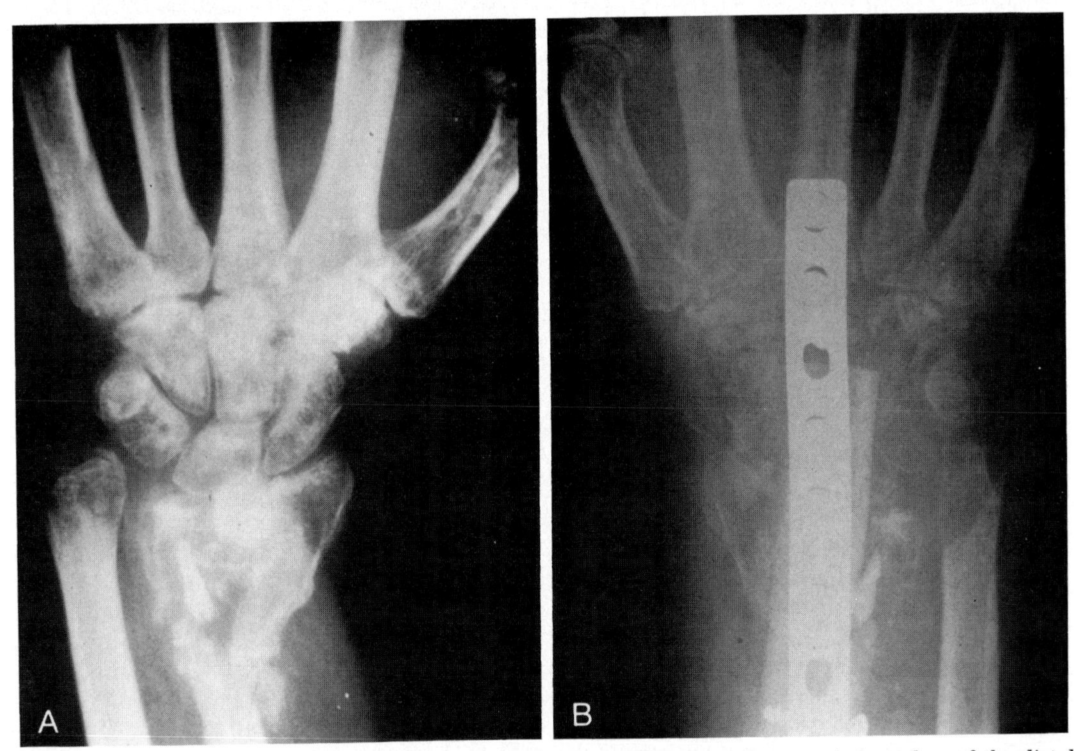

FIGURE 40–4. *A*, Preoperative wrist of a young manual laborer showing traumatic bone loss of the distal radius and disruption of the articular surface. *B*, Wrist of the same patient after arthrodesis using a 3.5-mm compression plate.

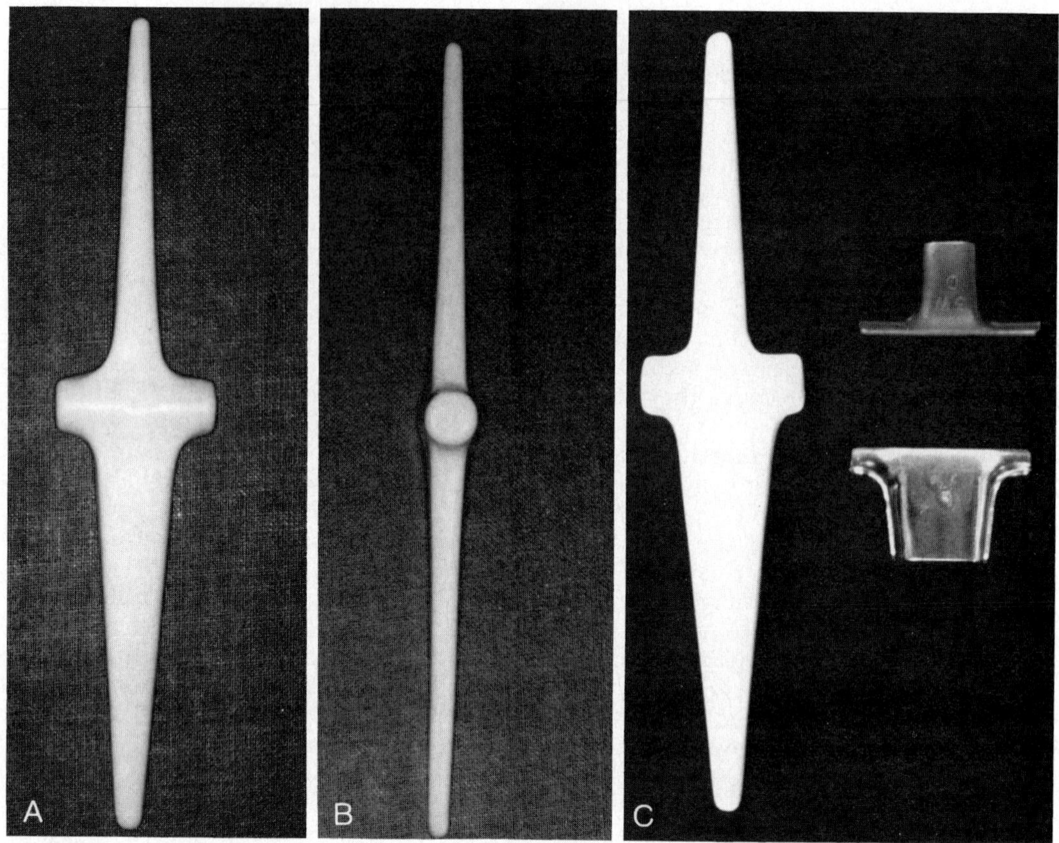

FIGURE 40–5. *A* and *B*, Anteroposterior and lateral views of the Swanson silicone interpositional wrist arthroplasty. *C*, Silicone implant with titanium grommets.

the bone edges of the medullary canal,[7, 11] titanium metal bone liners (grommets) have been introduced to improve durability (Figs. 40–5C and 40–6). Theoretically, they act as shielding devices to protect the implant from sharp bone edges.[23] In an experimental model, Peimer[28] has shown, however, that the tear rate and tear location within the prosthesis are similar with or without grommets.

The flexible implant is not a total prosthesis but should be considered a resection arthroplasty with interposition of a silicone rubber spacer. The spacer helps maintain an adequate joint space and overall wrist alignment, whereas a new capsuloligamentous system develops around the midsection of the implant. Cinefluorography studies indicate that motion not only occurs through the flexible midsection but also occurs as the stems (not fixed into bone) slide in and out of the intramedullary canal.[23]

Operative Technique (Swanson)

The wrist joint is exposed through the dorsal approach previously described. The dorsal capsuloligamentous structures are reflected as a single distally based flap. The scaphoid, lunate and triquetrum, which are often partially fragmented, are excised piecemeal employing a rongeur (Fig. 40–7A). The distal half of the scaphoid may be retained to help support the thumb. In resecting these carpal bones, care is taken to preserve the palmar radiocarpal ligaments and capsule. If capsular detachment occurs from either the radius or carpus, reattachment is necessary before final implant insertion. The proximal half of the capitate is excised, and the distal end of the radius is squared off perpendicular to its longitudinal axis. Just enough bone is resected to allow complete reduction of the carpus on the end of the radius,

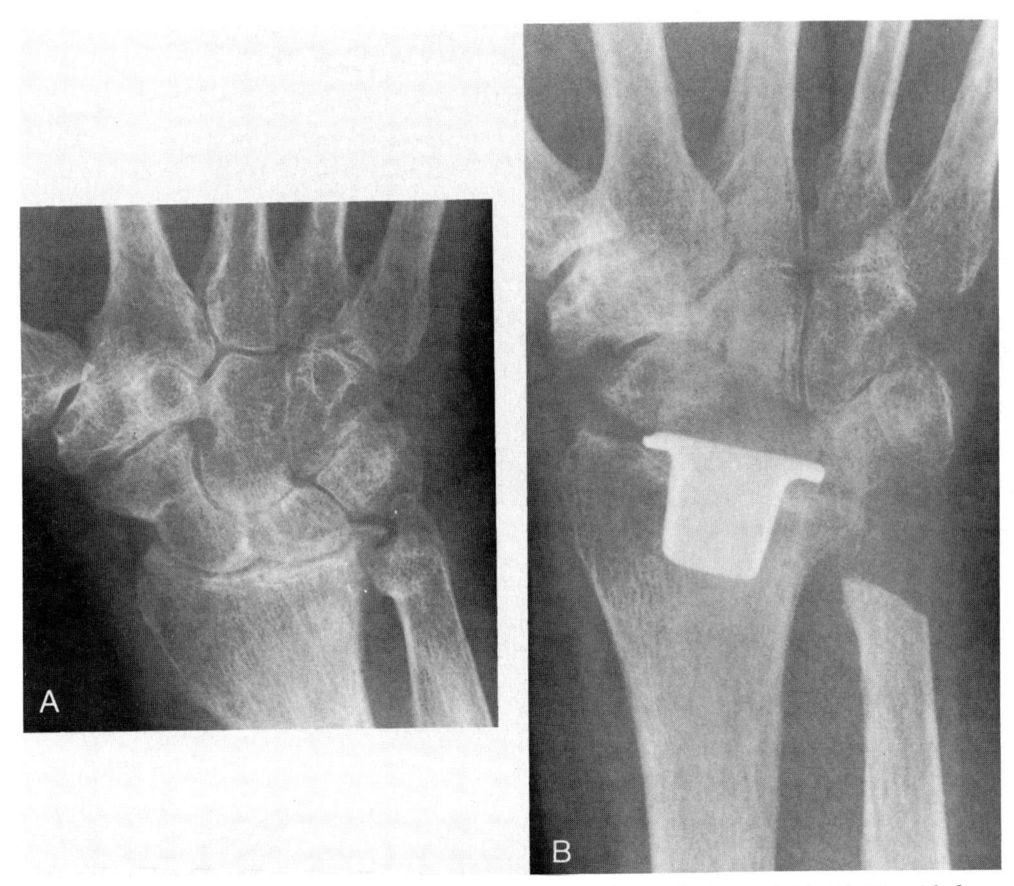

FIGURE 40–6. *A*, Preoperative radiograph of the wrist of a patient with rheumatoid arthritis with destructive changes involving the radiocarpal joint, the midcarpal joint, and the distal radial-ulnar joint. *B*, Radiograph following flexible interpositional arthroplasty using titanium grommets.

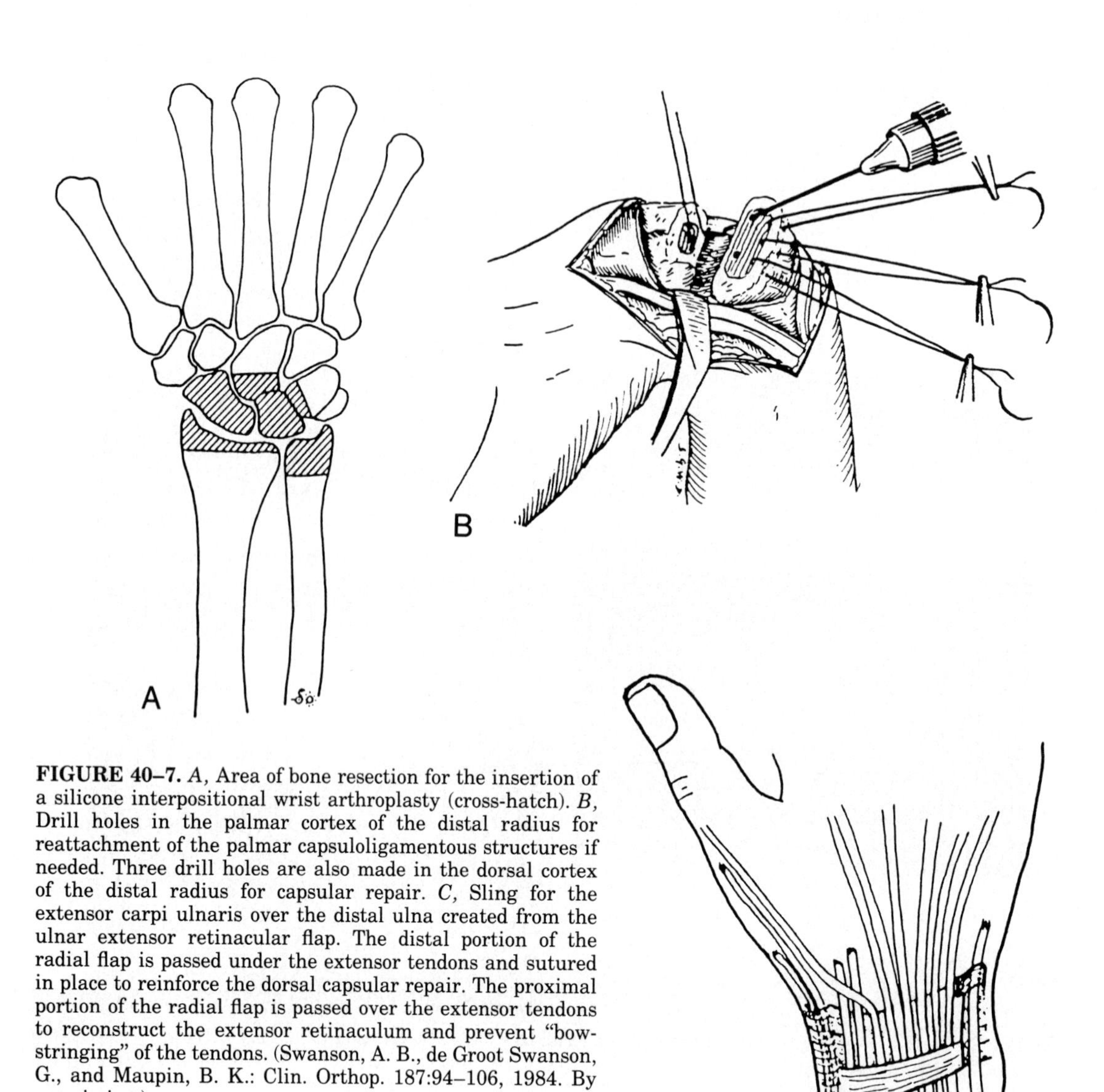

FIGURE 40–7. *A,* Area of bone resection for the insertion of a silicone interpositional wrist arthroplasty (cross-hatch). *B,* Drill holes in the palmar cortex of the distal radius for reattachment of the palmar capsuloligamentous structures if needed. Three drill holes are also made in the dorsal cortex of the distal radius for capsular repair. *C,* Sling for the extensor carpi ulnaris over the distal ulna created from the ulnar extensor retinacular flap. The distal portion of the radial flap is passed under the extensor tendons and sutured in place to reinforce the dorsal capsular repair. The proximal portion of the radial flap is passed over the extensor tendons to reconstruct the extensor retinaculum and prevent "bowstringing" of the tendons. (Swanson, A. B., de Groot Swanson, G., and Maupin, B. K.: Clin. Orthop. 187:94–106, 1984. By permission.)

allowing enough space for the implant. Approximately 1 to 1.5 cm of separation between the radius and carpus is needed. The carpus should be resected only as far distally as the proximal capitate, with any additional bone resected from the radius. The distal medullary canal is prepared first. A small thin broach or Kirschner wire is passed through the capitate into the medullary canal of the third metacarpal. If any doubt exists regarding the position within the medullary canal, a small Kirschner wire may be drilled out through the third metacarpal head with the proximal phalanx fully flexed. Alternatively, an intraoperative radiograph may be obtained (Fig. 40–8). A fine curette or an air drill is utilized for the final preparation of the canal.

The intramedullary canal of the radius is prepared by first defining the orientation of the canal with a small curette. Final preparation is done with a broach or an air drill. Trial implants are selected to determine the proper implant size. The proximal stem is first inserted into the medullary canal of the radius. The distal stem is then inserted into the third metacarpal. The largest implant that will fit without buckling is selected. This stem may require shortening if it protrudes more distally than the metaphyseal area of the third metacarpal.

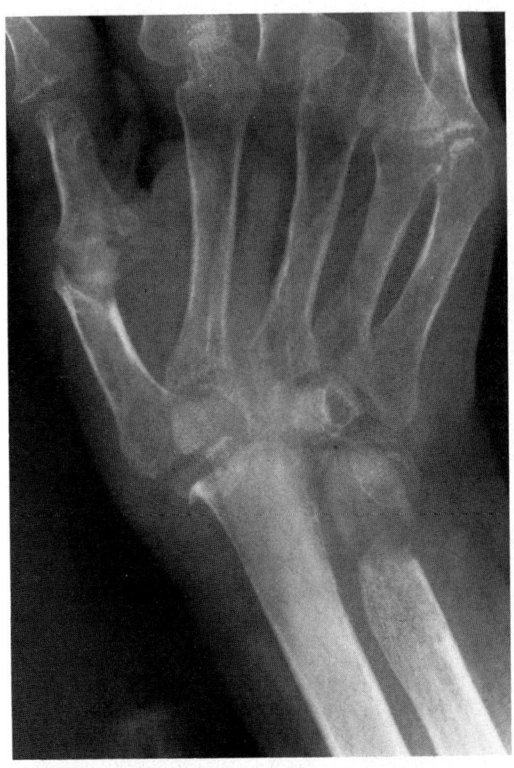

FIGURE 40–8. Radiograph of the wrist demonstrating a technical error during flexible implant insertion. The distal stem was placed into the soft tissues and not into the third metacarpal canal. Intraoperative confirmation of proper stem placement is recommended.

If titanium grommets are employed, the size corresponding to the selected implant size is employed. The distal grommet press-fits into the dorsal surface of the capitate. The proximal grommet inserts into the palmar side of the radius. Further preparation of the intramedullary canal may be required to allow a flush fit of the grommets. When the canal is prepared, it should allow a secure press-fit of the grommets with gentle pressure. A trial reduction with the grommets in place is again performed with special attention to assure no impingement of the distal grommet with the implant. Once proper sizing has been confirmed, the trial implant and grommets are removed.

If the palmar capsuloligamentous structures need repairing, two to three drill holes are made in the distal palmar radius or the palmar capitate, as needed. The palmar structures are repaired with a 3-0 nonabsorbable braided suture (Fig. 40–7B). Three drill holes are then made in the dorsal distal radius, and a 3-0 nonabsorbable braided suture is passed through these holes for later dorsal capsular repair. The grommets, if used, and the implant are then inserted with the no-touch technique. The proximal stem is first inserted into the radial canal. The distal stem is then inserted into the third metacarpal canal. The dorsal capsule is secured to the distal radius employing the previously placed sutures. The repair of the capsular structures is tested by moving the wrist through 30 degrees of extension and flexion and 10 degrees of radial and ulnar deviation. The distal retinacular flap is passed underneath the extensor tendons and utilized to reinforce the dorsal capsular repair (Fig. 40–7C). The distal ulnar step-cut flap is used to secure the extensor carpi ulnaris over the dorsum of the ulna. Any extensor tendon repairs or transfers are then completed.

The pull of the wrist extensors should

also be assessed. To help correct radial deviation of the wrist, the extensor carpi radialis longus may be transferred to the extensor carpi radialis brevis insertion by interweaving it with the brevis tendon, or it may be transferred even further ulnarly by interweaving it with the extensor carpi ulnaris tendon. The proximal extensor retinacular flap is then repaired over the extensor tendons to prevent tendon "bowstringing."

The skin is loosely closed over a subcutaneous drain, and a bulky dressing is applied incorporating either a long-arm splint or a sugar tong–like splint with the forearm maintained in supination. The dressing is removed in 3 to 5 days, and either a short-arm circular cast or thermoplastic splint is applied. If extensor tendons have been repaired, an "outrigger" with rubber band slings is incorporated to keep the fingers in extension. Wrist immobilization is continued for 6 weeks. Range-of-motion exercises are begun with only 50 to 60 degrees of total flexion and extension being the goal. A greater arc of motion has been associated with increased implant failure.

TOTAL WRIST ARTHROPLASTY

Following the success of total joint arthroplasty elsewhere in the body, Meuli[24] and Volz[34] each developed a prosthesis for total wrist arthroplasty in the early 1970s. Meuli's original design incorporated a ball-and-socket trunnion with two-stemmed metal proximal and distal components and an interposed polyethylene ball. The two stems of the distal component were originally inserted into the second and third metacarpals (Fig. 40–9).

Volz's original design had a two-stemmed proximal component with a polyethylene cup. The distal component also had two stems inserted into the second and third metacarpals. The articulating sur-

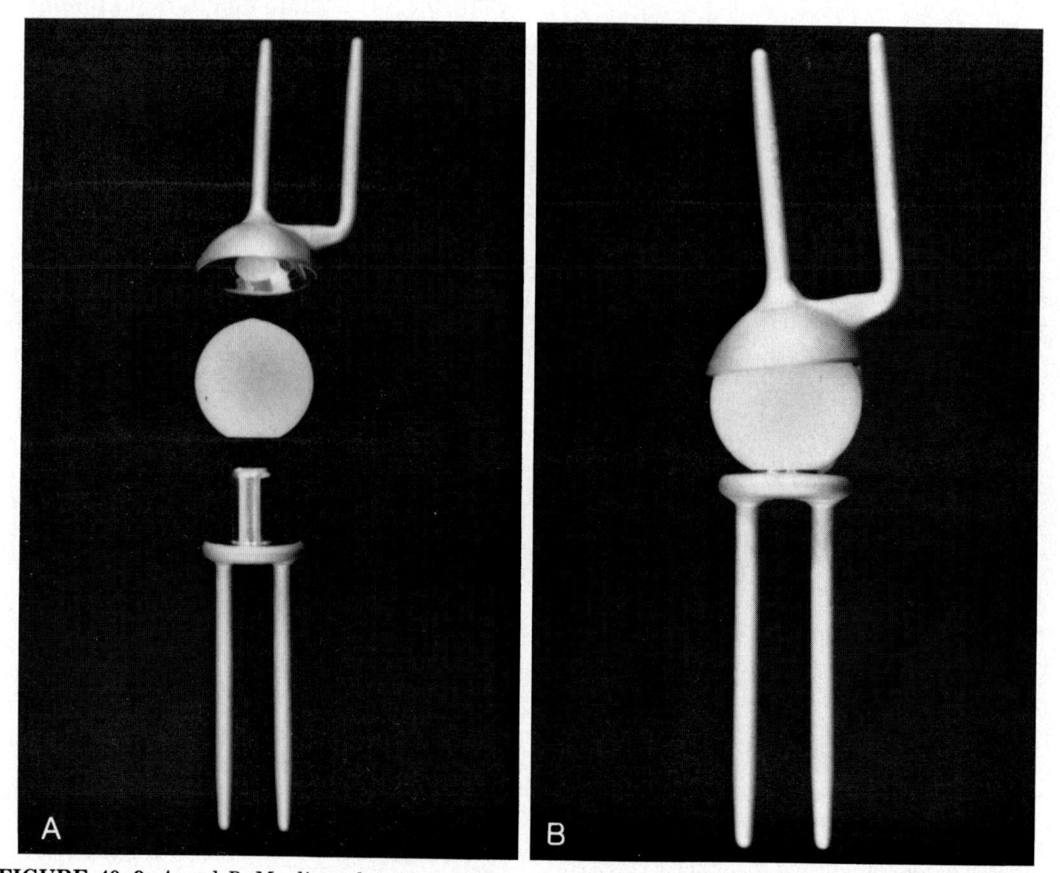

FIGURE 40–9. *A* and *B*, Meuli total wrist prosthesis. A polyethylene ball is interposed between distal and proximal metal components. The two stems of the distal component are offset in an attempt to better align the center of rotation of the prosthesis with the true wrist axis.

face of the distal component was not a true sphere but a segment of a torus with a larger radius of curvature for radial-ulnar deviation than for flexion-extension. The Meuli design functioned more as a true ball-and-socket joint, allowing triaxial motion.[24, 25] In contrast, the range of motion with the Volz design was more restricted, allowing 90 degrees of flexion-extension and 50 degrees of radial-ulnar deviation.

Although the Meuli design allows a greater range of motion, Beckenbaugh[3] has pointed out that the Volz design actually has more "play" between its distal and proximal components. Therefore, the Meuli design allows less dissipation of force across the articulation and thus transmits more of the force to the intramedullary stems.

Problems with the initial design of both of these prostheses related primarily to maintaining a balanced wrist alignment.[4, 10, 21] Each design incorporated a distal component with a stem in the second and third metacarpals, centering the radial-ulnar deviation axis between the two. Because the prosthetic center of rotation is radial to the normal wrist's center of rotation,[37] many patients developed ulnar deviation deformities owing to increased moment arms of the ulnar wrist tendons. The prosthetic center of rotation was also more dorsal than that of the normal wrist, increasing the flexion moment arm. Thus, some patients developed both ulnar deviation and flexion deformities. Modifications in both designs have attempted to approximate the normal wrist axis more closely (Fig. 40–10).[3, 26, 36]

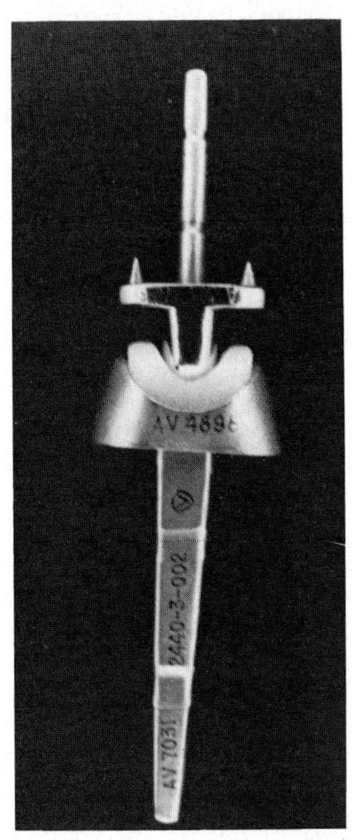

FIGURE 40–10. Volz total wrist prosthesis. The single-stem distal component is a modification of an earlier double-stemmed component in an attempt to better align the prosthesis axis. (Taleisnik, J.: The Wrist. New York, Churchill Livingstone, 1985. By permission.)

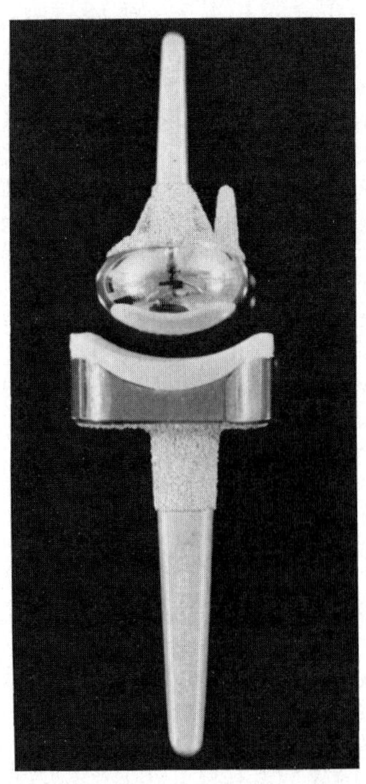

FIGURE 40–11. Biax total wrist prosthesis. The articulating surface forms an ellipsoid with a larger radius of curvature for radial-ulnar deviation than for flexion-extension. The periarticular surfaces of the distal and proximal stems are porous coated.

Beckenbaugh and Linscheid[5] introduced a design called the Biax total wrist prosthesis (Fig. 40–11). The distal articulating surface forms an ellipsoid. The radius of curvature for radial-ulnar deviation is larger than that for flexion-extension—closely approximating that of the normal wrist.[37] The distal component has a long stem to fit into the third metacarpal and a short fixation stem to fit into the trapezoid for rotational stability of the distal component. The proximal component consists of a broad polyethylene-bearing surface set into a metal tray. The radial stem of the proximal component is offset both dorsally and radially to align both the radial-ulnar deviation axis and the flexion-extension axis close to that of the normal wrist. The periarticular surfaces of both the proximal and distal stems have been porous coated to enhance cement fixation and to improve stress distribution, especially in the proximal component.

The surgical procedure for the Biax total wrist prosthesis is similar to that for both of the newer designs of the Meuli and Volz prostheses. The surgical procedure for the Biax is described next.

Operative Technique (Beckenbaugh)

The wrist is approached dorsally, and the extensor retinaculum is elevated as previously described. The distal ulna is also exposed and resected as described. The dorsal capsule is elevated utilizing the T-shaped incision, and the carpus and distal radius are exposed. The remnants of the proximal carpal row are resected along with the head of the capitate employing a rongeur. The distal radius is resected perpendicular to the long axis of the radius with a power saw. The intramedullary canal of the third metacarpal is defined using a sharp awl or Steinmann pin driven through the capitate into the metacarpal. Presence within the third metacarpal intramedullary canal may be confirmed by inserting a blunt-tipped instrument down the medullary canal until it strikes the head of the metacarpal. The canal is progressively enlarged with a combination of the metacarpal rasp and larger pins. The medullary canal of the radius is then defined with a pointed awl or pin and the canal enlarged with a combination of a rongeur and radial rasp. Care must be taken in the preparation of the medullary canal both distally and proximally to ensure that components are maintained parallel to the transverse axis of the radius and hand.

Once the medullary canals have been prepared, the trial distal and proximal components without a porous coating are positioned and the wrist is reduced. The recommended tension between the two components is such that longitudinal pulling on the hand will distract the wrist 1 to 2 mm. The largest size possible is selected. Intraoperative radiographs are recommended to confirm the position of the trial components. The porous coating on the periarticular surfaces of the proximal and distal components is not accounted for by the trial implants and will result in a snug fit of the final components.

The trial components are removed, and three small drill holes are placed in the cortical bone of the distal radius for reattachment of the dorsal capsule. A 3-0 nonabsorbable suture is passed through each of these drill holes prior to final component insertion. A cancellous bone plug is inserted down the third metacarpal shaft, using the rasp to seat the plug. A proximal plug in the radius is not needed. Methyl methacrylate cement is mixed and injected with a 12-ml syringe into the medullary canals of the third metacarpal and radius. The distal component is seated first by using the appropriate size metacarpal driver. The proximal component with the appropriate radial driver is seated next. Care must be taken during seating to maintain appropriate rotational alignment of the components. Excess cement is trimmed, the wrist articulated, and compression maintained until the cement has set. Intraoperative radiographs may be made to confirm appropriate positioning and cement filling. The wrist is taken through a passive range of motion to assure that no impingement occurs between the prosthetic components and the remaining carpal bones. Any excess bone should be excised. The dorsal capsule is secured to the distal radius with the previously placed 3-0 nonabsorbable braided suture. The distal portion of the extensor retinaculum is placed underneath the extensor tendons. This step reinforces the dorsal capsule while maintaining the proximal portion over the extensor tendons and prevents tendon bowstringing. The skin is closed loosely over a drain. A bulky compression dressing is applied incorporating a long-arm splint or sugar tong–like splint.

The drain is removed in 1 to 2 days and long-arm immobilization continued for 2 weeks. The dressing is removed. Short-arm immobilization is continued for 2 more weeks. Additional immobilization is determined by the intraoperative range of motion. If the patient had only 10 to 15 degrees of flexion and extension, as little as 2 weeks of immobilization is recommended. If the patient had greater than 60 degrees of flexion and extension, the cast should remain for up to 8 weeks. Once immobilization is discontinued, gentle range of motion exercises are begun. A splint should be worn at night for an additional 6 weeks. The postoperative goal of range of motion should be approximately 40 degrees of flexion, 40 degrees of extension, and 10 degrees of radial and ulnar deviation.

RESULTS

Flexible Implant Arthroplasty

Early results with flexible implant arthroplasty have shown good relief of pain, maintenance of preoperative range of motion, and correction of deformity.[7, 11, 14, 31] However, 5 years postoperatively, 70 percent of patients have shown radiographic deterioration; of these, 20 percent have actual implant fracture (Fig. 40–12).[7, 11] All 71 patients in one study were noted to have subsidence of the prosthesis into the radius, carpus, or both with longitudinal wrist collapse.[7] In another study of 53 silicone rubber prostheses,[11] subsidence was noted in 70 percent, with settling of the implant into the distal radius, carpus, or both, and abutment of the remaining carpus on the distal radius. Prosthetic breakage was 9 percent, and the reoperation rate was 25 percent. In these patients, radiographic deterioration did not directly correlate with clinical failure, similar to arthroplasty of other joints. Despite the high radiograph deterioration rate, 60 percent of patients at 5 years maintained good clinical results.[7, 11] Postoperative range of motion cannot be expected to improve when compared with preoperative meas-

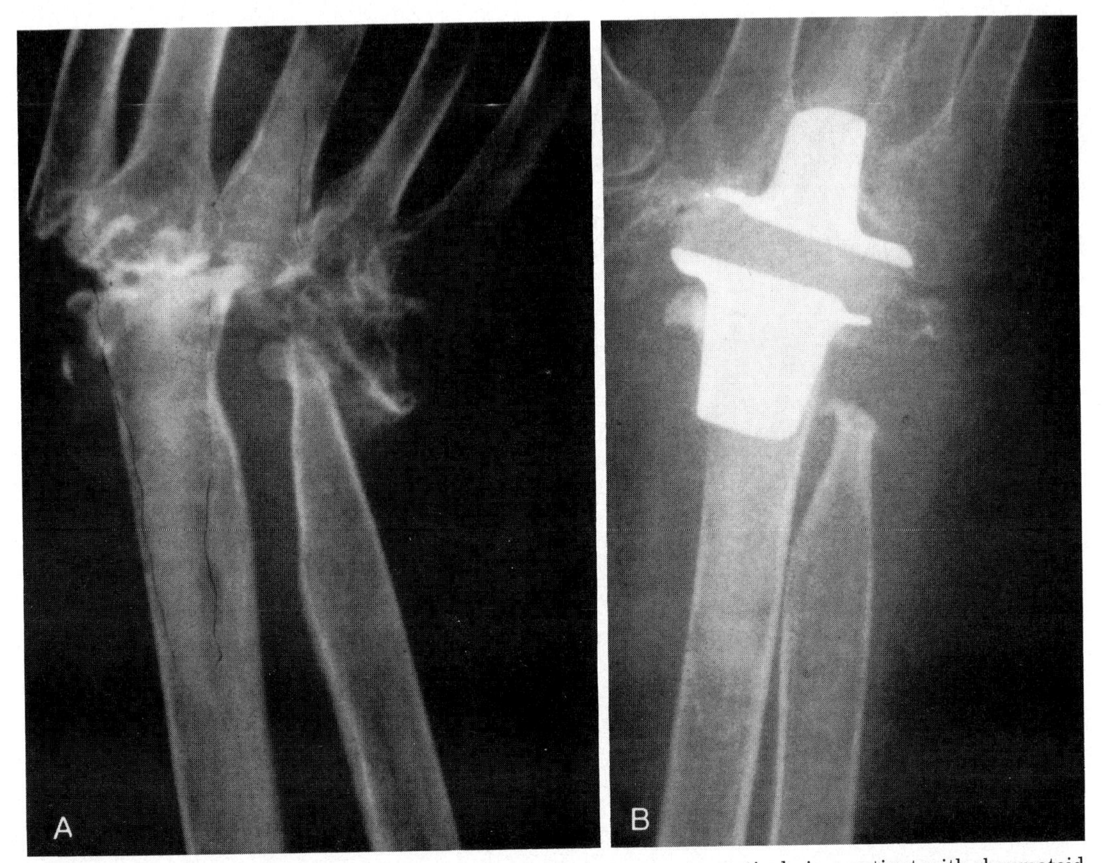

FIGURE 40–12. *A*, Flexible interpositional arthroplasty 4 years postoperatively in a patient with rheumatoid arthritis. Implant has fractured at the base of the distal stem with ulnar subluxation of the hand and wrist. *B*, Radiograph after revision arthroplasty with another flexible implant and titanium grommets.

urements, but the arc of motion is changed to a more functional range. No improvement in strength can be expected, partly because of finger involvement in many patients with rheumatoid arthritis.[35] Failures have been linked directly to heavy use and increased postoperative range of motion,[7] prompting recommendations for longer postoperative immobilization with the goal of less motion and improved stability.

Total Wrist Arthroplasty

Early follow-up data for total wrist arthroplasty have been similar to those for flexible implant arthroplasty in the ability of these procedures to relieve pain and maintain preoperative range of motion.[24, 34] Besides the initial complications related to doubled-stemmed distal components with the development of ulnar and flexion deformities, problems have related mainly to stem loosening and stress shielding of the distal radius.[4, 9] The incidence of stem loosening and stress shielding has been as high as 50 percent in patients with the Meuli prostheses.[23] Radiographic deterioration after total wrist arthroplasty has not been associated with significant pain, just as it has not after flexible implant arthroplasty. With palmar subluxation of the distal component, patients more often present with median nerve compression or flexor tendon ruptures (Fig. 40–13).[9] Loosening has not been as frequent with the Volz prosthesis,[9, 10, 21] possibly because it is less constrained functionally. However, an average of 3.7-mm bone resorption has occurred under the radial collar in 79 percent of cases and metacarpal component loosening has occurred in 24 percent. Good results have been reported in 60 percent of cases with both single- and double-stemmed distal components of the Volz design[10]; good results have been reported in 47 percent of patients with the double-stemmed distal component and 77 percent of those with the single-stemmed distal component.[10] The competence of the extensor carpi radialis brevis and the degree of correction of palmar and ulnar contracture have been two of the most important determinants of a final good result with the Volz design.[21]

FAILURES AND COMPLICATIONS

Results of revision of a broken silicone prosthesis with another implant have not been encouraging. In one study, four of 12 patients refractured the second prostheses; only four of the patients with second prostheses had adequate strength for activities of daily living.[7] Clinical experience with replacement of silicone prostheses with a total wrist is too limited to permit conclusions at this time. Dislocations of total wrist implants have been infrequent and may be treated by closed reductions in many cases.[9, 36]

Arthrodesis remains the standard revision procedure for failure of both silicone interpositional and total wrist arthroplasties. A bone graft is necessary and is usually obtained from either the lateral or medial surface of the ilium. A medial iliac graft, because of the cortical concavity, allows good positioning of the wrist and good cancellous bone contact with the freshened surfaces of the radius and carpus. Alternately, an iliac bone graft may be fashioned into the shape of a wrist prosthesis and inserted into the medullary canals of the radius and third metacarpal. Fixation may be obtained with an intramedullary Steinmann pin or external fixator.

Infections have been reported in less than 2 percent of cases.[9] When they occur, the implant is removed and the infection is cleared with appropriate debridement and antibiotics. The wrist may then be salvaged with an arthrodesis. Alternatively, the wrist may be left as a resection arthroplasty; however, clinical experience is limited with this technique. Unlike results for the lower extremity, the results of immediate or delayed implant exchange after infection are unknown.

SUMMARY AND CONCLUSIONS

Particular technical points are common to both interpositional and total wrist arthroplasties. Foremost is correction of the deformity. Frequently, longstanding flexion and ulnar deviation lead to profound soft tissue contracture. Adequate soft tis-

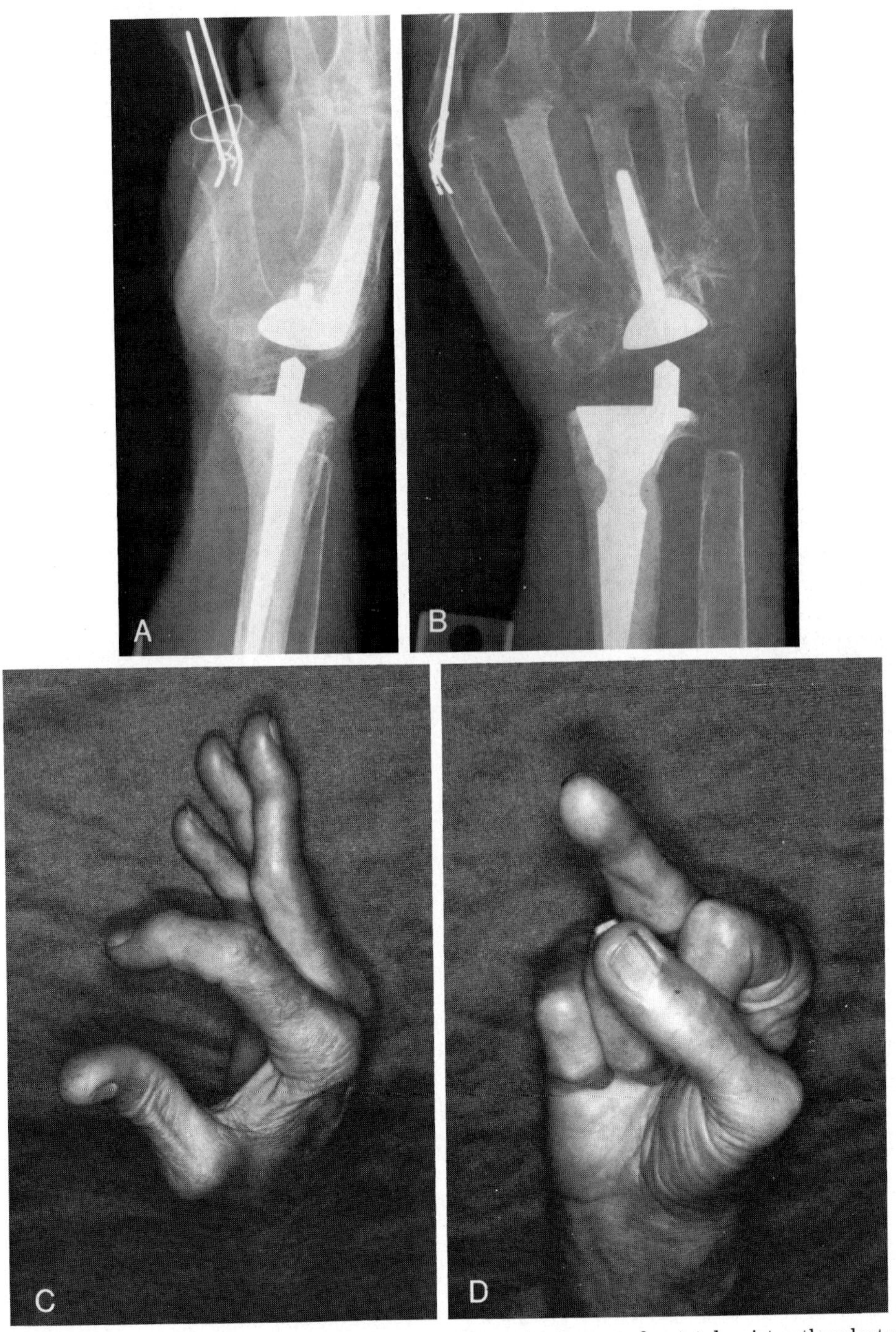

FIGURE 40–13. Lateral (*A*) and anteroposterior (*B*) radiographs 4 years after total wrist arthroplasty. *C* and *D*, Patient presented with inability to actively flex the long finger. Surgical exploration revealed an attritional rupture of the flexor tendons to this finger over the palmar edge of the implant.

sue release is mandatory, even requiring volar capsular release. Muscle-tendon rebalancing begins with inspection of the wrist extensors during initial dissection. A functional or reconstructed extensor carpi radialis brevis is essential. Other considerations for rebalancing include tenotomies of the flexor carpi ulnaris and palmaris longus tendons. Proper seating of the distal stem of a silicone rubber prosthesis in the third metacarpal and proper centering of a total wrist implant along the ulnar border of the distal radius decrease the likelihood of recurrent deformity, stress, and prosthetic failure.

Prosthetic design continues to evolve. Currently, the best candidate for a silicone rubber interpositional arthroplasty is a patient with inactive rheumatoid arthritis whose demands on the wrist are low. Total wrist arthroplasty may be indicated in the patient with good bone stock, a surgically correctable deformity, and a potential for balanced wrist mechanics. For the severely deformed or unstable wrist, we believe that total arthrodesis is a reliable procedure for producing a pain-free, well-aligned wrist. We continue to explore other reconstructive procedures, including radiocarpal synovectomy, distal ulnar resections or Suave'-Kapandji procedures, and limited wrist arthrodeses.

References

1. Agee, J. M.: Personal communication, 1987.
2. Albright, J. A. and Chase, R. A.: Palmar-shelf arthroplasty of the wrist in rheumatoid arthritis. J. Bone Joint Surg. 52:896, 1970.
3. Beckenbaugh, R. D.: Total joint arthroplasty. The wrist. Mayo Clin. Proc. 54:513, 1979.
4. Beckenbaugh, R. D. and Linscheid, R. L.: Total wrist arthroplasty: A preliminary report. J. Hand Surg. 2:337–344, 1977.
5. Beckenbaugh, R. D. and Linscheid, R. L.: Arthroplasty in the Hand and Wrist. Operative Hand Surgery, 2nd ed., vol. 1. Edited by D. P. Green. New York, Churchill Livingstone, 1988.
6. Berger, R. A., Crowninshield, R. D., and Flatt, A. E.: The three-dimensional rotational behaviors of the carpal bones. Clin. Orthop. 167:303–310, 1982.
7. Brase, D. W. and Millender, L. H.: Failure of silicone rubber wrist arthroplasty in rheumatoid arthritis. J. Hand Surg. 11A:175–183, 1986.
8. Brash, J. C. and Jamieson, E. B.: Cunningham's Textbook of Anatomy, 8th ed. New York, Oxford University Press, 1943.
9. Cooney, III, W. P., Beckenbaugh, R. D., and Linscheid, R. L.: Total wrist arthroplasty: Problems with implant failures. Clin. Orthop. 187:121–128, 1984.
10. Dennis, D. A., Ferlic, D. C., and Clayton, M. L.: Volz total wrist arthroplasty in rheumatoid arthritis: A long-term review. J. Hand Surg. 11A:483–490, 1986.
11. Fatti, J. F., Palmer, A. K., and Mosher, J. F.: The long-term results of Swanson silicone rubber interpositional wrist arthroplasty. J. Hand Surg. 11A:166–175, 1986.
12. Fitzgerald, J. P., Peimer, C. A., and Smith, R. J.: Distraction resection arthroplasty of the wrist. J. Hand Surg. 14A:774–781, 1989.
13. Gilford, W. W., Bolton, R. H., and Lambrinudi, C.: The mechanism of the wrist joint with special reference to fractures of the scaphoid. Guy's Hosp. Rep. 92:52–59, 1943.
14. Goodman, M. J., Millender, L. H., Nalebuff, E. A., and Philips, C.: Arthroplasty of the rheumatoid wrist with silicone rubber: An early evaluation. J. Hand Surg. 5:114–121, 1980.
15. Hollingshead, W. H.: Anatomy for Surgeons, 2nd ed., vol. 3. New York, Harper & Row, 1969.
16. Hooper, J.: The surgery of the wrist in rheumatoid arthritis. Aust. N.Z.J. Surg. 42:135, 1972.
17. Johnston, T. B. and Whillis, J.: Gray's Anatomy: Descriptive and Applied, 30th ed. New York, Longmans, Green, 1949.
18. Kaplan, E. B.: Functional and Surgical Anatomy of the Hand, 2nd ed. Philadelphia, J. B. Lippincott Co., 1965.
19. Kauer, J. M. G.: The collateral ligament function in the wrist joint. Acta Morphol. Neerl. Scand. 17:252, 1979.
20. Kulick, R. G., Defiore, J. C., Staub, L. R., and Ranawat, C. S.: Long-term results of dorsal stabilization in the rheumatoid wrist. J. Hand Surg. 6:272, 1981.
21. Lamberta, F. J., Ferlic, D. C., and Clayton, M. L.: Volz total wrist arthroplasty in rheumatoid arthritis: A preliminary report. J. Hand Surg. 5:245, 1980.
22. de Lange, A., Kauer, J. M. G., and Huiskes, R.: Kinematic behavior of the human wrist joint: A roentgen-stereophotogrammetric analysis. J. Orthop. Res. 3:56–64, 1985.
23. Lichtman, D. M.: The wrist and its disorders. Philadelphia, W. B. Saunders Company, 1988.
24. Meuli, H. C.: Arthroplastie du poignet. Ann. Chir. 27:527–530, 1973.
25. Meuli, H. C.: Arthroplasty of the wrist. Clin. Orthop. 149:118, 1980.
26. Meuli, H. C.: Meuli total wrist arthroplasty. Clin. Orthop. 187:107–111, 1984.
27. Nalebuff, E. A. and Millender, L. H.: Arthrodesis of the rheumatoid wrist: functional evaluation of a modified technique. Orthop. Rev. 1:4–16, 1972.
28. Peimer, C. A.: Personal communication, 1989.
29. Ruby, L. K., Cooney, III, W. P., An, K. N., et al.: Relative motion of selected carpal bones: A kinematic analysis of the normal wrist. J. Hand Surg. 13A:1–10, 1988.
30. Sarrafian, S. K., Melamed, J. L., and Goshgarian, G. M.: Study of wrist motion in flexion and extension. Clin. Orthop. 126:153–159, 1977.
31. Swanson, A. B., de Groot Swanson, G., and Maupin, B. K.: Flexible implant arthroplasty of the radiocarpal joint—surgical technique and long-term study. Clin. Orthop. 187:94–106, 1984.

32. Taleisnik, J.: The ligaments of the wrist. J. Hand Surg. 1:110–118, 1976.
33. Taleisnik, J.: The Wrist. New York, Churchill Livingstone, 1985.
34. Volz, R. G.: The development of a total wrist arthroplasty. Clin. Orthop. 128:180, 1976.
35. Volz, R. G.: Total Wrist Arthroplasty: A Clinical and Biomechanical Analysis. American Academy of Orthopaedic Surgeons Symposium on Total Joint Replacement of the Upper Extremity. Edited by A. E. Inglis. St. Louis, C. V. Mosby Company, 1982.
36. Volz, R. G.: Total wrist arthroplasty: A clinical review. Clin. Orthop. 187:112–120, 1984.
37. Youm, Y., McMurtry, R. Y., Flatt, A. E., and Gillespie, T. E.: Kinematics of the wrist. I. An experimental study of radial-ulnar deviation and flexion-extension. J. Bone Joint Surg. 60:423, 1978.

CHAPTER 41

Arthroplasty in the Hand

LARRY K. CHIDGEY
PAUL C. DELL

METACARPOPHALANGEAL JOINT

Anatomy

The metacarpophalangeal joint is a condyloid joint formed by the ovoid head of the metacarpal and the elliptic cavity of the base of the proximal phalanx. The joint is surrounded by the capsule, radial and ulnar collateral ligaments, accessory collateral ligaments, and fibrocartilaginous volar plate. The radial and ulnar collateral ligaments originate from a depression in the subcapital area of the distal metacarpal. Their insertion is at the palmar corner of the base of the proximal phalanx. The accessory collateral ligaments originate from the collateral ligament proper, fanning out to insert into the volar plate. The fibrocartilaginous volar plate has a strong insertion to the palmar aspect of the base of the proximal phalanx, thinning out proximally to a flexible membranous origin from the base of the metacarpal neck. The adjacent volar plates and metacarpophalangeal joints are interconnected by the deep transverse metacarpal ligament. The first annular ligament originates from the palmar surface of the volar plate and encircles the flexor tendons.

As the extensor digitorum communis tendons join the dorsal hood at the level of the metacarpophalangeal joint, transversely oriented fibers (the sagittal bands) arise from the tendon margins. The sagittal bands pass palmarly around the metacarpal head and the base of the proximal phalanx, forming a sling to insert into the volar plate. The extensor digitorum communis tendon has no strong dorsal insertion into the proximal phalanx. Only in occasional specimens are a few fibers found extending from the under surface of the tendon into the dorsal joint capsule. These inconstant, flimsy fibers probably play more of a role in centralizing the tendon than in actually extending the proximal phalanx.

The extensor tendon has a moment arm of about 1 cm for extension of the metacarpophalangeal joint.[9] Therefore, any tension on the extensor tendon will produce an extensor moment at the metacarpophalangeal joint even if the tendon crosses other joints more distally before inserting.[10] As tension increases in the extensor digitorum communis tendon, the sagittal bands shift from a perpendicular to a more parallel position, lifting the proximal phalanx into extension. The tendons of the interosseous and lumbrical muscles form the lateral bands at either side of the metacarpophalangeal joint. Transverse fibers from the lateral band arch over the dorsum of the proximal phalanx distal to the sagittal bands and superficial to the extensor digitorum communis tendon. The transverse fibers serve as the primary flexors of the metacarpophalangeal joint through a lasso effect, as tension is exerted in the intrinsic muscle. Distal oblique extensions from the lateral bands continue distally to form elements of the extensor mechanism of the interphalangeal joints. This envelope of interconnecting fibers with multiple muscle contributions circumferentially around the finger has been termed a "torque tube."[1] The circumferential integrity of this torque tube is essential to normal metacarpophalangeal function.

Biomechanics

The metacarpophalangeal joint has classically been described as having three axes: flexion-extension, abduction-adduction, and rotation. Agee and Hollister[2] described the metacarpophalangeal joint as having two axes of rotation, which better defines the true movement of the joint. A flexion-extension axis is transverse through the metacarpal head at the origin of the collateral ligaments. The other axis (cone axis) traverses the metacarpal head obliquely in a palmar direction along a line in approximately 60 degrees of flexion relative to the longitudinal axis of the metacarpal. Brand[9] has likened the movement of the proximal phalanx around this cone axis to that of an umbrella (Fig. 41–1). With the finger extended, attempted abduction-adduction more closely approximates an arc following the surface of an open umbrella. As the tip of the finger approaches the thumb for pulp-to-pulp pinch, the finger can be rocked around this oblique axis with the proximal phalanx following the surface of a partially closed umbrella. A nearly completely closed umbrella is simulated by bringing the proximal phalanx in line with the cone axis. In this situation, pure rotation is possible. The interosseous muscles are in the ideal position to control motion around this cone axis. During pulp-to-pulp pinch, the interosseous muscles provide dynamic stability to the partially flexed proximal phalanx, especially during fine manipulation. Present implant designs have been targeted

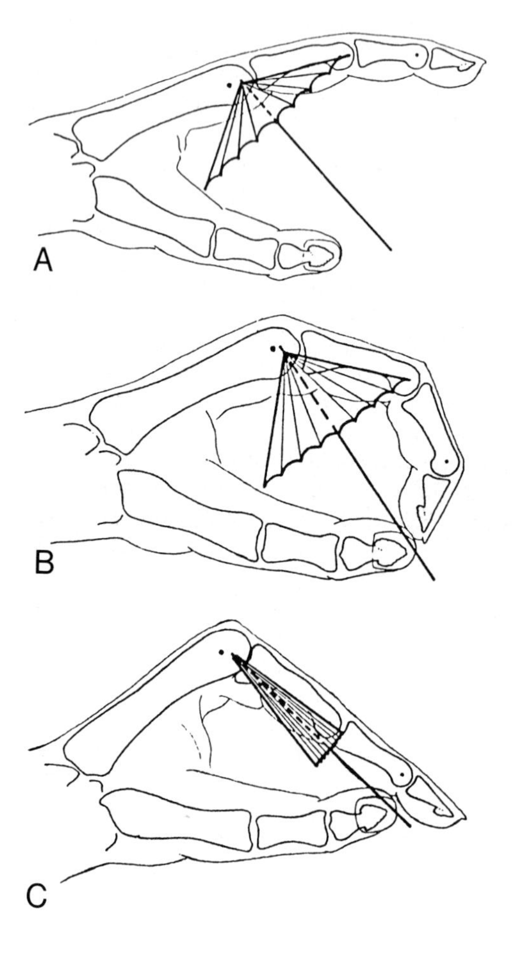

FIGURE 41–1. *A,* The longitudinal cone axis is oriented approximately 60 degrees to the axis of the metacarpal. Lateral deviation of the extended finger follows an arc about this axis similar to that of the surface of an umbrella. *B,* With tip-to-tip pinch, the pulps are along the cone axis, providing increased stability during fine manipulation. *C,* In full metacarpophalangeal joint flexion, the longitudinal axis of the proximal phalanx is aligned with the cone axis and pure rotation is possible. (Brand, P. W.: Clinical Mechanics of the Hand. St. Louis, C. V. Mosby Company., 1985. By permission.)

to restore the flexion-extension axis; however, they cannot possibly restore a patient's sense of stability with fine manipulation without this cone axis being taken into consideration.

Surgical Approaches

Transverse Approach

A transverse incision is made over the dorsal aspect of the hand at the level of the metacarpal heads (Fig. 41–2B). Distal and proximal blunt dissection for several centimeters is required to fully mobilize the skin flaps. Particular care is taken to preserve the large dorsal longitudinal veins lying in the valleys between the metacarpal heads. The dorsal apparatus is fully exposed, and the extensor tendon, which is often dislocated into the ulnar valley, is identified. Intrinsic tightness is addressed by excising the ulnar transverse and oblique fibers[18] (Fig. 41–3A). The ulnar sagittal bands are incised, permitting the dorsal apparatus to be reflected radially, exposing the capsule (Fig. 41–3B). A longitudinal incision in the capsule exposes the joint (Fig. 41–3C). Alternately, after ulnar intrinsic release, the joint capsule may be exposed by making an incision radial to the extensor digitorum communis tendon and incising the sagittal bands, the transverse fibers, and a portion of the oblique fibers. Proponents of the radial approach point out that this incision allows imbrication of the redundant dorsal apparatus after implant insertion, re-establishing and tightening the sagittal bands. However, longstanding ulnar subluxation of the dorsal apparatus leads to soft tissue contracture, preventing centralization of the tendon without ulnar release.

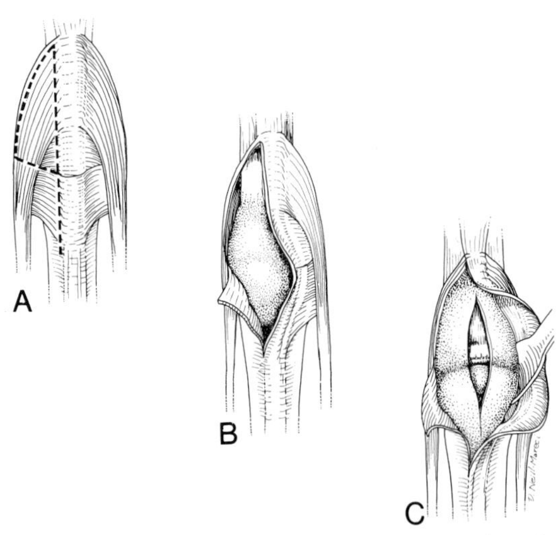

FIGURE 41–3. *A,* Intrinsic tightness may be addressed by excising the ulnar transverse and oblique fibers, allowing centralization of the extensor digitorum communis tendon. *B,* The joint capsule is exposed by incising the ulnar sagittal band along the ulnar margin of the extensor digitorum communis tendon and reflecting the extensor apparatus radially. *C,* A longitudinal incision in the capsule exposes the joint.

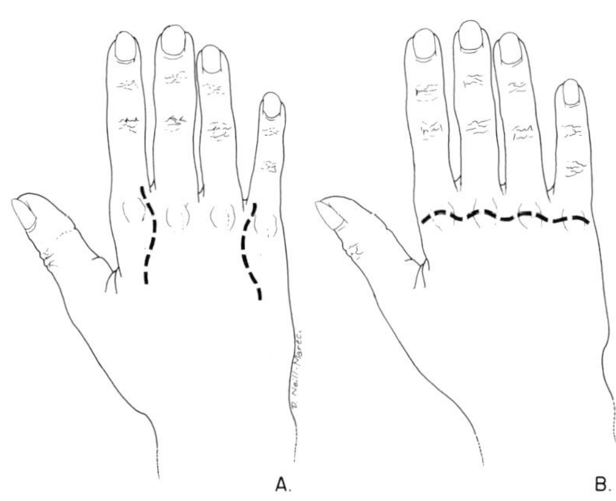

FIGURE 41–2. *A,* Preferred longitudinal skin incision for approaching the metacarpophalangeal joints. Preservation of the dorsal longitudinal veins and cutaneous nerves lying between the metacarpal heads is simplified with this approach. *B,* Transverse skin incision for approaching the metacarpophalangeal joints.

Following an ulnar incision, the radial elements of the dorsal apparatus may be reefed to centralize the tendon. One of us (PCD) routinely makes an ulnar incision. The other (LKC) places the incision dependent upon the degree of soft tissue contracture. A radial incision is made when the ulnar aponeurosis is only mildly contracted. However, with significant ulnar-sided contracture, the extensor tendon cannot be centralized without an ulnar release. In this situation, after implant insertion, the radial portion may be repaired to the ulnar aponeurosis followed by suturing of the extensor tendon to the repaired hood as suggested by Beckenbaugh and Linscheid.[4]

Longitudinal Approach

To expose the index and long fingers' metacarpophalangeal joints, a longitudinal incision is centered between the index and long fingers starting 1.5 cm distal to the metacarpophalangeal joint level and extended proximally 4 cm (Fig. 41–2A). To expose the ring and little metacarpophalangeal joints, an identical longitudinal incision is centered between these two metacarpal heads. Blunt dissection mobilizes the skin adequately, permitting excellent exposure of adjacent joints. Preservation of the dorsal longitudinal veins and cutaneous nerves lying between the metacarpal heads is simplified with this approach. We have noticed a significant reduction in postoperative swelling since employing this preferred longitudinal approach.

Indications for Arthroplasty

Destructive changes of the metacarpophalangeal joint are most commonly caused by rheumatoid arthritis and may be associated with profound proximal and distal joint imbalance. Arthroplasty is indicated for patients with painful metacarpophalangeal joint destruction unresponsive to medical management. Alternately, some patients have impaired hand function secondary to soft tissue imbalance, with minimal discomfort. In this situation, metacarpophalangeal arthroplasty may improve overall hand function as well as aesthetics. However, if the joint can be fully corrected passively and joint destruction is absent radiographically, soft tissue releases and rebalancing should be considered rather than arthroplasty. Intrinsic tightness may be addressed by excision of the ulnar and, as needed, the radial transverse and oblique fibers. Frequently, the extensor digitorum communis tendon needs to be formally centralized.

The metacarpophalangeal joint contributes 77 percent to the total finger flexion arc.[21] Restricted metacarpophalangeal joint motion significantly impairs hand function, making arthroplasty and maintenance of motion highly desirable. However, previous infection may preclude implant arthroplasty. Alternative surgical options include soft tissue arthroplasty[16, 33, 34] and arthrodesis. Arthrodesis may be considered in the index finger of a young, heavy laborer who needs a strong pinch. The joint should be fused in approximately 40 degrees of flexion to provide pulp-to-pulp pinch between the index finger and thumb.

Before undertaking metacarpophalangeal joint reconstruction in the rheumatoid patient, the surgeon should thoroughly assess the flexor and extensor tendons as well as the joints proximal and distal to the metacarpophalangeal joint. Symptomatic wrist, elbow, and shoulder involvement should be addressed appropriately. Imbalance of the wrist extensors, particularly volar subluxation of the extensor carpi ulnaris, may lead to a radially deviated wrist and hand, with weak or absent ulnar deviation. As part of a zigzag collapse deformity, the metacarpus shifts radially and the metacarpophalangeal joints fall into more ulnar deviation.[26, 27] Clearly, if the metacarpophalangeal joint arthroplasties are subjected to these uncorrected forces, ulnar deviation will recur rapidly. If the wrist is passively correctable without advanced radiocarpal disease, the extensor carpi radialis longus tendon is transferred to the centralized extensor carpi ulnaris tendon. Alternately, arthrodesis of the radius to the lunate and perhaps the scaphoid balances the wrist while simultaneously addressing a destroyed radiocarpal joint. Both of these procedures can be undertaken at the same operation as metacarpophalangeal joint arthroplasties. Furthermore, wrist deformity significantly affects the excursion of the flexor and extensor tendons at the metacarpophalangeal joint. Advanced wrist deformity may alter the moment arms of the tendons so that minimal force may be transmitted to the metacarpophalangeal joints and impair the functional results of metacarpophalangeal arthroplasties.

Flexor and extensor tendon function may be adversely affected by tenosynovitis, adhesions, or rupture.[15] Failure to correct these problems will compromise results of metacarpophalangeal arthroplasty. The extensor tendons of the ring and little fingers and the extensor pollicis longus tendon are most frequently attenuated by dorsal subluxation of the distal ulna and Lister's tubercle, respectively. The flexor tendons, particularly to the index and middle fingers, are frequently ruptured by carpal disease involving the scaphotrapezial joint. As described by Nalebuff,[25] flexor tendon ruptures should be addressed prior

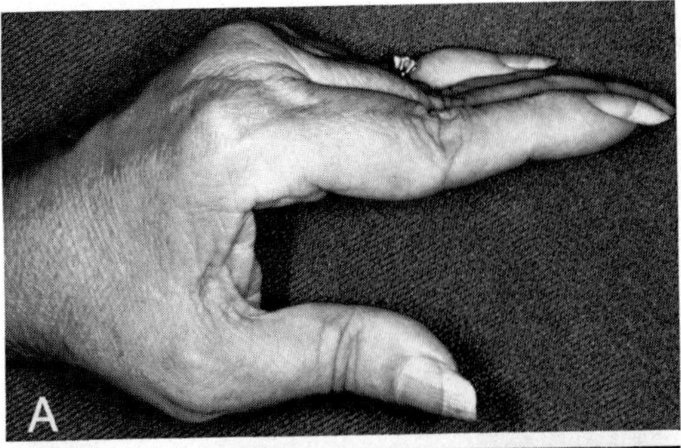

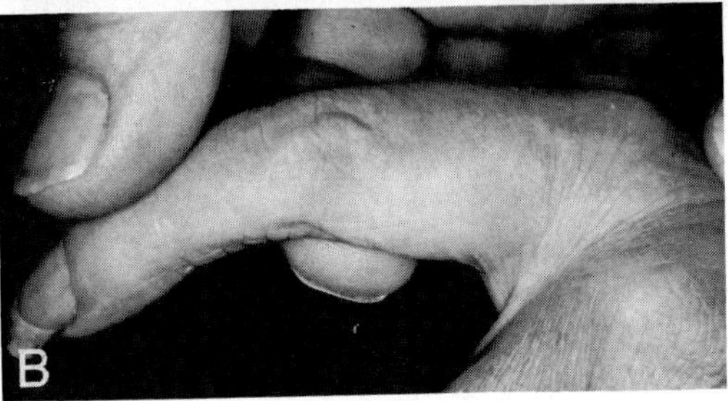

FIGURE 41–4. *A,* Hand of a patient with rheumatoid arthritis with "swan-neck" deformity of the proximal interphalangeal joints in addition to metacarpophalangeal joint destructive changes. *B,* Intrinsic tightness is demonstrated by limited flexion of the proximal interphalangeal joint while the metacarpophalangeal joint is maintained in extension. Proximal interphalangeal joint flexion improves as the metacarpophalangeal joint is flexed to relax the intrinsic tendons. An intrinsic tendon release is required during metacarpophalangeal arthroplasty.

to metacarpophalangeal joint arthroplasty, but attention to extensor tendons may be better delayed until passive metacarpophalangeal joint motion is restored. After metacarpophalangeal arthroplasty has restored adequate passive motion through dynamic splinting, extensor tendon repairs or, more appropriately, transfers may be performed. Proximal interphalangeal joint deformities may also need to be managed in conjunction with metacarpophalangeal joint arthroplasty. Soft tissue procedures (Fig. 41–4) or arthrodesis (Fig. 41–5) for boutonniere and swan neck deformities may be performed simultaneously with metacarpophalangeal joint arthroplasty.

Flexible Implant Arthroplasty

In the late 1960s, Swanson[29] developed a silicone rubber implant for the hand, available in ten sizes (sizes 00 through 8) (Fig. 41–6). The implant is designed as an adjunct to resection arthroplasty and relies on encapsulation to help maintain alignment. The implant is not fixed into the medullary canal. Flexion-extension occurs both through the hinged portion of the implant and through the gliding of the implant within the medullary canal.[29] Because of the high tear rate on the bone edges of the medullary canal, titanium metal bone liners (grommets) have been introduced to help shield the implant. Insufficient clinical data are available at this time to determine whether the grommets will decrease prosthetic failure.

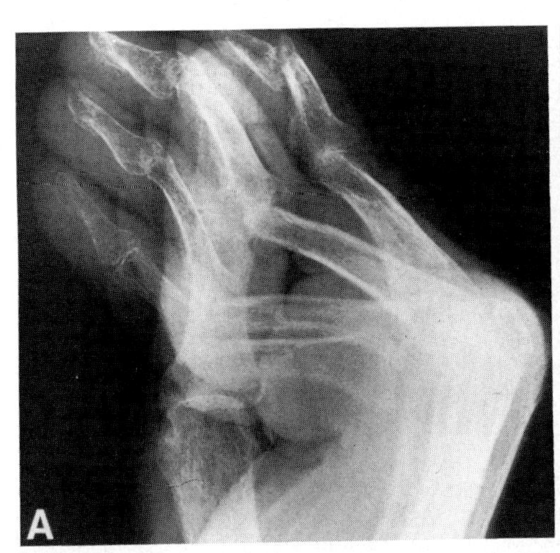

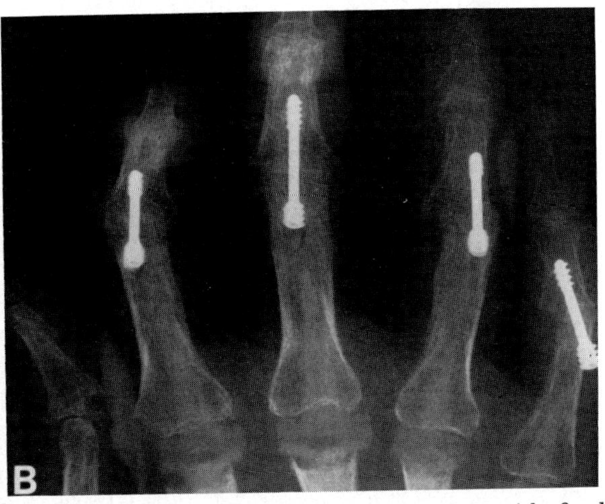

FIGURE 41–5. *A,* Lateral radiograph of the hand of a patient with rheumatoid arthritis with fixed (uncorrectable passively with metacarpophalangeal joint both flexed and extended) "swan-neck" deformity of the proximal interphalangeal joints. *B,* Radiograph following metacarpophalangeal joint arthroplasty and arthrodesis of the proximal interphalangeal joints in a more functional position. Both metacarpophalangeal and proximal interphalangeal joints were addressed during the same surgical procedure.

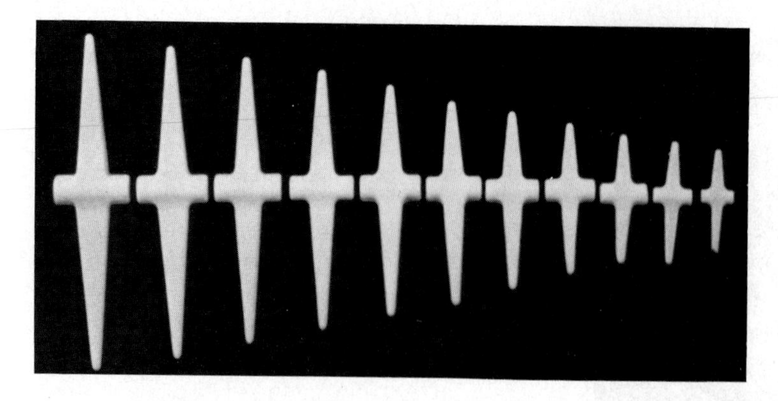

FIGURE 41–6. Swanson silicone implants for flexible interpositional arthroplasty are available in 10 sizes from 00 to 8.

Operative Technique (Swanson)

The metacarpophalangeal joints are exposed through either the transverse or preferably longitudinal skin incisions, and the dorsal apparatus is reflected as previously outlined. A longitudinal midline incision is made in the capsule, and radial and ulnar flaps are developed. Dissection continues circumferentially, detaching the collateral ligaments at their metacarpal origin. Care should be exercised to preserve these soft tissue flaps for later reconstruction. An adequate synovectomy is performed to expose the metacarpal and phalangeal articular surfaces. The metacarpal head is osteotomized at the metaphyseal flare with a power saw (Fig. 41–7A). The osteotomy site is situated near the origin of the collateral ligaments and should be palmarly angulated 10 to 15

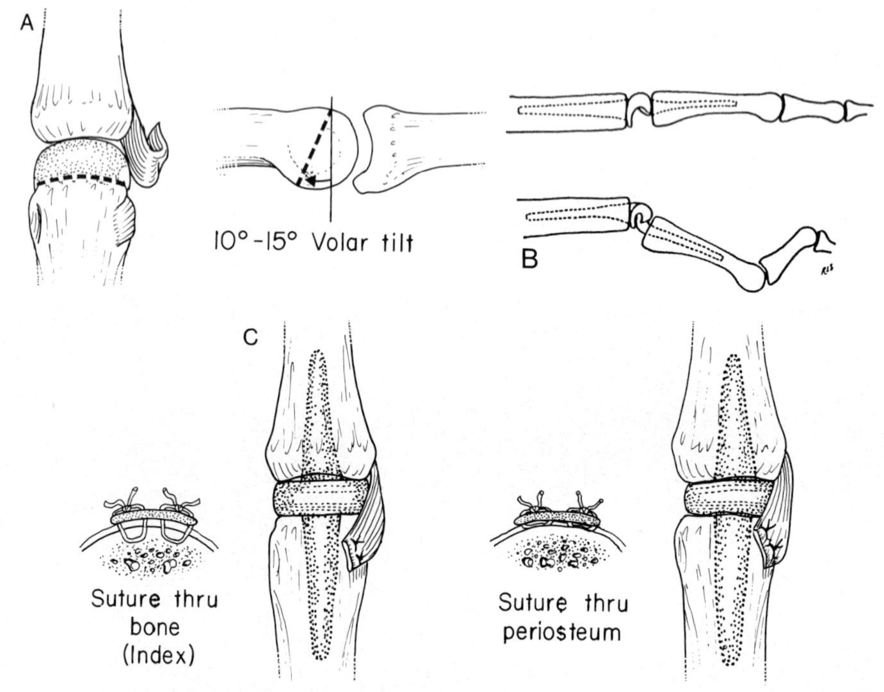

FIGURE 41–7. *A,* The metacarpal head is osteotomized near the origin of the collateral ligaments and should be angulated palmarly 10 to 15 degrees to facilitate implant flexion. *B,* With the trial implant in place, the joint is fully extended. The metacarpal and proximal phalanges should remain well aligned. Evidence of subluxation, bony impingement, or volar buckling indicates that further soft-tissue or bone resection is needed. (Swanson, A. B.: J. Bone Joint Surg. 54A:435–455, 1972. By permission.) *C,* In the index metacarpal, two small holes are made dorsoradially at approximately 3 to 4 mm from the osteotomy site for reattaching the radial cuff of soft tissue. In the other three digits, the radial cuff of tissue is sutured dorsoradially to periosteal soft tissue proximal to the osteotomy.

degrees to facilitate implant flexion. After metacarpal head excision, the synovectomy is completed. The base of the proximal phalanx must now be mobilized and exposed, a difficult task when the proximal phalanx is subluxated or dislocated palmarly with significant soft tissue contracture. These soft tissues can be released sequentially as necessary to completely expose the base of the proximal phalanx and realign it with the metacarpal. The volar plate should be released from the neck of the metacarpal with a Freer elevator. An ulnar intrinsic release was described as part of the surgical approach to the joint, but occasionally an excision of the radial transverse and oblique fibers is necessary. In the little finger, the abductor digiti quinti is routinely incised. However, passive alignment of the joint may require release of the flexor digiti quinti as well. The last muscle attachment is preserved as frequently as possible to provide flexion strength. An attempt is made to preserve the subchondral bone of the proximal phalanx to give support to the implant. If the base of the proximal phalanx is severely eroded dorsally secondary to joint subluxation, it should be resected perpendicular to the long axis of the proximal phalanx.

Frequently, metacarpophalangeal joint motion has been restricted for a protracted time with decreased flexor tendon excursion, possibly resulting in subsequent adhesions of the flexor tendons to each other and the surrounding sheath. Adequate postoperative tendon excursion is essential for a favorable result and must be confirmed at surgery. After mobilization of the base of the proximal phalanx, distraction may be performed to expose the flexor tendons for inspection. If the volar plate has been released from its insertion on the metacarpal, this maneuver often provides adequate exposure of the flexor tendons. When additional exposure is needed, a longitudinal incision in the volar plate may be performed. A small nerve hook is placed around each of the flexor tendons. They are pulled into the wound and adequate excursion is confirmed. If exposure is inadequate through this dorsal approach or excursion cannot be confirmed, a transverse palmar incision should be made over the proximal border of the A1 pulley at this time to establish tendon excursion.

The medullary canals of both the proximal phalanx and metacarpal are shaped with a blunt-tipped burr in a rectangular fashion. The implant trials are used to select the proper size. The largest implant possible should be chosen. The joint should then be fully extended with the trial implant in place and should demonstrate no evidence of subluxation, bony impingement, or volar buckling, all of which indicate that further soft tissue or bone resection is needed (Fig. 41–7B). If titanium grommets are to be utilized, additional preparation of the medullary canal may be required to accomplish a secure press-fit. The distal grommet fits dorsally into the proximal phalanx; the proximal grommet fits palmarly into the metacarpal. The implant size corresponding to the grommet should be selected; although, in rare situations, an implant size smaller than the grommet size may be selected. The trial implant is removed, and the wound thoroughly irrigated.

Prior to final implant insertion, any required soft tissue rebalancing is completed. In the index metacarpophalangeal joint two small holes (0.09 mm) are made in the dorsoradial aspect of the metacarpal approximately 3 to 4 mm from the osteotomy site (Fig. 41–7C). A 4–0 braided nonabsorbable suture is placed through the radial cuff of soft tissue and passed through the metacarpal holes but not tied. This step will help to resist the strong subluxing force of the thumb during pinch activities, which could lead to a hyperpronation deformity. If insufficient radial collateral ligament substance is present, the radial collateral ligament should be reconstructed using the radial portion of the volar plate as described by Swanson[28] (Fig. 41–8). The grommets, if used, are press-fit into position. The final implant is inserted, utilizing the no-touch technique. In the index finger, the previously placed suture is tied, maintaining the finger in slight supination, full extension, and slight radial deviation. After implant insertion in the other three digits, the radial cuff of tissue is sutured to periosteal soft tissue dorsoradially in the metacarpal joint proximal to the osteotomy (see Fig. 41–7C). The long, ring, and little fingers should be maintained in full extension and slight radial deviation during this step. We have found that bony attachment tends to lessen flexion, al-

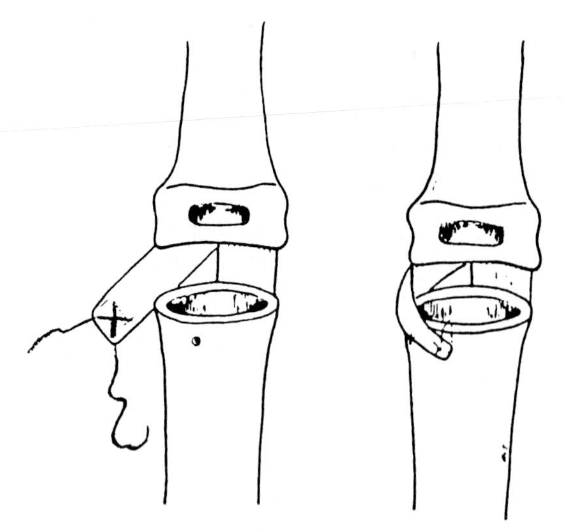

FIGURE 41–8. The radial portion of the volar plate may be used to reconstruct the radial collateral ligament in the index finger if insufficient tissue is present. (Swanson, A. B.: J. Bone Joint Surg. 54A: 435–455, 1972. By permission.)

though it provides more stability for pinch. If enough capsule is present, it is repaired over the implant, maintaining corrected finger posture. The extensor aponeurosis repair and extensor tendon centralization are then completed as previously outlined. With severe deformity of the metacarpophalangeal joint combined with swan neck deformity of the proximal interphalangeal joint, suturing the central tendon directly into the dorsal base of the proximal phalanx through drill holes will centralize the tendon and concentrate extensor force at the metacarpophalangeal joint while decreasing the extensor force at the proximal interphalangeal joint. Skin closure is completed over a drain, followed by application of a compression hand dressing that incorporates splints to maintain the metacarpophalangeal joints in extension and slight radial deviation.

At 3 to 5 days postoperatively the hand is placed in a thermoplastic splint with dynamic extension outriggers (Fig. 41–9). The outriggers are positioned so that they provide an extension and radial deviation force to the proximal phalanx. Force coupling is helpful to protect the supinated index posture. Active and active-assistive exercises are begun, concentrating on a range of motion from 10 to approximately 70 degrees of flexion. Frequently, we alternate dynamic flexion splints with extension outriggers to obtain this arc. If the proximal interphalangeal joints are freely mobile, they may need to be splinted in extension with small static splints while the metacarpophalangeal joints are exercised to concentrate all flexor and extensor forces at the arthroplasty. For 6 weeks postoperatively, dynamic splinting is used during the day and resting splints at night to maintain the metacarpophalangeal joints in extension and radial deviation. Splints are worn full time. At 6 weeks, daytime splinting may be discontinued but nighttime splinting should continue for 8 weeks.[23]

Total Arthroplasty

Since initial attempts to replace the metacarpophalangeal joint with a metallic hinged prosthesis in the 1950s and 1960s,[11, 13, 14] a total metacarpophalangeal joint prosthetic design leading to uniformly good results has yet to be found. Problems with implant fracture, implant migration, bone erosion, and loosening have plagued every prosthesis. A report of up to 20 years of follow-up data on Flatt's metallic hinged prosthesis revealed stem perforation of the metacarpal in 44 percent of implants and perforation of the proximal phalanx in 59 percent.[6] The prosthesis failed through the

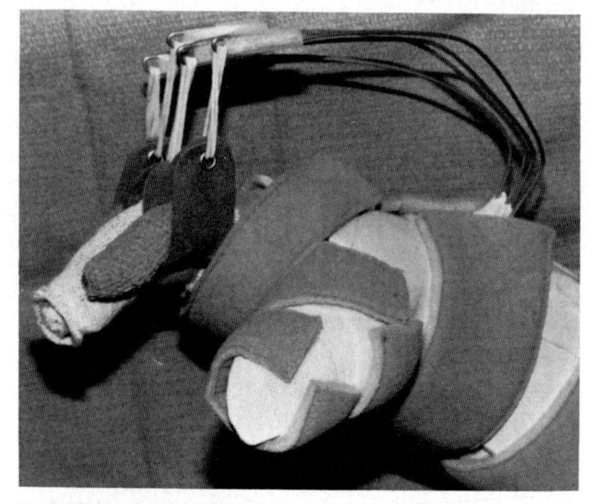

FIGURE 41–9. Following metacarpophalangeal joint arthroplasty, the hand is placed in a thermoplastic splint incorporating dynamic extension outriggers. These outriggers are positioned to provide an extension and a radial deviation force to the proximal phalanx. Exercises are begun concentrating on a range of motion from 10 to approximately 70 degrees of flexion.

prongs or at the screw in 47 percent of implants, and recurrent ulnar deviation was observed in 58 percent. A number of later designs have incorporated a metallic component that articulates with a polyethylene component cemented into the medullary canal of the metacarpal and proximal phalanges (e.g., the Steffee, St. Georg-Buchholz, Schultz, and Strickland prostheses). Similar problems with implant fracture, implant migration, and implant loosening have led to unpredictable results. Until total metacarpophalangeal joint arthroplasty provides consistent results comparable with those of flexible implant arthroplasty, these implants are best reserved for medical centers with staffs with a large amount of experience in joint arthroplasty of the hand.

Clinical and Radiographic Outcome

Clinical results with flexible interpositional arthroplasty have generally been satisfactory.[5, 7, 24, 25, 28, 32] The spectrum of deformity is so varied in patients with rheumatoid arthritis that some reviewers have suggested that individual patient comparisons as well as comparisons between various studies are impossible.[25] Despite these variations in individual patients, some generalizations have held up through several clinical studies.[5, 7, 24, 28, 32] Overall, subjective patient satisfaction has been between 70 and 80 percent. Objective improvement has been variable, but some generalizations may also be made in this area. The active range of motion can be expected to increase only slightly and to show some mild deterioration with time. Studies with follow-up intervals from 2.5 to 5 years have shown an active range of motion of approximately 40 degrees.[5, 7, 24, 32] Although the active range of motion shows minimal improvement, the arc of motion is in a more extended position and thus is believed to be more functional. Extension lags in these same studies have ranged between 10 and 20 degrees. Some recurrence of ulnar drift has also been found in 40 to 50 percent of patients, although rarely does the recurrent ulnar drift exceed 30 degrees.

In none of these studies has an increase in power grip or pinch strength been demonstrated despite pain relief in more than 70 percent of patients. Despite the subjective impressions of 80 percent or more of the patients that their hand function had significantly improved, one study found no significant objective improvement over preoperative values.[7] Aesthetic improvement was reported by over 80 percent of patients. Perhaps some patients equated improved hand function with their overall satisfaction with improved aesthetics.

The fracture or tear rate of the implant has been related to the type of silicone employed in implant construction. When first introduced, the silicone elastomer had a fairly low resistance to tearing. Clinical reports about this early prosthesis showed a fracture rate over 20 percent.[7] With the introduction of the newer high-performance silicone implant, the fracture rate has been reduced to between 0 and 5 percent (Fig. 41–10).[5, 32]

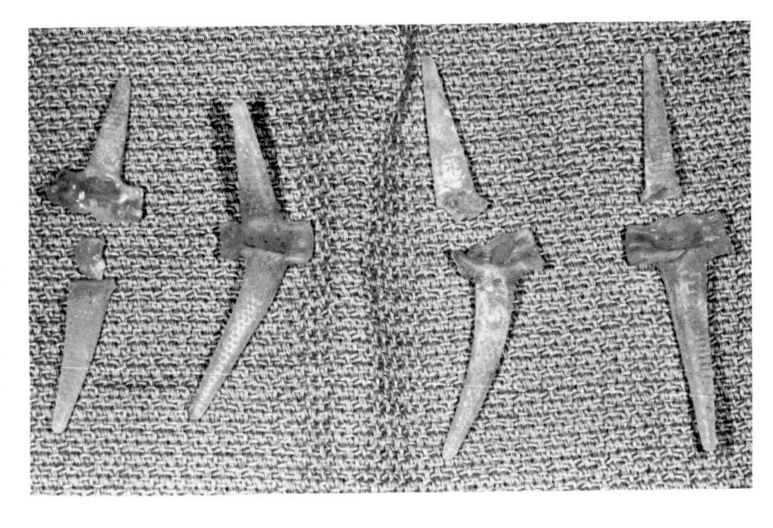

FIGURE 41–10. Silicone implants harvested from all four metacarpophalangeal joints of a patient with rheumatoid arthritis 6 years after arthroplasty. The patient was having increasing symptoms of pain and recurrence of ulnar and palmar subluxation. Of the four implants, three were found to be fractured. New silicone implants were inserted during the same surgical procedure.

Most of our implant failures occur in patients with a strong mobile thumb stressing a reconstructed index metacarpophalangeal joint. Replacement of the fractured index prosthesis and the addition of grommets with proper soft tissue balancing have not alleviated this problem. Currently, we believe that it is preferable to provide greater index stability than metacarpophalangeal motion in these patients. Occasionally, we immobilize this joint for 3 to 4 weeks before initiating motion in an attempt to allow greater collagen maturation.

Radiographic changes in the bone have been represented by both bone resorption and bone formation about the implant. Cortical erosions have been identified in 40 to 100 percent of patients, whereas bone production has been noted in 35 to 50 percent.[7, 17] Bone production may rarely progress to bony ankylosis. Radiographic bony changes have correlated poorly with clinical result.

Failures and Complications

Implant fracture has not correlated directly with clinical result. Many patients with fractured implants continue to have pain-free motion and stable joints. This finding relates to the original purpose of the silicone implant to act as a spacer around which a new capsuloligamentous structure forms. Once this structure has matured, fracture of the implant may not compromise overall joint function. Therefore, a fractured implant needs to be revised only if symptoms are produced or if it has resulted in significant deformity.

Infection rates have been reported to be less than 1 percent.[24] Infection of an implant often involves only one joint despite multiple metacarpophalangeal arthroplasties in the same hand. In general, removal of the implant combined with several days of antibiotic administration is sufficient to clear the infection.[25] The implant may be left out, converting the metacarpophalangeal joint to a resection arthroplasty with favorable function expected. This outcome relates to the tight capsuloligamentous envelope that has formed around the implant and is similar to the reason why some patients with fractured implants continue to do well. Alternatively, the implant may be replaced following resolution of the infection, or an arthrodesis of the joint may be performed.

Because the metacarpal head has been previously excised, arthrodesis of the metacarpophalangeal joint after failed flexible implant arthroplasty results in shortening of the digit unless an interpositional bone graft is used. A cortical cancellous iliac bone graft may be fashioned into the shape of the implant and inserted into the medullary canals of the metacarpal and proximal phalanx, with the wider waist portion of the graft maintaining finger length. Fixation may be secured with K-wires or a dorsal 2.7-mm mini-fragment plate.

Summary

Flexible interpositional arthroplasty of the metacarpophalangeal joint generally improves the aesthetic appearance of the hand, alters the arc of metacarpophalangeal motion, and satisfies the patient. Associated joint imbalance and tendon function must be evaluated simultaneously and treated. The objectives should be a stable index metacarpophalangeal joint for thumb pinch and well-aligned long, ring, and little joints with an arc of motion of 10 to 70 degrees. Implant fracture does not necessitate replacement unless recurrent ulnar-volar displacement of the finger is prominent.

INTERPHALANGEAL JOINTS

Anatomy

The proximal interphalangeal joint is a bicondylar joint formed by the two condyles at the distal end of the proximal phalanx and the corresponding concavities of the base of the middle phalanx. The major plane of motion is flexion and extension, but because the surfaces are not completely congruous, a small amount of rotation and translation is permitted, thus allowing for adaptability to irregular surfaces during grip. The axis of rotation is oblique and is not perpendicular to the longitudinal axis of the phalanx.[19] This oblique axis orientation results in a helicoid motion during flexion and extension so that the finger tips converge during flexion to the base of the thumb. The collateral ligament system of the proximal interphalangeal joint has two major components[8] (Fig. 41–11). The proper collateral ligament originates from the proximal phalanx and inserts more palmarly on the middle phalanx. The accessory collateral ligament, also called the suspensory ligament, originates from both the proximal phalanx and the palmar margin of the proper collateral ligament itself. The accessory collateral ligament then fans out and inserts along the lateral margin of the volar plate. The volar plate is a fibrocartilaginous structure with a strong distal attachment to the palmar lateral corner of the middle phalanx and a thinner intervening central distal attachment. Proximally, the volar plate splits into two tails that have been likened to a swallow's tail. Each tail takes origin from the proximal phalanx just medial to the origin of the A2 pulley. The vincular arterial vessels pass dorsal to the two tails to supply the flexor tendons. Dorsally, the capsule is relatively thin and confluent with the overlying extensor mechanism. The lateral bands and extensor digitorum communis tendon contribute to the central slip, which inserts distally into the middle phalanx.

Proximal interphalangeal joint stability is contributed by the collateral ligament system, the volar plate, and the bony articulation itself. Under axial loading by the tendons, the joint is compressed and has some intrinsic stability attributable to the bicondylar arrangement. Bowers and colleagues[8] have studied the contribution of the proper collateral ligament, the accessory collateral ligament, and the volar plate to joint stability. The joint is stabilized by the proper collateral ligament when the finger is flexed more than 60 degrees. In terminal extension, the joint is stabilized by the accessory collateral ligament and volar plate. Between these ranges, the joint has up to 10 degrees of lateral tilt with passive stressing before the proper collateral ligament becomes taut.

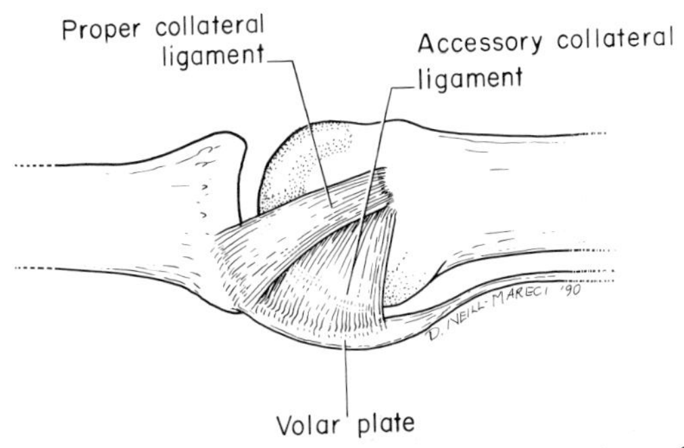

FIGURE 41–11. The collateral ligament system of the proximal interphalangeal joint has two major components, the proper collateral ligament originating and inserting onto bone and the accessory collateral ligament inserting along the lateral margin of the fibrocartilaginous volar plate.

The distal interphalangeal joint is a bicondylar joint with some similarities to the proximal interphalangeal joint. The proper and accessory collateral ligaments contribute to lateral stability with a volar plate resisting hyperextension. The volar plate differs from that at the proximal interphalangeal joint in that the swallow tails proximally blend into the A4 pulley and have no direct insertion into bone.[20] Additionally, the flexor digitorum profundus tendon blends with the volar plate as they both insert into the palmar aspect of the distal phalanx.

Biomechanics

The interphalangeal joints are a major component of the kinematic chain making up the finger. Littler and Thompson[21] have divided the flexion-extension path into two distinct components: the first involves metacarpophalangeal joint motion, whereas the second component involves interphalangeal joint motion. The proximal interphalangeal joint contributes 85 percent of the interphalangeal motion, whereas the distal interphalangeal joint contributes 15 percent. Consequently, preservation of proximal interphalangeal joint motion is far more critical than that of distal interphalangeal joint motion.

Analysis of interphalangeal joint motion cannot be considered in isolation but must be assessed in relation to the proximal and distal joints. The importance of the interrelationship between the joints in a kinematic chain and the influence of overlying tendon moment arms have been emphasized by Brand.[9] The importance of moment arms in understanding finger kinematics is best illustrated by an example. Suppose an external force is applied to the distal pulp of the finger in such a direction as to try and extend the distal interphalangeal joint (Fig. 41–12). This force can be resisted by tension on the flexor digitorum profundus tendon. The external force will have a moment arm of approximately 2.0 cm at the distal interphalangeal joint. This value is in contrast to the profundus moment arm of only 0.5 cm at the distal interphalangeal joint. Therefore, the profundus muscle must contract with a force four times greater than the external force to maintain equilibrium. Tension on the profundus tendon not only influences the distal interphalangeal joint but each joint it crosses during its path to the distal phalanx. The external force will also have a moment on each of the more proximal joints. This same external force will have a moment arm of approximately 5.5 cm at the proximal interphalangeal joint, whereas the profundus tendon has a moment arm of only 0.75 cm. Therefore, 7.33 (5.5/0.75) times the external force must be applied at the proximal interphalangeal joint level to maintain equilibrium. Only four times the external force is applied through the profundus at the distal interphalangeal joint to maintain equilibrium. Therefore, the remaining force must be supplied by the flexor digitorum superficialis tendon to maintain proximal interphalangeal equilibrium.

If for some reason the superficialis is inadequate, the finger will assume a swan neck deformity. In this situation, as the proximal interphalangeal joint hyperextends, the patient may attempt to prevent hyperextension through further tension on the profundus, providing further flexion at the distal interphalangeal joint. Another common cause of swan neck deformity in rheumatoid arthritis is initiated at the metacarpophalangeal joint level. Metacarpophalangeal joint synovitis and soft tissue changes often result in the extensor tendons sliding off the dorsal aspect of the metacarpophalangeal joint into the intermetacarpal valley. This change greatly reduces the moment arm of the extensor tendons at the metacarpophalangeal level. As the patient attempts to extend the metacarpophalangeal joints, the extensor force is transmitted to the proximal interphalangeal joint. Over time, this increased extensor force stretches the static palmar restraining structures, resulting in proximal interphalangeal joint hyperextension. This entire process may be exacerbated by proximal interphalangeal joint synovitis.

The boutonniere deformity (flexion of the proximal interphalangeal joint and hyperextension of the distal interphalangeal joint) is another common finger deformity seen secondary to both trauma and rheumatoid arthritis. The primary pathology involves the proximal interphalangeal joint. Through traumatic disruption or attenuation associated with synovitis, loss of the central tendon results in a major decrease in the extensor moment at the proximal interphalangeal joint. The lateral bands have a very small moment arm at the proximal interphalangeal joint,[9] but for a period of time they may be sufficient to prevent flexion of the proximal interphalangeal joint, as long as the bands stay in their anatomic position. The triangular ligament, which maintains normal dorsal position of the lateral tendons, may be dis-

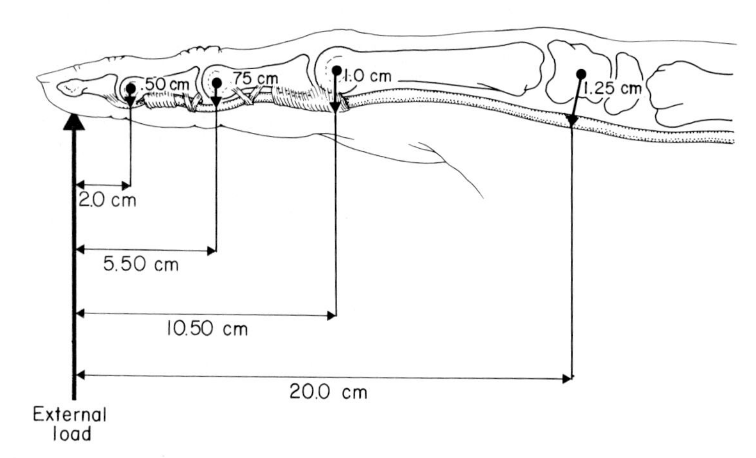

FIGURE 41–12. The moment arm of an external force applied to the finger tip increases disproportionately at each of the more proximal joints compared with the flexor digitorum profundus moment arm. Numbers represent moment arms in centimeters. (Modified from Brand, P. W.: Clinical Mechanics of the Hand. St. Louis, C. V. Mosby Company, 1985.)

rupted initially or may stretch with time, resulting in palmar migration of the lateral tendons. Migration of the lateral tendons further decreases their extensor moment arm. With continued pull of the flexors, a flexion deformity develops at the proximal interphalangeal joint. Attempts at extension result in the lateral tendons concentrating all of the extensor force at the distal interphalangeal joint. With time, the static constraints to hyperextension are attenuated, resulting in a hyperextension deformity at the distal interphalangeal joint level. These are a few examples of soft tissue and tendon pathology requiring correction for successful interphalangeal arthroplasty.

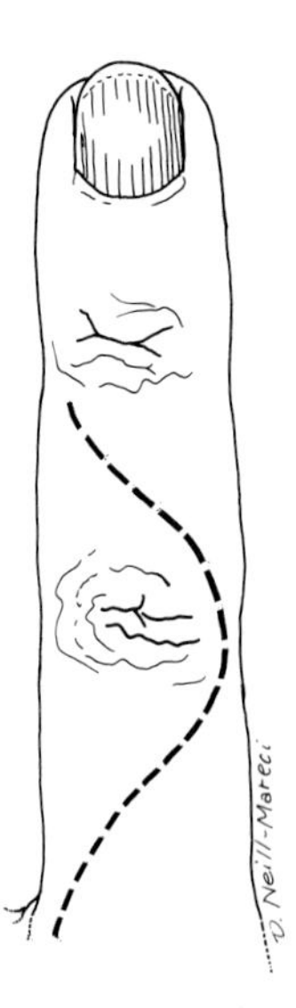

FIGURE 41–13. The incision for proximal interphalangeal joint arthroplasty is modified in fixed "swan-neck" deformities. A curved dorsal incision with an oblique limb over the middle phalanx is selected. The proximal portion may be closed, leaving the distal portion of the wound open to allow full flexion with no skin tension.

Surgical Approaches

Proximal Interphalangeal Joint

Dorsal Approach. A straight dorsal longitudinal incision is made over the proximal interphalangeal joint. This incision is modified in fixed swan neck deformities in which the contracted dorsal skin may limit joint flexion after reconstruction. In this situation, a curved dorsal incision with an oblique limb over the middle phalanx is used (Fig. 41–13). The proximal portion may be closed and the distal portion of the wound left open to allow full flexion with no skin tension. The extensor mechanism is then exposed. A longitudinal incision down the center of the central extensor tendon is made to the level of the central slip insertion onto the middle phalanx. The extensor mechanism may be retracted to each side for exposure of the joint. Alternatively, the central slip may be detached from its insertion into the middle phalanx and reattached after implant insertion through drill holes. If the extensor tendon is detached, postoperative motion must be restricted to allow healing, making this method less attractive.

In swan neck or boutonniere deformities of the proximal interphalangeal joint, the changes in the extensor mechanism must be corrected. With a swan neck deformity, a longitudinal incision is made on each side of the central tendon, and the conjoined lateral tendons are mobilized so that with joint flexion they will slide laterally and palmarly (Fig. 41–14). A step cut in the central tendon may be necessary to permit repair in a lengthened position after implant insertion. In a boutonniere

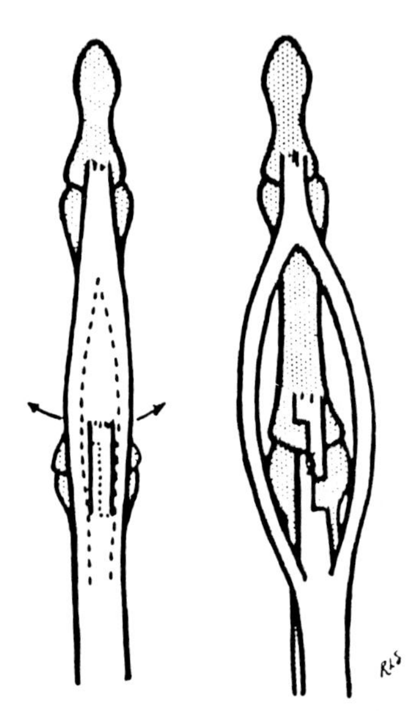

FIGURE 41–14. In "swan-neck" deformity, the changes in the extensor mechanism must be corrected. A longitudinal incision is made on each side of the central tendon, and the conjoined lateral tendons are mobilized. A step-cut in the central tendon may be necessary to permit repair in a lengthened position after implant insertion. (Swanson, A. B.: J. Bone Joint Surg. 54A: 435–455, 1972. By permission.)

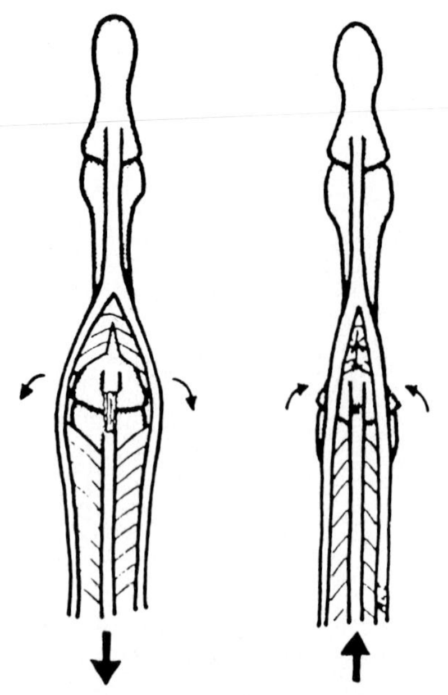

FIGURE 41–15. In a boutonniere deformity the central tendon is advanced and reattached through drill holes into the middle phalanx. The lateral tendons are mobilized from their contracted palmar position by a longitudinal incision along the palmar border. In severe boutonniere deformities, the lateral tendons may be sutured to each other over the dorsal aspect of the joint. (Swanson, A. B.: J. Bone Joint Surg. 54A: 435–455, 1972. By permission.)

deformity, the central tendon is detached from its insertion into the middle phalanx and advanced to be reattached through drill holes in a shortened position (Fig. 41–15). The lateral tendons are mobilized from their contracted palmar position by a longitudinal incision along the palmar border of the lateral tendon, allowing them to move dorsally. The central slip may be insufficient in severe boutonniere deformities, requiring central slip reconstruction. One reconstructive option is to suture one lateral tendon to the other over the dorsal aspect of the joint. The distal interphalangeal joint should then be checked for any residual extension contracture. If present, the extensor tendon overlying the midportion of the middle phalanx should be divided and the distal joint manipulated.

Lateral Approach. A midlateral longitudinal incision is centered over the proximal interphalangeal joint (Fig. 41–16).[22] The incision is placed on the ulnar side of the joint for the index, long, and ring fingers and on the radial side for the little finger. The retinacular ligament is incised along the palmar border of the lateral tendon and the tendon retracted dorsally. The collateral ligament is divided in its midsubstance. The volar plate is incised distally to a point slightly beyond the midline of the finger. The joint is dislocated laterally, with the opposite intact collateral ligament acting as a hinge.

Palmar Approach. A palmar zigzag incision is centered over the proximal interphalangeal joint and blunt dissection carried through the subcutaneous tissue to expose the flexor sheath. A flap incision is

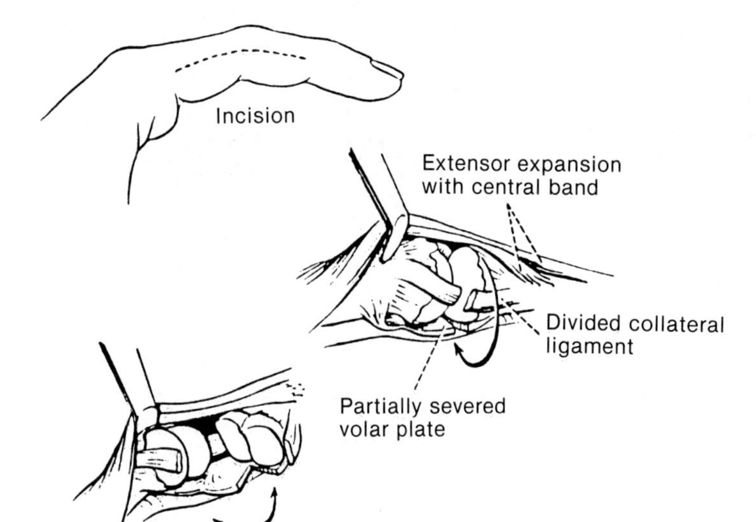

FIGURE 41–16. A midlateral longitudinal incision has been described to approach the proximal interphalangeal joint. The collateral ligament is divided in its midsubstance. The joint is dislocated laterally with the opposite intact collateral ligament acting as a hinge. (Lipscomb, P. R.: J. Bone Joint Surg. 49A: 1135–1140, 1967. By permission.)

made through the flexor sheath incorporating the A3 pulley. The flexor tendons are retracted laterally, exposing the volar plate. A distally based flap incision is made in the volar plate, permitting the joint to be hyperextended and dislocated. Partial release of the collateral ligaments proximally may be needed to fully dislocate the joint.

Distal Interphalangeal Joint

A dorsal T-shaped incision is made over the distal interphalangeal joint, with the transverse portion of the incision kept just proximal to the germinal nail matrix (Fig. 41–17A). The extensor tendon is exposed and divided approximately 5 mm proximal to the distal interphalangeal joint, carefully preserving the insertion into the distal phalanx. Dorsal marginal osteophytes are removed with a small rongeur, and the joint surfaces are exposed by fully flexing the joint. Alternately, a dorsal H-shaped incision may be selected (Fig. 41–17B). The transverse limb lies in the skin creases over the distal interphalangeal joint with midlateral radial and ulnar extensions. Proximal and distally based flaps are elevated to expose the terminal tendon. Joint exposure is identical to that described for the T-shaped incision.

Indications for Arthroplasty

Arthroplasty of the proximal interphalangeal joint is indicated in patients with painful joint destruction secondary to rheumatoid arthritis, degenerative arthritis, or post-traumatic arthritis in which soft tissue procedures alone are unable to restore function. Implant arthroplasty of a joint must take into consideration the proximal and distal joints as well. In concomitant involvement of the metacarpophalangeal joint and the proximal interphalangeal joint, restoration of balance in the kinematic chain is difficult, and arthroplasty of both joints becomes less reliable. Therefore, arthroplasty for the metacarpophalangeal joint should be considered in combination with an arthrodesis of the proximal interphalangeal joint. Implant arthroplasty of the proximal interphalangeal joint has been most successful in isolated joint involvement. For patients with disability of both the index and long fingers who require heavy use of the hand, Swanson and associates[30] have recommended that fusion of the index proximal interphalangeal joint in 20 to 40 degrees of flexion be combined with implant arthroplasty of the proximal interphalangeal joint of the long finger. In this way, the individual can use the fused index finger for strong pinch activities and still retain motion at the long finger proximal interphalangeal joint for grip activities. These investigators believe also that maintaining flexion in isolated proximal interphalangeal joint involvement of the ring and small fingers is important in grasp activities and that implant arthroplasty is indicated. In their review of proximal interphalangeal joint arthroplasties, they found a high incidence of recurrent hyperextension in implant arthroplasty for swan neck deformities and concluded that proximal interphalangeal arthroplasty is contraindicated in most swan neck deformities.

Implant arthroplasty for isolated involvement of the proximal interphalangeal joint of the index finger should be approached with caution. A strong radial collateral ligament is required to resist ulnar deviation during pinch activities and should be assessed preoperatively. A collateral ligament reconstruction will be required if it is inadequate. Swanson and coworkers[30] believe that strong pinch activities can be transferred to the long finger and that patients appreciate maintenance of proximal interphalangeal motion in the index finger. Others believe that arthrodesis of the index proximal interphalangeal joint is preferred in most patients to maintain a strong index-to-thumb pinch.

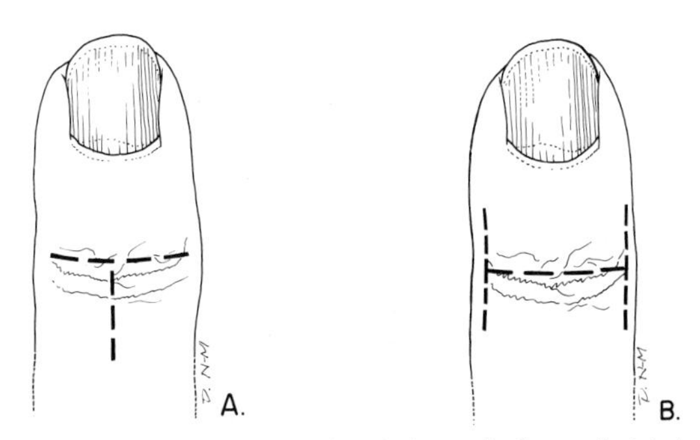

FIGURE 41–17. The distal interphalangeal joint may be approached through a dorsal T-shaped incision *(A)* or an H-shaped incision *(B)*.

Implant arthroplasty of the distal interphalangeal joint is rarely indicated; this joint occupies a very small percentage of the total arc of finger motion.[21] Arthrodesis is a reliable procedure at this joint level and results in minimal functional deficit.

Flexible Implant Arthroplasty

Operative Technique (Proximal Interphalangeal Joint)

The incision and joint exposure are carried out as previously described. We prefer the dorsal approach and use either a straight longitudinal or curvilinear incision. Care is taken to leave the central tendon insertion and collateral ligaments intact, if possible. If the collateral ligaments must be detached, it is preferable to detach them from the proximal side. They should later be reattached to bone. After the extensor tendon incision is made, the joint may be flexed and the two halves of the extensor tendon retracted to each side. A transverse cut with approximately 20 to 30 degrees of palmar bevel is then made across the neck of the proximal phalanx in the region of the metaphyseal flair. The palmar bevel helps prevent bony abutment during flexion between the proximal and middle phalanx (Fig. 41–18). The cartilage is removed from the middle phalanx along with any osteophytes, but an attempt is made to preserve the subchondral bone. In severe fixed deformity, the transverse cut in the proximal phalanx may need to be carried out first and the condyles of the proximal phalanx removed to allow flexion of the joint. The proximal and middle phalanges must be passively aligned, often requiring release of the collateral ligaments and the palmar plate in severe deformity. The base of the middle phalanx may also need to be resected. The medullary canals of both the proximal and middle phalanges are prepared using a blunt-tipped burr. The implant is then selected. An implant of size 0, 1, 2, or 3 is usually required for proximal interphalangeal arthroplasty. An implant of appropriate size should show no signs of impingement in its midsection with the joint extended.

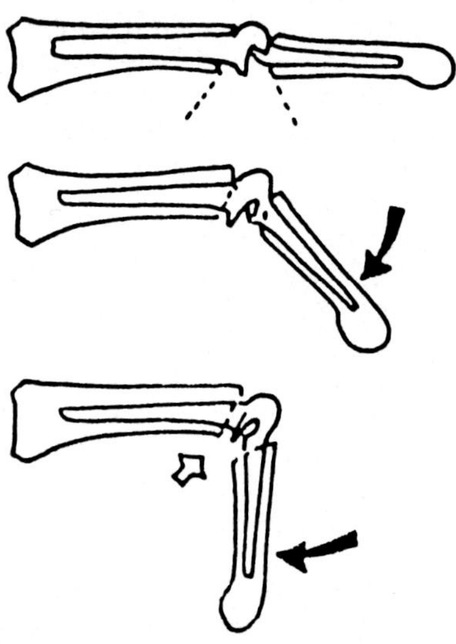

FIGURE 41–18. The proximal phalanx osteotomy should have a palmar bevel to prevent bony abutment and implant impingement with flexion. If the middle phalanx requires an osteotomy, this one should be beveled as well. (Swanson, A. B.: J. Bone Joint Surg. 54A: 435–455, 1972. By permission.)

In some cases, the implant with an appropriately sized midsection has stems that are too long. They may be cut off. The ends of the stem should be approximately 1 mm shorter than the reamed canal to allow adequate gliding during flexion and extension. Prior to insertion of the final implant, appropriate drill holes should be made for reattachment of the collateral ligaments and central tendon and 3–0 nonabsorbable sutures placed. In lateral deviation deformities, the collateral ligament should be reefed on the weak side. If the collateral ligament is found to be insufficient, reconstruction should be undertaken combining the existing collateral ligament with the accessory collateral ligament and a portion of the palmar plate, as described for metacarpophalangeal arthroplasty. The structure should be sutured to the dorsolateral portion of the proximal phalanx through drill holes. The final implant is inserted and the collateral ligament repair completed. The central tendon is then repaired. The joint should be taken through a range of motion. Full passive extension should be achieved as well as 70 degrees of passive flexion. The skin is closed using interrupted 5–0 nylon sutures over a small drain. A bulky hand dressing is applied to maintain the involved proximal interphalangeal joints in extension.

A modification of Swanson's postoperative plan as proposed by Thompson[31] has given successful results. The involved proximal interphalangeal joints are maintained in extension full time for 2 weeks, after which time gentle active flexion exercises are started. Between exercise sessions, a removable static splint is worn to maintain the proximal interphalangeal joints in extension. The static extension splint is maintained between exercise programs and during sleep for 6 weeks postoperatively. Thereafter, the splint may be worn only at night as long as full extension can be maintained during the day. If an extensor lag develops, intermittent daytime splinting between exercise sessions should be continued for 2 additional weeks. Extension splinting at night should be continued for 3 to 6 months. Use of the hand for light activities without the splint may be started at 6 to 8 weeks after surgery.

Operative Technique (Distal Interphalangeal Joint)

The distal interphalangeal joint is exposed dorsally as previously outlined. The joint is acutely flexed to expose the articular surfaces. The dorsal portion of each collateral ligament may have to be incised to fully flex the joint. The head of the middle phalanx is cut transversely with a small oscillating saw or a rongeur (Fig. 41–19). The remaining osteophytes are removed with a rongeur as well as the articular cartilage of the distal phalanx. The medullary canal is then reamed with a blunt-tipped burr. A trial implant of appropriate size is selected. The most common sizes are 0 to 00. The implant should show no signs of buckling with full extension. The final implant is inserted using the no-touch technique and the extensor tendon repaired with 4–0 nonabsorbable suture. An extension splint is applied across both the proximal interphalangeal and distal interphalangeal joints for the first 2 weeks postoperatively. The distal interphalangeal joint is then splinted for an additional 2 weeks full time. Gentle active flexion exercises may then be started with full time extension splinting between exercise sessions. At 6 weeks postoperatively, splinting can be discontinued during the day but nighttime splinting continued for 3 months postoperatively. If an extensor lag develops, intermittent daytime splinting between exercises should be continued for 2 more weeks.

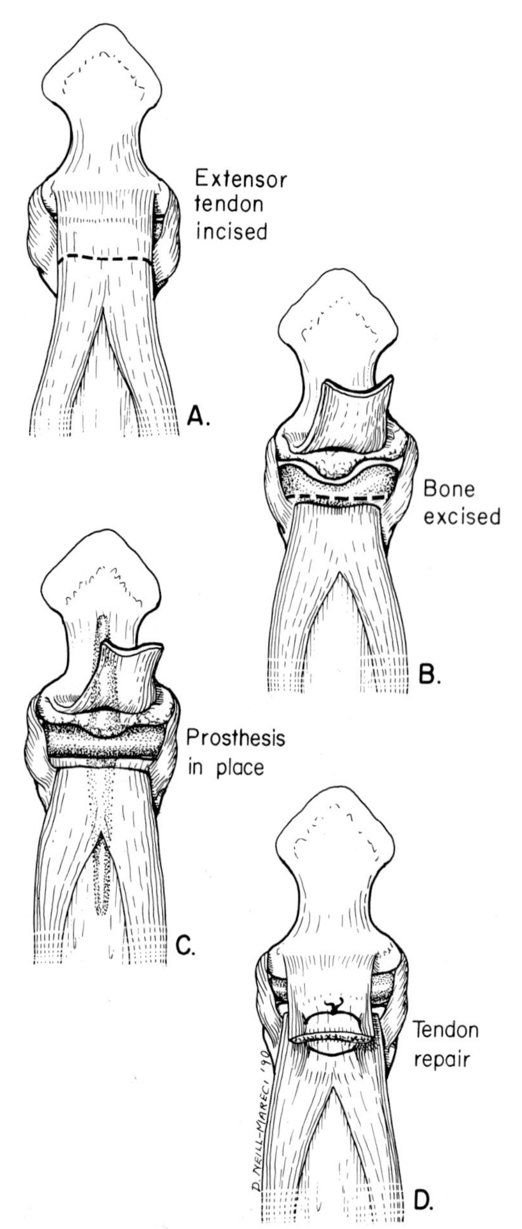

FIGURE 41–19. Steps in distal interphalangeal joint arthroplasty are shown. *A,* After skin incision, the extensor tendon is incised 5 mm proximal to the joint. *B,* The distal portion of the middle phalanx is then excised. *C,* After medullary canal preparation, the appropriate size implant is placed. *D,* The extensor tendon is repaired.

Total Arthroplasty

Total joint arthroplasty of the interph langeal joints has been associated problems similar to those related to metacarpophalangeal joint total arthroplasty. Initial reports of patients with metallic hinged prostheses showed a high rate of implant failure, loosening, and migration.[11, 13] Other attempts at cemented prostheses have included the Biomeric implant, which consists of a flexible elastomer hinge bonded to a central titanium core (Fig. 41–20). A high rate of implant fracture was reported. Currently available cemented implants, such as the Steffee prosthesis, have also proved unpredictable. These implants, like those involved in metacarpophalangeal total arthroplasty, are best restricted to medical centers with staffs with considerable experience in joint arthroplasty of the hand.

Clinical Outcome

After proximal interphalangeal joint arthroplasty, most patients obtain good pain relief with modest increases in motion.[28, 30] Many patients have no increase in motion, but the arc of motion is placed in a more functional range. Complete pain relief has been noted in 98.3 percent of patients.[28, 30] A range of motion of 40 to 60 degrees can be expected. If adequate attention is given to the collateral ligaments, stability is also

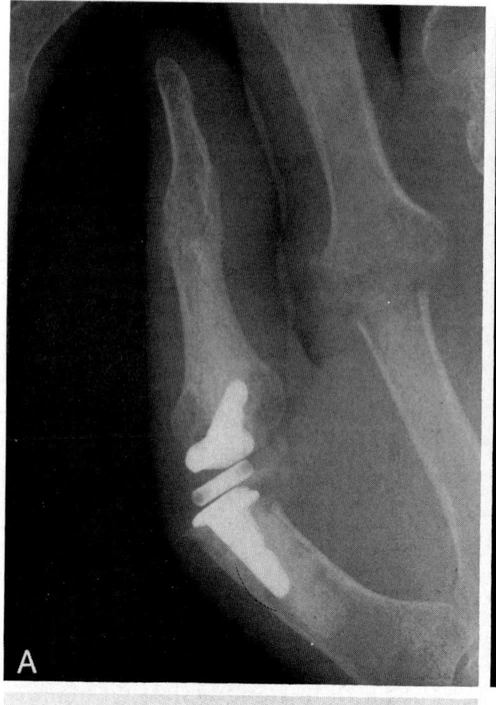

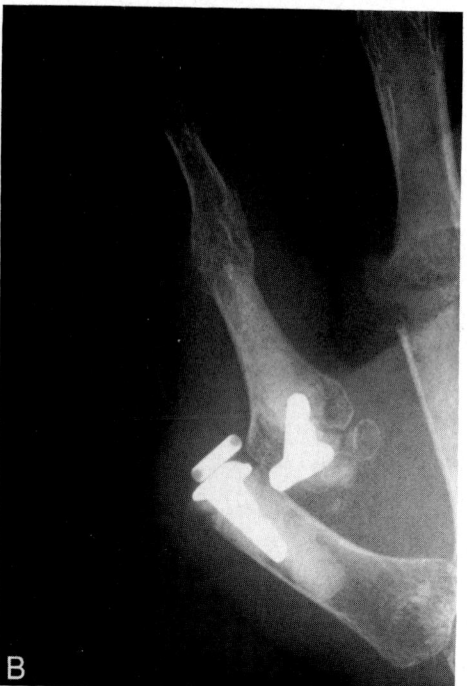

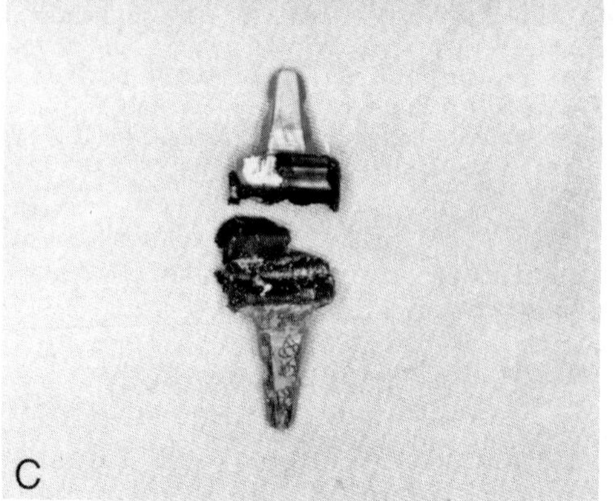

FIGURE 41–20. *A,* Radiograph of a patient with rheumatoid arthritis with a Biomeric implant inserted into the metacarpophalangeal joint of the thumb. *B,* Radiograph several years postoperatively showing fracture of the implant and dislocation of the metacarpophalangeal joint. *C,* Fractured implant after removal. The implant fractured through the flexible elastomer. Similar problems have been frequent with implant placement at the proximal interphalangeal joint.

reliably established. Ulnar deviation of more than 5 to 10 degrees has been noted in only 3.7 percent of patients.[28, 30] Radial angulation has not been a problem.

Implant fracture has been reported in 5.2 percent of patients in series incorporating both the old silicone elastomer as well as the higher performance silicone (Fig. 41–21). It is assumed that the fracture rate will be less when the results with high performance silicone alone are examined. Because recurrence of swan neck deformity has been found in 21 percent of patients, Swanson and colleagues believe that implant arthroplasty at the proximal interphalangeal joint for swan neck deformity is rarely indicated.[30]

Although pathology of the distal interphalangeal joint is more commonly treated by arthrodesis, in appropriately selected patients good pain relief and improved aesthetics can be expected with implant arthroplasty. Two studies, both with approximately 5 years of follow-up data, have shown active range of motion of approximately 30 degrees with an extensor lag of 12 degrees.[12, 35] Although pinch strength was not found to be increased over that measured preoperatively, most patients reported that dexterity had improved.

Failures and Complications

Postoperative bone overgrowth has been noted in 4.2 percent of implants.[30] It has progressed to bony ankylosis in a few patients (Fig. 41–22). Infections have been rare—reported in only 0.36 percent of patients.

A failed flexible interpositional arthroplasty may be salvaged through insertion of another implant or, more commonly, through arthrodesis. The finger can be shortened to achieve bone-to-bone contact and fixation achieved with K-wires, a Herbert screw,[3] or a 2.0-mm minifragment plate. Alternatively, finger length may be maintained by fashioning a cortical cancellous interposition graft in the shape of an implant and inserting the bone stems into the medullary canal of each phalanx, with the wider waist of the bone graft maintaining length. Fixation may be achieved with K-wires or a 2.0-mm plate.

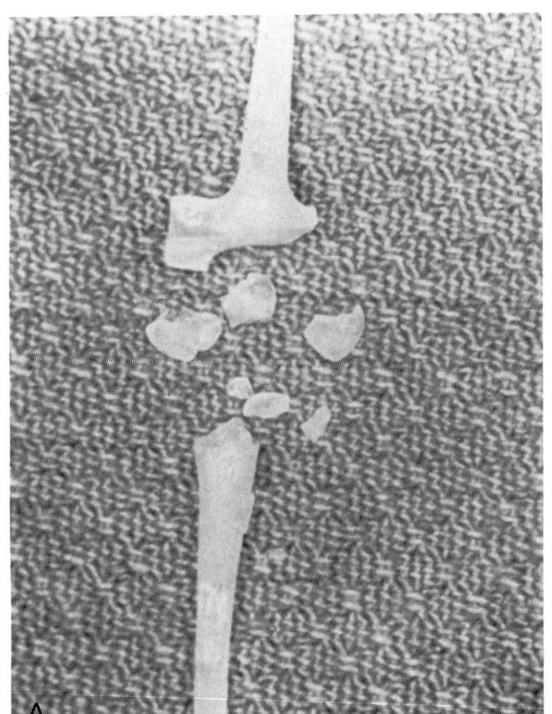

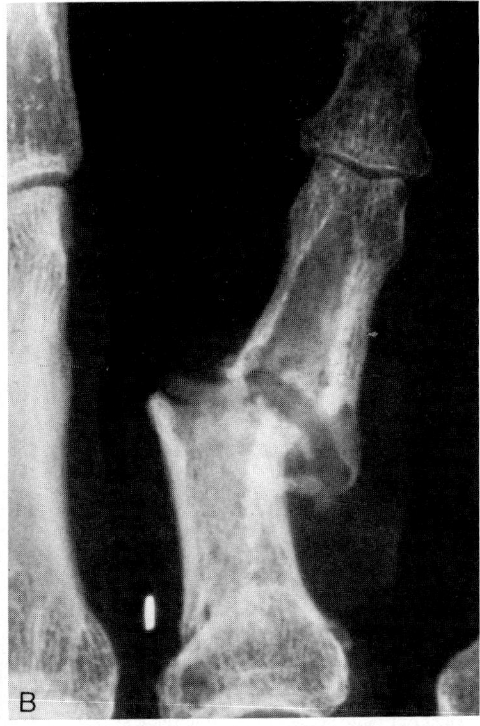

FIGURE 41–21. *A*, Fractured silicone implant removed 4 years after surgery in a patient with rheumatoid arthritis at the proximal interphalangeal joint. *B*, Radiograph of the same patient's proximal interphalangeal joint arthroplasty immediately before implant removal. Patient complained of increasing deformity and pain.

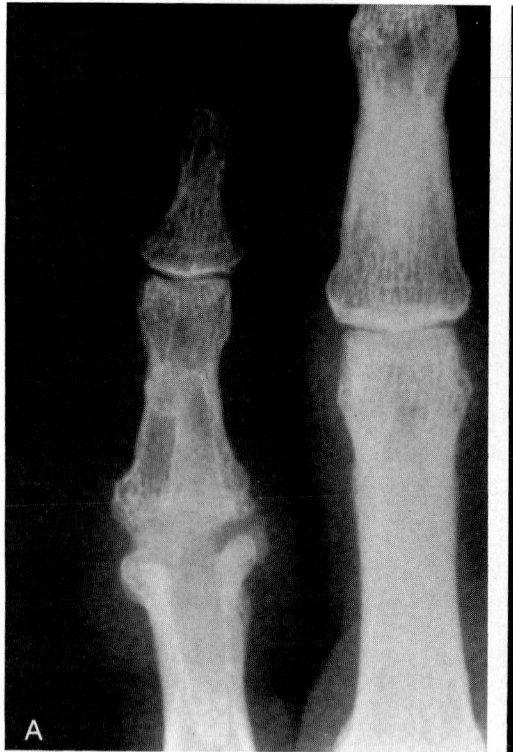

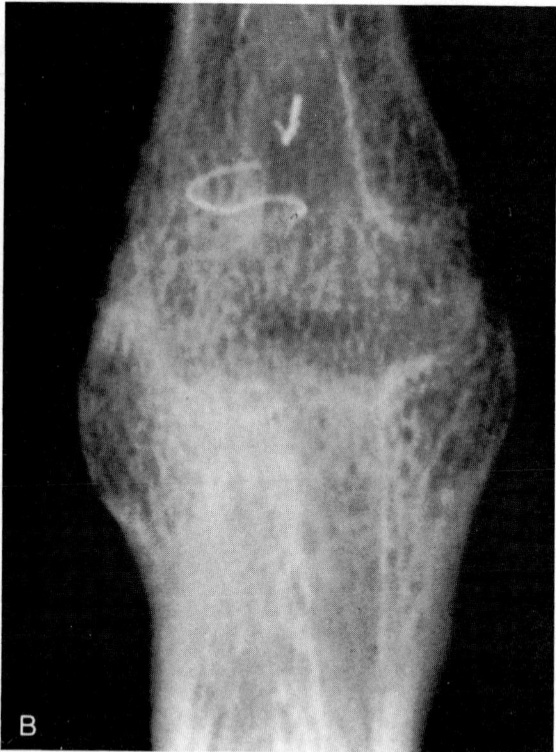

FIGURE 41–22. *A,* Radiograph of a patient with rheumatoid arthritis 2 years after proximal interphalangeal flexible interpositional arthroplasty with evidence of bony overgrowth. *B,* Radiograph of the same patient 3 years after arthroplasty showing complete bony ankylosis of the proximal interphalangeal joint with the implant still in place.

Summary

Although less frequently indicated than flexible interpositional arthroplasty of the metacarpophalangeal joint, in well-selected patients the results of arthroplasty of the interphalangeal joints may be equally satisfying. Single joint replacement has generally yielded more predictable results. As in the metacarpophalangeal joint, associated joint imbalance and tendon function must be evaluated and treated simultaneously.

References

1. Agee, J. M.: Personal communication, 1987.
2. Agee, J. M. and Hollister, A.: Personal communication, 1987.
3. Ayres, J. R., Goldstrohm, G. L., Miller, G. J., et al.: Proximal interphalangeal joint arthrodesis with the Herbert screw. J. Hand Surg. 13A:600–603, 1988.
4. Beckenbaugh, R. D. and Linscheid, R. L.: Arthroplasty in the hand and wrist. Operative Hand Surgery, 2nd ed. Edited by D. P. Green. New York, Churchill Livingstone, 1988.
5. Bieber, E. J., Weiland, A. J., and Volenec-Dowling, S.: Silicone-rubber implant arthroplasty of the metacarpophalangeal joints for rheumatoid arthritis. J. Bone Joint Surg. 68A:206–209, 1986.
6. Blair, W. F., Shurr, D. G., and Buckwalter, J. A.: Metacarpophalangeal joint arthroplasty with a metallic hinged prosthesis. Clin. Orthop. 184: 156–163, 1984.
7. Blair, W. F., Shurr, D. G., and Buckwalter, J. A.: Metacarpophalangeal joint implant arthroplasty with a silastic spacer. J. Bone Joint Surg. 66A: 365–370, 1984.
8. Bowers, W., Wolf, J. W., Nehil, J. L., et al.: The proximal interphalangeal joint volar plate. I. An anatomical and biomechanical study. J. Hand Surg. 5:79–88, 1980.
9. Brand, P. W.: Clinical Mechanics of the Hand. St. Louis, C. V. Mosby Company, 1985.
10. Brand, P. W., Thompson, D. E., and Micks, J. E.: The biomechanics of the interphalangeal joints. The Interphalangeal Joints. Edited by W. H. Bowers. New York, Churchill Livingstone, 1987.
11. Brannon, E. W. and Klein, G.: Experiences with a finger-joint prosthesis. J. Bone Joint Surg. 41A: 87, 1959.
12. Brown, L. G.: Distal interphalangeal joint flexible implant arthroplasty. J. Hand Surg. 14A:653–656, 1989.
13. Flatt, A. E.: Restoration of rheumatoid finger-joint function. Interim report on trial of prosthetic replacement. J. Bone Joint Surg. 43A:753, 1961.
14. Flatt, A. E.: Restoration of rheumatoid finger-

joint function. J. Bone Joint Surg. 45A:1101, 1963.
15. Flatt, A. E.: The Care of the Rheumatoid Hand, 3rd ed. St. Louis, C. V. Mosby Company, 1974.
16. Fowler, S. B.: Arthroplasty of metacarpophalangeal joints in rheumatoid arthritis. Proceedings of the American Society for Surgery of the Hand. J. Bone Joint Surg. 44A:1037, 1962.
17. Hagert, C. G., Eiken, O., Ohlsson, N. M., et al.: Metacarpophalangeal joint implants. I. Roentgenographic study on the silastic finger joint implant, Swanson design. Scand. J. Plast. Reconstr. Surg. 9:147–157, 1975.
18. Harris, C., Jr. and Riordan, D. C.: Intrinsic contracture in the hand and its surgical treatment. J. Bone Joint Surg. 36A:10–20, 1954.
19. Landsmeer, J. M. F.: Anatomical and functional investigation on the articulations of the human finger. Acta Anat. 25(Suppl 24):1–69, 1955.
20. Landsmeer, J. M. F.: Atlas of Anatomy of the Hand. Edinburgh, Churchill Livingstone, 1976.
21. Littler, J. W. and Thompson J. S.: Surgical and functional anatomy. The Interphalangeal Joints. Edited by W. H. Bowers. New York, Churchill Livingstone, 1987.
22. Lipscomb, P. R.: Synovectomy of the distal two joints of the thumb and fingers in rheumatoid arthritis. J. Bone Joint Surg. 49A:1135–1140, 1967.
23. Madden, J. W., De Vore, G., and Arem, A.: A rational postoperative management program for metacarpophalangeal joint implant arthroplasty. J. Hand Surg. 2:358–366, 1977.
24. Mannerfelt, L. and Andersson, K.: Silastic arthroplasty of the metacarpophalangeal joints in rheumatoid arthritis: Long-term results. J. Bone Joint Surg. 57A:484–489, 1975.
25. Nalebuff, E. A.: The rheumatoid hand: Reflections on metacarpophalangeal arthroplasty. Clin. Orthop. 182:150–159, 1984.
26. Shapiro, J. S.: The etiology of ulnar drive: A new factor. J. Bone Joint Surg. (Abstract) 50A:634, 1968.
27. Smith, R. J. and Kaplan, E. B.: Rheumatoid deformities at the metacarpophalangeal joints of the fingers: A correlative study of anatomy and pathology. J. Bone Joint Surg. 49A:31–47, 1967.
28. Swanson, A. B.: Flexible implant arthroplasty for arthritic finger joints: Rationale, technique and results of treatment. J. Bone Joint Surg. 54A: 435–455, 1972.
29. Swanson, A. B.: Flexible Implant Resection Arthroplasty in the Hand and Extremities. St. Louis, C. V. Mosby Company, 1973.
30. Swanson, A. B., Maupin, B. K., Gajjar, N. V., et al.: Flexible implant arthroplasty in the proximal interphalangeal joint of the hand. J. Hand Surg. 10A:796–805, 1985.
31. Thompson, J. S.: Interphalangeal joint arthroplasties. The Interphalangeal Joints. Edited by W. H. Bowers. New York, Churchill Livingstone, 1987.
32. Vahvanen, V. and Viljakka, T.: Silicone rubber implant arthroplasty of the metacarpophalangeal joint in rheumatoid arthritis: A follow-up study of 32 patients. J. Hand Surg. 11A:333–339, 1986.
33. Vainio, K.: Surgery of rheumatoid arthritis. Surg. Ann. 6:309–335, 1974.
34. Weilby, A.: Resection arthroplasty of the metacarpophalangeal joint a. m. Tupper using interposition of the volar plate. Scand. J. Plast. Reconstr. Surg. 11:239–242, 1977.
35. Zimmerman, N. B., Suhey, P. V., Clark, G. L., et al.: Silicone interpositional arthroplasty of the distal interphalangeal joint. J. Hand Surg. 14A: 882–887, 1989.

SECTION IX

LOWER EXTREMITY REPLACEMENT: THE ANKLE

CHAPTER 42

Total Ankle Arthroplasty

HARRY E. FIGGIE, III
ANTHONY S. UNGER
ALAN E. INGLIS
MATTHEW J. KRAAY
MARK P. FIGGIE

Total ankle arthroplasty is most successful in elderly patients who are sedentary or in patients who have systemic arthritis with advanced destruction of the tibiotalar joint. Because these patients often have arthritis in other lower extremity joints, maintenance of tibiotalar motion is beneficial. In young, heavy, or active patients, however, arthrodesis is the treatment of choice for degenerative arthritis or posttraumatic arthritis of the tibiotalar joint; isolated ankle fusion is durable, pain-free, and suitable for manual labor and prolonged standing (Fig. 42–1).[1, 5, 15] The gait (walking) pattern after ankle arthrodesis may be acceptable if compensatory increases in motion in the small joints of the foot maintain the normal center of gravity of the body relative to the axis of the knee, ankle, and foot, and dissipate forces distributed through the tibiotalar and tibiofibular joints.[1, 5, 15, 18]

Maintenance of tibiotalar motion is beneficial in patients with systemic arthritis because of the diffuse nature of this disease. A patient with rheumatoid arthritis frequently has changes in the hindfoot, midfoot, and forefoot. Ankle arthrodesis may lead to an unacceptable shifting of gait pattern stresses into the diseased joints of the foot, exacerbating pain and disability.

The quality of gait after total ankle arthroplasty is related to many factors including the condition of the patient, the strength of the gastrosoleus and anterior compartment muscles, the implant type and alignment, the fixation method, and the surgical approach.[6, 31] The ideal arthroplasty provides (1) a stable, pain-free ankle offering a minimum of 10 degrees of dorsiflexion and 20 degrees of plantar flexion; (2) satisfactory durability for normal activities of daily living; (3) minimal bony resection, and (4) inherent stability under normal loading conditions.

BIOMECHANICS

The bony axis of the ankle joint passes from the tip of the medial through the tip of the lateral malleoli. Therefore, this axis passes from a dorsoanteromedial position to a posterolateral and plantar position.[9, 14, 22] The ankle itself functions much like the knee—it is not a fixed hinge but has a series of instantaneous centers of rotation that take the form of a reversed letter C.[9, 23, 25, 28, 29] The tibiotalar joint undergoes both sliding and rolling in the ankle mortise in dorsiflexion and plantar flexion. The axis of the bony architecture of the ankle allows

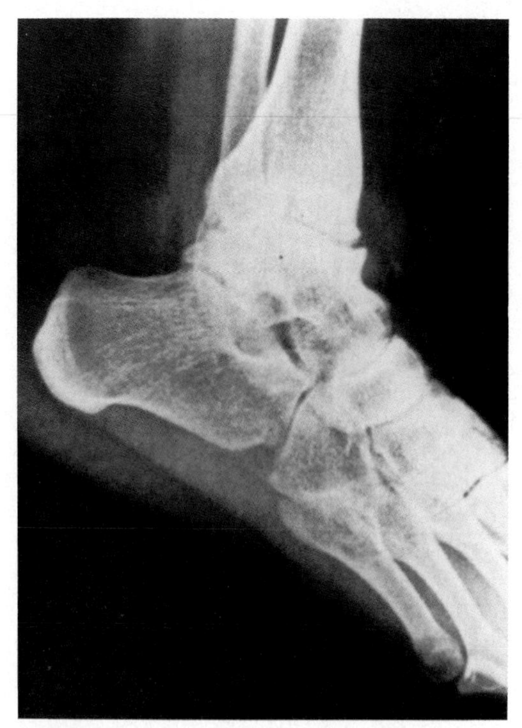

FIGURE 42–1. A patient with hemophiliac arthropathy who has primarily tibiotalar disease. This patient would be best treated with arthrodesis.

dorsiflexion to occur concurrently with abduction and plantar flexion to occur concurrently with adduction. Minimal inversion and eversion occur during the normal gait cycle. The normal ankle joint requires approximately 30 degrees of motion (10 degrees of dorsiflexion and 20 degrees of plantar flexion) during the normal gait cycle.[9, 22, 25, 29]

Ankle prostheses must allow for these motions; otherwise, excessive stresses are placed on the implant-bone interface or at the subtalar or midtarsal joints. The normal ankle joint accepts loads of four to five times body weight in the normal gait cycle.[29] Shear forces pass through the tibiotalar joint that are approximately 80 percent body weight. The surface area available in a normal ankle is adequate to accept these loads; the ankle is actually under lower loads per square centimeter than either the hip or the knee.[10, 29]

INDICATIONS AND CONTRAINDICATIONS

The best candidates for total ankle arthroplasty are patients with systemic arthritis who have low activity levels. This population includes patients with rheumatoid, psoriatic, and hemophiliac arthropathy or systemic lupus erythematosus. Patients with American Rheumatism Association functional class III or IV rheumatoid arthritis, who have extensive arthritis or ankylosis of the small joints of the foot, are also satisfactory candidates for implant arthroplasty but not for arthrodesis because of widespread disease (Fig. 42–2).

Studies indicate that total ankle arthroplasties with minimally constrained cementless devices may be useful in the management of patients with post-traumatic arthritis and avascular necrosis. Satisfactory preliminary results have been reported.[3, 13] Although most investigators believe that the procedure should not be done in a patient with aseptic necrosis of the talus and post-traumatic arthritis when the physiologic age is under 60 years, Buechel and coworkers[3] reported successful results with an average follow-up interval of 5 years.

Absolute contraindications to total ankle

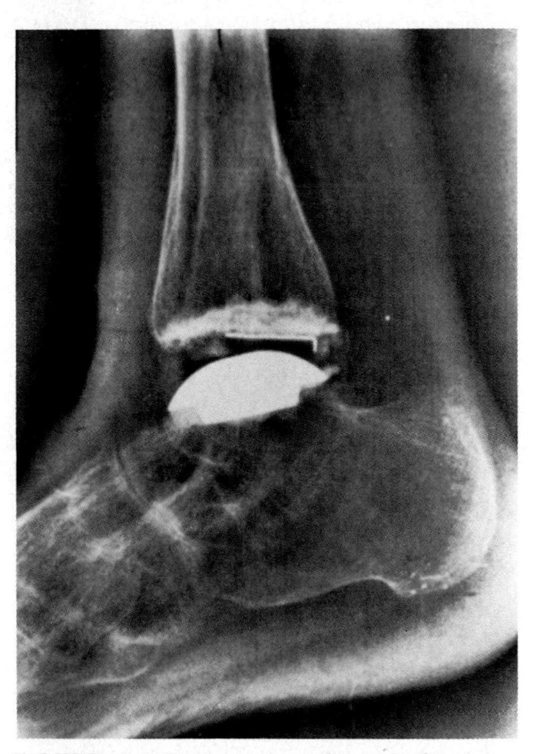

FIGURE 42–2. Postoperative radiograph of an American Rheumatism Association functional class IV ankle joint demonstrating diffuse subtalar ankylosis. This type of patient is a good candidate for ankle arthroplasty.

arthroplasty include local or remote sepsis, joint neuropathy, and neuromuscular disease with spasticity. Relative contraindications to total ankle arthroplasty are a physiologic young age; high activity level; obesity; and poor soft tissues especially with isolated tibiotalar post-traumatic arthritis or osteoarthritis. Most surgeons also consider failed arthrodesis and peripheral vascular disease to be contraindications to total ankle arthroplasty, although isolated satisfactory results for revision of failed arthrodesis have been reported.[3]

PREOPERATIVE ASSESSMENT

Careful preoperative assessment is essential for a successful ankle arthroplasty. The patient's neurovascular status, muscle balance, and skin condition should be evaluated. Preoperative vascular evaluation consists of noninvasive studies, such as Doppler ultrasonography, thermography, and flourescein testing. Arteriography is indicated if the arterial supply to the foot is deficient. Total ankle arthroplasty is contraindicated in severe peripheral vascular disease. If the foot is predominantly supplied by a single artery, special care must be taken to preserve the vessel. Some controversy exists about the surgical approach in such cases. Some surgeons avoid exposing the dominant vessel (e.g., using an anterior approach for a posterior tibial–dominated foot), whereas others expose and protect the dominant vessel. The reported series are too small to allow meaningful conclusions at this time.

The patient must be examined for neuropathy: flaccidity, spasticity, and sensory loss. When proprioception or sensation is absent, the possibility of a neuropathic joint must be investigated. Loss of proprioceptive feedback allows abnormal transmission of loads leading to early failure of the implant. Muscular imbalance causes large stress gradients and predisposes the patient to early implant failure. For this reason, peripheral polyneuropathy, stroke, and other muscle imbalances are also contraindications to implant arthroplasty.

If multiple surgical procedures are indicated, the order of priority for reconstruction is forefoot, hindfoot, and tibiotalar joint. A postoperative infection of the forefoot or hindfoot may lead to direct or hematogenous infection of the implant arthroplasty, possibly necessitating implant removal. In addition, a painful forefoot or subtalar joint prevents the patient from placing the foot in a plantigrade position and compromises rehabilitation. Muscular balance at the tibiotalar joint may require tendon transfer, a procedure that should be performed only after the foot is in its final reconstructive stage. We recommend that all forefoot and hindfoot surgery be performed prior to total ankle arthroplasty.

PREOPERATIVE TECHNICAL CONSIDERATIONS

Prior to arthroplasty, anteroposterior and lateral radiographs are obtained with the patient in the weightbearing position. The film includes a standard for magnification. Preoperative radiographs are done for two reasons: to assess preoperative varus/valgus deformity of the tibiotalar joint and to determine the center of rotation of the tibiotalar joint. Both are critical components of preoperative planning. The principle of total ankle arthroplasty is to restore alignment of the knee, ankle, and subtalar joint. Hindfoot malalignment should not be corrected at the time of ankle arthroplasty but beforehand.

Unlike the arthritic knee, the arthritic ankle is not affected by extensive ligamentous contracture. As a result, ankle arthroplasty may restore neutral alignment of the knee, ankle, and hindfoot without ligamentous recession. When deformities exceeding 20 degrees of varus or valgus are present, a local bone graft may be required for reconstruction rather than bone cuts alone to restore alignment. Ankle arthrodesis should be considered when multiple planes of malalignment are present or when body architecture necessitates oblique positioning of the joint line. The resection planes should (1) place the prosthetic joint line at or near the premorbid joint line, (2) restore the center of rotation of the prosthetic reconstruction at or near the premorbid joint centers, and (3) preserve maximum bone stock (Fig. 42–3).

The center of rotation of the ankle joint is best determined on the lateral radio-

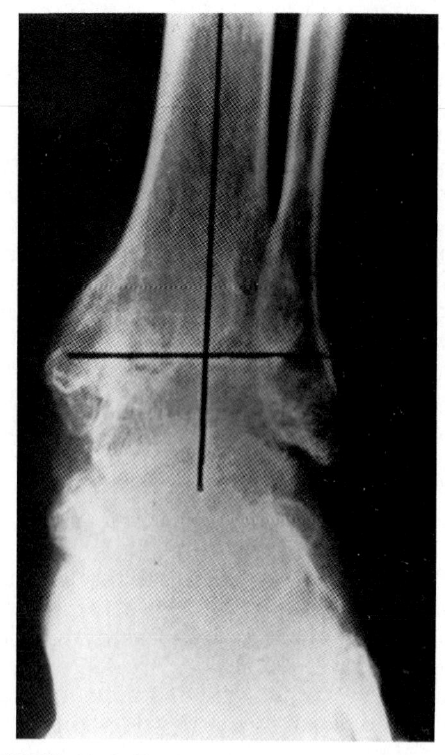

FIGURE 42–3. Preoperative anteroposterior radiograph indicating that bone resection is necessary to restore neutral alignment. (From Operative Orthopaedics. Edited by M. W. Chapman. Philadelphia, J. B. Lippincott Company, 1988. By permission.)

graph. After a midtibial shaft line is drawn, the center of rotation is identified by employing an overlay of concentric rings (Fig. 42–4). The rings are aligned with the radius of curvature of the talar dome in the lateral view. The center of rotation should fall within 5 mm of the midshaft line. The offsets from the cortex of the tibia to the center of rotation are then measured. The posterior cortex is used when a posterior surgical approach to the ankle is planned. The posterior cortex provides a reproducible offset for positioning the implant in the anteroposterior plane intraoperatively. Duplication of the exact center of rotation by arthroplasty is critical for success.

IMPLANT DESIGNS

The three major types of prostheses are incongruent, congruent, and anatomic.[26] Incongruent prostheses allow satisfactory motion in all planes with minimal constraint of these devices. However, they provide mobility at the expense of diminished loadcarrying capacity. Reduced capacity is a result of the small surface area for contact. These devices are also troubled by poor polyethylene-wear characteristics, early loosening, and inherent instability. Incongruent prostheses have several types of surfaces, including the trochlear, concave/convex, and convex/convex.

Congruent prostheses include the uniaxial prostheses, which have a high degree of inherent constraint. Motion is restricted to a single plane, and the ankle is made to function as a hinge. Although the device has better inherent stability than multiaxial prostheses, it is subjected to excessive torsional loads. The wear characteristics are better than those of a multiaxial joint because of wider load distribution and resistance to surface deformation. The primary variations of this type of prosthesis include the spheric (ball and socket), cylindric and conic styles and the spheroid or barrel-shaped devices.

Early results of total ankle arthroplasties utilizing minimally constrained bicondylar devices, i.e., anatomic prostheses, have been promising.[3, 13, 20] These devices offer inherent stability, and the bony axis can be placed in satisfactory alignment, mimicking the normal instant centers of the ankle. To date, no clinical or radiographic failure has occurred in devices im-

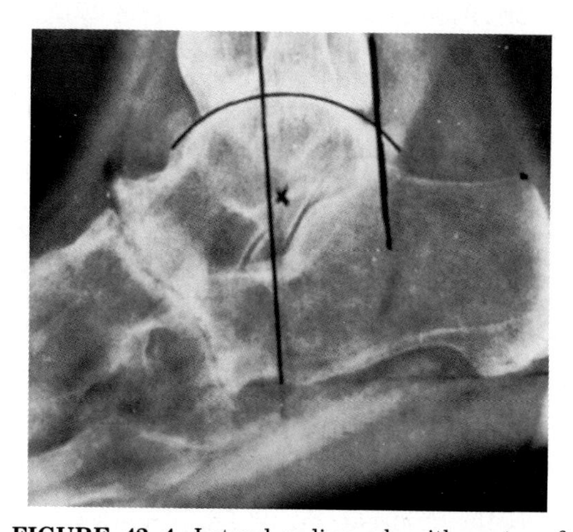

FIGURE 42–4. Lateral radiograph with center of rotation (*x*) identified by a concentric ring overlay. Implant positioning can then be determined from either the posterior cortex of the tibia or the insertion of the Achilles tendon into the calcaneus. (From Operative Orthopaedics. Edited by M. W. Chapman. Philadelphia, J. B. Lippincott Company, 1988. By permission.)

planted at the Hospital for Special Surgery and University Hospitals of Cleveland. No subsidence has been observed. The success of arthroplasty with this device appears to be highly dependent on restoration of anatomic alignment and optimization of component fit. In Buechel's series, one polyethylene-bearing failure and one deep infection occurred. The bearing failure was managed by revision of the polyethylene without removal of the device; the deep infection was salvaged by debridement and maintenance of the ankle joint in place. In neither series was tibial subluxation noted. The results of the more anatomic-style semiconstrained devices appear to be at least as good as those of the other minimally constrained devices, but further follow-up data are needed.[2, 7, 8, 10, 17, 19, 20, 24, 27, 30, 32]

Functional Results of Current Implant Designs

The early results of total ankle arthroplasty were decidedly inferior to those following hip, knee, shoulder, and elbow arthroplasties, partly because of the high loosening rates. Newton[19] reported 24-percent loosening and 40-percent failure rate in 50 patients followed 2 to 5 years. Herberts and associates[12] reported similar findings. Stauffer[27–29] and Stauffer and Segal[30] reported a 7-percent failure rate in 108 ankles at an average 4-year follow-up interval using the Mayo prosthesis. However, the number of patients with radiographic loosening was not discussed. Pipino and Calderale[21] have reported 60-percent satisfactory outcomes, with failures resulting primarily from tibial settling. Samuelson and Freeman[24] reported 70-percent satisfactory results in their first 75 patients with the Imperial College London Hospital prostheses. This experience contrasts with only 32 percent (13 of 41) reported by Bolton-Maggs and associates.[2] These investigators believed that the results with this prosthetic device were so poor that it should be abandoned.

Considerable disagreement exists about the benefits of ankle arthroplasty in patients with rheumatoid arthritis. Most workers agree with Lachiewicz and coworkers[16] who believe that the procedure is successful in this patient population. Lachiewicz and coworkers reported 100-percent good and excellent functional results with the Mayo prosthesis at an average 3-year follow-up period in 15 patients with severe rheumatoid arthritis. All patients improved significantly after surgery, and implant durability was satisfactory. However, results deteriorated somewhat by the 6.5-year follow-up evaluation, at which time 85 percent were rated as good or excellent. In all, 14 of 15 had radiolucent zones at the bone-cement interfaces. Of more concern, in 12 of the 14 devices with radiolucent zones, the talar components had tilted within the talar bones. Not all investigators are optimistic about the results of this procedure. Newton[19] reported unsatisfactory outcomes with total ankle arthroplasties in his series of ten patients with rheumatoid arthritis. His results were so poor that he concluded that the surgery should not be performed in this patient population.

Implants that provide a more normal anatomic load transmission appear to be associated with satisfactory outcomes. Inglis[13] communicated satisfactory clinical results, at an average of 5-year follow-up, without talar subluxation employing a custom-fit cementless device having a more anatomic bicondylar configuration. Buechel and associates[3] found no aseptic loosening in a mixed population of 23 ankles followed for an average of 5 years employing biologic fixation. To date, the resurfacing minimally constrained bicondylar devices that more closely mimic the normal kinematics of the ankle joint appear to be more durable than earlier prosthetic devices. They continue to function satisfactorily at intermediate follow-up periods and compare favorably with the nonanatomic devices previously described. For similar follow-up data reported to date, clinical outcomes are superior. The radiographic follow-up evaluations suggest a longer durability for these devices.

SURGICAL TECHNIQUE

Anterior Approach

The anterior approach for total ankle arthroplasty closely resembles that for an-

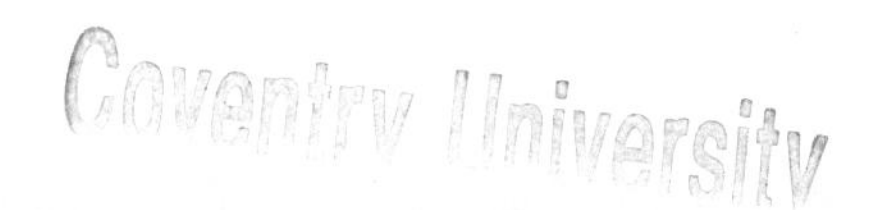

kle arthrodesis. With the patient supine on the operating table and the pneumatic tourniquet in place, a 15-cm incision is made from the base of the second metatarsal, carried proximally to the crest of the tibia. The incision is equidistant between the medial and lateral malleoli. Skin and subcutaneous tissues are divided sharply to the deep fascia, and the extensor retinaculum is opened longitudinally. The extensor hallucis longus and tibialis anterior muscles are identified and reflected medially. The extensor digitorum communis is reflected laterally. The neurovascular bundle is reflected laterally. Sharp dissection is used to enter the capsule of the ankle joint. Periosteal dissection is employed to identify the lateral malleolus and medial malleolus. Care is taken to preserve the deltoid and lateral collateral ligaments. Bennett retractors are placed subperiosteally around the medial and lateral malleoli.

At this time, Steinmann pins are placed parallel to the proposed cuts, approximately 2 cm proximal to the joint. After radiographs are taken to confirm position, attention is directed to the lateral malleolus, where a small longitudinal incision is made at the tip. The tip is resected distal to the origin of the fibular collateral ligament to prevent fibular/talar impingement. Parallel cuts are made in the tibia and on the talus with the Steinmann pins as guides. Minimal bone is removed from the talus so that the neck of the talus will not be violated (Fig. 42–5). The tibial saw cut is usually made 7 mm above the articular surface, with care taken to protect the medial malleolus. After the two parallel cuts have been made and the bone has been removed, sizing is performed with the appropriate spacing blocks. The largest prosthesis possible in the medial-lateral plane is selected. Tension should be balanced on the lateral and medial ligament complex, and 2 to 4 mm of overall laxity is ideal. The trial components are placed, and the ankle is put through full range of motion. If the components are placed too anteriorly, the implant arthroplasty will lack dorsiflexion; if too far posteriorly, the plantar flexion will be inadequate. At this point, trial components are removed and, if the prosthesis will be cemented, the bone is thoroughly cleaned by pulsating lavage. When cement fixation is employed, both components should be cemented simultaneously but the tibial component should be placed first. The foot is brought up to neutral position and the cement allowed to harden. When biologic fixation is applied, the tibial component is placed first. A drain is placed deep in the wound. The superficial fascia is closed with interrupted absorbable sutures, and the skin and subcutaneous tissues are closed in standard fashion. The ankle is placed in a well-padded soft dressing with a posterior splint.

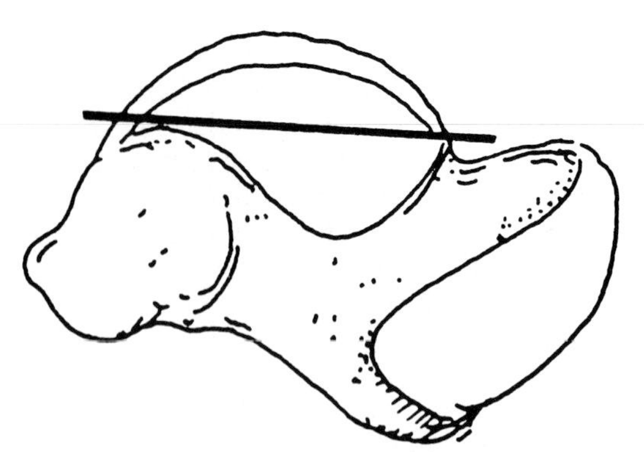

FIGURE 42–5. Level of cut on talus.

Posterior Approach

The posterior approach has been shown to be associated with fewer soft tissue and wound complications. This approach also offers wider exposure and visualization of the implant than the anterior approach. In addition, the center of rotation of the implant arthroplasty can be better assessed because the anatomy of the posterior cortex of the tibia and os calcis is constant.

After the patient is placed prone, draped in a sterile fashion, and a tourniquet is applied, a medial zig-zag incision is made, starting 10 cm proximal to the medial malleolus and parallel to the medial border of the Achilles tendon. The incision is brought down to the level of the insertion of the Achilles tendon (Fig. 42–6A). The crural fascia is identified and opened longitudinally (Fig. 42–6B). The plantaris tendon is identified and released off the insertion of the medial aspect of the os calcis. The deep posterior fascia is identified on the posterior aspect of the tibia, and the muscular flexor group is identified. Dissection is carried underneath the flexor tendons subperiosteally around the medial

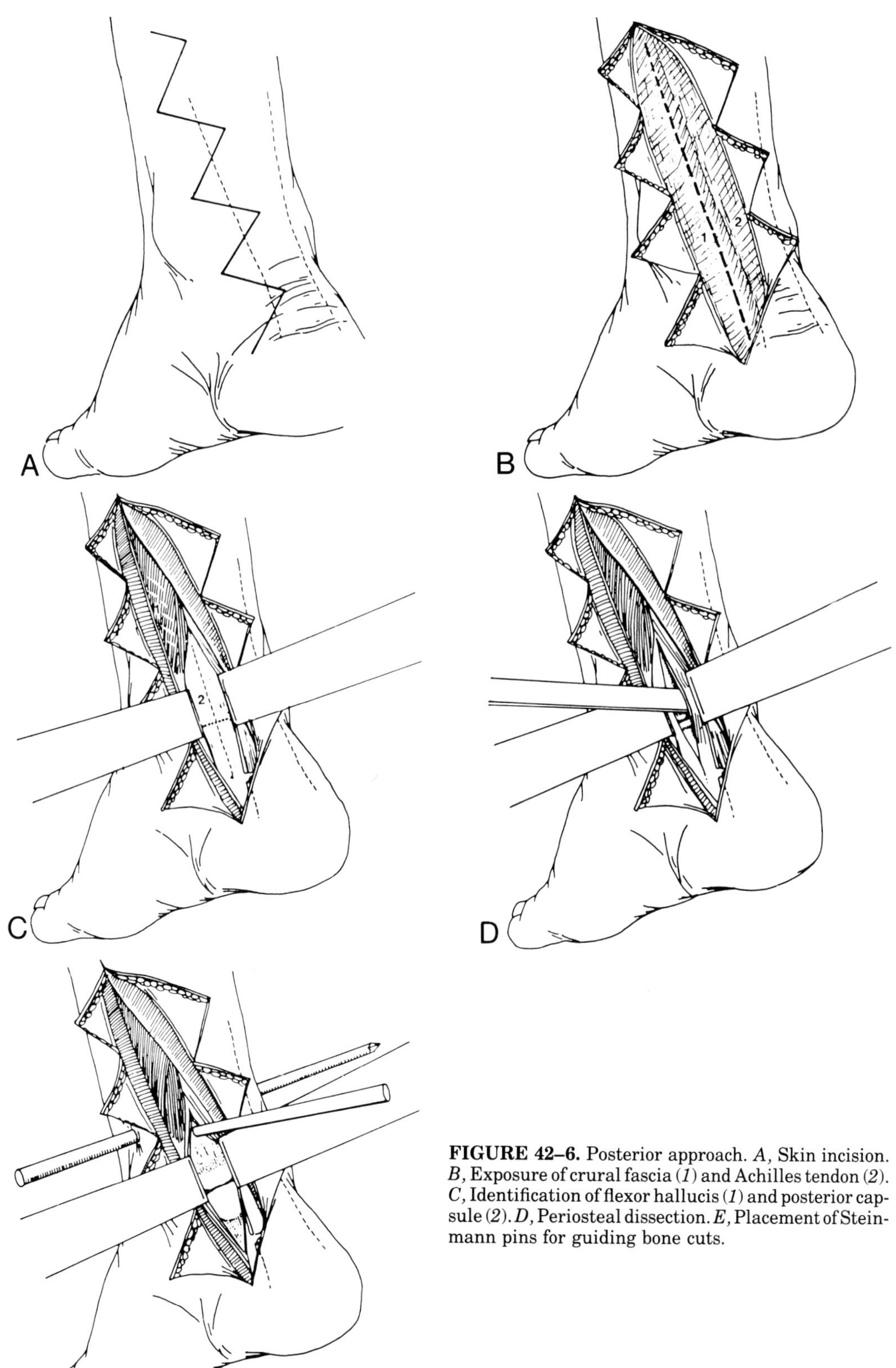

FIGURE 42–6. Posterior approach. *A,* Skin incision. *B,* Exposure of crural fascia (*1*) and Achilles tendon (*2*). *C,* Identification of flexor hallucis (*1*) and posterior capsule (*2*). *D,* Periosteal dissection. *E,* Placement of Steinmann pins for guiding bone cuts.

malleolus. This maneuver preserves the medial flexor group and neurovascular bundle. A Bennett retractor is placed medially around the malleolus (Fig. 42–6C). Approximately a fourth of the Achilles tendon may be taken down for better exposure. Subperiosteal dissection is carried laterally around the lateral malleolus, exposing the entire ankle joint (Fig. 42–6D). Steinmann pins are placed parallel to the proposed level of cuts, approximately 2 cm proximal to the distal tibial articular surface, and radiographs are obtained (Fig. 42–6E). A longitudinal incision directly over the lateral malleolus is made, and the tip is resected distal to the origin of the fibular collateral ligament to prevent lateral impingement. The orientation of the Steinmann pins with respect to the long axis of the tibia guides the angle of the tibial cuts in both planes. Care must be taken to remove bone off the tibia and not the talus. Removal of excessive talar bone can lead to damage of the talar neck with subsequent avascular necrosis or talar neck fracture.

After the cuts have been made, sizing is performed with the appropriate spacer blocks. Trial components are employed to assess the range of motion. If dorsiflexion or plantar flexion contractures remain, they are corrected by additional bone cuts or soft tissue balance. The center of rotation is assessed by either the bony landmark of the posterior cortex of the tibia or the insertion of the Achilles into the os calcis. Preoperative measurements are utilized to assess the position of the implant with respect to the center of rotation. The bony surfaces are thoroughly cleaned with a pulsating lavage if cement will be used.

Cement is pressurized into the bony surfaces with both components cemented simultaneously, but the tibial component is placed first. Excess cement is removed. The foot is then brought up to neutral position while the cement polymerizes. When biologic fixation is applied, the tibial component is placed first. The wound is irrigated thoroughly and closed in layers, with a drain placed deep in the wound. The deep fascia is closed with interrrupted absorbable sutures. Skin and subcutaneous tissues are closed in standard fashion with interrupted sutures. The ankle is placed in a well-padded dressing with a posterior splint.

POSTOPERATIVE CARE

After surgery, the repaired ankle should be kept elevated for 3 to 4 days. Suction should be continued until drainage ceases, usually 24 to 48 hours. As soon as the wound has healed, the ankle is placed in a short walking cast. When a cemented implant arthroplasty is performed, the patient may begin weightbearing to his or her level of tolerance. The cast is usually worn for 2 to 3 weeks. When cementless prostheses are implanted, 6 weeks of partial weightbearing are required.

Patients are discharged from the hospital when wound healing is complete and they are independent. Patients with cemented implants are first seen as outpatients at 2 to 3 weeks postoperatively for cast removal. Patients with cementless implants are seen at 6 weeks postoperatively. The patients then progress to full weightbearing as tolerated without restriction. Thereafter, patients return for follow-up evaluations every 3 months for the first year. Radiographs are obtained at each visit. The patient is then seen on a yearly basis.

COMPLICATIONS

Superficial wound infections, hematomas, and skin edge necroses are the most common complications following total ankle arthroplasties. Superficial wound infections should be managed with cast immobilization and antibiotic therapy until the wound has healed. Wound hematoma should be evacuated. Skin necrosis should also be managed with cast immobilization and antibiotic therapy. In the case of significant skin loss, skin coverage should be accomplished promptly with local or remote flaps or skin grafts.

Dislocation of the implant is a rare complication after total ankle arthroplasty, but the most common direction of dislocation when it occurs is posterior. Closed reduction and cast immobilization for 6 weeks are usually successful, but in rare cases open reduction is necessary. When chronic dislocation occurs owing to malalignment or muscular imbalance, the best treatment is 6 to 12 weeks of immobilization in a cast. If conservative treatment fails, revision arthroplasty with muscle balancing or ankle arthrodesis may be tried as a salvage procedure.

Fibular and medial malleolus impingement may occur after total ankle arthroplasty owing to malalignment or subsidence of the talar component. Talar subsidence results in loss of hindfoot height. Of the two complications, fibular impingement is more common—it is corrected by distal resection of the fibula to the level of the collateral ligament origin. Medial malleolar impingement is rare and should be treated by partial resection of the medial malleolus distal to the origin of the superficial deltoid ligament.

Deep infection is the most serious complication following total ankle arthroplasty. Evaluation of the infection consists of (1) technetium-, gallium-, or indium-labeled white blood cell scan, which separately or in combination may demonstrate local infection; (2) complete white blood cell count with differential; (3) aspiration arthrogram; and (4) erythrocyte sedimentation rate. The aspiration arthrogram may show implant loosening and provides joint fluid for culture. Increases in erythrocyte sedimentation rate or C-reactive protein are nonspecific markers for inflammation and therefore may not be very helpful in patients with systemic arthritis. When deep infection is found, the implant and cement should be removed. Revision for septic failure must always be performed as a two-stage procedure. The options include arthrodesis, resection arthroplasty, and revision total ankle arthroplasty.

STRATEGIES FOR REVISION

Revision of a failed component is difficult. Frequently, the bone stock in the talus and tibia have been compromised. The key consideration is usually the quality of bone stock available for reconstruction in the talus. If substantial amounts of the talar body have been lost or if the talar neck has been violated, either arthrodesis or resection arthroplasty should be performed. When satisfactory bone stock remains in the talus, total ankle arthroplasty as a revision procedure can be considered, although the indications are limited to patients with severe hindfoot disease and midfoot disease. In such patients, ankle arthrodesis would cause disabling shifts of loadbearing to the hindfoot and midfoot. If bone stock in the talus is deficient in a patient with severe midfoot and hindfoot arthritis, resection arthroplasty is indicated. The surgical approaches for revision total ankle arthroplasty, resection arthroplasty, and arthrodesis are identical to those previously described. When revision implant arthroplasty is contraindicated, arthrodesis or resection arthroplasty usually provides a satisfactory result.[27]

Arthrodesis or Resection Arthroplasty After Failed Total Ankle Replacement

For ankle arthrodesis or resection arthroplasty following failed arthroplasty, the skin incision and approach described previously are selected to expose the ankle implants. The tibial and talar components are taken out. All bone cement is removed from the cancellous bone. Frequently, this step leaves a 1- to 2-cm defect. When resection arthroplasty is performed, the tibia is centralized on the talus and held in position by a large Steinmann pin placed from the heel through the talus and into the tibia. The pin is removed 6 weeks postoperatively. After another 6 weeks, the cast is taken off. Resection arthroplasty is contraindicated when the medial or lateral malleolus is deficient.

When arthrodesis is elected, tricortical block graft and cancellous bone are taken from the ilium (Fig. 42–7A). The block graft is shaped to fit the contours of the ankle mortise. The foot should be in neutral position in both sagittal and coronal planes. After graft material is packed around the tricortical graft, the ankle joint is stabilized by either an external compression apparatus or internal fixation with cancellous screws (Fig. 42–7B). If the implants are being removed for infection, a two-stage procedure may be employed, with serial debridement performed until the infection is eradicated. Intravenous antibiotics are administered for 6 weeks. Two weeks after cessation of antibiotics, repeat

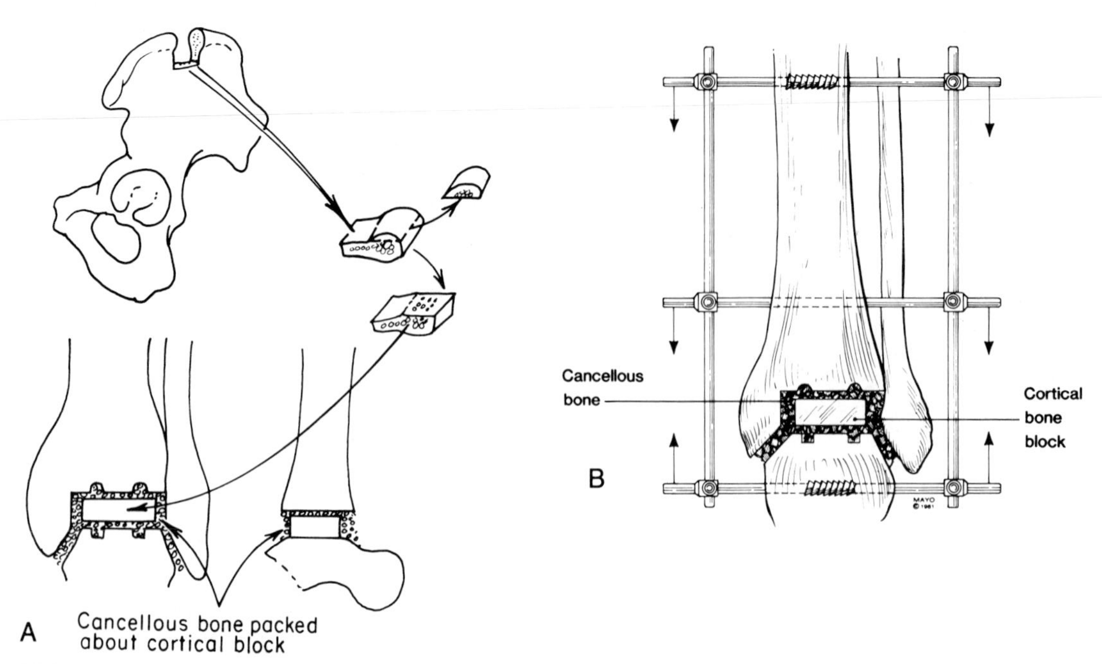

FIGURE 42–7. Technique of revision arthrodesis for failed total ankle arthroplasty. *A*, Tricortical graft taken from the iliac crest is shaped to occupy ankle mortise. Cancellous bone is packed around graft. *B*, External fixator is placed through talus and tibia with the foot in neutral alignment. (Stauffer, R.M.N.: Clin. Orthop. 170:186, 1982. By permission.)

aspiration is performed. Final revision is accomplished after culture findings are negative.

SUMMARY

Total ankle arthroplasty is a successful procedure in carefully selected patients. Implant arthroplasty should be limited to sedentary patients with multiple joint involvement. This procedure is not indicated for isolated tibiotalar arthritis in young active patients. The surgical technique is demanding, requiring careful selection of implant, thorough preoperative planning, and a patient who will comply with the postoperative regimen. The chief advantage of the operation is maintenance of motion in the tibiotalar joint in the severely compromised patient with systemic arthritis. Usually, this advantage outweighs any disadvantages of the procedure. The technology of ankle implant arthroplasty keeps changing, and the results of properly selected patients are improving.

Implant design is currently directed at minimizing bone stresses and improving stability while decreasing constraint. A metal-backed bicondylar implant meets needed design criteria while offering multiaxial motion. Biologic fixation of total ankle arthroplasty is desirable because the cancellous surface offers a good tissue bed and complete immobilization can be achieved. Also, current cement technique is poor. Clinical trials are currently under way of bicondylar variable center-of-rotation implants employing metal backing, variable joint height, and biologic fixation.

Current research is directed at improving alignment criteria, optimizing implant mechanics, and improving implant fixation to minimize subsidence. The objective of alignment is to balance the dorsiflexion and plantar flexion muscles while centralizing the implant to prevent excessive eccentric load because of the body's center of rotation, Finite element modeling is now under way to allow optimization of implant centers.

References

1. Adam, W. and Rand, C.S.: Arthrodesis of the hindfoot in rheumatoid arthritis. Orthop. Clin. North Am. 7:827–840, 1976.
2. Bolton-Maggs, B.G., Sudrow, R.A., and Freeman, M.A.R.: Total ankle arthroplasty: A long-term

review of the London Hospital experience. J. Bone Joint Surg. 67B:785–790, 1985.
3. Buechel, F.F., Pappas, M.J., and Iorio, L.J.: New Jersey low contact stress total ankle replacement: Biomechanical rationale and review of 23 cases. Foot Ankle 8:279–290, 1988.
4. Burge, P. and Evans, M.: Effect of surface replacement arthroplasty on stability of the ankle. Foot Ankle 7:10–17, 1986.
5. Charnley, J.: Compression arthrodesis of the ankle and shoulder. J. Bone Joint Surg. 33B:180, 1951.
6. Denottaz, J.D., Mazur, J.M., Thomas, W.H., et al.: Clinical study of total ankle replacement with gait analysis. A preliminary report. J. Bone Joint Surg. 61A:976–988, 1979.
7. Dini, A.A. and Bassett, F.H.: Evaluation of the early result of Smith total ankle replacement. Clin. Orthop. 146:228–230, 1980.
8. Evanski, P.M. and Waugh, T.R.: Management of arthritis of the ankle. Clin. Orthop. 122:110–115, 1977.
9. Frankel, V.H. and Nordin, M.: Biomechanics of the Ankle. Basic Biomechanics of the Skeletal System. Edited by V. H. Frankel and M. Nordin. Philadelphia, Lea & Febiger, 1980.
10. Greenwald, A.S.: Ankle Joint Mechanics. Ankle Injuries. Edited by I.G. Segal, D. Segal, and R.E. Leach. New York, Churchill Livingstone, 1983.
11. Groth, H.E., Shen, G.S., and Fagan, P.J.: The Oregon ankle: A total ankle designed to replace all three articular surfaces. Orthop. Trans. 1:86, 1977.
12. Herberts, P., Goldie, I.F., Korner, L., et al.: Endoprosthetic replacement of the ankle joint. A clinical and radiological follow-up. Acta Orthop. Scand. 53:687–696, 1982.
13. Inglis, A.E.: Personal communication, 1987.
14. Inman, V.T., Ralston, H.J., and Todd, F.: Human Walking. Baltimore, Williams & Wilkins, 1981.
15. Johnson, E.W. and Boseker, E.H.: Arthrodesis of ankle. Arch. Surg. 97:766, 1968.
16. Lachiewicz, P.F., Inglis, A.E., and Ranawat, C.S.: Total ankle replacement in rheumatology arthritis. J. Bone Joint Surg. 66A:340–343, 1984.
17. Lester, J.G.: The Mayo ankle arthroplasty. J. Bone Joint Surg. 65B:520–521, 1983.
18. Mazur, J.M., Schwartz, E., and Simon, S.R.: Ankle arthrodesis. Long-term follow-up with gait analysis. J. Bone Joint Surg. 61A:964–975, 1979.
19. Newton, S. E., III: Total ankle arthroplasty: Clinical study of fifty cases. J. Bone Joint Surg. 64A: 104–111, 1982.
20. Pappas, M., Buechel, F.F., and DePalma, A.F.: Cylindrical total ankle replacement. Surgical and biomechanical rationale. Clin. Orthop. 118:82–92, 1976.
21. Pipino, F., and Calderale, P.M.: PC ankle prosthesis. Five-year follow-up. Acta Orthop. Belg. 49:725–735, 1983.
22. Root, M.L., Orien, W.P., and Weed, J.H.: Normal and Abnormal Function of the Foot. Los Angeles, Clinical Biomechanics Corp., 1977.
23. Sammarco, G.J., Burstein, A.H., and Frankel, V.H.: Biomechanics of the ankle: A kinematic study. Orthop. Clin. North Am. 4:75–96, 1973.
24. Samuelson, K.M., Freeman, M.A.R., and Tukel, M.A.: Development and evolution of the ICLH ankle replacement. Foot Ankle 3:32–36, 1982.
25. Scolz, K.C.: Total Ankle Replacement. Foot Science. Edited by J.E. Bateman. Philadelphia, W.B. Saunders Company, 1976.
26. Spector, E.E.: Ankle implants. Clin. Podiatr. 1:225–235, 1984.
27. Stauffer, R.N.: Salvage of painful total ankle arthroplasty. Clin. Orthop. 170:184–188, 1982.
28. Stauffer, R.N.: Total joint arthroplasty—The ankle. Mayo Clin. Proc. 54:570–575, 1979.
29. Stauffer, R.N.: Total ankle joint replacement. Arch Surg. 112:1105–1109, 1977.
30. Stauffer, R.N. and Segal, N.M.: Total ankle arthroplasty: Four years' experience. Clin. Orthop. 160:217–221, 1981.
31. Unger, A.S., Inglis, A.E., Mow, C., and Figgie, H.E., III: Total ankle arthroplasty in rheumatoid arthritis: A long-term follow-up study. Foot Ankle 8:173–179, 1988.
32. Wiedel, J.D.: Total ankle arthroplasty with Smith prosthesis. Orthop. Trans. 1:154, 1977.

SECTION X

TUMORS

CHAPTER 43

Joint Reconstruction after Tumor Resection

DEMPSEY S. SPRINGFIELD

Only a few years ago, most patients with primary malignant tumors of the bone were treated with amputations. In the rare case, when the limb of a patient with a bone sarcoma was saved, the motion of the adjacent joint was usually limited or the joint was fused. This is no longer true—not only has limb salvage increased, but the motion of the joint has been saved and the extremities are, in general, quite functional.

ADVANCES IN RESECTION AND RECONSTRUCTION

In the past, the only limb salvage candidates were those few patients whose tumors were small and either confined to the bone or having a minimal extraosseous component. The joint usually was resected with the tumor, since most malignant tumors involve the metaphysis and epiphysis, and arthrodesis was performed. The three reasons for this procedure were as follows.

First, the surgeon was not able to define the extent of the tumor accurately before the operation. The imaging tests available—plain radiographs, angiograms, plain tomograms, and technetium bone scans—were of limited accuracy.[19] As a result, the prudent surgeon excised a large margin of surrounding normal tissue to be sure that all of the tumor cells were removed. Today, more accurate methods to define the extent of a sarcoma are available. Radiologists have diagnostic tools—computerized tomography (CT) and magnetic resonance imaging (MRI)—capable of defining the anatomic limits of a tumor and its relationships to vital structures. With CT, the surgeon can examine cross-sectional anatomy and define the exact extent of a sarcoma, which is a major improvement in the planning of most limb salvage procedures. The subsequent introduction of MRI was a further improvement in defining the anatomic extent of a tumor. These two tools have been instrumental in the successful salvage of a greater number of limbs.

The second reason that surgeons were more likely to amputate than to salvage tumor-involved limbs was the lack of adjuvant therapy. Surgical resection was the only treatment. If the surgeon failed to control the primary tumor, the patient invariably died. Now, more patients are candidates for limb salvage because of the availability of chemotherapy for bone sarcomas, especially osteosarcoma and Ewing's sarcoma. At first, chemotherapy was given only after surgery, but preoperative (neoadjuvant) chemotherapy is rapidly becoming the preferred method of initial management.[10, 21, 46] Although not yet proved, preoperative chemotherapy seems to improve the outlook for limb and joint salvage surgery.

The third reason why limb salvage is now more common is the availability of methods for reconstruction. Before limb salvage became routine, the surgeon usually had to develop a method of reconstruction for each patient or needed a prosthesis manufacturer to construct a customized prosthesis. In the past decade, extensive activities have been witnessed in both allograft transplantation and prosthetic material and design development. The possibility of a limb salvage resection has rekindled interest in developing bone banks so that surgeons can procure allografts for skeletal and joint reconstructions. Large-segment allograft bone with or without cartilage is available for reconstructing the major joints.[1, 2, 8, 17, 24, 29, 37, 47, 50, 51]

Although locally aggressive benign and malignant bone tumors are not common, when they do occur, surgical resection is usually necessary. Improved imaging studies, more routine preoperative adjuvant therapy, and better means of reconstruction have all contributed to the increase in limb salvage operations. The resections and reconstructions are technically difficult. The patient must be able to tolerate what are essentially two operations performed under the same anesthetic: the tumor resection and the reconstruction.

CLASSIFICATION OF PELVIC RESECTIONS

Numerous workers have discussed indications and techniques for pelvic resections. (See references 6, 9–14, 20, 25, 27, 28, 31, 38, 39, 41, 44, 45, 48, 53.) Enneking and Dunham[13] proposed a classification system for pelvic resections, grouping them according to similarities in reconstruction and ultimate function (Fig. 43–1). This classification system is simple and provides a common language to describe the type of resection. Because each type of resection results in different structural deficits, each group should be considered separately.

Only those pelvic resections that require removal of the acetabulum significantly affect the patient's function. Therefore, only when the acetabulum is resected should a reconstruction of the bony pelvis be considered. Resections of the ilium or pubis do not require bone reconstruction,

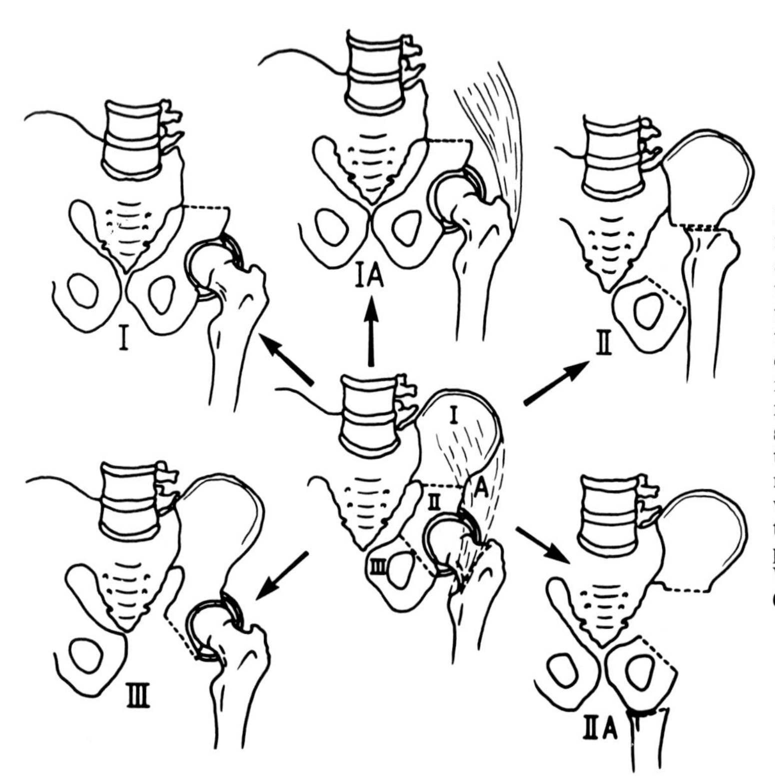

FIGURE 43–1. Types of pelvic resections proposed by Enneking and Dunham. Type I is the iliac wing only, type II is the periacetabular pelvis, and type III is the pubis and ischium exclusive of the acetabulum. The letter A indicates that the overlying muscle or the hip joint is resected as well. If more than one type are done together, both numbers are given, e.g., the iliac wing and periacetabulum with the hip joint is a type I and IIA pelvic resection. (Enneking, W.F.: J. Bone Joint Surg. 60A:732, 1978. By permission.)

as the patient is able to walk without external aids and function almost normally.

After a type I or type IA resection (iliac wing with or without the abductors), the patient will have a Trendelenburg limp, although it is usually minimal (Fig. 43–2). Transfer of the psoas insertion from the lesser trochanter to the greater trochanter is recommended when the psoas is not removed with the iliac wing. The transfer stabilizes the pelvis during stance and seems to improve gait (walking), although no gait analysis studies have been published. After the iliac wing resection has been completed, the psoas is released from its insertion on the lesser trochanter, taking care not to injure the femoral nerve. The psoas is separated from the iliacus muscle, and the distal tendon is pulled into the pelvis. The psoas can then be transferred and sutured onto the remaining abductor tendons near the greater trochanter. Immobilization in abduction for the initial 4 to 6 weeks after surgery is recommended. Although the transferred psoas loses motor strength and cannot abduct the limb against gravity, it does work well enough to improve the gait.

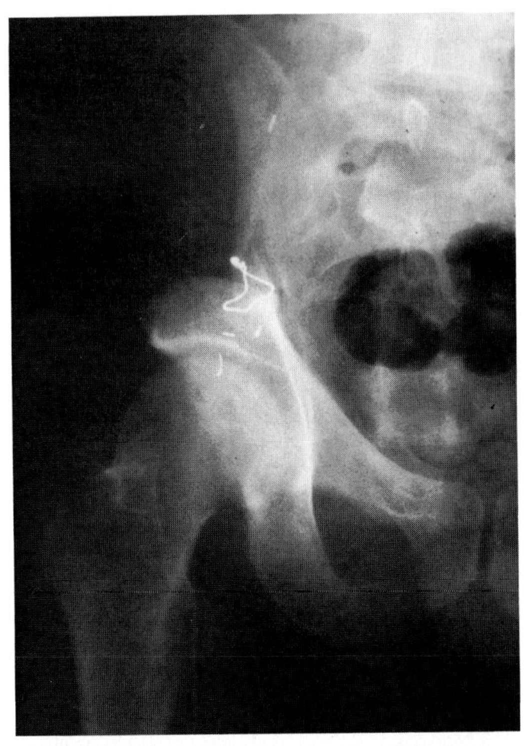

FIGURE 43–2. Anteroposterior view of the hip in a patient who has had the ilium resected. The wire closed the gap in the sciatic notch so that the sciatic nerve would not be trapped between the remaining ilium and sacrum. Patients who have undergone this procedure have varying degrees of limp. However, they need no external aids, and replacement of the ilium is not indicated. Strut grafts between the ilium and sacrum have been used but do not improve function and are rarely indicated.

Resection of the pubis (type III or IIIA) is often necessary for tumors in the pubis. Even if a portion of the medial acetabulum must be resected, it is rarely necessary to reconstruct the bony pelvis. The hip joint always remains stable as long as the ligamentum teres remains, and it usually is stable even when the ligaments have been excised. The hip joint should not be dislocated during resection of the pubis unless absolutely necessary. Dislocation increases the instability of the hip and the risk of subsequent dislocation or chronic subluxation. Afterward, a large inguinal hernia is present, but it is not usually symptomatic and needs no specific treatment.

RECONSTRUCTIONS AFTER ACETABULAR RESECTIONS

Although patients can walk after acetabular resections (type II), even without reconstruction (resection arthroplasty, flail hip), function is much better if the limb is stabilized.[3] At one time, the only stable reconstruction was arthrodesis or fibrous ankylosis. Now, the surgeon has a variety of choices for reconstructing the acetabulum.

The safest option is to leave the joint flail and not attempt a formal reconstruction.[10] This choice will result in satisfactory function and is best if the patient cannot tolerate additional surgery. A simple reconstruction can be done if the ilium has been transected through the superior acetabulum and the femoral head retained. The remaining ilium and femoral head are wired together, and a spica cast is applied.[13, 14] If all of the ilium and acetabulum have been resected but a portion of the pubis remains, the femur can be wired to the pubis. If the resection is greater but formal reconstruction is not done, the patient should be placed in skeletal traction, with the pin in the distal femur, for 6 weeks (Fig. 43–3). Some patients will be

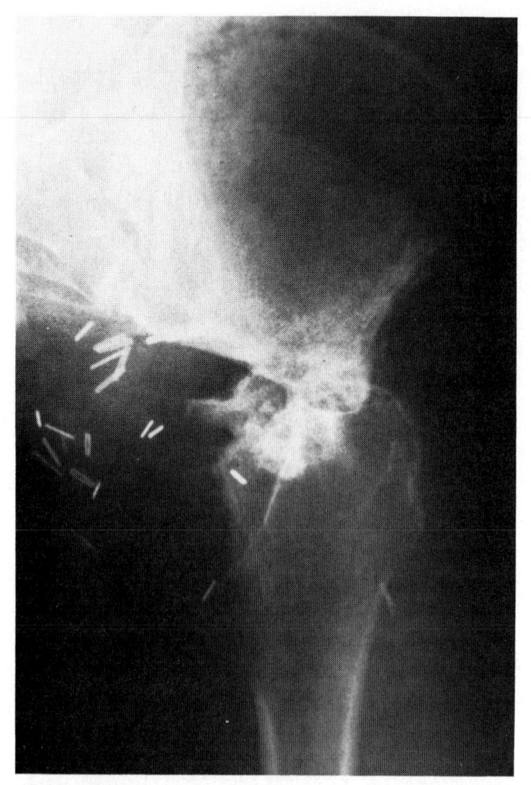

FIGURE 43–3. Anteroposterior view of the hip in a patient who had resection of the entire acetabulum, hip joint, pubis, ischium, and adjacent soft tissue (type IIA and IIIA). A reconstruction of the bone was believed to be contraindicated owing to previous irradiation. The patient was treated in skeletal traction for 6 weeks and then allowed to ambulate, first nonweightbearing with progression as tolerated. At 1 year, she was able to walk with one cane. When last evaluated, she had mild pain, excellent motion, and slight pistoning of the extremity on weightbearing.

able to walk with one crutch or a cane, but the limb undergoes piston-type movement with weightbearing, and most patients are not satisfied with this type of extremity.

If the entire hip joint has been resected or the entire ilium has been removed and the patient can tolerate further surgery, a formal reconstruction should be done. The reconstructive options include arthrodesis, autoclaved autogenous bone/prosthesis reconstruction, allograft replacement, allograft/prosthesis reconstruction, and saddle prosthesis. The greater the magnitude of the reconstruction, the greater the risk of complications, and the more important the reconstruction as a means of maintaining function.

An arthrodesis is difficult and requires months to heal, but the patient's function is excellent and activities are unrestricted once the arthrodesis is solid (Fig. 43–4). Even the patient in whom arthrodesis is attempted but stable fibrous ankylosis develops has better function than the patient with an unstable flail hip.[6, 10, 11, 14, 53]

Replacement of the acetabulum with either an allograft or a prosthesis has significantly improved the options for the surgeon and the patient. These reconstructions are difficult, however, and the complications are significant. Therefore, they should not be undertaken without a thorough understanding of the potential problems. After an allograft/prosthesis or autoclaved autogenous bone/prosthesis arthroplasty, the patient retains hip motion, although activity will have to be limited. This is an excellent reconstructive option for the more sedentary patient.

Custom-built prostheses have been utilized when only the acetabulum is resected

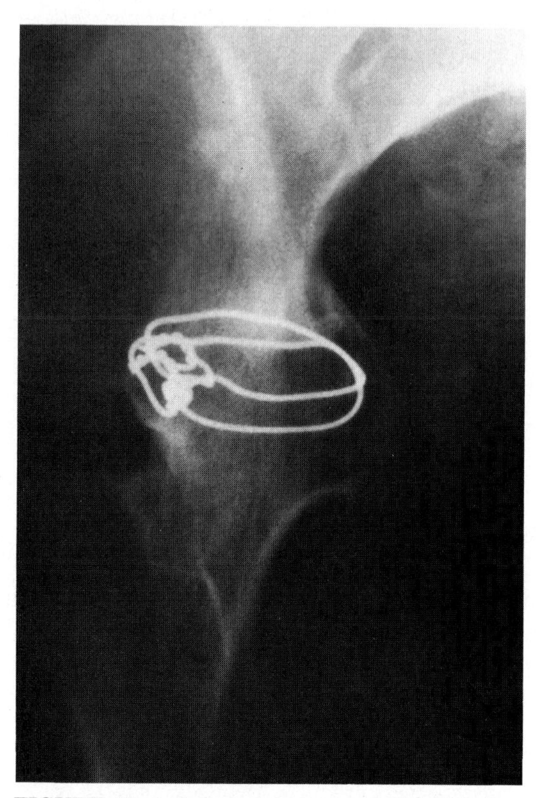

FIGURE 43–4. Anteroposterior view of the hip in a patient who had a resection of the acetabulum, ischium, and pubis (type II and III). The limb was shortened and the femoral head wired to the remaining ilium. The patient was placed into a hip spica cast for 8 weeks. The arthrodesis healed. The patient then wore a 1-inch heel lift, had no pain, and ambulated without external aids.

(type II). The saddle prosthesis, used mainly in Europe, is said to function well, but it has not been adequately evaluated.[42]

Arthrodesis

Arthrodesis with an intercalary allograft or autograft is probably the best option for the patient who can tolerate reconstruction and who needs a strong extremity. When more than 6 cm of bone has to be resected, as with an extra-articular hip joint resection (type IIA), arthrodesis without an intercalary graft would result in an excessively short limb. Intercalary allograft, which is fixed to the ilium and remaining femur with large plates, maintains the proper length of the extremity and helps obtain an arthrodesis. This reconstruction requires 2 to 3 additional hours of surgery, and postoperative rehabilitation is prolonged. The patient must be able to tolerate both of these, if this type of reconstruction is selected.

It is difficult to position the extremity properly during the operation—30 to 35 degrees of flexion, 0 to 5 degrees of external rotation, and neutral abduction-adduction. I have found a satisfactory, although somewhat crude, method. I position the patient on the operating table before "prepping" and draping and secure the pelvis. The extremity to be operated on is placed in the optimal position for an arthrodesis, and the position of the foot is carefully noted. When later positioning the extremity for the arthrodesis, the foot again is put in this position and held until the allograft, which has already been fixed to the distal femur, is rigidly fixed to the pelvis.

In a case in which the femoral head is retained and the ilium is resected immediately above the acetabulum (type II), the femoral head and proximal femur can be rigidly fixed to the ilium with a large plate. If a second plate can be added, the fixation will be more secure. If the patient is not cooperative postoperatively or if the fixation is not strong, a spica cast should be applied. Although it is often possible to achieve arthrodesis with minimal internal fixation and prolonged cast immobilization, a successful arthrodesis is more certain if rigid internal fixation is applied.

Early function is better if early ambulation is permitted. The patient can ambulate in the immediate postoperative period with crutches, bearing partial weight on the operated limb. The ipsilateral knee should be exercised early to decrease loss of knee motion, a common complication of arthrodesis of the hip, especially with major resections of proximal thigh muscles.

Graft/Prosthesis

If hip motion is to be retained, the acetabulum must be reconstructed. Some workers have advocated utilization of the resected ilium for the reconstruction.[18] The surgical technique is similar to replacement of the ilium with an allograft. The tumor is curetted on a separate sterile table in the operating room until no more tumor is visible. The remaining bone is autoclaved and replaced in the patient. A standard total hip replacement is used as the joint. The limited published results have been acceptable, but additional data are needed to establish the place of this reconstructive method.

Another option is to replace the resected acetabulum with an allograft hemipelvis and to replace the femoral head with a conventional hemiarthroplasty (Fig. 43–5). This type of reconstruction should not be thought of as an established method either—it will be another decade before the appropriateness of this technique will be known—but it is an option after tumor resection. Allograft hemipelvis has been most successful in the patient who does not require significant muscle resection (type II), but it can be done even when adjacent muscle must be resected (type IIA).

The size of the allograft hemipelvis should be close to the size of the patient's hemipelvis, although size is not as important in pelvic reconstructions as it is in distal femoral or proximal tibial reconstructions. After the tumor has been resected, the pelvic allograft is tailored until it is identical to the resected portion of the patient's pelvis. The remaining pelvis must be exposed in the operative field so that the allograft can be fixed to the host bone. Usually, the initial incisions must be extended and the soft tissues stripped off the remaining ilium and pubis. The allograft

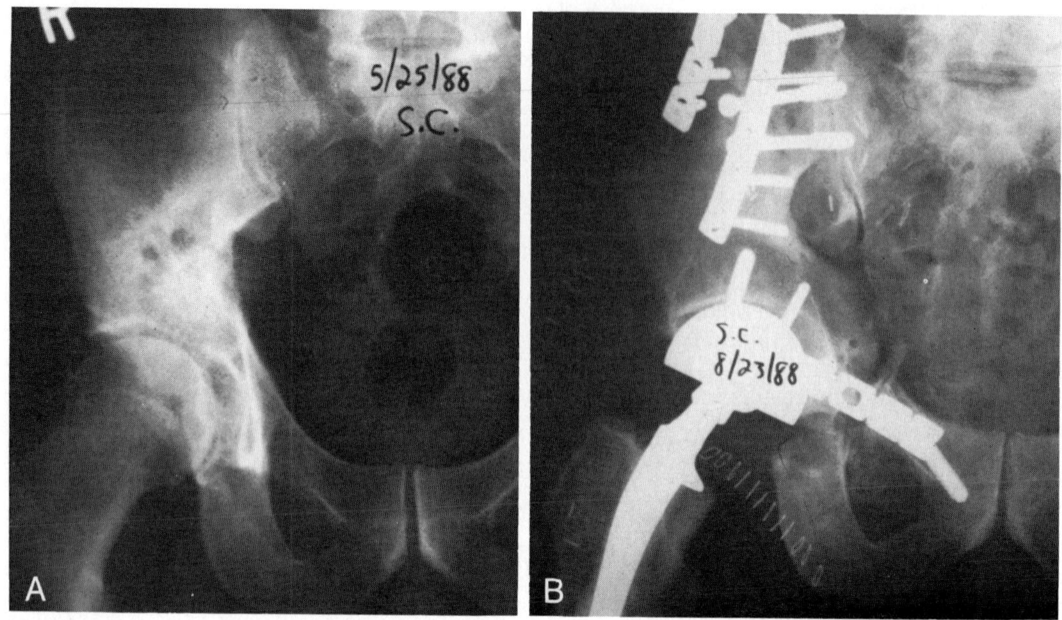

FIGURE 43–5. *A,* Anteroposterior view of the hip of a 52-year-old man who complained of groin pain. The lesion involved the superior and medial wall of the acetabulum and proved to be a low-grade angiosarcoma. On the computerized tomographic scan, the lesion appeared not to enter the hip joint. No evidence of metastatic disease was found. A surgical resection was done. *B,* Anteroposterior view of the reconstructed hip of the patient. A resection of the acetabulum and a portion of the ilium with the iliacus muscle was done (type IIA resection). A wide margin was obtained. The pelvis was reconstructed with an allograft. In such cases, fixation between the patient's bone and the allograft is difficult. Each case requires special consideration. The allograft's acetabulum was not the same size as the patient's acetabulum, and therefore a bipolar femoral endoprosthesis was implanted. At 2-year follow-up, the patient's allograft had healed and he walked without external aids.

is then placed into the defect and rigidly fixed to the remaining pelvis with plates. Pelvic reconstruction plates are useful, but stronger plates should also be inserted if possible. Interfragmentary screws can be helpful. A femoral head prosthesis of the proper size is selected and fixed into the proximal femur in a conventional manner. The prosthetic femoral head is reduced into the acetabulum. The hip abductors are attached to the allograft and to the abdominal muscles.

Strict bed rest is advised for the first 10 to 14 days. After this time, the patient is allowed out of bed on two crutches, with partial weightbearing. The initial physical therapy should be active-assisted motion to the ipsilateral knee and hip. The hip should be kept from adduction beyond 30 degrees of abduction for the first month, but it can be flexed early. Quadriceps and hamstring strengthening exercises are also begun early. Only after 5 to 6 weeks should the patient be encouraged to use the hip abductors, which should be well healed by this time. The allograft bone usually does not heal to the host bone for 6 to 9 months. It is best if the patient walks with two crutches and remains partially weightbearing, to protect the host-allograft junctions. Most patients are independent by the second month but remain on crutches for a year.

Custom Prostheses

An alternative to allograft reconstruction after pelvic resection is a custom pelvic prosthesis to replace a hemipelvis. The limited bone available for fixation makes a total prosthetic pelvis unlikely to be a long-term success.

Another prosthetic option is the saddle prosthesis.[42] A device that should be considered experimental, the saddle prosthesis was designed to replace the hip joint and salvage hip function in the patient who has had a major resection or excessive bone loss after failure of a total hip replacement (Fig. 43–6). Those surgeons who use the saddle prosthesis assert that it provides an

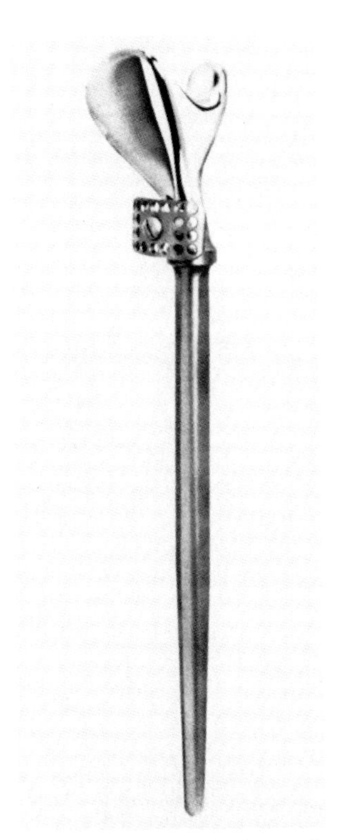

FIGURE 43–6. The "saddle" endoprosthesis manufactured by Link America, Inc. It has been used in Europe more than in North America. This endoprosthesis has been redesigned with an off-set at the collar.

excellent, stable, moving hip joint for patients with major pelvic resections that include the acetabulum or entire hip joint. Although the saddle prosthesis can replace the proximal femur or the entire femur in addition to the pelvis, use is more common in Europe than in the United States.

Initial reports of function were promising, but complication rates were high.[42] Recent design changes have been made. It will be some time before adequate experience with the saddle prosthesis has accumulated.

RECONSTRUCTIONS AFTER PROXIMAL FEMORAL RESECTIONS

Primary bone tumors in the proximal femur are relatively common, and they often are discovered before they have become so large that they involve the sciatic nerve posteriorly or the femoral artery anteriorly. The amputation that would be done to control a lesion in the proximal femur—hemipelvectomy—also stimulates the surgeon to consider limb salvage for patients with these tumors.[24, 26, 29, 43]

The reconstruction options after resection of the proximal femur include the following: (1) osteoarticular allograft replacement, (2) allograft/prosthesis composite replacement, (3) total prosthesis replacement, and (4) arthrodesis with intercalary autograft or allograft. The choice of the reconstruction procedure should be based on the patient's expectations and the surgeon's experience.

The older patient (over 65 years of age) is probably best treated with a prosthesis, because such a reconstruction allows the earliest weightbearing and shortest rehabilitation. The prosthesis should last 10 to 15 years if properly cared for. The younger patient, who is likely to outlive the expected life of a prosthesis, is probably better served with a biologic replacement. The allograft is a biologic replacement and at least has the potential to survive for the patient's lifetime. An additional advantage of the allograft is that it replaces the resected bone. If arthritic problems develop in a patient with an allograft, a conventional prosthesis can be employed. Arthrodesis is the best method of reconstruction for the patient who wants to be physically active and needs the strongest possible extremity. When the acetabulum must be resected along with the proximal femur, an allograft arthrodesis is an excellent method for reconstructing the limb (Fig. 43–7).

Allograft

A reconstruction with an allograft can be done either with or without a prosthesis. For an osteoarticular allograft, which does not include a prosthesis, the allograft femoral head should fit anatomically in the patient's acetabulum (Fig. 43–8). An allograft femoral head that fits into the acetabulum and is held by suction with direct lateral traction wears well and appears on the postoperative radiograph to be an anatomic replacement. When the femoral head does not fit, a hemiarthroplasty is recommended. A bipolar femoral head prosthesis may be utilized.

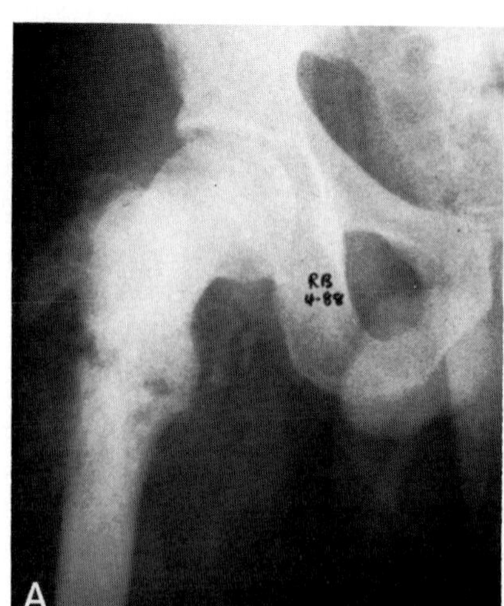

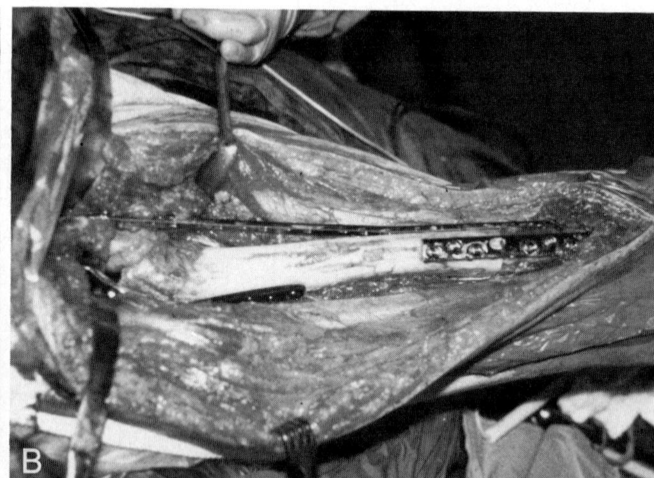

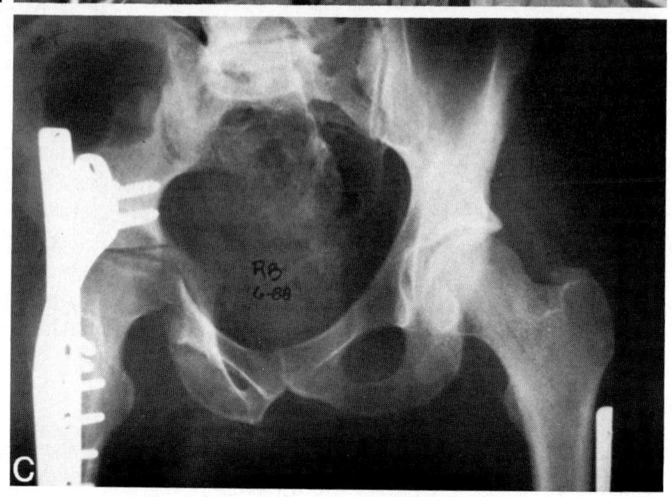

FIGURE 43–7. *A,* Anteroposterior view of a hip with a pathologic fracture through an osteosarcoma of the proximal femur. The initial evaluation revealed that the tumor invaded the hip joint but did not involve the major neurovascular structures. No metastases were found. The patient was treated with preoperative chemotherapy, and a limb salvage resection was done. Because of the extension into the hip joint, an extra-articular resection was necessary. The reconstruction is shown in *B* and *C*. *B,* Intraoperative photograph of the reconstruction shown in *C*. The patient's femoral head is to the left. A long intercalary allograft is between the distal femur and remaining ilium. The allograft is stabilized to the host bone with plates. *C,* Anteroposterior view of the reconstructed hip of the patient with a proximal femoral osteosarcoma whose radiograph is shown in *A*. The proximal femoral component was an allograft. The allograft and host bones were stabilized with plates (see *C*). The allograft-host junctions healed while the patient was on chemotherapy, but metastatic disease subsequently developed.

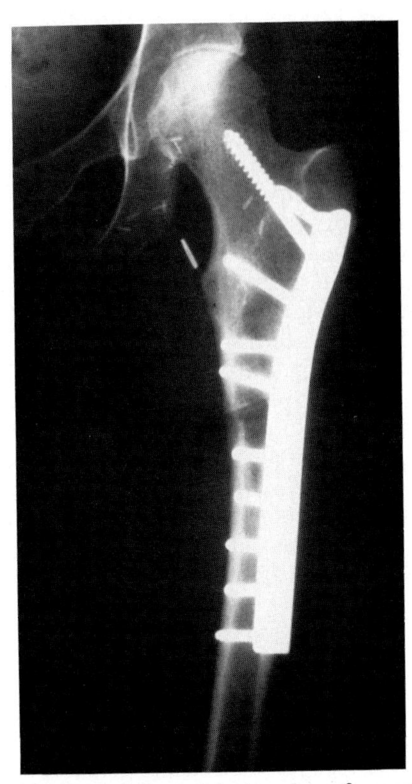

FIGURE 43–8. Anteroposterior view of an osteoarticular allograft of the proximal femur utilized to replace the proximal femur of a 27-year-old woman with a chondrosarcoma. This radiograph was taken 1 year after surgery. The junction of the allograft and host bone is between the fifth and sixth screws counting from proximal to distal. The bone healed well, and the patient walked with no limp and no external aids. The abductors were sutured to the allograft abductor tendons, which had been left attached to the greater trochanter of the allograft. These attachments seemed to heal well and offered a functional insertion of the muscle. In order to do an osteoarticular allograft of the femoral head, the surgeon must make certain that the allograft fits almost perfectly in the patient's acetabulum. Otherwise, a prosthesis should be selected to replace the femoral head. Thinning of the articular cartilage occurs, but the patient has no symptoms.

One of the advantages of an allograft reconstruction is that the length of the replacement part can be adjusted in the operating room. If the preoperative length of the extremity is to be unchanged, the allograft is cut to the same length as the resected segment. When the extremity needs to be lengthened or shortened, the allograft is prepared accordingly. After a trial reduction to check the length, the allograft is fixed with a large compression plate and screws to the patient's femur. At least eight cortices of the allograft should be held by screws. Some surgeons select a plate that extends the entire length of the allograft, but I confine the plate and screws to the diaphysis of the allograft segment. Proper rotation of the proximal allograft segment is important. The linea aspera of the allograft should line up with the linea aspera of the patient's femur, and 15 degrees of femoral neck anteversion should be present.

The femoral head is reduced after the allograft has been fixed to the patient's femur. The part of the hip capsule and the stump of abductor muscle tendon insertions that have been left on the allograft are sutured to the patient's remaining hip capsule and hip abductors, respectively. When possible, the patient's psoas tendon is sutured to the allograft's psoas tendon, but this step is not necessary for an excellent result.

When the femoral head does not fit the patient's acetabulum or when the acetabular cartilage is diseased, an allograft/prosthesis composite should be chosen (Fig. 43–9). The allograft can be prepared on a separate table by a second team of surgeons while the resection is being done. When the proximal femoral allograft is less than 200 mm, I choose a press-fit prosthesis with a 300-mm narrow stem. The allograft femoral neck is cut for the prosthesis chosen, and the canal is prepared with the appropriate reamers or broaches or both. The prosthesis is placed in the allograft femur so that the stem extends beyond the distal extent of the allograft. The allograft/prosthesis composite is positioned with the stem of the prosthesis in the canal of the femur. The proper rotation is obtained, and a trial reduction is done. If the composite is satisfactory, the hip is dislocated.

The allograft is fixed to the host bone with a large compression plate. The screws are angled to clear the stem of the prosthesis. In my opinion, intramedullary fixation alone is not adequate, but the combination of the small intramedullary stem and plate provides excellent fixation. The prosthesis is reduced and, if possible, the hip capsule is sutured around the neck of the prosthesis. The patient's hip abductors are sutured to the allograft's hip abductor tendons.

When the resection is greater than 250

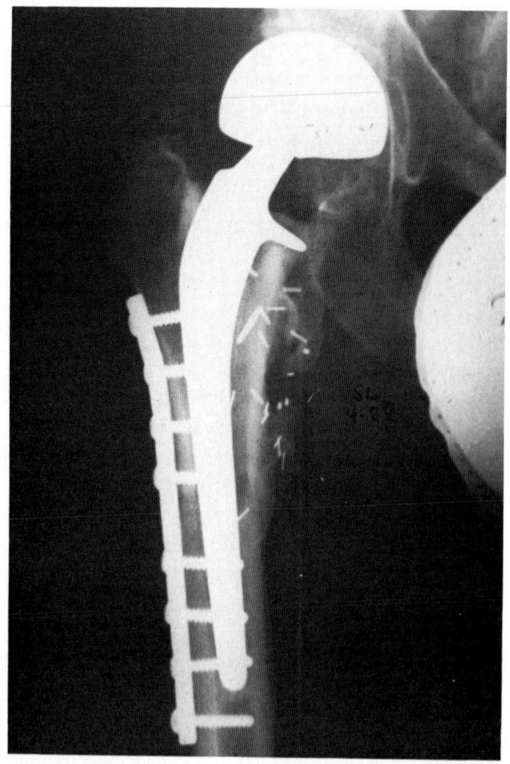

FIGURE 43–9. Anteroposterior view of an endoprosthetic/allograft composite replacement of a proximal femur. This type of reconstruction is employed when the allograft femoral head does not fit well in the patient's acetabulum or when preexisting degenerative arthritis occurs. The advantage of this composite is that it can be tailored to fit the patient intraoperatively rather than modifying tissues to fit the custom prosthesis. The abductors can be sutured to the greater trochanter for a more anatomic reconstruction, providing better function. The combination of a stem and plate to stabilize the junction of the allograft and host bone has worked well.

mm, a regular length stem bipolar prosthesis is appropriate. It can be cemented or press-fit. The shorter stem is employed with longer reconstructions to reduce any stress concentrations that might occur if the tip of the prosthesis were near the allograft-host junction.

The limb is kept in abduction for the first week postoperatively. The patient is then allowed to begin ambulation on two crutches, bearing only the weight of the limb on the operated extremity until the allograft-host bone junction is healed. A longer period of immobilization may be necessary if the repair of the abductor mechanism is insecure. The patient should not flex the hip beyond 90 degrees or adduct beyond neutral.

Active and active-assisted motion of the ipsilateral knee as well as quadriceps and hamstring strengthening exercises are important. The patient should not attempt active hip abduction for 6 weeks, at which time an exercise program to strengthen the abductor muscles may be started. This delay in exercising the hip abductors allows the host abductor tendons to heal to the allograft abductor tendons. Progress in strengthening and motion should be steady but slow.

It usually takes 6 to 9 months until the allograft-host junction is strong enough for the patient to begin to bear significant weight. I ask patients to restrict some activities permanently—jogging, aerobics, and racquet sports. However, bike riding, swimming, low-impact aerobics, and rowing are permitted.

Prostheses

Functional results have steadily improved as prosthetic hip joints have been redesigned and built with better materials. The early models had design flaws that led to frequent fatigue fractures, but these are not now a major problem. The differences among individual prostheses are minimal, but only longer follow-up data will tell whether they are significant.

Various customized, one-of-a-kind prostheses and modular, off-the-shelf prostheses are available to replace proximal femurs (Figs. 43–10 to 43–12). I select the totally customized prostheses more often than the modular types. The patients usually receive preoperative chemotherapy while the prosthesis is being made, and most can wait the 2 weeks now required for production. The modular systems have been significantly improved to the point that early results are as good as those with the totally customized devices.[8, 17, 50] The type of prosthesis is not as important as the quality of the resection and the postoperative rehabilitation.

The large prostheses have performed better than was originally predicted. With successful prosthetic replacement after resection of the proximal femur, the patient can expect excellent function almost as soon as the wound is healed. Within a month or two, most patients can walk with

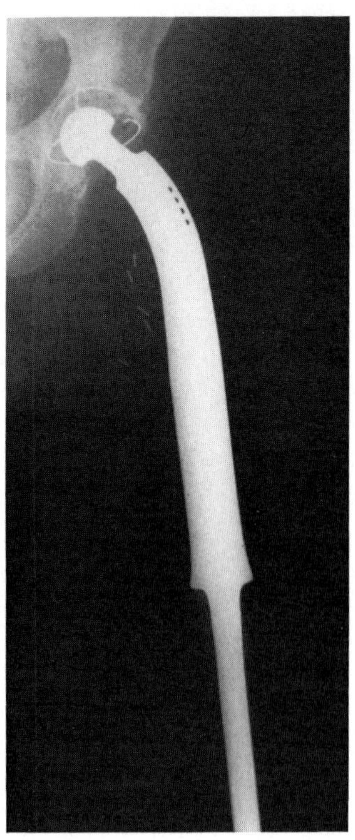

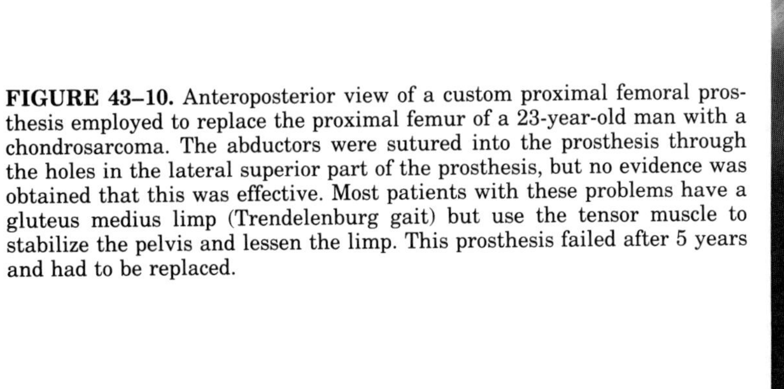

FIGURE 43–10. Anteroposterior view of a custom proximal femoral prosthesis employed to replace the proximal femur of a 23-year-old man with a chondrosarcoma. The abductors were sutured into the prosthesis through the holes in the lateral superior part of the prosthesis, but no evidence was obtained that this was effective. Most patients with these problems have a gluteus medius limp (Trendelenburg gait) but use the tensor muscle to stabilize the pelvis and lessen the limp. This prosthesis failed after 5 years and had to be replaced.

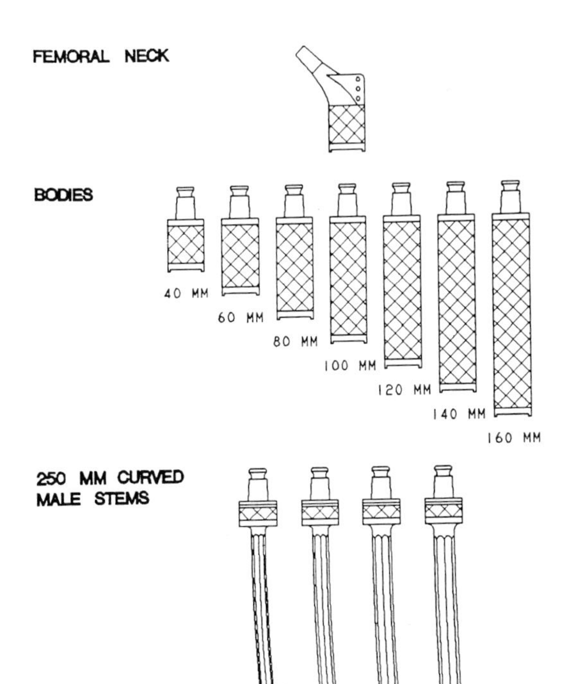

FIGURE 43–11. Example of a modular proximal femoral endoprosthetic system (Zimmer, Inc.). The modular system permits tailoring of the prosthesis during the operation.

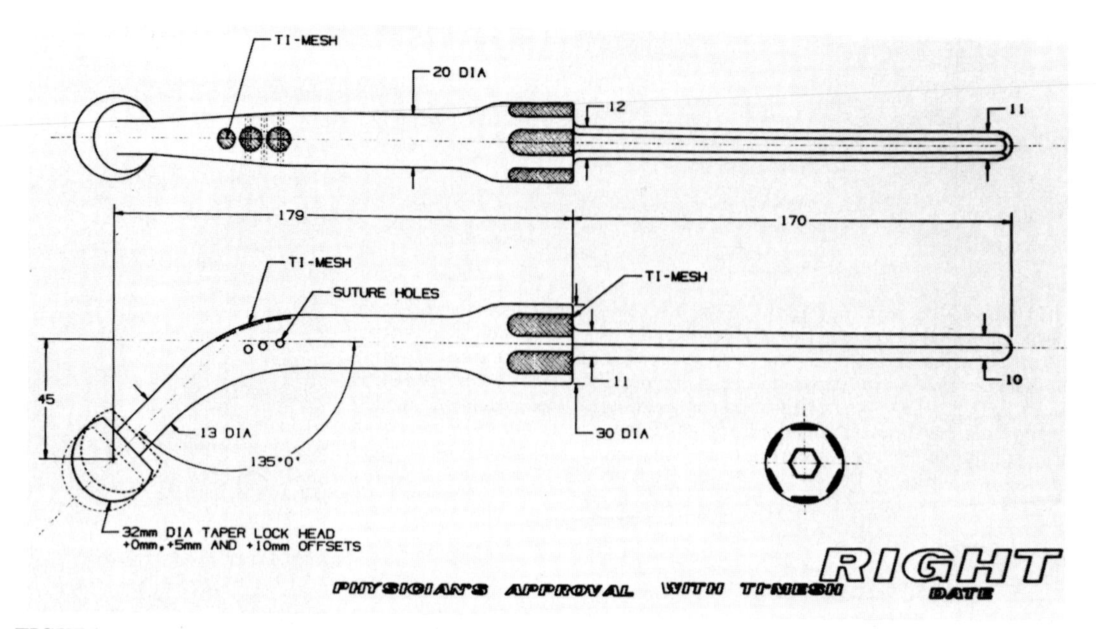

FIGURE 43–12. Preliminary drawing of a custom proximal femoral prosthesis (Techmedica, Inc.). The surgeon approves or changes the design. The prosthesis is then made.

a minimal abductor limp and no external aid. These results are in contrast to the results of allograft replacements, because the patient is not able to bear full weight until the allograft has healed, which takes 6 to 9 months.

The life expectancy of the prosthesis is inversely proportional to the activity of the patient.[8, 24, 50] The older patient who restricts activity can expect to have a functioning prosthesis for the remainder of life. However, the young patient will either have to dramatically restrict activity or will need a revision in 10 to 15 years. If a large prosthesis fails, it is more difficult to reconstruct the extremity because of the limited bone remaining.

The reconstructive techniques for a prosthesis are not difficult. Rotation to obtain the proper femoral neck anteversion and length of the extremity are the two main considerations. The femoral canal is reamed at least 2 mm larger than the prosthetic stem. The prosthesis is cemented into place. The prosthesis is reduced, and the wound is closed. The hip abductors should be sutured to the tensor fasciae latae while the extremity is held in 30 to 45 degrees of abduction. The patient can expect a minimal limp and little if any pain. A cane for walking minimizes stress on the prosthesis and may prolong its life.

The patient who has had a major resection will not be ready to start postoperative physical therapy as quickly as the patient who has had a routine hip replacement. I wait until the third or fourth day after surgery before having the patient start to walk. Because proximal thigh resections predispose the patient to loss of knee motion, physical therapy for the ipsilateral knee begins in the immediate postoperative period.

RECONSTRUCTIONS AFTER DISTAL FEMORAL RESECTIONS

The distal femur is the most common location of a tumor that requires resection. Reconstruction of the knee after a distal femoral resection is probably the most common limb salvage reconstruction. The distal femoral reconstruction has only to replace the bone and articulate with the tibia if motion is desired, but it does not have to provide an attachment for a major muscle group. Unlike other bones, the distal femur does not have a major muscle insertion, as does the tibia with the patellar tendon, the humerus with the rotator cuff, and the hip with the abductors. The demands on the femoral reconstruction therefore are much less than the demands on reconstructions at these other locations.

Function following reconstruction depends on the amount of soft tissue resection that has been done. The patient in whom only the bone has been resected, usually for a recurrent giant cell tumor of bone or intraosseous malignancy, is an excellent candidate for any of the available methods of reconstruction. A patient whose resection is extra-articular or includes the entire extensor mechanism is not a good candidate for an articulating reconstruction and is better served with an arthrodesis or rotationplasty reconstruction.[5, 15, 54]

The patient's demands for the extremity also must be considered. The sedentary patient, who will be sitting more than standing and who does not want to engage in strenuous physical activities, is an excellent candidate for an articulating reconstruction. The patient who wants to be physically active or whose lifestyle demands standing, walking, lifting, and similar activities is better served with an arthrodesis or rotationplasty. Amputation should not be overlooked as a means of "reconstruction." An amputee has excellent function. Amputation is the safest and quickest method of managing primary bone tumors.

Arthrodesis

Arthrodesis after major resection of the distal femur or proximal tibia has proved to be an excellent method of reconstructing a limb.[5, 15] Alternatives include an autograft or allograft to replace the resected bone and either an intramedullary rod or compression plates for fixation. Results of the various techniques are essentially the same.

Autogenous bone has the advantage of being safe, but it is of limited quantity and requires major additional surgery. Allograft is more available, but it carries a small risk of disease transmission. An advantage of intramedullary rod fixation is that it is "load sharing," and it does not require drill holes in the graft. However, an intramedullary rod requires exposure of the proximal femur and buttock, and these tissues may become contaminated if the margin of resection is inadequate. Plate fixation has the advantages of being rigid and requiring limited additional exposure, but drill holes in the grafts may act as stress risers. Another disadvantage of plate fixation is "load shielding." Each surgeon must weigh the pros and cons of these methods and choose the one that is best suited. My preference is allograft replacement and intramedullary rod fixation.

Arthrodesis with autograft is accomplished with the use of the ipsilateral or contralateral fibula, or both, and the hemicortex of the tibia. The hemicortex of the femur is utilized if the tibia rather than the femur has been resected.[15] The length of the resected specimen is measured before it is removed from the operating table. A segment of fibula 2 to 3 cm longer than the defect is harvested. If the defect is long and most of the fibula is required, the fibular head might be harvested with the shaft. This decompresses the peroneal nerve, and even with removal of the entire proximal fibula, significant knee instability does not result. In addition, a cortical graft 2 cm longer than the defect is obtained from the anterior tibia. The resected distal femur is then replaced by the fibular and tibial cortical grafts.

When an intramedullary rod is used, it is inserted retrograde up the femur and out the buttock. A spacer maintains the length of the defect. After the rod is driven antegrade into the tibia, the grafts are secured in place. For plate fixation, first a plate and then the grafts are secured in the femur and tibia. An additional plate is placed on the femur, grafts, and tibia. It takes at least a year for the grafts to heal and complete early remodeling. During this time, the patient is kept in a long leg brace, bearing partial weight and walking with two crutches.

When allograft replaces the resected segment, it is cut to the same length as the resected specimen and held between the femur and tibia. Either an intramedullary rod or two plates are needed for internal fixation. The postoperative management is the same as that with autogenous graft, although a brace is not needed if the fixation is rigid.

Osteoarticular Allograft

If any of the quadriceps, even just the rectus femoris, is retained after an intra-articular resection of the distal femur, an osteoarticular allograft reconstruction can be done. Osteoarticular allograft reconstructions are probably most appropriate in the young patient (Fig. 43–13). Although the articular cartilage of the fresh-frozen allograft is not normal, function is good. Eventually, degenerative arthritis develops, but by that time the allograft provides excellent stock for subsequent joint reconstructions. In contrast, reconstruction after failure of a large prosthesis is usually more difficult because of the limited remaining bone.

After resection has been completed, the allograft is cut to the proper length and fixed to the host bone with a large compression plate. The posterior cruciate ligament is repaired. The posterior capsule of the allograft is sutured, but not too tightly, to the remaining posterior capsule of the tibia with multiple interrupted, nonabsorbable sutures. The knee is allowed to extend just short of 0 degrees. The medial and lateral collateral ligaments also are repaired with interrupted, nonabsorbable sutures, which should be as tight as possible. The anterior cruciate ligament should be repaired, but it is not known whether this ligament heals. The extensor mechanism is sutured back in place, with the patella centralized as much as possible, based on the amount of resected tissue. Hamstring transfers usually do not help active extension, and they restrict flexion.

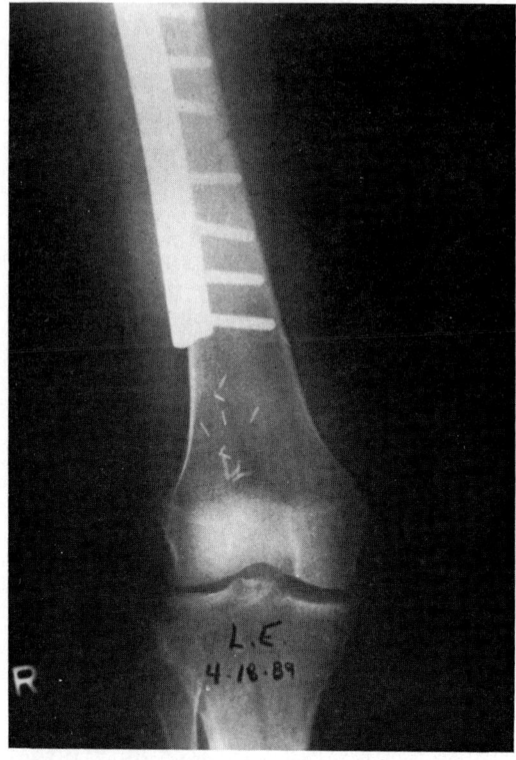

FIGURE 43–13. Anteroposterior view of a distal femur resected for a low-grade osteosarcoma involving the distal metaphysis. A fresh-frozen osteoarticular allograft replaced the resected bone. The patient had no muscle resected, and function was excellent. The allograft healed to the femur, and the patient ambulated without a limp. She will probably develop osteoarthritis in the knee within the next 15 years and need additional surgery, but a conventional total knee replacement can be done.

The extremity is placed in a long cast for 3 months, and the patient is allowed to ambulate on crutches, bearing minimal weight. When the cast is removed, the patient can begin to regain knee motion slowly. The joint should not be manipulated or vigorously stretched. The patient should continue to bear only minimal weight until the allograft appears on plain radiographic studies to be healed to the host bone, usually after 6 to 9 months.

The patient can expect to regain 90 degrees of motion in the knee and to ambulate without external aids. The knee is modestly unstable and does not tolerate strenuous activities well. I ask patients with osteoarticular allografts to use a cane whenever they walk more than a half mile and to refrain from activities that cause high stress to the lower extremities.

Although thinning of the allograft articular cartilage is common, clinical evidence of arthritis is rare until years after the allograft has been in place. When the joint wears out, joint replacement or arthrodesis can be done.

Prostheses

It was to salvage limbs in patients with distal femoral tumors that surgeons most needed large custom prostheses. Custom distal femoral prostheses have been routinely utilized for about 15 years.[49] The distal femur is an ideal bone to replace with a prosthesis because of the absence of significant tendon attachments. The only criteria are that the prosthesis replace the bone and articulate with the tibia. Also, the prosthesis must have built-in stability.

Initially, hinged prostheses were used, but rotating-hinge devices have been introduced of late (Fig. 43–14). Modular prostheses, which can be assembled in the operating room as needed, are available. The advantage of the modular prostheses is that the length can be adjusted at the last minute if necessary, whereas the length of custom prostheses cannot be adjusted. However, the dimensions of the custom device are exact for the patient, whereas those of the modular component are only close.

Some prostheses have porous coatings on the intramedullary stems. Bone grafting over the porous-coated portion is thought to result in a more biologic and more permanent fixation.[50] The principal problem with these prostheses has been late (after 10 to 15 years) loosening, fracture, and infection.

A patellar prosthesis can be employed, but I rarely choose this type. The articular surface of the patient's patella is usually normal.

Most distal femoral prosthetic devices have typical tibial components and are implanted in the tibia in the usual fashion. The femoral component is cemented into the femoral canal after it has been reamed to accept the stem of the prosthesis. As with osteoarticular allografts, hamstring transfers are rarely indicated.

Postoperatively, the patient who has had a prosthetic reconstruction can be rehabilitated quickly. I do not provide braces for these patients. Rather, they are allowed up on crutches with weightbearing as soon as they have recovered from the surgery, usually on the second or third postoperative day. Quadriceps strengthening is begun immediately, with straight leg raise exercises and active motion. The patient can expect to eventually have 95 to 100 degrees of motion and to walk without external aids. I ask all patients who have prostheses to use a cane when they walk more than a half mile and to refrain from running, but many patients are quite active.

Allograft/Prosthesis Composite

When an allograft is used with a conventional total knee replacement, the length of the resection can be tailored during the operation. The allograft is not cut until (1) the level of the resection has been finally determined and (2) the size of the joint has been adjusted with the prosthesis. The allograft is fixed to the host bone with a plate, and the prosthesis is implanted in a conventional manner utilizing bone cement.

RECONSTRUCTIONS AFTER PROXIMAL TIBIAL RESECTIONS

The proximal tibia is the second most common site to be salvaged by resection in

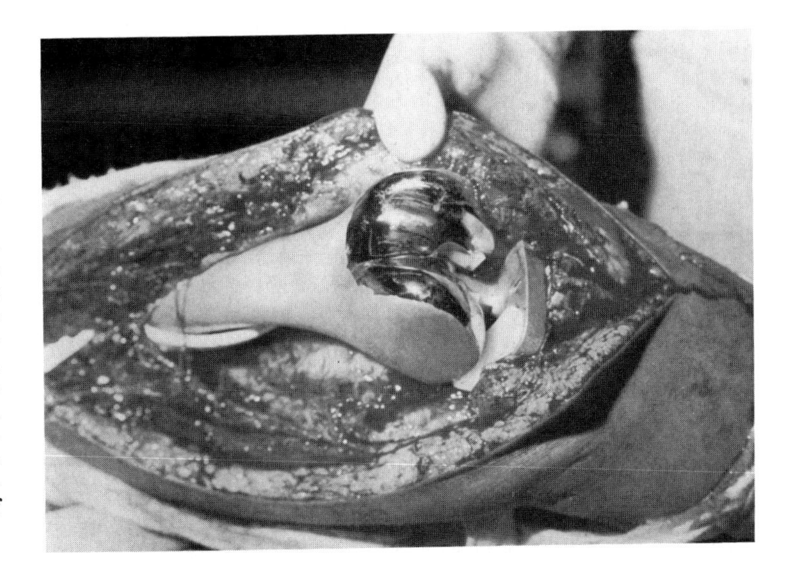

FIGURE 43–14. Intraoperative photograph of a custom distal femoral replacement with a rotating hinge-type total knee. This patient had an osteosarcoma in the distal femur but only a minimal amount of muscle had to be resected. She was ambulating without a limp within 6 weeks of surgery. She was without disease 5 years later and showed every indication of living a full life span. A replacement of this endoprosthesis if it fails will be difficult. When an endoprosthesis fractures or loosens and is not infected, an allograft/endoprosthesis composite is my choice of reconstruction.

cases of tumors of the bone. The indication for limb salvage and the demand on the proximal tibia make the procedure different from distal femur salvage. The patient with a proximal tibial tumor can have an above-knee amputation with a long stump, remain active, and undergo the best oncologic treatment possible. By contrast, the patient with a distal femoral tumor would have to have a hip disarticulation for a comparable operation. The stump is short if an above-knee amputation is done, and the oncologic treatment is somewhat compromised. Thus, amputation for a patient with a proximal tibial lesion is more acceptable than is amputation for a patient with a distal femoral tumor.[34]

When knee motion is maintained with either allograft or prosthesis, the patellar tendon must be securely attached to the tibia for good knee extension. It is difficult to reconstruct the tibial attachment of the patellar tendon. A significant portion of the tibia is not covered by muscle. Therefore, the coverage of a prosthesis or an allograft is more difficult, often requiring muscle flaps.

Arthrodesis

An arthrodesis for reconstruction after resection of the proximal tibia is essentially the same operation as an arthrodesis after resection of the distal femur. One of the grafts must be taken from the distal femur. The contralateral fibula often must be harvested, because a portion of the ipsilateral fibula is resected with the tibial tumor.[5, 15]

Osteoarticular Allograft

If an exact allograft match is not possible, the tibia can be minimally larger (up to 3 mm) than the femur in the medial to lateral direction. The allograft is fixed to the host bone, and the joint capsule and ligaments are repaired just as they are for a distal femoral osteoarticular allograft reconstruction. The principal difference is the reconstruction of the patellar tendon. The distal patellar tendon is left on the proximal tibia of the allograft and is sutured to the patient's remaining patellar tendon. The total length of the patellar tendon must be identical to what it was prior to the resection. If it is too long, the patella rides high, the tibia is more likely to sag posteriorly, and the extension is weak. If it is too short, the patella is too distal and regaining flexion is difficult. A crisscross stitch, with a nonabsorbable # 2 suture, connects the allograft tendon to the host tendon. When the cast is removed 3 months after surgery, the patellar tendon is strong enough to begin active exercises.

The patient can expect to have 95 degrees of motion and eventually to walk without external aids (Fig. 43–15). The knee will have minimal instability. I suggest the same restrictions as those for distal femoral osteoarticular allograft recon-

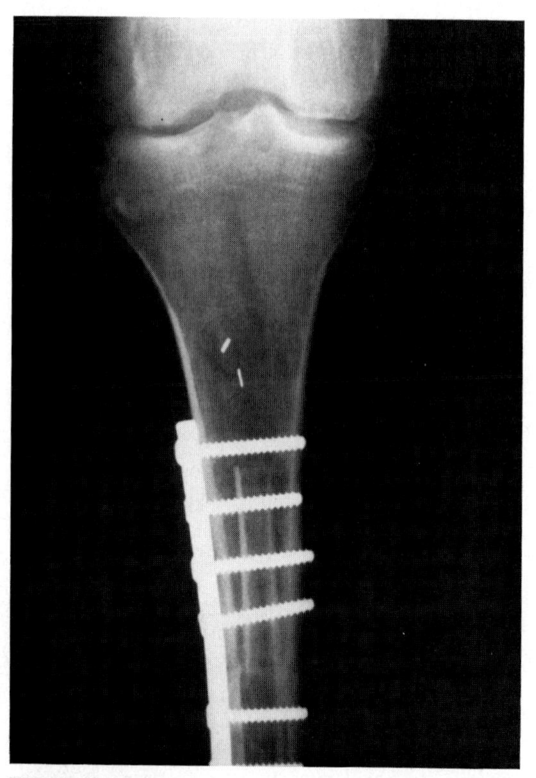

FIGURE 43–15. Anteroposterior view of the proximal tibia in a patient who had a recurrent giant cell tumor of bone at this site. The proximal tibia was resected, and a fresh-frozen osteoarticular allograft replaced the bone. The patient's patellar tendon was sutured to the allograft's patellar tendon. Care was taken to maintain the proper length of the patellar tendon. The proximal portion of the patient's fibula was resected with the proximal tibia. Therefore, an additional portion was removed and used as an intramedullary cortical graft. This is not usually done. Subsequently, the patient had active extension with less than 5 degrees of extensor lag.

structions—patients are not to engage in strenuous physical activities.

Prostheses

The excellent function and better surgical margins obtained with above-knee amputations and the more difficult surgical resection of a proximal tibial tumor help explain the limited experience with proximal tibial prostheses when compared with femoral prostheses. A custom prosthesis for reconstruction after resection of the proximal tibia is substantially different from that for the distal femur.

The patellar tendon insertion is critical to the function of the knee, and the tendon does not attach well to artificial materials. Numerous methods have been tried to overcome this difficulty. The nonbiologic means of attachment have not been satisfactory. Through a variety of methods, biologic material can be obtained for attachment of the tendon.[29, 30, 36, 40] These methods work reasonably well but add significant surgery to the reconstruction.

One method is to transfer one of the heads of the gastrocnemius anteriorly over the prosthesis and sew the patellar tendon to it. An alternative is osteotomy of the fibula, angling it anteriorly and medially so that it can act as a bony insertion for the patellar tendon. Kotz and associates[29, 30] believe that the proximal fibula provides a better insertion for the tendon and a more cosmetic appearance. With both of these methods, the knee should be immobilized for 6 weeks to allow complete healing of the reconstructed patellar tendon. Rehabilitation after immobilization should proceed slowly. It is less difficult to regain lost motion than to try to repair a ruptured patellar tendon.

A patient who has a prosthetic reconstruction can be mobilized early, starting within the first week. Knee flexion is restricted until the patellar tendon has had a chance to heal. Depending on the type of reconstruction, it may take 3 to 6 weeks, but by this time the knee should be moving well. The patient can expect full extension, at least passively, and flexion to 90 degrees. Few patients will have full active extension. Most will have a lag of 20 degrees.

Allograft/Prosthesis Composite

The principal value of combining an allograft and a prosthesis for reconstructing the extremity after the proximal tibia has been resected is to have a biologic insertion for the patellar tendon. The length of the reconstruction can be modified in the operating room, which makes it possible to adjust the resection as needed.

When an allograft/prosthesis composite is selected, the prosthesis should be an inherently stable device so that the reconstructed joint is stable. I prefer a rotating-hinge prosthetic knee. The prosthesis is fixed with bone cement, and the allograft is internally fixed to the host bone with a plate. Usually, the stem of the tibial component and the plate overlap. Short screws are employed in the portion of the plate that is at the level of the stem of the prosthesis. The patellar tendon is sutured to the allograft tendon with a # 2 nonabsorbable suture, using a crisscross stitch.

The patient who has an allograft/prosthesis composite reconstruction is initially placed in a long leg cast and walks bearing minimal weight for 8 to 12 weeks. Quadriceps tightening exercises can begin while the cast is on. Gravity-assisted flexion and gentle active extension are the initial exercises after the cast is removed. Crutches and minimal weightbearing are continued until the allograft has healed to the host bone, which usually takes 6 to 9 months. Patients can expect active flexion to within 5 degrees of full extension and flexion to at least 95 degrees.

If the union is not solid, as judged by the appearance on plain radiographic studies at 1 year, bone grafting is recommended.

When a patient who has had previous osteoarticular allograft reconstruction develops disabling degenerative arthritis, the reconstruction can be converted to an allograft/prosthesis composite (Fig. 43–16).

RECONSTRUCTIONS AFTER PROXIMAL HUMERAL RESECTIONS

Tumors around the shoulder have been resected without amputation since the early 1880s, but reconstructive experience

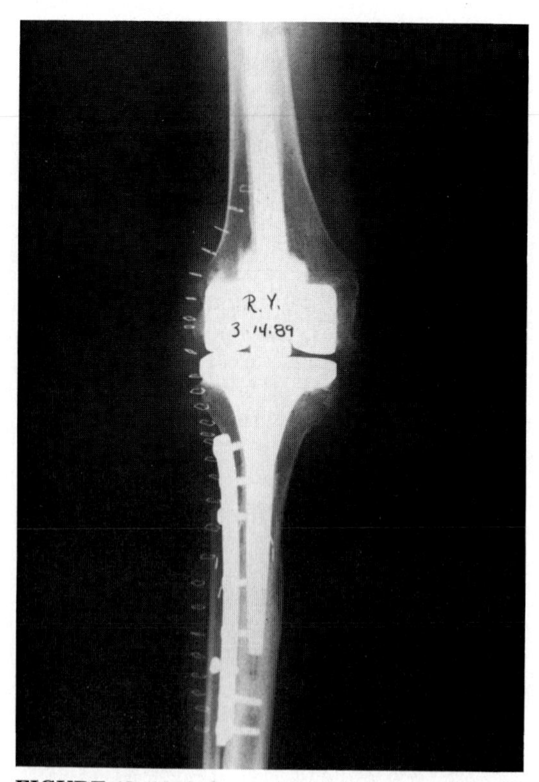

FIGURE 43–16. Anteroposterior view of an allograft/prosthesis composite reconstruction. The patient had an osteoarticular allograft 5 years before the total knee replacement for secondary osteoarthritis. An allograft/prosthesis composite replacement can be done as an initial reconstruction if degenerated articular cartilage occurs on the distal femur or if the match between the allograft and host articular surface is unacceptable (>5 mm).

after resection has been limited.[32] With suspension of the proximal humerus to the remaining clavicle or rib cage, the shoulder remains flail, and the patient is not able to control the extremity well without external support. If the entire scapula is resected, no satisfactory method stabilizes the shoulder. Scapular prostheses and allografts have not yet proven to be a benefit.[35] However, if the proximal humerus is resected, even if the shoulder joint is resected too, a reconstruction should be done to optimize the patient's function. When resection of the tumor does not require removal of the surrounding soft tissues or glenoid, shoulder motion can be preserved.

The choice of reconstruction depends on the patient's age and activity level. For the more physically active patient, arthrodesis is the reconstruction of choice. The patient with an arthrodesis can raise and hold heavy objects away from the body but cannot rotate the arm well. The patient with a prosthetic reconstruction does not have active abduction beyond 45 to 60 degrees and has little strength in abduction or flexion, but rotation of the arm and shoulder stability are excellent. The inability to securely attach the rotator cuff to the prosthesis is a significant limitation of prosthetic replacement. Nonetheless, a prosthetic reconstruction may be appropriate for an older patient. The ability to reconstruct the rotator cuff is an advantage of allograft reconstruction. With either an osteoarticular allograft or an allograft/prosthesis composite, the patient's rotator cuff can be sutured to the allograft rotator tendon, thus retaining the function of the rotator muscles. This maneuver greatly improves the motion of the shoulder, especially abduction.[33]

Arthrodesis

When arthrodesis is chosen as the method of reconstruction, the resected bone should be replaced unless less than 8 cm has been removed. If the arm will be shortened by more than 8 to 10 cm, an intercalary graft—either allograft or autograft—is selected to replace the resected proximal humerus and maintain normal arm length (Fig. 43–17).[52] Fibulae can be used as autograft, but they should be doubled, with two fibulae placed side by side. Single-fibula allografts or autografts often fracture during the healing process. When two fibulae are present, fatigue fractures will heal and lead to hypertrophy. Iliac crest bone graft may supplement the fibulae but is not essential for healing.

The most difficult aspect of the surgery is plate fixation on the scapula to rigidly immobilize the intercalary graft and remaining humerus. I bend a large compression plate so that it can be screwed to the spine of the scapula and the humerus while the arm is positioned in 35 to 50 degrees of abduction and 10 to 15 degrees of flexion. Rotation is not determined by the bend in the plate. The hand is positioned in the midline of the body, which allows excellent abduction and flexion. This maneuver also puts the hand in a useful position with regard to rotation and allows the arm to rest at the side.

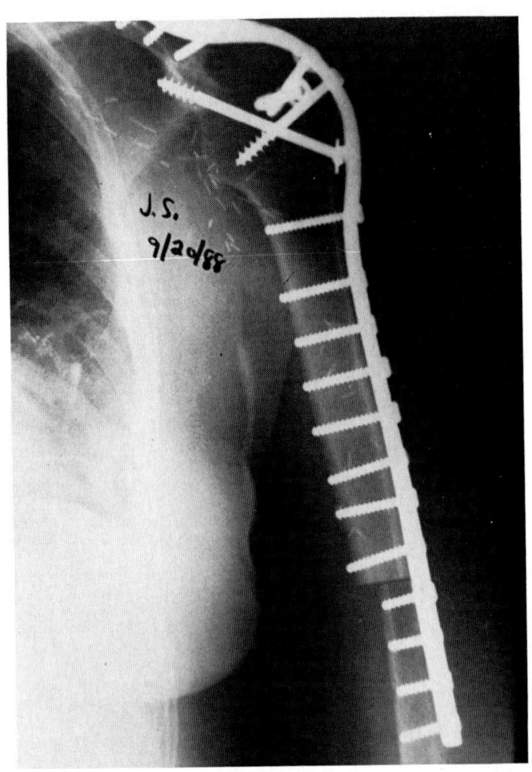

FIGURE 43–17. Anteroposterior view of the proximal humerus of a patient who had an allograft arthrodesis. The patient had a large osteosarcoma in the proximal humerus that required resection with most of the shoulder girdle muscles. An articulating reconstruction would have produced a flail shoulder, and the patient wanted a strong stable arm. A large compression plate fixed the allograft to the scapula and host distal humerus. Once the allograft heals in a case like this, the arm will function as in a standard arthrodesis. Complications with these complex shoulder arthrodeses have been more common than with standard arthrodeses. This problem is probably caused by the more radical surgery done in these patients who must have either extra-articular resections or resections of large portions of the surrounding muscles with the tumor.

A shoulder spica is applied postoperatively until the union is solid, unless the internal fixation is particularly strong.

Prosthesis

The advantage of a prosthesis is that the patient can function immediately and reasonably well.[1, 4, 7, 22, 46] The demands on the humerus are less than those on the lower extremities, and as a result failure has been less than that for prosthetic reconstruction of the lower extremity. However, although the rotator cuff can be sutured to the prosthesis, the fixation is less than ideal. If the resection is distal to the deltoid insertion, abduction is particularly poor (Fig. 43–18). A variety of methods have been tried to improve the attachments of the muscles to the prosthesis, but so far none have been satisfactory.

Rehabilitation after a prosthetic reconstruction of the proximal humerus depends on the extent of the soft tissue repair. If the muscle insertions have been repaired and they are not too tight when the arm is at the side, the arm can be placed in a sling for 10 to 14 days, and pendulum motion exercises can be performed. For repairs under tension, the arm should be held in abduction for 6 weeks.

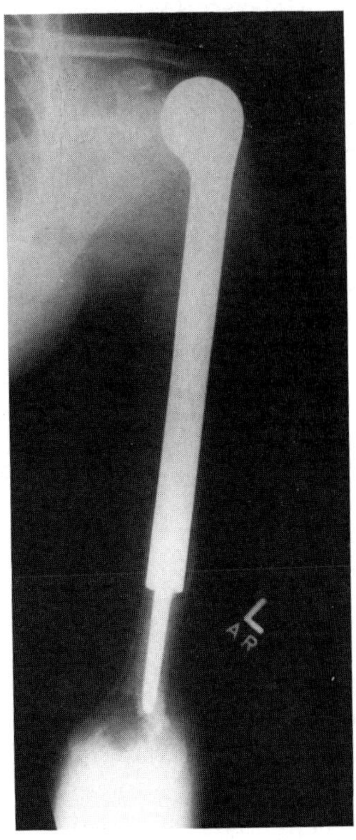

FIGURE 43–18. Anteroposterior view of a proximal humeral endoprosthesis. The patient had a resection of an osteosarcoma of the proximal humerus reconstructed with this custom device. She had excellent rotation and could raise her hand to her mouth, behind her head, and to the opposite axilla. She was unable to abduct or forward flex more than a few degrees, however.

Osteoarticular Allograft

Experience with osteoarticular allografts for the proximal humerus is limited, but they seem to function well (Fig. 43–19).[16] The patient's muscles can be repaired to the allograft's muscle insertions, including the rotator cuff insertion. These repairs heal well and enable the muscles to control the upper arm. When the surrounding soft tissues must be resected, an arthrodesis may be more appropriate, although some patients prefer to maintain rotation rather than have the abduction provided by an arthrodesis.

After the tumor has been resected, the allograft is cut to the same length as the resected portion of the humerus. The allograft is fixed to the host bone with a large compression plate, and the soft tissues are then repaired. The available muscles are sutured to the allograft insertions. The shoulder capsule of the allograft is repaired to the patient's shoulder capsule. The capsular repair should allow full abduction. The arm is held in maximum abduction for 3 months.

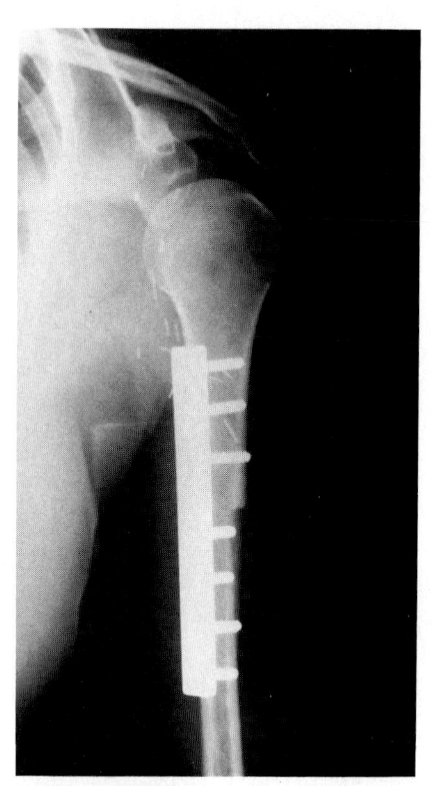

FIGURE 43–19. Anteroposterior view of the humerus in a patient who had a solitary renal cell metastasis 3 years after treatment of a primary kidney tumor. She underwent a fresh-frozen osteoarticular allograft reconstruction after resection of the proximal humerus. This patient was placed in a shoulder spica cast for 10 weeks with her arm in maximal abduction. The allograft healed to the humerus, and she subsequently had normal active abduction and forward flexion.

I put the patient in a shoulder spica preoperatively, then bivalve and remove the cast. At the completion of surgery before the patient is awakened, the spica is put back on, with the arm in the desired position. After 3 months the spica is replaced by an abduction splint, as the arm is brought down and motion is started. Once the arm can be brought to the patient's side, strengthening exercises are begun, gently and gradually. The patient is not allowed to lift weights over a few pounds until the allograft has healed to the host humerus, which usually takes about 6 months.

Allograft/Prosthesis Composite

The articular surface of the allograft functions well, and a prosthetic replacement usually is not needed, unless the patient has degenerative joint disease.[17, 53] The advantage of an allograft/prosthesis composite is that the rotator cuff tendons and the deltoid can be sutured to soft tissue attachments of the allograft. This provides fixation and retains more motion than is possible when a prosthesis is employed without the allograft.

The intramedullary stem of the prosthesis should be long enough to bridge the junction between the allograft and the host bone. In addition to the intramedullary stem fixation, a compression plate is utilized.

The shoulder should be immobilized in abduction for 8 to 12 weeks. As with the patient with an osteoarticular allograft alone, I immobilize the arm in a shoulder spica in maximum elevation for 3 months. This practice seems to improve final motion.

References

1. Bos, G., Sims, F., Pritchard, D., et al.: Prosthetic replacement of the proximal humerus. Clin. Orthop. 224:178–191, 1987.

2. Burrows, H.F., Wilson, J.N., and Seals, J.T.: Excision of tumors of humerus and femur with restoration by internal prosthesis. J. Bone Joint Surg. 57B:148–149, 1975.
3. Campanacci, M. and Capanna, R.: Closing Remarks. Limb Salvage in Musculoskeletal Oncology. Edited by W. F. Enneking. New York, Churchill Livingstone, 1987.
4. Campanacci, M., Cervellati, C., Gherlinzoni, F., and Capanna, R.: Endoprosthesis of the humerus: Description of a new Model and its application. Ital. J. Orthop. Traumatol. 8(1):59–65, 1982.
5. Campanacci, M. and Costa, P.: Total resection of distal femur or proximal tibia for bone tumors. J. Bone Joint Surg. 61B:455–463, 1979.
6. Capanna, R., Guernelli, N., Ruggieri, P., et al.: Periacetabular Pelvic Resections. Limb Salvage in Musculoskeletal Oncology. Edited by W. F. Enneking. New York, Churchill Livingstone, 1987.
7. Capanna, R., Mapelli, S., Ruggieri, P., et al.: Resection of the proximal humerus and I.O.R. modular prosthesis in the treatment of metastatic lesions. Ital. J. Orthop. Traumatol. 14(2):143–148, 1988.
8. Dobbs, H.S., Scales, J.T., and Wilson, J.N.: Endoprosthetic replacement of the proximal femur and acetabulum. J. Bone Joint Surg. 63B:219–224, 1981.
9. Dunham, W.K., Jr.: Acetabular Resections for Sarcoma. Limb Salvage in Musculoskeletal Oncology. Edited by W. F. Enneking. New York, Churchill Livingstone, 1987.
10. Eilber, F.R., Eckardt, J.J., and Grant, T.G.: Resection of Malignant Bone Tumors of the Pelvis: Evaluation of Local Recurrence, Survival, and Function. Limb Salvage in Musculoskeletal Oncology. Edited by W. F. Enneking. New York, Churchill Livingstone, 1987.
11. Eilber, F.R., Grant, T.T., Sakai, D., and Morton, D.L.: Internal hemipelvectomy. Cancer 43:806–809, 1979.
12. Enneking, W.F.: Local resection of malignant lesions of the hip and pelvis. J. Bone Joint Surg. 48A:991–1007, 1966.
13. Enneking, W.F., and Dunham, W.K.: Resection and reconstruction for primary neoplasm involving the innominate bone. J. Bone Joint Surg. 60A:731–746, 1978.
14. Enneking, W.F. and Menendez, L.R.: Functional Evaluation of Various Reconstructions after Periacetabular Resection of Iliac Lesions. Limb Salvage in Musculoskeletal Oncology. Edited by W. F. Enneking. New York, Churchill Livingstone, 1987.
15. Enneking, W.F. and Shirley, P.D.: Resection-arthrodesis for malignant and potentially malignant lesions about the knee using an intramedullary rod and local bone grafts. J. Bone Joint Surg. 62A:1039–1058, 1980.
16. Gebhardt, M.C., Roth, Y.F., and Mankin, H.J.: Osteoarticular allograft for reconstruction in the proximal part of the humerus after excision of a musculoskeletal tumor. J. Bone Joint Surg. 72A:334–345, 1990.
17. Gebhardt, M.C., McQuire, M.H., and Mankin, H.J.: Resection and allograft arthrodesis for malignant bone tumors of the extremity. Limb Salvage in Musculoskeletal Oncology. Edited by W. F. Enneking. New York, Churchill Livingstone, 1987.
18. Harrington, K.D., Johnston, J.O., Kaufer, H.N., et al.: Limb salvage and prosthetic joint reconstruction for low-grade and selected high-grade sarcomas of bone after wide resection and replacement by autoclaved autogeneic grafts. Clin. Orthop. 211:180–214, 1986.
19. Hudson, T.M., Haas, G., Enneking, W.F., and Hawkins, E.F.: Angiography in the management of musculoskeletal tumors. Surg. Gynecol. Obstet. 141:11–21, 1975.
20. Huth, J.F., Eckardt, J.J., Pignatti, G., and Eilber, F.R.: Resection of malignant bone tumor of the pelvic girdle without extremity amputation. Arch. Surg. 123:1121–1124, 1988.
21. Huvos, A., Rosen, G., and Marcove, R.C.: Primary osteogenic sarcoma. Pathologic aspect in 20 patients after treatment with chemotherapy, en bloc resection and prosthetic bone replacement. Arch. Pathol. Lab. Med. 101:14–18, 1977.
22. Imbriylia, J.E., Neer, C.S., and Dick, H.M.: Resection of the proximal one-half of the humerus in a child for chondrosarcoma. Preservation of function using a fibular graft and Neer prosthesis. J. Bone Joint Surg. 60A:262–264, 1978.
23. Jenson, J.S.: Resection arthroplasty of the proximal tibia. Acta Orthop. Scand. 54:126–130, 1983.
24. Johnsson, R., Carlsson, A., Kisch, K., et al.: Function following mega total hip arthroplasty compared with conventional total hip arthroplasty and healthy matched control. Clin. Orthop. 192:159–167, 1985.
25. Johnson, J.T.H.: Reconstruction of the pelvic ring following tumor resection. J. Bone Joint Surg. 60A:747–751, 1978.
26. Johnston, J.O.: Local resection in primary malignant bone tumor. Clin. Orthop. 153:73–80, 1980.
27. Karahar, E.O., Jr. and Korkala, O.L.: Resection of large tumors of the anterior pelvic ring while preserving functional stability of the hip. Clin. Orthop. 195:270–274, 1985.
28. Karakousis, C.P.: The abdominoinguinal approach in limb salvage and resection of pelvis tumors. Cancer 54:2543–2548, 1984.
29. Kotz, R., Pongracz, N., Fellinger, E.F., and Ritsch, P.: Uncemented Hinge Prostheses with Reinsertion of the Ligamentium Patellae. New Developments for Limb Salvage in Musculoskeletal Tumors. Edited by T. Yamamuro. Berlin, Springer-Verlag, 1989.
30. Kotz, R., Ritsch, P., and Trachtenbrodt, J.: A modular femur-tibia reconstruction system. Orthopaedics 9:1639–1652, 1986.
31. Lane, J.M., Duane, K., Glasser, D.B., et al.: Periacetabular Resections for Malignant Sarcomas. Limb Salvage in Musculoskeletal Oncology. Edited by W.F. Enneking. New York, Churchill Livingstone, 1987.
32. Linberg, B.E.: Interscapulo-thoracic resection for malignant tumors of the shoulder joint region. J. Bone Joint Surg. 10:344–349, 1928.
33. Malawer, M.M., Meller, I., and Dunham, W.K.: Shoulder Girdle Resections for Bone and Soft Tissue Tumors. New Developments for Limb Salvage in Musculoskeletal Tumors. Edited by T. Yamamuro. Berlin, Springer-Verlag, 1989.

34. Malawer, M.M. and Mettale, K.A.: Limb-sparing surgery for high-grade malignant tumors of the proximal tibia. Clin. Orthop. 239:231–248, 1989.
35. Mankin, H.J., Fogelson, F.S., Thrasher, A.Z., and Jaffer, E.: Massive resection and allograft replacement in the treatment of malignant bone tumors. N. Engl. J. Med. 294:1247–1255, 1976.
36. Mankin, H.J.: Personal Communication, 1990.
37. Marcove, R.C. and Rosen, G.: En bloc resections for osteogenic sarcoma. Cancer 45:3040–3044, 1978.
38. McLaughlin, R.E., Sweet, D.E., Webster, T., and Merrit, W.M.: Chondroblastoma of the pelvis suggestive of malignancy. Report of an unusual case treated by wide pelvic excision. J. Bone Joint Surg. 57A:549–551, 1975.
39. Milch, H.: Partial resection of the ischium. J. Bone Joint Surg. 17:166–171, 1935.
40. Missenard, G., Tomeno, B., Langlais, F., et al.: Total Knee Prosthesis After Upper Tibia Resection for Tumors. New Developments for Limb Salvage in Musculoskeletal Tumors. Edited by T. Yamamuro. Berlin, Springer-Verlag, 1989.
41. Mutschler, W., Burri, C., and Kiefer, H.: Functional Results after Pelvic Resection with Endoprosthetic Replacement. Limb Salvage in Musculoskeletal Oncology. Edited by W.F. Enneking. New York, Churchill Livingstone, 1987.
42. Nilsonne, A.: Limb-preserving radical surgery for malignant bone tumors. Clin. Orthop. 191:21–26, 1984.
43. O'Connor, M.I. and Sims, F.H.: Salvage of the limb in treatment of malignant pelvic tumors. J. Bone Joint Surg. 71A:481–494, 1989.
44. Radley, R.J., Liebig, C.A., and Brown, J.R.: Resection of the body of the pubic bone, the superior and inferior pubic rami, the inferior ischial ramus, and the ischial tuberosity. A surgical approach. J. Bone Joint Surg. 36A:855–858, 1954.
45. Rosen, G., Murphy, M.L., Huvos, A.G., et al.: Chemotherapy, en bloc resection, and prosthetic bone replacement in the treatment of osteogenic sarcoma. Cancer 37:1–11, 1976.
46. Ross, A.C., Wilson, J.W., and Scales, J.T.: Endoprosthetic replacement of the proximal humerus. J. Bone Joint Surg. 69B:656–661, 1987.
47. Salzer, M., Knahr, K., Sekera, J., and Braun, O.: Resection of Malignant Pelvic Bone Tumors. Limb Salvage in Musculoskeletal Oncology. Edited by W.F. Enneking. New York, Churchill Livingstone, 1987.
48. Shives, T.C., Sim, F.H., Pritchard, D.J., and Bowman, W.E.: Limb Salvage for Tumors about the Pelvic Girdle. Limb Salvage in Musculoskeletal Oncology. Edited by W.F. Enneking. New York, Churchill Livingstone, 1987.
49. Sim, F.H. and Chao, E.Y.S.: Prosthetic replacement of the knee and large segment of the femur or tibia. J. Bone Joint Surg. 61A:887–892, 1979.
50. Sim, F.H. and Chao, E.Y.S.: Segmental Prosthetic Replacement of the Hip and Knee. Tumor Prostheses for Bone and Joint Reconstruction. Edited by E.Y.S. Chao and J.C. Ivins. New York, Thieme-Stratton, 1983.
51. Steel, H.H.: Partial or complete resection of the hemipelvis. J. Bone Joint Surg. 60A:719–730, 1978.
52. Taminiau, A.H., Hooning van Duyvenbode, J.F., and Slooff, T.J.: Reconstruction of the proximal humerus with tibial autografts after resection of osteochondroma in adolescents. Clin. Orthop. 201:173–178, 1985.
53. Tomeno, B., Languepin, A., and Gerber, C.: Local Resection with Limb Salvage for the Treatment of Periacetabular Bone Tumors: Functional Results in Nine Cases. Limb Salvage in Musculoskeletal Oncology. Edited by W.F. Enneking. New York, Churchill Livingstone, 1987.
54. Winklemann, W.W.: Hip rotationplasty for malignant tumors of the proximal part of the femur. J. Bone Joint Surg. 68A:362–369, 1986.

Index

Note: Page numbers in *italics* refer to illustrations; page numbers followed by t refer to tables.

C

I

N

O

S

T